Trauma

Dose schedules are being continually revised and new side effects recognized. Oxford University Press makes no representation, express or implied, that the drug dosages in this book are correct. For these reasons the reader is strongly urged to consult the pharmaceutical company's printed instructions before administering any of the drugs recommended in this book.

Trauma

Edited by

Eugene Sherry

University of Sydney, Nepean Hospital

Lawrence Trieu

Concord Repatriation General Hospital, Sydney

John Templeton

Keele University

Assistant Editor

Jennifer Yuan

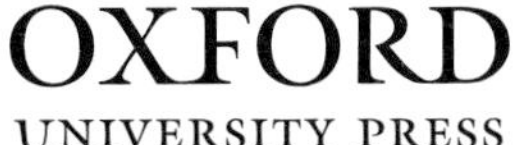

UNIVERSITY PRESS

OXFORD
UNIVERSITY PRESS

Great Clarendon Street, Oxford OX2 6DP

Oxford University Press is a department of the University of Oxford.
It furthers the University's objective of excellence in research, scholarship,
and education by publishing worldwide in

Oxford New York

Auckland Bangkok Buenos Aires Cape Town Chennai
Dar es Salaam Delhi Hong Kong Istanbul Karachi Kolkata
Kuala Lumpur Madrid Melbourne Mexico City Mumbai Nairobi
São Paulo Shanghai Singapore Taipei Tokyo Toronto

Published in the United States
by Oxford University Press Inc., New York

First published 2003

British Library Cataloguing in Publication Data

Data available

Library of Congress Cataloging in Publication Data

Data available

ISBN 0 19 263179 9

10 9 8 7 6 5 4 3 2 1

Typeset by Newgen Imaging Systems (P) Ltd., Chennai, India
Printed in Great Britain
on acid-free paper by
Bath Press, Bath, UK

Dedications

Cogito et seco

ES:

Dedicated to my glorious sons, Conor, Declan, and Tom

LT:

Dedicated to Hong Quach for her love, my parents Quang and Kim for their support, and my brothers Joseph, Nelson, and Jackson for their encouragement

Preface

Oxford University Press asked us to write a trauma book for the new millennium. We believe we have achieved this.

The twentieth century started with a major conflict in the Balkans and, tragically, it ended in the same way. This new century faces the spectre of terrorism. Conflict and its manifestations, as well as vehicle accidents, appear set to be with us well into the twenty-first century. The need for trauma specialists will not go away.

Modern medicine and surgery has become superspecialized and we often fail to understand each other's jargon. The aim of this text is to providing a way of uniting those of us who care for the victims of accidents or acts of violence, so that we can help ourselves to help our patients.

We have brought together a team of talented traumatologists from around the world to contribute to this book. The paper text is closely linked to the Internet by offering updates with WorldOrtho (www.worldortho.com), a niche orthopaedic and trauma content provider. We hope that it will find a place in every emergency department and trauma unit.

Enjoy this text and your good work; let us know how we can improve future editions. Send an email (esherry@bigpond.com) or a short text message (+61 414 185 238) to me (ES).

Key point

- Bookmark the WorldOrtho website, www.worldortho.com

ES University of Sydney, Nepean Hospital

LT Concord Repatriation General Hospital, Sydney

JT Keele University

December 2002

Acknowledgements

The editors would like to thank Richard Marley for his initiative and enthusiasm in starting and supporting this project. We would also like to acknowledge Dr Vlasios (Bill) Brakoulias who has supported the text with his remarkable and original line drawings, and Professor John Thomson who ably researched and supplemented Chapter 1. Thanks also to Kiet Trieu and Drs William Truong, Tai Khoa Lam, and Anh Huy Tang for their assistance in proofreading various chapters. The members of the Orthopaedic Department, University of Sydney, Nepean Hospital, have never hesitated to provide much of the raw clinical material for this text.

This is not my Body

(i)
This is not my body
or my blood

I shall not scream
for I have become
a sea of pain soaring
into the sky
filling the sun
and the moon
with blood

and I shall surrender
at last these
alien fragments
of jagged ivory
to the fission
of hidden
dancing stars
across a whiteness
I cannot touch

(ii)
was I once guided
by the stars
the moon
and the clouds
to heal the sky
and the sea?

now I cannot escape
from this cavernous
cold white room
where the dome of dense
white light whispers
at 3 a.m.
to the many glowed hands
- this is miracle
number ten

as we quietly
and tenderly renew
the fragmented precious
curves and lines
with pieces
of shining metal
and strings

while the fractured
soul is still
sleeping

Jenny Ma Wyatt (1998)

Contents

Contributors

Editors

Eugene Sherry
Department of Orthopaedic Surgery, University of Sydney, Nepean Hospital, Sydney, NSW, Australia

John Templeton
Emeritus Professor of Traumatic Orthopaedic Surgery, Keele University, UK

Lawrence Trieu
Concord Repatriation General Hospital, Sydney, NSW, Australia

Assistant editor

Jennifer R Yuan
Department of Surgery, Nepean Hospital, Sydney, NSW, Australia

Authors

Nanni Allington
Department of Orthopaedic Surgery, CHR La Citadelle, Liege, Belgium

Keith P Allison
North Staffordshire Hospitals NHS Trust, City General Hospital, Stoke-on-Trent, UK

Simon V Bariol
Department of Urology, Sutherland Hospital, Sydney, NSW, Australia

Peter Barry
Department of Surgery, Westmead Hospital, Sydney, NSW, Australia

Greg B.Bennett
Medical Division, Nepean Hospital, Sydney, NSW, Australia

David Bihari
Intensive Care Unit, St George Hospital, University of New South Wales, Sydney, NSW, Australia

James Branley
Department of Infectious Disease, Nepean Hospital, Sydney, NSW, Australia

Gary J Browne
New Children's Hospital, Westmead, Sydney, NSW, Australia

Ian Cameron
Rehabilitation Studies Unit, Department of Medicine, University of Sydney, Sydney, NSW, Australia

Daniel T Cass
Paediatric Trauma, New Children's Hospital, Westmead, Sydney, NSW, Australia

Alexandre K H Chao
Department of Vascular Surgery, Westmead Hospital, Sydney, NSW, Australia

Cholavech Chavasiri
Department of Orthopaedic Surgery, Faculty of Medicine, Siriraj Hospital, Mahidol University, Bangkok, Thailand

Alison L S Chiu
Department of Anatomy and Histology, University of Sydney, Sydney, NSW, Australia

Robin K C Choong
New Children's Hospital, Westmead, Sydney, NSW, Australia

Loretta B Chou
Division of Orthopaedic Surgery, Stanford University, California, USA

Lee Collins
Medical Physics Department, Westmead Hospital, Sydney, NSW, Australia

Roslyn Crampton
Senior Staff Specialist, Department of Emergency Medicine, Westmead Hospital, Sydney, NSW, Australia

Jonathan Curtis
Department of Neurosurgery, Royal North Shore Hospital, Sydney, NSW, Australia

Bella van Dalen
Department of Orthopaedic Surgery, Hevoziekenhuis Hospital, Almere, The Netherlands

Gordon Dandie
Department of Neurosurgery, Royal North Shore Hospital, Sydney, NSW, Australia

Michael Davis
Department of Intensive Care, St George Hospital, Sydney, NSW, Australia

Mark Dexter
Department of Neurosurgery, Westmead Hospital, Sydney, NSW, Australia

Geoffrey Donald
Department of Orthopaedic Surgery, Nepean Hospital, Sydney, NSW, Australia

Charles Eaton
West Palm Beach, Florida, USA

Jean R Edwards
Sexual Assault and Child Protection Service, Northern Sydney Area Health Service, Sydney, NSW, Australia

Andrew Finckh
Department of Emergency Medicine, St Vincent's Hospital, Sydney, NSW, Australia

John P Fletcher
Division of Surgery, Westmead Hospital, Sydney, NSW, Australia

Kerwyn Foo
Westmead Hospital, Sydney, NSW, Australia

Emma Green
Royal North Shore Hospital, Sydney, NSW, Australia

Kayvan Haghighi
Department of Surgery, Concord Repatriation General Hospital, Sydney, NSW, Australia

Michael A Hargraves
Department of Ophthalmology, Westmead Hospital, Sydney, NSW, Australia

Peter G Hayward
Nepean Hospital, Sydney, NSW, Australia

Antony F Henderson
St Vincent's Hospital, Sydney, NSW, Australia

Carolyn Hogan
Intensive Care Unit, Nepean Hospital, Sydney, NSW, Australia

Andrew J A Holland
Department of Academic Surgery, The Children's Hospital at Westmead, Sydney, NSW, Australia

Ke Huang
Department of Orthopaedic Surgery, Nepean Hospital, Sydney, NSW, Australia

Simon R Hutabarat
Department of Orthopaedic Surgery, The Canberra Hospital, Canberra, ACT, Australia

Balakrishnan Ilango
Department of Orthopaedic Surgery, South Manchester University Hospitals, Manchester, UK

Erica Jacobson
Department of Neurosurgery, Westmead Hospital, Sydney, NSW, Australia

Roland Jiang
Department of Surgery, Westmead Hospital, Sydney, NSW, Australia

Roy M Kimble
Department of Paediatric Surgery, Royal Brisbane Hospital for Children, Brisbane, Queensland, Australia

Clayton King
Rehabilitation Studies Unit, Department of Medicine, University of Sydney, Sydney, NSW, Australia

Robert Kirby
North Staffordshire Hospital, Stoke-on-Trent, UK

Mark Kohout
Department of Plastic and Reconstructive Surgery, Westmead Hospital, Sydney, NSW, Australia

Gawel Kulisiewicz
The Canberra Hospital, Canberra, ACT, Australia

Howard Lau
Department of Urology, Westmead Hospital, Sydney, NSW, Australia

Nicholas Lotz
Department of Plastic and Reconstructive Surgery, Royal North Shore Hospital, Sydney, NSW, Australia

Jenny Ma Wyatt
Department of Anatomical Pathology, Nepean Hospital, Sydney, NSW, Australia

Nicola Maffulli
Department of Trauma and Orthopaedic Surgery, Keele University School of Medicine, North Staffordshire Hospital NHS Trust, Stoke-on-Trent, UK

Damian McMahon
University Department of Surgery, The Canberra Hospital, Canberra, ACT, Australia

James Middleton
Rehabilitation Studies Unit, Department of Medicine, University of Sydney, Sydney, NSW, Australia

Dianna Milinkovic-Balog
Education Centre Against Violence, NSW, Australia

Paula J Mohacsi
Organ and Tissue Donation Co-ordinator, Northern Sydney Health, St Leonards 2065, Australia

Rhidian Morgan-Jones
University Hospital of Wales, Cardiff, UK

Henry Murray
Department of Obstetrics and Gynaecology, Nepean Hospital, University of Sydney, Sydney, NSW, Australia

Nicholas Neal
North Staffordshire Hospitals NHS Trust, Stoke-on-Trent, UK

Nhi Nguyen
Nepean Hospital, Sydney, NSW, Australia

Daniel J Prinsloo
North Staffordshire Hospitals NHS Trust, City General Hospital, Stoke-on-Trent, UK

Daniel Rahme
Department of Orthopaedic Surgery, Nepean Hospital, Sydney, NSW, Australia

Ray F Raper
Senior Staff Specialist, Intensive Therapy Unit, Royal North Shore Hospital, St Leonards 2065, Australia

Anthony D Redmond
Emeritus Professor of Emergency Medicine, Department of Orthopaedic Surgery, Keele University, Staffs, UK

Michael D Robertson
Mayo-Wesley Centre for Mental Health, Taree, NSW, Australia

John Rooney
Department of Orthopaedic Surgery, The Canberra Hospital, Canberra ACT Australia,

Jayanth Sundar Sampath
Department of Trauma and Orthopaedics, Blackburn Royal Infirmary, Blackburn, UK

Anthony Shakeshaft
Department of Surgery, University of Sydney, Nepean Hospital, Sydney, NSW, Australia

Kevin Smith
North Staffordshire Hospitals NHS Trust, Stoke-on-Trent, UK

Brian Spurrett
Department of Obstetrics and Gynaecology, University of Sydney, Nepean Hospital, Sydney, NSW, Australia

David Stanton
Department of Orthopaedic Surgery, Concord Repatriation General Hospital, Sydney, NSW, Australia

Rodney Studd
Department of Surgery, Concord Repatriation General Hospital, Sydney, NSW, Australia

Kourosh Tavakoli
Department of Plastic and Reconstructive Surgery, St Vincent's Hospital, Sydney, NSW, Australia

Peter Templeton
Leeds Teaching Hospitals NHS Trust, Leeds, UK

Peter Thomas
North Staffordshire Hospitals NHS Trust, Stoke-on-Trent, UK

Joseph Duc Huy Trieu
Concord Repatriation General Hospital, Sydney, NSW, Australia

Sameer Viswanathan
Concord Repatriation General Hospital, Sydney, NSW, Australia

Robyn Walker
Submarine and Underwater Medicine Unit, HMAS Penguin, Sydney, NSW, Australia

Patrick H Warnke
Department of Oral and Maxillofacial Surgery, University of Kiel, Germany

Julian White
Department of Toxinology, Women and Children's Hospital, North Adelaide, South Australia

Barry H Wilkins
Department of Intensive Care, New Children's Hospital, Westmead, Sydney, NSW, Australia

Stephen F Wilson
Rehabilitation Studies Unit, Department of Medicine, University of Sydney, Sydney, NSW, Australia

David Winlaw
Department of Cardiothoracic Surgery, St Vincent's Hospital, Sydney, NSW, Australia

Stephen Worrall
Department of Oral and Maxillofacial Surgery, St Luke's Hospital, Bradford, West Yorks, UK

Gary Yee
Department of Plastic and Reconstructive Surgery, St. George Hospital, Sydney, NSW, Australia

Medical illustrator

Bill Brakoulias
Westmead Hospital, Sydney, NSW, Australia

Abbreviations

ABC airway, breathing, and circulation
ABG arterial blood gases
ABI ankle–brachial index
ACF anterior cranial fossa
ACL anterior cruciate ligament
ADH antidiuretic hormone
ADI atlanto–dens interval
ADL activities of daily living
ADP adenosine diphosphate
ADR adverse drug reaction
AIO Ambulance Incident Officer
ANS autonomic nervous system
AO Arbetisgemeinschaft für Osteosynthesefragen (Association for the Study of Internal Fixation)
AP anteroposterior
APO apolipoprotein
ARDS Adult respiratory distress syndrome
ARS acute radiation syndrome
ASD acute stress disorder
ASDH acute subdural haematoma
ASIS anterior superior iliac spine
ATF anterior talofibular (ligament)
ATLS Advanced Trauma Life Support
ATP adenosine triphosphate
AVN avascular necrosis
AVPU alert, voice, pain, unresponsive
BAI blunt aortic injury
BBB blood–brain barrier
BCI blunt cardiac injury
BIPP bismuth iodoform paraffin paste
BSF basilar skull fracutre
CAGE cerebral arterial gas embolism
CBF cerebral blood flow
CBV cerebral blood volume
CCP cerebral perfusion pressure
CF calcaneofibular (ligament)
CHI closed head injury
CISC clean intermittent self-catheterization
CJD Creutzfeld–Jacob disease
$CMRO_2$ metabolic rate for oxygen
CMV cytomegalovirus
CNVM chorodial neovascular membrane
CPAP continuous positive airway pressure
CPK creatine phosphokinase
CPM continuous passive motion
CPR cardiopulmonary resuscitation
CSDH chronic subdural haematomas
CSF cerebrospinal fluid
CT computed tomography
CTE chronic traumatic encephalopathy
CVR cerebral vascular resistance
DAI diffuse axonal injury
DCI decompression illness
DCP dynamic compression plate
DCS dynamic compression screw
DDAVP deamino-D-arginine vasopressin
DEXA dual energy X-ray absorptiometry
DIC disseminated intravascular coagulation
DISI dorsal intercalary segment instability
DPL diagnostic peritoneal lavage
DSD detrusor–sphincter dyssynergia
DVT deep venous thrombosis
ECG electrocardiograph
EDH extradural haematoma
ESR erythrocyte sedimentation rate
$ETCO_2$ end-tidal carbon dioxide
FIM functional independence measure
F_IO_2 fraction of inspired oxygen
GCS Glasgow Coma Scale
GOS Glasgow Outcome Score
HO heterotopic ossification
HRR heart rate reserve
I&D incision and drainage
ICC intercostal chateter
ICP intracranial pressure
IDC indwelling catheter
II image intensifier

IM	intramedullary (nail, etc.)
IMF	intermaxillary fixation
IOFB	intraocular foreign body
IOP	intraocular pressure
IPPV	intermittent positive pressure ventilation
ISS	Injury Severity Score
IVF	*in vitro* fertilization
IVP	intravenous pyelogram
MAOI	monoamine oxidase inhibitor
MAP	mean arterial pressure
MAST	military antishock trousers
MCL	medial collateral ligament
MCP	metacarpophalangeal (joint)
MDI	multidirectional instability
MIO	Medical Incident Officer
MRA	magnetic resonance angiography
MRI	magnetic resonance imaging
MSE	mental state examination
MVA	motor vehicle accident
NAIR	National Arrangements for Incidents involving Radiation
NGT	nasogastric tube
NIBP	non-invasive blood pressure
NOE	naso-orbito-ethmoid (complex)
NSI	nutritional screening index
OPSI	overwhelming postsplenectomy infection
OR	odds ratio
ORIF	open reduction and internal fixation
OTT	orotracheal tube
PA	posteroanterior
P_aCO_2	arterial partial pressure of carbon dioxide
P_aO_2	arterial partial pressure of oxygen
PCA	patient-controlled analgesia
PCL	posterior cruciate liagement
PEEP	positive end expiratory pressure
PSIS	posterior superior iliac spine
PT	prothromin time
PTA	post-traumatic amnesia
PTF	posterior talofibular (ligament)
PTS	Paediatric Trauma Score
PTSD	post-traumatic stress disorder
PTT	partial thromplastin time
PVI	pressure–volume index
RDI	required daily intake
RICE	rest, ice, compression, and elevation
RM	repetition maximum
ROM	range of motion
RPT	refractory period of transmission
SAH	subarachnoid haemorrhage
SCH	subconjunctival haemorrhage
SCI	spinal cord injury
SCIWORA	spinal cord injury without radiological abnormality
SDH	subdural haematoma
SERPIN	plasma serine protease inhibitor
SGA	subjective global assessment
SIADH	Syndrome of inappropriate ADH secretion
$S_{jv}O_2$	jugular venous saturation
SMAS	superficial musculo-aponeurotic system
SPECT	single-photon emission computed tomography
SSD	silver sulfadiazine
SSEP	somatosensory evoked potentials
SSRI	selective serotonin reuptake inhibitor
TBI	traumatic brain injury
TCD	transcranial doppler ultrasonography
TENS	transcutaneous electrical stimulation
TFCC	triangular fibrocartilage complex
TLSO	thoraco-lumbar-sacral orthosis
TMJ	temporomandibular joint
TOE	transoesophageal echocardiography
TPN	total parenteral nutrition
tSAH	traumatic subarachnoid haemorrhage
TSCL	therapeutic soft contact lenses
VF	ventricular fibrillation
WHO	World Health Organization

1

CHAPTER 1

The trauma problem

EUGENE SHERRY

CHAPTER 1
The trauma problem

EUGENE SHERRY

Historical introduction

Trauma has a long and interesting history. The great medical writings of the past have, of necessity, been about injury. The Edwin Smith Papyrus, written between 3000 and 1600BCE, describes 48 cases of trauma from the head to the foot. The principles enshrined there are still pertinent today.

Hippocrates (460–370BCE) came from the tradition of Greek natural philosophers. His writings comprise 60 books (including *De Articularis*, a masterful account of the treatment of fractures and dislocations) from 430 to 330BCE. He systematized medicine, established medical science and introduced proper independence and social standing for the physician. Hippocrates said that war was the only proper training for a surgeon, and, as we shall see, many developments in trauma care have been prompted by military necessity.

The great Galen (129–199CE) was influenced by the work of Hippocrates and gained his vast experience as a gladiatorial surgeon in the Pergamon arena in Asia Minor. His writings (over 500 medical treatises, of which 83 have survived) dominated the theoretical basis of medicine for the next 1500 years. When he died, medical scientific enquiry—at least in Europe and around the Mediterranean—is said to have ceased for hundreds of years (Singer and Underwood 1962).

In the Byzantine era, the Christian church fathers assumed the care of crippled children and adults. Paul of Aegina (625–690) and Apollonius were influenced by Hippocrates and worked in Alexandria. The great Arab tradition of medicine—the medicine of later Greek antiquity—centred on Rhazes (850–932) and Avicenna (980–1036).

The great universities, hospitals and medical faculties of Europe (in Salerno, Paris, Oxford, Bologna, Montpellier, and Padua) were founded during the period known as the 'awakening' (tenth to twelfth centuries). Great hospitals, derived from the Roman *valetudinaria*, were established in Baghdad (the Bimaristan Al-Azudi in 981) and in London (St Bartholomew's in 1123, St Thomas's in 1200).

Ambroise Paré (1510–1590) was said to have revolutionized the treatment of war wounds while serving as an army surgeon and surgical adviser to several French kings. He noted the cleansing action of maggots on wounds, used windlass traction for femoral fractures, recognized cord compression in vertebral fractures, and saw in the modern era of prostheses and brace-making.

The 'age of the scientific revolution' in the seventeenth century saw the publication of William Harvey's *De Motu Cordis* (which described blood circulation), intravenous injections, and blood transfusions. But it was the insatiable and all-embracing intellectual enquiries of the great John Hunter (1728–93) which were to dominate surgical thinking from the eighteenth century until the present. Hunter established himself as an expert in comparative physiology and experimental morphology), trained the top surgeons and scientists of the day (including Jenner, Astley Cooper, John Abernethy, and two Americans of Civil War fame—John Morgan, founder of the first American Medical School at the University of Pennsylvania, and William Shippen), and wrote *A Treatise on the Blood, Inflammation, and Gunshot Wounds* (one of the best texts on trauma).

The period of colonial expansion by the major European powers (seventeenth to nineteenth centuries) introduced western concepts of surgical and trauma care as far away as Australia. Dominique Jean Larrey (1766–1842), Napoleon's surgeon, who personally performed over 200 amputations in one 24 hour period during the Russian campaign, considered all aspects of trauma care (sanitation, food supplies, transport, training of personnel) of the wounded soldier.

The nineteenth century was a time of social upheaval and intellectual development. Important medical developments included the introduction of anaesthesia by W.T.G. Morton in 1847, the publication of Virchow's *Cellular Pathology* in 1860, and from 1867 onwards antiseptic surgery based on the work of Pasteur and Lister. The principles of nursing care were established by Florence Nightingale on the basis of her experiences during the Crimean War (1853–56). She established sanitation, food services, clean water, laundry, cleaning, statistical data collection, and medical records. The American Civil War (1861–65) was probably the bloodiest war ever fought, with disorganized, chaotic, and ignoble medical services.

The major conflicts of the twentieth century necessitated improvements in trauma care, with understanding of metabolic care, fluid therapy, treatment of haemorrhagic shock, use of antibiotics, resuscitation, helicopter evacuation, electronic monitoring of patients, and refined anaesthetic services.

- World War I (1914–18) was characterized by the high incidence of gas gangrene in the trenches. The Inter-Allied Surgical Conference in Paris in 1917 established the rule for management of war wounds: debridement and delayed closure (unless <8 hours old). Motorized ambulances were introduced, Dakin's solution was used as an antiseptic, and penetrating abdominal injuries were explored.
- In World War II (1939–45) wounds were fully debrided and left open, and whole blood transfusions were used at the battle front. Antibiotics and intramedullary nailing of the femur (established by G. Kuntscher, 1900–72) were used for the first time, and air evacuation and special surgical units were introduced.
- From the Korean conflict (1950–53) arose the MASH unit (near the area of conflict), helicopter evacuation over rough terrain, vascular repair in limb injuries, further use of antibiotics, and recognition of early renal failure and treatment with haemodialysis.
- In the Vietnam War (1964–75) there was further use of helicopter evacuation, laboratory back-up in the field, and use of the artificial kidney.

It is worthwhile to look at the mortality from injury in these four conflicts to see how trauma services have developed (Table 1.1). Mortality has continued to decrease in more recent wars. The British–Argentine conflict over the Falklands in 1982 saw the widespread use of the field surgical team. This was a highly mobile team (surgeon, anaesthetist, resuscitation officer, four theatre technicians, blood transfusion, technician, clerk), which worked independently and was operational within 15 minutes. In Operation Desert Storm (the Gulf

Table 1.1 Surgical mortality for head, chest, and abdominal wounds (US Army)

War	Head	Thorax	Abdomen
World War I			
Cases	189	104	1816
% Mortality	40	37	67
World War II			
Cases	2051	1364	2315
% Mortality	14	10	23
Korean Conflict			
Cases	673	158	384
% Mortality	10	8	9
Vietnam War			
Cases	1171	1176	1209
% Mortality	10	7	9

War of 1991) there was a very low loss of American and allied troops (331 deaths, most non-combatant). This low mortality was due to rapid evacuation and excellent clinical care.

Future challenges

Murray and Lopez (1996) have highlighted the challenges ahead. There is little likelihood of an end to armed conflict, and economic development (or at least the number of motor vehicles) will continue to increase. Consequently, war and road traffic accidents, which in 1990 were respectively the 16th and 9th leading causes of disability-adjusted life years (a composite measure of the burden of a health problem), are expected to rise to 8th and 3rd respectively by the year 2020.

Trauma looks likely to remain the unsolved epidemic. Specialized care for trauma victims will be the way of the future, and the refinement of such care will depend upon innovation, inventions, and advances in medical science.

Although the challenges of the future seem daunting, they are not insurmountable. Many of our forebears faced and overcame greater problems with significantly fewer resources at hand.

Trauma in the USA

Murphy (1994) has provided a succinct overview of trauma epidemiology in the USA. Much of this data is from the National Centre for Health Statistics which publishes a yearly mortality report summarizing deaths in the USA (Table 1.2).

- Trauma is the leading health problem in the USA, with >140 000 deaths annually (147 891 in 1995) and the leading cause of years of potential life lost before age 65 (before cancer and heart disease) (NCHS 1995; see Table 1.2).
- Most injuries are probably preventable.
- One-third of the population sustain a non-fatal injury each year (most common cause of death <34 years).There were 59 127 000 injuries reported in 1995.

Table 1.2 10 leading causes of injury deaths in the United States, 1999 (all races, both sexes, 25–34 years age group)

Rank	Cause of death	Deaths
1	Unintentional motor vehicle traffic	6602
2	Homicide firearm	3048
3	Suicide firearm	2621
4	Unintentional poisoning	2355
5	Suicide suffocation	1323
6	Suicide poisoning	785
7	Undetermined poisoning	543
8	Homicide cut/pierce	467
9	Unintentional drowning	446
10	Unintentional fall	343

Source: National Vital Statistics System, NCHS, CDC http://www.cdc.gov/ncipc/osp/

- Trauma is the leading cause of lost work hours.
- One out of every eight beds in the USA is for trauma.
- Every year 80 000 people sustain severe brain/spinal cord injuries.
- The cost in 1988 was US$180 billion.
- Men are 2.5 greater risk than women.
- The death rate is highest in poor urban areas.
- More than half of motor vehicle accidents are alcohol-related.
- Over 90% survive their injury.
- 60% of deaths occur in the first 24 hours.
- The most highly injured group are 15–24 years, with motor vehicle accident causing >54% of injuries.
- Falls exceed motor vehicle accidents as the leading cause of non-fatal injuries (and cause 12 000 deaths/year; the elderly are at greatest risk).
- The rate of homicide death is 12.7/100 000 in USA (as compared with 2.7 in Australia,

2.4 in Italy,1.0 in Japan, and 0.8 in the UK).

- 75% of homicides were firearms related. Homicide is the leading cause of death for black males aged 15–24 years; and leading cause of occupational death in New York City and Los Angeles. Rosenberg and Fenley (1991) have identified biological (e.g. age, gender, psychiatric illness) and sociological factors to account for interpersonal violence in the USA. 'If current trends continue, by the year 2003 firearm deaths will surpass motor vehicle-related deaths as the leading cause of injury and death in the US' (Grossman 1998).
- Burns cause 6 000 deaths/year (death is from inhalation of carbon monoxide and toxic substances; alcohol and cigarettes are factors in house fires), lightning causes 80 deaths/year. However, there is decreasing incidence with education about smoking and alcohol use in bed, along with the use of fireproof clothing and bedclothes.
- There were 30 484 suicide deaths in 1992 (80% white males).

It is important to be aware of the trimodal distribution of deaths from trauma with regard to time. There are three peaks:

- *immediate:* half of all deaths, not possible to save, from massive head injury/brain stem injury/major cardiovascular event
- *early:* within first few hours, from torso trauma in these cases
- *late:* about 20% of all, from organ failure and sepsis, influenced by inadequate early resuscitation or care.

The concept of the 'golden hour' is used to describe the urgent need for the treatment of trauma victims within the first hour after injury. It is thought that morbidity and mortality are reduced if such care is started within this hour. This concept was developed by Trunkey (1983) and is the underlying philosophy of current trauma care.

Trauma in UK, Australia, Europe, Singapore, and the developing world

Trauma in the United Kingdom

Within the UK the supervision of emergency departments was the responsible of orthopaedic surgeons until in 1970 the Accident Services Review Committee indicated that from the staffing point of view, the orthopaedic solution had failed (consultant cover in emergency departments was nominal only). From 1971 the Joint Consultants Committee recommended that emergency departments be placed under the control of a consultant in accident and emergency medicine, with registrar training programmes. Fewer than 10% of UK orthopaedic consultants give musculoskeletal trauma as their major interest (only about a dozen surgeons out of >1000 practice primary and secondary trauma alone). In the UK, with a population of 55 million, there are about 900 000 musculoskeletal injuries each year, of which >100 000 are left with a significant disability (Oliver 1997). Only two units, Edinburgh and Oxford, have completely separated the management of acute injuries from elective practice. In Oxford the unit is staffed 24 hours a day by a resident consultant traumatologist. In Edinburgh the unit is staffed by a non-resident consultant. The Oxford consultants act as trauma team leaders in the emergency department, whereas the Edinburgh consultants triage through the emergency department consultants.

Trauma in Australia

The situation in Australia is similar to that in the USA for general injury and motor vehicle accident fatalities (Table 1.3) , but with significantly fewer firearms injuries and declining road fatalities, especially since 1989 (Federal Office of Road Safety, Australia) (Table 1.4), because of random alcohol breath testing and use of seatbelts and airbags. There are significant numbers of swimming pool fatalities involving children.

Table 1.3 Injury deaths in Australia, 1996

Mode of injury death	Age group (years)										
	0–4	5–9	10–14	15–24	25–34	35–54	55–64	65–74	75+	All ages	Age adjusted
Motor vehicle accidents	4.5	3.2	4.3	21.0	12.5	8.8	9.4	10.8	21.8	10.8	10
Swimming pool	2.3	0.4	0.2	0.7	0.6	0.6	0.4	0.5	0.4	0.6	
Drug-related (all)	0.2	0.1	0.1	1.7	3.5	2.3	0.5	0.6	1.2	1.7	1
Firearm/missile			0.1	0.4	0.1	0.2	0.3	0.1	0.1	0.2	
Excessive temperatures						0.1		0.5	0.9	0.1	
Exposure/neglect/ hunger/thirst							0.1		0.1		
Strike/struck by object or person					0.5	0.4	0.3	0.4	0.5	0.5	0.2
In sports				0.1							
Explosion						0.1	0.1		0.2		
Electric current	0.1	0.2	0.2	0.3	0.3	0.3	0.4	0.2	0.1	0.2	
Suicide (all)			1.1	14.7	16.1	15.1	12.3	10.5	11.5	11.2	10
Unarmed fight/ brawl IPV				0.1	0.6	0.2	0.1	0.2		0.2	
Firearm IPV	0.2	0.2	0.2	0.6	0.8	0.6	0.7	1.1	0.2	0.6	
Cutting/ stabbing IPV	0.1	0.1		0.9	1.0	0.6	0.3	0.4	0.2	0.5	
Child battering/ maltreatment	0.5										
Medical misadventure, complications	0.1			0.2	0.2	0.3	0.7	2.1	2.8	0.5	

IPV, interpersonal violence.

Adapted from National Injury Surveillance Unit, Australia. http://www.nisu.flinders.edu.au/welcome.html

State, year of death registration, counts, rates per 100 000 population, age group and sex; rates for cells with case counts less than 4 have been suppressed.

Trauma in Europe

The overall rates for death from motor vehicle injury for Europe are similar to those in Australia and the USA. There are lower rates in smaller countries (the Netherlands and the UK) and where driving safety laws, such as compulsory seatbelts and lower permitted blood alcohol levels for driving, were introduced earlier (Sweden).

Table 1.4 Australian road fatalities, 1981–97

Year	Drivers	Passengers	Pedestrians	Motorcyclists[a]	Pedal cyclists[b]	Total[c]
1981	1279	889	629	424	94	3321
1982	1237	850	591	482	88	3252
1983	1034	689	512	410	103	2755
1984	1036	756	541	390	90	2822
1985	1143	763	538	404	83	2941
1986	1134	730	537	405	78	2888
1987	1095	737	493	359	79	2772
1988	1144	776	548	323	87	2887
1989	1122	781	501	299	98	2801
1990	935	634	420	262	80	2331
1991	910	554	343	248	58	2113
1992	815	570	350	197	41	1974
1993	859	513	331	203	45	1953
1994	809	501	367	190	59	1928
1995	874	491	398	204	48	2017
1996	869	499	351	193	57	1970
1997	777	429	329	176	52	1766

[a] Motorcyclists includes both riders and pillion passengers.

[b] From 1989, this figure includes both bicycle riders and pillion passengers.

[c] Total includes road users not separately classified.

Trauma in Singapore

Trauma has been the leading cause of death in Singapore for over 40 years (Iau *et al.* 1998). Over half of trauma deaths are from motor vehicle accidents, <3.5% from assault, but there are no gunshot injuries (stiff legal penalties have almost abolished private ownership of firearms in this country). Although 77.6% are unavoidable, 25% have been found to be potentially or frankly preventable. Even in a small island city-state 50 km long, with five government general hospitals, the policy of 'scoop and run' before stabilization (airway management, stabilize fractures, and fluid resuscitation) should be abandoned.

Trauma in the developing world

There is a growing epidemic of trauma in the developing world which has been noted by orthopaedic surgeons working in these areas. Motor vehicle accidents are now the third highest cause of death (Cumming 1998). Factors include the large number of pedestrians and cyclists (many living below the poverty line) involved in these accidents; overcrowding of public transport; poor maintenance of roads; few speed restrictions; and the underdeveloped medical management and treatment of trauma. In addition, non-fatal trauma which occurs at home (poor vision from cataracts may be a significant factor) and in the workplace.

Table 1.5 Motor vehicle accidents and people killed or injured in 1996 in Europe (injury rate and death rates in parentheses)

	Population (M)	Number of accidents	Number of accidents (per 100 000 people)	Number of deaths	Number of deaths (per 100 000 people)	Number injured	Number of injuries (per 100 000 people)
Denmark	5.251	8080	153.8754	514	9.788611	9810	186.8215
Finland	5.116	7274	142.1813	404	7.896794	9299	181.7630
France	66.8665	125 406	187.5468	8080	12.08377	170 117	254.4128
Germany	94.084	373 082	396.5413	8758	9.308702	493 158	524.167
Italy	57.333	183 415	319.9117	6193	10.80180	264 213	460.8393
Netherlands	20.5645	11 561	56.21824	1180	5.738043	11 966	58.18765
Norway	4.37	8779	200.8924	255	5.835240	12025	275.1716
Portugal	9.92	49 265	496.6229	2100	21.16935	66627	671.6431
Sweden	8.837	15 321	173.3733	537	6.07672	20810	235.4871
UK	62.288	235 939	378.7872	3598	5.776393	316 704	508.451

Courtesy of Dr D. Van der Peet.

Natural disasters can be a major cause of trauma, although there is little data on this subject (see Chapter 3).

Prevention

W Haddon, the first Director of the US National Highway Traffic Safety Administration, formulated a conceptual approach to injury prevention (essentially host/vehicle/environment) (Haddon 1972):

- Prevent the creation of hazards (limit firearms sales, e.g. handgun control in Australia in 1997).
- Reduce the number of hazards.
- Prevent the release of a hazard (child-proof medication holders) or modify its release.
- Separate hazards from hosts in terms of space and time (traffic overpasses to prevent congestion).
- Use material barriers (screens).
- Modify basic qualities of hazards (airbags).
- Make hosts more resistant to damage.
- Counter damage already present (first aid training).
- Stabilize, repair, and rehabilitate the injured.

This is covered by three basic strategies:

- *Education and persuasion:* Public education campaigns with intention of altering behaviour; such as driver education about fatigue and alcohol/drug use, use of seatbelts and airbags (not often successful where compliance is required, e.g. putting on seatbelt versus automatic triggering of airbag).
- *Legal regulation of behaviour:* To protect individual and others exposed such as speed restrictions, which decreases injury rate (Kloeden *et al.* 1998), use of helmets, and alcohol restriction.
- *Automatic protection:* Car manufacture standards include glare reduction, braking systems, seatbelts, head restraints, collapsing steering

columns, puncture-resistant gas tanks, child restraints; building better and safer highways with divided highways and break-away light poles; water sprinklers in buildings. All such measures need to be subjected to cost–benefit analysis (how much to spend, how to spend it and how to make the service available).

Such measures can be further reduced to four steps:

1 Define the problem.
2 Identify causes and risk factors.
3 Develop and test interventions.
4 Implement interventions and evaluate their impact.

Haddon's approach has been hailed among the greatest public health achievements of the century, and has reduced road mortality in the USA to one-third of what it was in the 1950s. In contrast, the Americans have made little progress in reducing gun-related violence.

References

Cumming WJ (1998) *World Orthopedic Concern Newsletter* 76: 1–3.

Federal Office of Road Safety, Australia. http://www.dot. gov.au/ For further information, email: forsstats@dot.gov.au.

Grossman MD (1998) Introduction to trauma care. In: AB Peitzman *et al.* (ed) *Trauma manual*. Lippincott-Raven, Philadelphia, Pa.

Haddon W (1972) A logical framework for categorizing highway safety phenomena and activity. *Journal of Trauma* 12: 297.

Iau PTC, Ong CL, Chan ST (1998) Preventable trauma deaths in Singapore. *Australian and New Zealand Journal of Surgery* 68: 820–825.

Kloeden CN, McLean AJ, Moore VM, Ponte G (1998) Travelling speed and the risk of crash involvement. http://raru.adelaide.edu.au/speed/.

Murphy JT (1994) Epidemiology of trauma. In: Lopez-Viego MA (ed) *The Parkland Handbook trauma handbook*. Mosby, St. Louis, Mo.

Murray CJL, Lopez AD (1996) Evidence-based health policy—lessons from the global burden of disease study. *Science* 274: 740–743.

NCHS (1995) Vital Statistics System. National Center for Health Statistics; http://www.cdc.gov/nchs/nvss.htm

Oliver C (1997) Trauma column. In: WorldOrtho; www.worldortho.com.

Rosenberg ML, Fenley MA (1991) *Violence in America: a public health approach*. Oxford University Press, New York, NY.

Singer C, Underwood EA (1962) *A Short History of Medicine*, 2nd edn. Oxford University Press, Oxford.

Trunkey DD (1983) The trimodal distribution of death after injury. *Scientific American* 249(2): 28–53.

2

CHAPTER 2

Resuscitation and assessment of the severely injured patient

DAMIAN McMAHON AND GARY J BROWNE

CHAPTER 2
Resuscitation and assessment of the severely injured patient

DAMIAN McMAHON AND GARY J BROWNE

Resuscitation of the injured patient is the restoration of 'normal physiology', with the end point being successful delivery of oxygen to tissues, especially the brain and the heart. The injured patient may have traumatic pathology, which inhibits this perfusion of vital organs. The term *trauma resuscitation* describes the period of intense medical intervention and discovery, by clinical examination and imaging modalities, which identifies and corrects these problems, salvaging life and limb.

Restoration of physiology (resuscitation) and assessment of injury are synchronous events in the acutely injured patient. The successful trauma resuscitation requires coordinated, methodical and structured approach to the assessment and ongoing correction of physiology. It is a dynamic and continuous process, requiring repeated reassessment.

The Advanced Trauma Life Support Course (ATLS)/Early Management of Severe Trauma Course (EMST), run by the American College of Surgeons and Royal Australasian College of Surgeons respectively, provides a structured framework for the priorities of a trauma resuscitation. It is strongly recommended that all physicians caring for acutely injured patients attend this course. It should be mandatory that all trauma team members have undertaken such instruction.

Commonly in larger hospitals a trauma team approach is advantageous. This chapter presents a team-orientated approach to trauma resuscitation. The trauma team is a multidisciplinary group, available around the clock, with skills to attend to the patient's multiple needs simultaneously. The team plan of care should still adhere to the principles espoused by ATLS. The trauma team resuscitation should be well rehearsed. Anything that is worthwhile doing requires practice—a trauma resuscitation is no exception.

Trauma resuscitation is a time-critical medical intervention. The term 'golden hour' was coined to emphasize the need for rapid assessment and management. For some patients it is the golden minute; for others a longer period of time is allowed before their injuries will, if undetected or untreated, inflict morbidity or even loss of life and limb. Our ability to recognize the most severely injured patients occurs only at the end of our assessment process. Therefore it is important to react to all potentially seriously injured patients as if they are indeed so—promptly, but in the orderly fashion outlined below. In that way the team will most expeditiously evaluate the current patient, and enhance their ability to deal with a patient for whom the seconds do count. Just like sporting teams, trauma teams play as they train. A non-critical resuscitation is an opportunity for the team to practice an efficient, controlled and correctly ordered assessment and management, the experience to be used when a patient really does need it.

Key point

- Successful trauma resuscitation requires a coordinated, methodical, and structured approach.

Phases of resuscitation

Trauma resuscitation consists of several overlapping phases: pre-hospital, primary survey, secondary survey, definitive care and tertiary survey, and finally rehabilitation, the key points of which are summarized in Table 2.1. Each will be considered in turn.

Pre-hospital phase

The pre-hospital phase is just the first step in the continuum of care for the seriously injured patient that ultimately ends with return to the previous level of function.

Debate about the merits of 'scoop and run' versus 'stay and play' modes of pre-hospital care are often discussed in overly simplistic terms. The important elements of pre-hospital phase are retrieval or extraction of the patient, airway maintenance, control of external haemorrhage, fluids for shock, immobilization, and transport to the nearest appropriate institution. This may not necessarily be the nearest hospital. Communication with the receiving hospital is a key element of pre-hospital care.

The history of the mechanism of injury is as important in trauma resuscitation as in any area of medical care. This knowledge allows the prediction of possible injuries and the focusing of examination and imaging on suspected injuries. Use whatever clues (clothing, etc.) are available to you. Wherever possible details of pre-injury co-morbidity should be gleaned, especially current medications. Anticoagulant use is just one important example.

Pre-hospital reports of deranged physiology (e.g. hypotension, tachycardia) should be regarded as true and a signal to search for the reason. Minimization of the potential for life-threatening injury in newly

Table 2.1 Summary of the phases of trauma care

Phase	Key points
Pre-hospital care (without delay)	Extraction, maintain airway, control bleeding, transport, notification MIST handover
Primary survey (30 seconds)	Airway with cervical spine control Voice, airway patency Breathing Breath sounds, trachea, percussion Circulation Pulse, pulse pressure, heart rate ECG leads, pulse oximetry, blood pressure cuff Disability GCS Pupil responses Check spinal cord function Exposure Initial radiographs Urinary and gastric tubes
Secondary survey (unhurried, thorough)	Top-to-toe examination Determine need for further radiographs or other imaging Announce care plan
Definitive care	Operating theatre/intensive care/general ward/discharge
Tertiary survey (next day)	Creation of an injury problem list with identification of each specific managing physician

arrived patients who superficially look uninjured is a natural reaction, but it should be resisted.

The transition from pre-hospital phase to primary survey, the *handover*, is a very important step. Successfully done, it sets the tone of the resuscitation—controlled, orderly, quiet. Pre-hospital details can be transferred to the trauma team succinctly under the headings of mechanism of injury, suspected injuries, vital signs, and treatment given (MIST).

The report should be delivered before the patient is moved on to the resuscitation bed. Unless the patient is *in extremis*, with closed chest compression in progress for example, the trauma team should all listen to the handover from the pre-hospital carers. It should conclude in less than 30 seconds, and then the patient is moved over to the resuscitation trolley for the primary assessor to begin. Further details of pre-hospital care should be asked after satisfactory completion of the primary survey.

Key points

- The pre-hospital to hospital handover—MIST.
  - mechanism of injury
  - suspected injuries
  - vital signs
  - treatment given.

It is best to be sceptical about interhospital transfers, not to believe the transferring hospital. The patient should be treat like a fresh arrival, and a full assessment repeated. The transferring hospital may have missed injuries, and the patient's condition may have deteriorated during transport.

Primary survey

The primary survey is the rapid initial evaluation to detect life-threatening injury. It should be completed as rapidly as possible. The mantra of airway, breathing, circulation, disability, exposure (ABCDE) should always be adhered to, because it imposes the correct priorities. As each trauma pathology is uncovered and treated, return to the beginning of the primary survey and repeat the assessment. The basic skills required for a successful resuscitation are highlighted here; details of the practical skills are contained elsewhere.

Key point

- Find the injury before it finds you!

A. Airway

Immobilize the cervical spine with a hard collar if one is not already in place. Speak to the patient. Ask them to speak back. Listen for patency, voice, stridor, and inspect for foreign body and soft tissue injury. Open the airway and inspect for soft tissue swelling, foreign bodies, and loose teeth. Look at the neck.

Correct problems by basic support of delivering oxygen by mask, suction of airway, chin lift, and jaw thrust. If these fail, advanced airway support with oropharyngeal airway (if tolerated) should be tried. If these manoeuvres fail to clear the airway, or the patient is not breathing spontaneously, then a definitive airway must be assured by endotracheal intubation. Nasotracheal intubation is an alternative in spontaneously breathing patients without significant facial injury. The role of laryngeal masks in trauma airway management is emerging, but yet to be clearly defined.

Definitive airway management is most commonly required for upper airway injury or coma. Coma may be due to shock or brain injury. Confirmation of tube position is confirmed by multiple methods. Remember in the profoundly shocked patient no end tidal carbon dioxide may be detected. Skill in endotracheal intubation is mandatory for a trauma team member.

Clearly the airway takes priority over the potentially undiscovered cervical spine injury. However, the cervical spine should be maintained in the neutral position during endotracheal intubation and stabilized by inline traction. Skill in maintaining in-line cervical spine immobility during endotracheal intubation is mandatory for a trauma team member (Fig. 2.1). This is an example of the role of the fourth doctor in the team—kneeling behind the left shoulder of the patient and maintaining in-line cervical traction by pulling, which is always easier than pushing. The front section of the hard collar should be removed once the traction is in place. This permits easier cricothyroid pressure, allows easier intubation and saves time should a surgical airway be required.

Rapid sequence induction may be required for the best attempt at endotracheal intubation. If two attempts by the most experienced airway doctor have failed to produce endotracheal intubation and other manoeuvres fail to maintain the airway adequately, then a surgical airway is required. This is an uncommon situation, but if the most skilled team member has been unsuccessful in intubating the patient repeated attempts are unlikely to be rewarded. A surgical airway may be improvised with a large-bore needle cricothyroidotomy and provision of high-flow oxygen. Skill in obtaining a surgical airway is mandatory for a trauma team member.

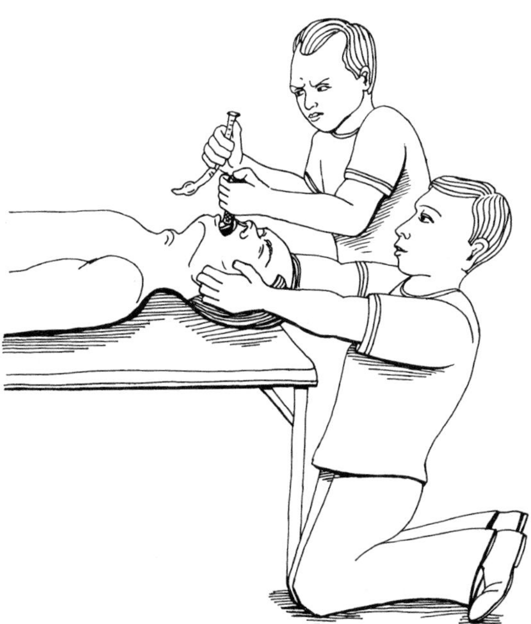

Figure 2.1 Maintaining in-line cervical spine immobility while intubating.

It should be possible to complete the primary survey down to D (disability) before definitive airway management to obtain the most complete primary survey.

Key point

- Skill in obtaining a surgical airway is mandatory for a trauma team member.

B. Breathing

Listen to breath sounds, check the trachea position. Tension pneumothorax is a clinical diagnosis based on the absence of breath sounds and a trachea deviated away from that side. It is a physiological diagnosis when accompanied by hypotension secondary to mediastinal shift and obstruction of venous return. It demands immediate needle thoracostomy in the secondary intercostal space. Sadly, it is still seen on chest radiograph! Other conditions recognized in the chest at this stage are open chest wounds, pneumothorax, and haemothorax.

If the patient is not in immediate physiological compromise it is prudent to take a chest radiograph before intubating the appropriate hemithorax. Skill in needle thoracostomy and chest tube thoracostomy is mandatory for a trauma team member.

Pulse oximetry is a valuable adjunct in monitoring the injured patient. It is of limited use when peripheral perfusion is poor, but high values usually mean airway, breathing, and circulation are intact.

Resist the temptation to stick your finger in a chest wound! Your clinical examination and chest radiograph will determine the presence of a pneumothorax. This means the chest cavity has been violated. Sticking your digit in a wound will only increase the likelihood of there being a pneumothorax. Do not put the chest tube, when required, through the chest wound.

Key point

- Skill in needle thoracostomy and chest tube thoracostomy is mandatory for a trauma team member.

C. Circulation

Placing a hand on the femoral or brachial pulse and observing pulse rate, pulse pressure, respiratory rate, and mental status can rapidly assess the circulation. The carotid is often shielded by a collar and the radial is prone to diminution in cold weather and shock. Broad categories of absent, weak or thready, and good should be reported and responded to. Numerical values of heart rate can be obtained from monitoring equipment once the patient is connected to leads and of blood pressure from automatic blood pressure cuffs, both of which are attended to by nursing staff.

Hypotension may be masked until over 30% of circulating blood volume has been lost. Tachycardia demands a search for blood loss, especially in the younger patient. Other signs of blood loss are thirst, cool clammy skin, and tachypnoea. Pre-hospital reports of hypotension or tachycardia should be regarded as real and not dismissed. Remember: find the injury before it finds you via circulatory collapse. Think: this patient is bleeding. Other clues to blood loss are the sweaty clammy patient, pale and cool extremities, and the patient reporting thirst. Usually the search for potential sites of haemorrhage sufficient to cause haemodynamic instability is limited to just five places: external, the chest, the abdomen, the pelvis, and the extremities. The retroperitoneum is the significant exception. Brain injury does not cause hypotension.

External blood loss may be reported from the scene or be clinically obvious. Scalp bleeding is a potent source of haemorrhage and should be controlled by surgical clips. Other sites of external blood loss should be controlled by pressure. The chest radiograph will declare significant intrathoracic bleeding. Compare the two lung fields carefully—an increased opacity in one hemithorax compared to the other may represent a litre or two of blood in the pleural space, layered, as the patient lies recumbent. Differentiation between this and extensive pulmonary contusion is usually possible. Likewise the pelvic film will declare significant disruption of the pelvic ring sufficient to cause major blood loss. If this is present the volume of the pelvis may be reduced by wrapping a sheet firmly around the pelvis or applying a MAST suit. Application of external fixation, emergently with a C-clamp or more definitively with iliac crest pins and a cross-pelvis bar (see Chapter 20), complement these first aid measures. This is the occasion when an orthopaedist can be life saving. On occasion pelvic haemorrhage may require angiographic embolization to aid haemorrhage control. Extremity fracture, especially fracture of shaft of femur, can produce major haemorrhage but be fairly obvious clinically. Application of external splinting devices such as the Hare traction device should be considered part of the resuscitation process, and early placement is effectively giving the patient a blood transfusion, as it may obviate the future need for transfusion. Skill in rapid application of external traction devices is mandatory for a trauma team member. All other major bleeding sites except the abdomen can be promptly, if crudely, discounted as major bleeding points. The abdominal cavity should be tapped to exclude the presence of significant intra-abdominal bleeding. Skill in performing diagnostic peritoneal lavage (DPL) is mandatory for a trauma team member. Aspiration of frank blood means laparotomy, as does 100 000 RBC/ml. Increasingly a focused abdominal sonogram (FAST), performed for trauma, will replace DPL as the principal modality for detecting intra-abdominal bleeding.

Key points

- Where is the bleeding? Think chest, abdomen, pelvis, extremity, and external.
- Skill in rapid application of external traction devices is mandatory for a trauma team member.
- Skill in performing DPL is mandatory for a trauma team member.

If there is shock, and no evidence of bleeding externally, on the chest (chest radiograph), the pelvis (plain radiograph), extremities (especially femur), then the abdominal cavity needs to be definitively tested for bleeding with either DPL or FAST. Good though many surgeons believe they are, laying a hand on the abdomen cannot exclude the presence of intra-abdominal bleeding. Only in the haemodynamically stable patient should a CT scan of the abdomen be entertained (Table 2.2). The retroperitoneum is the exception.

If shock is present it should be corrected by stopping the bleeding and volume resuscitation begun. The choice of fluids is discussed below. Volume resuscitation is best accomplished by two large-bore (14G) peripheral intravenous cannulas. The antecubital fossa provides the most reliable site. Flow through a tube is inversely proportional to its length and directly proportional to its radius to the fourth power. A 16G cannula is the minimum size that should be entertained during a trauma resuscitation. Skill in obtaining large-bore peripheral intravenous access is a mandatory skill for a trauma team member. Central venous cannulation need only be attempted when arms are missing, or after failed peripheral cannulation or tenuous peripheral cannulation. The femoral vein is the preferred site, given the constancy of the anatomy and the ability to cannulate this vessel rapidly even in a patient without cardiac output. Using a Seldinger wire technique a thick 8Fr rapid infusion catheter can be introduced. Short and thick is better than long and thin. Subclavian and jugular veins are a secondary alternative for this reason. However, if an intercostal catheter is already *in situ* that side should be chosen. Skill in obtaining a femoral central venous catheter is mandatory for a trauma team member. Rarely, all the above attempts fail and venous cutdown is used as a last resort.

Table 2.2 Where's the blood?

Site	Action
External	Look!
Chest	Chest radiograph
Pelvis	Plain pelvis radiograph
Extremity	Look!
Abdomen	DPL, FAST

A brief word on the military antishock trouser (MAST). Despite cries against its use, the MAST has a limited but defined role. It should be applied to in the field to shocked, bluntly injured patients in whom transport time will be >20 minutes, especially where there is a suspected severe pelvic or long bone fracture. Patients being transported from community or non-trauma hospitals without resources for angiographic embolization or immediate skeletal fixation of severe pelvic fractures should also have the MAST suit applied. The suit should be inflated when systolic blood pressure falls to <90 mmHg. However, in the trauma resuscitation the MAST must not interfere with venous access or patient assessment, and if inflation of the MAST produces respiratory distress it should immediately be deflated and diaphragm rupture suspected.

Key points

- Skill in obtaining large-bore peripheral intravenous access is a mandatory skill for a trauma team member.
- Skill in obtaining a femoral central venous catheter is mandatory for a trauma team member.

D. Disability

Assessment of neurological disability requires determination of a coma score, a check of pupils, and integrity of the spinal cord. The assessment is straightforward. Speak clearly to the patient, asking them to respond with their name and to grasp your fingers. Note the eye, motor, and voice response. Do not place your fingers in the patient's hand and ask them to squeeze. An involuntary response may be noted, giving the patient a higher score. If there is no response check the response to painful stimulus. Again note the eye, motor, and voice response. Establish a Glasgow Coma Score (GCS) (Table 2.3). Check the pupils. Lastly, in the responsive patient, ask them to wiggle their toes, an efficient check of spinal cord function.

The GCS dictates the patient's further management. For example, a score <8 demands definitive airway management. A score of 13 or less demands a CT scan of the brain. Later on, the score also may change the management and disposition of the patient.

Remember that a low coma score may be a consequence of hypoperfusion. Resuscitation of the circulation always takes priority over resuscitation or assessment of the brain. The haemodynaically unstable patient should never be taken to the CT scanner without adequate assessment and stabilization of the airway, breathing, and circulation.

Ingrained belief that analgesia limits ability to measure coma score often leads to avoidance of appropriate narcotic administration. Even in the time it takes to draw up drugs, an assessment of disability can be made. Sympathetic narcotic delivery, titrated against the patient's needs, will not interfere with disability assessment.

E. Exposure

Never assume all the potential injuries are observed. Completely disrobing the patient and checking for

Table 2.3 Glasgow Coma Score (with modification for children)

Eye opening (E)		
4	Spontaneous	
3	To speech	
2	To pain	
1	No response	
Best motor response (M)		
6	Spontaneous (obeys commands)	
5	Localizes pain	
4	Withdraws to pain	
3	Abnormal flexion to pain (decorticate posture)	
2	Abnormal extension to pain (decerebrate posture)	
1	No response	
Best verbal response (V)		
	Adult	*Child*
5	Orientated	Social smile, orients to sound, follows objects, coos, uses jargon, converses. Interacts appropriately with environment
4	Confused/disoriented	Consolable cries. Aware of environment; unco-operative interactions
3	Inappropriate words	Inappropriate persistent cries, moans, inconsistently aware of environment/inconsistently consolable
2	Incomprehensible sounds	Agitated, restless, inconsolable cries. Unaware of environment
1	No response	No response
(E+M+V) = coma score		

all potential injury is part of the discipline required to evaluate the patient efficiently. Except for a haemodynamically stable patient with a GCS of 15 plus, have no compunction in cutting clothing off. For those with extremity injury this is often the kindest thing to do. After all items of clothing have been removed, traction splints can be applied. Failure to remove undergarments is often a telling sign of an inadequate examination of the acutely injured patient.

The log roll of the patient can be done now, or as part of secondary survey. If the patient's injuries permit, now, with all the trauma team members present to assist, is often the best time to log roll the patient to complete the exposure. Examination of the back includes lifting the leg to check for perineal injury and a rectal examination to check for anal tone and, less importantly, high-riding prostate gland and rectal blood.

Insertion of urinary and gastric catheters is also part of the primary phase of assessment and resuscitation.

Imaging in the primary survey is limited to, in this order, a plain chest radiograph, plain pelvis radiograph, and lateral cervical spine plain radiograph. In penetrating injury trajectory determination equals injury identification, so all wounds should be marked with a radio-opaque marker. Paperclips are ideal for this. The initial chest radiograph, pelvis, and lateral cervical spine films may be taken now before beginning the secondary survey, so they can be developed and inspected as the secondary survey is progressing. Ideally in penetrating trauma the chest radiograph should be an erect film to optimize the chance of revealing haemo- or pneumothorax. Remember that the chest radiograph is a component of both the B and the C evaluation, the pelvis radiograph part of the C, and the lateral cervical spine part of the D.

The primary survey should uncover immediately life-threatening problems. At the completion of the primary survey the team leader/assessor can often make a determination of the need for transfer to another facility.

Shock and its management

Until this point we have implied that in trauma hypotension and shock are due to loss of circulating blood volume. Other important causes are

- Tension pneumothorax.
- Cardiogenic shock secondary to blunt cardiac injury (rare), cardiac tamponade (rarer), and air embolus (rarer still). Acute myocardial infarction is important in the elderly trauma patient and may have been the initiating event.
- Neurogenic shock: Brain injury does not cause shock. High spinal cord injury produces a sympathectomized patient, with peripheral vasodilatation and thus hypovolaemia. Both neurogenic and haemorrhagic shock should be initially treated with volume resuscitation. Failure to respond to volume resuscitation indicates ongoing blood loss or neurogenic shock. In selected cases alpha-adrenergic agents may be beneficial to impose vascular tone. There is no role for their use in the initial management of haemorrhagic shock.
- Septic shock: It is very uncommon for an acutely injured patient to present with septic shock.

Key point

- Non-bleeding causes of shock are tension pneumothorax, spinal cord injury, and cardiac injury.

Standard resuscitation guidelines are based on laboratory studies of controlled haemorrhage. Many trauma patients, especially penetrating trauma patients, have ongoing bleeding. Aggressive fluid resuscitation before control of bleeding may increase mortality by increasing blood loss and haemodilution. In animal models of uncontrolled haemorrhage aggressive fluid resuscitation produced a worse outcome than no treatment at all, which was worse than restricted fluid resuscitation. The early use of blood was beneficial. Delaying fluids until definitive control of haemorrhage in the operating theatre has been trialed clinically with improved survival. Enthusiastic adoption of this concept has led to the idea that any resuscitation is harmful.

Optimal resuscitation can be likened to keeping a water tank sufficiently full so that the tap on the side of the tank works (i.e. perfuses vital organs especially brain, heart, and kidneys). For the penetrating trauma patient keeping the tank full, or a full intravascular compartment, will only result in ongoing loss until the hole is repaired surgically. For bluntly injured patients the situation is more complicated as the sites of loss are multiple and many, if not all, may be sufficiently small as to be not amenable to surgical control (Fig. 2.2) During the time spent evaluating the patient and determining the presence or otherwise of surgically correctable bleeding points, what should the level of the tank be? And what if an interhospital transfer extends the time to surgical control, for example?

Thus resuscitation of the bluntly injured patient does not nicely fit the model of uncontrolled bleeding. The most appropriate end point for restricted fluid resuscitation remains to be determined. Ideally in the initial phases resuscitation should be limited to that required to maintain an adequate blood pressure, not a normal blood pressure, while a search for and correction of surgically manageable bleeding sites is undertaken. This is the Goldilocks principle of not too much, not too little, but just enough to maintain the circulation without over-resuscitating. If no overt bleeding point is found the resuscitation can proceed to more conventional normalization of vital signs, with production of urine providing golden evidence of adequate tissue perfusion.

The initial choice of fluids in the shocked patient should be crystalloid, as a bolus given as rapidly as possible. The subsequent choice depends on the response to the initial bolus. Those that manifest only a transient or no rise in blood pressure will need blood in addition to crystalloid. No response to the initial bolus suggests a 30–40% loss of circulating blood volume. The choice of blood, cross-matched, type specific, or type O packed cells again depends on the response to the crystalloid resuscitation. Any patient who does not have a rapid restoration of vital signs is highly likely to require a transfusion, and the earlier the best blood (cross-matched) can be delivered to the resuscitation area the quicker it can be given when required. Blood products (platelets, fresh frozen plasma) will be required in the exsanguinating patient. Administration of type O packed cells should be a signal to request these additional products and avoid any delay in delivery.

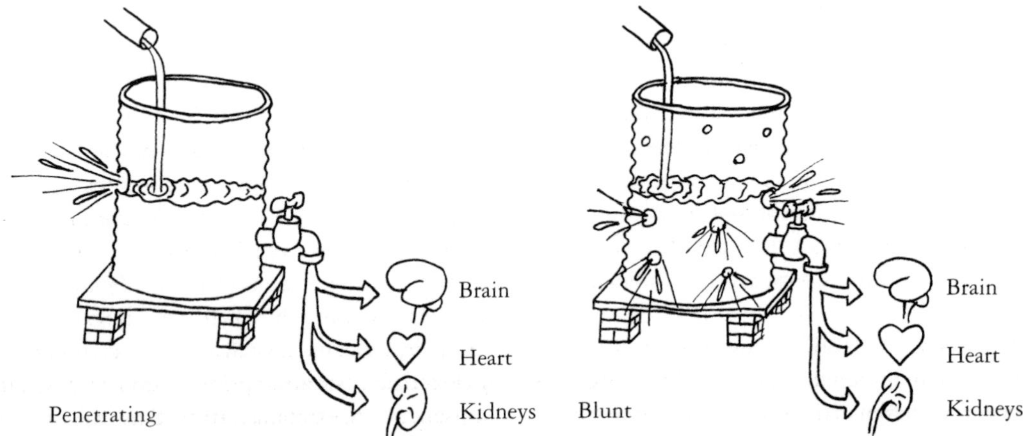

Figure 2.2 The two tanks. Penetrating versus blunt trauma.

Determination of end points for resuscitation of patients in shock

The shock state is a manifestation of an imbalance between oxygen supply and demand. Initial efforts at resuscitation focus on stabilizing the patient's vital signs. Implicit in the management of shock is restoration of circulating volume and haemorrhage arrest. Normalization of heart rate, blood pressure, and urine output may be all that is needed. Despite resuscitation some patients may manifest evidence of hypoperfusion of vital organs and may require therapy that can be guided initially by following the base deficit or levels of serum lactate. Serial arterial blood gases are mandatory in monitoring response to resuscitation in the shocked patient. If shock persists, invasive monitoring of gastric pH and oxygen delivery may be helpful to guide further volume management. These latter interventions are beyond the scope of the initial phases of care, and best followed in the intensive care setting.

Conflicting physiological data can arise during the resuscitation phase. In those patients more invasive monitoring may be required, such as arterial lines, central venous pressure transduction, and urinary bladder pressure measurement. Elderly patients are a good example, where a failing cardiac pump may manifest signs of volume overload when in fact hypovolaemia exists. The value of a Swann–Ganz catheter in this circumstance is supported by clinical investigation.

Avoiding hypothermia

Resuscitating the shocked patient requires not only restoration of circulating blood volume and haemorrhage arrest but also avoidance of hypothermia. Hypothermia is the enemy when salvaging the exsanguinating patient and can produce a vicious downward spiral that results in death. Hypothermia is mostly iatrogenic, secondary to the delivery of large volumes of fluid below core body temperature, and is rarely environmental. Once core temperature falls, especially <33°C, the coagulation proteins fail to function, more bleeding ensues, more fluid resuscitation is required, and hypothermia worsens. In the exsanguinating patient loss of circulating coagulation proteins and platelets exacerbates this problem and they additionally need to be replaced.

Hypothermia may be minimized by pre-warming the resuscitation area, covering the patient as rapidly as possible after examination with warm blankets or reflecting foil, delivering pre-warmed crystalloid (from a heating cabinet or microwave) and when blood is required delivering it through a blood-warming device. A high-flow fluid warmer is a useful adjunct. Installing a radiant lamp in the roof over the usual site of the patient trolley is another effective method of passively avoiding hypothermia.

Key point

- The best way to treat hypothermia is to prevent it.

The simple act of measuring core temperature, especially early in the resuscitation phase, is a powerful way of reminding the team of the dangers of hypothermia and the steps required to minimize it.

When to stop the resuscitation

It is important to be able recognize those patients who are dead and those who are very nearly dead. If a patient arrives with closed chest compressions in progress and no spontaneous cardiac output, i.e. no palpable pulse, they are dead. If there has been only a short period of time since the loss of a palpable pulse, no more than 10 minutes, and there is a narrow complex organized ECG rhythm (determined by quickly connecting the patient to a monitor or using defibrillator paddles), then the patient is very nearly dead. The narrow ECG complex is evidence that the heart is not yet hypoxic. The patient will almost certainly die but a series of manoeuvres are indicated, in the vain hope of salvaging traumatic cardiac arrest. Continuing closed chest compression alone or attempting a cardiac resuscitation is useless in the trauma setting. Securing an airway, inserting bilateral needle thoracostomies, a rapid 2 litres of crystalloid and a needle pericardiocentesis are indicated in blunt trauma patients. Unless cardiac output is restored at this point, the resuscitation should be ceased.

If there has been penetrating injury to the torso then an emergency left chest thoracotomy is indicated. With the left chest opened in the fourth or fifth rib interspace with a rib retractor first the pericardial sac is opened, then the aorta clamped, and if bleeding the pulmonary hilum or lung segment clamped. Unless cardiac output is restored at this point the resuscitation should be ceased. Emergency or resuscitative thoracotomy, indeed all invasive procedures, carries some risk to the team and should not be undertaken in an already dead patient. The trauma team must contain a member with sufficient surgical skills to complete the in-chest procedures, and an operating theatre on standby, before emergency thoracotomy is contemplated.

If pulses are lost during the resuscitation phase the same sequence should be followed.

Secondary survey

The secondary survey describes the thorough top-to-toe examination of the patient that is carried out after the primary survey and any interventions required have taken place. The importance of completing the primary survey before beginning the secondary survey, including exposure, cannot be emphasized enough. The secondary survey needs to be unhurried and thorough.

Before beginning the secondary survey it is useful to remind the examiner of the mechanism of injury. The patterns of injury will vary. For example, a pedestrian will manifest cross-diaphragm injury, with observable head and leg injuries increasing the chance of occult chest and abdominal injury. For patients with penetrating wounds, trajectory determination equals injury identification. To explain this further—a consideration of what might have been injured by a projectile or impaling object allows an estimation of what might be injured, followed by ruling in or ruling out injury to those suspected areas by thorough clinical examination or imaging.

Key point

- For penetrating injury, trajectory determination equals injury identification.

Special attention should be paid to the head. Facial bone fractures, base of skull fractures, rhinorrhea or otorrhea, ocular injuries, and scalp lacerations need to be sought by careful systematic examination.

Special attention should be paid to examining the neck again during the secondary survey, as it lies hidden under a hard collar. The potential for painful injuries, such as multiple rib fractures, or fracture of shaft of femur, to mask or distract from injury in other areas should be remembered. Thus the threshold for imaging areas of the body should be lowered if a distracting injury is present, thereby reducing the chance of a missed injury.

It is certainly possible to suspect intra-abdominal injury on examination, but our ability to exclude abdominal injury is limited. This is especially so in those with depressed conscious state, elderly people, and those with distracting injuries. The threshold for CT scanning the abdomen should be lower in these patients. The threshold should also be lower in those patients in whom repeated clinical examination is not possible, such as those under operative fixation of an extremity fracture.

The stabbed stay stabbed. Do not remove objects impaling the patient, such as knives, even in a 'stable' patient. Impaling objects should be removed in an operating theatre where the consequences can be rapidly dealt with.

During the secondary survey all the areas for which plain films are required should be noted, ideally on a white board. At the end of the secondary survey, should no more pressing priorities exist, then the radiological survey should be completed.

Key point

- Mark all penetrating wounds with a paper clip when performing radiographs.

- Remember painful injuries can mask or distract from injury in other areas.

At the completion of the secondary survey the team leader should announce to the team the priorities of care and the next sequence of care, e.g. plain films of the wrist and ankle, or transfer to the CT scanner. This begins the transition from resuscitation to definitive care phase and should again be accompanied by complete written and oral handovers of care if required.

Tertiary survey

The tertiary survey is the repeat examination conducted on the admitted patient, usually the next morning after admission. The clinical examination, essentially a repeat of the primary and secondary survey from the day before, coupled with interpretation of all radiographs, should allow a complete injury summary to be recorded in the patient's hospital record. Any areas of injury not suspected the day before should have appropriate radiographs taken.

The routine performance of the tertiary survey is a powerful method of preventing missed injuries, particularly injuries such as extremity fracture in the unconscious patient. Although often minor in the current context of the patient, if left untreated these injuries, can be a significant source of longer-term disability for the patient and litigious annoyance for the doctor.

Key points

- Phases of resuscitation: pre-hospital, primary survey, secondary survey, definitive care and tertiary survey, and rehabilitation.
- Remember the ABCDEs of primary survey.
- Secondary survey involves an unhurried, thorough top-to-toe examination of the patient and occurs after primary survey and intervention.
- Tertiary survey can detect missed injuries.

Summary of the phases of trauma resuscitation

Pre-hospital (without delay)

- extraction, maintain airway, control bleeding, transport, notification
- MIST handover.

Primary survey (30 seconds)

- airway with cervical spine control (A)
  - voice, airway patency
- breathing (B)
  - breath sounds, trachea
- circulation (C)
  - pulse, pulse pressure, heart rate
  - ECG leads, pulse oximetry, blood pressure cuff
- disability (D)
  - GCS
  - pupil responses
  - spinal cord function
- exposure (E)
- initial radiographs
- urinary and gastric tubes.

Secondary survey (unhurried, thorough)

- top-to-toe examination
- determine need for further radiographs or other imaging
- announce care plan
- prepare definitive care site (operating theatre/intensive care/general ward/discharge).

Definitive care

- operating theatre, intensive care, acute care admission
- includes handover

Tertiary survey (next day)

- creation of an injury problem list with identification of each specific managing physician

- rehabilitation
- discharge.

Stress response

A working knowledge of the stress response is important to help understand the physiological impact of major trauma on the patient, especially as it applies to the initial phases of resuscitation. Hormones, the autonomic nervous system, and locally released agents such as cytokines produce a cascade of interactions to produce a host of responses that follow a recognized pattern, the depth and duration of which is variable. The initial response is aimed at maintaining adequate delivery of substrate, especially oxygen, to the organs. This can begin immediately after injury. The initial phase is characterized by the release of catecholamines and vasoactive hormones, with increases in heart rate, cardiac contractility, and cardiac output. Peripheral and splanchnic vasoconstriction occurs and extravascular fluids are mobilized to maintain blood volume. Blood glucose levels rise, free fatty acids are mobilized, and a peripheral leukocytosis is noted. The initial phase, the ebb, gives way to the flow phase as metabolic emphasis shifts to providing substrate for healing. It can be difficult to separate the ebb phase of the stress response from the ongoing consequences of inadequate resuscitation.

Death from major trauma can occur immediately, or early (often due to exsanguination) or be delayed for weeks and then be a consequence of multiple organ failure. This last peak of deaths represents a major consequence of an exaggerated altered body metabolism in response to trauma, the ongoing impact of inadequate resuscitation, or indeed both providing ongoing stimulus for a profound stress response. This hypermetabolic state, characterized as the systemic inflammatory response syndrome (SIRS), can lead to a syndrome of multiple organ dysfunction (MODS), which is responsible for late trauma deaths.

Trauma response

Organization of the trauma resuscitation area

Organization before the patient's arrival

An area dedicated to the resuscitation of the trauma patient should be established, usually as part of the emergency department. The area should be removed from the more general areas of the emergency department, be in close geographic proximity to the operating suite, and be secure so that access by non-medical personnel (family, friends, media, other combatants) can be limited. Easy access to the radiology suite with CT scanning and the intensive care unit are desirable.

The dedicated space must be large enough to allow the team to function while performing any of the procedures necessary during trauma resuscitation. A well-lit room with mobile light sources is ideal. Provision of overhead radiant heating sources and individual room ambient temperature control to prevent hypothermia should also be included.

Communication in the trauma resuscitation room is essential, and is enhanced by use of a white board marker to record pre-hospital details and the current on-call team, a podium for the nurse scribe to work, and telephones with extensions separate from the other functions of the emergency department.

Equipment and placement

Placement of equipment in the trauma resuscitation room should be carefully considered to maximize functionality and make the best use of he space available. Only a minimal amount of equipment should be stored in the work area.

Universal barrier precautions

The body fluids of any trauma patient should be considered a potential infective agent. Eyewear and gloves are mandatory, and a mask, impervious gown, and overshoes provide additional protection. On a practical note, the routine wearing of barrier precautions will reduce laundry costs. These items should be available in a designated area, ideally at the entrance to the resuscitation area.

Remember the golden rule: protect yourself before the patient. Those few moments needed to don protective garb rarely influence the ultimate outcome for the patient, and indeed produce the mindset for a controlled, practised trauma response.

Another barrier should be thought of at this moment. Wearing a lead gown under the waterproof overgown, or slipping a lead gown on at the completion of the primary survey, allows the resuscitation to proceed while the initial radiographs are being performed. The assessor can proceed to the secondary survey and the proceduralist continues with urethral catheterization while the chest radiograph is being done, for example.

Key point

- Protect yourself before the patient.

Trauma team members

Ideally the trauma team should assemble, decide on roles, and be positioned before the patient's arrival. Those few moments of introductions, assignment of roles, and establishment of the leadership role are vital. The composition of the trauma team will vary from one institution to another (Fig. 2.3). Establishing a rapport with the nursing staff, and acknowledging their sometimes vast experience, is very important. Learn and use first names. Where a full response is possible, the ideal team would be:

- *Nurse 1:* The principal nurse who will have prepared the room before the patient's arrival and will accompany the patient until definitive care. Should begin the resuscitation standing on the patient's left side, ready to connect the patient to monitoring immediately on transfer to the resuscitation trolley.
- *Nurse 2:* The proceduralist nurse, who in addition to drawing the initial bloods is ready to set up any trays required for interventions.
- *Nurse 3:* The historian or scribe. Will also facilitate communication with other areas of the hospital such as the operating theatre and blood bank. Need not necessarily be a nurse.
- *Doctor 1:* The team leader. Stands at the foot of the bed.
- *Doctor 2:* The primary assessor. Stands at the patient's right side, stethoscope at the ready.
- *Doctor 3:* The airway. Stands at the patient's head, controlling the airway. Must never leave that station until directed to do so by the team leader.
- *Doctor 4:* The proceduralist.

The various medical roles need not be limited to particular specialties but each team member must have the skills to fulfil tasks directed to them.

- *Radiographer:* Stands off to one side, with universal precautions on. May have already placed a radiography plate on the resuscitation trolley to facilitate a rapid chest radiograph.
- *Wardsman:* Stands at the ready, especially to rapidly dispatch blood for cross-matching. Useful too for the combative patient.
- *Blood bank technician:* Responds to the call for the trauma team with an enquiry after 10 minutes to determine the likelihood of the need for an operating theatre.
- *Operating theatre nurse in charge:* Responds to the trauma team call with an inquiry after 10 minutes to determine the likelihood of the need for an operating theatre.
- *Nursing supervisor:* Assesses the resources the patient will require and if necessary calls the extra staff required.

In smaller hospitals the first medical responder will be required to fill all roles. Nursing support and

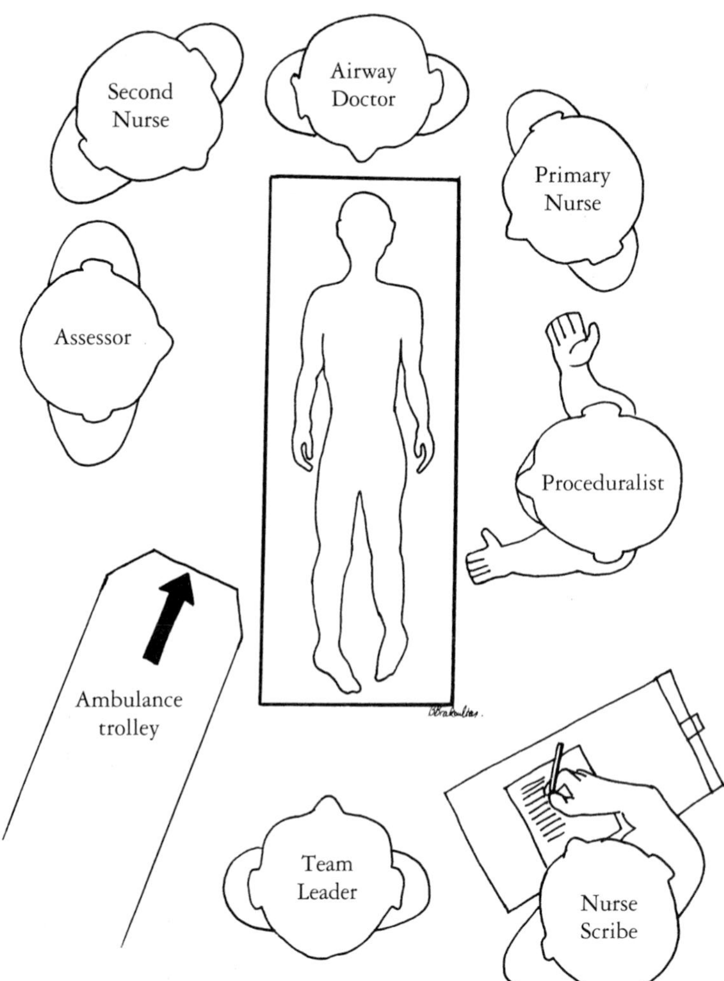

Figure 2.3 Trauma team members.

experience is invaluable in these circumstances. The resuscitation should then proceed along ATLS/EMST lines. Should a second responder arrive, then that person should be assigned to be the airway doctor until the primary survey is completed. Only with a full complement of nurses and doctors can a team leader have the luxury of stepping back to the patient's feet and directing the team.

Trauma team and team leadership

The clinical priorities of trauma resuscitation, as taught in the ATLS course, consider the steps in a longitudinal manner. A begets B, which begets C: this is considered a vertical resuscitation and entirely appropriate when only one or two physicians can attend the patient. However, in the modern trauma receiving hospital a team is activated to respond to the priorities of the acutely injured patient. In a well-drilled team multiple facets of the assessment and interventions required to continue the resuscitation may be carried out simultaneously. This is summarized in Figs 2.4 and 2.5.

The horizontal trauma resuscitation requires all team members to have well-defined roles, appropriate to the skills of each person. The team needs to be lead by the most senior clinician in the team. The leadership of the team is the single most important element of a successful trauma resuscitation. This usually works best with the team leader standing at the foot of the bed beside the nurse scribe, while another team member conducts the primary survey. Direction to team members should be given in a strong clear voice, addressing them by name so there can be no ambiguity about who has been assigned a particular task. Assessment findings should be communicated back to the team leader and scribe nurse in an equally clear voice. Control of noise levels during a resuscitation is a marker of a smooth-running resuscitation. The hype and noise levels featured in TV trauma resuscitation represent poor examples of how a patient might be rapidly assessed and resuscitated. Shouting or addressing team members by anything other than their name should not be condoned. During a time-critical trauma resuscitation there is often little room to debate. Clinical priorities are made by the most experienced clinician who is also leading the team, and dissent from decisions should be reserved for after the event. One trap for the team leader, as the most experienced clinician, is to be drawn in to the resuscitation, especially to perform procedural tasks. This may result in a loss of focus and lack of direction of the resuscitation. However, on occasion the team leader must undertake procedural tasks. Another important skill for the team leader is to tactfully reassign procedural tasks when it becomes clear the person asked to do the task, e.g. inserting a large-bore intravenous cannula, is not handicapped by lack of expertise. An exception to the most senior person being the team leader might be when an in-training clinician is given an opportunity to lead the team, with the more senior clinician participating and offering advice.

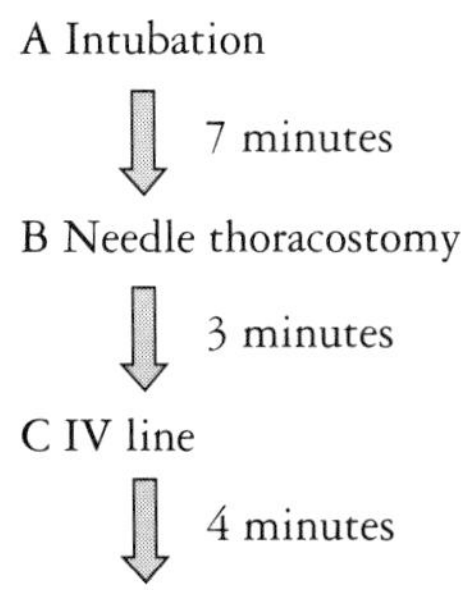

Figure 2.4 Vertical resuscitation.

An important task for the team leader is to ensure, along with the nursing staff, that all team members have adequate barrier precautions. No staff should be allowed inside the box that surrounds the patient without donning protective gear. Identifying unprotected staff is an effective way of establishing oneself as the team leader.

No member of the team should leave the resuscitation area without clearing it with the team leader. At an appropriate point in time, when it is clear that a patient does not have pressing priorities and after the primary survey has been completed, the team leader may chose stand down the team. Non-essential team members should be invited to return to their other duties outside the trauma resuscitation. Barrier precautions may be relaxed.

Trauma resuscitation is not a spectator sport. The team leader must firmly control the hubbub from onlookers, and on occasions direct non-essential staff to leave the trauma resuscitation area. Senior staff are often guilty of this behind-the-scenes noise, which only distracts from the job at hand.

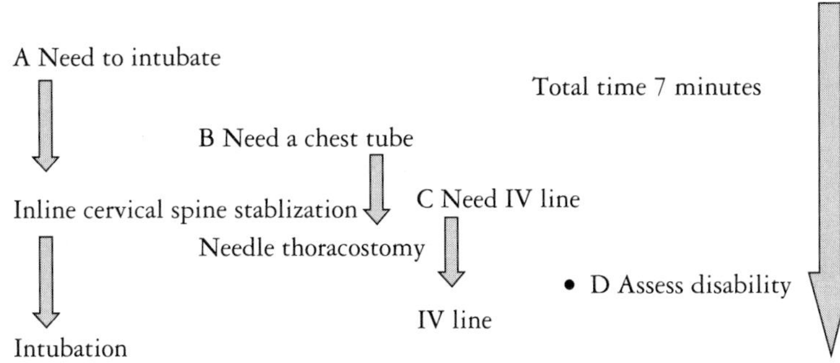

Figure 2.5 Horizontal resuscitation (simultaneous activity by different trauma team members).

The trauma team members should be drawn from suitably skilled physicians from the fields of surgery, emergency medicine, anaesthesia, and critical care. Other clinical disciplines, especially general practitioners in smaller hospitals, need to be involved. The trauma team must always include a surgeon or their designated representative, the surgical registrar. This permits timely response from the surgical teams in critical situations. If the surgeon is not present their representative should notify the surgeon that trauma resuscitation is about to take place, even before the patient arrives. This will ensure maximal responsiveness, as it is easier to stand a surgeon down than to scramble to locate and free one from other responsibilities should that be required. That ingrained desire to 'present' the patient with a complete clinical summary on initial registrar-to-surgeon contact should be resisted. There is value in having junior resident staff and medical students attached to surgical teams or to the emergency department act as team members at trauma resuscitation. They can perform simple procedures, but more importantly they will, as they mature clinically, be more ready to assume their roles in the team trauma resuscitation situation.

Activation of the trauma team should be by predefined criteria appropriate to each hospitals staffing and trauma caseload. Many criteria for team activation have been advocated, but the important issue is to develop criteria and then modify them according to the local experience. There is no place for a 'wait and see' approach. This risks losing valuable moments. The trauma team should be activated whenever a patient fits the predefined criteria. An overtriage rate of 50%, that is with no time-critical injuries, is considered acceptable to capture those patients who truly do have them. Even if the patient does not have time-critical injury most trauma team activations lead to admission to hospital. In addition, the non-critical resuscitation is a golden opportunity for the team to practise, without life-and-death pressure, the rapid assessment and transfer to definitive care needed on other occasions. Overtriage has led to enthusiasm for a two-tiered response based on the patient's pre-hospital physiology. Two-tiered responses are well tried and have much to recommend them as a judicious use of hospital personnel and resources, especially where there is a sophisticated trauma response. A two-tiered system should always contain the flexibility to upgrade rapidly to a full team response when required.

Trauma team members should be aware of the experience and skill of their nursing colleagues, and be sensitive to their 'suggestions' during the resuscitation. These suggestions, based on extensive experience, are nearly always appropriate.

For hospitals with a sufficient volume of major trauma cases and a well-established quality assurance process, real-time videotaping of trauma resuscitations and subsequent review is an invaluable tool for improving team performance.

The more often the trauma team is activated, the more seamless the team functioning will be. Therefore, paradoxically, for the smaller hospital where only a small complement of trauma responders might be drawn together, there is an even greater burden to prepare for the arrival of the major injured patient. For example, in a country hospital where a time-critical injury may only arrive once every 3 months, careful planning, dry or mock resuscitations, and a critical debrief of the response after the arrival of such a patient assume an even greater importance than in larger institutions. Call and back-up arrangements to provide the largest support possible should be worked on. In the institutions training such as that afforded by ATLS/EMST courses will increase confidence by the trauma care provider that they gave the best possible care for the patient with the resources available. Hospitals in smaller communities often work under the added pressure of at least one team member knowing the injured patient.

Finally, even with the best trauma responses patients will die. It is inevitable. It can be emotional. Again the team leader must lead: reassure all the team members of the value of their contribution, leave a review of performance until the dust has settled, contact the coroner or medical examiner, and seek out family or next of kin.

Trauma systems

Trauma systems describe a co-ordinated response to major injury in a defined geographic region that permits prompt access to optimal care. The essence of trauma systems is delivering patients to facilities with the resources to deal with that particular patient. This inevitably requires bypass of some hospitals sometimes. Trauma systems have shown a capacity to reduce death and disability, and enhance equity of access for both urban and rural patients to optimal care. Optimal care includes all phases of the management of injury—pre-hospital, resuscitation, definitive care, nd rehabilitation.

Development of a trauma system is a political process as much as it is medical, because it determines how resources are allocated and where. A trauma system has many components, including leadership and political will, continuous planning and development, adequate financing, public education and injury prevention, and efficient communication networks. Above all, a trauma system details where in a healthcare system the injured patient should be. Different levels of care within a trauma system have different facility and personnel requirements. Once designation and accreditation of trauma centres is undertaken there is a requirement for periodic review to ensure compliance with the agreed standards.

Paediatric resuscitation

(see also Chapter 28, Resuscitation and stabilization of the seriously injured child).

Key differences between adults and children in response to injury

Successful paediatric trauma management of the injured child depends on an understanding of the unique characteristics of children's anatomy, physiology, development, and psychology (Table 2.4).

Table 2.4 Unique characteristics of paediatric anatomy and physiology

Anatomical/physiological characteristic	Clinical relevance
characteristic	
Small body size	Injuring forces dissipate over small body mass, resulting in high frequency of multiple organ injuries
High ratio of body surface to mass	Places child at risk of hypothermia or dehydration
Relatively large size of head	Places child at particular risk of head injury
Compliant, elastic paediatric skeleton	Injuries to internal organs commonly seen without external signs of trauma or fracture, e.g. pulmonary contusions without rib fractures
Blood volume is 80 mL/kg	Guides intravenous resuscitation
Airway characteristics	
Large tongue, small mouth	Tongue easily obstructs airway
Epiglottis less stiff	may obscure glottis during intubation
Larynx more cephalad and anterior	risk of oesophageal intubation
Cricoid cartilage narrowest part of airway	Uncuffed endotracheal tubes are used in children <8 years old to avoid mucosal pressure necrosis
Trachea is short	Risk is intubation of right main bronchus

It is important to anticipate and be prepared, with a full range of equipment and to the availability of expertise, to assist with more difficult procedures or radiological interpretation, as necessary.

Children, especially small infants, are generally more vulnerable to hypoxia in the presence of the hypercatabolic state after trauma, because of a high basal metabolic rate, reduced functional residual capacity, increased work of breathing, and a high oxygen consumption. They are also prone to hypoglycaemia because of limited glycogen stores and to hypothermia because of immature thermoregulation and relatively large surface area, with greater loss of water and heat. Children in a rather cold environment may therefore become hypothermic, which may exacerbate the shock. If these factors are not considered or prevented early on, the injured child may remain physiologically decompensated.

There is wider dissipation of impacting force over less body mass in small children, making multiple injury more common. Their reduced muscle bulk gives little protection to underlying organs and parenchyma. Children are therefore more likely to have underlying visceral injuries rather than overlying bony injuries. These injuries may take some time to become evident. Abdominal injuries are typical of this, and may not present until 3–4 hours after a child's arrival in the Accident and Emergency department, the child eventually developing hypovolaemic shock.

Key points

- After trauma children as compared to adults are more prone to:
  - hypoxia
  - hypoglcyaemia
  - visceral injuries.

Important differences between children and adults are the normal ranges for vital signs (heart rate, respiratory rate, and blood pressure). Vital signs are dependent on age, development and size, and the environment and situation, and may not necessarily represent underlying pathology. The upper and lower limits, given in Table 2.5, are clearly defined and if breached should immediately raise concern. The rules of thumb in Table 2.6 can be a helpful guide.

Children, particularly small infants, have small airways with poorly developed cartilage which tend to collapse, a large occiput, and an infantile anteriorly placed high-lying larynx—all predisposing to upper airway obstruction. They also have a small mouth with a large tongue, which can cause relative airway obstruction. All of these factors can lead to imminent airway obstruction in a small infant even with minimal injury, and render intubation more difficult. Minute ventilation, a function of both tidal volume and respiratory rate, is increased through an increase in respiratory rate.

Table 2.5 Normal vital signs[a]

	Pulse rate (min^{-1})	Systolic BP (mmHg)	Respiratory rate (min^{-1})	Urine output ($mL\ kg^{-1}\ h^{-1}$)
Infant	95–160	>60 and <110	30–60[b]	>1
Pre-school child	80–140	>70 and <110	20–30	>1
Older child	70–120	>80 and <120	18–25	>0.5
Adolescent	60–100	>90 and <135	12–20	>0.5

[a] These figures are a guide only. Values at the extremes or outside these ranges should be interpreted in the light of the full clinical examination. A 'normal' value does not exclude significant illness in any individual.

[b] Infants may normally breathe up to 60/min, but RR > 40 is abnormal in presence of other respiratory symptoms and signs.

Table 2.6 Rules of thumb

Systolic blood pressure[a]	80+(2 × age in years) for children ≥1 year of age
Blood volume	<2 years of age = 100 mL/kg; ≥ 2 years of age = 80 mL/kg
ETT size (internal diameter in mm)	Age in years/4 + 4 for children ≥1 year of age
Position of ETT	
Length (cm at incisor teeth)	Age in years/2 + 12 for oral tube (age+10 for age 1–5)
Length (cm at nostril)	Age in years/2+16 for nasal tube (age+13 for age 1–5)
Weight	8 + (2 × age in years) for children ≥ 1 year of age

[a]Diastolic BP should be approximately 2/3 systolic BP. A BP fall >10 mmHg is significant.

ETT, endotracheal tube.

Therefore an unexplained increase in respiratory rate must be treated with greatest respect because it may reflect metabolic decompensation from uncontrolled shock. The infantile larynx is anteriorly placed and higher in the neck, at around the C2–C3 level. Cuffed endotracheal tubes are recommended after 8 years of age. Children also tend to have a collapsible chest wall with poorly developed, easily fatiguable muscle. Babies rely on diaphragmatic breathing and any compromise of diaphragmatic movement can precipitate respiratory failure. It is therefore important in a seriously injured child to consider venting the stomach and reducing the quantity of gastric contents to prevent diaphragmatic splinting. Infants <6 months of age also tend to be nose breathers and even simple nasal obstruction can cause apnoea; hence it is very important to have suction available.

Children have less contractile tissue per unit of myocardium (and a fixed stroke volume) and therefore cardiac output is limited by heart rate. Cardiac output is high in infants who have high energy (and oxygen) consumption and are operating high on the ventricular function curve. Although cardiac output falls in an almost linear fashion as blood volume is depleted, systolic blood pressure is sustained, even with 30% or more blood loss, because of increased vascular resistance secondary to peripheral vasoconstriction; diastolic blood pressure is elevated with a narrow pulse pressure. Cardiac output is rate dependent, so persistent tachycardia in a seriously injured child must be assumed to represent hypovolemia.

Children have a relatively short neck, making evaluation and immobilization of the cervical spine difficult.

Children are afraid of being hurt; they are also afraid of the unknown and often are very disturbed by the general air of panic and confusion that usually surrounds an emergency. Their behaviour in this situation may be inappropriate, with emotional withdrawal or regression to an earlier developmental level. The approach needs to be developmentally appropriate and recognize the importance of the family unit in both accidental and non-accidental injury.

Key points

- Children are more prone to airway obstruction because of the anatomy of the skull.
- Cardiac output in children is limited by heart rate.

Injury patterns unique to children

Children have many patterns of injury that are unique and easily overlooked, particularly in the case of multisystem injury. Although injury is often diffuse rather than localized, leading to more serious system pathology and a greater morbidity and mortality rate, it must be emphasized that the initial resuscitation period in the injured child is very much a respiratory rather than a circulatory phenomena. When managing the injured child the treating physician must be aware of the association between a child's size, mechanism of injury, and potential injuries likely to result. When a child is hit by a car the femur is at the level of the bumper, the child's trunk is often at the level of the bonnet of the car, and as a result of the impact with the car the child is always thrown with the head landing on the road. This association of femur, chest, and head injury is known as Waddell's triad. In this way timely intervention for the multiply injured child can be anticipated and planned. Non-accidental injury is an all-too-common problem that must be considered in a multisystem injured child.

Head injury

Head injury is the leading cause of death amongst all childhood victims of injury. Children sustain a disproportionately large number of head injuries, although their survival rate for these injuries is better than that of adults. In the case of multiple trauma they tend to have severe diffuse brain injury with variable outcome. Up to 80% of children dying of multiple trauma have a head injury, for the following reasons:

- head to body ratio larger
- less myelination
- thinner, more compliant cranial bones.

Raised intracranial pressure is more commonly seen than space-occupying lesions. In the case of young babies and infants these can occur together, and non-accidental injury needs to be considered. An open fontanelle does not protect against increased intracranial pressure.

Spinal cord injury

Injury to the spinal cord is being reported with increasing frequency in childhood multiple trauma. There are characteristics of the child's spinal cord and differences in the types of injuries sustained that lead to important differences in the pattern of injuries seen. Many spinal injuries involve the upper cervical spine, although lower injuries are now being increasingly reported. The following characteristics contribute:

- relatively large, heavy head
- weak neck musculature
- hypermobility and laxity of ligaments and joint capsules
- natural fulcrum for flexion at the C2–C3 and C3–C4 levels
- horizontal orientation of articular surfaces.

Spinal cord injury without radiological abnormality (SCIWORA) occurs almost exclusively in children. A strong association exists between childhood lumbar spine injury and lap seatbelts found in many motor vehicles. These lumbar injuries may be intraspinous (Chance) fractures but are frequently associated with other intra-abdominal injuries (including left acute traumatic diaphragmatic hernia).

Extremity injuries

The bones of the extremities tend to deform rather than fracture, although fractures are common and are associated with multiple trauma. Fractures are the most frequent injury missed in the child with multisystem injuries, because of the higher incidence of incomplete or complete but non-displaced fractures. The pattern of extremities injuries in children can be attributed to a number of factors:

- cortical bone is highly porous and easily disrupted
- periosteum is resilient, elastic, and vascular
- radiological diagnosis is difficult
- healing is rapid and non-union rare
- ligamentous injury is rare
- remodelling is in the plane of the fracture
- ischaemic injury can occur.

Thoracic injury

The presence of thoracic injury in children is a strong marker of severe and multisystem trauma. When thoracic trauma has occurred there is an 80% chance that other systems have been severely injured. The risk of physiologic derangement from thoracic injuries is high in children because underlying organs are often affected. Injury to the heart and great vessels is rare in children. This pattern of injuries is due to a number of factors:

- greater elasticity of bony and cartilaginous chest wall (lower incidence of fractured ribs and sternum, and flail chest)
- kinetic energy is more readily transmitted to underlying parenchyma (high incidence of pulmonary contusion, pneumothorax, haemothorax, or any combination)
- compensatory ability in the presence of pericardial or pleural collections is limited.

Pneumothorax in children is often a silent but lethal abnormality that requires a high index of suspicion on the part of the managing clinician. If a tension pneumothorax is suspected and vital signs rapidly deteriorate, management (by insertion of a chest tube under aseptic technique; Fig. 2.6 and see page 724) must be prompt.

Abdomen

Abdominal injury is common in paediatric trauma, with the lap seatbelt as a major cause. It is especially common in children with multiple trauma and a well-recognized association in children with non-accidental injury. Abdominal tenderness, distension and symptomatic haematuria are clinical clues. The most common injuries are to solid organs such as liver and spleen, followed by bowel and pancreas. This pattern of injuries is due to a number of reasons:

- solid organs have little protection
- kinetic energy readily transmitted to parenchyma
- small size predisposes to multiple injury.

One important consideration when assessing the abdomen is to remember the well-known axiom 'the stomach is always full' (Fig. 2.7). This is never so true as in the injured child, and unexpected emesis can be life threatening. Most commonly, however, gastric stasis which impedes venous return and splints the diaphragm can lead to cardiopulmonary compromise. Venting the stomach with an orogastric tube easily prevents this.

Pelvic injuries are mostly fractures and occur in pedestrian accidents. They behave differently from adult pelvic fractures, with less haemodynamic compromise. However, they are an important marker of multisystem injury and should trigger a search for other injuries.

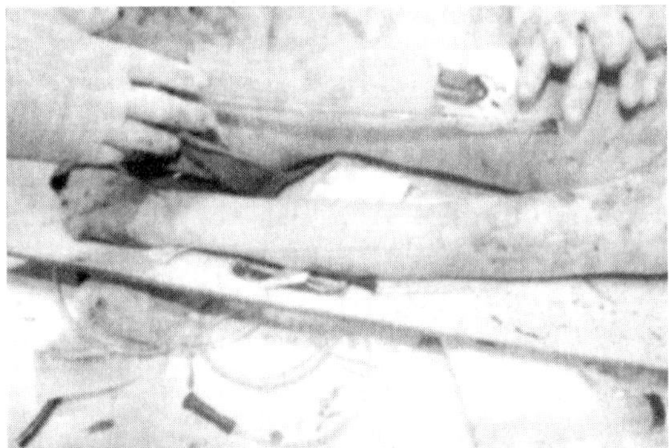

Figure 2.6 Insertion of a chest tube.

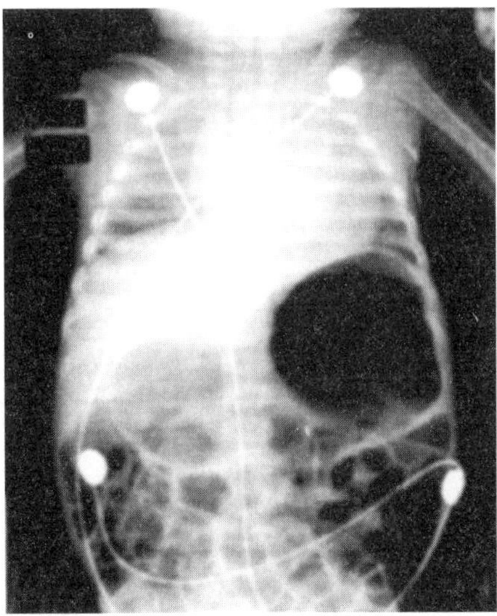

Figure 2.7 Radiograph of full stomach.

Conclusion

Resuscitation is an ongoing process, on through to the definitive management phase. Just like the transition from pre-hospital to resuscitation phase, the transition to definitive care should be accompanied by the formal handover of the care of the patient with a succinct, preferably written, summary of events thus far. Dedicated medical record sheets encourage the recording of the trauma resuscitation in the manner in which it occurred—pre-hospital, primary survey, secondary survey, imaging results, investigation results, and injury summary.

Throughout the resuscitation and assessment phase the care providers need to keep an eye on the big picture—what are the patient's injuries and what is the highest priority? Investigation should never impede resuscitation. Transfer to definitive care, especially the operating theatre, should not be delayed by lower priority concerns. The lack of a precise diagnosis should not stop you treating the patient (Table 2.7).

Table 2.7 The golden rules of trauma resuscitation

Protect yourself before the patient
Seek the injury before it finds you
Practice makes perfect—treat every resuscitation with the same degree of care
Trauma resuscitation is a team sport—and the team leader is captain, coach, and referee
Treat the problem—don't make a precise diagnosis
For penetrating injury—trajectory determination equals injury identification

Key point

- Treat the patient, do not make a diagnosis.

The joy of trauma care remains. At the end of a trauma resuscitation you will have had the satisfaction of working as a team. Many patients will survive their injury in spite of what you did. But occasionally you will be rewarded with the tangible satisfaction that the co-ordinated, timely assessment and intervention assembled for that patient has limited the morbidity of injury, and spared life or limb. That makes it all worthwhile.

Further reading

Colquhoun MC, Handley AJ, Evans T (eds) (2000) *ABC of resuscitation*. BMJ Books, London.

Mattox K, Feliciano DV, Moore EE (1999) *Trauma*, 4th edn. McGraw-Hill, New York.

Maull KI, Cleveland HC, Feliciano DV (1995) *Advances in trauma and critical care*. Mosby-Year Book, St Louis.

Mistovich JJ, Werman HA, Benner RW, Margolis GS (1997) *Advanced cardiac life support*, 2nd edn. Prentice Hall, Englewood Cliffs, NJ.

Peitzman AB, Rhodes M, Schwab CW, Yealy DM (1998) *The trauma manual*. Lippincott-Raven, Philadelphia.

3

CHAPTER 3

Disaster medicine

ANTHONY D REDMOND

CHAPTER 3
Disaster medicine

ANTHONY D REDMOND

Traditionally, disasters are divided into 'natural' and 'man made'. However, the pressures on the poor to live in areas prone to earthquake and flood, and the power of the rich to protect themselves, suggests to many that all disasters are ultimately man made. In 1988 an earthquake in Armenia killed more than 25 000 people. One year later, an earthquake of similar magnitude struck California USA; it killed 300, and this number largely because building regulations had been illegally ignored.

The vulnerability of the affected population can contribute as much to the disaster as the triggering event, and poverty constitutes the greatest vulnerability. This also compounds the other vulnerabilities associated with poverty—environmental degradation, poor land use, and rapid population growth. The death rate from disaster is six times higher in richer than in poorer countries and therefore, not surprisingly, more than 90% of victims of 'natural' disaster in the latter part of the twentieth century lived in Asia and Africa.

A disaster may be referred to as 'simple' where the infrastructure remains intact and 'complex' where resources have been compromised. In some countries resources are always compromised and any disaster is complex. Events may also be described as 'compound', which is another term for 'complex'. Of more obvious meaning, and therefore of more use, are the terms 'compensated' and 'uncompensated'. These descriptions may describe the whole of the event or more commonly a phase within the event. It is important to recognize that although many disasters are characterized by an initial overloading of the local services some events may be compensated for in the short term but a system may decompensate later, and often when wider attention for the incident has moved on.

Key points

- It may be that all disasters are ultimately man made.
- A disaster may be referred to as 'simple' where the infrastructure remains intact and 'complex' where resources have been compromised.

The overwhelming of local resources will trigger the need for triage. Three or four multiply injured patients presenting to a small rural emergency department may overwhelm available resources, at least for a while. A single critically ill or injured patient will overwhelm an under-prepared department. A very large number of patients with relatively minor conditions will overwhelm the best prepared.

Whether an incident tips over into a disaster rests in the balance between the size of the event measured in the number or complexity of casualties and the ability of the doctor, institution, region, or nation to respond adequately. This ability will be determined by training, preparedness, and pre-existing and residual resources. It is the failure to respond adequately, and to be overwhelmed, that characterizes a disaster.

Major incidents

The term 'major incidents' is generally used for those events that could potentially threaten an institution but are compensated for without collapsing into a disaster.

A number of definitions are in use. A major incident may be defined as any emergency that requires the implementation of special arrangements by one or more of the emergency services, health service, or local authority. It may also be defined as an incident where the number, severity, or type of live casualties, or the location of the incident, requires extraordinary resources. However, even events involving large numbers of dead, especially when there are no survivors at all, can still represent a very special and often very difficult major incident and in the public's mind may be the very worst kind. A major incident may also be defined as any occurrence that presents a serious threat to the health of the community or disruption to the service, or causes such numbers or types of casualities as to require special arrangements to be implemented by hospitals, ambulance services, or health authorities.

Common to all definitions is the concept of a very unusual event that requires an extraordinary response. Not all major incidents involve trauma. Chemical and nuclear accidents create major incidents of often huge proportions, but do not usually require the input of a surgeon. Some involve the services of specialist surgeons, for example when there are a large number of burns.

Key point

- The term 'major incident' is generally used for an event that could potentially threaten an institution but is compensated for without collapsing into a disaster.

Prepare, practice, and have a plan

The response to a single critically injured patient probably represents an institution's best response to a stressful event. Major incidents can be seen as progressively larger versions of this scenario. As performance is unlikely to get better in a major incident, an institution has a daily reminder of its best response to a major incident in its response to a major trauma. The range of injuries and problems that occur simultaneously in a severely injured patient require the co-ordinated response of a multidisciplinary team who have been trained and appropriately equipped. So it is for a major incident, albeit in a more complex setting. As the number of casualties grows, so must the response, expanding to involve the whole of the hospital and at times neighbouring institutions. In the largest of catastrophes national and even international assistance may be required. The principles throughout remain the same, however, with senior staff supervising the work of others, agencies continuously communicating with each other, and casualties being repeatedly triaged as the evolving incident changes their priority for treatment within the overall scheme of things. To have any chance of getting a major incident right you must first get a major trauma right.

In planning for major incidents many authors and institutions plan their response on the number of 'minor' and 'major' casualties they could cope with. However, a word of caution is necessary. Until a patient has been assessed and examined the severity of their injury may not be fully appreciated, and a large number of patients of any severity all arriving at once will place considerable strain on even the best of emergency departments. In fact a hospital's capacity for treating severe casualties will be limited by the number of intensive care beds available at that time, or that can be vacated or staffed within a very short time.

Planning must prepare doctors and institutions to co-operate and not compete. A realistic appreciation of the capacity to cope will allow early and safe onward transfer of casualties and as wide a distribution as possible. Critically, if inappropriate overtriage of patients to one institution has occurred, staff at that institution must recognize the need to transfer on whenever possible.

A trauma system that usually directs severely injured patients past smaller hospitals towards a specialist trauma centre must not be misused to direct all patients to the centre in a major incident. All the hospitals within the system must share the burden of the response, but with the trauma centre taking special responsibility for those with the most complex injuries.

Key points

- The response to a single critically injured patient probably represents an institution's best response to a stressful event.
- Until a patient has been assessed and examined the severity of their injury may not be fully appreciated and a large number of patients of any severity all arriving at once will place considerable strain on even the best of emergency departments.

Plans

Plans must be discussed and agreed within the emergency department, then outwards from there. Each department in the hospital must sign up to them with staff understanding their responsibility to be familiar and up-to-date with plans for a major incident. Procedures should be discussed and agreed with all relevant external agencies, with the ambulance service playing an integral part at every stage.

Plans must be based on the familiar. Plans that involve staff moving their activities to another location, however nearby, will inevitably create unnecessary tensions and confusion or be ignored—adding further to the confusion. Staff should work in areas and roles with which they are most familiar. When distressed we all gain comfort from the familiar, and a major incident is not the time to learn new skills.

A comprehensive major incident plan should be available to all departments and staff should be required to read it before taking up their appointment and at least yearly thereafter. The plan should identify roles, not individual personalities who may be unavailable on the day of the incident. Who might fill these roles can of course be indicated, but the most important function of the plan is to identify the key roles that must be filled by those available. As people more appropriate to a specific role become available they can take over. The plan must illustrate and emphasise the need for flexibility.

- Each member of staff should be given an action card for their role in a major incident and a full file of action cards be available in the emergency department at all times.
- Training for major incidents can take several forms, but should involve all staff at least at some stage.
- The simplest and most repeated exercise should be a communications exercise, whereby staff are called unannounced to establish the likely strength of the immediate response on any given occasion. If carried out about once a year this will remind staff to stay in touch with the hospital when on call.
- Key members of staff can engage in a tabletop exercise with members of the emergency services and other potentially receiving hospitals. This helps establish how patients might be distributed across a region.
- Individual departments can run through their procedures and 'walk through' patients to familiarize themselves with the dynamics of patient throughput and where they will be working come the event.
- An institution should envisage a full-scale practice every 5 years or so. If carried out not too frequently but involving all staff it can quickly highlight the strengths and weaknesses of current arrangements and remove some of the mystery that often surrounds these events.
- Those who may potentially be involved in on-site care should exercise regularly with the emergency services to ensure they have some experience of the realities of working out of doors and in difficult circumstances.
- In the UK there is a major incident medical management and support course (MIMMS) which all doctors who might be involved at a senior level in a major incident should attend.

Debriefing

It is important that such extraordinary events are concluded with an occasion for all those involved to have an opportunity to relate their contribution and learn from the contributions of others. In this way the collective knowledge of the institution grows and individuals are made to feel a part of the overall effort. All staff should be thanked by those in charge. This is also an opportunity to identify anyone who may have been psychologically traumatized by the event.

Counselling

Psychological support should be offered confidentially to all those involved, but in practice psychological sequelae will be minimized if staff are adequately trained and equipped, put to work in areas appropriate to their skills, and tasked to a level appropriate to their training and qualifications.

Alert procedure

The alert procedure is usually activated by the ambulance service but may be instigated by the police. At times the unheralded flood of patients into the emergency department causes the hospital itself to declare a major incident. It is important that an incident is formally declared, as failure to so do even in the face of the obvious will lead to confusion and unnecessary delay in mobilizing further resources. It is better to declare an incident and stand down than to begin mobilizing resources too late.

In the UK the standard format is as follows:

- major incident—standby
- major incident declared—activate plan
- major incident cancelled—stand down
- major incident—casualty evacuation complete.

Pre-hospital

Hospitals must be prepared to provide support to the emergency services at the scene of an incident. Those likely to be required must be adequately trained and equipped for the event. The delivery of safe and appropriate medical care in the pre-hospital setting is increasingly recognized as a speciality in its own right. Training courses are available in the UK with specialist examinations in immediate medical care held by the Royal College of Surgeons of Edinburgh (DipIMC RCSEd) and a diploma in the medical care of catastrophes from the Society of Apothecaries of London (DMCC).

An essential component of safe and effective pre-hospital medical care is a recognition of the place of doctors in the overall scheme of things. In large-scale disasters, safety, shelter, food, and water will take priority over medicine. In lesser events safety and rescue will still take priority. Doctors must truly appreciate that they are part of a team, and a team of which they are unlikely to be the overall leader.

There are recognized tiers of command during a major incident:

- *Bronze* is operational and describes the medical teams involved with the on-site care of casualties or the hands-on care of patients in the hospital.
- *Silver* is tactical and refers to the on-site incident officers who control activity at the scene and the triage officers at the hospital.
- *Gold* is strategic and describes medical directors of the ambulance service and hospitals.

The emergency services will establish inner and outer cordons at the scene. The outer will exclude all but official personnel and the inner will circumscribe the rescue area itself.

Medical Incident Officer

The most senior doctor at the scene will be designated the Medical Incident Officer (MIO). The task of the MIO is to carry out triage of the casualties in association with the most senior ambulance officer—the Ambulance Incident Officer (AIO). At the scene the police and sometimes the army will be in overall charge. On arrival the MIO will locate the command and control centre and report to the police officer in charge. The MIO needs to wear highly visible and fire-resistant clothing, including a helmet. He or she will be clearly labelled as a doctor and at all times carry and show on demand a recognized official ID.

In the UK, the ambulance service are in charge of the on-scene medical response. The MIO must quickly report to and stick with the AIO and as a team they will supervise and direct the despatch of casualties. They will decide in which order they will leave the incident and to which hospital they will be taken. This latter function is as important as the former. It is imperative that a balance is struck between despatching patients to the most appropriate hospital for their needs and not dangerously overloading one or more institutions. These decisions are made jointly between the AIO and the MIO.

It is the duty of the ambulance service in the UK to provide communications facilities for the medical team, but an appropriately equipped and trained team will already have their own.

The ambulance service will establish a casualty clearing station where the medical team will be based and carry out triage.

The fire service is in charge of the rescue. In addition, it is their responsibility to establish decontamination facilities. Medical staff must only enter buildings or other areas after receiving clear and recent permission from the fire service to so do. Equally, the fire service will decide who is contaminated and when they are decontaminated.

In addition to performing triage the MIO will supervise mobile medical teams and communicate regularly with all the receiving hospitals.

Mobile medical team

Ideally the mobile medical team will be drawn from supporting and not receiving hospitals. The members of these teams should be identified beforehand to allow for appropriate training. They should be familiar with the equipment they will be carrying and wear full safety clothing including a helmet.

Key point

- Ideally the mobile medical team will be drawn from supporting and not receiving hospitals.

Hospital response

In overall medical control of the incident will be a senior doctor who is not directly involved in treatment or triage. This will usually be the medical director of the institution or their deputy. Someone must assume this role until a designated person arrives. Alongside the chief executive of the institution and the director of nursing they will take their place in the designated control room. They will liaise closely with the police and triage officers. A member of the administrative staff must be tasked very early on to deal with the media, who should be kept informed by regular and punctual briefing sessions and well away from the treatment areas.

The immediate response to a major incident will involve those staff already in the building and rostered to be on call. The calling in of additional staff should be controlled and the plan should clearly indicate where they rendezvous. To avoid crowding out the emergency department this should be a designated place near to but separate from where the casualties arrive. Arriving staff should be registered and provided with a tabard that identifies their grade and speciality and given special documentation packs. These should contain a unique set of pre-numbered notes and pathology request forms. This will allow for a rapid register of the patients, even without names. Included in the pack is a property bag, again pre-numbered.

When preparing staff for a major incident it should be emphasized that staff all ready on duty or on call are likely to cope initially, and that additional help will be required some hours later and certainly by the next day. The excitement of wishing to be involved at the start should be tempered by a sense of responsibility to supporting the longer-term needs of the victims.

The hospital switchboard is the most important area in a major incident and staff must protect it.

If an incident has occurred and you are off the premises, do not ring in to the switchboard. Ideally, wait by the number you have already given to the switchboard for such an emergency. Staff already in the building should bypass the switchboard whenever possible by using direct dial facilities or commandeering pay phones—which can be converted to direct dial in an emergency by prior arrangement with the phone company.

Individual departments can assist by arranging their own cascade system for call out: an initial call from the department initiates a further cascade of calls from the recipient, and so on. The use of pagers can further relieve the burden on the telephone switchboard. Internal communication can be greatly facilitated by the use of 'runners', and this is a good use of unqualified volunteers.

Mobile phones are potentially of great use, but the local cell can quickly become blocked with the weight of traffic. The media in particular dominate their use and will ring their news desk then keep the line open for as long as possible to protect their own access to the cell. This problem can be overcome by initiating *access overload*. Recognized agencies can gain prior approval from the government and confidential access code words to limit access to the local cells to certain approved mobile numbers.

All routine work must stop as soon as an incident is declared. Urgent consideration should be given to the transfer of patients to other institutions to make room for the reception of casualties. With modern transport facilities one's imagination must stretch to considering securing the assistance of institutions far away from one's own. At all costs one must resist the temptation to see the event as special only to you and one in which you will cope at all costs. In developed countries there is often little need to compromise the care of patients in this way, even in the face of a major incident, if one involves all the resources in an area and sometimes in a country. Furthermore, although the initial reception of casualties may last only a few hours their ongoing surgical management may consume the human and physical resources of a hospital for months.

Coincidental emergencies unrelated to the major incident may still present to the hospital, usually unannounced. These have to be absorbed into the triage process regulating the wider incident and take their place in the overall priorities identified by the triage officers.

Key point

- All routine work must stop as soon as an incident is declared.

Chief triage officer

The chief triage officer will usually be the consultant or specialist in charge of the emergency department, or the most senior doctor in the department until he or she arrives. A guiding principle throughout disaster management is to avoid precious commodities such as senior experienced personal being captured by and therefore lost to a single patient. Rather, such people should stand back a little, prioritize the casualties, and supervise and direct the work of the less experienced. The chief triage officer places themselves at the door of the emergency department and all casualties will pass before them. By applying a quick triage sieve, casualties will be divided into categories 1, 2, and 3:

- category 1 will go into the resuscitation bay
- category 2 will go into the major treatment areas
- category 3 will be directed away from the main treatment areas to a designated minor area.

The senior doctor in each of these areas will perform further triage to identify further priorities within patient groups or within treatment needs for an individual patient.

Staff will be organized into teams assigned to individual patients and given clear instructions by a designated team leader. All staff should wear large clear tabards that identify their grade and speciality. In the confusion of a major incident it is important that senior doctors know at first glance the resources available to them, and do not overtask the less experienced. Instant identifiability of staff also acts as an extra protection against the unwelcome intrusion of the media.

Surgical triage officer

Once patients that might require surgery have been identified by the emergency department staff they will be referred to the surgical triage officer. Again this should be a designated senior member of staff. Rather than operate themselves, the surgical triage officer will identify the type and limitations of surgery to be carried out and the order in which patients are to be treated.

Triage

The purpose of triage is to do the most for the most. It is a job for the most senior person available. Triage needs to be done quickly but repeated continuously. It will be done first where the casualty is found, repeated on scene at the casualty clearing station, repeated when the casualties are despatched, carried out on arrival at the receiving hospital, repeated prior to surgery or other treatment, and continuously updated until the patient is removed, discharged, or dies.

From the French verb *trier* meaning to sort, the word is used to describe the process whereby casualties are sorted into priorities. This process is an extension of the triage process whereby a severely injured patient is surveyed to identify those conditions that require treatment before others. An individual's injuries are triaged and priority given first to airway problems, then breathing problems and circulation (the familiar ABC routine). Some injuries may be so minor that treatment can be delayed, or so severe that no treatment can be offered. Just as in a multiply injured patient you can't treat every injury first, so triage is performed when the number of those requiring treatment exceeds the number of those available to treat.

No discussion of triage is complete without mention of Baron Dominique Jean Larrey, Surgeon Marshall of Napoleon's Imperial Guard. It is he who is credited with recognizing the importance of prioritizing patients for surgery, sorting through the chaotic jumble of patients left in the aftermath of battle to rescue first those most likely to benefit from early treatment and—it has to be said—to be most likely to be fit to return to the battle. His belief in the power of early surgery led him to break with battlefield tradition and rescue patients directly from the field of battle rather than waiting till darkness brought a break in hostilities and cover for the rescue. The theatre of war still provides us with the basic models, and unfortunately repeated practical demonstrations, for developing and improving triage systems. Perhaps the greatest lesson from these experiences has been that priorities for the individual patient change as the condition and number of other casualties changes. Triage is dynamic and continuous.

Triage involves rapid, repeated, and authoritative decision-making. It is therefore a job for the most experienced. When resources of skill are limited, the greatest good for the greatest number may best be achieved by tasking your most experienced worker to identify those most in need of treatment and identify to the less skilled those procedures (and no more) they should perform.

Unfortunately there are two triage 'systems' in widespread use, although they are really different names for more or less the same thing. The P system refers to priorities: P1 is immediate priority; P2 urgent priority, and P3 delayed priority. The T system refers to treatment: T1 immediate treatment, T2 urgent treatment, and T3 delayed treatment. The T system also includes a T4 category—expectant. Patients in this category would receive immediate treatment in normal circumstances but the severity of their condition is such that the likelihood of survival is so small that the greatest good for the greatest number dictates that resources are nor 'wasted' on their care and they are set aside in favour of those who will clearly benefit from immediate care. Such decisions require great experience and maturity. Whoever makes such decisions will have to live with the consequences—unlike the patient. These decisions must be constantly revisited. The first triage scan might very well reveal few patients in need of immediate lifesaving care, so a T4 patient moves up the scale to T1. It takes maturity to accept the consequences of what appears to have been a now avoidable delay and greater maturity to act appropriately when a more 'deserving' case appears. In fact the need for T4 decisions is rare in civilian practice but not uncommon in war, particularly with regard to gunshot wounds to the head. However, large-scale disasters in remote and poor areas of the world will pose similar triage challenges to members of rescue teams.

Key points

- Triage categories:
  - life threatening, immediate care required
  - urgent care within 6 hours
  - delayed
  - dead
  - expectant.

Conventionally triage category 1 is colour coded red, triage category 2 yellow, and category 3 green. The dead are coded white and expectant blue.

The triage category is determined by applying the ABCs of resuscitation, commonsense, and experience.

For example, patients with airway obstruction tension pneumothorax or similar airway emergency are category 1, as are patients with very severe haemorrhage. Common sense applies. Patients who can walk and talk are not category 1, and are unlikely to be category 2. Respiratory rate and capillary refill require no special equipment and can be done quickly, in the field and in the dark. On first pass a patient who makes no respiratory effort in spite of a basic airway manoeuvre is dead and put to one side. These rapid assessments of walking, talking, respiratory effort, and appearance constitute the initial triage sieve.

Attempts have been made to standardize triage methods by putting numbers on decisions to make a triage scoring system. The advantages of such development lie in consistency between operators and more meaningful audit. However, the fundamental nature of a disaster or major emergency is that it is unusual, and the greatest defence against the threat of the unusual is flexibility. The Triage Revised Trauma Score (Table 3.1), adapted from the established hospital trauma score, has been used by paramedics in the USA to help standardize the direction of patients to specialist trauma centres. It may have a place in larger incidents but is generally untried in this area. However, having completed all the components a drop of 1 point in any of the three final categories is significant and although the score runs from 1–12 the three major triage categories are represented only by the final three scores, i.e.

- triage category 1 = TRTS 1–10
- triage category 2 = TRTS 11
- triage category 3 = TRTS 12.

The triage category should be recorded on a card that is appropriately coloured, clearly visible, and capable of being updated. The most practical is probably the cruciform (Cambridge) card.

Table 3.1 Triage Revised Trauma Score

	Measurement	Score
Respiratory rate (breaths/min)	10–29	4
	>29	3
	6–9	2
	1–5	1
	0	0
Systolic blood pressure (mmHg)	>90	4
	76–89	3
	50–75	2
	1–49	1
	0	0
Glasgow Coma Score (GCS)	13–15	4
	9–12	3
	6–8	2
	4–5	1
	3	0

Chemical and radiation

Incidents involving chemical and radiation contamination may not involve the surgeon, but if there is coincidental injury the surgeon must be familiar with the protocols in force at such times. Ideally decontamination is completed at the scene under the supervision of the fire service.

Casualties are decontaminated in a 'warm zone' and proceed to a 'clean zone' prior to transport. Nevertheless, contaminated patients may still arrive at hospital. As part of their major incident preparedness institutions should either have a portable decontamination unit comprising a shower from which washings can be gathered, or have arrangements already in place to secure a special unit from the fire brigade. Copious water is usually appropriate for washing, with the exception of certain chemicals such as phosphorus. If decontamination has to be carried out in hospital do not allow the water to drain into the mains but keep the washings for later safe disposal.

Potentially contaminated casualties must be directed along isolated and clearly demarcated 'contaminated' to 'clean' pathways. There must be protective clothing and airways protection for staff. Staff in these areas are lost to the rest of the unit and will themselves need to be decontaminated after they have finished. It is a difficult but important triage decision to calculate the number of staff that can be 'sacrificed' in this way. Whether resuscitation can ever precede decontamination is a triage decision for the moment and to be taken by the most senior of doctors. The needs of one individual are clearly being matched against the needs of another and in effect the needs of those others who may be denied treatment if the contaminated helper is taken out of action.

Incidents involving radiation follow similar guidelines. Certain hospitals with medical physics departments on site will be designated to receive these casualties and have special arrangements already in place. However, radiation-contaminated casualties can appear at any department and all should be familiar with the National Arrangements for Incidents involving Radiation (NAIR) or their own national equivalents.

Disasters

There is no definitive cut-off point between a major incident and a disaster, and sometimes the terms are used interchangeably. However, in general a disaster is an incident where the authorities are failing to cope and look unable to cope for the foreseeable future. This failure may be as a result of the scale of the incident, a lack of preparedness, or an increased vulnerability. Many of the worst disasters occur as a result of all three. The difference between the size of the disaster and the scale of the response determines the impact of the disaster.

There is no generally agreed definition of a disaster, but authorities would recognize it as the result of a vast ecological break down in the relationship between humans and their environment, a serious and sudden event (or slow, as in drought) on such a scale that the stricken community needs extraordinary efforts to cope with it, often with outside help or international aid.

The top 10 killers in terms of 'natural disasters' are illustrated in Table 3.2. Many of the worst disasters involve the mass migration of people and require the skills of public health and primary care doctors. Certain disasters involve large-scale injury and so involve surgeons. When offering aid to a stricken country, respond only to a specific request from a recognized and authoritative body and ensure you will be self-sufficient. This will ensure your skills are quickly matched to the needs of the victims, complement the work of others, and do not divert precious resources to meeting your needs rather than those of the victims.

Key point

- Disaster is the result of a vast ecological break down in the relationship between humans and their environment, a serious and sudden event (or slow, as in drought) on such a scale that the stricken community needs extraordinary efforts to cope with it, often with outside help or international aid.

Table 3.2 Types of disaster ranked by mortality 1947–80

Type of disaster	Number of deaths (thousands)
Tropical cyclones, hurricanes, typhoons	499
Earthquakes	450
Floods other than those associated with hurricanes	194
Thunderstorms and tornadoes	29
Snowstorms	10
Volcanoes	9
Heatwaves	7
Avalanches	5
Landslides	5
Tidal waves (tsunamis)	5

Earthquake

The threat of an earthquake lies in its power to collapse structures. The death toll is therefore higher if an earthquake happens at night when most people are in their homes. The combination of entrapment and injury limits the severity of injury that can be survived until rescue and evacuation to adequate surgical services can be achieved. The victims of severe injuries to the head and chest usually die before rescue and evacuation. Most rescue is carried out within 2–3 hours of the initial shock and accomplished by those in the earthquake area. However, it can be some time before further rescue and evacuation as the response is invariably hampered by damage to roads, buildings and communications; sadly, survival from entrapment is rare beyond 2 days. The surgeon is therefore most likely to be dealing with skeletal trauma, severe soft tissue injury, and occasionally abdominal injury. The work comes largely within the province of orthopaedic and plastic surgeons, with the support of intensive care specialists to manage the metabolic problems that accompany prolonged crush. In practice the bulk of injured survivors have peripheral limb injuries. Three times as many people are likely to be injured in an earthquake as are killed by it. These events therefore place an enormous burden on a region's and often a nation's surgical services. Furthermore, those treating the victims of an earthquake are removed for treating coincidental injury and disease. The impact of an earthquake on a vulnerable country can be immense, and surgeons should look to what help can be offered across regions and even across nations.

Despite intense media concern, the unburied dead rarely pose a threat to health. The evidence to date is that threats to public health most often come from the mass migration of people, usually into temporary camps—a factor shared with the majority of disasters including the greatest of them all, war.

Trauma surgery may also be required in the aftermath of tsunami and floods as they destroy buildings and produce injury. Deforestation in poorer areas has increased the risk of landslides and corresponding injury. Erupting volcanoes pose a greater threat of injury than burns, as a result of structural damage, rock falls, and frantic attempts to escape. Consideration should be given to the potential for respiratory problems among those injured in a volcanic eruption, including adult respiratory distress syndrome (ARDS) in the perioperative period if there has been a significant exposure to volcanic ash.

Complex emergencies

When a disaster occurs in an area already involved in civil conflict the UN refers to it as a 'complex emergency'. The commonest combination is the mass migration of people into refugee camps as a consequence of civil war in the area.

Armed conflict

Wars and other conflicts remain a major source of death and injury and, like disasters of all kinds, affects the poor more than the rich. Once again the poor of Africa and Asia bear the greatest burden.

Table 3.3 Department of peace and conflict research Uppsala University Sweden—battle related deaths in major conflicts 1990–1995

	1990	1991	1992	1993	1994	1995
Europe	74	6–10 K	11.2–21.4 K	14.2–42 K	1.5 K	1–33 K
Middle East	>3.4 K	>16 K	3.3–4.0 K	3–4 K	4.8–12 K	3.25–5.5 K
Asia	>15 K	>16 K	14–60 K	23.5–35 K	6.3–15 K	>6.2 K
Africa	33.5 K	37 K	14–40 K	25 K	25–35 K	15 K
Americas	6–7.5 K	3.2–6.2 K	>5.4 K	>3.4 K	>1.4	>1.7 K

Land mines

The World Health Organization has estimated that the conflict in the former Yugoslavia alone had already caused more than 5000 mine-related amputations by 1995, and the toll is still rising. It is estimated that 110 million land mines are scattered across 64 countries and the ICRC estimates they kill or maim 2000 people each and every month.

Battlefield injuries

Military surgeons are trained in recognizing and managing the special and difficult features of injuries incurred on the field of battle. Civilian surgeons may still face these injuries when acts of terrorism bring battlefield injuries to city streets or when they volunteer or are called upon to practice in a war-torn area. The following must be firmly born in mind.

- Wounds are inevitably and significantly contaminated.
- Damage is widespread with involvement often distant to the site of wounding.
- Mortality is inversely related to the time from wounding to treatment.
- The overwhelming priority is early and thorough wound excision.
- The risk of wound infection will be reduced by delayed primary closure.
- Abdominal contamination and sepsis may be controlled by the judicious use of colostomy.
- Vascular repairs are best done early.
- Internal fixation of bone is best avoided.

The greatest threats posed by battlefield injuries relate to their inevitable contamination and the delay to surgery. When faced with battlefield injuries, early antibiotic cover should be commenced, with penicillin (5 megaunits intramuscularly 6 hourly) remaining the mainstay of early therapy. Serious infection will only be controlled or prevented by surgery, and in particular by early and adequate excision. Meticulous attention should be paid to tetanus prevention, with tetanus toxoid given routinely. Gas gangrene has been a scourge of war since ancient Greece, and pathogenic spore-bearing organisms continue to contaminate wounds and threaten the lives of soldiers. *Clostridium welchii* is the commonest organism, but wounds are usually contaminated with a mixture that also includes *C. oedematiens*, *C. septicum*, *C. histolyticum*, and *C. sporogenes*. Delay in treatment is the most significant factor in its development. Its presence is usually heralded by the sudden onset of severe pain. Oedema and serosanguinous exudate develop, with the extent of deep tissue involvement not always reflected in the appearance of the overlying skin. Early and extensive debridement up to amputation is required.

Battlefield analgesia is best achieved with morphine. Diluting 10 mg of morphine in 10 ml of saline allows the surgeon to repeatedly administer small amounts to ease the pain and distress without compromising the airway.

The role of intravenous fluid replacement in such circumstance can be unclear. If evacuation of the casualty will be rapid, safe, and guaranteed then fluid resuscitation can proceed along standard Advanced Trauma Life Support Course (ATLS) guidelines. However, increasing the blood pressure before haemostasis has been secured can dislodge fragile clot and increase haemorrhage—a source of concern when intravenous fluid replacement was introduced in World War I. If the casualty and yourself are entrapped, then fluid replacement will have to be reduced to a level that maintains a radial pulse. If a prolonged entrapment is envisaged then later renal dialysis may have to be traded for an early but short-lived elevation of the blood pressure.

Gunshot wounds

Bullets damage tissues with the energy they liberate, directly injuring the tissues they strike and indirectly injuring surrounding and sometimes distant tissues if the energy release is great enough. The energy transferred in this way is proportional to the movement of the bullet through the tissues as it *tumbles* (rolls forwards) and *yaws* (spins about its long axis). The mass, shape, and type of bullet—or indeed any missile—all contribute to its energy potential, although the most important factor is likely to be its *velocity*.

In low-energy transfer injuries the energy available for release is all absorbed by the tissues the missile strikes. Its threat to the victim therefore lies in the importance of the structures it hits. This threat is obviously increased when the bullet fragments on impact, either by accident or by design. Missiles of low velocity (<300 m/s) are most likely to produce this effect.

High-energy transfer injuries are most likely to occur when a high-velocity missile generates so much energy that on impact its release will spread its effects away—sometimes far away—from the point of wounding. The local effect of this massive release of energy on impact is a cavitation of tissues at the point of wounding, creating a hole 10–15 times the size of the missile. The speed of the missile is such that this cavitation will occur after the bullet has moved on (and often out of the body) leaving a hole that expands rapidly to tear and stretch tissue then collapses inwards with further destructive effect. All this takes place in less than a second. The external evidence may be deceptive when all the energy has been contained within, but the formation of the cavity will have sucked in large amounts of contaminated debris including clothing, soiled skin, and earth, creating a massive injury behind a small wound.

The treating doctor is unlikely to know the type or indeed the speed of the missile. Furthermore, relatively slow moving missiles may be designed to give up large amounts of energy on impact and high velocity bullets may act as low velocity missiles when they lose energy in flight or ricochet before or after entry. The safest option is to assume the missile was high velocity and investigate accordingly.

Blast injuries

Explosions from shells, grenades, mortars, and bombs produce devastating injuries on the battlefield and increasingly in the streets. Injuries are the result of the direct effect of penetration by the fragments of the exploding device and the often more damaging effect of the rapidly expanding explosive gas and air. Most explosive devices have a hard, usually metal casing which fragments to produce very many high-velocity and high-energy transfer penetrating injuries. The explosive itself converts rapidly to an expanding gas. The first effect of this is to produce a positive expansive phase where a blast shock wave travelling at 3000 m/s spreads outwards. In a confined space the wave will be reflected back on itself, increasing its potential for harm. The speed of expansion falls off quite quickly, reducing the area of harm around blasts in the open air. Anyone likely to be exposed to these incidents should be aware that a blast shock wave moves like a sound wave and will go round walls. It also travels better and further in water. The shock wave is followed by a short negative phase where debris may be sucked in, after which there is a mass movement of air producing the so-called blast wind. This is produced as the expanding gases of the explosive device displace an equal volume of air. It is the blast wind that causes most tissue damage, including evisceration and amputation. The explosion will accelerate any materials within the device itself (nails, ball bearings) producing high-energy transfer missiles and produce further devastating injury by accelerating fragments of furniture and masonry. The human body is generally more vulnerable to injury from fragments accelerated by the blast than to the blast itself. Where the body is particularly vulnerable is at the interface between tissue and air. The tympanic membrane is the most vulnerable in this regard, and will rupture under forces of about 0.5 kg/cm^2. Of more concern is haemorrhage and oedema into pulmonary alveoli (blast lung), and at higher pressures injury to the gas-containing gut. The likelihood of pressure damage to the lung and abdomen is reduced when the blast occurs outside. Treating surgeons should be aware that blast lung may not become manifest until 12 hours after injury. Confusion may precede overt hypoxia and haemoptysis, with ultimately the development of an ARDS-like syndrome.

Finally, the explosion is exothermic and will produce burns, directly if the victim is near enough, and indirectly from secondary fires.

Cold injuries

The field of battle is an inhospitable place even when the guns are silent. Hypothermia can occur, but more commonly prolonged exposure to the cold, wet, and wind, particularly for relatively immobile combatants, will produce localized injuries to the limbs, most commonly the feet (immersion foot). Such injuries were a familiar feature of the trenches of World War I, hence their other name of 'trench foot'. When cold injury progresses to freezing it produces 'frostbite'. In general the best treatment for cold injury to a limb is rapid rewarming by immersion in warm water (40–42°C). If there is coincidental hypothermia then temporary cooling of the limb may be required to delay thawing until it can take place at normal body temperature.

Cold injury to limbs provokes numbness, pallor, or blue discoloration with induration, swelling, and decreased movement. Avoid a potentially more damaging cycle of thawing–freezing–thawing by rewarming the limb in an environment where further cold injury will be avoided.

Rewarming limbs is painful, and adequate analgesia (often morphine) will be required. Aspirin can be added for its analgesic but also antiplatelet activities. The vasodilatory effects of alcohol are a useful excuse for its administration.

Finally, avoid early amputation. The power of a limb to recover from cold injury is much greater than might be suggested by its early appearance. Providing there is no infection, any decision about amputation can be delayed until its need is obvious.

The hidden casualties of war

Women and children suffer dreadful consequences of war. Violent rape and mutilation may bring the woman to the care of a surgeon, and children's height makes them particularly vulnerable to the effects of land mines. Moreover, the breakdown in the usual system of medical care means that conditions that were easily treated in peacetime become life threatening and disabling with the neglect and isolation of war. Curable cancers become fatal without early medication, and diabetes claims a mortality not seen for generations in the west. When there is a break in hostilities or civilians escape the war zone the surgeon may very well be faced with hip and other fractures unreduced and untreated, and cancers at a late stage in their development. Sadly, when the war is over the work of the surgeon may only be beginning.

Further reading

Advanced Life Support Group (1995) *Major incident medical management and support—the practical approach*. BMJ Publishing Group, London.

ACS (1997) *Advanced trauma life support manual. Preparations for disaster*. American College of Surgeons, Chicago, USA, pp 409–410.

Baskett PJ, Weller R (1987) *Medicine for disasters*. John Wright , Bristol.

Cahill K (ed.) (1993) *A framework for survival: heath human frights and humanitarian assistance in conflicts and disasters*. Council on Foreign Relations, New York.

Champion HR, Sacco J, Copes WS *et al.* (1989) A revision of the trauma score. *Journal of Trauma* 29: 623–629.

Dufour D, Kromann Jensen S, Owen-Smith M *et al.* (1990) *Surgery for victims of war*, 2nd edn. International Committee of the Red Cross, Geneva.

EU Directive (1996) *Safety standards for the protection of health of workers and the general public against the dangers arising from ionising radiation*. European Union, Brussels.

Masellis M, Gunn SWA (1992) *The management of mass burn casualties and fire disasters*. Kluwer, London.

Moreau M, Gainer PS, Champion HR (1985) Application of the trauma score to the pre hospital setting. *Annals of Emergency Medicine* 14: 1049–1054.

Noji EK (1997) *The public health consequences of disasters*. Oxford University Press, New York.

Prescott MV, Redmond AD (1999) Mass casualty and major disaster planning. In: (eds) *Intensive care medicine*. BMJ Publications, London, pp 312–321.

Redmond AD (1999) Disaster medicine. In: *Pre Hospital medicine*. Arnold, London, pp 619–630.

Shah BV (1983) Is the environment becoming more hazardous? Global survey 1947–80. *Disasters* 7: 202–209.

Sherriff H, Wallin C (1989) The Cambridge Casualty Card—a triage card for multiple casualties. *Journal of the British Association for Immediate Care* 12: 30–3.

Wallace WA, Rowles JM, Colton CL (1994) *Management of disasters and their aftermath*. BMJ Publishing Group, London.

4

CHAPTER 4

Nutritional support of the critically injured patient

MICHAEL DAVIS AND
DAVID BIHARI

CHAPTER 4

Nutritional support of the critically injured patient

MICHAEL DAVIS AND DAVID BIHARI

Many patients who are severely injured from an episode of trauma are unable to eat. There are many reasons for this, not least a physical inability. Even those less severely injured patients who are physically able may not eat enough to support their metabolic state. Hospital food is notoriously unappealing, and the injury-associated pain together with the pain relief (usually opioids) may be such to cause marked anorexia and nausea. Metabolic deficits are difficult to make up, and their influence on the natural history of the injury depends very much on the underlying nutritional state of the individual. It is important for the medical attendants to address this issue early on in the post-injury period.

Key point

- Many patients who are severely injured from an episode of trauma are unable to eat.

Metabolic response to trauma

The metabolic response to injury involves a number of well-described events triggered and influenced by various mediators. A catabolic state ensues designed to mobilize substrates that can be used by those regions of the body involved in the recovery from injury. This results in fat mobilization, hyperglycaemia, salt and water retention, and net protein breakdown (Meguid *et al.* 1974, Oppenheim *et al.* 1980, Weissman 1990, Winmore 1991). Fever, tachypnoea, tachycardia, and a raised white cell count are the usual clinical correlates. Collectively this is known as the stress response; more recently the term systemic inflammatory response syndrome (SIRS) has been used (AMCP/SCCM 1992).

Key point

- A catabolic state ensues designed to mobilize substrates that can be used by those regions of the body involved in the recovery from injury.

Mediators of the metabolic response

The mediators of the stress response can be broadly divided into two groups

- those that are released from stimulation of the neuroendocrine axis, i.e. hormones
- those with a primary immunological function, such as cytokines.

The response is complex, however, involving the release of multiple mediators that are interconnected by amplification loops and negative feedback signals (Winmore 1991, Grimble 1996).

Key point

- Mediators are neuroendocrine and immunological.

Neuroendocrine axis

Hormones are released from afferent neuronal stimulation and also via cytokine release at the site of

Table 4.1 The stress response to injury

Hormone	Response to stress	Effect
Catecholamines: adrenaline noradrenaline dopamine	Increased levels	Increased heart rate, increased oxygen consumption, redistribution of bloodflow, glycogenolysis, gluconeogenesis, inhibition of insulin release, peripheral insulin resistance, lipolysis
Cortisol	Increased levels via increased pituitary ACTH secretion	Gluconeogenesis, proteolysis, alanine synthesis, insulin resistance, increased sensitivity of adipose tissue to lipolysing hormones, anti-inflammatory
Glucagon/insulin	Increased levels of both but the insulin level is inappropriately low for the level of hyperglycaemia, i.e. increased glucagon/insulin ratio	Gluconeogenesis, glycogenolysis, lipolysis
Growth hormone	Transient increase	Counter-regulatory, anabolic effects
Somatomedin C (IGF-1)	Decreased level	Mediates growth hormone function
ADH, renin, aldosterone, angiotensin	Increased levels	Salt and water retention
T3	Decreased	Sick euthyroid syndrome
T4	Decreased or normal	
rT3	Increased	
TSH	Normal	

Table 4.2 Metabolic effects of cytokine production

Fever
Anorexia
Nitric oxide and free radical generation
Altered copper, zinc, and iron metabolism
Enhanced antioxidant defences
Muscle proteolysis
Lipolysis
Gluconeogenesis

injury. A list of the major hormones involved in the stress response and their effects is seen in Table 4.1.

Cytokines and other mediators

Cytokines are a group of proteins or peptides released from a variety of cells in response to injury. They influence the immune response, as well as producing widespread metabolic changes (Grimble 1996) (see Table 4.2). Cytokines may be considered pro-inflammatory or anti-inflammatory. Some pro-inflammatory cytokines such as interleukins (IL)-8, IL-1 and tumour necrosis factor (TNF)-α lead to the production of nitric oxide and other oxidant molecules which may damage the host. Furthermore, cytokines such as IL-1 and TNF-α induce further production of IL-6 and of themselves. Excessive or inappropriate production of cytokines has been associated with increased morbidity and mortality. Other cytokines such IL-4 and IL-10 are anti-inflammatory and inhibit production

Table 4.3 **Cytokines and other inflammatory mediators**

Cytokines		Other mediators	
Pro-inflammatory	**Anti-inflammatory**	**Pro-inflammatory**	**Anti-inflammatory**
Tumour necrosis factor	Interleukin-4	Platelet activating factor	Prostaglandin E2
Interleukin-1	Interleukin-10	Leukotriene B4	
Interleukin-6		Thromboxane A2	
Interleukin-8			
Interferon γ			

of IL-1 and TNF-α. A list of cytokines and other immune mediators is shown in Table 4.3.

Alteration of the stress response

The value of the stress response is evident by the poor outcome of sympathectomized and adrenalectomized animals when starved. However, a prolonged stress response with production of cytokines is believed to contribute to the occurrence of multiple organ failure (Beal and Cerra 1994). The challenge lies in modulation of the stress response to the advantage of the host. This may be achieved by diminishing or preventing the signal at four levels:

1 the initial stimulus
2 gene transcription and translation of the cytokines
3 stimulation of effector cells
4 transduction of the cell signal.

Clinically this has been attempted with variable effect using glucocorticoids (Bone *et al.* 1987), monoclonal antibodies to cytokines (Fisher *et al.* 1996), immune enhanced enteral nutrition (Atkinson *et al.* 1998, Houdijk *et al.* 1998), early excision of burnt tissue, and gut decontamination (Winmore 1991). Nevertheless, it is clear that the form of an individual's stress response reflects not only the severity and nature of the injury sustained but also the underlying genotype of that individual. Our understanding of the genes controlling the stress response is in its infancy but already various forms of polymorphism for TNF production in septic states has been reported (Stuber *et al.* 1996, Westendorp *et al.* 1997). The concept of protective or destructive sets of 'trauma genes' has been introduced to explain the individual susceptibility to an injury of a given severity.

Key point

- It is clear that the form of an individual's stress response reflects not only the severity and nature of the injury sustained but also the underlying genotype of that individual.

Assessment of nutritional status

Malnutrition may occur in trauma patients both from the catabolic state induced as part of the stress response and from periods of inadequate intake that occur during treatment, e.g. surgery. Consequently this may lead to critical loss of body mass and function. Malnourished patients have a greater chance of developing complications whilst undergoing treatment (Chandra 1983, Windsor and Hill 1988). This has led to the term nutrition-associated complications (NAC) (Detsky *et al.* 1984a,b). These complications include death, sepsis, abscess formation, pneumonia, wound healing difficulties and respiratory failure (Detsky *et al.* 1984, 1994, Windsor and Hill 1988a).

The aim therefore of nutritional assessment is essentially threefold:

- assess the risk of morbidity and mortality from malnutrition
- identify the cause(s) of malnutrition in the patient
- assess if the patient would benefit from nutritional support.

Assessment of nutritional status can be divided into two components:

- analysis of changes in body composition
- analysis of alteration in physiological function.

The increased risk of NAC is thought to be caused more by functional impairment rather than changes in body composition (Windsor and Hill 1988b), but there is clearly a correlation between the two components (Detsky *et al.* 1994).

Traditionally many of the tests to assess nutritional status have focused on measurement of body composition (Table 4.4). Although these tests have been used successfully to predict morbidity and mortality, they often only provide a single snapshot of nutritional status at the moment of measurement. Furthermore, they can be expensive and time consuming to perform. A more dynamic and practical test is the subjective global assessment (SGA) (Baker *et al.* 1982, Detsky *et al.* 1987). This is a clinical test encompassing historical, symptomatic, and physical parameters (Jeejeebhoy 1998). It attempts to identify malnourished patients who are at increased risk of medical complications and would benefit from nutritional therapy. It has been shown to be a better predictor of complications than traditional methods of nutritional assessment (Detsky *et al.* 1984a, 1987). The components of this technique are shown in Fig. 4.1. Once applied, the patients are characterized into one of three groups:

- well nourished
- moderate or suspected malnutrition
- severe malnutrition.

The characterization is a subjective one. Equivocal information is given a lesser weighting than more definitive data to arrive at the final judgement.

Table 4.4 Measurement of body composition

Body mass index
Anthropometry
Creatinine-height index
Isotope dilution
Bioimpedance analysis
Dual-energy X-ray absorptiometry
Whole-body counting and neutron activation
CT
MRI

Key point

- A more dynamic and practical test is the subjective global assessment (SGA).

Nutritional requirements in the trauma patient

Energy requirements

The existing body cell mass is the major determinant of the total caloric requirement (Cerra *et al.* 1997). This may be either estimated or measured directly. The practice of matching energy input with energy expenditure remains controversial for a number of reasons. First, there is often poor utilization of administered nutrients in stressed catabolic patients (Long *et al.* 1976, Hill and Church 1984). Secondly, the excess administration of energy, particularly as carbohydrate, can stimulate metabolism leading to an increased production of carbon dioxide. The increased carbon dioxide may

History

1. Weight change and height:
   Current height____ cm, weight____ kg
   Overall loss in past 6 months: ____ kg, ____ %
   Change in past 2 weeks (use + or –): ____ kg, ____ %
2. Dietary intake change (relative to usual intake) or no change
   Duration = ____ days
   Type: suboptimal solid diet
   Hypocaloric liquids
   Starvation
   Supplement: (circle) nil vitamin, minerals
3. Gastrointestinal symptoms that persisted for >2 weeks
   None
   Nausea
   Vomiting
   Diarrhoea
   Pain at rest on eating
4. Functional capacity
   No dysfunction
   Dysfunction duration = ____ days
   Type: Working suboptimally
   Ambulatory but not working
   Bedridden
5. Disease and its relation to nutritional requirements
   Primary diagnosis: ______________
   Metabolic demand (stress):
   No stress
   Moderate stress
   High stress (bums, sepsis, severe trauma)

Physical status

(for each trait, specify: 0 = normal, 1 = mild deficit, 2 = established deficit)

Loss of subcutaneous fat
Muscle wasting
Oedema
Ascites
Mucosal lesions
Cutaneous and hair changes

Figure 4.1 Features of the subjective global assessment (SGA) system (derived from Detsky *et al.* 1987).

subsequently cause respiratory failure or ventilatory dependency in patients with marginal respiratory reserve. Finally, there is evidence that a hypocaloric nutritional regimen in the early post-traumatic period may be associated with an improved outcome (Zaloga and Roberts 1994, Battistella *et al.* 1997). Administering 25–35 kcal (105–145 kJ) per kg of body weight appears adequate for most patients.

Key points

- The existing body cell mass is the major determinant of the total caloric requirement.

Sources of energy

The three dietary sources of energy are carbohydrate, lipid, and protein. Traditionally protein or nitrogen requirements have been considered separately, and are often not included in the overall energy intake.

Carbohydrate

Glucose is the predominant source of carbohydrate and is metabolized by all body tissues including the brain. It is also required for protein anabolism. Glucose usually accounts for 30–70% of total caloric intake, i.e. 2–5 g/kg per day. Excess glucose administration results in lipogenesis and increased carbon dioxide production (Wolfe *et al.* 1980).

In the early post-traumatic period insulin may be required, particularly in diabetics, to keep blood sugar levels within normal physiological limits. This is due to the relative insulin deficiency for the level of hyperglycaemia seen in the stress response (Weissman 1990). Furthermore, since hyperglycaemia is a potent inhibitor of neutrophil function, maintaining normoglycaemia is an important priority.

Lipid

Lipid provides more energy per unit mass than carbohydrate (9.3 kcal/g compared with 4.1 kcal/g). It is important for the function of lipid-soluble vitamins, cell wall integrity, and prostaglandin synthesis.

The amount that lipid should contribute to the total caloric intake is not known. Indeed, one study (Battistella *et al.* 1997) showed an improved outcome, lower infection rate, and a reduced period of respiratory failure if lipid was withheld in trauma patients requiring total parenteral nutrition (TPN). Furthermore, there is considerable *in vitro* evidence of immunosuppression associated with the available intravenous lipid preparations (Robin *et al.* 1989, Seidner *et al.* 1989, Gogos *et al.* 1990, Atkinson and Bihari 1994) and some *in vivo* evidence (Freeman *et al.* 1990). Throughout the late 1980s and 1990s, as a consequence of pharmaceutical advances improving the stability of lipid in the 'three in one' TPN solutions, lipid has accounted in general for 15–30% of total daily caloric intake delivered by the intravenous route. Intravenous nutrition delivered via a peripheral vein ('peripheral TPN') has used even higher proportions (up to 70–80%) so as to reduce the osmolality and hence venous toxicity of the TPN solution (Kolhardt *et al.* 1994).

What type of lipid to use for nutrition is also not clear. However, omega-6 polyunsaturated fatty acid triglycerides should contribute at least 7% of total caloric intake to prevent essential fatty acid deficiency (Cerra *et al.* 1997). Fish oils such as the omega-3 fatty acids have generated much interest because of their ability to moderate the stress response in experimental models (Teo *et al.* 1991). A decreased number of infections and reduced length of stay has been shown in trauma patients (Bower *et al.* 1995) and in general intensive care patients (Atkinson *et al.* 1998) when given feeds containing omega-3 fatty acids. However, no difference in overall mortality was demonstrated and the fact that the feeds contained other immune enhancing components (arginine and purine nucleotides) makes it difficult to interpret the exact role of the omega-3 fatty acids. A theoretical advantage for the use of medium-chain triglycerides is that they may be absorbed from the small intestine independent of pancreatic lipase.

Protein

Protein or nitrogen intake should be sufficient to allow protein synthesis and promote nitrogen retention rather than being used as a source of energy due to inadequate intake of other caloric sources. This is usually achieved with 1.2–1.5 g/kg per day, or 15–20% of total caloric intake. In the past, a reduction in dose was considered necessary if the blood urea nitrogen or blood ammonia was rising together with a clinical encephalopathy. Nowadays, the widespread availability of haemodiafiltration for the treatment of renal failure and the recognition that withholding nitrogen only exacerbates endogenous breakdown have changed this view.

The ideal composition of the nitrogen source is not clear. Obviously it must include some quantity of essential amino acids and preferably an amount of non essential amino acids, but the precise quantities of each are undetermined (Table 4.5). Blood, plasma, and albumin are poor sources of nitrogen as they must first be catabolized into their constituent amino acids and they do not contain all the essential amino acids.

A lot of attention has focused on the use of particular amino acids such as glutamine, arginine or the branched chain amino acids. These are essential amino acids, which if given in relatively greater amounts than other amino acids (i.e. >0.5 g/kg per day) improve nitrogen balance and protein synthesis in trauma patients (Vente *et al.* 1991). A difference in outcome has yet to be demonstrated, however. Glutamine is a non-essential amino acid, which has stimulated interest for its role in enhancing immunity and preventing muscle loss in critically ill patients (O'Leary and Coakley 1996). Indeed, an early report has shown a lower frequency of pneumonia, sepsis, and bacteraemia in trauma patients who received glutamine-supplemented enteral nutrition

Table 4.5 Essential and non-essential amino acids

Essential	Semi-essential	Non-essential
Isoleucine	Cysteine	Arginine[1]
Leucine	Histidine	Alanine
Lysine	Tyrosine	Proline
Methionine		Aspartic acid
Phenylalanine		Glutamic acid
Threonine		Serine
Tryptophan		Glycine[a]
Valine		

[a] Considered 'non-essential' in health but may become 'essential' during periods of metabolic stress.

(Houdijk *et al.* 1998). However, this reduction in infection rate did not translate into a reduction in duration of ventilation or length of stay in the intensive care unit, so its clinical relevance is doubtful. Arginine is another non-essential amino acid, the role of which in nitric oxide synthesis, urea synthesis, and immune function has also attracted much interest (Cerra *et al.* 1997). As previously mentioned, it has been used together with omega-3 fatty acids and purine nucleotides (derived from yeast RNA) as part of an enteral nutrition immune enhancing regimen. This regimen has been shown to decrease infections and length of stay in trauma and other critically ill patients (Bower *et al.* 1995, Atkinson *et al.* 1998), although once again no change in mortality was seen. A meta-analysis of immune enhancing enteral nutrition using this regimen is now available and supports the view that the combination of immune enhancing nutrients has a positive effect on clinical outcome (Beale *et al.* 1999). Elemental feeds provide protein in the form of free amino acids or peptides. They are expensive and offer no advantage over standard feeds in trauma patients (Mowatt-Larssen *et al.* 1992).

Key point

- The branched-chain amino acids, if given in relatively greater amounts than other amino acids, improve nitrogen balance and protein synthesis in trauma patients.

Water and electrolytes

The normal adult daily water requirement is 30–35 mL/kg, although additional losses from diarrhoea, upper gastrointestinal losses, sweating, and fever must be considered. Ideally this water is given as part of the normal feeding regime. However, the electrolyte content of the nutritional regimes can differ, as well as the electrolyte requirements of individual patients. Thus, frequent measurement of electrolytes is usually required until the nutritional regime is stabilized to prevent physiological dysfunction. The normal adult electrolyte requirements are shown in Table 4.6.

Table 4.6 Adult electrolyte requirements

Electrolyte	Adult daily allowance (mmol/kg)
Sodium	1.0–2.0
Potassium	0.7–1.0
Calcium	0.1
Magnesium	0.1
Phosphorus	0.4

Vitamins and trace elements

The exact requirements of micronutrients are not yet determined, but they have many important roles and deficiency can result in serious illness or physiological dysfunction. Vitamins are important for optimal utilization of nutritional components. A list of vitamin requirements is shown in Table 4.7. Trace elements also must be considered; zinc, for example, is lost rapidly in critical illness (Shenkin 1986). It is an important component in many enzymes and deficiency results in hair loss, skin rashes, poor wound healing, and infections. A list of trace element requirements as recommended by the Australian Society of Parenteral and Enteral Nutrition (AuSPEN) is shown in Table 4.8.

Key point

- The exact requirements of micronutrients are not yet determined.

Growth hormone and other anabolic hormones

There has been much interest in the use of anabolic hormones to manipulate the stress response of trauma and thereby reduce morbidity. Growth hormone has been shown to increase net protein synthesis and improve nitrogen balance when infused into burned patients (Gore *et al.* 1991). However, early reports of randomized control trials in critically ill

Table 4.7 Normal values of blood and urinary vitamin levels

Vitamin	Units	Normal	Deficient
Retinol	μg/dL	10–100	<10
25-Hydroxy D	μg/dL	0.8–5.5	<0.7
1,25-Dihydroxy D	μg/dL	2.6–6.5	
α-Tocopherol	μg/dL	7.0–20.0	<5
Blood thiamine	μg/dL	2.5–7.5	<1.7
Urine thiamine	μg/g creatinine	>66	<27
Blood riboflavin	μg/dL	10–50	<10
Urine riboflavin	μg/g creatinine	>79	<27
Plasma vitamin B_6	μg/dL	>5.0	<2.5
Urine vitamin B_6	μg/g creatinine	>20	<20
Serum niacin	μg/dL	300–600	<300
Urinary N_1-methylnicotinamide	mg/d	2.2–9.4	<0.5
Ascorbic acid	mg/dL	0.4–1.5	<0.3
Plasma biotin	ng/dL	30–74	
Urinary biotin	μg/d	6–50	<6
Carotenoids	μg/dL	80–100	
Vitamin B_{12}	pg/mL	205–867	<140
Folic acid	ng/mL	3.3–20	<2.5

Table 4.8 Recommendations for trace elements

Trace element	24 hour dose	Comments
Zinc	30 μmol	Increased zinc supplements may be required with diarrhoea, or increased losses from ileostomy, fistula, or stoma
Copper	16 μmol	Increased copper supplements may be required with abnormal gastrointestinal fluid loss. Reduced copper supplements should be given in presence of liver or biliary tract disease
Manganese	8 μmol	Reduced manganese supplements should be given in the presence of cholestasis
Iodine	0.4 μmol	Povidine-iodine may be a significant source of iodine
Chromium	0.4 μmol	
Iron	20 μmol	
Selenium	1.5 μmol	Supplements of selenium may not be required in short-term parenteral nutrition. In long-term parenteral nutrition additional supplementation with selenium may be required
Molybdenum	0.2 μmol	

Source: Australian Society of Parenteral and Enteral Nutrition.

patients have shown a higher mortality in the treatment group. Similarly insulin, testosterone, and IGF-1 have all been shown to restore anabolism in stressed patients but their clinical effect is yet to be evaluated (Ferrando 1999).

Enteral versus parenteral nutrition

The enteral route is the preferred route for nutrition, for a number of reasons. First, there is the economic consideration. It has become clear that feeding by the enteral route is more cost-effective than TPN (Frost and Bihari 1997). Secondly, there may be a reduced incidence of gastrointestinal bleeding (Pingleton *et al.* 1983) associated with its use, but this has been difficult to document. However, more importantly a number of recent studies have shown a decreased septic morbidity in trauma and other critically ill patients fed enterally as opposed to via the parenteral route (Moore *et al.* 1989, 1992, Kudsk *et al.* 1992). One physiological mechanism has been postulated to explain these observations: the gut relies on adequate supply of oxygen and nutrients to maintain normal structure and function. Animal studies (Goodlad *et al.* 1988, Heyland *et al.* 1993) suggest that TPN may be associated with loss of mucosal integrity and immunological function. It has been suggested that these changes might lead to bacterial translocation and the passage of endotoxin into the systemic circulation (Baue 1993). This may result in SIRS and ultimately single or multiple organ failure (MOF).

A common criticism of enteral feeding is the inability to meet the estimated nutritional requirements of the patient. This is due to a number of reasons, such as impaired gastric emptying or feed absorption, diarrhoea, or fasting for procedures. However, the use of specific feeding protocols and aggressive instigation of prokinetic agents results in a greater volume of food delivered (Adam *et al.* 1997, Frost *et al.* 1997). TPN, however, can be increased easily to meet nutritional goals. Interestingly, a study by Moore and Jones (1986) demonstrated a similar nitrogen balance and caloric intake in patients fed by the enteral route compared to those receiving TPN, and another study (Adams *et al.* 1986) actually demonstrated an improved nitrogen balance in enterally fed patients. Additionally, a study in children with burns showed better nitrogen balance, less bacteraemia, and improved survival in those fed enterally compared to those fed intravenously (Alexander *et al.* 1980).

Key point

- The enteral route is the preferred route for nutrition.

Enteral nutrition

Access to the gastrointestinal tract

A list of the methods of access to the gastrointestinal tract for enteral nutrition is given in Table 4.9. The nasogastric route is relatively contraindicated in trauma patients with suspected or known base of skull fracture, owing to the risk of intracranial placement. In all other patients it is the preferred route as it is better tolerated than the oral route. The complication rate from insertion of nasogastric feeding tubes is relatively low but risks include nasopharyngeal bleeding and trauma, sinusitis, oesophageal perforation, and tracheobronchial misplacement.

Table 4.9 **Routes of delivery for enteral nutrition**
Orogastric
Nasogastric
Nasojejunal/nasoduodenal
Percutaneous gastrostomy
Surgical jejunostomy
Percutaneous jejunostomy

If nasogastric aspirates remain large despite the use of prokinetic agents (cisapride, erythromycin) then a fine-bore nasojejunal tube should be considered. These can be inserted blindly with the help of prokinetic agents or with the use of gastroscopic or radiographic guidance.

Many trauma patients undergo a laparotomy as part of their management. This provides the opportunity for placement of a percutaneous jejunostomy. This is particularly useful in the trauma patient as it bypasses the problem of gastroparesis often seen soon after these patients arrive in the intensive care unit. Many studies have shown that needle catheter jejunostomies inserted in patients with abdominal trauma allow successful early feeding with minimal complications (Moore *et al.* 1981, Jones *et al.* 1989). Percutaneous gastrostomy performed via endoscopy is usually reserved for patients requiring long-term enteral nutrition.

Timing of enteral nutrition

The timing of the initiation of enteral nutrition seems to be important. It has been hypothesized that feeding very early after trauma attenuates the stress response and leads to improved patient outcome. Indeed animal studies show that early enteral nutrition, compared to delayed enteral nutrition, is associated with greater wound strength after abdominal surgery (Zaloga *et al.* 1992) and a reduction in the metabolic response to injury (Mochizuki *et al.* 1984). Additionally very early (<2 hours) enteral nutrition in burns patients is associated with a reduced metabolic response (Chiarelli *et al.* 1990). However a randomized trial in blunt trauma patients comparing early and delayed enteral feeding failed to confirm these findings (Eyer *et al.* 1993). It showed no difference in the metabolic response, complications or mortality between the two groups.

It has also been hypothesized that bowel rest associated with delayed enteral nutrition is associated with gastrointestinal mucosal atrophy and loss of the mucosal barrier function (Minard and Kudsk 1994). This leads to bacterial translocation and possible exposure to endotoxin. As previously noted, a number of studies have showed the feasibility of early enteral nutrition in trauma patients. Several of these studies have shown a reduction in septic complications when early enteral nutrition was compared to delayed (>5 days) enteral feeding (Alexander 1999). Similarly, a study of head injured patients randomized to early (<36 hours) or delayed (3–5 days) feeding showed a decreased number of infections and reduced length of stay in the early fed group (Grahm *et al.* 1989). Thus, it is generally accepted that enteral nutrition should be started as soon as the trauma patient is fully resuscitated with a stable cardiovascular system.

Total parenteral nutrition

TPN is associated with an increased risk of infectious complications related to the direct immunosuppressive effects of the TPN solutions plus additional catheter-related complications. Furthermore, it does not provide the benefit of maintaining gastrointestinal structure and function that enteral nutrition does. Therefore it should only be used whenever enteral nutrition is not feasible (e.g. total small bowel resection) or requires supplementation. The numbers of patients receiving TPN are dwindling as intensive care physicians and surgeons have become more aware of the complications associated with this form of nutritional support. Nowadays, it is used in fewer than 15% of patients who require long-term support in the intensive care unit.

The benefits of TPN have been difficult to demonstrate. One large study (Buzby *et al.* 1991) suggested it should be limited to patients who are severely malnourished, and a recent meta-analysis (Heyland *et al.* 1998) failed to demonstrate any mortality advantage in surgical or critically patients. The meta-analysis did suggest, however, that there may be a reduction in nutrition-associated complications in patients who were initially malnourished, but the quality of the studies demonstrating these improved outcomes were somewhat doubtful. The obvious advantage for the parenteral route for nutrition is the ease of achieving nutritional goals. It has to be

Table 4.10 Common complications of total parenteral nutrition

Catheter complications (e.g. pneumothorax, infection, thrombosis)
Fluid overload
Electrolyte imbalance
Hyperglycaemia
Rebound hypoglycaemia
Vitamin deficiencies
Trace element deficiencies
Essential fatty acid deficiency
Hyperammonaemia
Liver dysfunction
Metabolic acidosis

remembered of course that TPN has been used successfully for long periods in that small minority of patients unable to receive enteral nutrition, but careful monitoring is required in order to prevent complications (Table 4.10).

Key point

- TPN should only be used when enteral nutrition is not appropriate or requires supplementation.

Conclusion

Although starvation is not an option in the care of the critically ill, trauma patient, controversy still surrounds the route and timing of nutritional support together with the exact nature of the formulation of nutrition delivered. Nowadays, parenteral nutrition is out of fashion, primarily because of its cost and the lack of efficacy studies in the critically ill trauma population. On the other hand, there does appear to be evidence emerging that early enteral nutrition, that is feeding established within 48 hours of admission to the intensive care unit, either using a surgical jejunostomy or the more simple nasogastric tube (in combination with prokinetics) is associated with improvements in outcome. Similarly, there are now a number of studies emphasizing the benefits of using specific immune enhancing nutrients—glutamine, arginine, omega-3 fatty acids, and purine nucleotides. It appears likely that nutritional support with one of these enhanced enteral formulations will become the standard of care for the critically injured trauma patient in the intensive care unit.

References

Adam S, Batson S *et al.* (1997) A study of problems associated with the delivery of enteral feed in critically ill patients in five ICUs in the UK. *Intensive Care Medicine* 23: 261–266.

Adams S, Dellinger EP, Wertz MJ *et al.* (1986) Enteral versus parenteral nutritional support following laparotomy for trauma: a randomized prospective trial. *Journal of Trauma* 26: 882–891.

Alexander JW (1999) Is early enteral feeding of benefit? *Intensive Care Medicine* 25: 129–130.

Alexander JW, MacMillan BG, Stinnett JD *et al.* (1980) Beneficial effects of aggressive protein feeding in severely burned children. *Annals of Surgery* 192: 505–517.

AMCP/SCCM (1992) American College of Chest Physicians/Society of Critical Care Medicine consensus conference. Definitions for sepsis and organ failure and guidelines for the use of innovative therapies in sepsis. *Critical Care Medicine* 20: 864–874.

Atkinson S, Bihari D (1994) Enteral nutrition in intensive care: no more 'gastrointestinal neglect'. *Current Medical Literature, Anaesthesiology* 8: 3–6.

Atkinson S, Sieffert E, Bihari D (1998) A prospective, randomized, double-blind, controlled clinical trial of enteral immunonutrition in the critically ill. *Critical Care Medicine* 26: 1164–1172.

Baker JP, Detsky AS, Wesson DE *et al.* (1982) Nutritional assessment: a comparison of clinical judgement and objective measurements. *New England Journal of Medicine* 306: 969–972.

Battistella FD, Widergren JT, Anderson JT *et al.* (1997) A prospective, randomized trial of intravenous fat emulsion administration in trauma victims requiring total parenteral nutrition. *Journal of Trauma* 43: 52–60.

Baue AE (1993) The role of the gut in the development of multiple organ dysfunction in cardiothoracic patients. *Annals of Thoracic Surgery* 55: 822.

Beal AL, Cerra FB (1994) Multiple organ failure syndrome in the 1990s; systemic inflammatory response and organ dysfunction. *JAMA* 271: 226–233.

Beale R, Bryg D, Bihari D (1999) Immunonutrition in the critically ill; a systematic review on clinical outcome. *Critical Care Medicine*.xx, xx, pp in press.

Bone RC, Fisher CJ Jr, Clemmer TP *et al.* (1987) A controlled clinical trial of high dose methylprednisolone in the treatment of severe sepsis and septic shock. *New England Journal of Medicine* 317: 653–658.

Bower RH, Cerra FB, Bershadsky B *et al.* (1995) Early enteral administration of a formula (Impact) supplemented with arginine, nucleotides, and fish oil in intensive care unit patients: Results of a multicenter, prospective, randomized, clinical trial. *Critical Care Medicine* 23: 436–449.

Buzby GP, Blouin G, Colling CL *et al.* (1991) Perioperative total perenteral nutrition in surgical patients: the Veteran Affairs Total Parenteral Nutrition Cooperative Study group. *New England Journal of Medicine* 325: 525–532.

Cerra FB, Benitez MR, Blackburn GL *et al.* (1997) Applied nutrition in ICU patients: a consensus statement of the American College of Chest Physicians. *Chest* 111: 769–778.

Chandra RK (1983) Nutrition, immunity, and infection: present knowledge and future directions. *Lancet* i: 688–691.

Chiarelli A, Enzi G, Casadei A *et al.* (1990) Very early nutrition supplementation in burned patients. *American Journal of Clinical Nutrition* 51: 1035–1039.

Detsky AS, Baker JP, Mendelson RA *et al.* (1984a) Evaluating the accuracy of nutritional assessment techniques applied to hospitalized patients: Methodology and comparisons. *Journal of Parenteral and Enteral Nutrition* 8: 153–159.

Detsky AS, Mendelson RA, Baker JP, Jeejeebhoy KN (1984b) The choice to treat all, some, or no patients undergoing gastrointestinal surgery with nutritional support: a decision analysis approach. *Journal of Parenteral and Enteral Nutrition* 8: 245–253.

Detsky AS, McLaughlin JR, Baker JP *et al.* (1987) What is subjective global assessment of nutritional status? *Journal of Parenteral and Enteral Nutrition* 11: 153–159.

Detsky AS, Smalley PS, Chang J (1994) Is this patient malnourished? *JAMA* 271: 54–58.

Eyer SD, Micon LT, Konstantinides FN *et al.* (1993) Early enteral feeding does not attenuate metabolic response after blunt trauma. *Journal of Trauma* 34: 639–644.

Ferrando AA (1999) Anabolic hormones in the critically ill. *Current Opinion in Clinical Nutrition and Metabolic Care* 2: 171–175.

Fisher C, Agost JM, Opal SM *et al.* (1996) Treatment of septic shock with tumour necrosis factor: Fc fusion protein. *New England Journal of Medicine* 334: 1697–1702.

Freeman J, Goldmann DA, Smith NE *et al.* (1990) Association of intravenous lipid emulsion and coagulase-negative staphylococcal bacteremia in neonatal intensive care units. *New England Journal of Medicine* 23: 301–308.

Frost P, Bihari D (1997) The route of nutritional support in the critically ill: Physiological and economical considerations. *Nutrition* 13: 58S–63S.

Frost P, Edwards N, Bihari D (1997) Gastric emptying in the critically ill—the way forward? *Intensive Care Medicine* 23: 243–245.

Gogos CA, Kalfarentzos FE, Zoumbos NC (1990) Effect of different types of TPN on T lymphocyte subpopulations and NK cells. *American Journal of Clinical Nutrition* 51: 119–122.

Goodlad RA, Plumb JA, Wright NA (1988) Epithelial cell proliferation and intestinal absorptive function during starvation and refeeding in the rat. *Clinical Science* 74: 301.

Gore DC, Honeycutt D, Jahoor F *et al.* (1991) Effect of exogenous growth hormone on whole-body and isolated-limb protein kinetics in burned patients. *Archives of Surgery* 126: 38–43.

Grahm TW, Zadrozny DB, Harrington T (1989) The benefits of early jejunal hyperalimentation in the head-injured patient. *Neurosurgery* 67: 729–735.

Grimble RF (1996) Interaction between nutrients, pro-inflammatory cytokines and inflammation. *Clinical Science* 91: 121–130.

Heyland DK, Cook DJ, Guyatt GH (1993) Enteral nutrition in the critically ill patient: a critical review of the evidence. *Intensive Care Medicine* 19: 435–442.

Heyland DK, MacDonald S, Keefe L *et al.* (1998) Total parenteral nutrition in the critically ill patient- a meta-analysis. *JAMA* 280: 2013–2019.

Hill GL, Church J (1984) Energy and protein requirements of general surgical patients requiring intravenous nutrition. *British Journal of Surgery* 71: 1–9.

Houdijk APJ, Rijinsburger ER, Jansen J *et al.* (1998) Randomised trial of glutamine-enriched enteral nutrition on infectious morbidity in patients with multiple trauma. *Lancet* 352: 772–776.

Jeejeebhoy KN (1998) Nutritional assessment. *Gastroenterology Clinics of North America* 27: 347–369.

Jones TN, Moore FA, Moore EE *et al.* (1989) Gastrointestinal symptoms attributed to jejunostomy feeding after major abdominal trauma—a critical analysis. *Critical Care Medicine* 17: 1146–1150.

Kolhardt SR, Smith RC, Kee AJ (1994) Metabolic evaluation of a 75% lipid/ 25% glucose high nitrogen solution for intravenous nutrition. *European Journal of Surgery* 160: 335–344.

Kudsk KA, Croce MA, Fabian TC *et al.* (1992) Enteral versus parenteral feeding: Effects on septic morbidity after blunt and penetrating abdominal trauma. *Annals of Surgery* 215: 503–511.

Long CL, Kinney JM, Gieger JW (1976) Nonsuppressibility of gluconeogenesis by glucose in septic patients. *Metabolism* 25: 193–200.

Meguid MM, Brennan MF, Aoki TT *et al.* (1974) Hormone-substrate interrelationships following trauma. *Archives of Surgery* 109: 776–783.

Minard G, Kudsk KA (1994) Is early feeding beneficial? How early is early ? *New Horizons* 2: 156–163.

Mochizuki H, Trocki O, Dominioni L *et al.* (1984) Mechanism of prevention of postburn hypermetabolism and catabolism by early enteral feeding. *Annals of Surgery* 200: 297–308.

Moore EE, Jones TN (1986) Benefits of immediate jejunostomy feeding after major abdominal trauma- A prospective randomized study. *Journal of Trauma* 26: 874–881.

Moore EE, Dunne EL, Jones TN (1981) Immediate jejunostomy feeding- Its use after major abdominal trauma. *Archives of Surgery* 116: 681–684.

Moore FA, Moore EE, Jones TN *et al.* (1989) TEN versus TPN following major abdominal trauma-reduced septic morbidity. *Journal of Trauma* 29: 916–923.

Moore FA, Feliciano DV, Andrassy RJ *et al.* (1992) Early enteral feeding, compared with parenteral, reduces postoperative septic complications: The results of a meta-analysis. *Annals of Surgery* 216: 172–183.

Mowatt-Larssen CA, Brown RO, Wojtysiak SI, Kudsk KA (1992) Comparison of tolerance and nutritional outcome between a peptide and a standard enteral formula in critically ill hypoalbuminemic patients. *Journal of Parenteral and Enteral Nutrition* 16: 20–24.

O'Leary MJ, Coakley JH (1996) Nutrition and immunonutrition. *British Journal of Anaesthesia* 77: 118–127.

Oppenheim WL, Williamson DH, Smith R (1980) Early biochemical changes and severity of injury in man. *Journal of Trauma* 20: 135–140.

Pingleton SK, Hadzima SK (1983) Enteral alimentation and gastrointestinal bleeding in mechanically ventilated patients. *Critical Care Medicine* 11: 6–13.

Robin AP, Arain I, Phuangsab A *et al.* (1989) Intravenous fat emulsion suppresses neutrophil chemiluminesce. *Journal of Parenteral and Enteral Nutrition* 13: 608–613.

Seidner DL, Masioli EA, Istfan NW *et al.* (1989) Effects of long chain triglyceride emulsions on reticuloendothelial system function in humans. *Journal of Parenteral and Enteral Nutrition* 13: 614–619.

Shenkin A (1986) Vitamin and essential trace element recommendations during intravenous nutrition: theory and practice. *Proceedings of the Nutrition Society* 45: 383–390.

Stuber F, Petersen M, Schade U (1996) A genomic polymorphism with the tumour necrosis factor influences plasma tumour necrosis factor-α concentrations and outcome of patients with severe sepsis. *Critical Care Medicine* 25: 381–384.

Teo TC, Selleck KM, Wan JM *et al.* (1991) Long term feeding with structured lipid composed of medium chain and N-3 fatty acids ameliorates endotoxic shock in guinea pigs. *Metabolism* 40: 1152–1159.

Vente JP, Soeters PB, Meyenfeldt MF von *et al.* (1991) Prospective randomised double-blind trial of branched chain amino acid enriched versus standard parenteral nutrition solutions in traumatized and septic patients. *World Journal of Surgery* 15: 128–133.

Weissman C (1990) The metabolic response to stress: An overview and update. *Anesthesiology* 73: 308–327.

Westendorp R, Langermans J, Huizinga T *et al.* (1997) Genetic influence on cytokine production and fatal meninogococcal disease. *Lancet* 349: 170–173.

Winmore DW (1991) Catabolic illness: Strategies for enhancing recovery. *New England Journal of Medicine* 325: 695–702.

Windsor JA, Hill GL (1988a) Risk factors of postoperative pneumonia: the importance of protein depletion. *Annals of Surgery* 208: 209–214.

Windsor JA, Hill GL (1988b) Weight loss with physical impairment: a basic indicator of surgical risk. *Annals of Surgery* 207: 290–296.

Wolfe RR, O'Donnell TF, Stone MF *et al.* (1980) Investigation of factors determining the optimal glucose infusion rate in total parenteral nutrition. *Metabolism* 29: 892–900.

Zaloga GP, Roberts P (1994) Permissive underfeeding. *New Horizons* 2: 257–263.

Zaloga GP, Bortenschslager L, Black KW *et al.* (1992) Immediate postoperative enteral feeding decreases weight loss and improves healing after abdominal surgery in rats. *Critical Care Medicine* 20: 115.

5

CHAPTER 5

Head injuries

GORDON DANDIE, JONATHAN CURTIS, AND MARK DEXTER

CHAPTER 5

Head injuries

GORDON DANDIE, JONATHAN CURTIS, AND MARK DEXTER

Head trauma encompasses a wide spectrum of injury severity, and it is without doubt the most prevalent and feared cause of long-term morbidity in the trauma patient. In terms of loss of function to the individual and cost to the community, the impact of head injuries is massive worldwide. It is one of the leading causes of death in children and young adults.

This chapter deals with aspects of head injury in adults. Paediatric head injury is in many ways a different condition and is dealt with in Chapter 30.

Key point

- The impact of head injuries is massive worldwide.

Epidemiology

Definition

Head-injured patients exhibit a wide spectrum of injury patterns and severity, ranging from trivial scalp lacerations to grossly disruptive, fatal brain injuries. The *International Classification of Diseases* requires multiple rubrics to adequately describe head injuries (WHO 1992). An all-encompassing definition is difficult and would be of limited usefulness. Optimum definitions derive from a combination of clinical and historical features. A history of blunt or penetrating trauma to the head, usually followed by a period of altered consciousness, and the presence of physical evidence of trauma, form the basic operational components of a head injury. A head injury may therefore be defined as the application and consequence of an external mechanical insult to the scalp, skull, and intracranial contents.

Classification

Multiple classification systems exist for head injuries. The primary event may be described in terms of the anatomical structures involved and patterns of injury, or by the nature of the biomechanical stresses involved. Clinical, radiological, and pathological grading systems may be used to stratify the severity of a head injury.

Anatomical classification

Primary head injuries can be classified anatomically into three categories: scalp and bony injuries, focal intracranial injuries, and diffuse intracranial injuries (Table 5.1).

- *Scalp injuries* vary from minor abrasions to extensive degloving injuries, but their magnitude correlates poorly with the degree of intracranial pathology. *Bony injuries* may be of the cranial vault or base of skull and occur with or without underlying brain injuries. Fractures may be linear or comminuted, depressed or undisplaced, closed or compound. Diastasis, another form of bony injury, refers to traumatic opening of suture lines.
- *Focal intracranial injuries* are defined as macroscopically visible parenchymal damage limited to a well-defined area. They may be extra-axial, such as subdural or extradural

Table 5.1 Anatomical classification of primary head injuries

Skull fractures	Focal brain injuries	Diffuse brain injuries
Vault linear depressed	Contusion coup contrecoup intermediate	Concussion mild classic
Basilar	Haemorrhage or haematoma epidural subdural intracerebral petechial	Diffuse axonal injury

From Gennarelli and Meaney with permission (1996).

haematomas, or intra-axial. Examples of the latter include cerebral contusion and intracerebral haemorrhage.

- *Diffuse intracranial injuries* reflect widespread brain dysfunction, often in the absence of macroscopically evident damage, and result from a combination of mechanical and physiological disruption of neurones, and vascular injuries.

Key points

- Primary head injuries are classified anatomically into three categories: scalp and bony injuries, focal intracranial injuries, and diffuse intracranial injuries.
- The Glasgow Coma Scale is a standardized and widely used system for grading severity of head injuries.

Biomechanical classification

Head injuries may be produced by direct contact with an object, by inertial acceleration-deceleration forces, or by some combination of these (Table 5.2). This is discussed in greater depth below.

Table 5.2 Mechanistic types of head injuries

Contact injuries	Head motion injuries
Skull deformation injuries	*Skull–brain relative motion*
Local skull bending	Subdural haematoma
Skull fracture	Contrecoup contusion
Epidural haematoma	Intermediate coup contusion
Coup contusion	
Skull volume changes	*Brain deformation*
Vault, basilar fracture	Concussion syndromes
Contrecoup contusion	Diffuse axonal injury
Shock wave propagation	Intracerebral haemorrhage
Intracerebral haemorrhage	Tissue tear haemorrhage

From Gennarelli and Meaney with permission (1996).

Grading of head injuries

Traumatic brain injury may be graded in terms of severity using a number of clinical grading systems. The most widely used of these is the Glasgow Coma Scale, which derives a GCS score from 3 to 15 based on components of the neurological examination (Teasdale and Jennett 1974, Randell and Chesnut 1997). Best responses are recorded for eye opening, speech, and motor function, and the points tallied (see Table 2.3, p. 18). Knowledge of the timing of examination is also important. The most accurate GCS score is that obtained immediately after resuscitation. For children, a modified GCS is used. This caters for an age-appropriate verbal response and is also scored out of 15. By using this uniform, reproducible system, repeated examinations provide a clear guide to any change in the patients' condition. It also enables unambiguous communication between clinicians regarding the level of injury.

Because the GCS provides a standardized method of describing the clinical status of a patient, it has become the basis of an arbitrary stratification of the head injuries into mild (GCS 13–15), moderate (GCS 9–12), and severe (GCS 3–8) (Borzuk 1997).

The CT appearance in head trauma may also be graded. This gives a radiological correlate of injury severity, and has predictive value for outcome. It is particularly useful in diffuse head injuries. A widely used international classification system is based on the initial CT appearance (Table 5.3). The status of the mesencephalic cisterns, the degree of midline shift present, and the presence of a mass lesion are quantified. Diffuse brain injuries are stratified into four categories. Complete effacement of the basal cisterns and midline shift >5 mm in the absence of a surgical mass define a subset of patients in whom the risk of development of severe intracranial hypertension and a fatal outcome is significantly higher (Toutant *et al.* 1984, Marshall and Eisenberg 1991).

Pathological grading following autopsy examination is used for ongoing research into head trauma and for epidemiological data collection.

Table 5.3 Diagnostic categories of types of abnormalities visualized on CT scanning

Category	Definition
Diffuse injury I (no visible pathology)	No intracranial pathology seen
Diffuse injury II	Cisterns present 0–5 mm contusions or midline shift seen
Diffuse injury III (swelling)	Cisterns compressed or absent
Diffuse injury IV (midline shift)	Midline shift >5 mm
Evacuated mass lesion	Any lesion evacuated surgically
Non-evacuated mass lesion	High or mixed density lesion not evacuated surgically

From Marshall and Eisenberg with permission (1991).

Key points

- The Glasgow Coma Scale is a standardized and widely used of grading severity of head injuries.

Incidence

Traumatic head injuries present a major public health issue globally. In developed countries trauma is the leading cause of death under the age of 45 and accounts for 10–20 deaths per 100 000 population annually (Jennett 1996, Palmer 1998). In the USA, >100 000 patients suffer varying degrees of disability each year (Palmer 1998). The economic repercussions are vast. In the USA alone, the annual cost of head injuries in terms of healthcare burden and loss of productivity exceeds US$25 billion (Borzuk 1997). Overall, 70–80% of patients seeking medical attention have mild head injuries. The remainder are divided equally into moderate and severe grades. Head injuries are responsible for almost half of trauma deaths, and they account for most of the long-term morbidity (Jennett 1996).

Key points

- The majority of head injuries are minor with the remainder divided between moderate and severe grades.
- The economic repercussions of head injuries are great.

Geographical features

In terms of overall incidence and distribution of causes, extreme variation is seen both internationally and within geographically adjacent areas. This is illustrated by population studies showing markedly higher admission rates for head injuries in populous inner city areas, where assaults are prevalent, compared with predominantly rural areas where vehicular injuries are usually implicated and overall incidence of head injuries is low (Table 5.4).

Age differences

The major impact of head injuries in all countries is on the younger population, typically 15–35 year olds (Jennett 1996). Age-specific mortality rates also peak in the elderly population, particularly in those >70 years of age (Kraus *et al.* 1984). As a group they are involved in falls more frequently and often sustain significant injuries resulting in disability. There is also a high incidence of head injury in the very young, particularly those aged under 15 years (Brookes *et al.* 1990), but the great majority of these are mild. Overall they form the largest subgroup of age-specific attenders in emergency departments (Jennett 1996).

Table 5.4 Distribution of causes of head injury (%) in different locations based on hospital admission

Location	Motor vehicle accidents	Falls	Assaults
USA (overall)	49	28	5
Olmsted	47	29	4
Bronx	31	29	33
Chicago (city, Black)	31	29	40
Australia	53	28	–
Scotland	24	39	20
France	60	32	1
Spain	60	24	–
Taiwan	90	5	–
Johannesburg	37	4	38–45

From Jennett with permission (1996).

Gender differences

For most age groups worldwide there is an overwhelming male predominance in head injuries, of the order of 2 : 1 (Kraus *et al.* 1984). The effect is less at either extreme of the age spectrum.

Genetics

Recent research has shown an association between a polymorphism of the apolipoprotein E (APO E) gene and outcome from head injury (Teasdale *et al.* 1997).

Apolipoprotein E is synthesized by reactive astrocytes and participates in the reparative response to acute brain injury by transporting lipids to regenerating neurons. Of the three isoforms of this protein in humans, APO E e4 is the least active in promoting repair, and may in fact be detrimental by promoting the deposition of amyloid. Teasdale *et al.* found patients with the APO E e4 allele were more than twice as likely as those without APO E e4 in their genotype to have an unfavourable outcome 6 months after head injury.

Patients with the APO E e4 polymorphism and who have a history of head injury are also at increased risk of developing Alzheimer's disease (Mayeux *et al.* 1995).

Key points

- Apolipoprotein E e4 is correlated with unfavourable outcome after head injury.

Aetiology

Causes of head injury

Motor vehicle accidents are the most significant cause of head injuries worldwide, followed by falls and assault. Alcohol usage contributes to many of these. The relative contributions and incidence trends are, however, highly location-specific (Table 5.4).

Vehicular accidents

Motor vehicle accidents predominate as a cause of severe head injury. In most cases, a vehicle occupant is injured. When pedestrians are involved they tend to sustain multiple injuries. Recent trends in developed countries suggest a reducing incidence of vehicular-related severe head injury (Table 5.5). The improved mortality rates correlate with the development of safer automobile design, improved traffic control, legislation to improve compliance with safety measures (e.g. wearing seatbelts) and public prevention campaigns. One such preventive campaign targets the use of alcohol, with widespread random breath testing. The effect has been highly significant in the UK (HMSO 1995). In contrast to this is the sustained high incidence of severe head injury from motor cycle accidents in places like Taiwan, where traffic control is less vigorous. Here road traffic accidents account for 90% of all head injury admissions and vehicular deaths rose from 31 per 100 000 in 1977 to 37 per 100 000 in 1987 (Lee *et al.* 1990). Comparatively, in the UK road deaths per 100 000 have decreased from 11 in 1980 to 7 in 1993. Other developed countries show similar trends (Table 5.5).

Table 5.5 Road deaths per 100 000 population: recent trends in developed countries

	1980	1985	1993
France	21	20	17
Australia	24	18	
USA	23	19	16
Canada	23	16	
Japan	10	10	11
The Netherlands	13	11	8
UK	11	9	7

From HMSO with permission (1995).

Falls

Falls are a particularly significant aetiological factor for head injury in elderly people, who are generally more frail and poorly mobile, and in whom righting reflexes are impaired. Very young, unsupervised toddlers who fall from a low height also comprise a substantial group. A head injury cause by a fall is more likely to require neurosurgical intervention than a head injury sustained in a motor vehicle accident. This is illustrated in Table 5.6.

Assault

Assaults are a major cause of admission for head injury in densely populated urban areas, particularly where large ethnic cultures coexist. In the New York Bronx or inner city Chicago up to 40% of significant head injuries are assault related. Assaults comprise almost half of all head injury admissions in Johannesburg, but barely contribute to admissions in France. Head injuries caused by gunshot wounds are also significant in the USA where they account for about 1 in 20 of these admissions (Sosin *et al.* 1989).

Recreational and occupational accidents

Occupational and recreational accidents are also prevalent, and related injuries each account for about 10% of head injury admissions (Baker *et al.* 1994).

Table 5.6 Approximate percentage of patients who may require surgery (excluding mild injuries)

	Not in coma		Comatose	
	Motor Equal	Unequal	Motor Equal	Unequal
Vehicular	20	40	20	30
Non-vehicular	40	70	60	80

From RACS with permission (1992).

Biomechanics of head injury

The biomechanics of head injury are complex because of the unique anatomical configurations of the brain being suspended in the bony cranium, and the head being connected to the trunk by the highly flexible cervical spine.

The two main forms of mechanical loading which result in tissue deformation, and thereby injury, are *contact loading* and *inertial loading* (motion or acceleration/deceleration forces) (Gennarelli and Meaney 1996). An impact to the head can result in both contact and inertial loading in varying degrees, but inertial loading can also occur without an impact to the head, such as deceleration of the head when a force is applied to the thorax of a moving person.

Each form of mechanical loading produces specific types of injuries, as indicated in Table 5.2. As can been seen from this table, contact loading produces injuries by local skull bending, skull volume changes, and shock wave propagation. Inertial loading produces injuries by relative motion between the skull and brain, and brain deformation.

The imparted energy from contact or inertial loading produces tissue deformation, and if this strain distorts the tissue beyond its functional or structural tolerance, an injury will result (Gennarelli and Meaney 1996). Tissue deformation can occur in the form of tension, compression, or shearing forces. The degree of injury produced depends on factors such as the amount of force applied, the rate of its application and the mechanical properties of the tissue.

Key point

- Motor vehicle accidents combined with alcohol are the leading cause of severe head injuries.

Pathology

Primary injury

Tissue deformation resulting from forces acting at the moment of impact constitute the primary injury. Impact and inertial forces are responsible in varying degrees for the different types of primary injuries (Table 5.2).

Scalp and skull injuries

All degrees of scalp injuries are commonly seen in the head-injured patient. Their importance lies both in the need for an adequate inspection and repair, and more importantly, in their role as a marker for potential underlying pathology. There is, however, only poor correlation between the presence of scalp injuries and intracranial pathology. A general knowledge of the anatomy is most helpful.

The scalp consists of five layers; skin, a dense connective tissue layer, the galea aponeurotica, a loose connective tissue layer, and the pericranium. The sensory nerves and arteries travel primarily in the layer of dense connective tissue. The arterial adventitia is intimately blended with the surrounding dense connective tissue, so that lacerated vessels are held open and may haemorrhage significantly (Welch and Boyne 1991). The venous drainage accompanies branches of the external carotid artery superficially, but there is also deep, transcranial drainage to the venous sinuses via emissary veins. The first three layers are intimately connected and can move freely over the pericranium, because of the loose connective tissue layer. Surgically they are considered as one layer (Bhattacharya *et al.* 1982).

Lacerations vary enormously in nature and extent, depending on the type and direction of forces applied. They may be small and superficial, or complex, stellate lesions involving most of the scalp. Scalp hair often obscures significant injuries.

Depending on the location, *scalp contusions or haematomas* may have great clinical significance and help direct the clinical and radiological examinations. Periorbital haematomas, often called 'racoon eyes' when present bilaterally, may reflect a fracture of the base of skull through the anterior cranial fossa. Similarly, post-auricular bruising (Battle's sign) usually reflects a petrous fracture of the base of skull. This sign may take days to develop.

Avulsion or degloving injuries represent a more severe type of the scalp injury. They occur when an appropriately directed force strips the mobile aponeurotic layer off the pericranium, the plane of cleavage being through the loose areolar connective tissue. Scalp vessels traversing this space may be torn, producing a subgaleal haematoma. In children, this is a potential cause for hypovolaemia.

The presence of a *skull fracture* reflects the degree of energy imparted at impact. They are found in 80% of all fatal head injuries (McCormick 1997). As discussed above, they may be open or closed, linear or depressed, and their presence greatly increases the likelihood of coexisting intracranial pathology. Fractures occur where local deformation of the vault exceeds regional bony tolerance. The nature of the fracture depends on the magnitude of the force applied, and also on the site impacted and the area over which the force is applied. Thin plated bone, such as that found in the pterional region, is far more susceptible to fracturing than is buttressed bone.

Linear fractures are a result of the outwards bending of bone at a distance from the impact site. The fracture line then takes the path of least resistance, usually running towards the point of contact. They are usually closed or 'simple' fractures. *Depressed skull fractures* occur when contact forces are sufficiently concentrated. They are generally deemed to be significant when a fragment is displaced to a depth greater than the thickness of the skull. The degree of comminution and placement of bony fragments is highly variable. *Compound injuries* are defined by the presence of an overlying scalp laceration or by fracture extension through a nearby air sinus. If there has been a dural tear, the chance of infection is increased significantly.

Basilar skull fractures (BSF) are fractures through the base of the skull, and may involve the anterior, middle, or posterior cranial fossae. They are usually extensions of cranial vault fractures and frequently follow, but are not limited to, occipital or mandibular impacts. Pneumocephalus in the absence of a cranial vault fracture is essentially diagnostic of BSF. A subtype of BSF fracture is the *hinge fracture*. If the fracture line traverses the dorsum sellae, a transverse hinge fracture is produced. In this case the carotid canal is usually opened, and the tegman tympani is also frequently involved. A haemotympanum is a common accompaniment. Carotid dissections may also complicate this type of fracture.

Cranial nerves may be directly damaged in BSFs. Fractures of the cribriform plate and anterior cranial fossa (ACF) may cause olfactory and optic nerve injuries. With this type of fracture, there is also a risk that insertion of a nasogastric tube may lead to intracranial placement, with disastrous consequences (Wyler and Reynolds 1977). Petrous temporal bone involvement may lead to facial or vestibulocochlear nerve injury. Otorrhea or rhinorrhea of cerebrospinal fluid (CSF) may result if the dural membrane is torn.

Diastasis refers to the traumatic opening of suture lines. This is most commonly seen at the coronal or lambdoid suture. A *growing fracture* occasionally occurs when lacerated dura is wedged between the sides of a calvarial fracture, producing a leptomeningeal cyst. This tends to enlarge with time. They are predominantly a feature of head injury in children and are seen most often in the parietal region.

Key points

- Scalp injuries are commonly seen with intracranial head injuries, however there is poor correlation between the presence of scalp injuries and intracranial pathology.
- 'Racoon eyes' present bilaterally may reflect a base of skull fracture through the anterior cranial fossa.

Focal lesions

Extradural haematomas (EDH) result from bleeding between the calvarium and dura mater. Meningeal vessels that groove the inner table of bone are usually implicated. The bleeding is typically arterial but the venous sinuses may also be implicated. The classic location is the temporoparietal region and results from middle meningeal artery disruption. However, about 18% occur in the anterior or posterior cranial fossae, and 10% are parasagittal (Jamieson and Yelland 1968). An overlying fracture is noted in about 90% of adults (Zimmerman and Bilaniuk 1982). Other intracranial pathology is expected in a third of patients (Blumberg 1998). Historically, only 20% of patients with traumatic EDHs follow a clinical course that includes a lucid interval (Jamieson and Yelland 1968).

Subdural haematomas may be classified as acute, subacute, or chronic, depending on the temporal profile of the lesion. Those presenting within 3 days of an injury are acute. Traumatic acute subdural haematomas (ASDHs) are seen in approximately 30% of severe head injuries. They are a poor prognostic sign, and, depending on the timing of surgical evacuation, have mortality rates up to 90% (Seelig *et al.* 1981). Most occur ipsilateral to the side of trauma, but about a third are contralateral (Lanksch *et al.* 1979). They are also frequently associated with skull fractures. There are two types of ASDH. The first type usually occurs in the context of a severe, diffuse type of traumatic brain injury and is continuous with contused, lacerated brain. The other type is a result of ruptured superficial cerebral bridging veins that traverse the subdural space on their way to a venous sinus. They usually collect over the convexity but may also occur in the interhemispheric fissure and along the tentorium. The prognostic significance of ASDHs relates to the presence of both regional and global ischaemia, and unilateral hemispheric swelling, which is highly variable and is not related to the thickness of the haematoma (Bullock and Teasdale 1990).

Subdural haematomas are classified as chronic when they are present for >3 weeks. However, the causative head injury is often very mild and in about 50% of cases a history of trauma is denied (Blumberg 1998). Important predispositions are age and underlying cerebral atrophy, particularly in alcoholics. Extensive brain distortion may be seen in the absence of a raised intracranial pressure (ICP) when there is atrophy. Pathologically, a fibrovascular neomembrane develops at the margins of the haematoma. This begins on the dural surface and may give rise to repeated microhaemorrhages. When there have been delayed recurrent haemorrhages, lamination of the haematoma may be evident. The membrane may also be calcified.

Subacute subdural haematomas may be defined arbitrarily as lesions presenting between 3 days and 3 weeks after trauma. Their pathology shares features of both acute and chronic subdurals.

Subdural hygromas are thought to be caused by a traumatic tear in the arachnoid membrane, which allows for the passage of CSF into the subdural space. Their prevalence in the head-injured patient is of the order of 6% (Blumberg 1998). They may be under high or low pressure, but usually resolve spontaneously. The radiological appearance of hygromas approximates that of a chronic SDH, but they are of lower density on CT.

Contusions are another type of focal injury. They are cortical bruises of the neural parenchyma, and usually affect the crown of a gyrus. If they occur at the site of impact a *coup lesion* is produced. They result from direct disruption of cortical tissue and tearing of surface vessels. The final result is localized haemorrhage or necrosis. Complicated contusions or 'lacerations' involve disruption of the pial membrane and variable white matter disruption.

In moderate to severe injuries global skull shape changes may occur, which, in addition to differential brain and skull movement during acceleration, create foci of low pressure sufficient to cause tissue disruption. When this leads to contusions opposite the site of impact, a *contrecoup lesion* is produced. However, regardless of the injury, frontal and temporal locations are the most common sites affected (Adams *et al.* 1980).

Intraparenchymal haemorrhage refers to focal haematomas >2 cm in size, deep to the cortical surface. This contrasts with areas of haemorrhagic contusion where blood diffuses into adjacent neural parenchyma. They are a result of deep vascular injury, and usually effect the frontal or temporal lobes where characteristic 'lobar' haemorrhages are produced. The basal ganglia are an uncommon site. The overall prevalence in severe head injuries is up to 1–3%, and in most cases they are accompanied by cortical contusions or an ASDH (Rivano *et al.* 1980). They are associated with hypoperfusion to adjacent brain, and in general a poor prognosis.

Intraventricualar haemorrhage is commonly associated with severe head injuries. This may result either from shearing of subependymal veins, from retrograde passage of subarachnoid blood, or from extension of an intracerebral haemorrhage. A frequent radiological feature of this type of haemorrhage is a blood fluid level in the occipital horns. In general it is a poor prognostic sign.

Key points

- Focal lesions include extradural haematomas, subdural haematomas, subdural hygromas, contusions, intraparenchymal haemorrhages, and intraventricular haemorrhages.
- Subdural haematomas may be classified as acute, subacute, or chronic, depending on the temporal profile of the lesion.

Diffuse injuries

The brain may be damaged even without an impact. This occurs in impulsive loading, where pure inertial forces are applied to the brain. These may be translational, angular, rotational, or a combination. Under the influence of these forces differential movement of the skull and dura occurs relative to the brain, and also within different regions of the brain parenchyma. The resulting damage may be focal or diffuse. Axonal disruption and microvascular injury are the pathological hallmarks. Traditionally they have been associated only with the high-velocity injuries seen in motor vehicle accidents, but they are now a recognized complication of falls and blunt assault injuries.

Diffuse axonal injury (DAI) is so named because of the presence of widespread damage to axons throughout the brain and brainstem. It is usually seen in the context of severe, high-speed traumatic brain injury where angular and rotational forces are causative. This type of injury accounts for roughly a third of deaths from head injury and most of the persistent neurological deficits seen in survivors (Teasdale and Graham 1998). The effect depends on the direction of the force applied and on local gyral geometry. It tends to be more severe if it occurs in the coronal plane. At a microscopic level axonal bulbs or retraction balls are seen with various degrees of parenchymal dehiscence (Blumberg 1998). Sites particularly susceptible include:

- internal capsule
- corpus callosum
- pontomedullary junction
- superior cerebellar peduncles
- subcortical white matter
- other areas of the brainstem.

The best macroscopic and radiological markers of DAI are haemorrhage in the corpus callosum and in one or both superior cerebellar peduncles. Grading is to some extent predictive of outcome and, as discussed above, an internationally recognized grading system has been formulated on the basis of CT appearance (Table 5.3).

Trauma is the most common cause of subarachnoid haemorrhage. On CT scan it is seen as high-density change in the sulci, major fissures, or basal cisterns. The multiple potential sites of origin for the haemorrhage include damaged pial vessels, extensive intraventricular haemorrhage, and haemorrhagic cortical contusions. The significance of this type of injury lies in the potential difficulty in distinguishing it with certainty from an aneurysmal source of haemorrhage, and the potential for developing communicating hydrocephalus as a delayed complication.

Primary brainstem lesions include contusions, shearing injuries, and various 'rents' or separations. They typically occur as part of a diffuse brain injury. Brainstem contusions are often associated with basilar fractures, usually of the clivus, and may coexist with superficial lacerations. Pontomedullary tears or rent is another brainstem lesion characteristic of severe trauma. They are most often due to marked hyperextension of the head and neck and rarely occur without a skull or upper cervical spine fracture (McCormick 1997). Other well-recognized injuries to the brainstem include tears and separations of the mesencephalic–pontine and spinal–medullary junctions. These injuries are lethal, and fortunately uncommon.

Key points

- The brain may be damaged even without an impact, through inertial forces.

Vascular injuries

Vascular injuries are a common feature of head injuries involving significant inertial forces, such as high-speed motor vehicle accidents, but may also be seen in less severe types of trauma. They may be classified as parenchymal or extraparenchymal and can effect all types of vessels, including dural sinuses (Table 5.7).

Traumatic aneurysms are a well-known complication of head injury, and may occur on branches of the external and internal carotid arteries. They are usually 'false' and result from complete mural rupture with organized surrounding haematoma. Superficial middle cerebral branches are the most common sites involved, followed by peripheral branches of the anterior cerebral artery (McCormick 1997). When major vessels at the base of the brain are involved, the distinction between traumatic and non-traumatic causation is difficult. Certain angiographic features, such as location away from branch points and absence of a definable neck, suggest the former.

Table 5.7 Classification of traumatic vascular injuries

Intraparenchymal	
Focal	Contusions Intracerebral haemorrhage Subarachnoid haemorrhage
Multifocal	Combinations of above
Diffuse	Widespread petechial microhaemorrhages
Intracranial and extraparenchymal	
Bridging vessels	Acute subdural Chronic subdural
Vessels adjacent to skull bones	Extradural haematoma
Circle of Willis and intracranial vertebral and carotids	Thrombosis Dissection Fistula
Extracranial	
Cervical vessels	As above Subintimal haemorrhage

From Blumberg with permission (1998).

Lesser forms of arterial disruption such as arterial dissection are more common, and may complicate all grades of head injury. Pathologically there is tearing of the intimal lining and variable disruption of the other vessel wall components. Exposure of subendothelial tissues and altered local haemodynamics predisposes to thrombosis. This may give rise to distal emboli or cause complete occlusion.

All segments of the internal carotid artery may be affected, but the extracranial portion above the bifurcation is the most common site. Traumatic vertebral dissections usually involve the distal extracranial portion of the artery between the axis and base of skull (Zee and Go 1998). Symptoms vary from a low-grade head or neck ache to massive stroke, but in many patients they are asymptomatic.

Lacerations to the dural sinuses, or thrombosis, usually results from penetrating injuries or depressed skull fractures. Traumatic carotid-cavernous fistulas occur in 1–2% of patients with severe head injuries (McCormick 1997). They are usually associated with a base of skull fracture, particularly those affecting the sphenoid bone.

Key points

- Vascular lesions such as traumatic aneurysms are well known complications of severe head injury.

Secondary injury

Secondary brain injury is the term used for all cerebral insults that follow the primary injury. It may result directly from the pathophysiological processes initiated by the primary insult, or it may be due to the extraneous effects of trauma such as hypoxia or systemic hypotension. The major forms of secondary injury seen are hypoxia, hypotension, disordered cerebral blood flow, and the commonly related pathologies of cerebral oedema and raised ICP. They may act in isolation, but more commonly there is a combination of interacting mechanisms that contribute to the secondary insult in a given patient. The importance of these secondary injuries lies in their potential for prevention, and reversibility.

Hypoxia

Hypoxic insults are known to significantly worsen outcome in traumatic brain injuries, and hypoxia is present in almost 50% of fatal head injuries (Chesnut *et al.* 1993). In the early post-injury phase, it is the most prevalent form of secondary insult.

A normally functioning cerebral vasculature is highly sensitive to hypoxia, and responds to this by vasodilatation, thereby increasing cerebral blood flow and maintaining oxygen delivery (Fortune *et al.* 1992). This is illustrated in Fig. 5.1, which demonstrates the usual increase in cerebral blood flow and oxygen delivery seen with hypoxia for any given P_aCO_2, in the non-head-injured patient. However, in the setting of a traumatic brain injury there is amelioration of this protective effect, and profound vulnerability to hypoxia. The major causes of hypoxia in the trauma patient are respiratory dysfunction resulting in asphyxia or inadequate ventilation, and impaired oxygen delivery. Another significant cause of relative or absolute hypoxia is increased metabolic demand, where energy expenditure exceeds oxygen dependent production. Seizures are one such cause of increased metabolic demand, and may result in complete consumption of cellular energy.

Physiologically, hypoxia is defined as an arterial partial pressure of oxygen (P_aO_2) <60 mmHg. At this level of P_aO_2 and below, the haemoglobin saturation with oxygen rapidly declines, causing a reduction in the arterial oxygen content. The end result is impaired oxygen delivery and a low tissue oxygen tension. As a result, there is cellular conversion from aerobic to anaerobic metabolism and reduced total energy production. Tissue damage will result if the insult is of sufficient severity or duration.

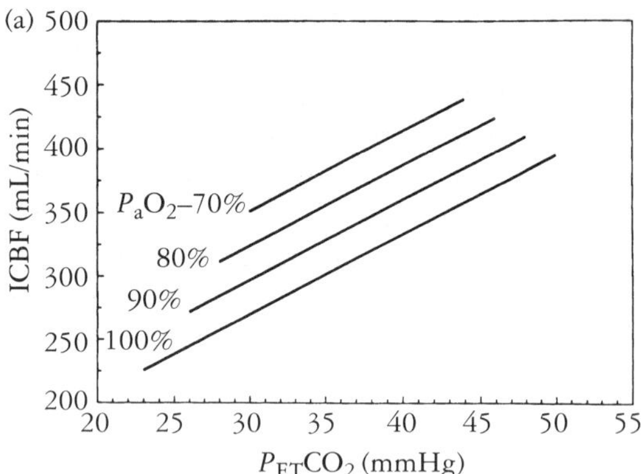

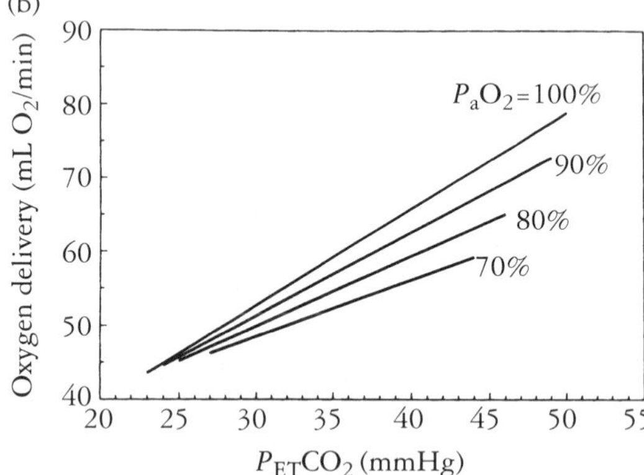

Figure 5.1 Increase in (a) cerebral blood flow and (b) oxygen delivery seen with hypoxia for any given P_aCO_2, in the non head-injured patient. (Popp *et al.* (1997) with permission)

The cellular effects of hypoxia are complex and varied, and are best understood in terms of the basic physiology. For normal neuronal survival and function, a continuous supply of energy in the form of adenosine triphosphate (ATP) is essential. The basic building blocks for this are adenosine diphosphate (ADP), oxygen, and glucose, and of these it is the ADP that is usually the limiting substrate. The production of ATP may take place either in the cytoplasm, where the anaerobic glycolytic pathway occurs, or in the mitochondria, where the critical oxygen-dependent respiratory chain enzymes reside and where the Krebs cycle takes place. The latter aerobic pathway is far more powerful, but requires a critical level of tissue oxygen tension. An important by-product of the former pathway is lactate and hydrogen ions. This means that in hypoxic conditions where oxygen is lacking, but where glucose and other substrate supplies are unaltered, ATP production occurs predominantly via the anaerobic glycolytic pathway, resulting in acidosis and disturbed cellular function (Siesjo 1992). In particular, there is inhibition of phosphofructokinase, a key enzyme in the glycolytic pathway, and widespread protein conformational change and dysfunction (Popp *et al.* 1997). With disruption of anaerobic pathways and the further depletion of energy levels, there is a degradation in all areas of cellular homeostasis, and in particular, transmembrane ion gradients. The main primary active transport system is the Na–K ATPase. It is electrogenic and highly energy dependent, and through the generation of the transmembrane Na^+ gradient it provides the energy for many of the secondary active transport systems, such as the Na–H^+ and Na–Ca^{2+} exchangers. In hypoxic conditions, where energy stores are depleted, there is a progressive failure of this pump and a loss of the Na^+ gradient (Popp *et al.* 1997). This leads to the accumulation of intracellular Na^+ and a reduced drive for Na^+-dependent secondary active transport systems. There is intracellular acidosis and accumulation of calcium. This in turn leads to the activation of Ca^{2+}-dependent proteases, resulting in cellular organelle and membrane injury, and further amplification of the process.

Key points

- Hypoxic insults significantly worsen outcome in traumatic brain injuries.

Cerebral blood flow and hypotension

A critically low cerebral blood flow may result from any cause of systemic hypotension or raised ICP, and profoundly influences outcome in the head-injured patient. The effect depends on the nature and severity of the insult.

Under normal conditions there are effective and highly sensitive physiological control systems operating to maintain adequate and appropriate global and regional cerebral blood flow (CBF), to compensate for fluctuations in blood pressure and brain activity. The normal CBF is approximately 55 mL/100 g per minute. Regional flow is also closely coupled to metabolic demand, such that in normal conditions there is a linear dependence of CBF on metabolic rate for oxygen ($C_{MR}O_2$). About half of the $C_{MR}O_2$ is for baseline cellular function and the remainder represents consumption for neural activity (Popp *et al.* 1997). The coupling process is not fully understood but is mediated in part by a number of vasoactive metabolites such as adenosine, K^+, or H^+ (Phillis 1989).

Cerebral perfusion pressure (CCP) is defined as the difference between mean arterial pressure (MAP) and ICP:

$$\text{CPP} = \text{MAP} - \text{ICP}$$

CCP represents the driving pressure for cerebral perfusion and estimates cerebral blood flow. In normal conditions the cerebrovascular circulation is autoregulated to maintain a constant cerebral blood flow over a wide range of CPPs. This range typically extends from a lower limit of 50 mmHg to an upper limit of 150 mmHg (see Fig. 5.2). Within this range, only transient deviations of CBF occur before these vascular regulatory mechanisms re-establish the steady state. At each end of the autoregulation range, the relationship of CBF to CPP becomes passive and linear.

The CBF may be described in terms of the CPP and the cerebral vascular resistance (CVR):

$$\text{CBF} = \text{CPP/CVR}$$

In the maintenance of a steady state CBF, the pivotal autoregulatory mechanism is an alteration in the CVR. This must be in the same direction and to the same degree as the CPP, either by vasodilatation or vasoconstriction of resistance vessels. In this way there in constancy of cerebral blood flow, as illustrated by the 'normal autoregulation' curve in Fig. 5.2. Another very important parameter is the cerebral blood volume (CBV). According to the Monro–Kellie doctrine (see below), blood is one of the three dependent intracranial volume components that influences ICP. As such, the vascular

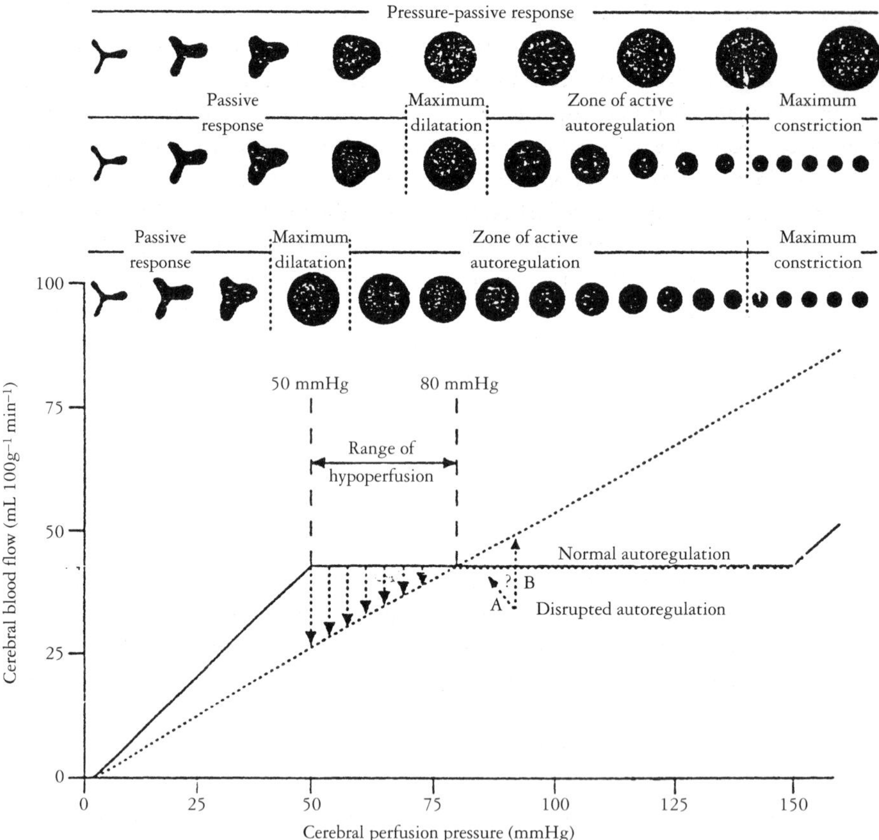

Figure 5.2 Autoregulation of the cerebrovascular circulation over a range of CPPs. (Reproduced from Chestnut *et al.* (1997), with permission).

response to changing CPP, whether it be vasoconstriction or vasodilatation, will lead directly to changes in CBV and indirectly to changes in ICP.

Traumatic brain injury frequently disrupts both the normal dependence of CBF on metabolic rate, and the normal independence of CBF on CPP, but the response is partial and heterogeneous (Obrist *et al.* 1984).

Of particular concern is the loss of autoregulation. In the context of trauma, a brain which has already suffered a primary mechanical injury becomes profoundly vulnerable to a further insult from systemic hypotension, because of an inability to maintain cerebral blood flow in the face of a falling CPP. In fact, hypotensive insults in severe head injuries are associated with a doubling of mortality and markedly increased morbidity (Chesnut *et al.* 1993). The pathology is consistent with a partial disruption to the vascular regulatory system and a resetting of the lower limit of autoregulation to a higher level (Bouma *et al.* 1992). There is a loss of active vasodilatation and an extension of the lower pressure-passive response, above which autoregulation commences.

The end result is a variable degree of cerebral hypoperfusion and ischaemia for the lower range of CPP values that would normally have been considered adequate (see Fig. 5.2, curve A). This helps explain the devastating effects of even transient episodes of hypotension (Chesnut *et al.* 1993), and the rationale behind the clinical goal in the head-injured patient of maintaining a CPP > 70 mmHg (Lang and Chesnut 1995). The theoretical response to a complete loss of autoregulation, with a purely pressure-passive change in CBF in response to variations in CPP, and its effect on CBV, is also seen in Fig. 5.2 (curve B).

Uncoupling of metabolism and CBF also occurs in about 50% of patients after severe head injury (Bhattacharya *et al.* 1989), and this may occur independently of autoregulatory dysfunction. In the first 4–8 hours after head injury, there is often a period of sustained global hypoperfusion. Figure 5.3 demonstrates the reduction in CBF seen during this period. Values <20 mL/100 g per minute are considered ischaemic (Chesnut *et al.* 1993), and are frequently seen. On the basis of nuclear medicine SPECT and Xe-enhanced CT studies, it is also evident that regional ischaemic zones exist around intracranial haematomas and contusions (Schroder *et al.* 1995). Evacuation of accessible haematomas however ameliorates this effect. After the acute phase of global hypoperfusion, there is usually a phase of relative or absolute hyperaemia, with CBF being maintained either within the normal range or above it, despite a reduced metabolic rate for oxygen. The mechanism may involve increased levels of lactate and a disruption of the normally vasoactive H^+ and K^+ coupling pathways (Desalles *et al.* 1987).

A clinically useful parameter for assessing the adequacy of CBF is the jugular venous saturation ($S_{jv}O_2$). It is a measure of cerebral venous oxygen content (C_vO_2). Using the Fick principle, the $C_{MR}O_2$ and CBF may be quantified:

$$C_{MR}O_2/CBF = (C_aO_2 - C_vO_2)$$

Normal arterial–venous oxygen content differences are 50–75 mL O_2 per litre of blood. High levels of $S_{jv}O_2$ result in a small arterial–venous oxygen content difference and indicate an inappropriately high level of CBF for the $C_{MR}O_2$, as is commonly seen after traumatic brain injury. Conversely, a low $S_{jv}O_2$ saturation indicates insufficient blood flow relative to the cerebral metabolic rate.

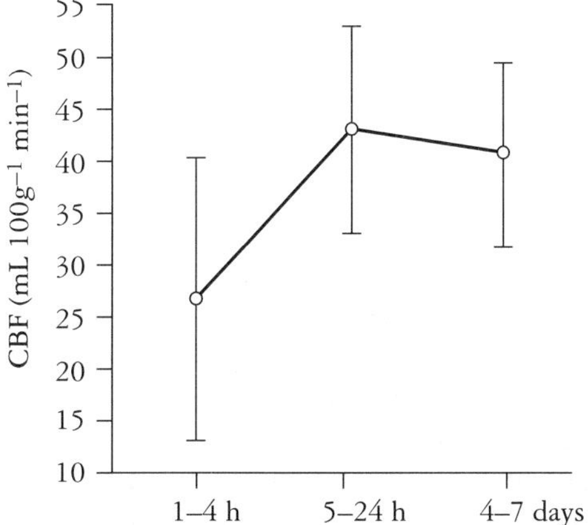

Figure 5.3 Reduction in cerebral blood flow. (Reproduced from Marion *et al.* (1991), with permission.)

As discussed above, the CBF is also normally highly sensitive to the arterial P_aCO_2 and P_aO_2, with appropriate increases in hypercapnoeic and hypoxic conditions (Fig. 5.1). Within the normal physiological ranges, the CBF increases 2–4% for each unit increase in P_aCO_2 and 2% for each percent of arterial oxygen desaturation (Fortune *et al.* 1992). In hypoxic conditions the reactive vasodilatation permits a higher CBF and improved oxygen delivery. However, in the head-injured patient this response is severely blunted in magnitude and is also of much shorter duration, leaving the patient extremely vulnerable to even transient episodes of hypoxia. The vascular regulation seen with changes in the P_aCO_2 are primarily mediated by extravascular H^+ concentration, so that an increase in H^+ concentration is accompanied by an increase in resistance vessel diameter (Heistad and Kontos 1983). Similarly, there is vasoconstriction and reduced CBF in hypocapnoeic conditions. The limit to this response is $P_aCO_2 = 20$ mmHg, at which point the effect of ischaemic-driven vasodilator metabolites overrides the vasoconstrictor response. Temporally, the effect persists until extravascular H^+ levels normalize. In normal conditions this happens within 16 hours. After head trauma the carbon dioxide reactivity of CBF is generally preserved, making hyperventilation an effective short-term tool in the treatment of intracranial hypertension. To avoid ischaemia from hypocapnoeic vasoconstriction, the P_aCO_2 is generally kept above 27 mmHg and if $S_{jv}O_2$ is being monitored, values >50% are usually accepted.

In response to a generalized reduction in cerebral perfusion pressures from hypotension, ischaemia is most severe in the boundary zones or 'watershed' regions of major arterial territories. Isolated arterial damage, as may occur in blunt or penetrating neck injuries or dissections, will lead to arterial territory ischaemia. Mixed forms of ischaemia are also commonly seen in the head-injured patient.

Cerebral oedema and raised intracranial pressure

The upper limit of normal adult ICP is 10–15 mmHg. In uninjured brains, pressures well above this are usually well tolerated. However, after severe head injuries, cerebral oedema and intracranial hypertension are poorly tolerated and are major causes of morbidity and mortality (Popp *et al.* 1997). For this reason an understanding of the pathophysiology involved is essential.

The intracranial compartment is a closed space housed by the bony calvarium and base of skull. The pressure inside is determined by the total volume of its three intracranial components: blood, brain and CSF. This is the Monro–Kellie doctrine (Mokri 2001). An increase in the volume of any one of these components will cause an increase in the ICP, once compensatory mechanisms are overcome and displaceable volume is depleted.

The buffering capacity for pressure changes is limited, and is largely mediated by redistribution of CSF, which normally contributes to about 10% of the intracranial volume (Popp *et al.* 1997). When pressures rise intracranially and CSF pathways are preserved, there is displacement of CSF to the extracranial spinal compartment and distension of the spinal dura. There is also an increase in CSF absorption. This is because the driving pressure, determined by the difference between ICP and venous pressure, is increased.

The extent to which an increase in volume results in increased pressure is called the *compliance*, and this value is pressure-dependent. As intracranial volume increases the compliance rapidly decreases.

The pressure–volume index (PVI) is another useful parameter and is measured as the change of volume required to increase ICP by a factor of 10. It is essentially independent of ICP. The relationship is as follows:

$$\text{PVI} = \text{change in volume}/\log(P_{\text{final}}/P_{\text{initial}})$$

A normal value is close to 25 mL (Maset *et al.* 1987). A low PVI indicates a loss of volume buffering capacity and therefore a low tolerance for any rise in ICP. It is frequently seen after traumatic brain injury, when a small increases in volume may result in a grossly elevated ICP. Serial values are far more significant than single measurements, but values <18 mL are generally considered pathological, and are predictive of protracted intracranial hypertension (Maset *et al.* 1987). The exponential manner in which ICP rises as a result of increased intracranial volume is illustrated in Fig. 5.4. The effect of a low PVI or reduced available buffering volume in decreasing compliance is also seen.

Cerebral oedema is a highly variable and potentially fatal response to head trauma. It may be focal or generalized. There are two major pathophysiological categories which may coexist: vasogenic oedema, resulting from a primary disruption to the blood–brain barrier and leading initially to extracellular accumulation of fluid, and cytotoxic oedema caused by cellular homeostatic dysfunction and resulting in intracellular accumulation.

Vasogenic oedema is a consequence of dysfunction of the blood–brain barrier. In the normal cerebral circulation the high density of vascular endothelial tight junctions and the absence of fenestrations form the so-called blood–brain barrier which permits only lipid-soluble particles to diffuse passively across the membranes. Transport systems are required for ionic particles, maintaining an intravascularly directed osmotic gradient.

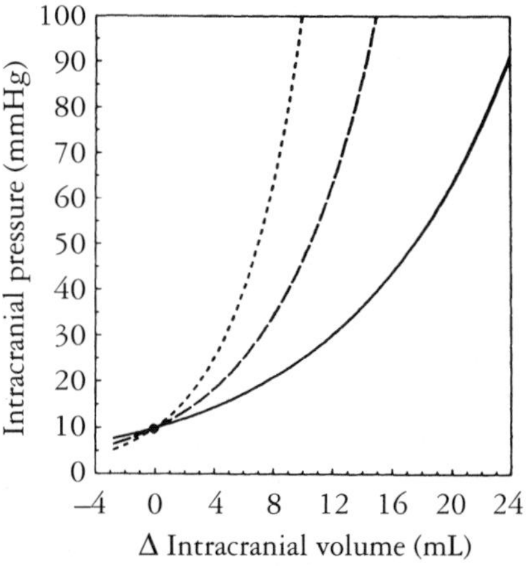

Figure 5.4 Exponential manner in which ICP rises as a result of increased intracranial volume. - - -, PVI=10 mL; – – –, PVI=15 mL; ——, PVI= 25 mL. (Reproduced from Popp *et al.* (1997), with permission.)

This inhibits the movement of water into the brain parenchyma. When the barrier is breached, the filtrate initially accumulates extracellularly, with a tendency to affect white matter preferentially. Venous or arterial pathologies may predominate.

In head-injured patients an arterial hyperaemic phase for cerebral blood flow is often seen, which usually peaks 24 hours after impact and increases the fluid flux across a disrupted blood–brain barrier (Bouma *et al.* 1992). Intravascular pressures are also increased when the venous return is compromised. Coexisting cardiac and pulmonary pathologies, such as cardiac tamponade and tension pneumothorax, are possibilities in the trauma patient. Life-threatening brain swelling may occur when there is significant cerebrovascular disruption. Treatment is directed at the correction of exacerbating factors and reversing the fluid shifts.

Cytotoxic or cellular oedema refers to the intracellular accumulation of fluid, and results from impaired cellular haemostasis. In this setting the blood–brain barrier is intact and there is a fluid shift from the extracellular to intracellular compartment. The pathology is multifactorial. One important process results from excessive uptake of potassium chloride following the post-traumatic rise in extracellular K^+. Hypoxia is also a significant factor, and, as outlined above, the metabolic derangements produced are diverse. Events pertaining more directly to cellular oedema include the conversion to anaerobic metabolism resulting in a breakdown of astrocyte glycogen macromolecules into multiple, osmotically active units of glucose; a loss of the full activity of the $Na–K^+$ ATPase with accumulation of intracellular Na^+ and disordered secondary active transport systems; and structural membrane damage, either directly or as a result of oxygen-free radicals. In combination these events lead to cell swelling and predispose to its deleterious secondary effects, including depolarization, activation of mechanosensitive Ca^{2+} channels, and the release of excitatory neurotransmitters. A further significant factor in the generation of cytotoxic oedema is a low serum osmolality. The latter may be iatrogenic, following inappropriate fluid administration, or may result from the syndrome of inappropriate ADH secretion (SIADH). Most vulnerable to all these changes are the astrocyte cell body and the neuronal dendrites, where swelling is preferentially focused (Popp *et al.* 1997).

After a head injury, each of the intracranial compartments may be expanded. Vasodilatation and extra-axial haematoma will affect the blood volume, there may be cerebral oedema or ICH to expand brain volume, and occasionally there may be obstructive hydrocephalus with dilatation of the ventricular system. These changes are partially absorbed by the available displaceable volume, and increased CSF absorption. But as the magnitude of the volume change increases and buffering capacity is overwhelmed, there is a decrease in intracranial compliance and early decompensation. The end result is a rise in ICP. At this early stage the elevated pressures can be easily normalized with hyperventilation and induced hypocapnoea, which causes vasoconstriction of intracranial feeding vessels and reduced blood volume.

As ICP increases and compliance decreases further, small volume changes lead to larger and more prolonged increases in pressure. *Plateau waves* (also known as Lundberg A waves) and other types of preterminal waveforms may be seen on the ICP monitor trace in this setting (Lundberg 1960).

Pathophysiology of neuronal injury

All degrees of neuronal injury are seen after head trauma. The outstanding feature, however, is the variable time course and the sequential pattern of cytoskeletal and metabolic derangements. Primary axotomy occurs at the time of impact and usually requires >20% strain in the neurolemma (Maxwell *et al.* 1997). Non-disruptively injured axons are exposed to a complex sequence of interacting events. The primary insult is to the cytoskeleton, with focal disruption of neurofilaments and a loss of axoplasmic neuronal transport. Traumatic depolarization may occur at this stage, with consumption of remaining energy supplies and release of excitatory neurotransmitters. Local axonal swelling and loss of cellular transmembrane homeostasis also occur. A critical event is the influx of calcium with the activation of destructive phospholipases and generation of oxygen free radicals. This leads to irreversible membrane damage and further release of damaging neuroexcitatory transmitters, of which glutamate is the most widely implicated.

Clinical assessment

Assessment of the head-injured patient is an ongoing process from the initial point of contact through to the completion of definitive management. At any time during this period the pathological sequelae of head injury may gradually or suddenly become clinically manifest. It is therefore crucial to initially obtain an accurate *baseline assessment* as a reference point for gauging improvement or deterioration in the patient's condition. This will enable prompt changes in management to optimize neurological recovery. This baseline assessment is also important as it remains the most useful indicator of the patient's prognosis.

Assessment of the head-injured patient is also a flexible process, as the ability of the patient to participate in the history and examination varies from full co-operation to amnesia to combative to unconscious. It is therefore useful to develop a comprehensive, systematic approach which can be tailored to the various clinical situations that present themselves.

History

The information to compile a history of the trauma and the patient's resulting symptoms often has to be obtained from a variety of sources. These may include the patient, various witnesses present at the time of the injury, and ambulance staff.

The time of injury is important as the starting point of the clinical timeline, and governs how long most patients with mild head injuries will be observed prior to discharge. It is often most easily obtained from the time the ambulance service was contacted (on the ambulance report). The mechanism of injury is also important in helping determine the severity and pattern of pathology after head injury. Factors such as the speed of motor vehicles involved, the height of falls, or the size and mass of objects, striking the head should be ascertained. The use of seatbelts or helmets (if applicable) should also be determined. These details also serve to alert the physician to possible inconsistencies between the reported cause and severity of the patient's injuries, which may suggest a preceding neurological event, or a desire to cover up an assault.

It is important to identify whether the patient suffered a loss of consciousness. The period of loss of consciousness is difficult to obtain, as anxious bystanders vary in their ability to recall this information, so an estimate is usual. It is useful to find out the patient's condition at the scene of the trauma, whether there was any period of airway obstruction or cyanosis, hypotension and the initial GCS score from the ambulance report. This can then be compared to the condition in the emergency department, again providing a temporal profile of the patient's neurological progress.

Information about the patient's premorbid status is sometimes available from family or friends. The patient may already have an established neurological deficit, may be taking anticoagulants or antiplatelet medication, or may chronically abuse alcohol and have concomitant cerebral atrophy or a coagulopathy. It is also important to think about the sequence of events. It is not uncommon for a preceding neurological event to result in an accident or fall and subsequent head injury. Use of alcohol or recreational drugs before the trauma is important to ascertain, as these can mask the patient's true level of neurological function. If the patient has been intubated before retrieval, medications for sedation and paralysis during the transfer should be identified as these can also change the clinical picture.

It is important to find out if the patient has suffered a post-traumatic seizure before assessment, as the postictal state can be prolonged and again mask the patient's true level of neurological function.

If the patient is able to communicate, a more conventional symptom review can then proceed. Headache, nausea, vomiting, dizziness, blurred vision, and photophobia are common after even mild head injury and may persist for weeks (*post-concussion syndrome*). They may also represent *meningism*, the irritation of the meninges by the presence of extravasated blood such as an extradural or subdural haematoma. Clinically this may be associated with the presence of nuchal rigidity (neck stiffness).

As spinal injury is often associated with head injury, it is important to ask about neck and back pain. Patients may also be able to identify specific areas of motor loss or sensory loss.

It is also useful to quantify the period of post-traumatic amnesia (PTA) in conscious patients. This is usually done by asking the patient what is the first thing they remember after the trauma, for example the paramedics arriving at the scene, or waking up in hospital. A patient who remains unable to recall events and exhibits poor short term memory for new information is said to be 'still in PTA'. Often patients still in PTA will perseverate questions, despite the dutiful efforts of staff to answer them.

Key points

- A satisfactory history may require a number of sources such other than the patient such as witnesses and ambulance officers.
- Time of injury, mechanism, factors such as vehicle speed and used of seatbelts, loss of consciousness, pre-morbid medical history, seizure activity, back and neck pain, and PTA are important.

Examination

The system for examination described below can be applied, with appropriate modification, to all patients with head injuries. Those with severe injuries associated with multiple trauma will require the full sequence, but for patients with milder injuries whose vital observations are stable the primary survey and resuscitation may be reduced to a mental checklist.

Primary survey and resuscitation

The primary tenets of airway, breathing and circulation (ABC) are critical in assessment of the trauma patient, and no more so than in the head-injured patient. Hypoxia and hypotension are major contributors to secondary brain injury and poor patient outcomes, and therefore must be reversed as soon as possible. Management of the ABC is usually commenced in the field by modern paramedic services. If intubation is indicated it should be performed with due concern for the haemodynamic and ICP effects of airway manipulation (Walls 1993). It is important to remember the possibility of occult spinal injury in the unconscious patient, and precautions should be adhered to from the outset. Most patients will have been transferred to hospital with a rigid cervical collar and spinal board. The collar should be checked for proper fit, and if removed to enable intubation, the neck should be maintained in neutral alignment manually (without traction) until the collar is replaced.

It important to pay close attention to the ventilation of the head-injured patient and vital to maintain a normal P_aCO_2. Hypoventilation and resultant hypercapnoea cause cerebral vasodilation and an increase in ICP. Hyperventilation and resultant hypocapnoea cause cerebral vasoconstriction and potential hypoperfusion. In the absence of signs of intracranial hypertension (neurological deterioration not explained by extracranial causes or evidence of transtentorial herniation) a P_aCO_2 range of 35–40 mmHg is recommended (Randell and Chesnut 1997).

Traditionally a systolic blood pressure of <90 mmHg was considered to represent hypotension in multiple trauma patients, but it is now considered important to maintain a mean arterial pressure (MAP) >90 mmHg to ensure an adequate cerebral perfusion pressure in the head-injured patient (Bullock *et al.* 1996). This translates to a target systolic blood pressure of >120 mmHg.

Dysfunction of the neurological system is assessed next. Perfunctory observations such as the AVPU approach (alert, voice, pain, unresponsive) are of little value to ongoing assessment or communicating with neurosurgical colleagues, especially if the patient is subsequently intubated before a more thorough neurological examination can be performed. A GCS assessment (Table 2.3) can be performed rapidly with practice, and may alert the physician to lateralizing signs early in the assessment. Pupil size and reaction can also be rapidly assessed without the aid of a torch in a properly lit resuscitation area.

The patient should be fully exposed and a 'space blanket' applied to ensure a thorough surface examination while maintaining core temperature. Intravenous access should be secured and fluids infused as appropriate. Blood is collected for laboratory analysis (arterial blood gases, full blood count, electrolytes, urea, creatinine, coagulation profile, serum glucose, and blood alcohol level) and cross-matching. The patient is connected to appropriate equipment to monitor pulse, blood pressure, electrocardiography, and oxygen saturation. If the patient is intubated, end tidal carbon dioxide should be monitored. An indwelling catheter (IDC) is inserted, unless there are signs of possible urethral trauma. A nasogastric tube (NGT) is inserted, unless there are signs of possible basal skull fracture (see below).

Usually the components of the primary survey and resuscitation are attended to simultaneously by a trauma team.

Secondary survey

During the secondary survey, assessment is periodically interrupted to enable the acquisition of chest, lateral cervical spine, and pelvic radiographs.

A more comprehensive neurological examination can be undertaken if the patient is stable after the primary survey and resuscitation phase. The scope of this examination will obviously depend on the patient's ability and willingness to participate. Co-operative patients (mild head injuries) can be fully assessed for dysfunction of higher centres, cranial nerves, motor system, and sensory system. Unconscious patients require a more truncated approach. This includes interpretation of the vital signs: pulse, blood pressure and respiratory rate. Bradycardia is often an indicator of neurological involvement. Associated with hypertension (*Cushing's reflex*), it is a late sign of brainstem compression, whereas associated with hypotension, it suggests spinal cord injury with loss of sympathetic vasomotor tone. Respiratory pattern depends on the level of the central nervous system affected, with Cheyne–Stokes breathing, hyperventilation, agonal (irregular) respiration, and finally apnoea occurring as injury progressively affects lower portions of the brainstem (Plum and Posner 1980). The GCS should again be assessed, although an unconscious patient will by now be intubated for airway protection and should only be assigned a score of 1 for verbal response. Similarly, patients with significant periorbital swelling may only score 1 for eye-opening response. The patient should not be hypoxic or hypotensive, and the effects of paralytic and sedative medications should be allowed to wear off, to ensure an accurate GCS (Marion and Carlier 1994). The pupils should be checked for size and reaction to light. Unilateral dilatation and sluggish or absent reaction to light (a "blown pupil") occurs when herniation of the medial temporal lobe (uncus) through the tentorial notch compresses the third cranial nerve and indicates severely raised ICP. This must be distinguished from traumatic mydriasis which is usually earlier in onset and associated with external evidence of orbital trauma, and the conscious state of the patient does not fit the diagnosis of severe head injury. If both pupils are fixed and dilated, the patient has central tentorial herniation due to extremely raised ICP. Meiosis associated with a Horner's syndrome can signify a carotid artery injury. An afferent pupillary defect, as detected by paradoxical dilatation during the swinging torch test, signifies optic nerve damage which may result from a fracture affecting the optic canal. Pinpoint pupils are usually due to opiates. The resting eye position is also easily assessed. Frontal lobe lesions can cause ipsilateral conjugate gaze deviation, whereas pontine lesions can cause contralateral conjugate gaze deviation. Frequently, however, patients with a reduced level of consciousness exhibit a dysconjugate gaze. The fundi should be examined to check for intraocular pathology and papilloedema. Mydriatic eye drops should be avoided to enable ongoing pupillary assessment. Motor functions (tone, movement to stimulation, reflexes) should be assessed be to identify any localizing signs. These may obviously be affected if neuromuscular paralytic agents are still active. Brainstem reflexes are usually only performed if the patient's prognosis is deemed to be so poor that withdrawal of active intervention is being considered.

The rest of the secondary survey proceeds from head to toe. Examination of the head involves checking the scalp for lacerations and haematomas. This is best done by palpation, as lesions can be easily hidden by hair or blood. Lacerations should be carefully explored with a gloved finger to check for underlying fractures. Arterial haemorrhage should be controlled by artery forceps, ligation, or pressure until definitive suturing can be performed. The orbital margins should be palpated for steps which may signify a fracture. The presence of a periorbital haematoma is usually due to external trauma if it extends beyond the margins of the orbit, but if it is confined to the margins of the eyelids it is most likely due to blood tracking through the orbit from an anterior base of skull fracture, a sign referred to as 'raccoon eyes'. There may also be associated subconjunctival blood extending to the posterior limits of the sclera which has tracked through the orbit. Infraorbital paraesthesia should be excluded; if present and associated with extraocular muscle entrapment it is indicative of a blowout fracture of the floor of the orbit. The nose is examined for clinical signs of fracture and septal haematoma. If the latter is present it should be evacuated to prevent ischaemic septal perforation. CSF rhinorrhoea can be difficult to detect at the initial assessment, especially in the presence of epistaxis, but when found denotes an anterior base of skull fracture. The 'target sign' may help distinguish at the bedside if CSF is present. Later, samples can be collected to analyse for glucose or β_2-transferrin. The ears should be examined for haemotympanum and otorrhoea of blood or CSF, which indicate a temporal base of skull fracture. It is important to check whether blood in the external auditory canal has trickled in from other facial or scalp lacerations. *Battle's sign* is bruising visible over the mastoid process and is also indicative of a base of skull fracture. The face should be inspected for swelling (possible underlying fractures) and symmetry (facial nerve palsy secondary to temporal bone fracture, although this usually develops late). The patient's bite should be assessed to check for possible mandibular fractures and loose or missing teeth. Movement of the upper dentition is attempted to detect Le Fort type maxillary fractures.

The neck is then examined. Until the presence of cervical spine injury has been excluded both clinically and radiologically (see below) the patient should remain in a properly fitted hard collar. It is important to realize that these orthoses do not prevent movement of the spine; they serve to remind the patient and clinicians to maintain a neutral spinal alignment. A combative head-injured patient may require sedation and intubation to achieve this aim. In the co-operative patient the hard collar may be loosened and gentle palpation performed to assess for tenderness. Crepitus due to subcutaneous emphysema suggests an airway injury. The carotid arteries should be palpated and auscultated, as bruits can signpost arterial dissection.

The chest, abdomen, pelvis, and limbs are then examined as outlined in other chapters.

The patient is then 'log-rolled' to permit examination of the back. This manoeuvre requires a minimum of three people to enable synchronous rotation of the head, trunk, and lower limbs whilst maintaining the total spine in neutral alignment. Vertebral palpation is carried out to detect tenderness or step deformities. A sensory level may be detected. A digital rectal examination is also performed to check sphincter tone and anal sensation.

At the completion of the secondary survey it is important to reassess the patient's ABC to ensure resuscitation is on track.

Herniation syndromes

A space-occupying lesion, such as an expanding haematoma, or generalized cerebral swelling, if allowed to progress, will eventually cause displacement of brain parenchyma from one compartment of the skull to another. This *brainshift* results in compression of structures and causes typical clinical syndromes. The presence of these signs in a head-injured patient represent severe intracranial hypertension, and must be treated with the utmost emergency if rapid, irreversible brainstem injury and death are to be avoided.

Lateral tentorial herniation results from a lateral supratentorial lesion causing movement of the uncus inferiorly through the tentorial notch. The resultant compression of the midbrain causes a decrease in the level of consciousness, compression of the oculomotor nerve at the free edge of the tentorium causes ipsilateral pupillary dilatation and loss of reaction to light, compression of the cerebral peduncle causes contralateral weakness, and compression of the posterior cerebral artery can cause ischaemia leading to homonymous hemianopia (although this is usually first detected on CT scanning rather than clinically). Occasionally the opposite cerebral peduncle is compressed against the contralateral tentorial edge causing ipsilateral weakness, and thus producing a *false localizing sign*. The indentation of the opposite peduncle can be seen macroscopically at autopsy and is called *Kernohan's notch*.

Post-traumatic central tentorial herniation often follows untreated lateral tentorial herniation or is the result of massive cerebral swelling. As a result, the patient is usually already unconscious and the upward gaze palsy due to pressure on the tectum is not assessable. The pupils may initially be small (pontine pupils) before becoming fixed and mid-sized. Traction on the infundibulum can produce diabetes insipidus.

Tonsillar herniation (*coning*) in the context of head injury is usually a progression of central tentorial herniation. Displacement of the cerebellar tonsils through the foramen magnum compresses the medulla and rapidly leads to respiratory arrest.

The degree of urgency in managing a patient with clinical signs of brain herniation cannot be overstated. The patient has an ischaemic brainstem and every minute counts until this situation is reversed.

Vascular injuries

The most important factor in assessing for traumatic vascular lesions is a high index of suspicion, as head-injured patients obviously have a number of other reasons for their altered clinical state. The hallmark finding is a delayed onset of neurological dysfunction. The delay is often hours to days after the injury, and after onset the abnormalities may fluctuate. The dysfunction is due to cerebral ischaemia and its specific effects reflect the vessel involved. Carotid lesions will exhibit anterior cerebral and middle cerebral territory symptoms and signs, including hemiparesis, hemisensory loss, and dysphasia (Stahmer *et al.* 1997). Vertebral lesions exhibit cerebellar and brainstem abnormalities in varying degrees, including vertigo, ataxia, nystagmus, dysathria, and cranial nerve palsies.

A patient who is sufficiently alert may also complain of unilateral neck pain or headache, and usually there are no external signs of trauma in these regions.

Carotid lesions may be associated with an incomplete Horner's syndrome (meiosis and partial ptosis) due to involvement of the sympathetic fibres of the internal carotid artery plexus (Stahmer *et al.* 1997). An audible carotid bruit may also be detected on the affected side.

A patient who has developed a traumatic arteriovenous fistula usually complains of an audible whooshing noise, which is synchronous with the pulse and most noticeable when resting in bed at night. An audible bruit may be evident on auscultation of the scalp. An orbital bruit is usually indicative of a carotid-cavernous fistula. Depending on the extent of haemodynamic changes in the venous system, these can progress to the development of chemosis, pulsatile exophthalmos, ophthalmoplegia and even visual loss.

Investigations

Plain radiographs

The skull radiograph has largely become redundant in the investigation of head trauma, having been supplanted by CT scanning. Plain skull radiographs are performed to detect skull fractures, but can be difficult to interpret because of the confusing vascular grooves and suture lines that are sometimes present.

In isolation, a non-depressed fracture rarely requires treatment, so the rationale for detecting the presence of a fracture is to determine if the patient has an increased risk of underlying intracranial pathology, which may lead to subsequent deterioration in their condition. The yield of skull radiographs in this regard is very low. A review of reported series encompassing >22 000 patients with head injury undergoing plain skull radiographs showed 3% had fractures. Of these, 91% had no intracranial pathology (Masters *et al.* 1987).

Even if a fracture is detected on skull radiograph, its predictive value of the patient having a haematoma or deteriorating is no better than careful neurological examination (Feuerman *et al.* 1988). Thus clinical grounds alone are sufficient to determine which patients warrant discharge, observation, or CT scanning (see below) and skull radiographs are therefore not usually indicated.

CT scanning

A non-contrast CT scan has become the primary investigation of the head-injured patient. The widespread availability of this technology has significantly improved the outcome of patients with intracranial pathology (Servadei *et al.* 1988). The images can also be sent via teleradiology from rural hospitals for remote neurosurgical consultation.

CT has many advantages: it is a non-invasive procedure, it can be performed rapidly (especially on the latest machines), it is able to localize acute intracranial haematomas accurately, it can show the presence of anatomic shift and hydrocephalus, it can adequately assess skull and facial fractures, it can detect small amounts of pneumencephaly, and it can localize metal foreign bodies (Zee *et al.* 1996).

Skull fractures and suture diastases are detected on specific bone windows (Fig. 5.5a). Although linear fractures that run horizontally and depressed fractures at the vertex may be difficult to detect on axial slices, they should be apparent on the scout view. Coronal reconstructions can be produced if doubt still exists. Fractures that involve air sinuses or the mastoid air cells will usually exhibit fluid levels. Pneumencephaly is easily distinguishable as sharply defined areas of 'black' within the intracranial compartment (Fig. 5.5b).

(a)

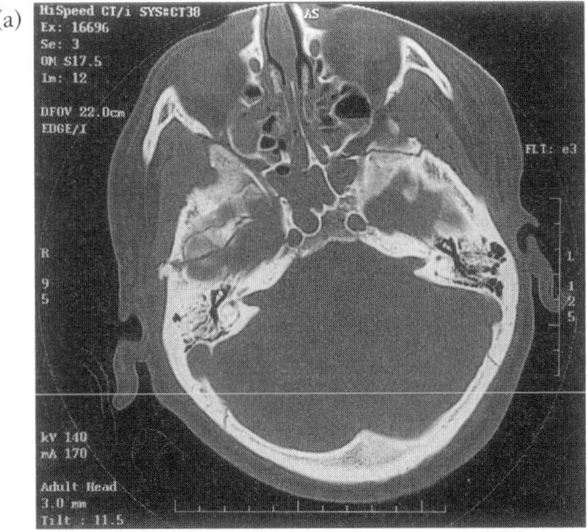

(b)

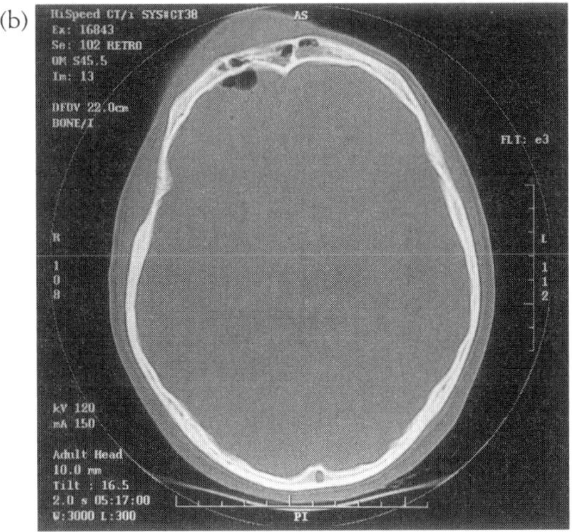

Figure 5.5 (a) Skull fractures and suture diastases are detected on specific bone windows. (b) Pneumencephaly is easily distinguishable as sharply defined areas of 'black' within the intracranial compartment.

Focal extra-axial and intra-axial lesions are detected on the soft tissue windows. Extradural haematomas appear as biconvex areas of hyperdensity adjacent to the skull, often closely associated with a fracture (Fig. 5.6). They usually do not cross suture lines. The presence of hypodense regions within a

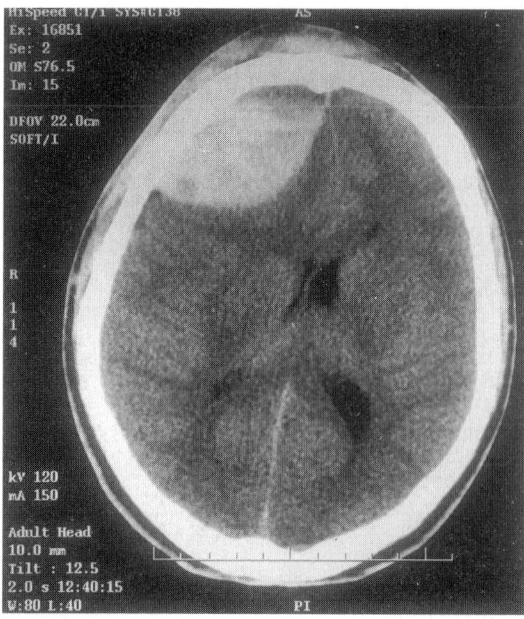

Figure 5.6 Extradural haematomas appear as a biconvex areas of hyperdensity adjacent to the skull, often closely associated with a fracture.

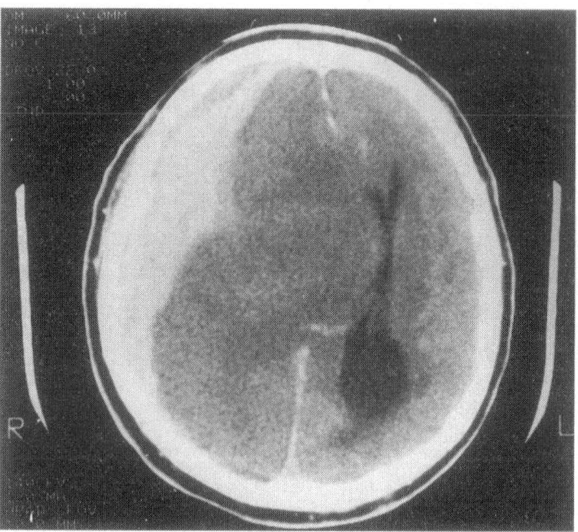

Figure 5.7 Acute subdural haematomas classically appear as a crescent-shaped hyperdensity which follows the convexity of the cortical surface.

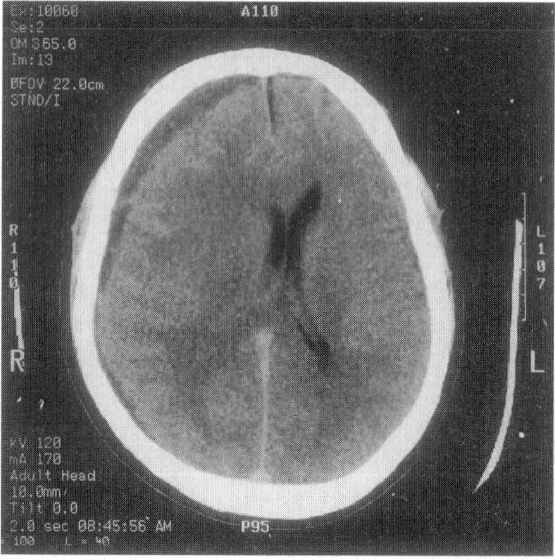

Figure 5.8 Chronic subdurals appear hypodense.

hyperdense extradural collection is said to represent active bleeding (Greenburg *et al.* 1985). An ASDH classically appears as a crescentic shaped hyperdensity which follows the convexity of the cortical surface (Fig. 5.7). They are often associated with underlying brain injury and thus the degree of mass effect and midline shift is often greater than that expected due to the haematoma alone (Zee and Go 1998). Subacute subdural haematomas often appear isodense with the brain parenchyma and may be difficult to detect on plain CT. Chronic subdural haematomas appear hypodense (Fig. 5.8). Occasionally lamination of the haematoma is evident if an acute bleed has occurred into a chronic subdural haematoma. The membrane of a chronic subdural haematoma may eventually show calcification.

Subdural hygromas have a similar appearance to chronic subdural haematomas, although they may appear darker. MRI can be used to better differentiate between these entities.

Traumatic subarachnoid haemorrhage is a common finding on CT following head injury. It appears as a hyperdensity in the subarachnoid spaces (fissures, sulci, or basal cisterns) in varying amounts (Fig. 5.9).

Cerebral contusions maybe haemorrhagic or non-haemorrhagic and usually occur on the surface or within the brain parenchyma. They are frequently located adjacent to areas where the inner surface of the

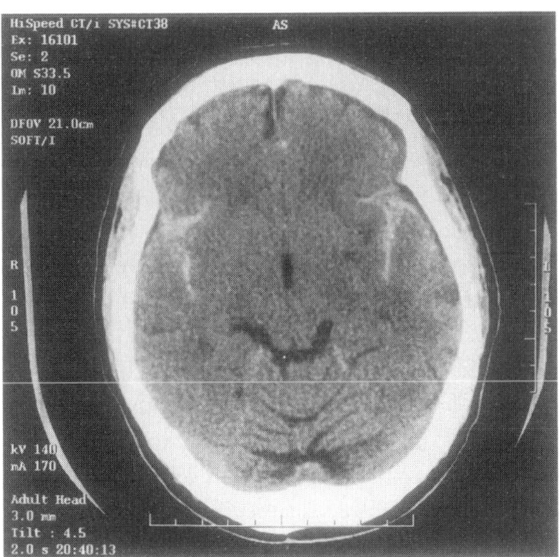

Figure 5.9 Traumatic subarachnoid haemorrhage is a common finding on CT after head injury. It appears as a hyperdensity in the subarachnoid spaces.

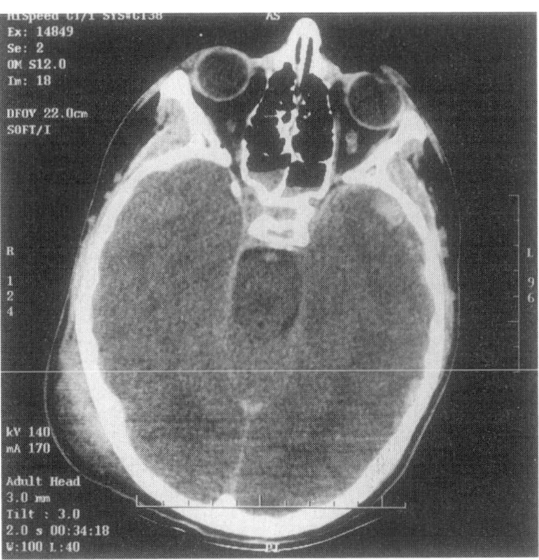

Figure 5.10 Haemorrhagic contusions have an associated hyperdense lesion within them.

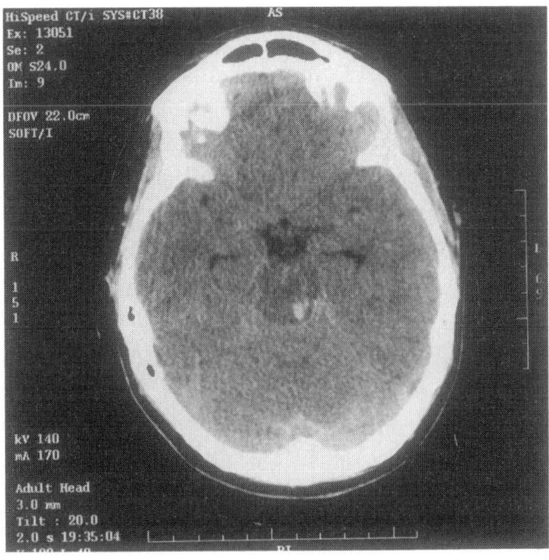

Figure 5.11 In more severe degrees of diffuse axonal injury, hyperdense lesions may be detected in the corpus callosum and rostral part of the dorsolateral pons.

skull is irregular, for example the floor of the anterior cranial fossa and the sphenoid ridge. Non-haemorrhagic contusions appear as circumscribed areas of hypodensity on CT, with a variable degree of local mass effect. Haemorrhagic contusions have an associated hyperdense lesion within them (Fig. 5.10).

Intraventricular haemorrhage appears as a hyperdensity within the ventricular system. Usually a small intraventricular haemorrhage will settle in the occipital horns while the patient lies supine on the CT table. Large amounts of intraventricular clot can obstruct the CSF pathways and produce hydrocephalus.

Diffuse axonal injury is not usually evident on CT. There may be multiple small focal hypodense lesions visible in the white matter, or small hyperdense petechial haemorrhages. In more severe degrees of diffuse axonal injury, hyperdense lesions may be detected in the corpus callosum and rostral part of the dorsolateral pons (Fig. 5.11).

Generalized cerebral swelling maybe indicated by widespread loss of definition of the subarachnoid and ventricular spaces. Midline shift is easily measurable on CT and herniation can also be readily detected. Vascular compression maybe evident as loss of grey/white differentiation in vascular territories. Occasionally an area of hypodensity in a large vessel such as the basilar artery may alert the viewer to the presence of a dissection and subsequent thrombosis.

Indications for emergency burrholes

Patients with a decreased level of consciousness and signs of brainstem dysfunction generally have a poor prognosis, but some can make good recoveries if an extra-axial haematoma is found and evacuated rapidly via craniotomy. Exploratory burrholes are a sensitive method for detecting extra-axial haematomas with negligible morbidity (Andrews *et al.* 1986). This technique has become largely redundant with the advent of CT scanning, although there remain some situations in which they are indicated, if a delay in obtaining a CT on a patient with suspected herniation is anticipated. These indications include the need to perform an urgent laparotomy on a hypotensive multiple trauma patient (Thomason *et al.* 1993), injuries in remote geographical locations, and delayed availability of a scanning room or staff.

The side for initial exploration is determined by (1) the side of pupillary dilatation, (2) if both pupils are dilated, the side that first dilated, (3) the side with external signs of injury, (4) the left side (dominant hemisphere in most people) (Greenberg 1997). The sequence for placing burrholes is ipsilateral temporal, contralateral temporal, ipsilateral frontal and parietal, contralateral frontal and parietal, ipsilateral and contralateral posterior fossa. Figure 5.12 shows the suggested sites for burrholes and a method for converting the scalp incisions into a 'trauma flap' for subsequent craniotomy.

Magnetic resonance imaging

MRI is of limited use in the initial assessment of acute head injury. The reasons for this include limited availability on an urgent basis, prolonged acquisition times for the images, and limited ability to monitor patients while in the scanner because of equipment cannot function properly in the strong magnetic field. The ability of MRI to delineate bony injury is poor, and in addition, its ability to detect acute haemorrhage for the first 3 days is markedly less than that of CT (Snow *et al.* 1986).

After 3 days, however, the superior anatomical and pathological resolution and multiplanar ability of MRI do afford it some utility. It is better at detecting the presence of small extra-axial collections and non-haemorrhagic contusions than CT. Lesions in the posterior fossa which may be obscured by bone artefact on CT are often clearly evident on MRI. Re-haemorrhage into chronic subdural collections is more apparent, and differentiation of chronic haematomas from hygromas is also superior with MRI.

MRI and magnetic resonance angiography (MRA) are also useful in detecting vascular injuries involving extracranial and intracranial vessels. MRI is particularly sensitive in detecting the mural haematomas associated with dissections (Figure 5.13).

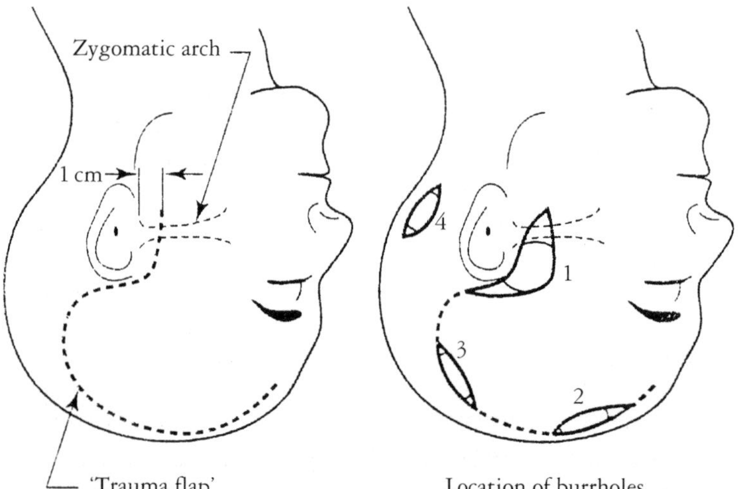

Figure 5.12 Suggested sites for burrholes and a method for conversion of the scalp incisions into a 'trauma flap' for subsequent craniotomy. (Reproduced from Greenberg *et al.* (1997) with permission.

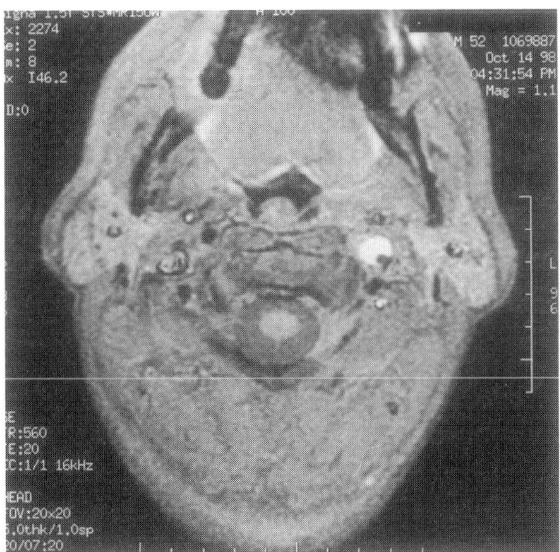

Figure 5.13 MRI is particularly sensitive in detecting the mural haematomas associated with dissections.

Late follow-up MRI is also used to confirm the presence and extent of structural damage resulting from head injury, as an aid to prognostication.

Assessment of cerebral perfusion

Although MRI and MRA are increasingly being used to screen for vascular lesions after head injury, cerebral angiography remains the gold standard for defining the nature and extent of these lesions, and their effect on cerebral perfusion. A dissection of the carotid or vertebral artery usually appears as a tapering of the intravascular dye column to either occlusion or a narrowed lumen extending a variable distance, the *string sign* (Fig. 5.14). Dissection of the internal carotid artery usually begins around 2 cm above the bifurcation, and vertebral injuries usually involve the distal extracranial segment of the vessel (Stahmer *et al.* 1997). An intimal flap, double lumen, thrombus, or distal embolic occlusion may also be apparent. Extracranial and intracranial traumatic aneurysm formation is also well defined by cerebral angiography. Angiographic features that help distinguish traumatic from congenital (berry) type aneurysms include location away from branch points, irregular contour of the aneurysm, absence of a well-defined neck, delayed filling and emptying, and more peripheral cortical locations (Giannotta and Gruen 1992).

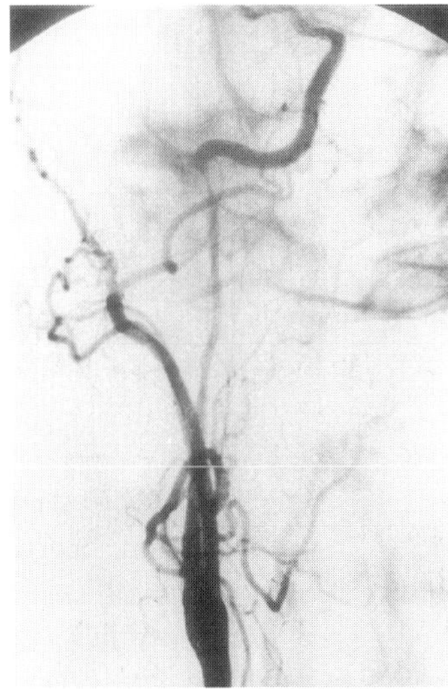

Figure 5.14 A dissection of the carotid or vertebral artery usually appears as a tapering of the intravascular dye column to either occlusion or a narrowed lumen extending a variable distance, the 'string sign'.

Carotid-cavernous and other traumatic arteriovenous fistulas are also best defined by cerebral angiography, and it is important that six-vessel angiography is performed to identify abnormal communications involving external carotid artery branches. The appearance of early venous drainage is the hallmark of these lesions.

Cerebral vasospasm following traumatic subarachnoid haemorrhage is also detected by angiography, with reported incidences ranging from 2% to 41% (Giannotta and Gruen 1992).

Transcranial doppler ultrasonography (TCD) is a commonly used non-invasive technique to monitor severely head-injured patients. Through serial measurement of extracranial and intracranial flow velocities in the internal carotid and middle cerebral arteries, conditions such as vasospasm, hyperaemia, hypoperfusion, impaired autoregulation and vascular (carbon dioxide) reactivity can be detected (Steiger *et al.* 1994).

Single-photon emission computed tomography (SPECT) scanning is a less commonly utilized method of evaluating cerebral perfusion and its regional variation.

Management

After rapid assessment and the commencement of resuscitative measures as required, ongoing management of the head-injured patient is determined by the severity of the injury. Patients are triaged according to their GCS score—mild (GCS 13–15), moderate (GCS 9–12), or severe (GCS 3–8)—and varying management algorithms are employed.

The patient, however, 'must be evaluated and managed on an individual basis and algorithms should be used to guide rather than to dictate management' (Fuerman *et al.* 1988). Multiple trauma patients may require further investigation, anaesthesia, and surgery for injuries to other systems, and this will influence the management paradigm. The confounding effects of alcohol intoxication must also be given due consideration and make the physician err on the side of caution (Gurney *et al.* 1992). Increasing usage of antiplatelet and anticoagulant medication, particularly in older patients, should also be taken into account. The availability and proximity of resources will also profoundly affect what can be achieved.

It is important to note that the patient's condition can deteriorate very quickly and therefore close neurological observation, and early response to clinical change, are paramount.

Mild closed head injury

The patient should be admitted to the emergency department and undergo hourly neurological observations for a minimum of 4 hours. They should remain 'nil by mouth' in case surgical intervention is required. CT scanning of the head should be undertaken if any of the indications listed in Table 5.8 are present. This approach will not identify all patients who would have abnormalities on CT, but should detect those with clinically significant abnormalities on CT and who may require neurosurgical intervention (Borzuk 1997, Miller *et al.* 1997). Skull radiographs may be obtained if the hospital does not have a CT scanner on site. If, however, the patient fulfils any of the indications for a CT of the head then they should be transferred to a suitable institution as soon as possible. A cervical spine radiograph series should be obtained if cervical pain or tenderness is present, or if confusion or intoxication obscures their evaluation. Simple analgesia can be tried (with a sip of water), but intramuscular or intravenous opiates may be required if the patient is vomiting or headache remains severe. Appropriate use of opiates will not affect the level of consciousness, but they should not be used (or needed) if the patient is intoxicated unless other major injuries, for example fractures, are causing pain. Antiemetics should be given if the patient is nauseated. Scalp lacerations must be explored, cleaned and sutured if present. Tetanus toxoid or immunoglobulin should be administered as indicated.

Table 5.8 Indications for CT Scan after Mild Head Injury.
Loss of consciousness > 5 minutes
Post-traumatic amnesia > 5 minutes
Deterioration in GCS
Persistent drowsness
Progressive or severe headache
Persistent nausea or vomiting
Focal neurological deficits
Suspected skull fracture
CSF leaf
Post-traumatic seizure
Multiple trauma (possibility of anaesthesia)
Late or second presentation to hospital

If after 4 hours observation the patient is normal or has only minimal symptoms (resolving headache, nausea, or dizziness), they may be considered for discharge. This should be into the care of a reliable companion who will stay with them and has been educated about the indications for returning the patient to hospital. Provision of a 'head injury card' with these indications listed is also useful. The patient should also be advised to attend a local general practitioner within 48 hours, or present to the next neurosurgical clinic, for a further review.

If, however, the patient meets any of the criteria listed in Table 5.9 they should be admitted for continued observation.

Table 5.9 Criteria for Admission following Mild Head Injury

Any of the following
Abnormal CT head
Inadequate care at home
Deterioration in GCS
Progressive headache
Persistent drowsiness
Persistent nausea and vomiting
Focal neurological deficits
Skull fracture
CSF leak
Post-traumatic seizure
Multiple trauma

Moderate closed head injury

After the history, primary survey, resuscitation, and secondary survey the management of this group of patients is similar to that described above, except that all patients undergo urgent CT scanning and neurosurgical consultation and are admitted for ongoing neurological observation. Intubation of restless or combative patients should be seriously considered to enable safe and artefact-free scanning.

- If the scan is normal, the patient is treated expectantly with appropriate supportive measures. Most will improve within hours. If their GCS has not improved to 14–15 within 12 hours, a further scan is indicated (Stein and Ross 1992).
- If the scan is abnormal and a fracture or intracranial lesion requires surgical intervention (see below), the patient should be prepared for theatre. Postoperatively they will be transferred to the neurosurgical intensive care unit.
- If the scan is abnormal, it should be repeated in 12–24 hours or sooner if neurological deterioration occurs.

Consideration should also be given to insertion of an ICP monitor, especially if the patient will require prolonged anaesthesia or ventilation for chest injuries, their neurological status worsens, or serial CT examinations show progression of intracranial lesions (Fearnside and McDougall 1998).

As the patient improves, the frequency of neurological observations can be decreased. All patients should have a repeat CT scan 48–72 hours after trauma to exclude the development of delayed intracranial pathology (Stein *et al.* 1993). Patients with late deteriorations in their GCS should be thoroughly assessed for medical causes (sepsis, hypoxia, electrolyte disturbances, hypoglycaemia, drug toxicity, metabolic disturbances) as well as intracranial causes (vascular injury, haematomas, swelling, seizures, hydrocephalus, meningitis/cerebral abscess).

Severe closed head injury

After a brief history, the importance of the primary survey (especially the ABC) and resuscitation cannot be overemphasized in this group of patients. All patients with a GCS of 8 or less require intubation for airway protection and precise control of oxygenation and ventilation. The blood pressure must be restored as rapidly as possible, preferably to a MAP >90 mmHg, with volume replacement and pressors if necessary (Randell and Chesnut 1997). The secondary survey is then quickly performed. Once initial assessment is complete, adequate sedation should be maintained during transfers and until the patient is stabilized in intensive care. Muscle relaxants may also be required.

If the patient has signs of raised ICP (progressive neurological deterioration unexplained by extracranial causes, or transtentorial herniation signified by a blown pupil or motor posturing) then a rapid bolus of intravenous mannitol should be given (1 g/kg). It should not be given as a prophylactic measure because of the possibly deleterious effect of the osmotic diuresis on volume replacement. Hyperventilation should also be avoided as prophylaxis, and is only considered appropriate as a final effort when other measures have failed to reverse the clinical signs of intracranial hypertension. In this circumstance a P_aCO_2 range of 30–35 mmHg should be adhered to (Randell and Chesnut 1997).

An urgent CT scan should then be obtained. If the patient has signs of intracranial hypertension and is haemodynamically stable, this should take priority over all other investigations including deep peritoneal lavage. If there will be a delay in obtaining the CT, consideration of urgent cranial exploration is warranted. If the patient has signs of intracranial hypertension and is haemodynamically unstable such that emergency procedures on other systems are required, simultaneous or immediately consecutive cranial exploration for an intracranial lesion should be performed. It is important to remember, however, that fluctuating pupillary signs can occur due to intermittent brainstem hypoperfusion during attempts to resuscitate patients with uncontrolled blood loss.

If the scan reveals an intracranial lesion requiring immediate surgery, the patient should be transferred to the operating theatre. If surgery is not required, the patient is transferred to the intensive care unit.

For prevention of early seizures, the patient is usually loaded with an intravenous anticonvulsant.

All patients with severe head injuries should have an ICP monitor inserted as early as possible, usually immediately after the scan unless an urgent craniotomy is required first. If surgery for other injuries is necessary, a monitor can be inserted simultaneously. Several methods of ICP monitoring are available, including placement of a pressure transducer in communication with the subdural, intraparenchymal, or intraventricular compartment. Insertion of an external ventricular catheter has the added benefit of enabling drainage of CSF to be used as a therapeutic option in the treatment of intracranial hypertension.

Ongoing management in intensive care and the treatment of specific pathologies associated with head injury are discussed below.

Scalp lesions and skull fractures

Scalp lesions

Injuries to the scalp as a result of head trauma vary enormously in severity: from mild abrasions, localized haematomas, and simple lacerations to stellate lacerations, degloving injuries, or avulsion of scalp tissue. Because of the rich vascular supply of the scalp, lacerations tend to bleed profusely and large amounts of blood can become congealed among the hair, often obscuring the position and extent of tissue damage. Careful inspection and palpation of the entire scalp is therefore required, and this may necessitate log-rolling the patient to access the occipital region if the cervical spine has not yet been 'cleared'. If a scalp laceration or degloving injury is present this should be covered with a sterile-saline soaked pad held in position with a crepe bandage, until time is available for definitive repair. Infrequently, persistent arterial bleeding may demand the application of an artery forceps or judiciously placed suture before this, although most scalp haemorrhage is controllable with a compression bandage.

Most scalp lacerations can be sutured in the emergency department. Shaving of the hair is not usually required. The area should be liberally washed with an antiseptic solution and the wound edges infiltrated with local anaesthetic. The laceration may be explored with a sterile-gloved finger for evidence of a fracture or foreign material. Large arterial vessels may require ligation. Copious irrigation of the wound with antiseptic solution, followed by sterile saline, via a syringe should then be performed. Debridement of apparently non-viable tissue should be undertaken with extreme caution, as the rich vascularity of the scalp rescues much of this tissue and it is easy to end up with a defect that will require more extensive surgery to repair. The scalp can be sutured in a single 'through and through' layer using a monofilament suture material such as nylon. Interrupted sutures are preferred to continuous ones, because of the lesser risk of skin-edge necrosis. If skin staples are to be used, an absorbable suture such as polyglycolic acid should be used first to approximate the galea aponeurotica. Sutures can be removed after 7 days.

If there is significant contamination of the wound, extensive degloving, tissue loss preventing simple primary closure, or cosmetically significant wounds (such as gravel or tyre rubber 'tattooing'), the neurosurgical or plastic surgery team should be consulted regarding management. Significant scalp injuries may require skin grafting, transposition flaps, pedicle flaps, or re-implantation to repair defects.

Infrequently, scalp haematomas in elderly patients can exhibit sufficient pressure to cause ischaemia of the overlying scalp. These haematomas require evacuation through a small incision which is then sutured and a compression bandage applied. It should be noted that the pinna of the ear can be made ischaemic by head bandages being too tight. Cotton padding can be positioned behind the pinna before application of the bandage to prevent this.

Closed skull fractures

Undisplaced fractures of the skull convexity include linear fractures, suture diastases (separation of a suture line), and comminuted (stellate) fractures. If the overlying scalp is intact, these fractures require no operative management. They do, however, indicate the need for investigation for underlying intracranial pathology. An asymptomatic patient with a linear fracture who has an otherwise normal CT scan can be discharged into the care of a reliable companion.

Compound skull fractures

Linear skull fractures associated with a small scalp laceration usually require only careful cleaning and closure of the wound as described above. Open comminuted fractures with free bone fragments should be explored and debrided in the operating theatre. Removal of contaminated bone fragments, and often dural repair, may be required.

Depressed skull fractures

Depressed skull fractures are only considered significant if the outer table of the depressed portion is below the level of the inner table of the normal skull. This is usually evident on axial bone window CT scans, although occasionally coronal reconstructions of the CT data may be necessary to adequately elucidate the extent of bone depression. Indications for surgical exploration and elevation of a closed depressed fracture are cosmetic deformity (particularly involving the forehead or orbital rim), underlying brain or dural injury, underlying haematoma with mass effect, underlying air sinus fracture, or compression of an underlying venous sinus. If a venous sinus is involved, surgery can be fraught with difficulty if the sinus has been lacerated by a bone fragment.

Open depressed fractures should always be urgently explored and debrided, owing to the risk of infection. Hair and debris can become wedged between the bone fragments, which should be completely removed. If the dura has been breached, bone and debris should also be cleared from the underlying brain and a watertight dural repair performed. The bone is usually discarded, and a delayed cranioplasty will be necessary.

Traumatic leak of cerebrospinal fluid

In isolation, base of skull fractures do not require any intervention. It is the associated injuries to traversing nerves, vessels, and adjacent air sinuses that may warrant attention. If the latter are associated with a dural laceration, a fistula between the subarachnoid space and air sinuses, mastoid air cells, or middle ear may be formed and a traumatic CSF leak results. Unless sealed, this provides a route for intracranial infection. The presence of a dural laceration is often heralded by evidence of pneumocephaly on the CT scan. In one reported series of head injuries, 7% had base of skull fractures, 2% developed CSF leaks, and 0.5% contracted meningitis. The majority of leaks were apparent within 48 hours, most of the others occurred within 3 months, but a few were delayed months to years before their onset (Lewin 1966).

CSF otorrhea occurs with fractures of the temporal bone, either through the mastoid air cells and an external auditory canal laceration or through the middle ear and perforation of the tympanic membrane. The vast majority of these leaks settle in a few days without the need for surgical intervention. The patient should be admitted and an earpad applied to the affected side to monitor the volume of leakage. Prophylactic antibiotics should not used, because of the risk of superinfection. The external auditory canal should only be cleaned by an ear, nose, and throat surgeon and follow-up auditory and vestibular testing should be arranged for 6 weeks after discharge from hospital.

CSF rhinorrhea results from base of skull fractures entering the paranasal air sinuses or the middle ear with passage of CSF through the eustachian tube. This form of traumatic CSF leak is less likely to heal of its own accord. The patient should be admitted and a nasal bolster applied to monitor the volume of leakage. Again, prophylactic antibiotics should not used because of the risk of superinfection. A lumbar drain may be inserted to divert CSF at a rate of 5–10 mL/hour, although this is controversial as it may promote entry of bacteria through the fistula and increase the risk of infection. Non-surgical management is usually attempted for 1–2 weeks, but if the leak persists the exact location of the fistula is usually sought with CT cisternography or radioisotopic studies, and surgical repair undertaken. Depending on the site of the leak, a transsphenoidal or intracranial approach may be utilized to repair the dural defect.

Cranial nerve lesions

- Base of skull fractures involving the cribriform plate often cause anosmia due to shearing of the traversing *olfactory fibres*. Management is expectant, with a poor prognosis for improvement. The patient will also complain of a reduction in the taste of food.
- The *optic nerves* can be damaged by fractures involving the apex of the orbit and optic canal. Surgical decompression does not improve the recovery rate and therefore management is again expectant, unless deterioration occurs after the initial insult.
- The *abducens nerve* can be injured by clival fractures. Management is expectant.
- The *facial nerve* can be injured in temporal bone fractures (especially with the less common transverse pattern of fracture), leading to a partial or complete lower motor neurone facial palsy. Most lesions recover with time, and expectant management is most commonly employed. The use of steroids and decompressive surgery remain controversial. Facial nerve grafting can be utilized to treat permanent lesions.
- The *vestibulocochlear nerve* can also be damaged by transverse temporal bone fractures. Management is expectant.

Focal intracranial lesions

Extradural haematoma

The classical presentation of head-injured patients with an EDH involves an initial period of loss of consciousness due to the initial impact, followed by a 'lucid interval' before they again lapse into unconsciousness as the haematoma expands. Only a minority of cases actually present this way, however, and the pattern described is certainly not pathognomonic for extradural collections. The patient may remain conscious or unconscious, depending on the severity of any underlying brain injury and the size of the haematoma. EDHs are very uncommon in older patients owing to greater adherence of the dura to the inner table of the skull with increasing age.

The treatment for EDH is urgent craniotomy, evacuation of the blood clot, and control of the source of haemorrhage (usually a branch of the middle meningeal artery or vein, less commonly a dural venous sinus). Burrholes are insufficient for this purpose. In remote areas or when urgent burrhole exploration is undertaken, the hole in the skull can be enlarged with bone nibblers to enable some decompression of the solid clot before transfer for definitive neurosurgical care. Haematomas that are <5 mm in thickness may be managed non-operatively, but given their propensity to enlarge in a delayed fashion, close observation in a neurosurgical unit and serial CT scanning is advisable.

Acute subdural haematoma

ASDH are more common in older patients because cerebral atrophy increases the risk of tearing cortical bridging veins, and are the most common haematoma associated with falls. There is also a greater likelihood of significant underlying brain injury associated with ASDH, which tends to obscure the relative contribution of the haematoma to the patient's clinical condition, as well as adversely affect outcome.

Subdural haematomas that are 5 mm or less in thickness can usually be managed without surgical evacuation, but again, close observation in a neurosurgical unit and serial CT scanning to ensure resolution and not expansion is required. The management of haematomas >5 mm in thickness depends on the clinical state of the patient. A small ASDH in a patient with no neurological deficit may be followed with serial CT scans until it liquefies, and then drained via a burrhole. However, small haematomas can be deceptively voluminous if spread out widely over the convexity. In patients with severe underlying brain injury even small-volume clots can add significantly to raised ICP problems and should be evacuated via urgent craniotomy. Generally all ASDH >10 mm in thickness or associated with >5 mm of midline shift should be urgently evacuated via a craniotomy and the source of bleeding controlled. An ICP monitor should also be inserted during the procedure, as many patients will have elevations in ICP following surgery.

Chronic subdural haematoma

Chronic subdural haematomas (CSDH) tend to occur in older patients and are often the result of very minor head trauma weeks to months before presentation. Symptoms vary from headaches or confusion to hemiparesis.

Treatment is drainage via burrhole with or without placement of a subdural drain. Craniotomy and removal of the haematoma membranes is unnecessary and adds to the morbidity in a generally elderly patient population.

Subdural hygromas are traumatic subdural collections of CSF due to laceration of the arachnoid. Symptomatic lesions are treated with burrhole drainage.

Intracerebral haematoma

The management of traumatic intracerebral haematomas is guided by the size of the haematoma and the clinical condition of the patient. Patients with small haematomas may be followed with close neurological observation and serial CT scanning. Haematomas causing significant mass effect and midline shift or contributing to elevations in ICP should be evacuated via craniotomy. This also applies to large cerebral contusions.

Raised intracranial pressure

The indications for insertion of an intracranial monitoring device in head-injured patients have been discussed above. The ICP is considered elevated if the patient's pressure is consistently >20 mmHg, and therapeutic measures should be instituted to try and prevent secondary brain injury from reduced cerebral perfusion pressure. These therapeutic measures tend to be categorized as general measures, first line treatments, and second line treatments.

General measures for the maintenance of a normal ICP after head trauma obviously include surgical evacuation of any extra- or intra-axial haematomas with significant mass effect. The greater the elevation in a patient's ICP due to generalized cerebral swelling, the smaller a haematoma has to be to contribute significantly to reducing cerebral compliance. Elevation of the head of the bed by 15–30° is recommended to displace CSF into the thecal sac and facilitate cerebral venous outflow. This manoeuvre is controversial, however, owing to the possibility of a paradoxical increase in ICP in the presence of decreased cerebral compliance (Durward *et al.* 1983). On balance, it appears useful but the effect on ICP should be carefully observed in each patient. It is important to avoid compression of venous outflow through the neck by ensuring that tracheotomy tapes and cervical collars are not too tight and that the neck remains in reasonably neutral alignment.

Ventilation should be controlled to maintain a normocapnic range of 35–40 mmHg. It should be remembered that positive airway pressure from mechanical ventilation is transmitted to the intracranial cavity through the mediastinal structures and therefore can influence ICP, but generally a positive end expiratory pressure (PEEP) of 5–15 cm H_2O is tolerable (Frank 1993). A normotensive blood pressure should be maintained. Hypotension will reduce the CPP, which will cause reflex vasodilation, increased CBF, increased cerebral blood volume, and increased ICP if autoregulation remains intact, or will cause reduced CBF and ischaemia if autoregulation has been lost. Hypertension can exacerbate cerebral oedema if autoregulation is impaired or the blood–brain barrier is disrupted in the injured brain. The patient should also be kept normothermic, as fever has a detrimental effect on ICP by increasing cerebral blood flow and cerebral blood volume.

Adequate sedation is important for patients on ventilators to prevent coughing and 'fighting the ventilator' by breathing against its breaths, both of which increase intrathoracic pressure and reduce cerebral venous outflow. Short-acting benzodiazepines such as midazolam are often used for this purpose. Pain is also an important factor in stimulating CBF, CBV, and ICP. Multiple injuries, surgical sites, and airway irritation from the endotracheal tube will all contribute to the patient's discomfort and adequate analgesia is therefore also very important. Narcotics such as morphine are commonly used.

First line treatments of raised ICP include heavy sedation to reduce cerebral metabolism and therefore reduce required CBF and CBV. Hypotension is a potential complication with increased sedation. Drainage of CSF via an external ventricular drain is an effective way of reducing intracranial volume and improving compliance. Drainage should be intermittent rather than continuous, to enable close monitoring of sudden rises in ICP. Generally, opening the drain for 5 minutes up to 4 times per hour is sufficient. Intermittent boluses of an osmotic diuretic such as mannitol can be utilized to draw water from the interstitial space into the intravascular space. Mannitol is also believed to assist oxygen delivery by improving the rheological characteristics of the blood. A typical regimen is 100 mL of 20% mannitol solution repeated 6 hourly. Careful attention must be paid to electrolyte and fluid balance during this treatment and the therapy is discontinued when the serum osmolality is above 310 mosmol/L. Loop diuretics are also useful as an adjuvant to osmotic therapy, particularly in controlling the associated increase in intravascular volume. Frusemide (furosemide) is generally used. Non-depolarizing neuromuscular paralysing agents can be used to facilitate mechanical ventilation by improving chest wall compliance and lowering mean airway pressures. Again these tend to be used intermittently, to avoid the complications of prolonged neuromuscular paralysis (Frank 1993).

Second line treatments are utilized when the above measures fail to consistently maintain an ICP of $<$20 mmHg. Precipitous rises in ICP, or an ICP that is difficult to control, should be investigated with further CT scanning to exclude a surgically correctable lesion. Second line treatments include barbiturate coma. High-dose barbiturates lower the ICP by reducing the cerebral metabolic rate and therefore the CBF. The complications can be significant, however, particularly hypotension and increased susceptibility to infection. Generally, following a loading dose, an infusion of barbiturate such as thiopentone or pentobarbital is titrated to 'burst suppression', which involves continuous EEG monitoring to confirm suppression of cerebral electrical activity.

Hypothermia is also an effective means of reducing cerebral metabolism and ICP (Metz *et al.* 1996). Patients are usually cooled to a core temperature of 34–36°C via a 'cooling blanket', but it is important they are sufficiently sedated.

An increasingly utilized treatment for raised ICP is CPP management (Rosner *et al.* 1995). This involves maintaining the MAP above the threshold required to ensure the CPP is $>$70 mmHg (CPP = MAP $-$ ICP) with careful intravascular volume control and vasopressors as necessary.

Hyperventilation to reduce the P_aCO_2 to a range of 25–35 mmHg is now considered a final effort to control ICP, and can only be utilized for short periods before physiological tolerance develops.

Other methods used for control of severe intracranial hypertension include decompressive craniectomy with or without partial lobectomy. Indomethacin has also been shown to be an effective agent in reducing ICP (Harrigan *et al.* 1997), and can be administered rectally. Lignocaine (lidocaine) boluses can also be used to control blood pressure and ICP surges during procedures in the intensive care unit which may cause airway irritation.

Seizures

Seizures within the first 48 hours of a head injury are common and do not necessarily foreshadow the occurrence of later seizures. Approximately 2% of people suffering head injury will go on to develop post-traumatic epilepsy. In those surviving a severe head injury, the risk of epilepsy is 10–15% (Hauser 1990). Seizures in the early period following head injury are believed to contribute to secondary brain damage by increasing metabolic demands, raising the ICP, and excess release of neurotransmitters (Schierhout and Roberts 1998).

It appears that the presence of extravasated blood in the brain parenchyma contributes to the pathogenesis of post-traumatic epilepsy. The iron in haemoglobin is a potent epileptogenic agent, and the ability of the brain's chelating agents to neutralize its effect may be overcome if enough blood is present after trauma.

To try to prevent the development of post-traumatic epilepsy, and reduce the negative impact of early seizures, prophylactic anticonvulsants have been widely used in treating head-injured patients. However, clinical trials have shown that although anticonvulsant usage reduces the incidence of seizures in the first week after injury by 73%, there is no reduction in the incidence of late seizures (Temkin *et al.* 1990). It is also unclear whether preventing early seizures actually improves outcome (Schierhout and Roberts 1998).

At present it therefore appears reasonable to use prophylactic anticonvulsants in cases of severe head injury for the first week after injury and then cease. Phenytoin is most commonly used as it can be administered intravenously. A skin rash occurs in approximately 4% of patients and necessitates a change of anticonvulsant. Monitoring of serum concentrations and liver function tests is required, as well as periodic full blood counts.

Patients who develop late seizure activity (post-traumatic epilepsy) require education about the implications of epilepsy, such as inability to drive until after a prescribed seizure-free period, and risks of swimming alone, climbing ladders, etc.

Traumatic subarachnoid haemorrhage

Traumatic subarachnoid haemorrhage (tSAH) is the most common pathological finding following head injury. In patients with severe head injuries, the incidence of tSAH on CT is up to 39% (Eisenberg *et al.* 1990). The presence of tSAH has also been shown to be independently associated with a significant worsening of prognosis. Patients with severe head injuries and evidence of tSAH have a twofold increase in mortality (Eiseberg 1990), and a twofold increase in unfavourable outcome at 6 months (European Study Group 1994), compared to those patients without tSAH.

There is increasing evidence that the prognostic significance of tSAH is partly related to its association with vasospasm. Other trauma admission CT findings associated with the development of vasospasm include subdural and intraventricular haemorrhage (Martin *et al.* 1995). Vasospasm is one of the many causes of cerebral ischaemia, a major contributor to secondary brain injury. Angiographic studies from the pre-CT era, and more recently, transcranial Doppler studies report the incidence of post-traumatic vasospasm to be 20–40%. The timecourse of vasospasm associated with tSAH is similiar to the vasospasm witnessed after aneurysmal SAH, with an onset around day 2 and peak around days 10–14 after injury.

Head-injured patients without vasospasm appear to be twice as likely to have a favourable outcome as those with vasospasm (Martin *et al.* 1995). This has led to increasing vigilance for post-traumatic vasospasm with serial transcranial Doppler examinations and routine angiography of patients with tSAH. Confirmed vasospasm is treated in a similar manner to that related to aneurysmal SAH. Several trials appear to show an improved outcome using the calcium channel blocker nimodipine prophylactically in head-injured patients with tSAH (Kakarieka 1997a,b).

Vascular lesions

The main hurdle in treating traumatic vascular lesions associated with head injury is recognizing the problem when it occurs. Diagnosis is delayed in most cases. This has been compounded by the advent of CT scanning replacing angiography as the mainstay of head injury investigation.

In cases of thrombosis or dissection of neck or intracranial vessels, the aim of treatment is to prevent completed stroke. The type of therapy utilized depends on the pattern of clinical presentation, the neurological status of the patient and the duration of their deficits. Patients in a stable clinical state are usually treated medically with anticoagulation followed by antiplatelet therapy and follow-up angiography to assess for resolution or progression of the lesion. Patients with a fluctuating or evolving neurological deficit may require mild hypertensive therapy or interventional radiological procedures such as intra-arterial thrombolysis or stenting. Occasionally surgical procedures such as endarterectomy, ligation, vascular reconstruction, or extracranial–intracranial bypass may be warranted.

Traumatic intracranial aneurysms often present with delayed subarachnoid haemorrhage and thus conservative treatment has a high mortality rate. Various endovascular and open surgical techniques can be utilized to repair these lesions.

Carotid-cavernous fistulae require treatment if they cause progressive proptosis, ophthalmoplegia, or visual loss. Usually transarterial or transvenous embolization is successful in closing the arteriovenous communication. Dural arteriovenous fistulae are most frequently asymptomatic, but they can be responsible for progressive headaches, neurological deficits, and SAH and may require endovascular treatment in such circumstances.

Intensive care of head-injured patients

The intensive care unit is where ongoing resuscitation, critical monitoring and maintenance of physiological homeostasis, and recognition and treatment of the sequelae of severe head injury occur. The prime aim is to prevent secondary brain injury and rescue salvageable brain tissue. This role includes optimum ventilation and prevention of chest infections in the unconscious patient. Blood pressure control, maintenance of an adequate intravascular volume and haemoglobin, and prevention of coagulopathies are also vital. Fluid and electrolytes must be carefully monitored, as imbalances can result from the development of SIADH, cerebral salt wasting syndrome and, less commonly, diabetes insipidus after head trauma.

The monitoring of ICP and medical treatment of raised ICP (see above) is also a key task of the intensive care unit. An increasingly used technique is continuous monitoring of $S_{jv}O_2$ in an effort to match cerebral blood flow with cerebral oxygen consumption (Cruz 1998).

Other important facets of the management of head-injured patients include provision of adequate nutrition, prophylaxis against DVT, skin care to prevent pressure areas, and the early management of increasing tone to prevent contractures.

Continuing research into the pathophysiology of brain trauma has shown that primary brain injury is not an immediate, irreversible process, but that the initial event sets in train a neurochemical cascade which eventually causes the 'primary injury'. This window of opportunity has led to increased efforts to find therapies to attenuate or reverse this pathological cascade and thus salvage neuronal tissue. Compounds such as calcium channel blockers, calpain inhibitors, excitatory amino acid antagonists, free radical and lipid peroxidation inhibitors, inflammation cytokine inhibitors, and neurotrophic factors are currently being evaluated (McIntosh *et al.* 1997).

Penetrating head injury

Penetrating head injuries can be further classified as missile and non-missile injuries. Missile injuries include those caused by bullets and shrapnel, and their incidence is increasing in civilian settings. Non-missile injuries can be caused by a variety of implements including knives, screwdrivers, arrows, spears, axes, rocks, and pens.

Missile injuries

The primary injury caused by a missile involves the scalp, skull, and brain. There are two main biomechanical effects that produce damage to the brain tissue.

- First, the passage of the missile causes a direct crush injury that creates a permanent cavity along its pathway through the parenchyma.
- Secondly, a pressure wave caused by the projectile leads to a rapid expansion and contraction of the tissues around the pathway, referred to as temporary cavitation. This results in a stretch injury which may damage tissue and blood vessels distant to the missile's pathway.

Secondary injury follows, including oedema and raised ICP which can exacerbate ischaemic damage. Respiration can also be affected, with variable periods of apnoea occurring immediately after the injury contributing to hypoxic injury. This is believed to be due to distortion of the brainstem at the time of impact. Coagulation disorders are also common, including disseminated intravascular coagulopathy, due to the release of brain tissue thromboplastin.

Late complications of missile injuries include CSF leaks, infection and abscess formation, traumatic aneurysm formation, seizures, and migration of retained bullet fragments.

The initial assessment and resuscitation of the patient with a penetrating head injury due to a gunshot wound is similar to that of the patient with a closed head injury, but with special consideration of the following points. The scalp should be shaved to assist detection of entry and exit wounds and control of bleeding points. Tetanus immunization status should be checked and tetanus toxoid with or without immunoglobulin given as required. Prophylactic antibiotics to cover gram-positive and gram-negative organisms should be commenced. Due to the increased incidence of post-traumatic seizures following missile injuries, prophylactic anticonvulsants are usually recommended, at least in the short term. The CT scout view and bone windows are the most useful in determining the location of retained missile fragments. Strong consideration of angiography is warranted if the missile has passed anywhere near a major intracranial artery. The timing of angiography is often delayed because of the urgent need for operative intervention.

Prognosis following penetrating head injury due to a missile is predominantly determined by the level of consciousness on admission: 94% of patients with a GCS <8 die (Benzel *et al.* 1991). Other factors indicating a worse prognosis include the pathway of the bullet traversing both hemispheres, multiple lobes, or a ventricle, and if the injury was sustained in a suicide attempt.

Because of the relatively poor prognosis in many of these injuries, the indications for surgery are controversial. A useful published protocol suggests surgery be performed on (a) patients with a GCS 9–15, (b) patients with a GCS 6–8 in whom the missile has not traversed both hemispheres, multiple lobes on the dominant side or through a ventricle, and (c) patients with a GCS 3–5 with a large extra-axial haematoma (Graham *et al.* 1990). The aims of surgery are to debride necrotic scalp, bone fragments, and necrotic brain tissue; remove haematomas and control bleeding; remove accessible bullet fragments; repair violated air sinuses; and achieve a watertight dural closure.

Non-missile injuries

The main difference with this form of injury is that the penetrating object is often left protruding from the cranium. In this situation the implement should be stabilized *in situ* until removal in theatre can be accomplished. Again, consideration of angiography should be cardinal.

Key point

- Penetrating head injuries can be further classified as missile and non-missile injuries.

Outcomes

Prognosis of head injury

The outcome from a head injury is often described with the aid of an outcome scale. The simplest and most widely used is the Glasgow Outcome Scale (Jennett and Bond 1975). The clinical state of the patient is often assessed, using this scale, at 3 months or 6 months, although given the propensity of these patients to continue improving for 1–2 years, later assessments may be more accurate.

Reliably predicting the outcome of head-injured patients, particularly those classified with severe injuries, has long been an objective of researchers and clinicians, with a view to withdrawing prolonged and expensive treatment from patients who ultimately will not benefit. A number of factors have been shown to correlate with poor outcome, including low post-resuscitation GCS, older age of the patient, pupillary abnormalities, the presence of hypoxia or hypotension prior to definitive treatment, traumatic subarachnoid haemorrhage, and inability to control ICP (Eisenberg *et al.* 1991, Vollmer *et al.* 1991, Kakarieka 1997a,b). However, the ability to select patients who will definitely have poor outcomes in the early phases of assessment and treatment remains an inexact science.

The mortality rate from head trauma climbs as the patients' post-resuscitation GCS (an indicator of severity of the primary injury) falls. The Traumatic Coma Data Bank results showed that patients with an initial GCS of 3 had a 78% mortality rate, whereas those with a GCS of 8 had an 11% mortality rate. Overall results for patients with severe head injuries (GCS 3–8) were good recovery 26.5%, moderate disability 16.4%, severe disability 15.6%, vegetative 5.2%, and dead 36.3% (Eisenberg *et al.* 1991).

Elderly patients who sustain a head injury have higher rates of morbidity and mortality than younger patients with similar injuries. The progressive increase in morbidity and mortality with age becomes most apparent beyond the age of 55 (Vollmer *et al.* 1991). This adverse effect of age on outcome appears to be related to intrinsic changes in the ability of the brain to recover from pathological insults as a result of the ageing process. It is independent of extrinsic factors such as mechanism of injury, non-neurological complications following injury, or premorbid systemic illness (Vollmer *et al.* 1991).

Key point

- The Glasgow Outcome Scale is the most commonly used scale to describe outcome from a head injury.

Post-concussion syndrome

Approximately 75% of all head injuries are mild (Kraus and Nourjah 1988), and up to 50% of these patients will suffer some form of post-concussion syndrome (Mandel 1989), a constellation of symptoms and signs which may occur in varying degrees after mild head injury.

The sequelae of mild head injury include headaches, cranial nerve symptoms, psychosomatic complaints, and cognitive impairment. Rare sequelae of mild head injury include subdural and EDHs, seizures, transient global amnesia, tremor, and dystonia (Evans 1992). The most common symptoms are headaches, dizziness, irritability, decreased concentration, memory problems, and sensitivity to noise.

The mainstay in treating post-concussion syndrome is reassuring the patient and family that the symptoms are not unexpected, and educating them about the condition. Symptom control with specific therapies may be required.

The majority of patients have significantly improved by 3 months, and 85–90% will have a full recovery by 1 year (Borzuk 1997). If symptoms persist beyond 1 year, the patient is described as having persistent post-concussion syndrome (Rutherford *et al.* 1978). Risk factors for persistent post-concussion syndrome include age >40; female gender; lower educational, intellectual, and socio-economic level; alcohol abuse; prior head injury;

multitrauma; serious other illness; and ongoing litigation (Edna and Cappelen 1987, Evans 1992). Controversy continues about what percentage of these patients are malingerers.

Brain death criteria

The mortality rate of severe head injury remains approximately 36%. Not infrequently these patients reach the point of non-survival while their respiratory function is supported artificially in an intensive care unit. It may then be necessary to establish that brain death has occurred so that futile treatment may be discontinued. If the patient is a candidate for organ donation and consent is obtained to harvest tissues, it is usually a legal requirement that certification of brain death has been performed by at least two medical practitioners in accordance with local laws. Brain death is established by determining the presence of irreversible coma and irreversible loss of brainstem reflexes and respiratory centre function, or by demonstration of the cessation of intracranial blood flow (ANZICS 1998).

The clinical criteria for confirming the presence of brain death are:

- an appropriate period of observation is required
- certain preconditions must be satisfied before clinical testing of brainstem function is undertaken
- clinical testing verifies the absence of brainstem function.

A minimum total period of observation of 6 hours is recommended to show irreversibility beyond all doubt. During this period the patient should be documented to have a GCS of 3, non-reactive pupils, absent gag and cough reflexes, and no spontaneous respiratory efforts. Preconditions that must be satisfied prior to clinical testing include; a diagnosis consistent with progression to brain death, exclusion of coma due to drugs or poisoning, exclusion of metabolic causes of coma, exclusion of hypothermia (core temperature >35°C) and intact neuromuscular conduction (ANZICS 1998). Suggested clinical testing of brainstem function should include response to painful stimuli in cranial nerve distribution, pupillary response to light, corneal reflexes, gag reflex, cough reflex, oculovestibular reflexes, and respiratory function in presence of an adequate stimulus (ANZICS 1998). This last clinical test is usually performed following preoxygenation. The ventilator is then stopped whilst oxygen is administered to the airway and the arterial PCO_2 is allowed to rise >60 mmHg. This represents an adequate stimulus to spontaneous ventilation, during which the patient must remain apnoeic. All of the above reflexes must be absent to certify brain death.

If the above clinical criteria cannot be met, three- or four-vessel cerebral angiography may be used to demonstrate absent intracranial blood flow (both anterior and posterior circulation) following the minimum period of observation of 6 hours (Greenberg *et al.* 1997).

Sport-related head injury

Concussion

Concussion is an alteration in mental status produced by trauma that may or may not involve a loss of consciousness. It is characterized by confusion and amnesia, which may begin immediately after the injury or develop several minutes later (Greenberg *et al.* 1997).

Minor head injuries resulting in concussion are extremely common in contact and impact sports. Most football fans will have witnessed a player who, after a knock to the head, gets to his feet dazed and takes a while to register where he is, or runs in the wrong direction, or appears poorly co-ordinated and fumbles a pass. Initial symptoms are those of mild head injury—headache, nausea and vomiting, dizziness, and confusion. Persisting symptoms represent the post-concussive syndrome and can last for days to weeks; persistent headache, poor concentration, memory problems, irritability, photophobia, tinnitus, anxiety, depression, and sleep disturbance.

The American Academy of Neurology has graded concussion into three levels and produced recommendations to guide physicians as to when to allow athletes suffering each grade of concussion to return to competition (Greenberg *et al.* 1997).

- Grade 1 concussion is defined as transient confusion, no loss of consciousness, and symptoms/mental status abnormalities resolve in <15 minutes.
- Grade 2 concussion involves transient confusion, no loss of consciousness, and symptoms/mental status abnormalities lasting >15 minutes.
- Grade 3 concussion refers to any loss of consciousness, either brief or prolonged.

An athlete who suffers a concussion should be immediately removed from the competition and assessed at frequent intervals. If they have returned to normal by 15 minutes (grade 1), the athlete may return to play. If a grade 2 injury or further grade 1 injury is sustained, they should be removed from the contest and not resume sport until they have been asymptomatic for a full week. If a grade 3 or a second grade 2 injury is sustained, the athlete should remain out of competition until asymptomatic for 2 weeks. A second grade 3 injury should see the competitor resting at least 1 asymptomatic month. Those suffering a grade 2 or 3 injury should be assessed by a neurologist or neurosurgeon before resuming their sport. Persisting symptoms warrant investigation with CT or MRI scanning, and any abnormality detected terminates the athlete's season (Greenberg *et al.* 1997).

Second impact syndrome

Second impact syndrome refers to the precipitous events which may follow a second head injury that is sustained before symptoms associated with a previous head injury have had time to resolve (Cantu 1998).

The most common situation in which closely repeated head injuries are likely is sport. Reported cases of second impact syndrome follow a general pattern: an athlete suffers an initial head injury, the severity of which may vary from grade 1 concussion to the presence of cerebral contusions, and following this has post-concussive symptoms such as headache, nausea, vomiting, visual disturbances, or cognitive problems. Before the symptoms have settled the athlete returns to participation in the sport and suffers a further head injury, which may again be very mild. The athlete then often appears dazed for a few seconds to minutes before suddenly collapsing, becoming deeply comatosed, dilating both pupils, and exhibiting respiratory failure (Cantu 1998). Many of those affected die either before or despite intensive medical care. At autopsy the usual findings are massive cerebral oedema and transtentorial or tonsillar herniation. Loss of autoregulation and resultant cerebral vascular engorgement are believed to be the pathophysiological mechanism behind the extreme cerebral swelling and rapidly ensuing brainstem failure.

Prevention is the best cure for this dangerous condition. It is important that all cases of concussion are identified, and athletes must not be allowed to practice or compete until at least 1 week after all post-concussive symptoms have resolved, no matter how long this takes (Cantu 1998). It is also suggested that athletes with persistent symptoms should have a CT scan of the head (Saunders and Harbaugh 1984). Education of athletes, coaches, and parents about the risk of second impact syndrome is also critical, so that pressure to perform is not unduly exerted on those who are perceived to have suffered only a minor 'knock to the head'.

Chronic traumatic encephalopathy

Chronic traumatic encephalopathy (CTE) refers to a spectrum of neurological injury caused by repetitive head trauma. It is most frequently observed in professional boxers, and there is a clear relationship between the number of bouts fought and the development of CTE (Ryan 1998).

Repetitive blows to the head cause an accumulation of neuropathological changes. These include compromise of the blood–brain barrier, loss of neuronal reserve and cerebral atrophy, diffuse axonal injury, loss of pigments and neurons in the substantia nigra, repeated contusions and gliosis, loss of Purkinje cells in the cerebellum, an increased incidence of cavum septum pellucidum with larger fenestrations, development of neurofibrillary tangles, and amyloid deposition (Mendez 1995). A recent study has suggested that individuals who carry the Apo E e4 allele in their genotype are at increased risk of developing dementia pugilistica (the severest form of CTE), through the association of this allele and an increase in amyloid deposition following acute head injury (Jordan *et al.* 1995).

The clinical manifestations of CTE range from mild motor, cognitive, and psychiatric abnormalities through to dementia pugilistica. The majority of affected boxers exhibit the mild, non-progressive end of the spectrum. This is characterized by dysarthria, tremor, mild lack of co-ordination, decreased attention, and emotional lability. A small minority of boxers progress to dementia pugilistica. This syndrome includes advanced parkinsonism, cerebellar dysfunction, slow mentation, amnesia, disinhibition, decreased insight, and occasionally overt psychosis (Mendez 1995).

Measures suggested to diminish the risk of progressive CTE include preventing commencement of the sport at a young age, limiting the number of bouts fought, discouraging amateurs from turning professional, and stricter medical supervision of the sport (Mendez 1995). There is also an increasing call from medical societies to ban boxing altogether.

References

Adams JH, Scott G, Doyle LS (1980) The contusion index: a quantitative approach to cerebral contusions in head injury. *Neuropathol Appl Neurobiol* 6: 319–324.

Andrews BT, Pitts LH, Lovely MP *et al.* (1986) Is computed tomographic scanning necessary in patients with tentorial herniation? *Neurosurgery* 19: 408–414.

ANZICS (1998) *Recommendations concerning brain death and organ donation*, 2nd edn. ANZICS Working Party on Brain Death and Organ Donation Report. Australian and New Zealand Intensive Care Society, Edgecliff, NSW.

Baker SP, Fowler C *et al.* (1994) Head injuries incurred by children and young adults during informal recreation. *American Journal of Public Health* 84: 649–52.

Benzel EC, Day WT, Kesterson L *et al.* (1991) Civilian craniocerebral gunshot wounds. *Neurosurgery* 29: 67–72.

Bhattacharya JP, Marmarou A, DeSalles AA *et al.* (1989) Cerebral blood flow and metabolism in severely head-injured children. Part 1: Relationship with GCS score, outcome, ICP, and PVI. *Journal of Neurosurgery* 71: 63–71.

Bhattacharya V, Sinha JK, Tripathi FM (1982) Management of scalp injuries. *Journal of Trauma* 22(8): 698–702.

Blumberg PC (1998) Pathology of traumatic brain injury. In postgraduate neuropathology course material, University of Sydney.

Borzuk P (1997) Mild head trauma. *Emergency Medicine Clinics of North America* 15(3): 563–583.

Bouma GJ, MuizelaarJP, Bandoh K (1992) Blood pressure and intracranial pressure-volume dynamics in severe head injury: Relationship with cerebral blood flow. *Journal of Neurosurgery* 77: 360–368.

Brookes M, Macmillan R *et al.* (1990) Head injuries in accident/emergency departments. How different are children from adults? *Journal of Epidemiology and Community Health* 44: 147–151.

Bullock R, Teasedale G (1990) Surgical management of traumatic intracranial haematomas. In: Vinken PJ, Bruyn GW, Braakman R (eds) *Handbook of clinical neurology*, vol 13(57), Head injury. Elsevier Science, Amsterdam, pp. 249–298.

Bullock R, Chestnut RM, Clifton G *et al.* (1996) *Guidelines for the management of severe head injury*. Brain Trauma Foundation, New York.

Cantu RC (1998) Second-impact syndrome. *Clinics in Sports Medicine* 17: 37–44.

Chesnut RM, Marshell LF, Klauber MR (1993) The role of secondary brain injury in determining outcome from severe head injury. *Journal of Trauma* 34: 216–222.

Cruz J (1998) The first decade of continuous monitoring of jugular bulb oxyhemoglobin saturation: Management strategies and clinical outcome. *Critical Care Medicine* 26: 344–351.

Desalles AAF, Muizelaar JP, Young HF (1987) Hyperglycemia, cerebrospinal fluid lactic acidosis and cerebral blood flow in severely head injured patients. *Neurosurgery* 21: 45–50.

Durward QJ, Amarcher AL, Del Maestro RF *et al.* (1983) Cerebral and cardiovascular responses to changes in head elevation in patients with intracranial hypertension. *Journal of Neurosurgery* 59: 938–944.

Edna T-H, Cappelen J (1987) Late post concussion symptoms in traumatic head injury: An analysis of frequency and risk factors. *Acta Neurochirurgica* 86: 12.

Eisenberg HM, Gary HE, Aldrich EF *et al.* (1990) Initial CT findings in 753 patients with severe head injury. A report of the NIH Traumatic Coma Data Bank. *Journal of Neurosurgery* 73: 688–690.

Eisenberg HM, Jane JA, Luerssen TG *et al.* (1991) The outcome of severe closed head injury. *Journal of Neurosurgery* 75: S28–S36.

European Study Group (1994) European Study Group on Nimodipine in Severe Head Injury. A multicenter trial of the efficacy of nimodipine on outcome after severe head injury. *Journal of Neurosurgery* 80: 797–804.

Evans RW (1992) The postconcussion syndrome and the sequelae of mild head injury. *Neurologic Clinics* 10: 815–847.

Fearnside M, McDougall P (1998) Moderate head injury: A system of neurotrauma care. *Australian and New Zealand Journal of Surgery* 68: 58–64.

Feuerman T, Wackym PA, Gade GF *et al.* (1988) Value of skull radiography, head computed tomographic scanning, and admission for observation in cases of minor head injury. *Neurosurgery* 22: 449–453.

Fortune JB, Bock D, Kupinski AM *et al.* (1992) Human cerebrovascular response to oxygen and carbon dioxide as determined by internal carotid artery duplex scanning. *Journal of Trauma* 32: 618–628.

Frank JI (1993) Management of intracranial hypertension. *Medical Clinics of North America* 77: 61–75.

Gennarelli TA, Meaney DF (1996) Mechanisms of primary head injury. In: Wilkins RH, Rengachary SS (eds) *Neurosurgery*, 2nd edn. McGraw-Hill, New York, NY.

Giannotta SL, Gruen P (1992) Vascular complications of head trauma. In: *Complications and sequelae of head injury*. American Association of Neurological Surgeons. Rolling Meadows, IL.

Graham TW, Williams FC, Harrington T *et al.* (1990) Civilian gunshot wounds to the head: a prospective study. *Neurosurgery* 27: 696–700.

Greenberg MK, Alter M, Ashwal S *et al.* (1997) Practice parameter: the management of concussion in sports. *Neurology* 48: 581–5.

Greenberg MS (1997) Exploratory burr holes. In: *Handbook of neurosurgery*, 4th edn, Greenberg Graphics, Lakeland, FL.

Greenburg J, Cohen WA, Cooper PR (1985) The 'hyper-acute' extra-axial intracranial haematoma: Computed tomographic findings and clinical significance. *Neurosurgery* 17: 48–56.

Gurney JG, Rivara FP, Mueller BA *et al.* (1992) The effects of alcohol intoxication on the initial treatment and hospital course of patients with acute brain injury. *Journal of Trauma* 33: 709–713.

Harrigan MR, Tuteja S, Neudeck BL (1997) Indomethacin in the management of elevated intracranial pressure: a review. *Journal of Neurotrauma* 14: 637–650.

Hauser WA (1990) Prevention of post-traumatic epilepsy. *New England Journal of Medicine* 323: 540–542.

Heistad DD, Kontos HA (1983) Cerebral circulation. In: Shepherd JT (ed) *Handbook of Physiology*: Section 2: The cardiovascular system. American Physiological Society, Bethesda, Md.

HMSO (1995) *Report of transport road accidents Great Britain 1994. The casualty report.* HMSO, London.

Jamieson KG, Yelland JDN (1968) Extradural haematoma: Report of 167 cases. *Journal of Neurosurgery* 29: 13–23.

Jennett B (1996) Epidemiology of head injury. *Journal of Neurology, Neurosurgery and Psychiatry* 60: 362–369.

Jennett B, Bond M (1975) Assessment of outcome after severe brain damage. A practical scale. *Lancet* 1: 480–484.

Jordan BD, Kanik AB, Horwich MS *et al.* (1995) Apolipoprotein E e4 and fatal cerebral amyloid angiopathy associated with dementia pugilistica. *Annals of Neurology* 38: 698–9.

Kakarieka A (1997a) Review on traumatic subarachnoid hemorrhage. *Neurological Research* 19: 230–232.

Kakarieka A (1997b) *Traumatic subarachnoid haemorrhage.* Springer, Berlin.

Kraus JF, Nourjah P (1988)The epidemiology of mild uncomplicated brain injury. *Journal of Trauma* 28: 1637–1643.

Kraus JF, Black MA, Hessol N *et al.* (1984) The incidence of acute brain injury and serious impairment in a defined population. *American Journal of Epidemiology* 119: 186–201.

Lang EW, Chesnut RM (1995) Intracranial pressure and cerebral perfusion pressure in severe head injury (review). *New Horizons* 3(3): 400–409.

Lanksch W, Grumme TH, Kazner E (1979) *Computed tomography in head injuries*. Springer, New York, N.Y., pp. 34, 68.

Lee ST, Louis TN *et al.* (1990) Features of head injury in a developing country-Taiwan (1977–1987). *Journal of Trauma* 30: 194–199.

Lewin W (1966) Cerebrospinal fluid rhinorrhea in nonmissile head injuries. *Clinical Neurosurgery* 12: 237–252.

Lundberg N (1960) Continuous recording and control of ventricular fluid in neurosurgical practice. *Acta Psychiatrica Neurologica Scandinavica* 36S: 1–93.

Mandel S (1989) Minor head injury may not be 'minor'. *Postgraduate Medical Journal* 85: 213–225.

Marion DW, Carlier PM (1994) Problems with initial Glasgow Coma Scale assessment caused by prehospital treatment of patients with head injuries: Results of a national survey. *Journal of Trauma* 36: 89–94.

Marshall FL, Eisenberg HM (1991) A new classification of head injury based on computerised tomography. *Journal of Neurosurgery* 75: S14–S20.

Martin NA, Doberstein C, Alexander M *et al.* (1995) Posttraumatic cerebral arterial spasm. *Journal of Neurotrauma* 12: 897–901.

Maset AL, Marmarou A, Ward JD *et al.* (1987) Pressure-volume index in head injury. *Journal of Neurosurgery* 67: 832–840.

Masters SJ, McClean PM, Arcarese JS *et al.* (1987) Skull X-ray examinations after head trauma. *New England Journal of Medicine* 316: 84–91.

Maxwell WL, Polvishock JT, Graham DL (1997) A mechanistic analysis of non-disruptive axonal injury: A review. *Journal of Neurotrauma* 14(7): 419–440.

Mayeux R, Ottman R, Maestre G *et al.* (1995) Synergistic effects of traumatic head injury and apolipoprotein e4 in patients with AD. *Neurology* 45: 555–557.

McCormick WF (1997) Pathology of closed head injury. In: Wilkins RH, Rengachary SS (eds) *Neurosurgery*, 2nd edn, Vol III. McGraw-Hill, New York, pp. 2639–2665.

McIntosh TK, Garde E, Saatman K *et al.* (1997) Central nervous system resuscitation. *Emergency Medicine Clinics of North America* 15: 527–550.

Mendez MF (1995) The neuropsychiatric aspects of boxing. *International Journal of Psychiatry in Medicine* 25: 249–262.

Metz C, Holzschuh M, Bein T *et al.* (1996) Moderate hypothermia in patients with severe head injury: Cerebral and extracerebral effects. *Journal of Neurosurgery* 85: 533–541.

Miller EC, Holmes JF, Derlet RW (1997) Utilizing clinical factors to reduce head CT scan ordering for minor head trauma patients. *Journal of Emergency Medicine* 15: 453–457.

Mokri B (2001) Monro–Kellie hypothesis: applications in CSF volume depletion. *Neurology* 56(12): 1746–1748.

Obrist WD, Langfitt TW, Jaggi JL *et al.* (1984) Cerebral blood flow and metabolism in comatose patients with acute head injury. Relationship to intracranial hypertension. *Journal of Neurosurgery* 61: 241–253.

Palmer JD (1998) The epidemiology of head injuries. *Current Medical Literature, Neurology* 14(2): 31–36.

Phillis JW (1989) Adenosine in the control of the cerebral circulation. *Cerebrovascular and Brain Metabolism Review* 1: 26–54.

Plum F, Posner JB (1980) *The diagnosis of stupor and coma*, 3rd edn. FA Davis, Philadelphia.

Popp AJ, Feustel PJ, Kimelberg HK (1997) Pathophysiology of traumatic brain injury. In: Wilkins RH, Rengachary SS (eds) *Neurosurgery*, 2nd edn, Vol III. McGraw-Hill, New York, pp. 2623–2637.

Randell M, Chesnut MR (1997) The management of severe traumatic brain injury. *Emergency Medicine Clinics of North America* 15(3): 581–603.

RACS (1992) Trauma Committee, Royal Australasian College of Surgeons. *Early Management of Severe Trauma (EMST) Course Manual*. RACS, Melbourne, Victoria.

Rivano C, Borzone M, Carta F *et al.* (1980) Traumatic intracerebral haematomas: 72 cases surgically treated. *Journal of Neurosurgery* 24: 77–84.

Rosner MJ, Rosner SD, Johnson AH (1995) Cerebral perfusion pressure: Management protocol and clinical results. *Journal of Neurosurgery* 83: 949–962.

Rutherford WH, Merret JD, McDonald JR (1978) Symptoms at one year following concussion from minor head injuries. *Injury* 10: 225.

Ryan AJ (1998) Intracranial injuries resulting from boxing. *Clinics in Sports Medicine* 17: 155–167.

Saunders RL, Harbaugh RE (1984) The second impact in catastrophic contact-sports head trauma. *JAMA* 252: 538–539.

Schierhout G, Roberts I (1998) Prophylactic antiepileptic agents after head injury: a systematic review. *Journal of Neurology, Neurosurgery and Psychiatry* 64: 108–112.

Schroder ML, Muizilaar JP, Bullock MR *et al.* (1995) Focal ischaemia due to traumatic contusion documented by sTable xenon CT and ultrastructural studies. *Journal of Neurosurgery* 82: 966–971.

Seelig JM, Becker DP, Miller JD *et al.* (1981) Traumatic acute subdural haematoma. Major mortality reduction in comatose patients treated within four hours. *New England Journal of Medicine* 304: 1511–1518.

Servadei F, Piazzi G, Seracchioli A *et al.* (1988) Extradural haematomas: An analysis of the changing characteristics of patients admitted from 1980 to 1986: Diagnostic and therapeutic implication in 158 cases. *Brain Injury* 2: 87–100.

Siesjo BK (1992) Pathophysiology and treatment of focal cerebral ischaemia. Part I Pathophysiology. *Journal of Neurosurgery* 77: 337–354.

Snow RB, Zimmerman RD, Gandy SE *et al.* (1986) Comparison of magnetic resonance imaging and computed tomography in the evaluation of head injury. *Neurosurgery* 18: 45–52.

Sosin DM, Sachs JJ, Smith SM (1989) Head injury associated deaths in the United States from 1979–1986. *JAMA* 262: 2251–2255.

Stahmer SA, Raps EC, Mines DI (1997) Carotid and vertebral artery dissections. *Emergency Medicine Clinics of North America* 15: 677–695.

Steiger H-J, Aaslid R, Stooss R *et al.* (1994) Transcranial doppler monitoring in head injury: Relations between type of injury, flow velocities, vasoreactivity and outcome. *Neurosurgery* 34: 79–86.

Stein SC, Ross SE (1992) Moderate head injury: a guide to initial management. *Journal of Neurosurgery* 77: 562–564.

Stein SC, Spettell C, Young G *et al.* (1993) Delayed and progressive brain injury in closed-head trauma: radiological demonstration. *Neurosurgery* 32: 25–31.

Teasdale GM, Graham DI (1998) Craniocerebral trauma: Protection and retrieval of the neuronal population after injury. *Neurosurgery* 43(4): 723–738.

Teasdale G, Jennett B (1974) Assessment of coma and impaired consciousness: A practical scale. *Lancet* ii: 81–84.

Teasdale GM, Nicoll JAR, Murray G *et al.* (1997) Association of apolipoprotein E polymorphism with outcome after head injury. *Lancet* 350: 1069–1071.

Temkin NR, Sureyya SD, Wilensky AJ *et al.* (1990) A randomized, double-blind study of phenytoin for the prevention of post-traumatic seizures. *New England Journal of Medicine* 323: 497–502.

Thomason M, Messick J, Rutledge R *et al.* (1993) Head CT scanning versus urgent exploration in the hypotensive blunt trauma patient. *Journal of Trauma* 34: 40–45.

Toutant SM, Klauber MR, Marshall LF (1984) Absent or compressed basal cisterns on first CT scan: ominous predictors of outcome in severe head injury. *Journal of Neurosurgery* 61: 691–694.

Vollmer DG, Torner JC, Eisenberg HM *et al.* (1991) Age and outcome following traumatic coma: why do older patients fare worse? *Journal of Neurosurgery* 75: S37–S49.

Walls RM (1993) Rapid-sequence intubation in head trauma. *Annals of Emergency Medicine* 22: 1008–1013.

Welch TB, Boyne PJ (1991) The management of traumatic scalp injuries: report of cases. *Journal of Oral and Maxillofacial Surgery* 49(9): 1007–1114.

WHO (1992) *Manual of the international statistical classification of diseases, injuries and causes of death*, 10th revision. World Health Organization, Geneva, Switzerland.

Wyler AR, Reynolds AF (1977) An intracranial complication of nasogastric intubation: Case report. *Journal of Neurosurgery* 47: 297–298.

Zee CS, Go J (1998) CT of head trauma. *Neuroimaging Clinics of North America* 8(3): 525–539.

Zee CS, Segall HD, Destian S *et al.* (1996) Radiologic evaluation of head trauma. In: Wilkins RH, Rengachary SS (eds) *Neurosurgery*, 2nd edn. McGraw-Hill, New York, N.Y.

Zimmerman RA, Bilaniuk LI (1982) Computed tomographic staging of traumatic epidural bleeding. *Radiology* 144: 809–812.

6

CHAPTER 6

Soft tissue neck injuries

DANIEL J PRINSLOO AND KEITH P ALLISON

CHAPTER 6
Soft tissue neck injuries

DANIEL J PRINSLOO AND KEITH P ALLISON

This chapter aims to discuss the management of soft tissue neck injuries. A thorough review of current literature has been made to give the best available evidence base. This chapter is specifically directed away from the management of the cervical spine and spinal injury in trauma patients. Specific consideration of skin involvement in these injuries is also omitted here. These issues are dealt with in other chapters.

We refer mainly to penetrating neck injuries, but in our opinion the assessment and management of any neck soft tissue injury should follow a common pathway. Soft tissue injuries in the neck are difficult to assess and manage. This compact, important anatomical area contains a dense concentration of vital vascular, aerodigestive, and nervous system structures; many of which are not accessible to physical examination, and surgical exposure is a challenge. There has been a shift away from early aggressive operative management to a more selective and conservative approach, but controversy still exists (Demetriades *et al.* 1996).

Key points

- Soft tissue injuries of the neck are difficult to assess and to manage.
- Surgical exposure is a challenge.
- There is controversy regarding mandatory exploration or selective conservatism.

History

- The first documented treatment of vascular injury in the neck was by Ambrose Paré (1510–1590).
- In 1803, Fleming ligated a lacerated common carotid artery.
- In World War II, 851 cases of neck injury were reported with a 7% mortality. In Vietnam this rose to 15% (Read *et al.* 1988).
- In 1944 Bailey (see Ellis and Paterson-Brown 2001) proposed early exploration of all cervical haematomas on the basis of wartime experience.
- Fogelmann and Stewart (1956) reported a series of 100 patients showing a mortality of 6% in patients undergoing early neck exploration versus 35% for those for whom exploration is delayed. They advocated mandatory, early exploration of any wound penetrating the platysma.
- Subsequently the rate of negative neck explorations increased and the operative mortality fell, leading to a selective approach to management challenging this older dictum (Asensio *et al.* 1991).

Neck anatomy

The anatomy of the neck is unique, as it contains many vital structures representing the most important body systems. Traditionally an anatomical scheme for the neck uses triangles, each triangle containing different vital structures and coated by muscle, fascia, and skin. Classically the neck is divided into anterior and posterior triangles by the sternocleidomastoid muscle.

The anatomical structures in the neck structures are invested by two fascial layers:

- The *superficial fascia* lies just beneath the skin and encompasses the body of *platysma* (a thin superficial muscle that originates over the upper part of the thorax and passes over the clavicles across the neck and blends with the superficial musculo-aponeurotic system (SMAS) of the face).

- The *deep cervical fascia* can be subdivided into investing, pretracheal, and prevertebral layers.
  - the investing fascia encompasses the sternocleidomastoid, omohyoid, and trapezius muscles as it encircles the neck
  - the pretracheal fascia attaches to the thyroid and cricoid cartilages and blends with the pericardium in the thorax; it encloses the major neck viscera (thyroid gland, trachea and oesophagus)
  - the prevertebral fascia encompasses the prevertebral muscles and blends with the axillary sheath, which houses the subclavian vessels.

The carotid sheath is formed by all three components of the deep fascia.

Key point

- The neck contains structures representing many different systems.

The tight fascial compartmentalization of the neck structures limits external bleeding from vascular structures. This beneficial effect is countered by the dangers of bleeding within these closed spaces, which can compromise the airway.

Anatomy
Neck contains structure representing different systems: ◆ Cardiovascular ◆ Respiratory ◆ Digestive.

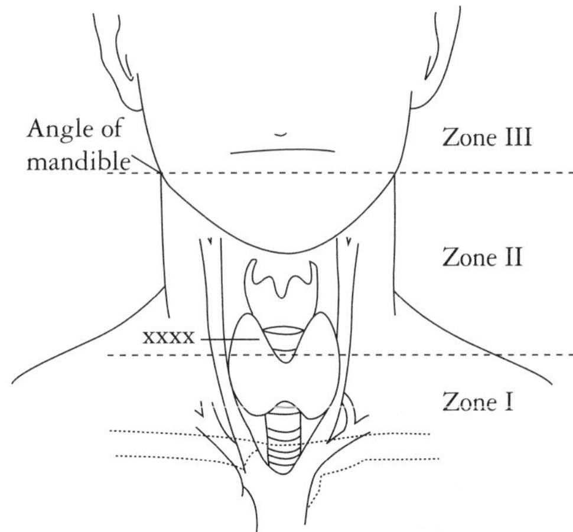

Figure 6.1 Anatomic zones of the neck. (Reproduced with permission from Feliciano *et al.* 1996.)

Penetrating neck injury is most commonly referred to in terms of zone of injury (Fig. 6.1, Table 6.1), rather than triangles. This is because this allows knowledge of the possible structures involved, the need for additional specialized investigations, surgery, and prognosis.

Mechanisms of injury

Neck injuries can be classified in different ways (Table 6.2). The anatomical site of injury and the related structures are vital, but the history, mechanism and pattern of injury also give important information and clinicians should get as much history as possible from pre-hospital carers or ambulance personnel.

Epidemiology

- The typical victim sustaining a penetrating neck wound is male in his late twenties (Miller and Duplechain 1991) The male : female ratio is 5 : 1 (Markey *et al.* 1975).
- Although one might expect the number of firearms injuries to have increased over the last 30 years, in fact firearms and stab wounds have increased at a comparable rate

Table 6.1 Anatomic zones of injury

Zone	Boundaries	Structures at risk
I	Clavicles inferiorly to the inferior aspect of the cricoid cartilage	Proximal common carotid, vertebral and subclavian arteries Major vessels of the superior mediastinum, apices of the lungs Oesophagus, trachea, and thoracic duct
II	Cricoid cartilage inferiorly up to the angle of the mandible	Carotid and vertebral arteries and internal jugular vein Larynx, trachea and oesophagus Vagus nerve, recurrent laryngeal nerve and spinal cord
III	Angle of the mandible to base of skull	Distal carotid and vertebral arteries Salivary glands, pharynx Spinal cord and cranial nerves IX–XII

Note: Some authors use the inferior border of the mandible as the upper boundary of zone II (Demetriades *et al.* 1997).

Table 6.2 Classification of neck injuries

Penetrating	Non-penetrating (blunt)
Low velocity	Road traffic accident
Stab wounds	Strangulation
Some gunshot and air pellet injuries[a]	Sport
High velocity	
Gunshot injuries[a]	
Blast/explosions	

[a] Shotgun blast from 2 m has a velocity of 300 m/s, compared with a rifle at 760 m/s. Kinetic energy imparted to wound = $1/2mv^2$.

(Markey *et al.* 1975, Saletta *et al.* 1976, Noyes *et al.* 1986).

- The most common site of injury is the anterior triangle of the neck.

Initial management

An airway, breathing and circulation (ABC) approach to all trauma patients has now become standard, thanks to the teaching of Advanced Trauma Life Support (ATLS). As part of this teaching, the assessment and immediate management of life-threatening problems go hand in hand in a stepwise progression. The presence of a bleeding neck wound should not detract from an airway injury: respiratory distress, stridor, and altered level of consciousness mandate emergency airway management (Walls *et al.* 1993). The importance of this process cannot be overemphasized too much; approximately 10% of patients with penetrating neck injuries present with airway compromise (Pate 1989), 25–40% have a vascular injury (10% carotid artery), and 10% have a respiratory tract injury.

Expeditious pre-hospital transfer, without intervention in the urban environment, gives the patient with life-threatening soft tissue neck injury the best chance of survival. Airway and respiratory care are paramount and early endotracheal intubation should be considered if patients present with symptoms of respiratory obstruction:

- restlessness
- stridor
- air hunger
- hoarseness
- tracheal tug
- retraction of supraclavicular, intercostals, or epigastric areas

- cyanosis
- inability to swallow and drooling
- Prophylactic intubation is preferred in as controlled a fashion as possible rather than emergency intubation, cricothyroidotomy, or tracheostomy.
- Patients should be assessed and initially treated in a Trendelenburg position in order to minimize the chances of air embolism.
- Direct pressure is used to control external haemorrhage. Vascular access should be attained, ideally on the contralateral side to the injury and blood is taken for cross-match of 6 units of packed red blood cells. If bleeding cannot be controlled by direct pressure, balloon tamponade may be attempted (Gilroy *et al.* 1992), but blind or non-selective clamping of vessels should be avoided to prevent further injury to structures.
- The insertion of a nasogastric tube at this early stage should be avoided to keep patient agitation to a minimum and to prevent bleeding which had previously been controlled.
- Demetriades *et al.* (1996) suggest an algorithm for evaluation of penetrating neck injuries (Fig. 6.2) There are other schemes based on findings in zones of the neck (Velmahos *et al.* 1994, Klyachkin *et al.* 1997). The basic aim is to have a fast and effective method of assessment, so that injuries are not missed and overtreatment avoided. A chart to aid the examination and recording of this type of injury has been proposed by Demetriades *et al.* (Fig. 6.3). Some authors feel that examination alone is sufficient in the assessment of zone II neck injuries; others feel that it is reliable in all zones (Velmahos *et al.* 1994, Demetriades *et al.* 1995, 1997, Jarvik *et al.* 1995, Kendall *et al.* 1998). We

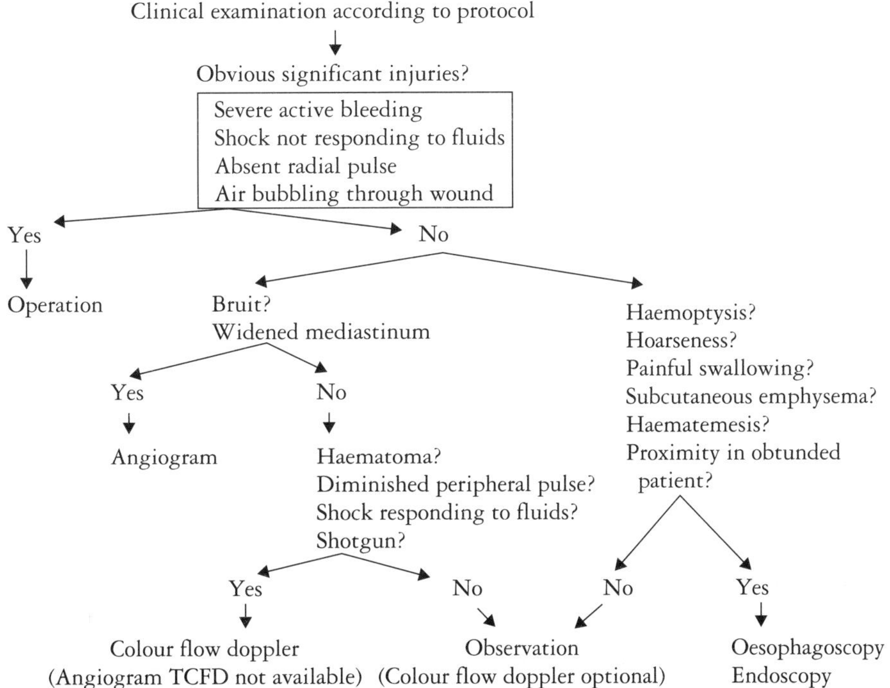

Figure 6.2 Algorithm for neck injury evaluation. (Reproduced with permission from Demetriades *et al.* 1996.)

A. Site of Injury
- ☐ Anterior neck triangle (anterior to SMS muscle)
- ☐ Posterior neck triangle (posterior to SMS muscle)
- ☐ Zone I (between clavicles and cricoid)
- ☐ Zone II (between cricoid and angle of mandible of skull)
- ☐ Zone III (between angle of mandible and base of skull)

Wound Tract
- ☐ Towards midline
- ☐ Towards clavicle
- ☐ Away from midline or
- ☐ Can't assess

B. Vascula Structures
1. Active bleeding: ☐ None, ☐ Minor, ☐ Moderate, ☐ Severe
2. Hypovolaemia: ☐ BP>100, ☐ BP 60–90, ☐ BP<60
3. Haematoma: ☐ None, ☐ Small, ☐ Moderate, ☐ Large, ☐ Expanding, ☐ Pulsatile
4. Peripheral pulses (compare with contralateral):
   Distal carotid: ☐ Normal, ☐ Diminished, ☐ Absent
   Superficial temporal: ☐ Normal, ☐ Diminished, ☐ Absent
   Brachial or radial: ☐ Normal, ☐ Diminished, ☐ Absent
5. Bruit: ☐ No, ☐ Yes if so, where ....)

C. Larynx/Trachea, Oesophagus
1. Haemoptysis (ask patient to cough): ☐ Yes, ☐ No
2. Air bubbling through wound? ☐ Yes, ☐ No (ask patient to cough)
3. Subcutaneous emphysema: ☐ Yes, ☐ No
4. Hoarseness: ☐ Yes, ☐ No
5. Pain on swallowing sputum: ☐ Yes, ☐ No
6. Haematemesis: ☐ Yes, ☐ No

D. Nervous System:
1. GCS: ☐ Eye response, ☐ Verbal response, ☐ Motor response
   Total GCS................
2. Localizing signs:
   Pupils:
   Limbs:
   Cranial nerves:
   Facial n. ☐ Normal, ☐ Abnormal
   Glossopharyngeal n. (check midline portion of soft palate): ☐ Normal, ☐ Abnormal
   Recurrent laryngeal n. (hoarseness. effective cough): ☐ Normal, ☐ Abnormal
   Accessory n. (lift the shoulder): ☐ Normal, ☐ Abnormal
   Hypoglossal n. (check midline position of tongue): ☐ Normal, ☐ Abnormal
   Spinal cord: ☐ Normal, ☐ Abnormal (specify)
   Horner's syndrome (myosis, ptosis): ☐ Yes, ☐ No
   Brachial plexus: median n. (fist): ☐ Normal, ☐ Abnormal
   radial n. (wrist extension): ☐ Normal, ☐ Abnormal
   ulnar n. (abduction/adduction of fingers): ☐ Normal, ☐ Abnormal
   musculocutaneous n. (flexion of forearm): ☐ Normal, ☐ Abnormal
   axillary n. (abduction of arm): ☐ Normal, ☐ Abnormal

Figure 6.3 Chart to aid the examination and recording of neck injuries. (Reproduced with permission from Demetriades *et al.* 1996.)

feel that this chart allows a methodical examination of the structures involved in penetrating neck injury and serves as a template for notes and research. Its universal adoption would allow better communication (Atta and Walker 1998).

Key points

- Use the ABC approach to emergency treatment.
- Direct pressure to control bleeding.
- Immediate transfer to hospital.
- Carry out a thorough clinical examination.
- Operate or investigate.

Investigations

On the basis of his experience in World War II, Bailey (1944) proposed mandatory neck exploration for all penetrating neck trauma that presented with a cervical haematoma. Fogelmann and Stewart (1956) suggested a policy of neck exploration for all injuries breaching the platysma. Unfortunately, although injuries were rarely missed this way, negative explorations of 30–89% were the result.

Investigations are becoming increasingly more sensitive, specific, and available (Table 6.3). They enhance our history taking and clinical examination, allowing a more selective approach to surgical exploration. This has to be balanced against the cost and morbidity of invasive investigations with a low yield in terms of changing management. A selective approach to management attempts to identify the patients who will benefit from early surgical intervention and those who can be managed conservatively.

Cervical spine precautions are rarely a necessity in patients with penetrating neck trauma, in the absence of neurological symptoms or signs (Kendall *et al.* 1998).

Operative management

Mandatory operation or selective conservatism?

Once the patient has been resuscitated and stabilized in the emergency department and the history and physical examination are complete; the surgeon has two options:

- to proceed to operation
- to investigate (see Table 6.3).

There is little argument about the immediate surgical management of patients with obvious symptoms and signs of major vascular or aerodigestive tract injuries. Immediate life-threatening features include:

- need for surgical airway
- expanding haematoma
- exsanguinating haemorrhage
- poorly controlled haemorrhagic shock
- haemomediastinum
- haemothorax.

Non-life-threatening features of involvement in soft tissue neck injury include:

- vascular injury in the haemodynamically stable patient
- upper aerodigestive tract lesions
- peripheral neurological deficit.

Clinicians advocating mandatory surgical exploration stress the following points:

- Immediate surgery prevents unnecessary delays in treatment.
- Physical examination is not reliable and potentially dangerous injuries may be missed (Ferguson *et al.* 1985, Timberlake *et al.* 1989, Apffelstaedt and Muller 1994).

Table 6.3 Investigation of neck injuries

Investigations available	Indications	Advantages and disadvantages
Plain lateral cervical spine radiograph	All patients	Quick, inexpensive, non-invasive assessment of bony structures and possible foreign bodies
CT	Stable patients with foreign body, laryngo tracheal or oesophageal injury suspected	Non-invasive Fast with newer technology (helical CT)
Angiography	Injury to all zones (I–III) in haemodynamically stable patients[a]	'Gold standard' vascular assessment but invasive, time consuming, morbidity 1.73%, mortality 0.03% (e.g. CVA)
Colour flow Doppler 4 (Demetriades *et al.* 1995, 1997, Ginzburg *et al.* 1996, Peter Corr *et al.* 1999)	Same as angiography	Non-invasive, similar sensitivity and specificity Dependent on user's expertise
MRI and angiography (James 1997)	Delayed onset vascular injury, Vascular intimal injury, Focal ischaemic symptoms, Postganglionic Horner's syndrome	Fast, no contrast required Not yet standard practice
Oesophagogram	Suspected upper digestive tract injury (dysphagia, subcutaneous emphysema, haematemesis,saliva from wound) High-velocity injuries	90% accuracy, non-invasive (Luntz *et al.* 1993)
Oesophagoscopy	Performed concomitantly with oesophagography	Invasive High sensitivity and specificity
Endoscopy (laryngoscopy and bronchoscopy)	Suspected laryngotracheal injury (respiratory distress, hoarseness, dyspnoea, subcutaneous emphysema, haemoptysis)	Invasive Accurate Require general anaesthesia (excepting fibre optic examination)

[a] Some authors advise in zones I and III only.

- No specialized diagnostic investigations are necessary if the neck is explored.
- Observation is expensive.
- Negative neck exploration is not associated with significant morbidity or mortality.
- Hospitalization and costs are not increased.

As already suggested in our section on special investigations, those clinicians opposed to mandatory exploration find that there is a high negative exploration rate, therefore making this approach expensive and increasing patient morbidity.

Asensio *et al.* (1991) have conducted an extensive review of current evidence and found that neither approach had been proved superior, so the controversy has yet to be resolved.

Surgical approach to the neck

- Exploration of the neck is through a standard incision along the anterior border of the sternocleidomastoid muscle extending from the angle of the mandible to the sternocleidomastoid junction (Fig. 6.4).
- An extension of the incision toward the origin of the sternocleidomastoid muscle may be made if the injury is located in zone III (Asensio *et al.* 1991).
- Other techniques to gain access to base of the skull injuries include anterior subluxation of the mandible (Dichtel *et al.* 1984) or lateral mandibulotomy (Fisher *et al.* 1984)
- The neck incision may also be extended as a supraclavicular incision for the management of zone I injuries.
- Further extension as a partial median sternotomy combined with an anterolateral thoracotomy may be useful in the management of zone I injuries.

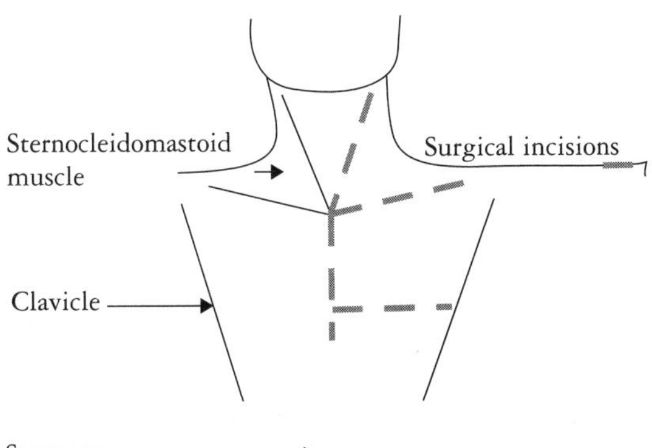

Figure 6.4 Surgical approach to the neck. Incisions are indicated by broad lines.

Management of specific structural injuries

Carotid artery

Carotid artery injuries account for about 22% of all cervical vascular injuries and are diagnosed in 6% of all penetrating neck injuries (Demetriades *et al.* 1997).

These are the most immediately life threatening of all soft tissue neck injuries as airway occlusion can occur due to bleeding contained within fascial planes.

Clinical presentations

- shock
- active external bleeding
- expanding haematoma
- absent or diminished pulses
- bruit
- neurological defects.

Investigations

- Zones I and II: angiography.
- Zone II angiography is more controversial, but can yield valuable information if it can be performed safely and quickly. It is here that good clinical examination and judgement are essential, as operative exploration will rarely miss carotid artery injury.
- Minor carotid injuries such as intimal tears and small false aneurysms are sometimes detected by angiogram or duplex ultrasonography.

Repair

- In the absence of neurological deficit, carotid artery repair must be performed whenever possible. Shunts are often used during the repair. Techniques of carotid artery repair are shown in Fig. 6.5.
- Carotid artery repair in the presence of neurological deficit is controversial because it was initially thought that restoration of blood

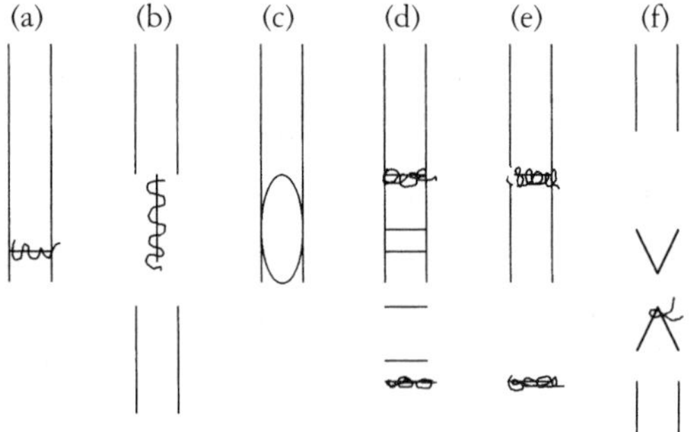

Figure 6.5 Techniques for arterial repair: (a) end-to-end anastomosis; (b) direct closure; (c) patch grafting; (d) synthetic material bypass grafting; (e) vein grafts—if an interposition graft is needed the saphenous vein is preferred; (f) vessel ligation.

flow might convert an ischaemic infarct to a worse haemorrhagic one. This was later discounted in favour of brain swelling as a cause. Most recent studies support re-establishment of blood flow in most patients with neurological deficit short of coma (Robbs *et al.* 1983, Ramadan *et al.* 1995). The presence of coma has a grave prognosis irrespective of operative management (Demetriades *et al.* 1989).

- Asymptomatic occlusion of the common or internal carotid artery may result in late local or neurological complications and should therefore be repaired whenever technically possible.

Subclavian vessels

Damage to the subclavian vessels is an uncommon injury with a high mortality rate. The prognosis of venous injuries is worse than that of arterial injuries because of air embolism and the inability of veins to contract and control bleeding.

Emergency treatment

Balloon tamponade is helpful to prevent exsanguinations.

Surgical approach

- Clavicular extension with retraction or partial excision of clavicle.
- Median sternotomy or left thoracotomy (for proximal injuries).

Repair

- Arterial injuries are best managed by simple repair, debridement and end-to-end anastomosis, or interposition graft (autologous vein or prosthetic material).
- Ligation of artery is only done in extremis as it is associated with claudication and subclavian steal syndrome.
- Subclavian vein is generally ligated unless repair can be done quickly without producing stenoses.

Jugular vein

The jugular veins are the most frequently injured vascular structures in the neck (Meyer *et al.* 1987). Injury presents in a similar way to carotid artery injuries. Operative management is by primary repair by lateral venorrhaphy, or ligation if repair is not feasible.

Vertebral artery

Injury to the vertebral artery is uncommon, but may be associated with injuries to other neck structures, most commonly spinal injury. Increasing numbers of these injuries are being elucidated with the increasing use of diagnostic angiography.

Management is usually by angiographic embolization, with surgery reserved for patients with severe active bleeding or when embolization fails.

Larynx and trachea

The main objectives of airway surgery are to re-establish a stable and sufficient airway and to obtain a good quality voice (Miller and Duplechain 1991).

Clinical presentation

- air escaping through the wound
- dyspnoea
- stridor
- haemoptysis
- subcutaneous emphysema

- hoarseness
- crepitation
- dysphonia.

Investigations

- laryngoscopy
- bronchoscopy
- oesophagoscopy.

Management of laryngeal injuries

Minimal laryngeal injury and undisplaced fractures are treated conservatively. Early repair gives a better outcome in terms of voice quality (Leopold 1983). Indications for surgery include:

- exposed laryngeal cartilage
- significant mucosal disruption
- arytenoids dislocation
- penetrating injury through larynx.

Management of tracheal injuries

Small wounds without tissue loss are treated conservatively (Ngakane *et al.* 1990, Sclafani *et al.* 1991). All other wounds are repaired primarily using interrupted non-absorbable sutures. The anastomosis should be well vascularized and tension free. The use of a tracheostomy to protect the repair is controversial because of the increased infection risk and related morbidity. If a tension-free anastomosis is not possible because of tissue loss, then musculofascial flaps or synthetic material are used for reconstruction (Miller *et al.* 1986).

Pharynx and oesophagus

Pharyngeal and oesophageal injuries are uncommon and therefore quite likely to be missed, resulting in severe complications (Demetriades and Stewart 1985, Feliciano *et al.* 1985).

Clinical presentation

- haematemesis
- odynophagia
- subcutaneous emphysema

Investigations

- plain radiographs may show intraluminal air
- oesophagogram (barium swallow)
- oesophagoscopy.

Repair

The repair should be carried out as soon as the patient is stable. Use absorbable sutures in one or two layers, and consider placing a muscle flap from one of the strap muscles or sternocleidomastoid over the repair (Miller and Duplechain 1991). The wound should be drained postoperatively.

In the case of an associated tracheal injury, an interposition muscle flap is valuable in helping to prevent tracheo-oesophageal fistula (Feliciano *et al.* 1985). In the case of extensive oesophageal injury, a cutaneous stoma should be created (Feliciano *et al.* 1985)

Neurological structures

The structures most commonly affected are the spinal cord or brachial plexus, but more extensive neurological injury created by cerebral ischaemia associated with major vessel damage (as mentioned previously) also fits into this group.

Peripheral nerve injuries include:

- vagus nerve
- phrenic nerve
- recurrent laryngeal nerve
- sympathetic chain.

Brachial plexus injuries are diagnosed and repaired during the initial exploration and other nerve injuries should be repaired where possible.

Parotid gland

An injury to the parotid is repaired by suturing parenchyma back together over a closed drainage system. If sialocoeles or fistulae develop after this, then aspiration and compression are preferred to further surgical intervention.

Sialocoeles from the parotid duct are more resistant to conservative management and may present with skin breakdown and fistula formation. These patients should be managed by total parenteral nutrition (TPN) with or without anticholinergic agents. Internal fistulization into the mouth is another possibility (Demetriades 1991).

Thoracic duct

Injury to the thoracic duct is rare, and usually associated with injury to the subclavian vessels. It may be missed at the initial exploratory operation and present postoperatively as a milky fluid leak in the drain fluid or a transcutaneous fistula.

Investigation of the fluid

- total serum protein >3 g/dL
- total fat content 0.4–4.0 g/dL
- triglyceride level >200 mg/dL
- alkaline pH
- lymphocyte predominance.

Management

Conservative management with TPN or low fat diet normally allows wound healing within 2 weeks (Fogli *et al.* 1993).

Prognosis following soft tissue injury of the neck

Historical reviews of deaths resulting from wounds of the neck in various wars reveal a mortality rate of 7–18% (Otis 1883, La Garde 1916, US Government 1927, Beebe and DeBakey 1952). With advances in resuscitation as well as specialized diagnostic technology, mortality rates today are 0–11%, regardless of the philosophy of mandatory or selective exploration (Markey *et al.* 1975).

References

Apffelstaedt JP, Muller R (1994) Results of mandatory exploration for penetrating neck trauma. *World Journal of Surgery* 18(6): 917–919.

Asensio JA, Valenziano CP, Falcone RE, Grosh JD (1991) Management of penetrating neck injuries. The controversy surrounding zone II injuries. *Surgical Clinics of North America* 71(2): 267–296.

Atta HM, Walker ML (1998) Penetrating neck trauma: lack of universal reporting guidelines. *American Surgeon* 64(3): 222–225.

Beebe GW, DeBakey ME (1952) *Battle Casualties: Incidence, Mortality and Logistic Considerations*.Charles C Thomas, Springfield, IL.

Demetriades D (1991) Surgical management of post-traumatic parotid sialoceles and fistulae. *Injury* 22(3): 183–184.

Demetriades D, Stewart M (1985) Penetrating injuries of the neck. *Annals of the Royal College of Surgeons of England* 67(2): 71–74.

Demetriades D, Skalkides J, Sofianos C, Melissas J, Franklin J (1989) Carotid artery injuries: experience with 124 cases. *Journal of Trauma* 29(1): 91–94.

Demetriades D, Theodorou D, Cornwell E III *et al.* (1995) Penetrating injuries of the neck in patients in stable condition. Physical examination, angiography, or color flow Doppler imaging. *Archives of Surgery* 130(9): 971–975.

Demetriades D, Asensio JA, Velmahos G, Thal E (1996) Complex problems in penetrating neck trauma. *Surgical Clinics of North America* 76(4): 661–683.

Demetriades D, Theodorou D, Cornwell E *et al.* (1997) Evaluation of penetrating injuries of the neck: prospective study of 223 patients [see comments]. *World Journal of Surgery* 21(1): 41–47.

Dichtel WJ, Miller RH, Feliciano DV, Woodson GE, Hurt J (1984) Lateral mandibulotomy: a technique of exposure for penetrating injuries of the internal carotid artery at the base of the skull. *Laryngoscope* 94(9): 1140–1144.

Ellis BW, Paterson-Brown S (2001) *Hamilton Bailey's emergency surgery*, 13th edn. Oxford University Press, Oxford.

Feliciano DV, Bitondo CG, Mattox KL *et al.* (1985) Combined tracheoesophageal injuries. *American Journal of Surgery* 150(6): 710–715.

Feliciano DV, Moore EE, Mattox KL (ed.) (1996) *Trauma*, 3rd edn. Appleton and Lange, Norwalk, CT.

Ferguson MK, Little AG, Skinner DB (1985) Current concepts in the management of postoperative chylothorax. *Annals of Thoracic Surgery* 40(6): 542–545.

Fisher DF Jr, Clagett GP, Parker JI *et al.* (1984) Mandibular subluxation for high carotid exposure. *Journal of Vascular Surgery* 1(6): 727–733.

Fogelmann MJ, Stewart RD (1956) Penetrating wounds of the neck. *American Journal of Surgery* 91: 581–581.

Fogli L, Gorini P, Belcastro S (1993) Conservative management of traumatic chylothorax: a case report. *Intensive Care Medicine* 19(3): 176–177.

Gilroy D, Lakhoo M, Charalambides D, Demetriades D (1992) Control of life-threatening haemorrhage from the neck: a new indication for balloon tamponade. *Injury* 23(8): 557–559.

Ginzburg E, Montalvo B, LeBlang S, Nunez D, Martin L (1996) The use of duplex ultrasonography in penetrating neck trauma. *Archives of Surgery* 131(7): 691–693.

Gray SW, Skandalis JE, McClusky DA (1985) *Atlas of Surgical Anatomy*. Williams and Wilkins, Baltimore, p. 15.

James CA (1997) Magnetic resonance angiography in trauma. *Clinical Neuroscience* 4(3): 137–145.

Jarvik JG, Philips GR III, Schwab CW *et al.* (1995) Penetrating neck trauma: sensitivity of clinical examination and cost-effectiveness of angiography. *American Journal of Neuroradiology* 16(4): 647–654.

Kendall JL, Anglin D, Demetriades D (1998) Penetrating neck trauma. *Emergency Medicine Clinics of North America* 16(1): 85–105.

Klyachkin ML, Rohmiller M, Charash WE, Sloan DA, Kearney PA (1997) Penetrating injuries of the neck: selective management evolving [see comments]. *American Surgeon* 63(2): 189–194.

La Garde LA (1916) *Gunshot injuries*. W Wood, New York, p. 204.

Leopold DA (1983) Laryngeal trauma. A historical comparison of treatment methods. *Archives of Otolaryngology* 109(2): 106–112.

Luntz M, Nusem S, Kronenberg J (1993) Management of penetrating wounds of the neck. *European Archives of Otorhinolaryngology* 250(7): 369–374.

Markey JC Jr, Hines JL, Nance FC (1975) Penetrating neck wounds: a review of 218 cases. *American Surgeon* 218(41): 77–83.

Meyer JP, Barrett JA, Schuler JJ, Flanigan DP (1987) Mandatory vs selective exploration for penetrating neck trauma. A prospective assessment. *Archives of Surgery* 122(5): 592–597.

Miller RH, Duplechain JK (1991) Penetrating wounds of the neck. *Otolaryngology Clinics of North America* 24(1): 15–29.

Miller RH, Lipkin AF, McCollum CH, Mattox KL (1986) Experience with tracheal resection for traumatic tracheal stenosis. *Otolaryngology – Head and Neck Surgery* 94(4): 444–450.

Ngakane H, Muckart DJ, Luvuno FM (1990) Penetrating visceral injuries of the neck: results of a conservative management policy. *British Journal of Surgery* 77(8): 908–910.

Noyes LD, McSwain NE Jr, Markowitz IP (1986) Panendoscopy with arteriography versus mandatory exploration of penetrating wounds of the neck. *Annals of Surgery* 204(1): 21–31.

Otis GA (1883) *Medical and surgical history of the war of rebellion*. US Government Printing Office, Washington DC.

Pate JW (1989) Tracheobronchial and esophageal injuries [published erratum appears in *Surgical Clinics of North America* 1989 Jun;69(3):following viii]. *Surgical Clinics of North America* 69(1): 111–123.

Peter Corr ATO, Carrim A, Robbs J (1999) Colour-flow ultrasound in the detection of penetrating vascular injuries of the neck. *South African Medical Journal* 89(6): 644–647.

Ramadan F, Rutledge R, Oller D *et al.* (1995) Carotid artery trauma: a review of contemporary trauma center experiences. *Journal of Vascular Surgery* 21(1): 46–55.

Reid JD, Weigelt JA, Thal ER, Francis H (1988) Assessment of the proximity of a wound to major vascular structures as an indication for arteriography. *Archives of Surgery* 123(8): 942–946.

Robbs JV, Human RR, Rajaruthnam P *et al.* (1983) Neurological deficit and injuries involving the neck arteries. *British Journal of Surgery* 70(4): 220–222.

Saletta JD, Lowe RJ, Lim LT *et al.* (1976) Penetrating trauma of the neck. *Journal of Trauma* 16(7): 579–587.

Sclafani SJ, Cavaliere G, Atweh N, Duncan AO, Scalea T (1991) The role of angiography in penetrating neck trauma. *Journal of Trauma* 31(4): 557–562.

Timberlake GA, Rice JC, Kerstein MD, Rush DS, McSwain NE Jr (1989) Penetrating injury to the carotid artery. A reappraisal of management. *American Surgeon* 55(3): 154–157.

US Government (1927) *Medical department of US Army in the World War*. US Government Printing Office, Washington, DC.

Velmahos G, Souter I, Degiannis E, Mokoena T, Saadia R (1994) Selective surgical management in penetrating neck injuries. *Canadian Journal of Surgery* 37(6): 487–491.

Walls RM, Wolfe R, Rosen P (1993) Fools rush in? Airway management in penetrating neck trauma [editorial; comment] [see comments]. *Journal of Emergency Medicine* 11(4): 479–480.

7

CHAPTER 7

Spinal injuries (cervical, thoracic, lumbar, sacral)

CHOLAVECH CHAVASIRI

CHAPTER 7

Spinal injuries (cervical, thoracic, lumbar, sacral)

CHOLAVECH CHAVASIRI

Spinal injuries occur most commonly in young men, resulting from motor vehicle accidents (42–56%), falls (19–30%), gunshot wounds (12–21%), sports (primarily diving, 6–7%), and miscellaneous causes (Kraus *et al.* 1975, Fine *et al.* 1979, Fife and Kraus 1986, Chavasiri and Chavasiri 1998b, Chavasiri and Unnanantana 1998). The initial evaluation and management of a patient with an injured spine starts at the scene of the accident. The correct procedure must be carried out to prevent further neurological deficit. Improved training of paramedical personnel, attention to immobilization, and careful patient transfer from the scene of the injury to hospital avoiding excessive movement of the affected site of the spinal injury, have resulted in a significant reduction of complete spinal cord injuries. A spinal column injury should be suspected until proved otherwise in all multiple trauma patients, especially in those who are unconscious or intoxicated, or have head and neck injuries. General patient assessment starts with initial patient evaluation and a carefully documented history and examination. This would include the mechanism of injury, the time that the injury occurred, and the time that the patient arrived at the hospital.

The idea of a spinal injury centre was first put into practice during World War II, at the Ministry of Pensions Hospital, Stoke Mandeville, England, under the supervision of Sir Ludwig Guttman in 1943 (Chavasiri and Unnanantana 1997). In time the concept of a spinal injury unit became well established throughout the world as a basis for successful treatment. In hospitals with spinal injury units, the proportion of complete injuries decreased from 65% to 46%, and overall mortality dropped from 20% to 9% (Tator *et al.* 1988, 1993).

Pathophysiology of spinal cord injury

The initial trauma causes primary injuries to the spinal cord. Immediately after the injury occurs, there is disruption of axonal transmission that may be caused by depolarization of axonal membranes secondary to failure of repolarization as a result of potassium leakage (Anderson 1985). The ischaemia caused by decreased spinal blood flow can cause further injury to the spinal cord (Fried and Goodkin 1971, Sandler and Tator 1976, Balentine 1978). Pathological examination of early stage trauma reveals greater injury to the grey matter than to the white matter (Ducker *et al.* 1971). Within a few minutes, petechial haemorrhages can be detected in the grey matter. By 30 minutes, neural haemorrhage and neuronal necrosis are seen centrally. Nerve fibres are swollen. By 4 hours, marked necrosis occurs in the grey matter and there is an increased necrosis of the oligodendroglia in white matter (Balentine 1978). By 8 hours, there is maximal axonal swelling and the beginning of axonal necrosis. The pathological examination reveals vesicular degeneration. The pathophysiology results from the depletion of adenosine triphosphate (ATP) stores, causing failure of calcium-dependent enzymes and membrane transport systems (Yashon 1978, Ikata *et al.* 1989, Jansen and Hanseboul 1989, Young 1993). This is followed by uncontrolled intracellular influx of calcium, which causes an overload of the mitochondrial calcium pump, leading to uncoupled oxidative phosphorylation and a further decrease in ATP production. Activation of calcium-dependent phospholipase A_2 breaks down membranes and releases arachidonic acid. Arachidonic acid decreases local spinal blood flow, causes release of lysosomal enzymes, mediates platelet aggregation, and generates peroxide free radicals. Disruption of cellular membranes by peroxidation and hydrolytic enzymes is thought to be an important factor in secondary spinal cord injury following trauma. Hence drugs which limit lipid peroxidation will be of great benefit in reducing secondary injury (Bracken *et al.* 1984, 1990, Anderson *et al.* 1988, Hall 1988).

Initial evaluation

Distinguishing between hypovolaemic and neurogenic shock (secondary to loss of sympathetic tone) is important. Bradycardia suggests that a neurogenic component is present, as opposed to tachycardia and hypotension which are associated with hypovolaemic shock. In general, treatment of hypovolaemia helps cord perfusion, although overhydration may increase cord swelling or cause pulmonary oedema. Swan–Ganz monitoring is helpful in this setting. Vasopressor medication may be needed to maintain normal blood pressure and sometimes atropine is required to increase heart rate in cases of severe bradycardia.

History and physical examination

A complete and documented history and physical examination must be conducted at the time of the initial hospital evaluation and this should be repeated with time. A general physical examination should be performed on all patients with spinal trauma for assessment of other associated injuries to organ systems or extremities (10–15% have associated major visceral disruption). Essentials of the physical examination include inspection and palpation of the neck through the sacrum. The patient should be rolled carefully into a semi-lateral position to identify skin abrasions. The spine is palpated to determine areas of tenderness, evidence of abnormal gaps between interspinous processes, step-offs, or sharp areas of kyphosis which will allow the immediate localization of the injury site as well as revealing the mechanism of injury and dictating the plan of management. It is important to evaluate the entire spine carefully; there is a 10–20% likelihood of contiguous or remote associated spinal fracture.

One of the most important issues is that each patient should receive a careful physical examination. The timing of the examination is important too. In particular, a meticulous neurological examination will document the lowest remaining functional level, assess for sacral sparing, or sparing of posterior column indicating an incomplete spinal cord lesion. This is essential.

Spinal shock (spinal cord concussion) may be evident if there is no function of the spinal cord, including motor, sensory and reflexes below the injury level, in the 24–72 hour period after the accident. If the bulbocarvenosus reflex is present (elicited by squeezing of the glans penis or tugging on the Foley catheter, or applying pressure to the clitoris which will in turn produce contraction of the rectal sphincter) the patient is then out of spinal shock.

It is important to carefully repeat the physical examination to detect any sparing of neurofunction, to determine if there is incomplete cord injury and if the patient is likely to recover. The results of the examination will influence the patient's management. A complete absence of distal motor or sensory function or perianal sensation, together with recovery of the bulbocarvenosus reflex, indicates a complete cord injury.

Once the patient has been identified as having a neurological injury in association with a cervical spine fracture, skeletal traction should be immediately applied to support the head and neck in an appropriate neutral alignment. Initial treatment with large does of methylprednisolone (30 mg/kg initially and 5.4 mg/kg per hour for the first

24 hours) has been shown to improve neurological recovery, but only if treatment is begun within the first 8 hours after the injury. Methylprednisolone is not effective if the spinal cord injury is in the area of the conus medullaris and nerve root.

Key points

- A thorough history and physical examination are essential.
- Other associated injuries are common and should be sought.
- If a neurological injury is identified early treatment with a large dose of methylprednisolone improves recovery.

Radiographic evaluation

Cervical spine

Any patient in whom a cervical spine injury is suspected should initially have lateral cross-table cervical radiography carried out in the emergency room. It is necessary to visualize the entire lateral part of the cervical spine by traction down shoulder. To reveal pathology at the cervicothoracic junction, the so-called swimmer's radiograph is necessary before the interpretation of cervical spine injury can be made. Otherwise pathology at the level of C7 and T1 may be overlooked.

The major features to be assessed on the lateral view are soft tissue swelling, bone fragmentation, and spinal canal size. The normal value for the ratio of canal diameter to body diameter is 0.8 or greater (Chavasiri and Chavasiri 1998a). There is not a strong correlation between neurological deficit and radiographic appearance. After that, anteroposterior, oblique, and open-mouth odontoid views can be obtained. The anteroposterior view is not very helpful in determining cervical spine injury except when the spine is grossly unstable. The opened mouth view will be helpful in visualizing pathology at C1–C2 (fracture C1, odontoid fracture, C1–C2 subluxation).

An oblique view with the X-ray beam at 45° off the vertical shows the pedicles and articular process well, and also subluxations (Fig. 7.1). A dynamic lateral radiograph (flexion/extension view) will determine ligamentous injury that is not apparent on the neutral view. It should be done by active range of motion and must not be passive; physician supervision is advisable when instability is suspected. Muscle splinting may prevent sufficient flexion for detection of posterior ligament injury, and repeat radiography a few days later is recommended.

(a)

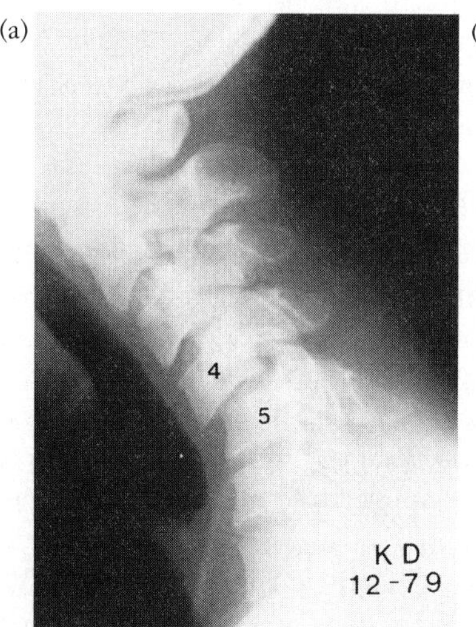

(b)

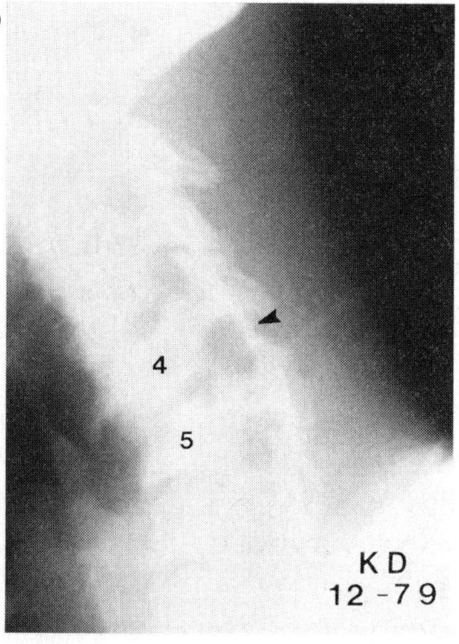

Figure 7.1 (a) Lateral radiograph showing anterior subluxation of C4 and C5. The vertebral displacement is approximately one-third of the vertebral body width. (b) Oblique radiograph demonstrating a fractured fifth cervical facet, allowing anterior subluxation.

Therefore, treatment depends on the bone radiography findings as well as on the pathology of the spinal injury.

The CT scan should be considered as an adjunct to plain radiographs. A CT scan may be helpful in defining injuries to the atlantoaxial complex, posterior rotating subluxation, and C1 ring fracture, and may be useful in assessing if there is bone in the canal. CT scanning clearly defines osseous anatomy and reveals the severity of osseous injury in more detail, so it is useful for assessing stability. Certain longitudinal fractures that are not seen well on plain radiographs (such as a non-displaced laminar fracture) may be defined well on CT scan, but it is much less sensitive for detecting fractures in the transverse plane (such as an articular process fracture).

MRI has advantages in demonstrating posterior ligamentous disruption, the pathology of the intervertebral discs, epidural haematoma, and canal compromise, and can more precisely define the extent of spinal cord injury.

The disadvantage of using MRI is that it cannot be used for patients who have cardiac pacemakers, ferromagnetic implants, or claustrophobia, and it is difficult for patients who require mechanical ventilation. Myelography alone is rarely indicated for the acute evaluation of spine trauma. It may be helpful in evaluating nerve root avulsions or suspected dural tears. CT enhanced with myelography is superior for localizing soft tissue compromise of the spinal cord.

Key point

- There may be poor correlation between radiological appearance and neurological deficit in cervical injuries.

Thoracic and lumbar spine

Imaging of the thoracic and lumbar spine is a less complex procedure than that of the cervical spine. Routine anteroposterior and lateral plain radiographs are part of the initial examination. The widening of soft tissue shadow at the area of the mediastinum is an important marker of upper thoracic fractures and the association of aorta injury (Bolesta and Bohlman 1991). The majority of acute thoracic and lumbar spine injuries are recognizable on the initial plain radiographs. A CT scan is indicated in the majority of patients with plain radiological evidence of injury. In a blinded study, orthopaedic surgeons and radiologists were only 50% accurate in distinguishing burst from compression fractures (Ballock *et al.* 1992).

The primary concern is to demonstrate the position of the vertebral body fragments, the integrity of the neural canal, and the relationship of the fragments to the spinal cord. It is essential to be aware that the upper four or five thoracic vertebrae are not routinely visible on the lateral radiograph of the thoracic spine because of the density of the superimposed shoulder. If the patient's condition permits, the Fletcher view provides an off-lateral projection of the upper thoracic segments by positioning one shoulder anterior and one posterior to the spine. Thus, the upper thoracic segments are projected obliquely between the rotated shoulder. When the true lateral view of the thoracic vertebrae is required, plain tomography or CT with sagittal or three-dimensional reformation is needed.

MRI is most commonly used in the patient in whom the fracture is not apparent but who has neurological deficit, or in the patient who has no correlation between the level of the fracture and neurological deficit. MRI can reveal injury to the posterior ligamentous complex.

Sacrum and coccyx

Acute injuries of the sacrum are most commonly associated with pelvic ring disruption. Isolated injuries of the sacrum and coccyx are uncommon. The sacral and coccygeal concavity make adequate visualization of all these segments on a single anteroposterior projection impossible. Consequently, in addition to the straight anteroposterior radiograph, the standard plain radiographic examination of the sacrum and coccyx must include rostrally and caudally angulated anteroposterior views, as well as a true lateral projection. The fracture can be identified by lateral polydirectional tomography or CT, or as an area of high radioactivity on a nuclear medicine scan.

Sacrococcygeal dislocation is difficult to diagnose radiographically because of the range of normal variation at this area and effects of pelvic delivery in women. Clinical correlation is important for these patients.

Classification of injury

Spinal injuries can be considered in the following categories: bone, soft tissue, and neural tissue (spinal cord and root). Spinal cord injuries are divided into complete (no function below a given level) or incomplete (with some sparing of distal function).

The most widely used system for evaluation of functional recovery is the Frankel scale, which consists of five grades (A–E), based on motor and sensory deficits.

Table 7.1 Frankel classification of spinal injury

Frankel grade	Function
A	Complete paralysis
B	Sensory function only below injury level
C	Incomplete motor function below injury level
D	Fair to good motor function below injury level
E	Normal function

Cervical spine injury

In patients with complete cervical spine injury, recovery of one nerve root level can be expected in 80%, and 20% will recover two additional functional levels. Patients with incomplete cord lesions are classified on the basis of the area of the spinal cord that has been the most severely damaged. The most frequent lesion is the *central cord syndrome* and most of these occur in elderly patients with pre-existing cervical spondylosis who sustain a hyperextension injury. The spinal cord is compressed anteriorly by the posterior osteophyte and posteriorly by the infolded ligamentum flavum. The area of the cord which is most injured is the central grey matter. This results in greater loss of motor function to the upper extremities than to the lower extremities with variable sensory sparing. The second most common cervical cord injury is the *anterior cord syndrome*, in which the damage is primarily in the anterior two-thirds of the cord sparing the posterior column (position sense, proprioceptive and vibratory sensation). Clinically these patients demonstrate greater motor loss than sensory loss (Table 7.1). It has the worst prognosis for recovery.

The *Brown–Sequard syndrome* is damage of the hemicord carrying ipsilateral motor loss and position/proprioception loss with contralateral pain and temperature loss. This usually occurs two levels below the insult. It is rare but has a good prognosis.

The very rare *posterior cord syndrome* consists of loss of deep pressure, deep pain, and proprioception, with otherwise normal cord function.

Isolated nerve root lesions can occur at the level of fracture, most commonly at C5 and C6, and are usually unilateral. The prognosis is favourable for recovery.

Upper cervical spine injury

Occipital condyle fractures

Fractures of the occipital condyle are rarely reported and usually occur in conjunction with C1 fractures. Because most of these injuries are the result of lateral bending and axial loading, they are relatively stable and can be treated by orthotic immobilization. However, if the injury is associated with instability of the occipitoatlantal joint, the treatment will require a cervico-occipital arthrodesis (Bohlman 1985).

Occipitoatlantal dislocations

Injuries of the occipitocervical joint are extremely rare. Patients with such injuries rarely survive. The diagnosis is easily overlooked on routine radiographs. The radiographic diagnosis is made from the lateral cervical spine roentgenogram made in neutral flexion-extension. The dens-basion relationship and Power's ratio are good tools in making the diagnosis (Fig. 7.2). A ratio of more than 1.0 suggests a posterior dislocation. In the normal lateral cervical spine view, the tip of the odontoid is in vertical alignment with the basion (Bailey 1952, Wholey *et al.* 1958, Evarts 1970, Wiesel and Rothman 1979, Georgopoulos *et al.* 1987). The normal distance between these two points in adults is 4–5 mm. However, it can be up to 10 mm in children and any increase in this distance is considered significant (Wholey *et al.* 1958, Weisel and Rothman 1979). The occipital condyles maye displaced anteriorly or posteriorly. The alar ligaments are avulsed from occipital condyles and the apical ligament is disrupted, as well as the tectorial membrane and posterior atlanto-occipital membrane (Eismont and Bohlman 1978). Incomplete injuries of the cervical cord at this level produce a quadriparesis with upper extremities involved more than the lower extremities, the so-called *cruciate paralysis* (Bohlman 1985). This lesion is highly unstable and is not amenable to conservative treatment.

One of the important considerations in the occiput C1 distraction injury is to avoid skull traction which may create overdistraction and cause further neurological deficit or death. Therefore a cervico-occipital arthrodesis is indicated after reduction of the fracture with slight traction. Halo cast immobilization is required after the orthodesis.

Atlas fracture

Injuries to the ring of C1 are secondary to compressive forces. The injury results in a spreading of the ring of C1 so in most cases is not associated with neurological damage.

Bilateral posterior arch fracture is usually seen on lateral cervical spine radiography. There is a 50% chance that another cervical spine injury is also present. A soft collar is probably sufficient for an isolated posterior arch fracture.

CT scans can detect anterior arch fracture, and dynamic lateral radiography reveals anterior hypermobility. The mechanism of the burst injury is described as four fracture lines, two in the anterior arch and two in the posterior arch (Fig. 7.3). The atlas fracture may be combined with a fracture of the lateral mass. Lateral displacement of the lateral masses more than 7 mm on the open mouth view represents rupture of the transverse ligament and potential instability of the C1–C2 complex (Fig. 7.4a). The measurement is the sum of the

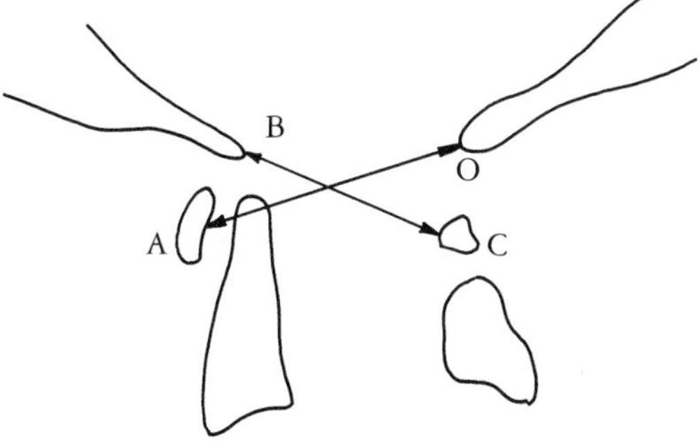

Figure 7.2 Powers' ratio is the ratio of the distance from basion (B) to posterior arch of the atlas (C) divided by the distance from opisthion (O) to anterior arch of C1 (A). A ratio >1 is indicative of instability.

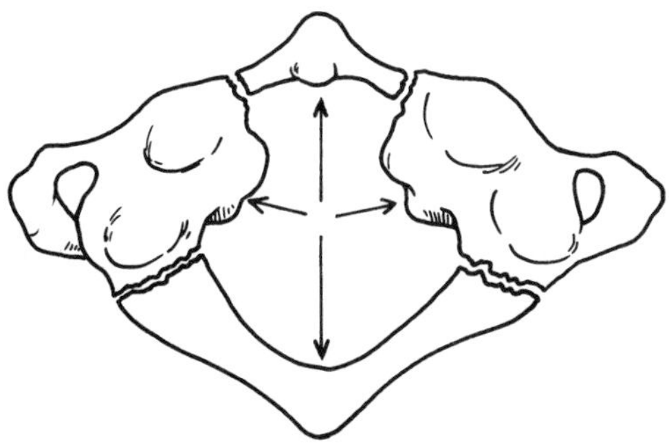

Figure 7.3 Jefferson's fracture is a burst fracture of C1 ring which has four fracture lines, two in the anterior arch and two in the posterior arch.

(a)

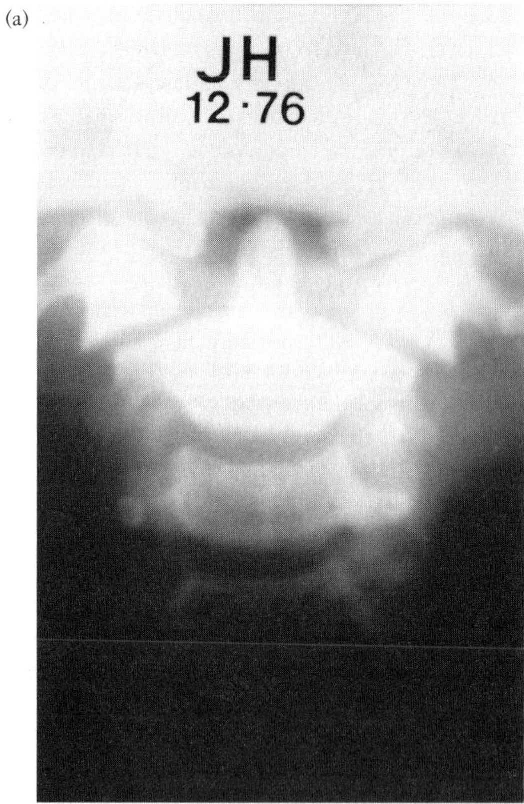

(b)

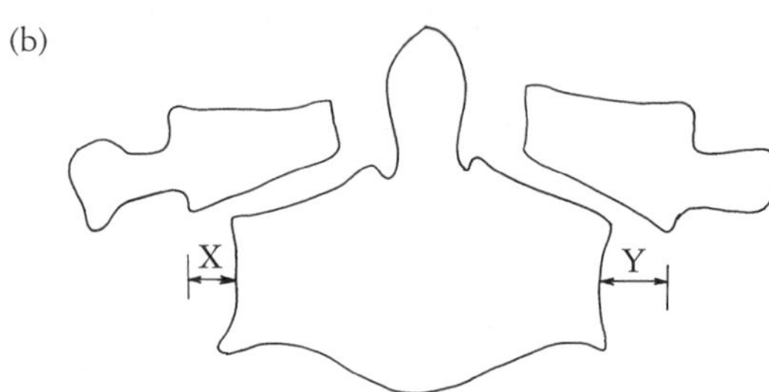

Figure 7.4 (a) Lateral mass fracture of the atlas. The open mouth view shows marked displacement of the lateral mass on both sides. (b) Fracture of atlas. If the displacement of the lateral mass of C1 is >7°mm, a transverse ligament disruption is suspected.

distance from the bilateral space of lateral mass of C1 to the outer borders of the axis in open-mouth view (Fig. 7.4b). Fracture of atlas rarely requires internal fixation except for those that are associated with tearing of the transverse ligament and atlantoaxial subluxation (Anderson and D'Alonzo 1974, Brashear *et al.* 1975). In these situation, it is better to apply a halo cast or vest, to allow the healing of the atlas. Test for instability should be carried out at 2–3 month intervals. Dynamic lateral radiography many reveal an atlanto–dens interval (ADI) >3 mm, and this indicates hypermobility. If at that time atlantoaxial subluxation persists with an ADI >5 mm, a posterior atlantoaxial arthrodesis is recommended. Posterior atlantoaxial dislocation is rare and requires arthrodesis after reduction in skeletal traction because of severe ligament disruption.

Atlantoaxial rotatory subluxations and dislocations

Rotatory dislocation at the C1–C2 articulation rarely occurs in adults and is significantly different when it occurs in children (Fielding *et al.* 1978a,b, Levine and Edwards 1989). Subluxations in children are usually related to viral infection, are almost always self-limited, and usually resolve with conservative treatment. The injury seen in adults usually occurs in a road traffic accident. The mechanism of injury is thought to be a flexion–extension injury or a relatively minor blow to the head (Wortzman and Dewar 1968). An open-mouth radiograph of this type of injury reveals asymmetrical space between the dens and the lateral mass of the C1 ring when compared to both sides. When the injury is more severe then the lateral mass of C1 overlaps the lateral mass of C2 on the affected side. That can be demonstrated on an open mouth radiograph, the so-called *wing sign* (Fig. 7.5).

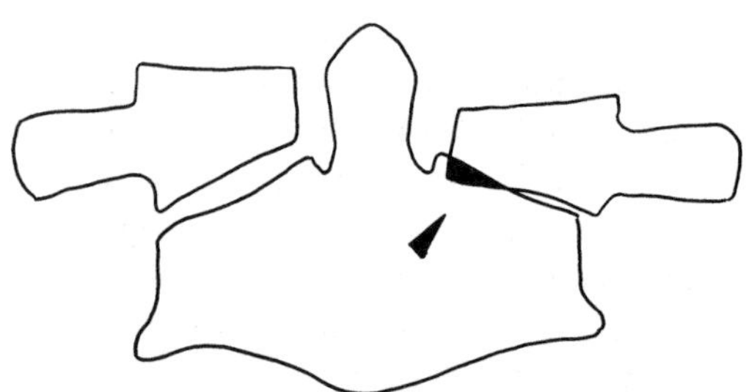

Figure 7.5 Open mouth view showing a wing sign. There is an overlaps of the lateral mass of C1 and C2 on the affected side.

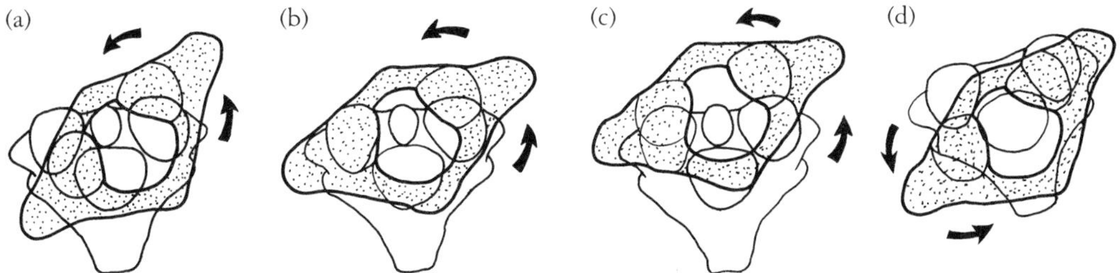

Figure 7.6 Classification of rotatory fixation of C1 and C2 by Fielding *et al.* (1978a): type I, rotatory fixation with no anterior displacement of the atlas and odontoid acting as a pivot; type II, rotatory fixation with disruption of transverse ligament and unilateral anterior displacement of one side of lateral of atlas and the opposite joint acting as a pivot (anterior displacement <3 mm); type III, rotatory fixation with disruption of transverse ligament and capsular ligament with anterior displacement <5 mm; type IV, rotatory fixation with posterior displacement; type V, frank rotatory dislocation.

The classification of these injuries was described by Fielding *et al.* (1978a) on the basis of radiographic appearance (Fig. 7.6). Levine and Edwards (1989) added the rotatory type of dislocation to this classification.

- Type I rotatory fixation is the most common. This is also known as Fielding and Hawkins type I and consists of partial capsular ligament disruption without transverse atlantal capsular ligament disruption. This type of injury occurs without anterior displacement at the atlas. The ADI is <3 mm and the transoral anteroposterior radiograph may show asymmetry between the C1 lateral mass and the dens.
- Type II is the second most common injury. It is associated with deficiency of the transverse ligament and unilateral anterior displacement of one lateral mass of atlas with the opposite intact joint acting as a pivot. The ADI is usually increased to 3–5 mm.
- Type III results from transverse atlantal ligament disruption as well as unilateral or bilateral capsular damage. If the subluxation is symmetric, no rotatory component is present but asymmetrical subluxation commonly occurs. The ADI is usually increased to >5 mm, and a wing sign may be seen on the anteroposterior radiograph.
- Type IV is a rare type of injury, with posterior displacement of the atlas noted on the axis, and includes damage to the dens.
- Type V, frank rotatory dislocation, is extremely uncommon (Jones 1984, Levine and Edwards 1986). The key to treatment is the early recognition of the injury. Although treatment is somewhat controversial, most authors agree that these injuries may be treated initially by halter or halo traction, but with caution against overdistraction. Supplementary manipulation with topical anaesthesia to the oropharynx can reduce a locked joint. If a satisfactory reduction can be obtained, halo immobilization for 3 months should be considered. If closed reduction cannot be obtained or maintained, open reduction and posterior wiring with a bone graft fusion is recommended.

Odontoid fractures

The overall incidence of odontoid fractures ranges from 7% to 14% of all cervical fractures (Crooks and Birkett 1944, Aymes and Anderson 1956, Nachemson 1959, Bohler 1965, Ryan and Taylor 1982) and they are usually the result of falls or motor vehicle accidents (Aymes and Anderson 1956, Apuzzo *et al.* 1978, Mouradian *et al.* 1978, Southwick 1980, Clark and White 1985). The exact mechanisms of injury remain unknown but probably include a combination of flexion, extension, and rotation (Alker *et al.* 1978, Mouradian *et al.* 1978, Bucholz and Burkhead 1978, Skold 1978). The dens is connected to the occiput and C1 by a number of tiny but important ligamentous structures. These ligaments are attached to the dens and allow for movement of the dens separate from the body of C2 in most fractures. This explains in part why this type of fracture is associated with problems of non-union. The second factor is the complex vascular anatomy of the dens. Fractures of the base of the dens are likely to cause damage to these vessels and create problems with healing. Another factor that may contribute to non-union is that the dens is almost completely surrounded by synovial cavities that make it almost entirely an intra-articular structure. When a fracture occurs, the first process of healing is haematoma formation. This haematoma formation is interfered with by the arachidonic acid of the synovial fluid surrounding the fracture. In the evaluation of a patient with a suspected odontoid fracture, it is important to rule out other cervical spine injury.

Anderson and D'Alonzo (1974) have classified these injuries into three anatomical types, on the basis of the level of injury.

- Type I fractures are the least common (5%). They are an oblique fracture through the upper end of the odontoid process and probably represent avulsion fracture of the alar ligament of one side of the tip of the dens. The evaluation should include a dynamic lateral view to rule out anterior subluxation of C1. A cervical collar for symptomatic management is usually sufficient.
- Type II fractures occur at the base of the dens. They are the most common (60%) and troublesome type, with the highest rate of non-union. The risk factors for non-union include older age (>40 years) (Apuzzo *et al.* 1978), initial displacement amount (>4–5 mm) (Apuzzo *et al.* 1978, Clark and White 1985), initial displacement direction (posterior worse than anterior), delay in diagnosis (>2 weeks) (Ryan and Taylor 1982), and redislocation in a halo vest.

  For the Type II odontoid fracture, generally accepted treatment alternatives include use of halo vest, posterior wiring and arthrodesis of C1–C2, and anterior C2 fixation. Initial attempted reduction and halo immobilization for 12 weeks is often successful if initial dens displacement is <5 mm, a good reduction can be maintained, and the patient is <50 years of age. Prolonged traction may lead to overdistraction and non-union. Patients with injuries that do not show an adequate reduction and those presenting more than 2 weeks after injury (Ryan and Taylor 1982) should be considered candidates for surgical stabilization by posterior atlantoaxial arthrodesis with wire and bone graft. This procedure has a 95% fusion rate. Anterior screw fixation of the dens has the potential advantage of preserving atlantoaxial motion. Before the screw can be used, the displacement of the odontoid fracture has to be brought into good alignment by traction. However, the procedure has several significant risks. A major concern is that the cancellous bone in the fractured dens fragment can be damaged by the thread of the screw and the interfragmentary compression of the screw may not occur. This can affect fracture healing. In addition, it is hard to demonstrate healing at the fracture site because of the size of the large screw compared to that of the dens fragment. If the C1 arch is also fractured, alternatives include using halo vest until the C1 arch is healed, then a posterior C1 and C2 arthrodesis if the dens is not healed, or anterior screw fixation of the dens, or Magrel type C1 and C2 posterior screw fixation and grafting. This is a technically demanding operation.
- In Type III fractures, the fracture plane passes through the vertebral body. Displaced, angulated fractures should be reduced in halo traction and held in halo vest immobilization for 12 weeks or until united. A cervical orthosis may be appropriate in some patients with stable, impacted fractures, particularly in elderly people. However, later problems of significant fracture displacement, angulation,

and non-union have been demonstrated, and these are more problematic than used to be thought (Clark and White 1985).

Bilateral pars interarticularis of C2 fracture (hangman's fracture)

Because the elongated pedicles are the thinnest portion of the bony ring of the axis and are additionally weakened by the foramen transversarium on either side, this area functions as a fulcrum in flexion and extension between the cervicocranium (skull, atlas, dens and body of axis) and the relatively fixed lower cervical spine, further enhancing the susceptibility of this area to injury (Brashear *et al.* 1975, Williams 1975). Francis and co-workers noted that approximately 31% of patients sustaining this injury have associated injury of the cervical spine (Francis and Fielding 1978, Francis *et al.* 1981). Forceful extension of an already extended neck is the most commonly described mechanism of injury, but other causes include flexion of a flexed neck and compression of an extended neck. A common classification is that proposed by Levine and Edwards (1985), which is essentially a modification of Effendi's radiographic systems (Effendi *et al.* 1981, Bohlman *et al.* 1982). This system is based on lateral cervical spine radiographs (Fig. 7.7).

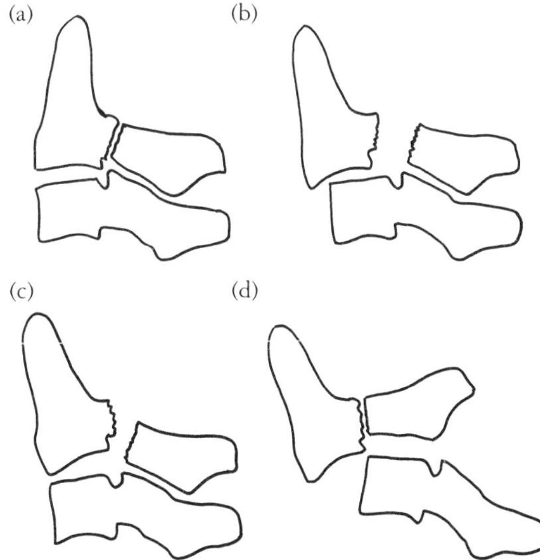

Figure 7.7 Classification of hangman's fractures: (a) type I is minimally displaced and no angulation; (b) type II is a fracture with both translation and angulation; (c) type IIA is a fracture with no translations, but severe angulation; (d) type III is combined with bilateral facet dislocation between C2 and C3.

- Type I is minimally displaced with no angulation and <3 mm of displacement, and may be treated in an extended or regular Philadelphia collar.
- Type II has significant angulation and translation and is typically treated with a halo vest for 12 weeks. In addition to the Type II fracture, the Type IIa has slightly or no translation but widening of the posterior part of the C2–C3 disc with traction and severe angulation of the fracture fragments. It should be treated in a halo vest. Halo traction may cause overdistraction of this injury.

  Type II injuries are usually treated conservatively, with halo or tong traction in extension for 5–7 days. If reduction is adequate with <4–5 mm of displacement or <10–15° of angulation, then a halo vest may be applied. If the reduction is inadequate, continued traction for 4–6 weeks is recommended, followed by further halo vest for an additional 6 weeks. In some cases, the halo vest may not maintain alignment and open reduction and internal fixation may be necessary to obtain and maintain reduction. The technique includes posterior oblique wiring, and screw fixation of the C2 posterior element to the C2 body.
- Type III has severe angulation, translation and also unilateral or bilateral facet dislocation at C2–C3.

  Type III fractures may occur with concomitant unilateral or bilateral facet dislocations and are also unstable. These type of injuries require surgery for facet reduction or stabilization.

Lower cervical spine (C3–C7) injury

Minor compression and avulsion fractures

Spinous process fracture ('clayshoveller's fracture')

The most common site for a spinous process fracture is at C7 and a sudden, single overload is the most likely cause. Treatment is usually symptomatic. Non-union at the fracture site is common.

Transverse process fracture

A transverse process fracture is an uncommon injury, caused by a muscle pull, and can be treated symptomatically.

Teardrop avulsion fracture

A teardrop avulsion fracture involves the anterior, inferior corner of the vertebral body, and is caused by hyperextension. A dynamic lateral radiograph can reveal hypermobility. A neck collar for a few weeks is probably appropriate.

Wedge compression fracture

A wedge compression fracture involves loss of vertebral body height anteriorly but does not involve the posterior wall. The posterior ligaments become taut when there is 25% loss of the anterior height. Compression of more than 50% without damage to the posterior wall may indicate posterior ligamentous instability. Fractures with up to 25% compression and intact posterior wall can be treated with orthosis. If late instability can be identified by lateral flexion/extension radiography, a posterior interspinous process wiring and bone graft should be considered.

Facet joint injuries

Subluxation and dislocation (unilateral or bilateral)

Subluxation and dislocation injuries include partial tearing of the posterior ligaments on the affected side(s) including the posterior portion of the disc. A lateral cervical spine radiograph may show anterior subluxation of the vertebral body above, and soft tissue swelling anteriorly, as well as a decreased amount of overlap of the articular processes. In the patient who has no neurological impairment, dynamic lateral radiographs under physician supervision may determine if there is hypermobility. Minimal subluxation is often treated with a Philadelphia-type collar for 6 weeks. There is a need for close follow-up to ensure that progressive subluxation does not occur: if it does, posterior wiring with bone grafting should be performed.

Unilateral facet dislocation

Unilateral facet dislocation involves forward rotation of one side of the vertebra about the contralateral facet joint and causes the vertebral body to subluxate approximately 25% of the anteroposterior body diameter (Fig. 7.8a). Two lateral masses of the dislocated vertebra may overlap partially on the lateral view radiograph, giving a 'bow-tie' sign (Fig. 7.8b). Clinically the patient may have torticollis. Patients who have sustained lower cervical spine injuries between the third cervical and first thoracic vertebrae with neurological deficit require immediate skeletal traction and attempted realignment of the spine to restore the spinal canal diameter. Restoration of spinal alignment is the first stage in decompression of the spinal cord (Bohlman *et al.* 1982). It is no longer believed that patients should have skeletal traction instituted over a period of days or weeks to attempt reduction of fractures and dislocations of the lower cervical spine with neurological deficit (Bohlman 1985). It is important to decompress the spinal cord as soon as possible, taking into account associated medical problems and other injuries. Treatment is by skeletal traction, gradually increasing the traction weight—5 kg to counter the weight head and an additional 2.5 kg for each level of cervical vertebra until the injury level is reached. Some authors have recommended that the maximum weight should be no more than one-third of body weight. This procedure requires close monitoring of the patient's neurological status

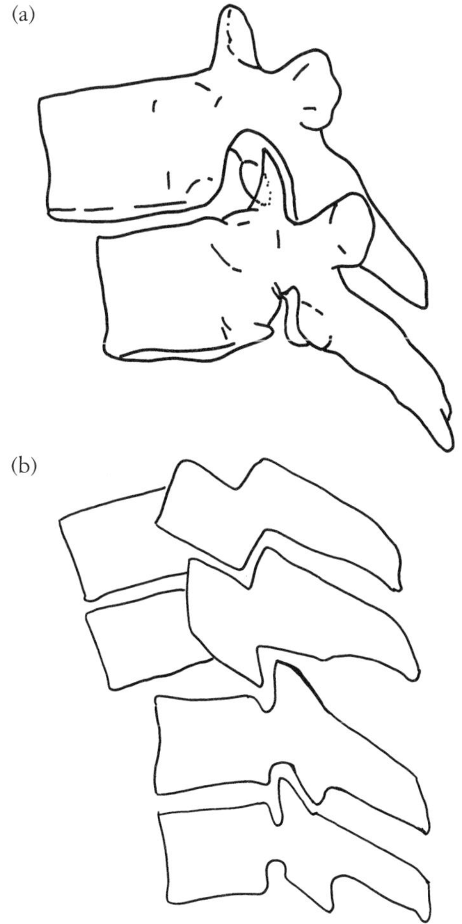

Figure 7.8 (a) Unilateral facet dislocation results in anterior translation of one vertebral body onto the adjacent lower body for approximately one-fourth to one-half of its anteroposterior diameter. (b) The two lateral masses of dislocated vertebra overlap partially on the lateral radiograph, giving a 'bow-tie' sign.

and must be performed in fully awake patients to avoid the problems of deterioration of neurological function. If close reduction is successful the weight should be reduced to 5 kg for a few weeks, and followed either by halo vest treatment for 3 months, or by posterior wiring and bone grafting. Because traction alone is often unsuccessful, some recent reports recommend gentle manipulation as an adjunct.

Author's preferred procedure

I have had a closure success rate of 40% using Gardner–Well tongs and gently manipulating them by hand, applying a distraction force as well as manually rotating the neck. The gentle flexion of the neck unlocks the facet. This procedure needs to be performed in fully alert and co-operative patients.

To determine disc rupture with this pathology, it has been recommended that MRI is used before reduction because some authors have reported a deterioration of neurological function after open reduction. However, in all these patients, this procedure was performed under general anaesthesia. It may be necessary to attempt reduction of flexion injuries and total dislocations with early institution of skeletal traction with no more than 25 kg (Fried 1974). If this fails within a few hours after injury, the patient is taken to the operating theatre where, under local anaesthesia, an open reduction and posterior wiring is carried out and iliac grafting is performed. The patient can be immediately ambulated in a halo vest to a sitting position the following day, and the rehabilitation programme can be begun.

Once open reduction and fusion have been performed, a cervical myelogram is carried out for assessment of the spinal canal for any protrusion of bone or disc fragments anteriorly.

Author's preferred procedure

I attempt closed reduction by gradually increasing the weight of skull traction in fully conscious and awake patients. I monitor the patient's neurological status by asking if they have any abnormal feelings or tingling sensations in their shoulder and arm during traction or gentle manipulation. If the patient has any abnormal feelings or sensations then the procedure must be stopped. If the recommended maximum weight of traction is reached and the reduction has not been successful then I perform gentle manipulation before deciding to perform open reduction and fusion.

It has been recommended that MRI should be carried out to show a herniated disc at the affected level before open reduction is performed. If there is a large rupture or a potential rupture of the disc into the spinal canal and compression of the spinal cord, anterior discectomy decompression, anterior reduction, and fusion is recommended. But if the anterior reduction is not successful, the posterior approach to perform partial facetectomy, reduction, and posterior bone graft will be needed.

There is an alternative method if preoperative MRI is not available or if the patient's status is not stable enough for this investigation to be performed. It is generally accepted that realigning the dislocated spine is the first method to decompress the spinal cord and achieve the best recovery. Open reduction can be performed via the posterior approach under local anaesthesia in the awake intubated patient. After partial facetectomy is completed and the patient has no abnormal feeling of tingling, then the reduction can be performed and the patient's neurological function monitored. If there is no deterioration of neurological function then the patient is allowed to have general anaesthesia to harvest bone from the iliac crest for posterior wiring and fusion.

Bilateral facet dislocation

Bilateral facet dislocation is usually associated with a high incidence of cord injury. There is approximately 50% anterior displacement of the upper vertebral body with respect to the lower on lateral radiography. This injury includes disruption of virtually all ligaments and the disc. MRI can demonstrate any protrusion of the disc and can help to predict if there is sufficient risk to warrant anterior discectomy before realignment. Initial treatment usually includes skeletal traction in an attempt to obtain reduction, which is usually successful. The amount of force needed is variable; up to one-third of body weight is frequently recommended. Neurological recovery may be improved with realignment. The usual treatment for this injury following reduction is posterior wiring and fusion. Halo vest management after closed reduction has also done, usually for 3 months. However, this needs close follow-up because ligament healing may not be sufficient to prevent late kyphotic deformity or redislocation.

For patients with complete cord injury with successful closed reduction, treatment with posterior wiring and fusion is recommended. Adding anterior decompression and fusion in cases of retropulsion of the middle column compresses the spinal cord and increases the chance of nerve root recovery.

Complex fractures

A fracture is described as complex when it includes damage to the vertebral body and posterior ligament complex.

Burst fracture

A burst fracture is caused by an axial load resulting in compression of the posterior vertebral body with retropulsion of bone fragments into the spinal canal. Treatment alternatives are prolonged traction until sufficient bone union occurs to sustain an axial compressive force, or anterior decompression and reconstruction with an anterior strut graft. Orthosis, including the halo vest, does not provide significant resistance to axial compressive loads. Traction alone may not produce adequate canal decompression.

Direct anterior decompression and strut graft is recommended in the patient with incomplete spinal injury where roentgenography reveals a mechanical compression to the spinal cord from an anterior bony fragment of the vertebral body. A halo vest is recommended for external immobilization for 6–8 weeks. Additionally, an anterior cervical plate may be considered, if the posterior ligament complex is disrupted, but this treatment is somewhat controversial.

The principal of treatment of spinal trauma is the need to preserve neurological function. This is certainly the most important factor if the patient has incomplete neurological deficit and the image shows mechanical compression from anterior body fragments. Neurological deficit and recovery is not correlated with the amount of canal compression. It has been shown that mechanical bone block can carry secondary compression to the anterior longitudinal vessels of the spinal cord so direct anterior decompression can increase spinal cord blood supply and promote the recovery of spinal cord function (Bohlman 1985).

Teardrop fracture-dislocation

The teardrop fracture-dislocation is very different from the teardrop avulsion fracture from a major compressive force, and there is much more disruption. A posteroinferior fragment encroaches into the canal and causes the paralysis that usually occurs. Anterior decompression and strut graft reconstruction is recommended.

Other fractures

Cervical fracture in ankylosing spodylitis

The fracture of the cervical spine in the patient with ankylosing spondylitis is an uncommon injury. However, it is commonly associated with spinal cord injury. The mechanism of spinal injury may be due to displacement of the fused spinal column as well as epidural haematoma. This type of fracture may be difficult to visualize on plain radiographs, because the site of injury commonly occurs at or near the cervicothoracic junction and there may be little or no displacement. Bone scanning or tomography may be necessary to confirm the diagnosis. Treatment options include halo traction, cervical orthosis (halo vest, stenooccipitomandibular orthosis), and internal fixation. Halo traction, if used, should be applied in the direction of the preexisting deformity. Alignment should be determined by periodic lateral cervical spine radiography.

Gunshot wounds

Gunshot wounds seldom cause sufficient osteoligamentous damage to require surgical treatment. A recent multicentre study assessing motor and sensory recovery and pain reduction revealed that bullet removal did not improve neurological recovery. Most of the injury was caused by the effects of the blast. Treatment with a broad-spectrum antibiotic to protect against infection is recommended, especially where there are cerebrospinal fluid leaks. However, there may be a role for removal of the compressive mass effect from the bullet in cases of incomplete spinal cord injury.

Vehicle acceleration and deceleration ('whiplash') injuries

Whiplash injuries are caused by the overstretching of a muscle or ligament and may result in pain, localized tenderness, and a decreased range of motion. Other symptoms may be present which are not clearly related to the pathophysiology, such as headaches, visual blurring, diplopia, nausea, vertigo, hoarseness, and jaw pain. Structures that may be involved include the cranial nerves, vestibular apparatus sympathetic nerve fibres, and oesophagus. There is controversy over whether the intervertebral discs are injured. The major mechanism of injury is the traffic accident when the car was hit from behind. Significant symptoms may be long lasting: 42% persist beyond 12 months, and 36% persist beyond 24 months. However, 88% of the first group were symptom free within the first 8 weeks. Initial presence of occipital headaches, suprascapular or arm symptoms, abnormal nerve root signs, and interscapular pain, usually indicate a poor outcome of recovery. Radiographs are frequently normal or reveal only loss of normal cervical lordosis.

The principles of treatment include short-term immobilization followed by gradual motion, nonsteroidal anti-inflammatory medication, careful but progressive muscle activation, and appropriate amounts of reassurance and encouragement.

Key points

- Major mechanism of injury is vehicular accident (hit from behind).
- Symptoms may be long lasting (beyond 24 months).

Upper thoracic fracture

Usually the upper thoracic vertebrae (T2–T10) are stable, thanks to the rib cage. The injury of the spine at this level is caused by severe violent trauma and is usually associated with neurological deficit. In general, mild compression fractures, gunshot wounds, and mild subluxation of the vertebrae are usually stable and can be treated by non-operative well-moulded orthosis. Sagittal slice fracture, burst fracture, and severe wedge-compression fractures are caused by more violent injury. The major indication for internal fixation and fusion of the fracture is in fracture-dislocation and in those patients who have had laminectomy without arthrodesis.

Bohlman *et al.* (1985) reviewed 218 patients with complete paraplegia who had fractures of the upper part of the thoracic spine. Of these, 184 with complete cord injury did not recover any significant neurological function regardless of the type of operative or non-operative treatment. Early anterior decompression, stabilization, and fusion will result in the best neurological recovery in patients with an incomplete cord injury. Although a costotransversetomy approach can be used, a transthoracic approach will allow better visualization of the spinal cord and the spinal column. Patients with paralysis for more than 48 hours without evidence of recovery of neurological function do not require any decompression procedure.

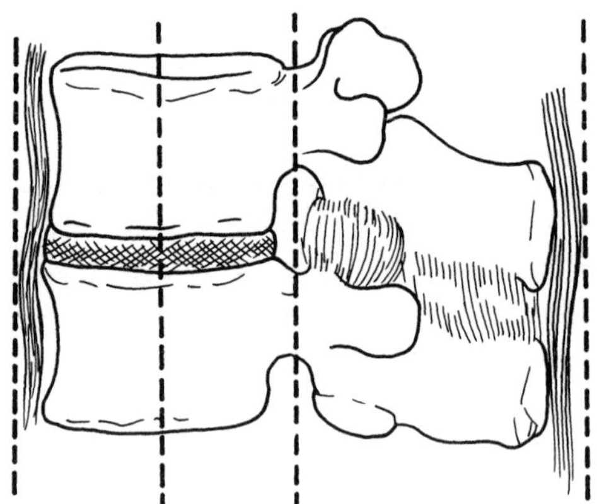

Figure 7.9 Denis's three-column concept of the spine. The anterior column consists of the anterior half of the vertebral body, anterior longitudinal ligament and anterior half of the disk. The middle column is composed of the posterior portion of the vertebral body and disk and posterior longitudinal ligament. The posterior column is the posterior ligamentous complex.

Thoracolumbar spine fracture

Denis (1984) proposed a three-column model of the spine, which has been widely accepted (Fig. 7.9). The middle column consists of the posterior longitudinal ligament, the posterior portions of the vertebral body, and the posterior annulus. Columns can fail individually or in combination by four basic mechanisms of injury—compression, distraction, rotation and shear. The resulting thoracolumbar spine injuries are of four major types.

Compression fractures

Compression fractures are a result of anterior or lateral flexion causing failure of the anterior column. The middle column remains intact and the injury rarely involves a neurological deficit. The posterior column may or may not be disrupted. The treatment depends on the status of the posterior elements. Non-operative treatment is preferred in those compression fractures where the amount of anterior compression is <40%, with <25–30° of kyphosis. If the anterior compression is >40% or more, or if the kyphosis >25–30°, or there is interference with the normal function of the posterior column, then initial posterior surgical treatment should be recommended.

Burst fractures

The essential feature of a burst injury is disruption of the anterior and middle columns with varying degrees of retropulsion into the neural canal, best identified on a CT scan. There may or may not be associated disruption of the posterior column (Fig. 7.10). There is a spreading of the posterior elements, seen on the plain anteroposterior radiograph of the spine as a widening of the interpedicular distance. Denis (1984) described five subtypes of unstable burst fractures: superior and inferior plate fracture; superior endplate fracture (the most common); lower endplate comminution; lateral collapse; and rotation.

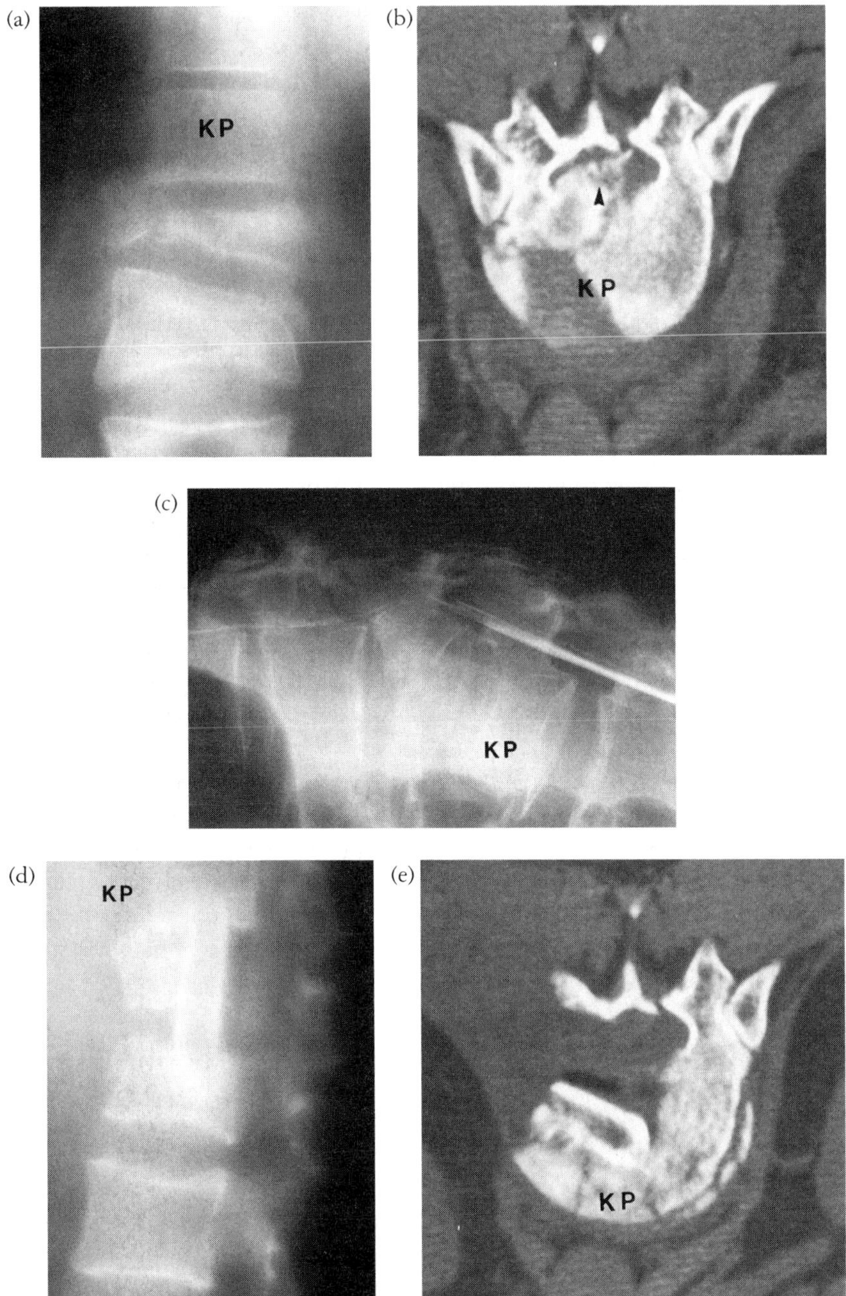

Figure 7.10 Denis's classification of burst fractures: (a) fractures of both end plates; (b) burst fracture with fracture of the superior end plate; (c) burst fracture with fracture of the inferior end plate; (d) burst fracture with rotation; (e) burst fracture with lateral bending.

The options for treatment depend on the severity of the injury. Management is based on the assessment of stability and the presence of a complete or incomplete neurological injury. The most important factors to be considered are the percentage of spinal canal compromise, the degree of angulation at the injury site, and the presence or absence of a neurological deficit. Treatment remains controversial. It is generally accepted that if the injured patient has no neurological deficit and canal compromise is <40%, there is no necessity for surgical decompression. If angulation is minimal, then these patients may be treated in a total contact thoraco-lumbar-sacral orthosis (TLSO) or hyperextension cast for at least 3 months. It has been demonstrated that the effectiveness of treatment usually results in kyphosis of 26.5° on average, with no correlation between kyphotic deformity and pain. The retropulsed fragments can gradually reabsorb with time, but late symptomatic kyphosis can be revealed with progressive deterioration of neurological deficit and there may be a need for late anterior decompression.

Initial surgical intervention is the preferred treatment in those patients with >40–50% of canal compromise, >25° kyphosis at the level of injury, and/or a neurological deficit. Decompression can be accomplished by posterior instrumentation via ligamentotaxis and should be performed within 2 weeks of the injury, otherwise soft callus around the fracture will prevent adequate reduction. Alternatively, this may be performed posterolaterally through the pedicle using the 'eggshell' technique or after resection of the pedicle. Instrumentation for two levels above and two levels below the affected fracture is accepted for the fracture at the thoracolumbar junction. The long rod and short fuse technique will provide the maximum effect of reduction by the mechanism of three-point effect with the long lever arm of the instrumentation (Chavasiri and Chavasiri 1998c). Care is needed to avoid overdistraction, especially when the fracture has disrupted the posterior ligaments. A double looped 1.2 mm wire passed around the spinous processes can act to prevent overdistraction. In addition, an intraoperative lateral spine radiograph is required. Prolonged immobilization of normal facets has been cited as a drawback to this technique. The pedicle screw and rods system is popular nowadays, extending only one level above and one level below the injury. It may be necessary to combine this with TLSO external immobilization for 1–2 months or with anterior fusion to provide axial support through the injured vertebrae. Problems of implant failure with resultant recurrent deformity and neural compression can occur, particularly if the normal spinal contour is not achieved. This is often not necessary in the lower lumbar and midlumbar spine, as more weight is carried through the posterior column of the spine.

Anterior decompression and strut bone graft fusion is indicated in patients with significant neural compression and incomplete neurological deficits. This is the best way to achieve adequate neural decompression. With the use of anterior instrumentation with strut bone grafts are usually indicated in those types of injury which have posterior element disruption. In any case anterior decompression using correct size of strut graft and good technique without anterior instrumentation can adequately decrease the occurrence of late kyphotic deformity. Bohlman (1976) reported that the result of late anterior decompression of the thoracolumbar spine can improve neurological function, and the patient will gain some grade of motor function, bowel and bladder control, and sexual function.

Distraction injuries

Chance fracture

A Chance fracture occurs due to distraction forces of the posterior and middle columns. This injury is usually secondary to seatbelt injury in someone wearing a seatbelt without a shoulder strap who is in a motor vehicle accident that produces a rapid deceleration over the belt. Initially there is posterior column failure, followed by progressive failure of the middle and anterior columns where the fulcrum of the injury is anterior to the vertebral column. The anteroposterior views will reveal a wide separation between the spinous processes. Treatment of pure osseous injuries consists of bed rest for a few weeks, followed by a total contact TLSO in hyperextension for 3–4 months and then assessment of stability by flexion/extension lateral radiographs. If non-operative treatment fails to achieve good stability of the injured spine, then surgical intervention using posterior compression instrumentation is recommended.

Flexion-distraction injuries

Flexion-distraction injuries are unstable, involving ligamentous disruption of the posterior elements and compression failure of the anterior column. Usually the fulcrum is at the middle column.

Fracture–dislocations

Fracture–dislocation injuries are considered to be highly unstable, because there is disruption of all three columns, and are often associated with neurological deficit, dural tears, and intra-abdominal injury. Complete dislocation or subluxation may occur, but some may reduce spontaneously. The majority of these patients require surgical treatment to realign the spinal column and to provide adequate posterior stabilization and decompression and allow early mobilization. There is rarely a role for primary anterior decompression. Anterior instrumentation alone is not sufficient to stabilize this type of injury because anterior screw fixation into the vertebral body is not rigid enough. There is also the disadvantage of the short lever arm mechanism of the implants.

Extension injuries

The mechanism of injury involves tensile forces applied to the anterior column and compression forces to the posterior elements. It may result in radiographic evidence of an anterior vertebral body avulsion fracture, as well as fractures of the spinous processes or laminae. These fractures are usually stable. These injuries can be treated with a flexion cast or orthosis for up to 12 weeks, depending on the patient's comfort.

Transverse process fracture

Fractures of the transverse processes are the result of direct blunt trauma or severe paraspinal muscle contraction. If there are multiple fractures of the transverse processes as the result of blunt trauma, associated intra-abdominal injuries and pelvic disruption are likely to be present.

Sacral fracture

Sacral fractures are often undiagnosed and untreated because radiographic diagnosis of this injury is difficult. Plain radiographs show only 30% of sacral fractures in most series. The Fugusion views are the best for the upper portion of the sacrum and can demonstrate injury to the foramen. Lateral radiographs can visualize a transverse sacral fracture. CT scanning demonstrates fracture lines and the severity of comminution in vertical type fractures of sacrum but is not so helpful in transverse sacral fractures. Denis *et al*. classified 236 cases of sacral fractures into zones.

- Zone I, the alar region, had 5.9% of patients with neurological deficit. There was occasional association with partial damage to the fifth lumbar root. The mechanism of injury frequently resulted from lateral compression. It is a stable fracture and usually treated with bed rest and early ambulation with partial weight bearing when symptoms permit.
- Zone II, or foraminal fractures, often resulted from vertical shear and 28.4% of those patients had some neurological finding, frequently associated with sciatica but rarely with bladder dysfunction. These fractures are usually stable and can be treated with bed rest and early mobilization. Sacral fractures in zone II associated with sciatica where the CT scan shows severe foraminal obstruction (75% occlusion) are best treated by foraminotomy.
- Zone III, the region of the central sacral canal, is frequently associated with saddle anaesthesia and loss of sphincter function (56.7% of

patients). Cystometry performed in conjunction with sphincter electromyography is most helpful in identifying fractures causing neurogenic bladder. When the fracture fragment is displaced and canal as well as foramen compression is evident, decompression via sacral laminectomy and foraminotomy at an early stage is recommended.

References

Alker GJ Jr, Oh YS, Leslie EV (1978) High cervical spine and cranio-cervical injuries in fatal traffic accidents. *Orthopedic Clinics of North America* 9: 1003–1010.

Anderson DK, Braughler JM, Hall ED *et al.* (1988) Effects of treatment with U-74006F on neurological outcome following experimental spinal cord injury. *Journal of Neurosurgery* 69: 562–567.

Anderson LD, D'Alonzo RT (1974) Fractures of the odontoid process of the axis. *Journal of Bone and Joint Surgery* 1663: 56A.

Anderson TE (1985) Spinal cord contusion injury, Experimental dissociation of hemorrhagic necrosis and subacute loss of axonal conduction. *Journal of Neurosurgery* 62: 115–119.

Apuzzo MLJ, Heiden JS, Weiss MH *et al.* (1978) Acute fractures of the odontoid process, An analysis of 45 cases. *Journal of Neurosurgery* 48: 85–91.

Aymes EW, Anderson FM (1956) Fracture of the odontoid process. *Archives of Surgery* 72: 377–393.

Bailey DK (1952) The normal cervical spine in infants and children. *Radiology* 59: 712–719.

Bailey JD (1978) Pathology of experimental cord trauma, II. Ultrastucture of axons and myelin. *Laboratory Investigations* 39: 254–266.

Balentine JD (1978) Pathology of experinebtal spinal cord trauma, I. The necrotic lesion as a function of vascular injury. *Laboratory Investigations* 39: 236–253.

Ballock RT, Mackersie R, Abitbol JJ *et al.* (1992) Can burst fractures be predicted from plain radiograph. *Journal of Bone and Joint Surgery* 74B: 147–150.

Bohler J (1965) Fractures of the odontoid process. *Journal of Trauma* 5: 386–390.

Bohlman HH (1976) Late progressive paralysis and pain following fractures of the thoracolumbar spine. *Journal of Bone and Joint Surgery* 728: 58A.

Bohlman HH (1985) Surgical management of cervical spine fractures and dislocations. *Instructional Course Lectures* 34: 163–187.

Bohlman HH, Ducker TB, Lucas JT (1982) Spine and spinal cord injuries, 2nd edn. In: Rothman RH, Simeone FA (eds) *The spine*. W.B. Saunders, Philadelphia..

Bohlman HH, Frechafer A, Dejak J (1985) The results of treatment of acute injuries of the upper thoracic spine with paralysis. *Journal of Bone and Joint Surgery* 67A: 360–369.

Bolesta MJ, Bohlman HH (1991) Mediastinal widening associated with fracture of the upper thoracic spine. *Journal of Bone and Joint Surgery* 73A: 447–450.

Bracken MB, Collins WF, Freeman DF *et al.* (1984) Efficacy of methylprednisolone in acute spinal cord injury. *JAMA* 251: 45–52.

Bracken MB, Shepard MJ, Collins WF *et al.* (1990) A randomized, controlled trial of methylprednisolone or naloxone in the treatment of acute spinal-cord injury, Results of the Second National Acute Spinal Cord Injury Study. *New England Journal of Medicine* 322: 1405–1411.

Brashear HR, Venters GD Jr, Preston ET (1975) Fractures of the neural arch of the axis, a report of twenty-nine cases. *Journal of Bone and Joint Surgery* 57A: 879–887.

Bucholz RW, Burkhead WZ (1978) The pathological anatomy of fatal atlantooccipital dislocations. *Journal of Bone and Joint Surgery* 60A: 279–284.

Chavasiri C, Chavasiri S (1998a) A study of Pavlov ratio in Thai people. *Siriraj Hospital Gazette* 50: 848–850.

Chavasiri C, Chavasiri S (1998b) Incidence of spinal injury in Siriraj hospital during 1996–1997. *Thai Journal of Trauma* 17: 22–24.

Chavasiri C, Chavasiri S (1998c) The efficacy of the Harrington distraction system vs pedicle screws and rod system for reduction of the cadaveric L1 burst fracture. *Thai Journal of Trauma* 17: 32–39.

Chavasiri C, Unnanantana A (1997) The first injury unit in Thailand. In: *WHO international seminar of prevention of spinal injury and rehabilitation*, 1997, Tokyo. WHO, Geneva.

Chavasiri C, Unnanantana A (1998) Outcome of the spinal injured patients at the first spinal injury unit in Thailand. *Siriraj Hospital Gazette* 50: 1–7.

Clark CR, White AA (1985) Fractures of the dens, A multicenter study. *Journal of Bone and Joint Surgery* 67A: 1340–1348.

Crooks F, Birkett AN (1944) Fractures and dislocations of the cervical spine. *British Journal of Surgery* 31: 252.

Denis F (1984) Spinal instability as defined by three-column spine concept in acute spinal trauma. *Clinical Orthopedics* 189: 65–76.

Denis F, Davis S, Comfort T (1988) Sacral fractures: an important problem. Retrospective analysis of 236 cases. *Clinical Orthopedics* 227: 67–81.

Ducker TB, Kindt GW, Kempf LG (1971) Pathological findings in acute experimental spinal cord trauma. *Journal of Neurosurgery* 35: 700–708.

Effendi B, Roy D, Cornish B *et al.* (1981) Fractures of the ring of the axis, A classification based on the analysis of 131 cases. *Journal of Bone and Joint Surgery* 63B: 319–327.

Eismont FJ, Bohlman HH (1978) Posterior atlantooccipital dislocation with fractures of the atlas and odontoid process, report of a case with survival. *Journal of Bone and Joint Surgery* 397: 60A.

Evarts CM (1970) Traumatic occipito-atlantal dislocations. Report of a case with survival. *Journal of Bone and Joint Surgery* 52A: 1653–1660.

Fielding WJ, Hawkins RJ, Hensinger RN, Francis WR (1978a) Atlantoaxial rotary deformities. *Orthopedic Clinics of North America* 9: 955–967.

Fielding WJ, Stillwell WT, Chynn KY, Spyropoulos EC (1978b) Use of computed tomography for the diagnosis of atlanto-axial rotatory fixation. *Journal of Bone and Joint Surgery* 59A: 37–44.

Fife D, Kraus J (1986) Anatomic location of spinal cord injury, relationship to the cause of injury. *Spine* 11(1): 2–5.

Fine PR, Kuhlemeier KV, DeVivo MJ *et al.* (1979) Spinal cord injury, An epidemiologic perspective. *Paraplegia* 17: 237–250.

Francis WR, Fielding JW (1978) Traumatic spondylolisthesis of the axis. *Orthopedic Clinics of North America* 9: 1011–1027.

Francis WR, Fielding JW, Hawkins RJ *et al.* (1981) Traumatic spondylolisthesis of the axis. *Journal of Bone and Joint Surgery* 63B: 313–318.

Fried LC (1974) Cervical spinal cord injury during skeletal traction. *JAMA* 229: 181.

Fried LC, Goodkin R (1971) Microangiographic observations of the experimentally traumatized spinal cord. *Journal of Neurosurgery* 35: 709–714.

Georgopoulos G, Pizzutillo PD, Lee M (1987) Occipito-atlantal instability in children, A report of five cases and review of the literature. *Journal of Bone and Joint Surgery* 69A: 429–436.

Hall ED (1988) Effects of the 21-aminosteroid U74006F on posttraumatic spinal cord ischemia in cats. *Journal of Neurosurgery* 68: 462–465.

Ikata T, Iwasa K, Morimoto K *et al.* (1989) Clinical considerations and biochemical basis of prognosis of cervical spinal cord injury. *Spine* 14: 1096–1101.

Jansen I, Hanseboul RR (1989) Pathogenesis of spinal cord injury and newer treatments, A review. *Spine* 14: 23–32.

Jones RN (1984) Rotatory dislocation of both atlanto-axial joints. *Journal of Bone and Joint Surgery* 66B: 6–7.

Kraus JF, Franti CE, Riggins RS *et al.* (1975) Incidence of traumatic spinal cord lesions. *Journal of Chronic Disease* 28: 471–492.

Levine AM, Edwards CC (1985) The management of traumatic spondylolisthesis of the axis. *Journal of Bone and Joint Surgery* 67A: 217–226.

Levine AM, Edwards CC (1986) Treatment of injuries in the C1–C2 complex. *Orthopedic Clinics of North America* 17: 31–44.

Levine AM, Edwards CC (1989) Traumatic lesions of the occipitoatlantoaxial complex. *Clinical Orthopedics* 239: 530–568.

Mouradian WH, Fietti VG Jr, Cchran GVB *et al.* (1978) Fractures of the odontoid, a laboratory and clinical study of mechanisms. *Orthopedic Clinics of North America* 9: 985–1001.

Nachemson A (1959) Fracture of the odontoid process of the axis, A clinical study based on 26 cases. *Acta Orthopaedica Scandinavica* 29: 185–217.

Ryan MD, Taylor TKF (1982) Odontoid fractures, A rational approach to treatment. *Journal of Bone and Joint Surgery* 64B: 416–421.

Sandler AN, Tator CH (1976) Review of the effect of spinal cord trauma on the vessels and blood flow in the spinal cord. *Journal of Neurosurgery* 45: 638–646.

Skold G (1978) Fractures of the neural arch and odontoid process of the axis, A study of their causation. *Zeischrift für Rechtsmedizin* 82: 89–103.

Southwick WO (1980) Current concepts review, Management of fractures of the dens (odontoid process). *Journal of Bone and Joint Surgery* 62: 482–486.

Tator CH, Duncan EG, Edmonds VE *et al.* (1988) Demographic analysis of 552 patients with acute spinal cord injury in Ontario, Canada, from 1948 to 1981. *Paraplegia* 26: 112–113.

Tator CH, Duncan EG, Edmonds VE *et al.* (1993) Changes in epidemiology of acute spinal cord injury from 1947 to 1981. *Surgical Neurology* 40: 207–215.

Wholey MH, Browner AJ, Baker HL Jr (1958) The lateral roentgenogram of the neck (with comments on the atlantoodontoid-basion relationship). *Radiology* 71: 350–256.

Wiesel SW, Rothman RH (1979) Occipito-atlantal hypermobility. *Spine* 4: 187.

Williams TG (1975) Hangman's fracture. *Journal of Bone and Joint Surgery* 57B: 82–88.

Wortzman G, Dewar FP (1968) Rotatory fixation of the atlantoaxial joint, Rotational atlantoaxial subluxation. *Radiology* 90: 479–487.

Yashon D (1978) Pathogenesis of spinal cord injury. *Orthopedic Clinics of North America* 9(2): 247–261.

Young W (1993) Secondary injury mechanisms in acute spinal cord injury. *Journal of Emergency Medicine* 11 (Suppl): 13–22.

8

CHAPTER 8

Brachial plexus injuries

PETER THOMAS,
GEOFFREY DONALD, AND
KAYVAN HAGHIGHI

CHAPTER 8

Brachial plexus injuries

PETER THOMAS, GEOFFREY DONALD, AND KAYVAN HAGHIGHI

The nerves which give sensation and control to the upper limb are all connected through the brachial plexus. Most brachial plexus injuries result in severe dysfunction of the arm and hand. In spite of advances in diagnosis and treatment, recovery in the majority of cases is still disappointing. The often catastrophic and permanent paralysis, numbness, and pain can have a devastating effect on a patient's ability to work and enjoy life. Optimum management of these injuries involves accurate diagnosis; repair or grafting of nerves which may recover; secondary operative treatment to stabilize joints by tendon transfer or arthrodesis; late tendon transfers to improve power; intensive rehabilitation; and pain management. When it is clear that an arm and hand will flail and remain numb, amputation will rid the patient of a useless limb and may allow for the use of a prosthetic arm or hand. The trauma surgeon must co-ordinate investigation and treatment by colleagues expert in imaging, neurophysiology, rehabilitation, pain management, counselling, and prosthetics. Patients with these devastating injuries require a great deal of support and encouragement. Operative surgery is of little use unless it is planned as part of a multidisciplinary approach.

Key point

- Most brachial plexus injuries result in severe dysfunction of the arm and hand.

Anatomy of the brachial plexus

The anterior grey columns contain the cells of the motor axons which pass via the anterior nerve root to the anterior ramus. These fibres, which are therefore postganglionic once they leave the cord, pass via the brachial plexus to the peripheral nerves in the arm and thence to the muscles. Sensory axons pass back up the peripheral nerves, through the brachial plexus, to the anterior ramus where they lie with the motor axons. They then pass into the dorsal nerve root where they are joined by sensory axons from the smaller posterior ramus. They then meet their cell bodies in the dorsal root ganglion where they synapse with preganglionic fibres which pass on through the dorsal nerve root to the cord. A lesion in or beyond the anterior ramus is therefore postganglionic: if the nerve root is torn out of the cord, the lesion is preganglionic.

The brachial plexus contains contributions from the anterior rami of the 5th, 6th, 7th, and 8th cervical and the 1st thoracic nerve roots after they have given segmental supply to the prevertebral and scalene muscles (Fig. 8.1). These nerve roots unite into three trunks: the 5th and 6th cervical form the upper trunk, the 7th cervical forms the middle trunk, the 8th cervical and the 1st thoracic the lower trunk. The trunks are located in the posterior triangle of the neck. They divide into anterior and posterior divisions which lie behind the clavicle. The upper two anterior divisions unite to form the lateral cord, the anterior division of the lower trunk forms the medial cord, and all three posterior divisions unite to form the posterior cord. In the axilla the three cords approach the first part of the axillary artery, envelop the second part, and give off branches around the third part. The roots lie between the scalene muscles, the trunks in the posterior triangle, the divisions behind the clavicle, and the cords in the axilla.

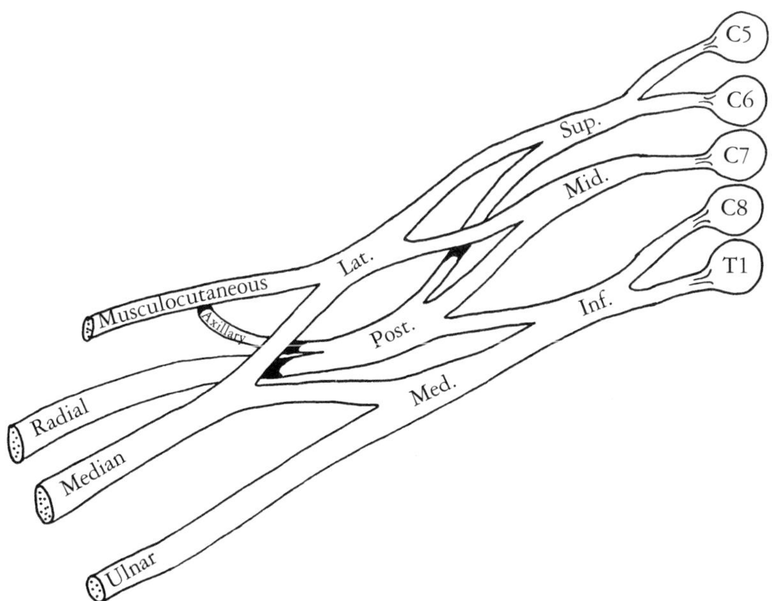

Figure 8.1 Anatomy of the brachial plexus.

Presentation

Acute injuries are caused by direct or indirect trauma. Direct trauma occurs in open injuries, indirect trauma usually in closed injuries. The commonest cause of closed trauma in Britain is a fall from a motorcycle. Brachial plexus injuries are more likely in any situation where an unprotected person is flung against something hard. They are more common in patients ejected from vehicles than in those who remain inside. The injury is usually a closed traction or avulsion of the brachial plexus or its roots. If the arm is forced downwards the damage may be confined to the upper roots or trunks. This will result in paralysis of the muscles of the shoulder girdle, with relative sparing of the muscles of the forearm and hand: the hand still works but cannot be placed or held in position. If the arm is forced upwards, the damage may be confined to the lower roots or trunks. This will result in paralysis of the muscles of the forearm and hand with relative sparing of the muscles of the shoulder girdle: the hand can be placed but will not work when it gets there.

Closed traction injuries can occur during a difficult delivery, when the baby will be found to have a paralysed arm at birth. Erb described the signs of a high root injury in neonates (Fig. 8.2) and Klumpke described those of injuries of the lower roots (Fig. 8.3). Traction injuries can also be iatrogenic. The dangerous 'Hippocratic' method of reducing a dislocated shoulder, by placing a foot in the axilla and pulling on the arm, can cause a traction injury as the plexus is stretched over the foot. Kocher's method is much safer.

The more severe traction injuries tend to be associated with fractures or dislocations around the shoulder girdle. The disruption of the bony skeleton allows wider displacement of the arm. Very severe traction injuries of this type are often associated with vascular injuries in the subclavian artery or its branches.

Penetrating injuries such as those caused by glass, knife, or shotgun can produce any combination of injuries to the plexus and surrounding structures.

The function of the brachial plexus may be compromised more slowly by pressure from something close by. A growing tumour, such as Pancoast's, can

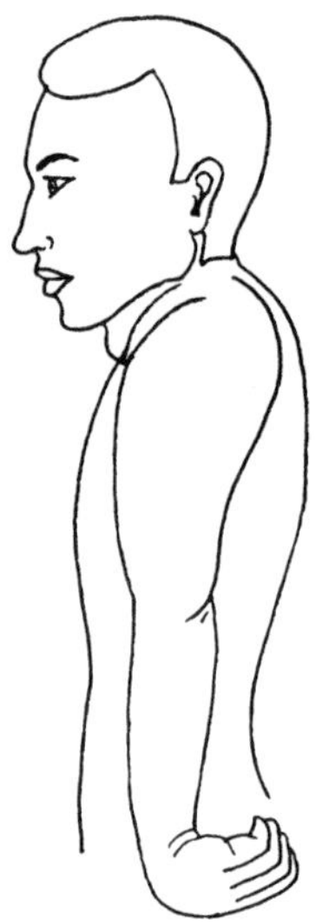

Figure 8.2 Erb's palsy (C5, C6).

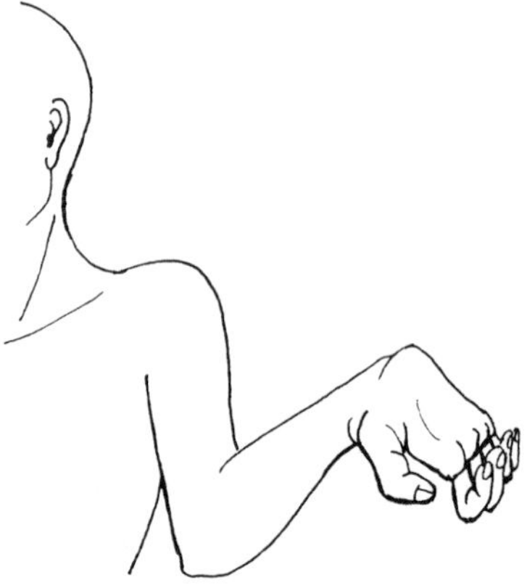

Figure 8.3 Klumpke's palsy (C8, T1).

press on the brachial plexus causing progressive dysfunction. A cervical rib or its fibrous analogue can irritate the brachial plexus stretched over it. Radiotherapy can cause fibrosis around the brachial plexus, resulting in progressive paralysis and pain.

Key point

- Direct trauma occurs in open injuries, indirect trauma usually in closed injuries.

Diagnosis

It is important to discover the exact mechanism of injury. In the conscious patient, weakness of one arm is usually obvious. Although it is often difficult in the acutely injured patient, a detailed neurological examination will usually allow one to delineate the extent of the brachial plexus lesion. An accurate record of these initial findings is also useful later. An improvement in the physical signs of a lesion, and the time over which this improvement occurs, may indicate whether it was a neurapraxia, an axonotmesis, or a neurotmesis.

- A *neurapraxia* is a 'concussion' of a peripheral nerve which usually recovers fully over hours or days.
- An *axonotmesis* is the name given to disruption of the axon within an intact enduneurial tube. This recovers over months as the axons grow back down the nerve at the rate of about 1 mm a day.
- The lesion is called a *neurotmesis* when part or all of the nerve is torn apart or cut through, disrupting all the structural elements. Unless repaired, a neurotmesis will not recover. Even when it is repaired carefully, the recovery from a neurotmesis is, at best, poor.

In the semiconscious patient a lack of spontaneous movement in one arm should make one suspicious of a brachial plexus injury, especially if a CT scan has excluded any intracranial cause for a hemiparesis.

Closed injuries in the unconscious patient are the most easily overlooked, but even here there can be useful signs. Denervated skin does not sweat, because the sudomotor fibres which control the sweat glands run with the sensory fibres to a particular dermatome. A brachial plexus lesion will disrupt a normal reflex arc. Reflexes should be elicited carefully.

The signs of Horner's syndrome are caused by loss of sympathetic innervation. The pupil is constricted on the affected side and there is loss of sweating on the same side of the head and neck. If the patient is able to open his or her eyes, unilateral ptosis will be observed. The sympathetic supply to these structures comes from preganglionic fibres which leave the lateral column of grey matter in the spinal cord and pass through the anterior ramus before leaving it in the white rami communicantes to the stellate ganglion. From there the postganglionic sympathetic fibres pass up towards the head. Horner's syndrome indicates avulsion of the 1st thoracic nerve root.

The acutely injured patient should be examined for any other injuries. If the brachial plexus injury is not associated with any other injury, then there is no indication for immediate surgery. The following investigations can then be planned:

- *Myelography* is useful for investigating nerve roots injuries. It demonstrates the post-traumatic pseudomeningocoels which form where the roots have been avulsed. The investigation must be delayed for a few weeks to allow the pseudomeningocoels to form. MRI scanning can give earlier information on the nerve roots and it can be combined later with myelography.
- *Nerve conduction studies* are not useful initially as they only confirm the neurological deficit found on physical examination. If there has been poor recovery over the first 3 months then nerve conduction studies become more helpful by showing where and whether recovery is occurring. Repeating a full neurological examination at regular intervals is the most useful way of mapping recovery.

Key points

- A brachial plexus lesion will disrupt a normal reflex arc.
- Horner's syndrome indicates avulsion of the 1st thoracic nerve root.
- Repeating a full neurological examination at regular intervals is the most useful way of mapping recovery.

Immediate surgical treatment

Immediate surgical treatment is indicated if the brachial plexus injury is associated with a penetrating injury, vascular injury, or bony injury requiring reduction with or without fixation. If the penetrating injury has been caused by something sharp—a knife, or glass—it is likely that the nerve lesions will be repairable by end-to-end anastomosis. Each lacerated nerve trunk is repaired with a fine non-absorbable interrupted epineural suture. There is no evidence that a more elaborate repair, such as repair of individual fascicles, confers any advantage. The suture is non-absorbable to induce the minimum tissue reaction in the nerve. The axillary artery lies within the brachial plexus. If a vascular surgeon intends to repair the vessels, it is vital that the nerves are repaired at the same time. Going in later would involve picking the vascular repair off the damaged plexus, a very difficult and dangerous task.

In a torn, ragged, or massive wound of the kind produced by a gunshot or chainsaw, for instance, a vascular injury in association with the brachial plexus injury is very likely. However, there is also likely to be tissue loss. The vascular repair will probably require vein grafts, and, for the reasons just given, the nerves will need to be repaired at the same time. Gaps in nerves will need to be filled with grafts too. Unfortunately, the best grafts are peripheral nerves taken from another part of the body. There is a short supply of suitable material. Any nerve which is harvested will leave a permanent deficit. The sural nerve is most commonly used first; this leaves numbness along the outer border of the foot. Very occasionally another limb or part of a limb requires primary amputation at the same time as grafts are needed for the primary treatment of the brachial plexus. In this unusual situation, peripheral nerves may be harvested from the amputated part. The nerve grafts are laid side by side to match the diameter of the nerve in which the gap is to be bridged. Each end of each graft is sutured with interrupted epineural stitches.

If there is a bony injury which requires reduction and stabilization, access to the brachial plexus may be gained while exposing the bone. A displaced fracture of the clavicle should be stabilized if associated with a brachial plexus injury. Access to the brachial plexus can be gained through this traumatic clavicular osteotomy.

Why shouldn't we explore the closed brachial plexus injury which is not associated with any of the concomitant injuries just mentioned? The reason is that even if the whole of the brachial plexus is explored acutely, the nature, site, and extent of the injury are often unclear. The damaged nerve trunks are usually found to be in continuity. Severe internal damage may extend over some distance. The only options are to leave alone or excise and graft. Which parts of the damaged nerve trunks should be excised and replaced with graft? It is usually impossible to say in a fresh traction injury. The site and extent of damage-in-continuity can only be assessed later by the degree and type of recovery measured clinically, and by nerve conduction studies. Excision of damaged nerve which might later recover would be a disaster and would waste valuable and scarce nerve graft.

When a nerve has been completely divided by a closed traction injury it is usually by an avulsion of the nerve roots from the spinal cord. This lesion cannot be repaired. The injury is preganglionic and will not recover even if the avulsed proximal end is sutured back into the spinal cord.

Key points

- If a vascular surgeon intends to repair the vessels, it is vital that the nerves are repaired at the same time.
- Suitable material for nerve grafts is in short supply; the sural nerve is most commonly used first.
- Excision of damaged nerve which might later recover would be a disaster.
- Avulsion of the nerve roots from the spinal cord cannot be repaired.

Physiotherapy and supportive treatment

Over the first few weeks after a closed traction injury of the brachial plexus, much needs to be done. The physiotherapist must endeavour to keep all the joints in the arm and hand fully supple, otherwise paralysed parts will quickly become stiff. This stiffness rapidly becomes irreversible and will compromise any later recovery of function. A flail arm will hang limply by the side, and the hand will become oedematous. This oedema will make the hand stiffer. The arm must be elevated when resting or carried in a sling when standing.

As patients become aware of the likely poor prognosis they will become anxious and depressed about what the future will hold for their employment, leisure, and social prospects. The help of a clinical psychologist familiar with these injuries is invaluable.

Key points

- The physiotherapist must endeavour to keep all the joints in the arm and hand fully supple.
- The help of a clinical psychologist is invaluable.

Planning of late surgical treatment

Clinical examination repeated every 4 weeks will demonstrate any recovery. If a preganglionic lesion is suspected, as a result of a Horner's syndrome for instance, an MRI scan or myelogram can be performed after about 4 weeks. If nerve root avulsions are found, there will be no recovery of nerve function. If the clinical examination and nerve conduction studies show progressive recovery then one should wait. If there is no recovery of a particular part of the brachial plexus then this should be explored and grafted after enough time has elapsed for any signs of recovery to begin: 6 months is a reasonable time to wait before considering exploration and grafting. In a totally flail limb, one complete peripheral nerve from the arm may be used to graft an extensive length of damage in the parts of the plexus which form other nerves. Deciding what to sacrifice to improve severely reduced function requires experience and care.

Tendon or muscle transfers may be used to restore the function of a paralysed muscle group. The principles of tendon transfer must be adhered to. It goes without saying that it is useless to transfer a paralysed muscle. A weak muscle will drop one MRC strength grade when transferred. The transferred muscle should, ideally, be phasic with the one it replaces; in other words, one should try to use a muscle which normally contracts at the same time as the one it is to replace or supplement. Flexor carpi ulnaris, for instance, is phasic with the finger extensors. Palpate your own flexor carpi ulnaris as you extend all your fingers strongly. It contracts phasically to stop the finger extensors from pulling the wrist into extension. The transferred tendon must have a similar excursion to the tendon it is supplementing or replacing. It must not be forced to go round too sharp a bend. Detaching it from its proper insertion should not reduce function more than the transfer will gain. Almost every muscle and tendon in the arm has been used in a reported successful transfer. Here are two examples:

- If the insertion of trapezius is detached from the acromion with a block of attached bone which is inserted into a groove cut in the outer aspect of the surgical neck of the humerus, the accessory nerve then supplies a muscle which abducts the shoulder.
- If the insertion of pectoralis major is detached and sutured to the proximal end of the biceps tendon, the elbow is now flexed by a muscle supplied by the lateral and medial pectoral nerves.

As these nerves come off the plexus between the trunks and anterior divisions, the transfer is only suitable for lesions of the cords or the posterior divisions.

Nerve transfers can improve function. The distal end of a functioning nerve is anastamosed to the proximal end of a nerve which has lost its proximal connection. Intercostal nerves can be used for transfers.

Stability of the upper limb can be improved by fusing one or more flail joints. The pectoralis major transfer just described only works well with a stable shoulder. If the shoulder is unstable as a result of weakness of the shoulder muscles, the transfer must be combined with a shoulder fusion. A fused shoulder allows the patient to control the position of the humerus with the shoulder girdle muscles. Fusion of the wrist helps to stabilize the hand in the absence of wrist flexor or extensors. This fusion also allows a functioning wrist flexor or extensor to be used as a transfer for improving hand function. The combination of fusions and transfers suitable for each patient will depend on their exact deficit and functional needs. Shoulder fusion combined with an elbow flexion transfer can restore useful function in a proximal brachial plexus lesion where the hand is spared.

Brachial plexus lesions often result in chronic pain with parasthesia in the limb, sometimes combined with phantom pain. Patients with these problems are often helped by visits to a specialized pain clinic where drug therapy can be combined with nerve block injections and psychological support with pain management strategies.

Key points

- Deciding what to sacrifice to improve severely reduced function requires experience and care.
- The principles of tendon transfer must be adhered to.
- Stability of the upper limb can be improved by fusing one or more flail joints.
- Patients are often helped by visits to a specialized pain clinic.

Prosthetics

The flail, insensate, and painful arm is the worst outcome of a complete brachial plexus lesion.

Supporting the limb with a brace can be helpful provided the shoulder has been fused. If elbow control can be gained with a tendon transfer, a wrist fusion can support the hand in an acceptable cosmetic position. Alternatively, a below-elbow amputation can allow the use of a better cosmetic prosthesis, provided elbow control exists or has been restored. Some patients still prefer to opt for trans-humeral amputation of the arm. Although with a transfer or fusion to control the shoulder it is possible to use a prosthesis, most patients tend not to. The purpose of the arm is to place the hand for sensory input and function. The pain, parasthesia, and sensitivity of the limb can make the wearing of a prosthesis uncomfortable. The purely cosmetic advantage of an artificial hand is often outweighed by the nuisance of it. Complex electropneumatic robotic limbs have been developed, but these still fail on the sensory side. Even when very accurate movement and placement of the artificial hand can be achieved, a 'blind' hand is not worth placing accurately.

Trauma surgeons sometimes consider brachial plexus injuries unrewarding to treat. If the final results are sometimes rather disappointing, this does not make these severely incapacitated patients less worthy of our best efforts. The best results of treatment are usually less spectacular than in many other types of limb injury, but the maximum possible return to function should still always be the aim.

Key points

- The flail, insensate, and painful arm is the worst outcome of a complete brachial plexus lesion.
- The maximum possible return to function should always be the aim.

Further reading

Carlstedt T, Grane P, Hallin R, Noren G (1995) Return of function after spinal cord implantation of avulsed nerve roots. *Lancet* 346(8986): 1323–1325.

Longmore J, Harvey J (1991) *Oxford handbook of clinical specialties*, 3rd edn. Oxford University Press, Oxford.

McMinn RMH (1994) *Last's anatomy, regional and applied*, 9th edn. Churchill Livingstone, Edinburgh.

Sherburn E, Kaplan S, Kaufman B, Noetzel M, Park T (1997) Outcome of surgically treated birth-related brachial plexus injuries in twenty cases. *Pediatric Neurosurgery* 27: 19–27.

Souza Neta E, Durand P, Sassolas F, Vial C, Lehot J (1998) Brachial plexus injury during cardiac catheterisation in children. *Acta Anaesthesiologica Scandinavica* 42: 876–879.

Tonkin M, Eckersley J, Gschwind C (1996) The surgical treatment of brachial plexus injuries. *Australian and New Zealand Journal of Surgery* 66: 29–33.

9

CHAPTER 9

Eye injuries

ANTONY F HENDERSON AND MICHAEL A HARGRAVES

CHAPTER 9
Eye injuries

ANTONY F HENDERSON AND
MICHAEL A HARGRAVES

Up to 10% of patients with facial trauma suffer significant injuries to ocular structures despite the eyes' many protective mechanisms, such as reflex lid closure, tear production, the cushioning effect of a retro-orbital fat pad, ocular deformation, and the protective bony orbital ridges. There are three main groups in the population who suffer eye trauma:

- The majority of patients are young men (males being affected four times more commonly than females) who are injured secondary to motor vehicle accidents, assaults, sports, and work-related injuries.
- Less commonly affected are small children who suffer ocular injuries owing to a combination of curiosity and immature motor skills.
- A third group consists of elderly people, suffering blunt ocular injuries from falls.

Current studies suggest a lack of awareness of potential ocular injury, with less than 50% of those patients with clinical signs potentially indicative of serious eye injuries actually receiving a formal ophthalmic examination.

Signs suggestive of serious ocular injury and indicating a need for ophthalmic assessment include subconjunctival haemorrhage, lid lacerations, diplopia, infraorbital anaesthesia, ptosis, and periorbital ecchymosis. Failure to recognize and act upon such signs may lead to exacerbation of ocular injuries.

This chapter outlines various ocular injuries classified according to the mechanism of trauma involved and will emphasize the signs that may indicate more serious ocular injuries. Important steps in diagnosis and management are discussed as well as investigative modalities such as ultrasound, which has reduced the need for exploratory surgery, with notes on surgical repair.

Assessment of ocular injuries

The assessment of ocular injuries is based on history, physical examination, and radiographic evidence. However, ocular injuries are rarely life threatening and treatment should be prioritized with respect to other life-threatening injuries.

History

A detailed history includes mechanisms involved, symptoms experienced, and general medical history. The history provides a good guide to the nature of the trauma and the probable injuries sustained.

Mechanism of injury

The magnitude and direction of forces involved will dictate the nature and extent of injury to the eye. Information of use includes the timing of injury, velocity, and nature of materials involved, blunt or projectile injury, and what protective eye wear was in place.

Symptoms

Decreased visual acuity is the most important symptom in eye injuries, but pain, blurred vision, discharge, tearing, diplopia, photophobia, floaters, flashing lights, or altered facial sensation are all of significance.

Ophthalmic history

The ophthalmic history should include any previous ocular history such as visual impairment, amblyopia, prior ocular trauma, whether contact lenses or spectacles are normally worn, family history of ocular disease, ophthalmic surgery, and ocular medications.

General medical and surgical history

The general history should include the patient's tetanus, hepatitis, and HIV status, and time of last oral intake.

Eye examination

The eyes should be examined in a systematic manner to avoid missing injuries.

Visual acuity is tested before eye manipulation or installation of mydriatics, and should be tested on each eye individually while occluding the other eye (test with glasses if normally worn). A Snellen chart is used. A patient who cannot read the largest letter on the chart should be asked to count fingers held up by the examiner. Failing this, hand motion perception is tested. If this cannot be detected then test light perception and light projection. The eyelids should be inspected for ecchymosis or lacerations, possible nasolacrimal system trauma, and levator injury. Palpation will reveal bony defects such as step-offs or depressions in the orbital rim. Hypoaesthesia in the distribution of the infraorbital nerve may be present in blowout fractures. The sensation in the ipsilateral cheek, upper lip, and upper gum should be tested. While the patient elevates the head and looks down, the eyelid should be everted to reveal foreign bodies or signs of trauma. The cornea should be examined for loss of clarity, irregularities, and foreign bodies, and the sclera for haemorrhages. An ophthalmoscope should be used. Fluoroscein dye uptake viewed with a cobalt blue light will demarcate corneal abrasions. The anterior chamber should be examined for blood, pus, or loss of depth; a thorough examination requires use of a slit-lamp. Pupil size, shape, symmetry, and direct/consensual pupillary responses should be inspected to detect an afferent pupillary defect. The swinging torch test should be performed. The irises should be inspected for iridodonesis (trembling of the iris during rapid eye movement due to poor iris support, e.g. lens subluxation). Ophthalmoscope examination can also demonstrate the presence or absence of the red reflex. Slit-lamp examination detects damage to the cornea, anterior chamber, iris, and lens. If a slit-lamp is unavailable, a simple pen light examination should be used to detect a hyphaema, corneal laceration, or shrunken globe. The visual field to confrontation should be noted. The face should be examined for fractures or cranial nerve palsies, and a general examination carried out for other significant injuries that may be more urgent. Photographs are often helpful for documentation.

Key points

- Clinical assessment of eye injuries involves a thorough history (mechanism of injury, symptoms experienced, past medical and ophthalmic history) and examination (visual acuity, eversion of eyelid, ophthalmoscopy, and slit-lamp examination).

Radiographic investigations

Plain films are useful for evaluating the orbits and sinuses, and detecting radio-opaque foreign bodies and air/fluid levels.

CT scan is the preferred imaging modality. An injury suspected on clinical grounds should be evaluated by CT imaging, whether or not plain radiographic films yield information: 1.5 mm cuts in the axial and coronal views are useful in evaluating orbital fractures, orbital rupture, emphysema, haemorrhages, and foreign bodies.

Ultrasonography is helpful in visualizing lens dislocation, vitreous haemorrhages, retinal detachment, and intraocular foreign bodies. This modality is contraindicated if the globe is perforated or ruptured.

MRI scanning is seldom used in the acute setting, but it is superior in viewing soft tissues.

Classification and types of injuries

Ocular injuries can be classified as closed or open (see Fig. 9.1).

- *Blunt injuries*: the eye wall does not have a full-thickness wound.
- *Open globe or penetrating injuries*: the eye wall has a full-thickness wound.

A blunt force causes a globe rupture and a sharp object causes a laceration at the site of impact.

Lacerations may be penetrating with a single entrance wound, or a perforating with an entrance and exit wound.

Types of injuries are illustrated in Fig. 9.2.

Superficial ocular injuries

Orbital haemorrhage

An orbital haemorrhage gives the appearance commonly known as a 'black eye'.

Ecchymosis and swelling

Ecchymosis and swelling to the orbital region may give rise to restricted eye movement and proptosis. These findings may make examination of the underlying structures difficult; however, more serious underlying injury such as an orbital fracture should be suspected.

Before investigating, the head should be elevated and topical anaesthetic drops instilled. Desmares lid retractors should be used to facilitate inspection of the globe. The eyelid should not be forced open. In uncomplicated cases the swelling resolves in 2–3 weeks. Treat with an ice pack, head elevation, and reassurance.

Subconjunctival haemorrhage

A subconjunctival haemorrhage (SCH) is a painless, bright red haemorrhage under the bulbar conjunctiva, which does not extend beyond the limbus. Typically the patient reports a prior coughing or vomiting episode, or has no recollection of preceding events. These haemorrhages may also be associated with hypertension or a bleeding disorder. An SCH associated with trauma and without a definable posterior border may be caused by blood tracking anteriorly from a basal skull fracture, and is an indication for CT of the skull. If an SCH is associated with pain on extraocular movement, underlying scleral perforation should be suspected. Once co-existing ocular injuries and hypertension

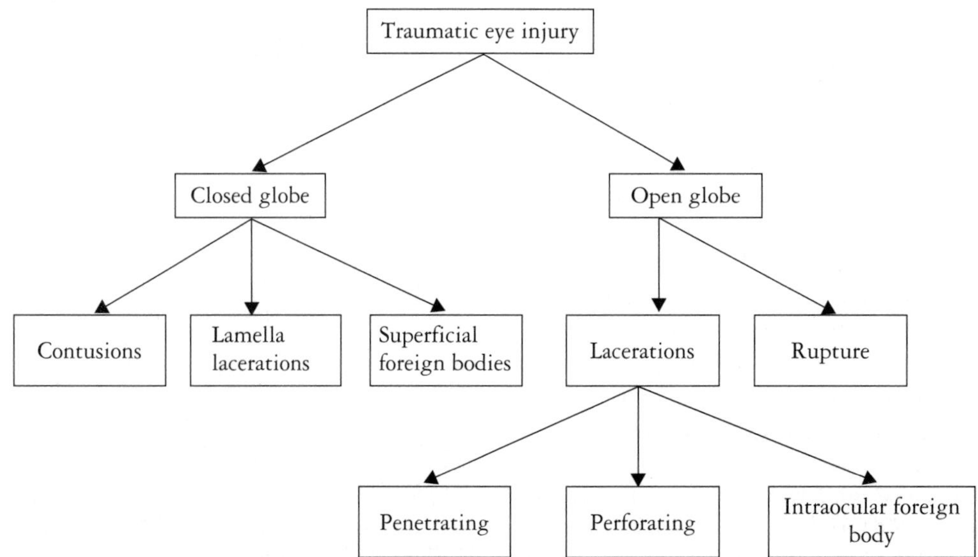

Figure 9.1 Classification of eye injuries.

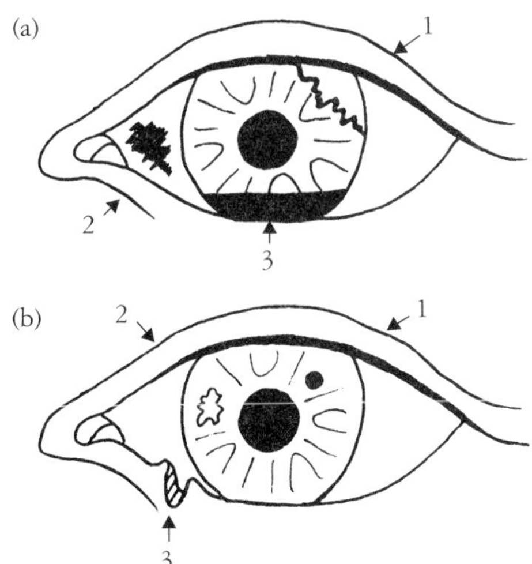

Figure 9.2 Types of eye injuries.
(a) 1. Iridodialysis; 2. Subconjunctival haemorrhage; 3. Hyphaema.
(b) 1. PErforation/penetration; 2. Corneal abbraisors; 3. Lower eye legment laceration.

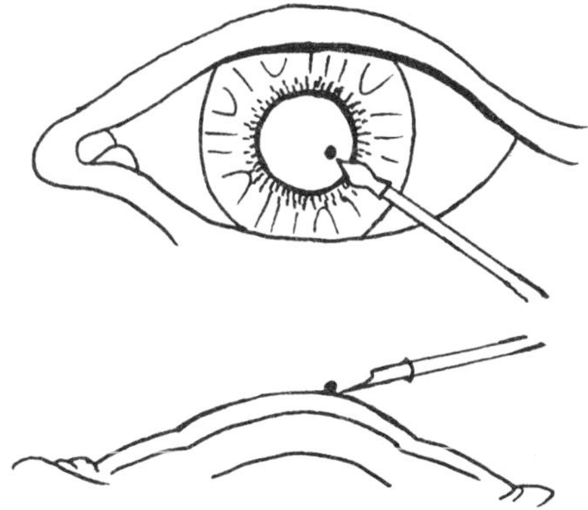

Figure 9.3 Corneal foreign bodies.

have been ruled out, no further treatment is necessary and resolution will occur within 2–3 weeks.

Corneal abrasions

A corneal abrasion is a focal loss of corneal epithelium following a blunt injury to the globe, caused for example by a fingernail, paper edge, foreign body, or contact lens. Symptoms may include pain, foreign body sensation, blurred vision, lacrimation, and photophobia. Slit-lamp examination with fluorescein dye is used to demarcate the size and position of the abrasion. The eyelids should be everted to exclude presence of a foreign body.

Contact lenses should not be worn during healing. Cycloplegics (2% cyclopentolate) may relieve blepharospasm. Antibiotics (chloramphenicol) for 4 days and daily review are required until the abrasion heals. Recurrent or persistent abrasions require ophthalmologic review.

Corneal foreign bodies

The foreign bodies most commonly found are metallic or glass particles lodging in the corneal surface as a result of grinding or hammering (see Fig. 9.3). Symptoms include pain, foreign body sensation, and lacrimation. Slit-lamp examination may reveal a foreign body; if metallic, it may be surrounded by rusty infiltrate.

Before treatment, 2–3 drops of local anaesthetic should be instilled. The foreign body should be prised off gently with a sterile 21G needle under slit-lamp magnification, with the patient focusing on a distant object and the operator's hand resting on the patient's cheek to reduce relative movement. Beware: repeated application of topical anaesthetic slows healing and may result in epithelial toxicity. Once the foreign body is removed, the remaining corneal abrasion is examined and treated with topical antibiotics and an eye patch. Multiple foreign bodies on the corneal surface may be more easily removed by irrigation or a cotton-tipped applicator soaked in local anaesthetic. Some deeply embedded inert foreign bodies such as non-leaded glass may be left in, as removal may lead to extensive scarring. In addition, deep foreign bodies should not be removed as removal may risk an aqueous leak. The eye should be covered with a protective metal shield and the patient referred for surgical management. If there is a suspicion of penetrating eye injury, careful inspection in the area of the conjunctival laceration is always required to rule out a scleral laceration or an intraocular foreign body. Dilated retinal examination is required to look for retinal damage or intraocular foreign body (IOFB). A CT scan (axial and coronal views) should be considered, to exclude an IOFB or a ruptured globe.

Conjunctival laceration

A conjunctival laceration is a superficial injury resulting from a sharp object, for example a rose thorn. It may produce symptoms of mild pain, eye redness, lacrimation, blepharospasm, or a foreign body sensation. SCHs are commonly present. Slit-lamp examination with white light may reveal a torn conjunctiva. The edge of the laceration stains brightly with fluorescein dye. Local anaesthetic is instilled and the conjunctiva is gently explored with a moist cotton swab, opened up and sclera exposed, to exclude possible perforation or scleral laceration. The conjunctiva has a protective rather than a structural role, which explains why conjunctival lacerations <1 cm heal without suturing. Lacerations >1 cm, or if Tenon's capsule has been torn, requires suturing with 6.0 or 8.0 absorbable sutures (Dexon or Vicryl) under topical anaesthetic. Topical antibiotics are required for 5–7 days and an eye patch for 24 hours. Follow-up for large lacerations is in 7 days. For full-thickness lacerations, see 'Ruptured globe'.

Corneoscleral lacerations

Corneoscleral lacerations are partial or full-thickness lacerations through the cornea or sclera. In adults they commonly result from work-related injuries involving small projectile fragments; in children, from injuries caused by pens, needles, or sharp toys. The patient may complain of decreased visual acuity, pain, or lacrimation. The globe should be handled cautiously to avoid applying pressure that might rupture a partial-thickness laceration or herniate the ocular content of a full-thickness laceration. If a ruptured globe is suspected, or if signs of perforation become apparent, then no further examination should be done. The eye is lightly padded and protected with a shield and the patient is prepared for further examination and repair in the operating theatre.

Partial-thickness laceration

A complete ocular and slit-lamp examination is required. Signs of perforations should be looked for (see 'Ruptured globe'). A drop of 2% fluorescein placed on the cornea over a possible entry site will become diluted by the issuing aqueous, turn green, and fluoresce (positive Seidel's test). Applanation tonometry may reveal hypotony. Inspection may reveal a shallow anterior chamber, pupil asymmetry, cataract formation, or lens capsule rupture.

The goals of treatment are to prevent infection, promote stromal healing, minimize scarring or surface irregularities, and prevent irregular astigmatism. Shallow lacerations are treated with cycloplegics (5% homatropine), prophylactic antibiotics (0.3% gentamicin), and a patch. Occasionally therapeutic soft contact lenses (TSCL) are used for 2–4 weeks until healing is complete. Long partial-thickness corneal lacerations accompanied by a wound gape are often sutured closed in theatre. Daily follow-up is required until healing is complete.

Full-thickness lacerations

Full-thickness lacerations that do not violate the limbus, do not have uveal or vitreous incarceration, are small (<3 mm), and are self healing (see 'Ruptured globe'). They may respond to non-operative measures such as TSCL to support the wound as it heals. Aqueous humour suppressants (acetazolamide, topical beta-blockers), antibiotics (0.3% ciprofloxacin) and cycloplegics (2% cyclopentolate) are used. Cyanoacrylate tissue adhesive is useful for non-self sealing puncture wounds <2 mm, or in the visual axis (sutures would impinge vision).

Eyelid lacerations

Eyelid lacerations require a complete ocular examination including a dilated retinal examination (Fig. 9.4). Suspicion of an orbital foreign body, ruptured globe or significant orbital trauma requires a CT scan (axial and coronal views with 1.5 cm cuts). Simple skin lacerations in the periorbital area are cleaned with povidone-iodine and the wound is irrigated with a syringe containing saline. Foreign bodies should be looked for. A surgical field should be isolated with sterile drapes and the eye covered

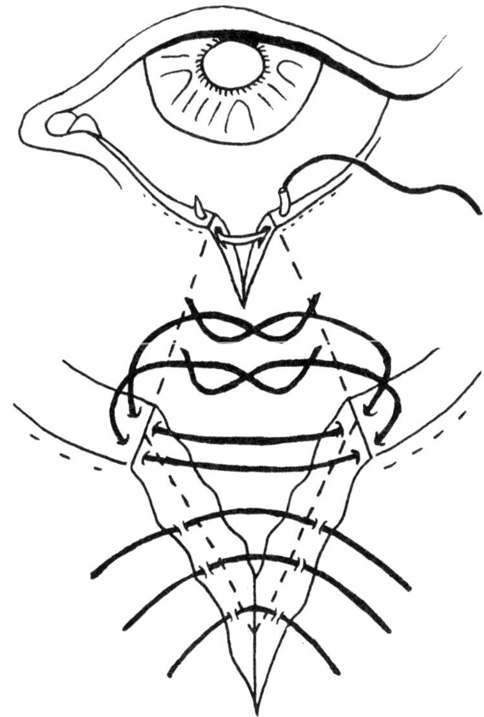

Figure 9.4 Eyelid lacerations.

with a protective shield. The various lacerations should be sutured as follows:

- Simple skin lacerations: Interrupted stitches under direct vision with fine non-absorbable 6.0 nylon. Sutures should be removed in 4 days.
- Deep lacerations of the eyelid: These are closed in two layers. Interrupted 6.0 absorbable sutures (Vicryl) are used to close the deeper tarsal layer without breaching the conjunctiva. The suture should be cut close to the knot.
- The superficial orbicularis and skin are closed with interrupted 6.0 non-absorbable sutures (nylon).

Eyelid margin lacerations must be accurately apposed to prevent deformity. Repair is carried out under sterile conditions using an operating loupe. Repair of the lid margin takes place before the skin repair. The lid margin is aligned using absorbable suture (6.0 Vicryl), which is passed subcutaneously through the orbicularis muscle and the tarsal plate. A single throw is placed to test correct alignment. Two further subcutaneous absorbable sutures (6.0 Vicryl) are placed in a similar way further away from the lid margin and spaced at regular intervals. Once tied, the suture ends are left long. The skin is sutured from the lid margin downwards (using two layers if the laceration is deep). The long ends of the three eyelid margin sutures are tied under the knot of the uppermost skin suture to prevent the suture ends from rubbing against the cornea. Topical antibiotics are applied and a course of systemic antibiotics in the case of contamination (dicloxacillin) or human/animal bites (cephalexin). Potentially contaminated wounds may benefit from a delayed wound closure of 2 days. Eyelid marginal sutures are removed in 10–14 days and skin sutures in 4–6 days.

Complex eyelid lacerations are those associated with severe ocular trauma (e.g. ruptured globe), the lacrimal apparatus, the levator aponeurosis producing ptosis, the superior rectus muscle exposing orbital fat, avulsion of the medial canthus tendon, or IOFB, and those involving extensive tissue loss or distortion of the anatomy. Treatment requires complex surgical repair.

Global ocular injuries

Intraocular foreign bodies

The presence of an IOFB must be excluded in all ocular injuries. A history of hammering metal on metal is highly suggestive. IOFBs cause ocular damage by disrupting the normal anatomy, introducing infection, scar tissue formation, and inflammatory reactions to the retained foreign body. Symptoms include pain or decreased vision. Clinically detectable signs may be absent, but if the history is highly suggestive of a penetrating injury, it is important not to cause further damage by doing a rigorous examination. Signs suggestive of a penetrating injury are hyphema, subconjunctival haemorrhage, irregular pupil, anterior or posterior segment inflammation, decreased intraocular pressure, or a hole in the iris seen by retroillumination. Under slit-lamp illumination, the anterior chamber and iris should be searched for a foreign body. An iris transillumination defect may be found by directing a small beam of light through the pupil and looking at the iris for a red reflex. The lens should be examined for disruption, cataracts, or IOFBs.

Investigations

Plain radiology is indicated for all ocular injuries involved in hammering or chiselling injuries involving metallic bodies (posteroanterior and lateral views) and CT scan or ultrasound for non-metallic bodies (MRI scan is contraindicated for metallic bodies).

Treatment

The patient should be transferred supine and kept nil by mouth. A protective shield should be placed over the involved eye and the contralateral eye covered with soft conjugate movement. In addition, tetanus prophylaxis should be noted, the entry site cultured, and intravenous antibiotics administered. Surgical removal of the IOFB is always indicated. Surgical repair involves suturing the entry site and the planned removal of the foreign body at a later date. Metallic foreign bodies require removal within 24 hours. Anterior foreign bodies are removed by corneal section and, if the lens is involved, lensectomy. Posterior foreign bodies are removed by forceps after a vitrectomy. Inert foreign bodies such as glass, stone, and plastics may not need removal but can simply be observed periodically for signs of inflammation.

Key points

- Do not cause further damage with a rigorous examination if clinical history is highly suggestive of penetrating injury.
- Radiography is indicated for all injuries involving metallic particles.

Ruptured globe

A ruptured globe is a full-thickness traumatic disruption of the sclera or cornea resulting from blunt forces causing an abrupt rise in intraocular pressure. It usually arises from work-related injuries, violence, or sports. The globe decompresses and ruptures through the weakest point—the insertion of the extraocular muscles or the corneoscleral junction. Diagnosis is usually obvious but may be occult. Symptoms and signs suggestive of globe rupture include pain, deceased visual acuity (a normal visual acuity is rarely present in a globe rupture), extensive SCH (often involving 360° of bulbar conjuctiva), a deep or shallow anterior chamber, hyphaema, low intraocular pressure (IOP) (but the IOP can be normal or high), irregular pupil, iridodialysis, cyclodialysis, lens subluxation, commotio retinae, retinal tears, vitreous haemorrhages, obvious corneal or scleral lacerations, or intraocular contents outside the orbit.

Treatment

A ruptured globe is an ophthalmological emergency. Further examination is avoided once the diagnosis of ruptured globe is made. Manipulation of the eye should be avoided, as pressure on the globe may risk extrusion of the intraocular contents and introduce infection. The eye should be protected with a shield and the patient kept nil by mouth. Treatment is with bed rest, systemic antibiotics (cephazolin and gentamicin) to prevent endophthalmitis, tetanus toxoid as necessary, antiemetics, analgesia (topical agents are contraindicated), and consent for the operative procedure.

Plain radiographs will detect radio-opaque metal foreign bodies and CT scan (axial and coronal sections 1.5 mm apart) is also useful. Radiolucent materials (wood and plastic) may be detected by MRI and may localize the rupture and exclude an IOFB.

Surgical repair involves exploration and repair of various damaged tissues according to a plan formulated before operating. Vitreous haemorrhages may predispose to proliferative vitreoretinopathy with scar formation and contraction. A vitrectomy can remove this stimulus and improve anatomical and visual outcome. Extensive injuries to the anterior segment may require secondary reconstruction. Enucleation is indicated as a last resort in the case of continued deterioration of the visual function. The various reconstructive procedures are beyond the scope of this book.

Orbital fractures

Orbital blowout fractures strictly involve only the orbital floor and spare the orbital rim. They are caused by direct impact of a blunt object just larger than the orbital rim (human fist, squash ball) forcing the eye back into the orbit, causing a sudden raise in the IOP and a blowout fracture at the weakest part of the orbit, the thin orbital floor. Herniation of the intraorbital contents into the bony defect may occur. Clinical features include pain (especially on attempted vertical eye movement, owing to entrapment of the inferior rectus and inferior oblique muscle). For the same reason there is restricted eye movement, particularly elevation and diplopia more marked on vertical gaze. There is paraesthesia around the cheek and upper lip below the eye due to damage of the infraorbital nerve and enopthalmos (measured by an exopthalmometer once swelling has subsided) due to orbital herniation into the maxillary sinus. Other signs may include epistaxis, eyelid oedema, and ecchymosis, and subcutaneous emphysema may occur on sneezing or nose blowing. Ophthalmological examination includes careful evaluation for rupture, hyphaema, or microhyphaema, traumatic iritis, retinal or choroidal damage. IOP should be measured. CT scan of the orbits and brain (axial and coronal views) is indicated if diagnosis is uncertain or surgical repair considered.

Treatment

Broad-spectrum oral antibiotics should be commenced, the patient instructed not to blow their nose, and ice packs applied to the orbit for 24–48 hours. Less severe cases are treated conservatively. Surgical repair at day 5–10 is indicated for more severe injuries, significant entrapment of soft tissues (persistent diplopia), or cosmetically unacceptable enophthalmos (>2 mm). Patients are followed up and monitored for the development of associated ocular injuries (e.g. orbital cellulitis, angle-recession glaucoma, and retinal detachment).

Medial wall orbital fractures are less common and may give rise to subcutaneous emphysema around the nose and eyelid. There is epiphora if the nasolacrimal duct is involved. Weakness of lateral eye movement and diplopia occur if the medial rectus muscle is entrapped. Plain radiographs may show herniated contents in the maxillary sinus and air in the orbit. CT scans provide more information. Treatment is with antibiotics to prevent orbital cellulitis, and eye padding. The patient should be instructed not to blow their nose until surgical correction is complete. Surgical correction is indicated if the medial rectus muscle is entrapped in the fracture.

Anterior segment injuries

Hyphema

Traumatic hyphaema is the presence of blood in the anterior chamber of the eye caused by tearing of small ciliary or iris vessels from blunt or penetrating injuries. They are classified according to the percentage of the anterior chamber filled with blood. A total hyphaema is often referred to as an 'eight ball hyphaema'. Symptoms include a dull ache and reduced visual acuity that improves as the blood settles. Layering of blood inferiorly in the upright patient is a sign. A force large enough to produce a hyphaema may cause other injuries, such as angle recession, lens subluxation, and peripheral retinal tears.

Complications include rebleeding (most commonly between 24 and 48 hours), elevated IOP (secondary to red blood cells obstructing the outflow canal of Schlemm), synechiae formation, and permanent corneal blood staining (facilitated by raised IOP).

Investigations

IOP should be measured using applanation tonometry (if it is very low, a ruptured globe should be suspected). B-scan ultrasound should be used to exclude retinal detachment.

Treatment aims to decrease risk of future bleeding, reduce complications, and screen for other ocular injuries. Most hyphemas spontaneously reabsorb within a week. Mydriatics are used to increase patient comfort and to prevent the formation of synechiae. Treatment is with antiemetics, mild analgesia, and avoidance of aspirin; the eye should be covered with a protective shield. Raised IOP (>25 mmHg) should be treated with topical beta-blockers (0.5% timoptol), acetazolamide, or intravenous mannitol if IOP >35 mmHg Treat. If the IOP remains high, the hyphaema should be treated surgically. Once the hyphema has cleared the drainage angle should be examined by gonioscopy to exclude recession. Some patients may require admission, but compliant patients with small hyphemas may be treated as outpatients. Treat with 1% atropine daily, slit-lamp examinations, and IOP measurement.

A sudden increase in pain or decrease in vision should alarm the patient to return for re-evaluation.

Traumatic iridocyclitis/uveitis

Iridocyclitis/uveitis—inflammation of the anterior chamber (iris and ciliary body)—can occur as a result of blunt trauma. Symptoms include pain, photophobia, and blurred vision. Inspection may reveal pupillary constriction secondary to spasm or a dilated pupil from traumatic mydriasis. Slit-lamp examination reveals perilimbal injection, white cells, and flare reaction. The IOP may be reduced if the inflamed ciliary body is producing less aqueous humour, or increased secondary to inflammatory obstruction of the draining trabecular meshwork. Other conditions associated with an anterior chamber reaction must be suspected, such as a traumatic corneal abrasion, traumatic hyphaema, and traumatic retinal detachment. Treatment is with cycloplegic agents (2% cyclopentolate) until inflammation subsides. Steroid drops (1% prednisone acetate) may be used. At 1 month ophthalmoscopy and gonioscopy should be performed to exclude angle recession and retinal breaks or disruption.

Traumatic mydriasis and miosis

Bruising and irritation of the iris sphincter can cause constriction. Small tears in the sphincter muscle fibres can cause dilatation. These defects may resolve over days or be permanent if the muscle fibres are damaged. Treatment is supportive and it is important to inform the patient of pupil asymmetry to avoid unnecessary investigations later.

Iridodialysis

Avulsion of the iris from its root, giving rise to separation of the iris from the sclera, may result from blunt trauma. No specific treatment is required, but ophthalmological referral is mandatory, as this condition may appear as a second pupil and can cause monocular diplopia, or the cosmetic defect may require surgical correction.

Traumatic glaucoma

Acute glaucoma may result from blunt injuries disrupting the canal of Schlemm and narrowing the angle of the anterior chamber. Lens swelling or dislocation can impede the outflow of aqueous humour and give rise to an acute elevation of IOP. Treatment is with miotics to increase the angle, topical beta-blocking agents (timolol), acetazolamide to decrease aqueous formation, and in the last resort mannitol.

Injuries to the lens

Traumatic cataract may result from a blunt or penetrating injury. Disruption of the lens capsule will cause the stromal cells to absorb fluid, swell, and cloud obscuring vision. Mild injuries lead to small anterior lens opacities that may not progress. More severe trauma may lead to either central posterior opacities which progress or peripheral lens opacities, which tend to be static. Treatment involves observing the cataract progression and allowing retinal pathology to settle for 6 months followed by lens replacement if sight is limited.

Lens subluxation or dislocation results from a severe blunt force applied to the globe in an antero-posterior direction causing stretching of the equatorial region and tearing of the zonule fibres. If more than 25% of these fibres are ruptured then the lens becomes unstable and may subluxate/dislocate into the anterior or posterior chamber. Anterior dislocation may give rise to acute angle closure glaucoma, and surgery is indicated. Posterior dislocation of the lens into the vitreous may be asymptomatic, and requires conservative treatment. A possible sign present is trembling or shimmering of the iris with rapid eye movements (iridodonesis). If it is complicated by secondary glaucoma, uveitis, vitreous inflammation, or cataract formation giving rise to visual loss, lens replacement will be necessary.

Posterior segment injuries

Vitreous haemorrhage

Haemorrhage in the vitreous may occur secondary to tearing of retinal vessels in blunt trauma. Retinal and choroidal tears must also be suspected. Symptoms include floaters, and dark streaks that move with the eye (blood in the vitreous humour). Signs include inability to view the fundus and loss of the red light reflex. Ultrasound and indirect ophthalmoscopy are used to evaluate the retina and choroid. Treatment is by head elevation, and ophthalmological referral. Delayed vitrectomy is indicated if blood does not resolve, to avoid scarring and retinal traction injury.

Choroidal rupture

Localized crescent-shaped tears in the choroid are a result of anteroposterior compression of the globe and occur in the posterior pole (crescenteric shape) or peripherally (radial shape). The patient may complain of decreased visual acuity. They are occasionally associated with macular oedema, and complicated by choroidal haematomas which may give rise to vitreous haemorrhages, or choroidal neovascular membrane (CNVM). Fluorescein angiography may confirm the choroid rupture or delineate a CNVM. There is no specific treatment other than observation. Should the patient complain of further loss of vision, or angiography delineates CNVM near the fovea, laser photocoagulation may be offered.

Commotio retinae (retinal contusion)

Retinal contusion may result from direct blunt trauma giving rise to the mechanical disruption of the retinal photoreceptors and diffuse retinal oedema. Symptoms may be decreased vision if oedema located near the macular or asymptotic. Fundoscopy reveals confluent areas of retinal whitening in which retinal vessels are clearly demarcated. Retinal detachment or retinal artery occlusion must be excluded. No specific treatment is required, and the contusion usually resolves spontaneously. Patients are re-examined in 2 weeks and instructed to return if they experience floaters, flashing lights, or decreased vision.

Retinal breaks, dialysis, and detachments

Breaks in the retina may occur after a penetrating or non-penetrating trauma to the globe. Forces produce a sudden deformation of the vitreous and retinal damage occurs in areas of strong adhesion, such as the anterior vitreous base. Retinal breaks may be horseshoe-shaped tears, which may lead to retinal detachment.

Retinal dialysis is the separation of the peripheral retina located, most commonly in the infra-temporal quadrant. Less commonly, it progresses to retinal detachment and often settles spontaneously. Breaks and dialysis progress to retinal detachment when vitreous fluid enters the subretinal space. Clinically this presents with floaters, photopsia, visual acuity loss (with macula involvement), and field reduction. Retinal breaks and dialysis are treated with photocoagulation as prophylaxis to retinal detachment. Scleral buckling surgery is indicated for breaks associated with retinal detachment.

Traumatic optic neuropathy

Avulsion of the optic nerve behind the optic nerve head results from the shearing forces from blunt trauma. There is little or no light perception. Examination reveals a total afferent pupillary defect, as shown by no direct or consensual response when light is shone in the affected eye, but an intact response when light is shone in the normal eye (Marcus Gunn sign). Fundoscopy reveals retinal infarction and large blot haemorrhages. The patient is informed of a poor visual prognosis.

Optic neuropathy may result from compression by haemorrhage, bone, or perineural oedema, and laceration of the nerve may result from bone fracture or foreign body. Clinically it presents with diminished visual acuity, especially colour, and exhibits a relative afferent pupillary defect. Fundoscopy shows retinal vein congestion and diminished retinal artery circulation. CT scan is used to detect a foreign body or to determine the cause of the neuropathy. Surgical intervention may be indicated with diminished visual acuity with neural decompression, but is only successful within the first few hours.

Key point

- Optic neuropathy is an ocular emergency. Successful recovery depends on early treatment by an eye surgeon.

Chemical injuries

Alkali injuries

Probably the most devastating injury to befall an eye is contamination with alkaline substances. These include caustics, concrete or cement, and ammonia-based liquids.

Such an injury, usually an industrial accident, represents a true ocular emergency. The pH is >8 and the chemical rapidly passes through the ocular tissues causing thrombosis and tissue necrosis. Pain is extreme and the associated blepharospasm makes treatment difficult.

Emergency treatment consists of immediate irrigation with whatever water is available. The eye is anaesthetized with tetracaine 0.5%, and irrigation is continued with normal saline until the pH approaches a neutral level. All particulate matter, such as concrete, must be removed from the fornices, under general anaesthetic if necessary.

Examination of the eye at this stage may show the white necrotic patches of the sclera and conjunctival fornices, together with clouding of the corneal stroma.

The appearance of a red injected eye is a good and healthy sign. The use of mydriatics and antibiotics is standard. The use of solutions containing ascorbic acid and steroids is controversial. Prognosis is generally poor.

Acid injuries

Acids cause much less devastating results than alkali injuries. The corneal epithelium coagulates and falls off, resulting in a large ulcer. The sclera remains viable. Treatment is basic and, in the main, recovery is good by comparison with alkali injuries.

Other chemical injuries

Many synthetic or acrylic compounds are now used in industry. In all cases treatment is similar and traditional. Water is ubiquitous as a means of treatment. Cyanoacrylate (superglue) causes a dramatic event, usually in children who, trying to remove the top of the tube, squirt the rapidly drying liquid into the eye. Fortunately the event cause relatively little injury as the glue does not stick to wet surfaces (cornea), but to the dry lid margins. Manual separation of the eyelids leaves the lashes in the coagulum but very little other damage.

Key points

- A chemical injures is an ocular emergency.
- First aid involves holding the eye open and irrigating with water.

Prognosis in ocular trauma

Patients exhibiting poor prognostic indicators should be informed of their diminished possibility of return of vision. The most important prognostic indicator is the visual acuity at initial assessment. Other poor indicators are presence of an afferent pupillary defect, blunt trauma, immediate loss of vision after the trauma, large scleral lacerations, and those extending more posteriorly. Penetrating air-gun injuries also have a poor prognosis.

Prevention

General ocular trauma, which includes home-related, work-related, and sport-related injuries, can impose a great burden on health service resources and the individual and can account for enormous direct and indirect costs. Direct costs include radiographs, blood tests, ambulance costs, legal costs, and staff salaries to all involved. Indirect costs can be estimated from number of days lost from school, work, training, or housework, for the patient and sometimes their family. The most effective way of reducing the incidence and severity of ocular trauma is its prevention, through the promotion of protective eye wear in the workplace and during sporting events. Sport has now become one of the most important causes of serious ocular injury in the UK (Pardhan *et al.* 1995). The use of protective eye wear in sporting events could potentially reduce the frequency of sport-related eye injuries by as much as 90% (Bell 1981). The use of laminated windshields and seatbelts decreases the incidence of penetrating eye trauma in motor vehicle accidents. The introduction of front seat airbags may further decrease the incidence of penetrating ocular trauma, but may increase blunt injuries. The use of protective eye wear remains at the discretion of the individual. Advice about the use of appropriate eye protection, in the form of posters depicting illustrations and statistics in strategic places as sporting venues and sport shops, and the availability of inexpensive, lightweight protective eye wear without visual field restriction, could all play a significant role.

Key point

- Many eye injuries are preventable. Simple measures such as education are usually all that is necessary.

References and further reading

Bell JA (1981) Eye trauma in sports: a preventable epidemic. *JAMA* 246: 156.

Cullom RD, Chang B (1994) *The Wills Eye Manual Office and Emergency Room Diagnosis and Treatment of Eye Disease*. Lippincott, Philadelphia.

Kuhn F, Morris R, Witherspoon CD (1995) A standardized classification of ocular trauma. *Ophthalmology* 103(2): 240–242.

Kuhn F, Halda T, Witherspoon CD (1996) Intraocular foreign bodies: myths and truths *European Journal of Ophthalmology* 6(4): 464–471.

Linden M, Renner G (1995) Trauma to the globe. *Emergency Medicine Clinics of North America* 13(3): 581–589.

Navon SE (1994) Management of the ruptured globe. *Ophthalmology Clinics* 12(4):71–84.

Pardhan S, Shalock P, Weatherill J (1995) Sport-related eye trauma: a survey of the presentation of eye injuries to a casualty clinic and the use of protective eye-wear. *Eye* 9 (Suppl): 50–53.

Pavan-Langston D (1985) Burns and trauma. *Manual of Ocular Diagnosis and Therapy*. Little Brown, Boston.

Pelletier C, Jordan D, Braga R (1998) Assessment of ocular trauma associated with head and neck injuries. *Journal of Trauma: Injury, Infection, and Critical Care* 44(2): 350–354.

Pieramici D, Sternberg P, Aaberg T (1996) Perspective: a system for classifying mechanical injuries of the eye (globe). *American Journal of Ophthalmology* 123(6): 820–831.

Ragge NK, Easty DL (1997) Trauma to the eye. *Immediate Eye Care* 12: 211–226.

Trieu L (1998) Eye and face. In: Sherry E, Stephen WF (eds) *Oxford Handbook of Sports Medicine*. Oxford University Press, Oxford, pp 180–195.

Varma R (1997) Trauma. *Essentials of Eye Care* 13: 479–500.

10

CHAPTER 10
Maxillofacial injuries

STEPHEN WORRALL

CHAPTER 10
Maxillofacial injuries

STEPHEN WORRALL

Facial trauma and its sequelae have been described since ancient times. The Edwin Smith papyrus (*c.* 1550 BCE) contains excellent descriptions of nasal and zygomatic fractures, the management of mandibular dislocations, and wound suture techniques. The diagnostic significance of bleeding from the nostrils and ears after a severe skull injury is also discussed; the existence of the dura and cerebrospinal fluid (CSF) were well known, even if their functions were not.

Maxillofacial fractures occur when the facial bones are subjected to forces that exceed their impact tolerance. The facial bones of females have lower impact tolerance levels than those of males. The impact force to the face in a 50 km/h (30 mph) collision is approximately 550 kg (1200 lb), which easily exceeds the fracture limits of most of the facial bones.

Key point

- Maxillofacial fractures occur when the facial bones are subjected to forces that exceed their impact tolerance.

Aetiology

In most countries, the commonest causes of civilian maxillofacial injuries are road traffic accidents (RTAs), assaults, accidental falls, sport, and industrial accidents. There are marked variations in the frequency of these aetiological factors both between and within different countries (Table 10.1). Much of this variation is the result of differing socio-economic, cultural, and environmental influences.

Table 10.1 The frequency of various aetiological factors as a percentage of all maxillofacial injuries in seven reported series from Australia, India, South Africa, Japan, and the UK

Reference	Simpson and McLean[a] (1995)	Sawhney and Ahuja (1988)	Khan (1988)	McDade *et al.* (1982)	Tanaka *et al.* (1994)	Telfer *et al.* (1991)	Hutchison *et al.* (1996)
Location	Adelaide	Chandigarh	Harare	UK	Tokyo	UK	UK
Date of study	1989–92	1982–83	1985–86	1979–80	1977–89	1987	1997
n	839	262	311	395	690	4305	6114
Assault	51.3	13	81.6	47	15.5	50.1	24
Fall/home	9.7	24		19.5	24.8		40
RTA	18.8	50	14.8	18	38.4	17.3	5
Sport or Other	20.2	13	3.6	15.5	21.3	32.6[b]	21
Unknown							9

[a] Adult maxillofacial injuries only.

[b] Includes accidental falls.

The incidence of maxillofacial injuries increased during the latter half of the twentieth century, and continues to increase. There was a 20% increase in the number of patients sustaining maxillofacial fractures in the UK between 1977 and 1987. Similar trends have been noted in other countries. In 1997, maxillofacial injuries accounted for over 4% of all attendances to UK accident and emergency departments. One-third of all major trauma victims (injury severity score >16) have associated maxillofacial injuries.

Road traffic accidents

Ever since the first fatal accident involving a motor vehicle in 1834, RTAs have been a major cause of maxillofacial injuries throughout the world. In the USA it has been estimated that the annual incidence of RTA-associated maxillofacial injuries requiring hospital treatment is 139 per 100 000 population. Maxillofacial injuries are the severest injuries sustained in 80% of RTAs and occur in approximately 80% of fatal RTAs.

Until relatively recently, RTAs were the commonest cause of maxillofacial injuries in most countries studied. This is no longer the case in several countries, as a result of improvements in road safety measures, particularly the compulsory wearing of seatbelts for vehicle occupants and crash helmets for motorcyclists, stricter drink-driving legislation, and continuing technological advances in vehicle and road design. However, RTAs still remain the commonest source of maxillofacial injuries in many countries, including India, Japan and Saudi Arabia, often as a result of drunken driving and speeding.

The introduction of compulsory seatbelt legislation in Sweden in 1975 led to a 28% reduction in severe maxillofacial fractures. A 25–72% reduction in maxillofacial injuries of all types was reported in the UK after the introduction of compulsory seatbelt legislation in 1983. It has been estimated that in the UK full compliance with seatbelt usage would result in a 53% reduction in fatalities and a financial saving of over £5 million per year from the reduction in maxillofacial injuries alone. Conversely, in countries where seatbelt compliance is poor, little or no reduction in vehicle occupant injuries has been observed.

Maxillofacial injuries sustained by restrained vehicle occupants most commonly arise as a result of facial contact with the steering wheel. Unrestrained front seat occupants are usually injured by facial contact with the windscreen, and unrestrained rear seat occupants (predominantly children), are most frequently injured by facial contact with the rear of the front seats.

Almost 40% of bicycle-related injuries sustained by children involve the maxillofacial area, and standard bicycle helmets offer little or no protection against maxillofacial injuries.

Key point

- The introduction of compulsory seatbelt legislation in Sweden in 1975 led to a 28% reduction in severe maxillofacial fractures.

Interpersonal violence

Assault is now the commonest cause of maxillofacial injuries in many countries. The number of maxillofacial injuries secondary to RTAs in the UK decreased by 34% in the 10 years between 1977 and 1987, but the number due to assaults increased by 47%. In Norway between 1970 and 1980 there was a 15% increase in assault-related maxillofacial injuries.

Numerous theories have been proposed to account for this trend. The two factors that have consistently been associated with increased levels of assault, and subsequent maxillofacial injuries, are excessive alcohol consumption and poor socioeconomic status, particularly male unemployment. In the UK in 1997 nearly a quarter of all maxillofacial injuries were caused by assaults, over half of which were alcohol related. Similar results have been found in Swedish and Norwegian populations. Young men aged 15–25 years are the commonest section of society to suffer assault-related maxillofacial injuries, particularly those in which alcohol is involved. The consumption of more than 7 units of alcohol in any 6-hour period by men in this age group substantially increases the risk of their being involved in interpersonal violence.

Accidental falls

The majority of maxillofacial injuries caused by accidental falls are minor cuts, abrasions, and bruises. Falls are a common source of facial injuries sustained by young children. In adults, over 10% of falls that result in a maxillofacial injury are associated with alcohol consumption. There is a strong clinical impression that a substantial number of maxillofacial injuries ascribed to accidental falls are actually secondary to an assault. Much of this 'misreporting' seems to involve women injured in the home. Non-accidental injuries to children are also often attributed to accidental falls by their perpetrator.

Key points

- Road traffic accidents, assaults, accidental falls, sport and industrial accidents are the commonest cause of maxillofacial injuries.
- The incidence of maxillofacial injuries continues to increase.

Classification

Maxillofacial injuries may involve the facial skeleton, the teeth, or the overlying soft tissues. Numerous classification systems have been described, and the majority concentrate on characterizing the pattern of facial fractures present. Soft tissue facial injuries may be superficial or deep, and either simple or complicated. Complicated wounds involve important underlying structures, such as named nerves, blood vessels, and ducts.

For classification purposes, the facial skeleton is traditionally divided into unequal thirds—upper, middle and lower—by two imaginary horizontal lines. The upper line passes between the two zygomatico-frontal sutures and the lower line passes along the occlusal plane and incisal edges of the maxillary teeth. Fractures of the maxilla, naso-orbito-ethmoid (NOE) complex, and zygomas are thus termed middle third fractures (Fig. 10.1).

The classification system proposed by Kelly *et al.* (1990) divides the face into upper and lower halves at the LeFort 1 level (see next paragraph). Each facial half is subdivided into two units. The *occlusal unit* consists of the teeth, palate and the alveolar processes of the mandible and maxilla. The *mandibular unit* consists of the remainder of the mandible. In the upper face the *cranial unit* is composed of the frontal and temporal bones laterally, and the frontal sinus and orbital roofs centrally. The *midfacial unit* is composed of the zygomas laterally, and the NOE complex centrally (Fig. 10.2).

Maxillary fractures are usually delineated according to the LeFort lines of weakness first described by the French surgeon René LeFort in 1901 as a result of his personal observations on the fracture patterns sustained by cadavers subjected to blunt facial trauma (Fig. 10.2). Although fractures sustained by patients are frequently comminuted or asymmetric, the simple LeFort description is helpful when conceptualizing complex facial fracture patterns and planning their subsequent management. Mandibular fractures can be readily classified according to the region of the bone involved (Fig. 10.3) and the simple numerical system devised by Henderson is a convenient

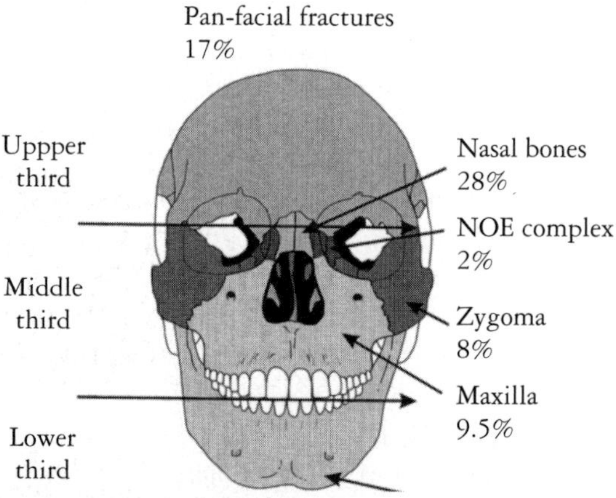

Figure 10.1 The three divisions of the facial skeleton and the frequency of facial fractures. Data adapted from Sawhney and Ahuja (1988).

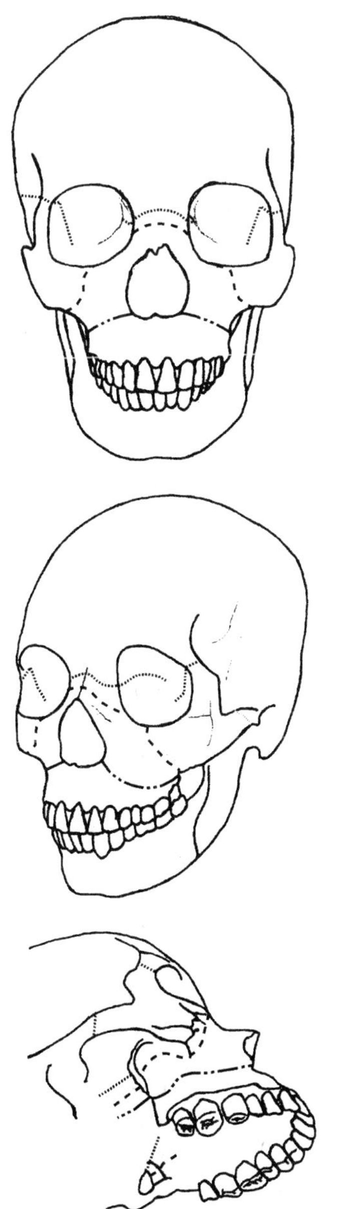

Figure 10.2 LeFort fracture lines. — - — -, Le Fort 1; - - - -, Le Fort 2; . . . ., Le Fort 3.

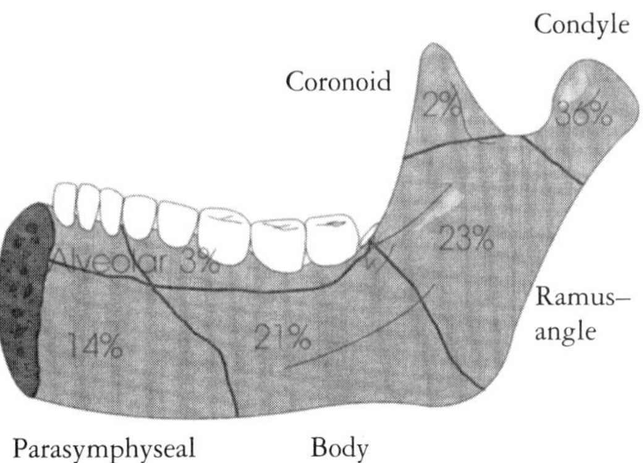

Figure 10.3 Frequency of mandibular fractures. From Luce (1984).

Table 10.2 Henderson's classification of malar fractures (1973, unpublished)

Type	Description of fracture
1	Undisplaced fracture at any site
2	Zygomatic arch fracture only
3	Tripod fracture—no distraction of zygomatico-frontal suture
4	Tripod fracture—distraction of zygomatico-frontal suture
5	Pure blow-out fracture of orbital floor
6	Isolated orbital rim fracture only
7	Comminuted fracture or other than any of the above

method for classifying zygomatic fractures (Table 10.2).

For routine day-to-day clinical use, the maxillofacial fracture classification system detailed in Table 10.3 is adequate. It enables the surgeon to produce an accurate description of the injured region and its severity, leading on to a logical treatment plan, and provides the trainee surgeon with a useful *aide memoire*. Cooter and David (1989) have refined this type of classification by the addition of an alphanumeric coding system, making it ideal for entry into a computer database. The system devised by Haug and Greenberg (1993), based on the AO/ASIF classification of mandibular fractures proposed by Spiessl (1989) is probably the most comprehensive currently

Table 10.3 A simple anatomical classification system for maxillofacial fractures

Site	Sub-site	Severity (applies to all sub-sites)	Treatment options (applies to all sub-sites)
Mandible	Condyle	Undisplaced	Conservative
	Coronoid/ramus	Minimally displaced	Closed reduction
	Angle	Severely displaced	Open reduction
	Body	Comminuted	
	Symphysis/parasymphysis		
	Dentoalveolar		
Maxilla	Le Fort 1–3		
Zygoma	Henderson type 1–7		
Nasal	Nasal bones		
	Naso-orbito-ethmoid		
	Naso-maxillary		
Orbit	Floor—impure		
	Medial wall		
	Lateral wall		
	Roof		
	Apex		
Cranial	Calvarium		
	Skull base		

available (Table 10.4). Using this classification a compound intraoral bilateral mandibular fracture with normal occlusion and involving the right angle and left condyle would be coded as:

Mn $F_{1L4}O_0S_1/F_{1L6}O_0S_0$

Although the extended AO/ASIF classification can readily transcribe even the most complex craniofacial fractures into 'surgical shorthand', it is arguably too complex for routine clinical use although it is a powerful tool for research and audit purposes.

Diagnosis

Full and accurate diagnosis of any maxillofacial injury requires a thorough clinical examination in order to elicit all the signs and symptoms present. Whenever possible it is important to obtain a clear history of the cause of the injury from the victim or eyewitnesses, particularly regarding the number and magnitude of the forces involved. A high-velocity impact from an RTA will produce a different and more severe pattern of injuries than those resulting from a single punch to the jaw. Where the clinical examination suggests the likelihood of a facial fracture, imaging studies will also be required to confirm the diagnosis and to fully assess its location and extent.

Examination

As a minimum precaution, protective surgical gloves must always be worn when examining or

Table 10.4 Extended AO/ASIF craniomaxillofacial fracture classification of Haug and Greenberg (1993)

Bone		Fragments		Location		Occlusion		Soft tissues	
Mandible	Mn	Incomplete	F_0	Precanine	L_1	Normal	O_0	Closed	S_0
		Single	F_1	Canine	L_2	Malocclusion	O_1	Open intraoral	S_1
		Multiple	F_2	Postcanine	L_3	Edentulous	O_2	Open extraoral	S_2
		Fragmented	F_3	Angular	L_4			Open intra/extraoral	S_3
		Avulsion	F_4	Supra-angular	L_5			Avulsion	S_4
				Condyle	L_6				
				Coronoid	L_7				
				Alveolar	L_8				
Maxilla	Mx	Incomplete	F_0	Separation through piriform aperture	L_1	Normal	O_0	Closed	S_0
		Single	F_1	Separation through ZMS	L_2	Malocclusion	O_1	Open intraoral	S_1
		Multiple	F_2	Separation through NMS/NFS	L_3	Edentulous	O_2	Open extraoral	S_2
		Fragmented	F_3	Alveolar	L_4			Open intra/extraoral	S_3
		Avulsion	F_4					Avulsion	S_4
Nasal	Na	Incomplete	F_0	Nasal tip	L_1			Closed	S_0
		Single	F_1	Entire nasal bone	L_2			Open intranasal	S_1
		Multiple	F_2	Nasal bone and frontal process of maxilla	L_3			Open cutaneous	S_2
		Fragmented	F_3	Nasal, ethmoid, frontal process of maxilla nasal spine of frontal bone	L_4			Open intranasal/ cutaneous	S_3
		Avulsion	F_4					Avulsion	S_4
Zygoma	Zm	Incomplete	F_0	Arch	L_1			Closed	S_0
		Single	F_1	Supra-arch	L_2			Open intraoral	S_1
		Multiple	F_2	Displacement of ZFS	L_3			Open extraoral	S_2
		Fragmented	F_3	Displacement of ZMS	L_4			Open intra/extraoral	S_3

Table 10.4 Continued

Bone		Fragments		Location	Occlusion	Soft tissues	
		Avulsion	F_4	Displacement of ZTS	L_5	Avulsion	S_4
				Orbital floor	L_6		
Frontal	Fr	Incomplete	F_0	Supraorbital rim	L_1	Closed	S_0
		Single	F_1	Anterior wall frontal sinus	L_2	Open intranasal	S_1
		Multiple	F_2	Posterior wall frontal sinus	L_3	Open cutaneous	S_2
		Fragmented	F_3	Floor frontal sinus	L_4	Open intranasal/cutaneous	S_3
		Avulsion	F_4			Avulsion	S_4
Other cranial	Cr	Incomplete	F_0	Sphenoid	L_1	Closed	S_1
		Single	F_1	Parietal	L_2	Open transcutaneously	S_2
		Multiple	F_2	Temporal	L_3	Avulsion	S_3
		Fragmented	F_3	Occipital	L_4		
		Avulsion	F_4				

NFS, naso-frontal suture; NMS, naso-maxillary suture; ZFS, zygomatico-frontal suture; ZMS, zygomatico-maxillary suture; ZTS, zygomatico-temporal suture.

treating any patient with a suspected maxillofacial injury. The clinical examination is divided into two parts, the *extraoral* and *intraoral* examinations. It is helpful to adopt a system of examination that is performed in an identical way on every patient, in order to minimize the risk of missing an occult injury. As always, thorough visual inspection should precede palpation. It is important to examine the entire head and neck meticulously if injuries such as occipital skull fractures and scalp lacerations are not to be overlooked.

The principle signs and symptoms of facial fractures are listed in Table 10.5. Not all of these will necessarily be present in every case. Soft tissue lacerations may transect important underlying structures such as nerves and arteries resulting in paraesthesia, paralysis, or profuse haemorrhage.

Key point

- As a minimum precaution, protective surgical gloves must always be worn when examining or treating any patient with a suspected maxillofacial injury.

Extraoral examination

The extraoral examination calls for careful and systematic inspection and palpation of the cranial bones, zygomas, orbits, maxillae, nasal bones, and mandible through the overlying soft tissues, starting peripherally and working centrally. Any swelling, bruising, tenderness, deformity, or crepitus should be identified and noted. Surgical emphysema is occasionally detected after zygomatic and orbital floor fractures if the patient has blown their nose. Patients with midface fractures should be advised not to blow their nose, to prevent this complication arising. Temporomandibular joint function is best assessed by simultaneously palpating both condylar heads and assessing for pain and symmetrical vertical and translatory movements.

Ocular abnormalities including subconjunctival haemorrhage, foreign bodies, reduced light and accommodation reflexes, reduced visual acuity, diplopia, ophthalmoplegia, enophthalmos, proptosis,

Table 10.5 Some signs and symptoms of maxillofacial fractures

Fracture site	Sign or symptom
Mandible	Pain Oedema Ecchymosis Drooling Sublingual haematoma Malocclusion Visible or palpable deformity Mental nerve paraesthesia (numb lower lip) Deviation on opening Bleeding from anterior wall of ear canal (condylar fracture)
Maxilla	Pain Facial deformity (long, flat, or dish face) Bilateral circumorbital ecchymosis and oedema Epistaxis Malocclusion Mobile maxilla—possible split palate Infraorbital nerve paraesthesia (numb cheek) Diplopia (with Le Fort 2 and 3 fractures) Opthalmoplegia (with Le Fort 2 and 3 fractures) Reduced visual acuity (with Le Fort 2 and 3 fractures)
Zygomatic complex	Pain Circumorbital ecchymosis and oedema Subconjunctival haemorrhage Flat cheek Infraorbital nerve paraesthesia (numb cheek) Limitation of mandibular opening (arch impinging on coronoid) Malocclusion Unilateral epistaxis Opthalmoplegia, diplopia, enopthalmos Reduced visual acuity
NOE complex	Dished in nasal bridge with saddle deformity Telecanthus Enopthalmos Shortened palpebral fissure
Anterior cranial fossa	Epistaxis ± CSF rhinorrhea Anosmia
Middle cranial fossa	Ecchymosis over mastoid process (Battle's sign) Bleeding from middle ear or posterior ear canal wall

and telecanthus must be actively sought in every case (see Chapter 9, 'Eye injuries'). Telecanthus is a feature of many, but not all, NOE fractures and results from disruption of the medial canthal ligament attachment. It can be extremely helpful to refer to a pre-injury photograph of the patient with a suspected NOE fracture in order to exclude an existing deformity and to help assess their normal intercanthal distance.

The zygomatic complex is best assessed from above and behind the patient. By placing the tips of the index fingers on the zygomatic buttresses and observing their relative positions, any facial asymmetry is readily identified. Enophthalmos or proptosis is similarly recognized by noting any asymmetry in globe or upper eyelid projection.

Cutaneous sensation over the distribution of the ophthalmic, maxillary, and mandibular divisions of the trigeminal nerve is assessed by the patient's response to a wisp of cotton wool lightly applied to the skin of the forehead, cheek and lower lip respectively. Facial nerve function is determined by asking the patient to furrow their brow, close their eyes tightly, purse their lips, and smile.

CSF rhinorrhea is indicative of a fracture in the region of the cribriform plate of the ethmoid, sphenoid, or frontal bones together with a tear in the overlying dura, and usually occurs within 24–48 hours of injury. The diagnosis is usually obvious from the clinical history and the typical appearance of a thin, glairy, serosanguinous nasal discharge that tends to form 'tram lines' on the facial skin as it evaporates and dries. If there is any doubt in the diagnosis, fluid should be sent for quantitative glucose analysis. Glucose levels >30 mg/100 mL are indicative of CSF, not nasal secretions. Glucose oxidase reagent strips should not be relied on as they not infrequently produce false negative results. Nasogastric tubes must not be inserted into patients with CSF rhinorrhea, as cannulation of the anterior cranial fossa via a disrupted cribriform plate is not unknown.

Key point

- Nasogastric tubes must not be inserted into patients with CSF rhinorrhea.

Intraoral examination

The intraoral examination involves inspection of the teeth and their occlusal relationship, together with the soft tissues of the oral cavity. A thorough knowledge of normal dental anatomy and the ability to recognize the abnormal is required for this aspect of the examination.

Fractures and luxation of the teeth are common after facial trauma, particularly in children, and can be extremely painful and distressing. All missing teeth must be accounted for. Where this is not possible a chest radiograph must be obtained to ensure that a missing tooth has not been inhaled.

Mandibular and maxillary fractures in dentate patients are usually associated with a malocclusion—the patient is unable to bite their teeth together normally. Edentulous patients with full dentures will similarly be unable to bring them together normally. Malocclusion must be specifically looked for in all patients who have sustained facial trauma.

With severely displaced fractures the malocclusion will be obvious and may be associated with a palpable or visible step deformity. In less severe displacements the malocclusion may be minimal and easily overlooked, but the patient will recognize its presence if specifically asked.

It should be appreciated that not all 'abnormal' occlusions signify an underlying fracture. Severe soft tissue injury may produce sufficient muscle spasm to prevent normal mandibular closure, and a temporomandibular joint effusion can produce a lateral open bite with deviation on opening. A 'malocclusion' may also be the patients' normal occlusion, as it is subject to substantial variation within the population. Approximately 80% of patients have a class 1 occlusion, 20% have a class 2 malocclusion, and only about 1% have a class 3 malocclusion. It is important to appreciate this fact, not only for diagnostic purposes but also to ensure correct treatment.

The maxilla should be gently manipulated to elicit any abnormal mobility. Hold the premaxilla between the index finger and thumb of one hand and palpate the nasal bridge and forehead with the palm of the other. Then pull the premaxilla gently forwards. Movement of the maxilla detectable intraorally suggests a LeFort 1 fracture; movement at the nasal bridge or forehead is indicative of a LeFort 2 or LeFort 3 fracture.

Key point

- Not all 'abnormal' occlusions signify an underlying fracture.

Imaging

Plain radiographs should be obtained on all patients suspected of having sustained a maxillofacial fracture (Table 10.6). A single 15° occipitomental view is sufficient for the initial assessment of all suspected midfacial fractures. If this initial 'scout' film indicates the possibility of a facial bone fracture then more specific views such as a submentovertex for zygomatic arch fractures and a true lateral view for nasal bone fractures can be obtained. Many emergency departments routinely take three or more 'facial bone' radiographs when screening for suspected midfacial fractures. These films account for some 1% of all radiographs taken in UK emergency departments. Reducing the screening radiograph to one view would result in considerable financial savings, and reduce the radiation dose to patients without adversely affecting their treatment.

Two views at right angles are required to adequately demonstrate a mandibular fracture. Ideally, these should be a Towne's view plus a panoramic tomogram. Panoramic tomography has the advantage of showing the entire mandible and facilitates the diagnosis of fractures of the body, ramus and condyles. However, most machines require the patient to be able to sit or stand upright, so this technique is not applicable to many cases of complex facial trauma and multiple trauma. Where panoramic tomography is unavailable or unobtainable, left and right oblique lateral views of the mandible are acceptable alternatives. Symphyseal fractures can easily be missed on extraoral views, owing to superimposition of the cervical spine. These fractures are often best demonstrated on an intraoral lower occlusal radiograph.

Table 10.6 Direct and indirect radiographic signs of facial fractures

Direct	Indirect
Demonstration of fracture lines	Asymmetry
Displacement of suture lines	Sinus opacification
Absence of normal anatomic structures	Air-fluid interface (fluid level)
	Air in soft tissues
	Malocclusion

CT has significantly improved the accuracy of diagnosing the pattern and extent of facial injuries and has become the standard of care for many complex facial fractures, especially those involving the orbits and NOE complex. CT readily differentiates between hard and soft tissues and can display distortion and displacement of bone, cartilage, muscle, and nerves. Its ability to display the myriad of fractures often present in middle third and orbital fractures, as well as the eye and its adnexae, is unparalleled. It is also extremely helpful in demonstrating the soft tissue oedema consequent on laryngeal trauma that can presage acute airway obstruction. Recent advances in CT hardware and software have lead to the development of systems that can manipulate cross-sectional CT data to produce three-dimensional images that are anatomically accurate to within 0.19 mm (0.28%). Three-dimensional reconstructions demonstrate spatial relationships that are not easily appreciated by studying conventional CT images facilitating both the diagnosis and treatment planning of complex cases, particularly middle third and orbital fractures. CT-acquired data can be used to fabricate solid three-dimensional models enabling preoperative model surgery and the construction of complex craniofacial implants. Because of the increased data acquisition time and radiation exposure three-dimensional imaging is less indicated in patients with minor dislocations and fractures, where it may actually be misleading.

If a CT scan is requested to exclude intracranial pathology in a patient with head and maxillofacial injuries, whenever possible the orbits, facial bones, and mandible should also be imaged. This can save valuable time later when definitive facial reconstruction is performed and can be extremely valuable in those cases where there is early simultaneous repair of both intracranial and maxillofacial injuries.

Key points

- Panoramic tomography has the advantage of showing the entire mandible and facilitates the diagnosis of fractures of the body, ramus, and condyles.
- CT has significantly improved the accuracy of diagnosing the pattern and extent of facial injuries and has become the standard of care for many complex facial fractures.

Significant associated injuries

The possibility of concomitant life-threatening injuries should always be considered during the examination of patients with maxillofacial injuries. Patients who have sustained fractures to facial bones with high tolerance levels such as the anterior mandible and supraorbital ridges are more likely to have associated major injuries than patients whose fractures are restricted to facial bones with low tolerances such as the NOE complex.

Head injuries

Many patients with maxillofacial injuries will have sustained a concomitant head injury. Overall, closed head injury (CHI), defined as a documented evidence of loss of consciousness and/or post-traumatic amnesia in the absence of a penetrating injury, affects approximately 20% of patients with facial fractures. Approximately 10% of patients with maxillofacial injuries will have a severe intracranial injury.

Laryngeal injuries

Fractures of the larynx may result from a high-velocity anterior impact to the laryngeal–hypopharyngeal region. This typically occurs in an RTA if the victim's throat strikes the dashboard or steering wheel. Laryngeal fractures can be single or comminuted and are nearly always occult, only declaring themselves when airway patency becomes compromised. It is important to have a high index of suspicion in any patient with superficial abrasions or lacerations to the anterior neck. Signs and symptoms include loss of the normal thyroid cartilage prominence, subcutaneous emphysema, hoarseness, a weak or absent voice, and stridor. Once the diagnosis has been confirmed by appropriate imaging studies. A secure airway must be established without delay. This is most safely and reliably accomplished by tracheostomy under local anaesthesia. Orotracheal or nasotracheal intubation is contraindicated, as both may produce further laryngeal bleeding and oedema rapidly leading to acute and life-threatening airway obstruction.

Cervical spine injuries

Damage to the cervical spine is associated with maxillofacial injuries resulting from high-velocity impacts such as RTAs and severe falls from height (see Chapter 7, 'Spinal injuries'). Middle third facial trauma is more likely to be associated with injuries in the area of C5–C7 whereas lower third facial trauma tends to produce C1–C4 injuries. It should be appreciated that in many combined maxillofacial–cervical spine injuries the facial injury may be restricted to minor soft tissue damage with no associated fractures of the facial skeleton.

All patients who have sustained a high impact maxillofacial injury should be assumed to have a concomitant cervical spine injury until proved otherwise. All patients at risk must have high-quality cervical spine views taken in two planes at right angles showing the entire cervical spine including the critical C7–T1 interface. Equivocal or sinister findings can be further imaged by CT. Whatever imaging studies are obtained, both they and the patient should be examined by an appropriate specialist and pronounced as normal before the cervical spine is 'cleared' and definitive treatment of the facial injuries performed.

Ophthalmic injuries

Damage to the eye or its adnexae occurs in as many as 90% of patients with a middle third facial fracture, with 12% of patients sustaining a severe ocular injury. All patients with facial injuries must be examined for an associated ophthalmic injury as part of their initial maxillofacial assessment (see Chapter 9, 'Eye injuries'). The most important predictors of significant ocular injury in the presence of a maxillofacial injury are decreased visual acuity, blowout and comminuted malar fractures, diplopia, and amnesia. A highly sensitive and specific scoring system based on these risk factors has been developed which is capable of identifying patients with maxillofacial injuries who require urgent referral to an ophthalmologist (Table 10.7). Visual acuity is the principle predictor of ocular damage and it must be formally assessed in all patients with midface injuries.

Rarely, a middle third facial fracture may involve the superior orbital fissure and the structures passing through it. From above downwards these are the lacrimal, frontal, trochlear, superior occulomotor, nasociliary, inferior oculomotor, and abducent nerves and the inferior ophthalmic vein. The signs and symptoms consequent on damage to these structures constitute the superior orbital fissure syndrome (Table 10.8). If the optic nerve is involved there will also be a reduction in visual acuity producing the orbital apex syndrome.

Table 10.7 Score sheet for determining which patients with facial injuries require referral to an ophthalmologist

Clinical feature	Score
Visual acuity	
6/6/or better	0
6/9–6/12	4
6/18–6/24	8
6/36 or less	12
No light perception	16
Malar fracture type	
Comminuted (type 7)	3
Blow-out (type 5)	3
Others	0
Motility abnormality	
Present (diplopia or squint)	3
Absent	0
Amnesia	
Retrograde + PTA	5
Absent	0

Add 1 if total score is 11 and female sex or age 30–39 years or RTA.

If total score = 0–4, do not refer; 5–11, routine referral; 12+, urgent referral.

From Al-Qurainy *et al.* (1991).

Carotid-cavernous fistula

Carotid-cavernous fistula is a rare but potentially life-threatening condition occurring in approximately 0.17% of patients with craniofacial trauma as a result of a tear in the wall of the siphon portion of the internal carotid artery within the cavernous sinus. Most cases are seen in patients with middle third fractures sustained in RTAs. The signs and symptoms include headache, pulsatile bruit, exophthalmos (possibly pulsatile), chemosis, ophthalmoplegia, and blindness. Urgent neurosurgical referral is required for the management of these cases, which have a cure rate of between 72–80%.

Key points

- Approximately 10% of patients with maxillofacial injuries will have a severe intracranial injury.
- In laryngeal injury, orotracheal or nasotracheal intubation is contraindicated.
- All patients who have sustained a high impact maxillofacial injury should be assumed to have a concomitant cervical spine injury until proved otherwise.

Table 10.8 Signs and symptoms of the superior orbital fissure syndrome

Periorbital oedema
Proptosis
Subconjunctival ecchymosis
Ptosis
Mydriasis
Opthalmoplegia
Absent direct light reflex
Preservation of consensual light reflex
Absent accommodation reflex
Absent corneal reflex
Paraesthesia/anaesthesia over forehead to vertex

- All patients with facial injuries must be examined for an associated ophthalmic injury as part of their initial maxillofacial assessment.
- Urgent neurosurgical referral is required for the management of carotid-cavernous fistula.

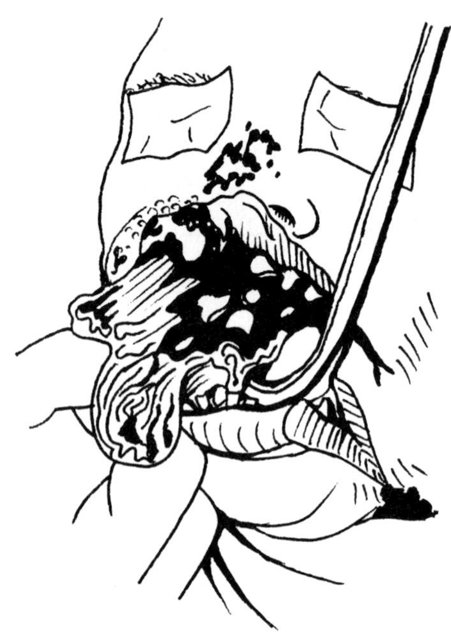

Fig 10.4 Extensive facial fractures and soft tissue injuries resulting in severe haemorrhage and airway obstruction. The airway is protected with a temporary tracheostomy (not visible).

Treatment

The timing of treatment can be divided into three phases: emergency (immediate), early (0–14 days after injury), and delayed (>14 days after injury).

Treatment goals include the preservation of life, sight, and speech; the restoration of normal function; and minimizing deformity. Accurate assessment of the nature and extent of the injuries, followed by their early and complete repair, is the best way to achieve these goals. The functional and aesthetic results after delayed reconstruction are seldom satisfactory, and are only acceptable when the management of associated life-threatening injuries must take priority.

Emergency treatment

The majority of maxillofacial injuries are minor cuts and abrasions, with less than 10% requiring hospital admission and operative treatment. Nonetheless, they can occasionally be life threatening as a result of airway obstruction or severe haemorrhage. Foreign bodies such as fragments of teeth, bone, dentures, and gastric contents may also occlude the airway. Middle third fractures can cause airway obstruction due to occlusion of the nasal airway resulting from backwards displacement of the facial skeleton or from torrential haemorrhage from torn blood vessels. Symphyseal and parasymphyseal mandibular fractures may result in loss of attachment of the extrinsic muscles of the tongue allowing it to fall backwards and occlude the oral airway (Fig. 10.4).

There is wide variation in the reported incidence of life-threatening bleeding after major maxillofacial trauma, although a figure of about 10% is probably representative. Severe haemorrhage after facial trauma, defined as a loss of 3 units of blood during the first 2 hours together with a drop in the haematocrit below 29%, is predominantly due to midface fractures, particularly LeFort 3 level fractures. Most bleeding after midface trauma originates from the external carotid system, particularly the maxillary artery, although the terminal branches of the internal carotid artery may also be involved. Bleeding from the lacrimal, frontal, and anterior and posterior ethmoidal arteries (all branches of the ophthalmic artery) can be extremely difficult to control, as these arteries are often damaged within their bony canals.

Airway

Securing and maintaining the airway is the first priority. Once protective gloves have been donned, and using a good light, the oral cavity is thoroughly examined for foreign bodies. A finger should be inserted along the side of the cheek to the back of the mouth and swept medially and forwards to dislodge any debris. This manoeuvre should be performed from both sides of the mouth. A large-bore sucker (plastic Yankauer) is used to aspirate any blood, mucus, and vomitus from the oral cavity and pharynx.

If the maxilla has been displaced posteriorly and is occluding the nasopharynx it should be disimpacted by hooking the index and middle fingers above and behind the soft palate and gently pulling forwards. If the tongue is falling backwards because it has lost its anterior attachment it should be retracted by a 0 gauge suture inserted through the dorsal surface some 2 cm posterior to the tip which is then pulled anteriorly and secured to the side of the face with surgical adhesive tape. If there is any doubt that a clear airway can be maintained, orotracheal intubation should be performed and the fashioning of a temporary surgical airway considered. These measures will protect the patients' airway, facilitate optimal tissue oxygenation, and minimize any secondary brain injury due to hypoxia.

Haemorrhage

Significant bleeding from middle third fractures usually manifests itself as persistent bilateral epistaxis and bleeding that 'wells up' in the oropharynx as it runs down from the back of the nasal cavity above.

After the maxilla has been disimpacted (if necessary), anterior and posterior nasal packs are inserted to tamponade the haemorrhage. A 12 gauge Foley catheter is inserted through each nostril along the nasal floor and gently pushed posteriorly. Extreme caution should be exercised in cases of suspected cribriform plate fracture. When the tip of the catheter becomes visible over the soft palate it should be pulled a short distance into the mouth to ensure that the balloon has passed through the choana. The balloon is inflated and the catheter pulled back through the nose until it impacts against the choana (Fig. 10.5). Ribbon gauze soaked in bismuth iodoform paraffin paste (BIPP) is then firmly packed into each nostril against the balloon until no more can be introduced. The two separate anterior nasal packs should be tied together in the midline. The Foley catheters are tied together over a gauze bolster to protect the nasal soft tissues while maintaining tension on their balloons. Alternatively, they can be secured using a Hollister umbilical cord clamp. Remember that the paraffin in BIPP can degrade the catheter balloons within 72 hours, causing them to deflate.

Anterior and posterior nasal packing occasionally fails to control the bleeding because of laceration of one or both maxillary arteries. In these circumstances

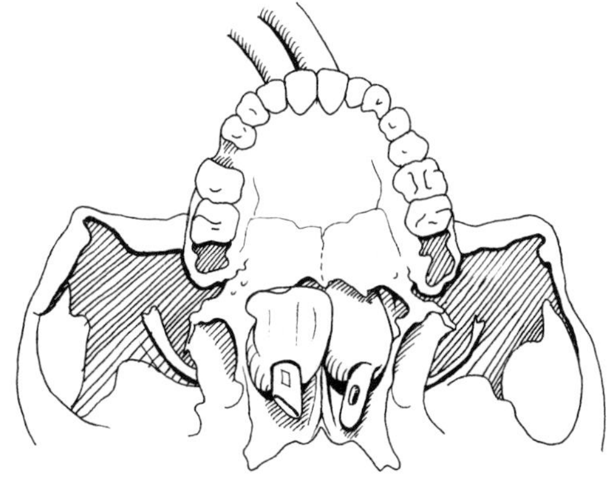

Figure 10.5 Postnasal packing using two inflatable balloon catheters. The balloons must be pulled forwards so that they occlude the choana.

the haemorrhage can usually be controlled by direct ligation or packing of the maxillary artery via a transantral (Caldwell–Luc) approach. Ligation of the external carotid artery in the neck as sole treatment for severe midface haemorrhage is seldom effective.

Bleeding from the facial soft tissue is best controlled by direct pressure until such time as definitive surgical exploration and vessel ligation can be performed. However, profuse bleeding from deep lacerations of the tongue, lip, or soft palate is seldom controlled by direct pressure. It may be possible to arrest such bleeding using artery clips or sutures in the emergency department, but care should be taken not to damage adjacent nerves and ducts.

Early treatment

Timing of treatment

The timing of the repair of maxillofacial injuries in patients with concomitant craniocerebral trauma is controversial. In many cases there is much to be said for performing the definitive repair of the facial fractures simultaneously with the neurosurgical repair of the intracranial injuries. This affords an ideal opportunity to use the same surgical approach (usually a coronal flap), and avoids the need for a second general anaesthetic. It has been shown that early repair of craniofacial fractures in patients with significant craniofacial trauma (ICP = 15 mmHg or greater) has no negative impact on survival and facilitates early rehabilitation. However, the overriding priority is to prevent further brain injury and patients with a high or unstable ICP should be subjected to the minimum surgical and anaesthetic insults in the first few days after their injury.

Although earlier treatment is usually desirable, particularly with compound fractures, there is a 7–10 day window of opportunity for the optimum treatment of mandibular fractures and even longer (14 days) for middle and upper third fractures. Providing the maxillofacial fractures are definitively managed within these times in patients with a favourable outcome assessment, the final functional and cosmetic results will not be compromised. This does not mean that the maxillofacial surgeon has no role to play during any early short neurosurgical procedures such as the placement of ICP monitoring devices or the evacuation of haematomas. This is an ideal time to fully assess the extent of the maxillofacial injuries and take impressions for study models if required. Discussion with the neurosurgeon at this time concerning placement of craniotomies or bone flaps can greatly facilitate future reconstruction. In particular, the maxillofacial surgeon should enjoin his neurosurgical colleague not to throw any bone away but to retain all fragments for future repair and reconstruction.

Key points

- Treatment of maxillofacial injuries is divided into emergency (immediate), early (0–14 days) and delayed phases (>14 days) following injury.
- The goals of treatment are to save life, preserve sight and speech, and minimize deformity.

Fracture fixation

Some of the various methods used to treat maxillofacial fractures are listed in Table 10.9. With the advent of internal fixation systems, particularly miniplates and reconstruction plates, the use of external fixation systems, with the exception of intermaxillary fixation, has a rapidly diminishing role in the management of maxillofacial fractures. Nonetheless, external fixation continues to have a role in the management of some grossly comminuted or infected fractures.

Likewise, although internal suspension wires are seldom indicated for definitive treatment, they are extremely useful for supporting and fixing Gunning splints and augmenting arch bar fixation in partially dentate jaws. It is important that surgeons who manage maxillofacial trauma are fully conversant with these more traditional fixation methods and not just the modern 'high-tech' plating systems (if the only tool in your toolbox is a hammer, every problem will look like a nail).

Intermaxillary fixation (IMF) involves securing the upper and lower teeth together in their normal

Table 10.9 Some fixation methods employed in the management of maxillofacial fractures

Type	Method
External fixation	
Intermaxillary fixation	Eyelet wire Arch bars Splints: cap, Gunning
Frames	Halo Levant Box Custom pin and rod systems
Fixators	Commercial devices Custom pin and rod systems
Internal fixation	
Non-rigid	Transosseous wires or sutures Suspension wires: circumzygomatic, circum-mandibular Kirschner wires
Semi-rigid	Transosseous miniplates (1.0–2.0 mm) or mesh
Rigid	Compression plates Reconstruction plates (2.7–3.0 mm) with bicortical screws Lag screws

pre-fracture occlusion. For many jaw fractures, if the teeth are placed in the correct occlusion the underlying bone of the mandible and/or maxilla will automatically assume its correct position and any contained fractures will be reduced and immobilized. However, this assumes that there has not been any significant disruption of the jaw–tooth interface. IMF alone is often sufficient treatment, but in many cases it will need to be augmented by some other method, typically open reduction and internal fixation (ORIF).

There are several methods of establishing IMF, but arch bars are arguably the best. One can use any of the commercially available prefabricated arch bars or, better still, a custom-made one cast by a maxillofacial technician on a model of the patient's dentition. The arch bar is secured to the mandibular and maxillary teeth by 0.4 mm or 0.5 mm stainless steel interdental wires and then the two arch bars are linked together by similar wires or orthodontic elastic bands, so establishing the IMF. Circumzygomatic and circum-mandibular wires can be used to augment the interdental wires where fixation is suboptimal because of multiple missing teeth.

If arch bars are not available IMF can be established via interdental eyelet wires. These are quick to apply, but they are not as versatile as arch bars although the incorporation of stainless steel buttons on to the eyelets enables them to be used with elastic IMF, which is not possible with the standard eyelet. One of the problems with both arch bars and eyelet wires is the risk of a 'sharps' injury. In high-risk cases IMF can be established by passing elastic bands around four bone screws from a 2 mm miniplate system screwed into the labial cortical plate of the anterior mandible and maxilla. Commercial systems are also available.

Despite its almost universal application in the management of maxillofacial fractures, there is a significant morbidity associated with the use of IMF. It restricts normal dietary intake resulting in significant weight and protein loss, reduces tidal volume, and increases the risk of aspiration of gastric contents should the patient vomit. The wires themselves are uncomfortable and damage the periodontal tissues. Postoperative IMF should be avoided wherever possible in patients who are malnourished or at risk of malnutrition (e.g. patients with eating disorders), epileptic, have severe breathing difficulties such as chronic obstructive airway disease or asthma, and where compliance is likely to be poor, as in alcohol and drug abusers.

External fixation systems such as halo, box, and Levant frames utilize the principle of craniomaxillary or craniomandibular fixation in order to immobilize facial fractures. Fractures of the midfacial, occlusal, or mandibular units are suspended from an intact and rigid cranial unit. In the case of isolated midface fractures they are sandwiched between the intact cranial unit above and mandibular unit below.

Box frames consist of four threaded bone pins screwed transcutaneously into the lateral supraorbital rims above and the body of the mandible below. The pins are then linked by two vertical and two horizontal bars by means of universal clamps. Other external systems are essentially variations of this scheme. Combinations of pins and bars can be used to build custom external fixation devices to support and control virtually any facial bone fracture.

The principle disadvantage with most, if not all, external fixation systems is that they involve closed fracture reduction usually guided by clinical observation of the occlusion and facial form. Because individual fractures are not visualized and anatomically reduced, there is a significant margin for error, particularly in re-establishing the correct facial projection after midface fractures. External frames are also cumbersome, unaesthetic, poorly tolerated, and prone to accidental dislodgement.

Miniplates have revolutionized the modern management of facial fractures by enabling precise anatomical reduction and fixation under direct vision (Fig. 10.6). True rigid fixation, which is only achievable with compression plate or lag screw systems, is associated with rapid bone healing by primary intention. Non-compression miniplates using monocortical screws are unable to produce true rigid fixation and are actually semi-rigid systems. However, in common use the term 'rigid fixation' usually refers to all types of small-plate osteosynthesis systems, both compressive and non-compressive, and is so used in this chapter.

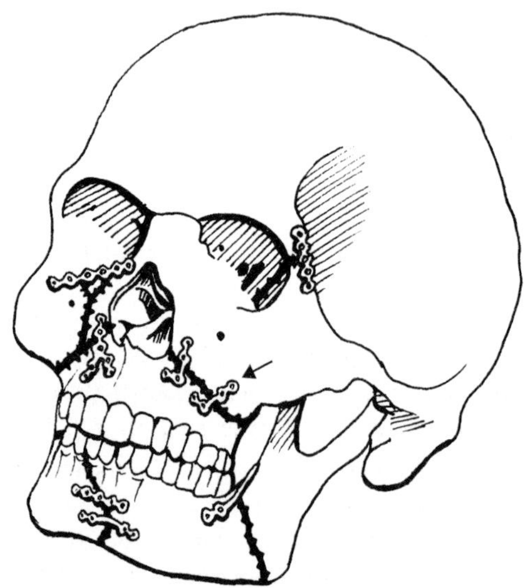

Figure 10.6 Model skull showing several common sites for the application of miniplates to fix fractures of the mandible, maxilla, and zygoma. Note the left buttress plate for stabilizing a fractured left zygoma (arrow).

By rigidly fixing the fractured segments together in their correct position, together with immediate bone grafting where significant skeletal defects exist, the three primary dimensions of facial bone reconstruction—facial width, facial height, and facial projection—can be restored. The requirement for external fixation is significantly reduced, as is the need for protracted postoperative IMF. The correct application of miniplates is a precise and exacting procedure unforgiving of errors in fracture reduction and immobilization, miniplate adaptation, and poor operative technique.

In all cases involving a fracture of a dentate jaw it is mandatory for the correct pre-fracture occlusion to be securely maintained in IMF while the miniplates are applied to the fracture sites. In many situations it is also necessary to initially reduce and control the fractures using stainless steel transosseous wires before achieving the final fixation with miniplates. A combination of transosseous wires, miniplates, and bone screws may be required to achieve the optimal reduction and fixation of complex fractures.

Nasal fractures

Nasal fractures are the commonest facial fracture reported in many published series. A history of blunt trauma to the nose, lateral deviation of the nasal bones or septum, visible or palpable deformity, epistaxis, ecchymosis, oedema, and small lacerations over the nasal bridge suggest the diagnosis.

It is important to examine the nasal cavities fully. This requires adequate suction, illumination, and a nasal speculum. Lacerations of the nasal septum, especially if sufficient to expose cartilage or bone, should be sutured with 5-0 or 6-0 plain catgut.

Septal haematomas must be evacuated in case they result in abscess formation or aseptic necrosis. Closed nasal fractures are best treated electively 5–6 days after injury to allow any associated swelling to resolve. Simple fractures of the nasal bones can often be treated by digital manipulation under local anaesthesia using lignocaine (lidocaine) by intranasal spray and external nasal infiltration with or without intravenous sedation.

Intranasal manipulation with Asch forceps is usually adequate treatment for a deviated or fractured nasal septum. The forceps blades are slid either side of the septum and pulled upwards and forwards to guide it into its midline position. If one or both nasal bones are displaced medially it may be necessary to use Walsham forceps to manipulate them laterally back into position. One blade is slid into the nose while the other (which should be covered with a piece of soft rubber tubing to protect the skin) is applied to the external surface. Using a gentle twisting and lifting movement the displaced nasal bone is repositioned. The nose is then gently packed with BIPP or Vaseline gauze for 24–48 hours and a closely adapted external nasal thermoplastic or plaster splint is applied and held securely with surgical adhesive tape for 7–10 days. Even with correct diagnosis and treatment the results of closed reduction are often disappointing, with approximately one third of patients having a persistent deformity.

Key point

- Simple fractures of the nasal bones can often be treated by digital manipulation under local anaesthesia.

Naso-orbito-ethmoid fractures

Fractures of the NOE complex involve the central midface, the nasal bones, the frontal processes of the maxilla, and the ethmoid bones and are arguably the most difficult of all facial injuries to treat successfully. Telecanthus is the principal deformity seen in NOE fractures. An intercanthal distance >35 mm is suggestive of a displaced NOE fracture, and a distance >40 mm is diagnostic. Telecanthus is invariably due to lateral and inferior displacement of the nasomaxillary buttress or fracture of a plate of bone in the region of the anterior lacrimal crest containing the insertion of the medial canthal ligament. It is unusual for the ligament itself to be divided or avulsed from the bone.

The aesthetic results of closed reduction and external fixation of NOE fractures are frequently disappointing. Optimal treatment of these fractures requires visualization of all fractures followed by ORIF. In the majority of cases a bicoronal flap together with the judicious use of local incisions and any conveniently situated lacerations provides the best access to the fracture sites. The bone fragment containing the medial canthal ligament insertion should be carefully identified, reduced in its correct position, and secured with miniplates or wires. If the tendon has been avulsed or is accidentally stripped off the bone, a transnasal canthopexy will be required to reattach it. Fine artery forceps are used to identify the tendon through a 4 mm vertical incision sited 3 mm medial to the medial canthus. The tendon is transfixed with a braided 3-0 wire or suture and passed transnasally on an awl posterior to the lacrimal fossa. The transnasal canthopexy rarely produces a perfectly natural appearance to the medial canthus, so accidental stripping of the medial canthal ligament off the bone should be avoided at all costs.

All other fractures are reduced and fixed and any defect >0.5 cm in the orbital floor or walls is bone grafted. Split cranial bone is ideal for this purpose. Wherever possible the bone grafts should rest on sound bone peripherally and be fixed with miniplates or transosseous wires. A dorsal nasal bone graft, which can be cantilevered off the frontal bone, will frequently be required to prevent a postoperative saddle deformity.

Fractures of the frontal sinus frequently coexist with NOE injuries and must be properly managed to reduce the risk of late complications such as CSF leak, meningitis, mucopyocele, and brain abscess. Displaced fractures of the anterior wall should be reduced and fixed with miniplates and immediate bone grafting as necessary. If the posterior sinus wall is intact and there is no evidence of a CSF leak it can be managed expectantly. If there is a significant posterior sinus fracture, especially with a concomitant CSF leak, the sinus should be cranialized and the dura neurosurgically repaired. Cranialization involves removing all fragments of posterior frontal sinus wall, stripping out all the remaining frontal sinus mucosa, and plugging the nasofrontal ducts with autogenous bone grafts. The insertion of a pericranial or similar flap may be indicated to separate the nasal and cranial cavities.

Zygomatic fractures

Significant inferior displacement of the zygomaticofrontal suture produces an antimongoloid slant due to a drop in the level of the lateral canthal ligament. Diplopia is often due to oedema in the extraocular muscles and usually settles within the first few days of injury. Diplopia that fails to resolve suggests an internal orbital fracture and requires further investigation. All patients with zygomatic fractures are at high risk of associated ocular injuries and must have a thorough ophthalmic assessment.

The zygoma tends to fracture at or near its three main articulation points—the zygomaticomaxillary suture, the zygomaticofrontal suture, and the zygomaticotemporal suture—producing what is commonly referred to as a *tripod fracture*. In reality they are quadrapod fractures because the zygomaticomaxillary buttress is also involved. Attaining an anatomical reduction at this latter site is fundamental to the management of unstable zygomatic fractures. Inadequate reduction and fixation at the zygomaticomaxillary buttress is responsible for much of the late deformity often associated with fractures managed by closed reduction or single point fixation at the zygomaticofrontal suture.

The indications for treating zygomatic fractures include correction of abnormalities in ocular position and motility, restoration of eye protection, relief of infraorbital nerve paraesthesia, improvement in mandibular opening, and the restoration of facial aesthetics. These indications are all relative and their importance varies with factors such as the patient's age and health. Hence many fractures are treated in young, fit, and healthy patients in order to restore their facial appearance, but this factor has a lower priority in the elderly or infirm.

Isolated zygomatic fractures associated with significant periorbital oedema and ecchymosis are best treated after a delay of 7–10 days. This not only allows time for the soft tissue swelling to settle and the degree of facial asymmetry to be accurately assessed, but it also provides an opportunity to obtain CT scans in cases of suspected internal orbital wall or floor fracture.

Closed reduction using a Gillies temporal approach is adequate treatment for most minimally displaced zygomatic fractures. After a 2–3 cm skin incision at 45° is made over the temple just anterior and superior to the pinna, the outer layer of temporalis fascia is divided. An instrument such as a Rowe or Bristow elevator can then be inserted below the fascia and under the zygomatic buttress. The depressed zygoma is elevated by firmly lifting the elevator in the opposite direction to the force that displaced it.

If the zygoma is unstable after closed reduction or if there has been any significant displacement the fracture(s) should be treated by ORIF using miniplates or transosseous wires. After elevation using a Gillies approach, all fracture lines and displaced sutures are visualized by means of appropriately placed cutaneous and mucosal incisions. A mucosal incision in the upper buccal sulcus gives excellent access to the zygomatic buttress facilitating accurate anatomical reduction and miniplate fixation. A buttress plate applied in this fashion is the most satisfactory way of preventing late zygoma sag and flat face deformity.

The zygomaticofrontal suture can be approached through a skin incision in the lateral eyebrow (which should not be shaved) or, more cosmetically, via an upper blepharoplasty incision. After anatomical reduction a miniplate is placed across the suture. Miniplate fixation at the zygomaticofrontal suture alone is often inadequate to resist displacing forces and consideration should be given to the application of an additional buttress plate.

Numerous approaches have been described to gain access to fractures of the infraorbital margin and internal orbit but they are all variations of the subciliary, infraorbital, or transconjunctival incisions. The subciliary incision affords excellent access to the lower half of the internal orbit and orbital margins. The incision is placed approximately 1 mm below the lower eyelashes and extended 1 cm laterally and inferiorly at the outer canthus. A thin skin flap is raised above the orbicularis occuli to the level of the inferior orbital rim. An incision is then made directly on to the bone of the anterior maxilla just below the rim so as to avoid opening the periorbita and avoiding the infraorbital nerve. Orbital rim fractures are best stabilized using low-profile or microplates.

Fractures of the orbital floor or walls often occur together with zygomatic fractures and are called *impure blowout fractures* (see Chapter 9, 'Eye injuries'). Isolated fractures of internal orbit are called *pure blowout fractures*. Pure blowout fractures can be caused by a direct blow to the globe by an object that is slightly smaller in diameter than the external orbital opening, causing a rapid rise in intraorbital pressure. An impact force of 2.08 J (equivalent to a 303 g weight dropped from 70 cm) is sufficient to cause a blowout fracture by this mechanism. Alternatively, a blow to the orbital rim can cause a shock wave that propagates along the floor of the orbit causing it to buckle and fracture without necessarily fracturing the rim itself. Orbital floor fractures may produce ophthalmoplegia and diplopia as a result of incarceration of the inferior rectus, inferior oblique, and periorbita (Fig. 10.7). Enophthalmos results from increased intraorbital volume, periorbita incarceration, and fat atrophy.

Simple, narrow internal orbital fractures can be treated by overlaying a thin sheet of silicone foam (Silastic) after retrieval of any prolapsed periorbita. The silicone must rest on sound bone all round and must not sag over the fracture. It should be cut to shape so that it lies passively just inside the orbital rim to which it can be secured by a few drops of cyanoacrylate tissue adhesive. Larger defects require bone grafts harvested from the skull, anterior

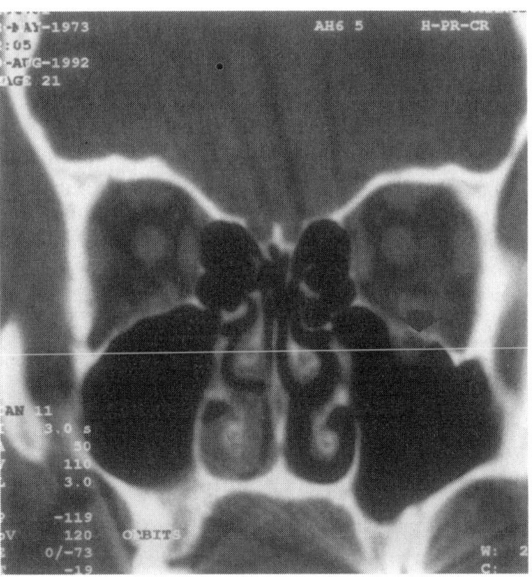

Figure 10.7 Coronal CT scan showing a left orbital floor fracture (arrow).

maxilla, or iliac crest depending on the volume required.

Retrobulbar haemorrhage is a rare but well recognized complication of midface, zygomatic, and orbital floor fractures and occurs after approximately 0.3% of zygomatic and orbital floor repairs. Its incidence is unrelated to the degree of surgical trauma. The usual cause is bleeding from a small branch of the infraorbital artery. The signs and symptoms include decreasing visual acuity, proptosis, diplopia, and pain. Failure to recognize and treat retrobulbar haemorrhage early is likely to result in permanent blindness. It is vital that all patients are assessed for this complication on presentation and at frequent and regular intervals postoperatively until discharge. Once the diagnosis is made, medical management should be instituted immediately and urgent arrangements made to return the patient to the operating theatre for orbital decompression. The orbit is explored, all bleeding is arrested, and any haematoma evacuated. If a graft was placed in the orbital floor it is removed, otherwise a defect is created in the floor to decompress the orbit.

The aim of medical management is to reduce intraocular pressure and so relieve pressure on the short posterior ciliary arteries which otherwise results in ischaemia of the optic nerve head.

The medical management of retrobulbar haemorrhage (doses for standard 70 kg adult without medical contraindications) consists of:

- 100–200 mL 20% intravenous mannitol
- 250–500 mg intravenous acetazolamide
- 1–3 mg/kg intravenous hydrocortisone.

Mandibular fractures

Mandibular fractures are traditionally described as being either vertically or horizontally favourable or unfavourable, depending on the propensity of the muscular forces acting upon the fractured segments to displace them from their normal anatomical position. Although the principle on which the description is based is useful the nomenclature is confusing because the terms 'horizontal' and 'vertical' refer to the direction from which the fracture is observed and not the direction of the fracture itself. The surgeon needs to assess whether the direction of the fractures and the direction of the muscular pull either side of them will result in adjacent segments being impacted or distracted. All other things being equal a simple, non-displaced 'favourable' fracture is likely to require less aggressive treatment than an 'unfavourable' one.

For patients with undisplaced favourable fractures who can easily bite into their normal pre-injury occlusion, and who are willing and able to comply with weekly clinical review, it may be permissible to adopt a conservative approach and prescribe a soft diet and analgesics. Minimally displaced fractures can frequently be managed by 4–6 weeks of IMF applied via arch bars or eyelet wires. ORIF is indicated for the majority of displaced fractures and minimally displaced fractures where IMF is contraindicated.

The most favourable site for internally fixing a fractured bone is where the tensile forces acting upon it are at their greatest. Champy *et al.* (1978) applied this 'tension band' concept to the internal fixation of mandibular fractures with miniplates. Tensional forces across a fracture at the mandibular angle are best resisted by a superior border miniplate, and the additional torsional forces acting across a fracture anterior to the mental foramen require the application of two miniplates approximately 5 mm apart.

After establishing IMF, access to the fracture is achieved via an incision in the labial or buccal sulcus approximately 5 mm below the mucogingival junction. A transbuccal approach using a trochar as a conduit for drills, screwdrivers, and screws facilitates plate application in areas with poor access, such as the posterior mandible. The IMF can be released when satisfactory fracture fixation has been achieved.

Occasionally, the access afforded by an intraoral incision is insufficient to enable full exposure and control of the fractured segments and an extraoral approach is required. For posterior mandibular fractures the incision should be placed approximately 3 cm below the lower border of the mandible in order to avoid damaging the marginal mandibular branch of the facial nerve. A submental incision is used for symphyseal and parasymphyseal fractures. In severely displaced or comminuted fractures the fragments should first be reduced and stabilized by transosseous wires prior to plate application. Lower border wires inserted via an elective extraoral approach are particularly helpful in controlling lingually displaced fractures.

Teeth in the line of fracture are best left *in situ*, provided that they are firm, not fractured, and have no associated periapical or periodontal infection, as they usually facilitate fracture localization and reduction.

In poorly compliant patients whose lifestyle and medical or social circumstances suggest that they are at high risk of further trauma, re-fracture, or postoperative infection, a strong case can be made for utilizing true rigid fixation to produce 'safe fixation'.

Fractures of the edentulous mandible present a different set of problems. In simple fractures in a non-medically compromised patient it is often possible to treat the fracture with IMF by means of

Gunning splints secured with circummandibular wires. However, in many cases IMF must be avoided and ORIF will be required. If there is sufficient bulk of mandible then miniplate osteosynthesis is the most satisfactory method but in atrophic mandibles compression or reconstruction plates may be required.

Fractures of the mandibular condyle have traditionally been managed either conservatively or by elastic IMF. Excellent functional outcomes are usually achieved with undisplaced or minimally displaced unilateral fractures managed this way. However, there is increasing evidence that closed reduction of severely displaced, severely telescoped, or dislocated fractures frequently results in an unsatisfactory outcome, particularly in bilateral cases. ORIF is indicated for this category of fracture, with persistent malocclusions after 3–4 weeks of elastic IMF. Early ORIF should be considered for bilateral fractures. The potential morbidity of ORIF for condylar fractures includes facial nerve paresis, which may be permanent, and avascular necrosis of the condylar head. It is thus not a procedure to be undertaken lightly or by an inexperienced surgeon.

Dislocation of the temporomandibular joint (TMJ) occurs if the condylar head is completely displaced from the glenoid fossa. In the majority of cases the condylar head moves anterior to the articular eminence. Posterior, lateral, and superior (central) dislocations are very rare. The clinical features include malocclusion (usually with an anterior open bite), TMJ pain, drooling, and dysarthria. Beware of misdiagnosing stroke or dementia in an elderly patient who has a dislocated TMJ. The diagnosis can be confirmed by a panoramic tomogram or lateral skull radiograph. While some dislocations reduce spontaneously (subluxations), many require manipulative or even operative reduction. In the majority of cases simple manipulation suffices. The patient should be seated with the operator standing behind them. The operator's thumbs (which should be wrapped in a gauze swab to protect them) are placed on the patient's lower molar teeth and the index fingers below the patient's chin. Slow, constant downward pressure is exerted on the molars while at the same time pulling upwards and backwards on the chin. The idea is to pull the condylar head onto the crest of the articular eminence and then slip it back into the glenoid fossa. Infiltrating the joint capsule with local anaesthetic before attempting to reduce the dislocation abolishes the neuromuscular reflex spasm maintaining the dislocation and significantly increases the success rate of the procedure. Occasionally, particularly with prolonged dislocations, intravenous sedation or general anaesthesia will be required before the dislocation can be reduced. Condylotomy, condylectomy, or mandibular osteotomy may even be required when manual reduction fails.

Key point

- Beware of misdiagnosing stroke or dementia in an elderly patient.

Maxillary fractures

The two nasomaxillary and zygomaticomaxillary buttresses maintain the relationship between the maxilla and the cranial base above and the mandible below. Correct anatomical reduction of these four anterior buttresses after a LeFort 1 maxillary fracture will ensure that the anatomical relationship between the midfacial, cranial, and mandibular facial units is correctly restored. Reconstruction of the posterior buttresses at the pterygoid plates is neither desirable nor necessary.

After the application of IMF the anterior buttresses are exposed via a horseshoe incision in the maxillary buccal sulcus extending from the first molar tooth on one side to its counterpart on the other. The maxilla is then degloved up to the infraorbital margins superiorly and the maxillary tuberosities posteriorly. All fractures are exposed and anatomically repositioned. Missing buttresses and significant defects are bone grafted using split calvarium. The buttresses and all fractures and bone grafts are then stabilized with miniplates.

A similar approach is adopted for LeFort 2 fractures. Access to the infraorbital rims and orbital floor can be increased by using a subciliary incision. Mobility of the maxilla in the region of the nasofrontal suture will require miniplate osteosynthesis to the frontal bone. Access to this region is via local incisions at the medial canthus, glabella, or a bicoronal flap. The management of LeFort 3 maxillary fractures is essentially the same as for panfacial fractures described in the next section.

Panfacial fractures

The reconstruction of a severe panfacial fracture may at first sight seem a daunting task, but it simply requires the surgeon to perform many of the individual facial fracture reductions previously described and then link them all together. However, the order in which the surgery is performed is crucial if predictably good results are to be obtained and mistakes minimized.

In the era of IMF and external fixation an 'inside-out' and 'bottom-up' approach was favoured, in which the reconstructed mandible acted as the primary template for the remainder of the facial reconstruction which then proceeded in a caudal to cranial direction. Unfortunately, closed fracture reduction and poor fragment control invariably led to errors in reproducing the normal facial width, height, and projection. With rigid fixation, correct spatial control of fractured facial bone fragments can be achieved. Table 10.10 details a treatment sequencing system for panfacial fractures. Not all fractures will require every step to be performed, but the order of treatment should be adhered to in all cases.

Table 10.10 Suggested sequencing scheme for the management of panfacial fractures

Order	Activity	Result achieved
1	Apply arch bars and IMF	
2	ORIF palatal fractures if present	Sets lower facial width
3	ORIF frontal bone and manage frontal sinus fractures	
4	Bone graft and /or pericranial flap to isolate nasal cavity from cranial cavity	
5	ORIF frontal bone to supraorbital bar	
6	ORIF orbital roof, medial and lateral orbital rims and ORIF all to supraorbital bar	
7	ORIF zygomatic arches	
8	ORIF infraorbital rim	Stabilizes NOE projection
9	ORIF zygomatico-frontal suture	
10	Bone graft orbital walls, floor and roof	Completes reduction of upper midface
11	ORIF mandibular fractures in sequential order: (a) ramus, (b) horizontal body	
12	ORIF condylar fractures	Completes reduction of lower face
13	ORIF Le Fort 1 level fracture at the pyriform and canine buttresses bilaterally	Links upper and lower face together

NOE, naso-orbito-ethmoid complex; ORIF, open reduction and internal fixation.

After Kelly *et al.* (1990).

Soft tissue injuries

Most facial abrasions and lacerations can be adequately managed under local anaesthesia by appropriately trained nursing or medical staff in a properly equipped emergency department. More extensive lacerations requiring >45 minutes to close are best managed in an operating theatre, and those involving named nerves, arteries and ducts are best dealt with under general anaesthesia. Fine, high-quality suturing requires fine, high-quality instruments and good illumination. It is unacceptable to attempt to repair facial lacerations using instruments designed for general 'casualty' use.

The fundamental aim in the management of all facial lacerations is to minimize scarring and its long-term cosmetic and psychological sequelae. The soft tissues can be considered as the 'fourth dimension' of facial reconstruction, and when associated with facial fractures they should be treated following early facial bone reconstruction as soft tissue that heals from a single insult over a correctly reconstructed facial skeleton provides the most natural facial appearance.

Most soft tissue injuries are suitable for immediate primary repair, but where there are associated life-threatening injuries and the patients' condition is unstable, wounds are best covered with sterile saline dressings which are changed frequently until such time as the patient's condition stabilizes and definitive repair can safely be undertaken.

Key point

- Most facial abrasions and lacerations can be adequately managed under local anaesthesia by appropriately trained nursing or medical staff in a properly equipped emergency department.

The margins of traumatic lacerations are often shelving, uneven, and of questionable viability. If good postoperative results are to be achieved they must be meticulously managed. Under appropriate anaesthesia, wounds are first thoroughly debrided using a suitable antiseptic solution to remove all foreign bodies such as dirt and glass. A soft sterile toothbrush or surgical scrub brush is very effective if used with care. Non-vital tissue should be judiciously excised, although irregular but otherwise viable wound margins are best not converted to a straight line. The extent of any tissue loss should be accurately assessed. Minor losses are inconsequential, but more significant ones, particularly if full thickness, may require immediate skin grafting or even flap repair.

Wounds should be closed in layers using absorbable sutures for the subcutaneous tissues such that all dead space is eliminated and the wound edges approximated. Final closure of the epidermis using a 5-0 or 6-0 gauge monofilament suture should evert the wound margins without tension. For the repair of facial lacerations in young children, or anyone for whom it is felt that co-operation with subsequent suture removal will be poor, excellent cosmetic results can be achieved using 6-0 plain catgut for epidermal closure. Evenly spaced adhesive suture strips applied at right angles to its long axis provide additional support for the wound. The application of a topical antibiotic such as 1% chloramphenicol ointment prevents desiccation and reduces wound infection.

Deep facial lacerations may transect the facial artery, the facial nerve, or the parotid duct. Lacerations around the medial canthus and nasomaxillary angle may involve the lacrimal drainage system. Facial lacerations involving any of these complications should be managed in an operating theatre under general anaesthesia. Under optimal conditions wounds should be thoroughly explored and any associated damage fully documented. The cut ends of any bleeding arteries should be fully exposed and ligated.

If a transected parotid duct is suspected the diagnosis can be confirmed by passing a fine catheter into the duct, gently infusing 3–4 mL of sterile saline, and observing for its emergence into the wound. Transected ducts should be repaired with interrupted 6-0 absorbable sutures over a plastic catheter stent to allow free drainage of saliva. The stent is sutured to the buccal mucosa alongside the parotid papilla and removed after 10–14 days.

Failure to recognize or adequately treat a transected duct will result in a sialocoele or salivary fistula, which can prove extremely resistant to treatment.

A laceration that involves the parotid duct may also involve the buccal branch of the facial nerve. If transection of a peripheral facial nerve branch is diagnosed, its repair should only be undertaken by a surgeon fully conversant with the local anatomy and skilled in the techniques of parotidectomy and microsurgery. If the transected branch is not readily identifiable via the laceration a formal superficial parotidectomy approach to the main trunk and its branches may be required before it can be located. Immediate microepineural repair using 9-0 monofilament sutures offers the best hope of preserving facial animation. The functional and hence aesthetic results of late repairs of undiagnosed facial nerve injuries are poor.

The nasolacrimal sac and duct and the superior and inferior canaliculi are at risk from facial fractures and lacerations in the region of the medial canthus and nasomaxillary angle. Obstruction to the lacrimal drainage system results in epiphora and dacrocystorhinitis. Transection of the inferior canaliculus or lacrimal sac can be confirmed by applying 1–2 drops of fluorescein to the lower fornix and observing for the dye in the wound. Repairs to the lacrimal drainage system, especially those involving the lacrimal sac and duct, can be complex and should be referred to a surgeon appropriately skilled in oculoplastic surgery. Significant ocular trauma must always be suspected in these injuries.

Maxillofacial injuries in children

Facial fractures in childhood are uncommon, accounting for approximately 5% of all facial fractures. In children <5 years of age the incidence is closer to 1%. Midface fractures in this age group are exceedingly uncommon, accounting for less than 0.5% of all facial fractures. The emergency management of facial injuries in children does not differ significantly from the methods previously described for adults. See Chapter 30, 'Paediatric head and maxillofacial injuries'.

Dental injuries

Fractures of the teeth, particularly the upper central incisors, are common. Approximately 35% of 9 year old children have experienced some type of dental trauma.

Compared to the severe injuries described elsewhere in this book, dental injuries might appear trivial. However, if not properly treated they can have a devastating impact on the child victim. Although the definitive management of dental injuries is the preserve of the dental surgeon, patients and their parents frequently contact a hospital emergency department for advice or treatment. Early and appropriate treatment significantly influences the prognosis for many dental injuries, relieves pain, and reassures anxious and concerned parents. Many of the common dental injuries and their emergency management are listed in Table 10.11.

If a patient, especially a child, has lost a tooth and it cannot be accounted for, a chest radiograph should be obtained to exclude its having been inhaled. Avulsed teeth have an 85–97% chance of being successfully replanted if treatment is timely and appropriate treatment is provided.

The root surface of avulsed teeth should not be handled but gently irrigated with running water for no more than10 seconds. If a tooth is allowed to dry out for an hour or more the periodontal ligament cells covering the root will die and replantation will be unsuccessful. The viability of the periodontal ligament cells can be maintained if the tooth is placed in a suitable medium within 20 minutes of injury. Periodontal ligament cells can remain vital for 2 hours in the patient's own saliva and for up to 6 hours in fresh milk. Water must not be used.

Once replanted, the tooth must be splinted and systemic antibiotics prescribed for 5–7 days. Splints can be fabricated from numerous materials. The simplest and probably the best method is to use a length of 0.7 mm diameter surgical/orthodontic wire secured to the tooth and its immediate neighbours with acid-etch composite cement. These materials are cheap and readily available. Alternatively, if there is access to a maxillofacial laboratory a custom-made

Table 10.11 Some types of dental injuries and their emergency treatment

	Type	Treatment
Crown fracture	Enamel	Smooth rough edges
	Dentine	Dress with calcium hydroxide paste and restore with acid-etch composite
	Pulp exposure: same day, small, clean	Irrigate with sterile saline and treat as for dentine fracture
	Pulp exposure: next day, large, dirty	Minimal pulpotomy to 2 mm below exposure then treat as for clean exposure
Root fracture	Coronal third	Reposition, check radiograph and splint for at least 2 months
	Middle third	Reposition, check radiograph and splint for at least 2 months
	Apical third	Reposition, check radiograph and splint for at least 2 months
Luxation injuries	Subluxation	Splint for 7–10 days if very mobile
	Lateral luxation	Reposition, compress socket and splint for 2–3 weeks
	Intrusion	If firm gently luxate to allow slight mobility no splint. If mobile leave alone
	Extrusion	Reposition and splint for 7–10 days
	Avulsion (immediate)	10 second rinse under cold water and replant in socket and splint for 7–10 days
	Avulsion (delayed)	Place tooth in patient's saliva or milk for transport then treat as for immediate avulsion

Adapted from Dewhurst *et al.* (1998).

vacuum-formed acrylic splint can be used. All patients who have sustained dental injuries, particularly fractures or luxations, require regular follow-up by their dentist or specialist restorative dental surgeon.

Key point

- Avulsed teeth have an 85–97% chance of being successfully replanted if treatment is timely and appropriate treatment is provided.

Facial fractures

Nasal fractures are the commonest facial bone fracture in children. The severity of injury may be underestimated because the significant soft tissue swelling that frequently accompanies these injuries often masks the deformity. Treatment is essentially similar to adult fractures but will need to be performed under general anaesthesia.

Mandibular fractures are the next most common facial bone fracture after fractures of the nasal skeleton. Many tend to be of the 'greenstick' type and can be successfully managed by either a soft diet and analgesics with frequent follow-up, or closed reduction. If there are sufficient teeth present IMF can be applied for 2–3 weeks, otherwise an acrylic splint can be fabricated on study models cast from dental impressions of the child's jaws and secured to the mandibular teeth with either dental cement or circum-mandibular wires.

ORIF is reserved for unstable or significantly displaced fractures. The same ORIF principles are used as for adult fractures but miniplate placement is complicated by the presence of the tooth buds in the body of the mandible which are at risk of damage from inappropriately placed screws. Small (1.0 mm) miniplates should be used in all but the largest children and placed near the lower border of the mandible. Because of the relative weakness of 1.0 mm miniplates compared to the standard 2.0 mm ones, fixation may need to be augmented with IMF or an acrylic splint.

The mandibular condyle in children has an exceptional capacity for growth and remodelling. Fractures of the mandibular condyle in children <12 years of age should be managed either conservatively with soft diet and analgesics or by elastic IMF if symptoms persist. Only in exceptional circumstances such as persistent pain or significantly reduced function should ORIF be contemplated. All children who sustain a condylar fracture require long-term follow-up to monitor mandibular growth and function.

Zygomatic and maxillary fractures can often be managed conservatively. Minimally displaced LeFort 1 fractures in young children can be treated with IMF for 2–3 weeks. Severe zygomatic, maxillary, and NOE fractures require ORIF and they should be managed along the same lines as adult fractures.

References

Al-Qurainy IA, Titterington DM, Dutton GN, Stassen LFA, El-Attar A (1991) Midfacial fractures and the eye: development of a system for detecting patients at risk of eye injury. *British Journal of Oral and Maxillofacial Surgery* 29: 363–367.

Champy M, Lodde JP, Scmitt R, Jaegar JH, Muster D (1978) Mandibular osteosynthesis by minature screwed plates via a buccal approach. *Journal of Maxillofacial Surgery* 6: 14–21.

Cooter RD, David DJ (1989) Computer-based coding of fractures in the craniofacial region. *British Journal of Plastic Surgery* 42: 17–26.

Dewhurst SN, Mason C, Roberts GJ (1998) Emergency treatment of orodental injuries: a review. *British Journal of Oral and Maxillofacial Surgery* 36: 165–175.

Haug RH, Greenberg AM (1993) Etiology, distribution and classification of fractures. In: Greenberg AM (ed) *Craniomaxillofacial Fractures*. Springer, New York, N.Y., pp. 1–19.

Hutchison I, Lawlor M, Skinner D (1996) Maxillofacial injuries. In: Skinner D, Driscoll P, Earlam R (eds) *ABC of Major Trauma*. BMJ Publishing Group, London, pp. 36–40.

Kelly KJ, Manson PN, Vander KC *et al.* (1990) Sequencing LeFort fracture treatment (organization of treatment for a panfacial fracture). *Journal of Craniofacial Surgery* 1: 168–178.

Khan AA (1988) A retrospective study of injuries to the maxillofacial skeleton in Harare, Zimbabwe. *British Journal of Oral and Maxillofacial Surgery* 26: 435–439.

Luce EA (1984) Maxillofacial trauma. *Current Problems in Surgery* 21: 1–68.

McDade AM, McNicol RD, Ward-Booth P, Chesworth J, Moos KF (1982) The aetiology of maxillo-facial injuries, with special reference to the abuse of alcohol. *International Journal of Oral Surgery* 11: 152–155.

Sawhney CP, Ahuja RB (1988) Faciomaxillary fractures in north India. A statistical analysis and review of management. *British Journal of Oral and Maxillofacial Surgery* 26: 430–434.

Simpson DA, McLean DA (1995) Epidemiology. In: David DJ, Simpson DA (eds) *Craniomaxillofacial Trauma*. Churchill Livingstone, Edinburgh, UK, pp. 85–99.

Spiessl B (1989) Classification of fractures. In: Spiessl B (ed) *Internal fixation*. Springer, New York, N.Y., pp. 152–159.

Tanaka N, Tomitsuka K, Shionoya K *et al.* (1994) Aetiology of maxillofacial fracture. *British Journal of Oral and Maxillofacial Surgery* 32: 19–23.

Telfer MR, Jones GM, Shepherd JP (1991) Trends in the aetiology of maxillofacial fractures in the United Kingdom (1977–1987). *British Journal of Oral and Maxillofacial Surgery* 29: 250–255.

11

CHAPTER 11

Chest injuries

DAVID WINLAW AND ANDREW FINCKH

CHAPTER 11
Chest injuries

DAVID WINLAW AND ANDREW FINCKH

Motor vehicle accidents and other deceleration injuries are the common causes of chest trauma. Early fatalities following severe trauma can be accounted for by injury to the chest and its contents. In patients surviving beyond 30 minutes, chest trauma may be unrecognized or its severity underestimated. Patients with isolated chest trauma and not *in extremis* at presentation are likely to survive, although their management may require aggressive investigation and treatment.

Major disruptions of the aorta, heart, and pulmonary vessels are associated with immediate death due to exsanguination. Injuries initially compensated for by peripheral vasoconstriction and tachypnoea—such as cardiac tamponade and haemo- or pneumothoraces—may subsequently cause a precipitous decline. Several hours after the initial injury, seemingly minor injuries may be associated with clinical deterioration, as is the case with lung contusion following blunt injury.

Key points

- MVAs and other deceleration injuries are the common causes of chest trauma.
- Major disruptions of the aorta, heart, and pulmonary vessels are associated with immediate death due to exsanguination.

Assessment of a patient with chest trauma

Assessment and initial management of injured patients should follow a described trauma protocol (ATLS/EMST) (RACS 1997). It is essential to obtain as much pre-hospital information as possible.

Key points

- pre-hospital information to seek (MIST):
  - mechanism of injury
  - injury sustained
  - signs evident at the scene
  - treatment to the point of arrival.

Severe chest injuries will be evident during the primary and secondary surveys and may necessitate early intubation, ventilation, and volume replacement. Eliciting tracheal deviation, observing chest wall movement, identifying obvious blunt or penetrating injury, as well as auscultation and percussion of the lung fields, are important parts of the initial survey.

Findings from physical examination, and possible explanations and associations are outlined in Table 11.1.

Isolated pneumothoraces occupying less than 40% of the pleural space are unlikely to compromise normal individuals. Tension pneumothorax should be suspected in any injured patient with respiratory distress. A high index of suspicion is required, as some of the 'classical' signs may be difficult to elicit in an acute situation. Intervention by needle thoracocentesis if *in extremis*—(14G hollow needle in second intercostal space, midlavicular line) or immediate insertion of an intercostal catheter (ICC) should be instigated if there is any clinical suspicion and not delayed until a chest radiograph is available. If a tension pneumothorax is

Table 11.1 Physical signs of chest injury

Clinical examination	Suspected diagnosis
Decreased chest wall movement	Pneumo ± haemothorax Tension pneumothorax
Tracheal deviation	Tension pneumothorax
Increased central venous pressure	Pericardial tamponade Tension pneumothorax
Scaphoid abdomen	Ruptured diaphragm with abdominal contents in the chest
Fractured sternum	Blunt cardiac injury (BCI)
Subcutaneous emphysema	Probable pneumothorax Major airway injury Oesophageal injury
Unequal pulses/blood pressures in arms	Aortic disruption due to blunt aortic injury (BAI)
Sucking chest wounds	Underlying lung laceration Open pneumothorax

diagnosed during the initial assessment, it should be treated before a radiograph is obtained, because the patient is likely to arrest due to cardiovascular compromise before the radiograph is taken, reviewed, and acted upon.

Key points

- Isolated pneumothoraces occupying less than 40% of the pleural space are unlikely to compromise normal individuals.
- Drainage of a suspected tension pneumothorax should be immediately performed, and not delayed by obtaining a confirmatory radiograph.
- Tension pneumothorax:
  - respiratory distress
  - decreased breath sounds
  - tracheal deviation
  - increased resonance to percussion
  - distended neck veins.

Investigations

Investigations required early in the assessment include a plain chest radiograph, assessment of oxygenation (pulse oximetry with or without arterial blood gases as indicated) and an ECG.

A history of smoking and significant co-morbidity (airways disease, asthma, and ischaemic heart disease) is important to elicit.

The initial chest radiograph is performed supine and over 1 L of blood may be present before this is evident, seen as a diffuse haziness over the entire lung field. This contrasts with an erect film where 200–300 mL of blood will be visible as blunting of the costophrenic angle.

Key points

- What to look for on the initial chest radiograph:
  - trachea—deviation
  - lungs—pneumothorax, contusion, lobar collapse

- pleural spaces—haemothoraces, pleural cap
- mediastinum—widening, aortic contour, shape of cardiac silhouette (see section on blunt aortic injury)
- bones—rib fractures, scapular fractures
- soft tissues—subcutaneous emphysema, swellings in the neck
- diaphragm—shape, position, and free abdominal gas.

Injuries to the chest wall and underlying lung

Fractured ribs, haemopneumothorax, flail chest, and pulmonary contusion result from injury to the chest wall and the underlying lung. Blood loss and hypoxia are the main concerns. Hypoxia may result from hypoventilation due to pain, increased work of breathing due to air or blood in the pleural spaces, large flail segments, lung collapse and ventilation/ perfusion mismatching.

Key point

- Blood loss and hypoxia are the main concerns.

Rib fractures

Fractured ribs are a common cause of pneumothorax, due to laceration of the underlying lung. First and second rib fractures are caused by extreme force and are commonly associated with major vascular injury (see 'Blunt injury to aorta'). Subdiaphragmatic injury, especially to the liver and spleen, may occur with fracture of lower ribs (especially ribs 7–9). When three or more adjacent ribs are broken in two or more places, instability results and the affected segment of chest wall moves paradoxically with respiration. This 'flail' segment increases the work of breathing, but the predominant problem is the underlying lung contusion.

Key points

- Fractured ribs are a common cause of pneumothorax.

Lung contusion

Lung contusion due to blunt injury is associated with significant force. Injury to the alveolocapillary membrane causes microhaemorrhages and fluid transudation, promoting the development of interstitial and alveolar fluid accumulation. This causes decreased compliance with the development of hypoxaemia. Contusion is commonly associated with haemopneumothoraces.

The patient's clinical condition may worsen after initial stabilization, as the effects of contusion worsen. Its onset may be insidious, with only mild chest wall bruising, tachycardia, and tachypnoea evident. Contusion appears as a patchy irregular alveolar infiltrate on chest radiograph but may not be apparent on the initial film.

Lung contusion may be difficult to differentiate from adult respiratory distress syndrome (ARDS). Contusion usually occurs earlier, however, is usually localized to the injured area affected (eg unilateral and lower or upper zones), and improves over 48–72 hours. ARDS tends to be more generalized, is later in onset and slower to resolve.

Key points

- The patient's clinical condition may worsen after initial stabilization.
- Lung contusion may be difficult to differentiate from ARDS.

Bleeding

Blunt and penetrating injury may cause disruption of chest wall vessels (intercostal and internal thoracic vessels) and damage to arteries and veins within the lung parenchyma. The resulting haemothorax and intrapulmonary haemorrhage is usually self-limiting. Lung tissue surrounding parenchymal vessels commonly tamponades the bleeding. Great vessel disruption should be considered with ongoing blood loss (see section on insertions of chest tubes, below).

Open pneumothoraces

Open chest wounds with underlying lung injury cause 'sucking' wounds (also known as an 'open pneumothorax'). When the communication between the lung and the atmosphere is more than two-thirds the diameter of the trachea, air will preferentially enter the wound rather than the trachea and neither lung will be effectively ventilated causing severe respiratory distress. Emergency treatment involves creating a flap valve using petroleum jelly gauze taped on three sides to allow air out but not in, together with formal ICC drainage of the pleural space.

Subcutaneous emphysema

Subcutaneous emphysema is caused by leakage of air into the tissues usually from lung injury at the site of a rib fracture. Pneumomediastinum such as that caused by a ruptured oesophagus may progress to subcutaneous emphysema over the neck and shoulders. Subcutaneous emphysema is a benign condition and does not in itself cause airway obstruction. Evacuation of the pneumothorax and treatment of the underlying injury is usually followed by rapid improvement.

Management guidelines for injuries to the chest wall and underlying lung

Patients with chest trauma require regular review of their cardiorespiratory status. Optimal management involves assessment of analgesic requirements and timely treatment of any clinical deterioration.

Analgesia options

Good analgesia allows the patient to cough to clear secretions and move in the bed without severe pain. It allows effective physiotherapy and promotes early recovery and reduces the likelihood of pneumonia. Table 11.2 is a guide to analgesic options.

Table 11.2 Guide to analgesic options

Oral	Paracetamol and codeine preparations
Parenteral	Intermittent narcotic (supplement with regular paracetamol)
	Patient-controlled narcotic dosing
	Narcotic infusion
Regional	Thoracic epidural Intercostal blocks

Patient-controlled analgesia (PCA) has advantages in the minimization of narcotic dosing and ensuring timely administration, i.e. before moving, for coughing etc. Standard ward admission is usually appropriate for this modality. Narcotic infusions require high dependency or intensive care level monitoring in most institutions. Thoracic epidurals are particularly useful in the management of flail chest and may reduce the requirement for intubation and positive pressure ventilation. Patients with thoracic epidurals require admission to a high dependency or intensive care unit, for monitoring of epidural effectiveness and safety.

Management of hypoxia

Continuous cardiorespiratory monitoring is required for at least 4 hours, for all patients requiring ICC insertion. During that time, it will become clear what intensity of nursing and medical care is required for ongoing management. In most institutions it will be a choice between a bed in a standard ward, a high dependency unit, or intensive care unit.

Supplemental oxygen, humidified if possible, should be titrated to oxygen saturation. This should be maintained at or above 92% and arterial blood gas measurements should be performed at least once in the first 2 hours to ascertain the P_aCO_2.

When the saturations fall below 90% or the P_aO_2 below 65 mmHg, oxygen delivery must be increased.

This may involve use of a higher F_iO_2, continuous positive airway pressure (CPAP) or consideration of intubation and positive pressure ventilation. Transfer to a higher intensity nursing and medical environment may be required. Repeated clinical assessment to exclude evolving problems (such as a new pneumothorax or worsening of lung contusion) should be undertaken. Remember both continuous positive airway pressure (CPAP) and intermittent positive pressure ventilation (IPPV) may cause or enlarge pneumothoraces and other barotrauma.

Key point

- Continuous cardiorespiratory monitoring is required for at least 4 hours.

Management of pneumothoraces

Traumatic pneumothoraces are treated by insertion of an ICC. Intramuscular narcotic analgesia is generally sufficient for patients with isolated pneumothoraces. Provided the lung fully re-expands after ICC insertion, the tube may be removed 24 hours after cessation of any air leak (bubbling on coughing) and another radiograph is performed after removal. Provided the lung is fully expanded on this film the patient may be discharged with oral analgesia on the same day.

Patients with severe lung injury undergoing general anaesthesia or transport, involving IPPV, may require 'prophylactic' ICC insertion. This is a reasonable approach if the risk of pneumothorax is considered high.

Management of haemothoraces

Traumatic haemothoraces should undergo drainage by ICC. Drain output should be monitored constantly and measured hourly. A total output of 1500 mL or drainage >200 mL/hour should prompt consideration of thoracotomy for haemostasis and evacuation of clot. This should also be considered when the haemothorax is incompletely cleared by ICC insertion, or the patient is haemodynamically unstable despite adequate fluid replacement in the absence of other injuries.

Key points

- Traumatic haemothoraces should undergo drainage by ICC.
- Consider thoracotomy when
  - total loss 1500 mL (blunt trauma)
  - drainage >200 mL/hour (blunt trauma)
  - initial output >1000 mL (penetrating trauma)
  - drainage >100 mL/hour (penetrating trauma)
  - haemodynamic instability (blunt and penetrating trauma).

The ICC should be removed 24 hours after drainage has ceased. Serous pleural fluid, up to 100 mL/day, will continue to drain after the blood has been completely cleared, but should not delay tube removal.

A word of caution on the management of small haemothorax and pneumothorax without ICC insertion

Rarely, small traumatic pneumothoraces may be observed without drainage. These patients need to be admitted to a monitored environment because of the risk of rapid pneumothorax expansion causing respiratory embarrassment and/or tension and should have a repeat chest radiograph 4–6 hours after admission.

Large amounts of blood left in the pleural space form a clotted haemothorax. Thoracotomy may be required to clear the pleural space and allow re-expansion of the lung. If this is not performed, a clotted haemothorax may progress to form a fibrothorax with the possibility of late chest wall deformities and trapped lung. Small haemothoraces (<15%) may be observed without drainage, but this requires repeat chest radiograph 4 hours after the initial film to detect any further accumulation of blood. A further chest radiograph is required one week after the injury to detect the development of a sympathetic effusion. This may occur as part of the inflammatory response to blood in the pleural space.

All haemopneumothoraces, and bilateral pneumothoraces should be drained, regardless of size.

Penetrating injury to the lung may be initially managed without open exploration when there is a small initial drainage (<400 mL after ICC insertion) but with a low threshold for thoracotomy if there is ongoing bleeding. Thoracoscopy is an alternative to thoracotomy in stable patients requiring exploration.

Key points

- Rarely, small traumatic pneumothoraces may be observed without drainage.
- All haemopneumothoraces and bilateral pneumothoraces should be drained regardless of size.

Antibiotics

It is recommended that 24 hours of antibiotics using a first-generation cephalosporin be used following insertion of an ICC (Barie *et al.* 1998).

Prophylactic antibiotics with extended gram-negative cover should be considered in smokers because of the increase in mucus production and stasis of secretions that occurs with cessation on admission.

Insertion of intercostal catheters

Insertion of an ICC can be a life-saving procedure, but guidelines should be followed for safe insertion. The sharp trocar is not used as part of standard ICC insertion because of the risk of causing further injury.

Site

The anterior axillary line in the fifth or sixth intercostal spaces is easily accessible and free of overlying muscle. Since the diaphragm is often elevated in trauma, as a result of either collapsed lung or increased intra-abdominal pressure, it is unwise to go below the level of the nipple.

Tube

Size 32 French tubes are the minimum acceptable size. Smaller tubes will not effectively drain large volumes of blood because clot obstructs the tube. Smaller tubes may be used for draining isolated pneumothoraces in stable patients. There is no place for fine 'pleurocath' or 'pleuovac' style catheters in major trauma, since they are too small to drain blood effectively, require a blind insertion technique, and kink easily.

Insertion

An aseptic technique is used. In conscious patients, local anaesthetic is infiltrated beneath the skin, into the subcutaneous tissues and over the rib. A 3 cm incision is made over the site of insertion directly through the dermis into the subcutaneous fat. Artery forceps are used to separate the intercostal muscles and localize the rib. The artery forceps are then pushed over the top of the rib (since the intercostal vessels run beneath the rib), through the intercostal muscles then the pleura, which 'gives way' with moderate pressure. Spreading the artery forceps then dilates this tract.

The operator confirms that the hole made in the chest enters the pleural space, by digital examination, sweeping the index finger in all directions. This confirms that there is a space for insertion of the chest tube, and that adhesions between lung and chest wall are not present at that site. It guards against the blind insertion of a tube directly into the lung, or into a high rising diaphragm or even the heart.

The chest tube is then inserted in the direction required—apically for air or basally for blood. The basal drain is directed by running the tube posteromedially around the chest wall. Drains pushed horizontally may lodge within a lung fissure, and incompletely drain blood and air. The tube is then connected to the underwater seal drain and secured to the skin with a suture and adhesive tape.

Low wall suction (–5 kPa, 10–20 cmH_2O) should be applied to all chest tubes except where major bronchopleural fistulae exist. In these circumstances, suction may increase the air leak without improving ventilation.

A chest radiograph should be performed following ICC insertion to confirm the position of the tube, and evacuation of air or blood as required. If a collection is incompletely drained, a further ICC may be required, usually at a different site. Where large blood loss is expected, two drains may be placed initially, one directed apically and one basally.

The chest drain is removed 24 hours after drainage of air (bubbling) has ceased or when daily drainage of serous pleural fluid is $<$150 mL. Suction should be disconnected before removal. Removal is performed in full inspiration and the wound is covered with petroleum jelly gauze followed by an occlusive dressing before expiration. Purse-string sutures may be used but are not necessary since the defect closes spontaneously within 24 hours, under an occlusive dressing. Furthermore, purse strings may give a poor cosmetic result because of hurried insertion, skin necrosis where they are pulled up, and propensity to infection.

Tracheobronchial and oesophageal injury

Major airways (such as trachea and bronchi) are injured in blunt trauma by rapid deceleration and shearing of more mobile bronchi from fixed proximal structures. Injury due to deceleration is usually within 2 cm of the carina or at the origin of lobar bronchi. Tracheal injuries in the neck are usually associated with direct trauma, e.g. neck struck by car dashboard.

Complete atelectasis of a lung, or pneumomediastinum (possibly with Hamman's sign or pericardial 'crunch' on auscultation) may be evident. Pneumomediastinum is also associated with injury to the pharynx, larynx, and oesophagus. Intrapleural bronchial injuries are associated with tension pneumothoraces, with massive air leak after tube insertion due to the bronchopleural fistula. More subtle injuries may require bronchoscopic evaluation if there is a high index of suspicion. A further clue may be the failure of supplemental oxygen to improve systemic saturations.

Tracheobronchial injuries are associated with oesophageal injuries in 25% of patients, and complicated in the early period by infection (pulmonary, mediastinal). Isolated oesophageal trauma is uncommon in blunt injury, although blows to the abdomen may cause linear tears in the lower oesophagus due to forced regurgitation of gastric contents. Management of the ruptured oesophagus involves delineation of the injury with a contrast study, drainage of any collection in the mediastinum and pleural space, and antibiotic treatment. Mediastinitis and empyema are potential complications.

In major airway trauma, the endotracheal tube cuff may be positioned beyond a tracheal injury. Double lumen endotracheal intubation may be required for more distal injuries. For a major tracheal disruption, a stoma may need to be fashioned from the distal end of the trachea to accommodate a tracheostomy tube.

Systemic air embolism is possible when there is a communication between a bronchus and pulmonary vein. This uncommon injury usually manifests with high-pressure IPPV, and is a cause of rapid deterioration often immediately following intubation. Another presentation is with neurological signs in the absence of head trauma. Froth in the blood gas syringe or haemoptysis may also be noted. The patient should be positioned head down and fluid resuscitated. Cardiac compression may be required, but emergent thoracotomy and securing of the vascular and bronchial injury is the only real means of treatment.

Key point

- Major airways (such as trachea and bronchi) are injured in blunt trauma by rapid deceleration and shearing.

Diaphragmatic injury

Diaphragmatic injuries due to penetrating and blunt trauma are common. Blunt trauma causes large defects, and 10% of pelvic fractures are associated with diaphragmatic rupture.

In blunt trauma, the sudden increase in intra-abdominal pressure causes a 'blowout' at the weakest point, the left posterolateral diaphragm (over 80%). The stronger right side is also 'protected' by the liver. Intra-abdominal contents—commonly colon, stomach, and spleen—may herniate into the chest, often not detected in multiply injured and ventilated patients. Difficulty in passing a nasogastric tube or the intrathoracic position of a successfully placed one may assist in the diagnosis. Diaphragmatic ruptures without herniation are difficult to demonstrate on CT scan, and diagnosis is often serendipitous, such as the appearance of abdominal lavage fluid in an ICC drainage bottle, or the appearance of a pneumoperitoneum on plain radiograph with coexisting thoracic trauma.

Diaphragmatic defects do not spontaneously close, regardless of the size, because of the pleuroperitoneal pressure gradient caused by respiration. If undetected in the early period, non-specific abdominal complaints due to intermittent herniation of abdominal contents may be the presenting symptom. Bowel obstruction and incarceration may also occur.

Operative closure and relocation of abdominal contents is required. The diaphragm may be approached from either the chest or the abdomen, and in a stable patient this may be performed laparoscopically.

Key points

- In blunt trauma, the sudden increase in intraabdominal pressure causes a 'blow out' at the weakest point, the left posterolateral diaphragm (over 80%).
- Diaphragmatic defects do not spontaneously close, regardless of the size.

Penetrating cardiac injury

Penetrating injuries to the heart are usually fatal, with less than 25% surviving to hospital. Those alive at presentation survive because the bleeding has slowed due to pericardial tamponade, which the patient is able to tolerate for a short time. It is wise to assume that any penetrating injury between the right midclavicular line and the left anterior axillary line involves the heart.

The anterior lie of the right ventricle makes it the most susceptible to injury, and is involved in over 40% of cases. The left ventricle is injured in over 30% of cases, the right atrium in 15%. The intrapericardial vessels and coronary arteries are infrequently involved (<5%).

Beck's triad of distended neck veins, hypotension, and muffled heart sounds is present in only 10–40% of patients. The venous pressure may not be elevated because of volume depletion, and muffled heart sounds are unreliable. Furthermore, other injuries such as blunt cardiac trauma and tension pneumothorax may also manifest these signs. In practical terms, haemodynamic compromise and an entry wound over the cardiac silhouette are all that are required to make a diagnosis of significant penetrating cardiac injury.

Knife and gunshot wounds are common causes of penetrating trauma, and in these conditions there is always an element of pericardial tamponade. Aggressive fluid resuscitation is required even when the filling pressures appear elevated, since this is initially the only way of increasing cardiac output. In shocked patients, emergency department thoracotomy is required.

It is rare for patients with penetrating cardiac injuries to be haemodynamically stable. In this event, pericardiocentesis may be performed and the drainage of even a small amount of blood may improve the patient's blood pressure, although this does nothing to address the injury itself. Echocardiographic confirmation of tamponade is desirable if available and time permits.

Key points

- Penetrating injuries to the heart are usually fatal.
- Beck's triad of distended neck veins, hypotension, and muffled heart sounds is present in only 10–40% of patients.

Technique of needle pericardiocentesis

Continuous ECG monitoring is required during needle pericardiocentesis. An aseptic technique is used. Purpose-built kits are available, containing a 16 or 18-gauge needle within a plastic cannula, at least 10 cm in length. Most central line insertion kits also have such a needle; alternatively, an 18 spinal needle may be used. The needle is inserted on the left-hand side, at the junction between the costal margin and the xiphisternum, at 45° to the skin, heading towards the left scapula.

Aspirate the needle as it enters the pericardial space, and withdraw it as fluid returns freely, leaving the cannula in place. If the needle touches the heart, ectopics or ST-T changes may appear on the ECG trace, and the needle should be withdrawn. An ECG monitoring lead may be attached to a metal pericardiocentesis needle, and when displayed as a V lead, may further assist in insertion.

If no blood is aspirated, then it is possible that the collection is clotted, that tamponade does not exist, or that the needle is incorrectly positioned. False positives may occur by aspiration of right ventricular blood if the needle is inserted too far. If time permits, echocardiography is useful to confirm the diagnosis and guide needle insertion. Pericardiocentesis is a difficult procedure often with an unsatisfactory outcome because of the blind nature of the procedure and operator inexperience. For this reason, either emergent thoracotomy or operative exploration is preferred for penetrating trauma.

Rarely, needle pericardiocentesis may be required in blunt trauma, when the patient does not respond to resuscitation and a suspicion of tamponade exists.

Technique of emergency room thoracotomy

Penetrating wounds of the chest with significant compromise, or rapid deterioration after arrival in the Accident and Emergency department with a penetrating wound are indications for emergency department thoracotomy. It is not useful for patients who have no signs of life after prolonged resuscitation (more than 15 minutes of CPR), or are multiply injured by blunt trauma.

The patient is intubated and fluid resuscitated whilst preparations are made for an anterolateral thoracotomy. After the chest is entered, ventilation is briefly ceased, the pericardium opened, and the injury identified. At that point, haemorrhage may be controlled by digital pressure, and fluid resuscitation should be continued. Relief of tamponade is usually associated with an improvement in haemodynamics, after which the cardiac injury can be repaired by direct suture.

A left anterolateral thoracotomy permits open cardiac massage, treatment of cardiac lacerations, and clamping of the descending thoracic aorta. Torrential lung bleeding may also be controlled through a thoracotomy. The best outcomes are for patients with isolated right ventricular lacerations and tamponade and a systolic blood pressure of 50 mmHg or more on arrival. Where the left ventricle or two cardiac chambers are involved, or tamponade is not present on opening, the prognosis is poor.

Blunt injury to the heart and sternal fractures

Severe cases of blunt cardiac trauma causing rupture of cardiac chambers result in immediate death due to tamponade and pump failure. Deceleration injuries, causing the heart to impact against the sternum and vertebrae, may cause injury to the myocardium, valvular structures, and pericardial attachments.

Acute valvular incompetence, usually affecting the aortic valve and less commonly the mitral valve, present with shock out of proportion to the degree of external injury. Acute regurgitation is poorly tolerated, although these injuries are uncommon as in most circumstances the myocardium absorbs most of the impact. This injury to the myocardium was previously known as 'cardiac contusion'. More recently it has been labelled blunt cardiac injury (BCI). The diagnosis and management of BCI, has been simplified as result of an evidence-based review of this condition (Pasquale *et al.* 1998).

The suspicion of BCI must be raised when there is evidence of direct trauma to the precordium (often caused by the steering wheel in a motor vehicle accident). BCI may manifest as ischaemic-like chest pain which is unrelieved by nitrate therapy, or failure to respond in a normal way to fluid resuscitation for other injuries.

All patients in whom blunt cardiac injury is suspected should have an ECG on admission. The ECG revealing potential BCI may show arrhythmia (especially ventricular ectopics and atrial fibrillation), ischaemia, heart block, and bundle branch block or non-specific ST changes. Patients with an abnormal ECG should be admitted for cardiac monitoring for 24 hours. If the admission ECG is normal, it is unlikely that blunt cardiac injury exists, and no further investigations are required after a 4 hour period of cardiorespiratory monitoring. Patients <55 years of age and without significant co-morbidity or other injury can be discharged from the emergency department after 4 hours. Older patients should be admitted and observed for 24 hours.

If the patient is haemodynamically unstable and BCI is suspected, then an echocardiogram should be obtained. This allows quantification of wall motion abnormalities, detects pericardial fluid collections, and confirms valvular competence.

It is unnecessary to perform cardiac enzyme analysis on patients in whom BCI is suspected. It is uncommon for creatine kinase-MB to be elevated in patients with a normal ECG. Although troponin assays are more specific and sensitive, their use does not significantly contribute to patient management since all unstable patients should undergo echocardiography and the ECG is a better screening test for stable patients.

Blunt cardiac injury is generally self-limiting, and specific complications are treated on their merits, such as anti-arrhythmic medication, or inotropes and intra-aortic balloon pumping for low output states.

Key points

- Use ECG as a screening test.
- Observe all for 4 hours.
- Admit and perform echocardiography on all with abnormal ECG or signs of BCI.
- Exclude other injury (fractured sternum, ruptured aorta).

Sternal fractures

Sternal fractures are a common cause of blunt cardiac injury, but clearly not all sternal fractures have BCI. If the admission ECG is normal, then it is not necessary to monitor these patients, nor is measurement of cardiac enzymes. These patients may require admission for analgesia, particularly in displaced bicortical fractures, but most patients with unicortical sternal fractures and normal admission ECGs may be safely discharged after 4 hours of cardiorespiratory observation. The majority of sternal fractures involve the upper or mid portion, and are associated with other injuries, especially rib fractures in 50% of cases.

Key points

- Sternal fracture management
  - lateral chest radiograph
  - identify displacement as a guide to magnitude of force
  - screen for BCI with ECG
  - echo those with abnormal ECGs
  - admit those requiring opiate pain relief
  - observe all for 4 hours
  - discharge those with minor discomfort only.

Great vessel injury

The great vessels are the major intrathoracic arteries and veins, principally the aorta and its branches, the pulmonary arteries, the vena cavae, and the subclavian vessels. Injury to these vessels accounts for 10–15% of MVA deaths, most of whom die at the scene or during transport. There is a high rate of death and serious complications in those surviving to hospital (Pasquale and Fabian 1998).

The most common injury is to the aorta, which is subject to shearing forces caused by the relative mobility of the arch and the fixed descending aorta. The tethering point is the ligamentum arteriosum, just distal to the origin of the left subclavian. In blunt aortic injury (BAI), over 80% of ruptures are at this point.

In patients who survive the initial injury, the aortic rupture is contained by a thin layer of aortic adventitia and surrounding haematoma, explaining the precarious nature of this condition and its propensity to complete rupture. In a recent series the overall mortality of patients with injuries including BAI, was 31%. Aortic rupture was the cause of death in 63% of these (Fabian *et al.* 1997).

Although significant force is required to cause this injury, 50% of patients have no other injuries and are quite stable, reinforcing the point that a high index of suspicion of BAI must be exercised (Table 11.3).

Key point

- There is a high rate of death and serious complications in those surviving to hospital.

Investigations for blunt aortic injury

The initial chest radiograph is often abnormal in BAI, and is a guide to the need for other investigations.

The most important findings are:

- a widened mediastinum
- loss of definition of the aortic knob
- downward deviation of the left main bronchus (normally 30° below horizontal) or rightward deviation of a nasogastric tube—both are due to displacement by periaortic haematoma

Table 11.3 Grounds for suspecting blunt aortic injury (BAI)

High speed deceleration or side impact, including MVAs and falls from more than 10 m
Multiple rib fractures or flail chest, particularly first and second rib fractures
Scapular fractures, since the scapular is normally well protected and a fracture is an indication of the force exerted
Sternal fractures
Fractures of the thoracic spine
Pulse deficits, due to compression of the lumen by peri-aortic haematoma
Hypertension, 150/100 in 75% of patients with ruptured aortas
Hypotension, due to intrathoracic blood loss, or large initial ICC drainage (750 ml)
Interscapular murmur, due to turbulent flow across injury, present in 30% of BAI
Anuria as a result of poor renal perfusion
Paraplegia, due to ischaemia of the spinal cord distal to injury

- loss (opacification) of the aortopulmonary window.

Less important signs include:

- a pleural cap, due to mediastinal haematoma tracking superiorly
- associated fractures of the first and second ribs
- rightward deviation of the trachea, usually at T4.

Interpreting mediastinal widening

If the mediastinum looks wider than normal following a high-risk accident, then this warrants further investigation. A subjective assessment of widening is more important than direct measurement. As a guide to typical values, if the mediastinum is >6 cm in width on an erect PA film, or 8 cm on a supine AP film, then mediastinal widening is probably present.

The chest radiograph is a screening tool for BAI. If there are any positive signs as listed above, then definitive tests must be performed (Table 11.4).

Key points regarding BAI

- Sensitivity = correctly identified true positives (ruptured aortas).
- Specificity = correctly identified true negatives (non-ruptured aortas).

If mediastinal haematoma is present on CT, BAI cannot be ruled out except by aortography. If helical CT shows a normal mediastinum, and there are no suggestive clinical signs, BAI is very unlikely, and an aortogram is not necessary (Pate *et al.* 1999).

Chest radiography is a good screening tool, although BAI may exist even with a normal chest radiograph and some centres advocate chest CT in all high-risk patients. In one such trial, over 40% of patients with angiogram-proven rupture had a normal mediastinum on chest radiograph (Demetriades *et al.* 1998).

Conventional (non-helical) CT systems are not recommended as investigations for BAI. They are

Table 11.4 Investigations for BAI

Aortography	Helical CT	TOE
High sensitivity ~92%	Highest sensitivity ~100%	Medium sensitivity ~80%
Highest specificity ~99%	Medium specificity ~83%	Low specificity ~80%
May assist in planning of surgical procedure if required	Mediastinal haematoma well demonstrated	Cannot examine entire aorta due to 'blind spot' over distal arch
Additional time required to transport patient to angiography suite	Patients often require CT examination of other areas	Allows examination of valves, cardiac function and pericardial space
Available at large centres	Widely available	Not widely available
Fast (once personnel available)	Fast (if modern scanner used)	Fast (once personnel available)
Invasive, contrast required	Not invasive, contrast required	Invasive, no contrast required Operator dependent
The 'gold standard'	A 'screening tool'	Developing role

For sensitivity and specificity for aortography and helical CT see Fabian *et al.* (1997).

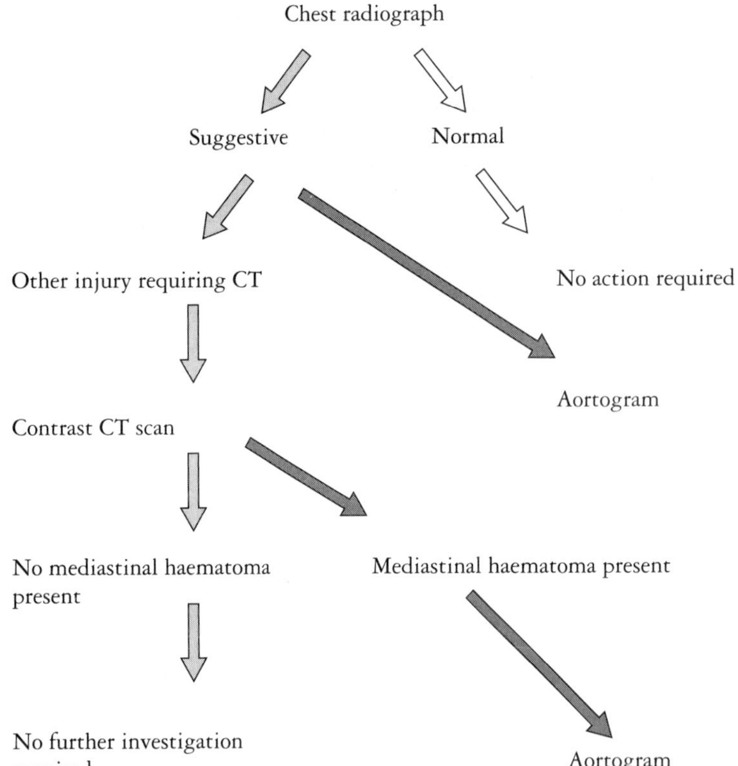

Figure 11.1 Algorithm for chest injuries.

significantly slower, and do not have the sensitivity or specificity of the newer machines.

A recommended approach is as follows (see Fig. 11.1):

- Patients with suspected aortic rupture on chest radiograph and no other injury undergo aortography as the first line of investigation.
- For patients with a chest radiograph suggestive of BAI and requiring other CT imaging (e.g. abdominal or head scan), perform a helical contrast CT of the chest as a screening tool.
- A CT finding of mediastinal haematoma prompts definitive evaluation by aortography. Although fractures of the vertebral column may cause mediastinal haematoma, it should be assumed that mediastinal haematoma is due to a ruptured aorta until cleared by aortography.
- Patients with normal CT scans of the chest, clearly demonstrating a normal sized mediastinum and intact contrast filled aorta, do not require aortography.
- Transoesophageal echo is not regarded as a definitive test, despite its obvious advantages.

This algorithm is summarized in Fig. 11.1.

Management of BAI

It is common for patients with BAI to be hypertensive, unless hypovolaemic because of other injuries. In stable patients, minimal volume replacement and maintenance of the systolic blood pressure <110 mmHg is preferred. A beta-blocker such as esmolol or metoprolol administered intravenously, and intravenous sodium nitroprusside as required, are used for this purpose (Fabian *et al.* 1998). Beta-blockade is preferred because of the reduction in aortic wall dP/dt, which is actually increased by dilators. Coughing and straining should be avoided by adequate sedation or paralysis particularly during insertion of nasogastric tubes or during intubation and insertion of a transoesophageal echocardiography (TOE) probe.

Frequently, transport to an institution with cardiothoracic surgical facilities will be required. Surgical repair of a ruptured aorta usually involves control of the aorta above and below the rupture and insertion of a vascular graft. There is a significant risk of paraplegia due to spinal cord ischaemia during surgical repair, particularly when the ischaemic time exceeds 30 minutes. To reduce this risk, some institutions perform the repair with cardiopulmonary bypass or use a bypass circuit from proximal to distal aorta, to maintain peripheral and possibly spinal perfusion. Systemic anticoagulation is usually required for these approaches and this may be contraindicated with concomitant injuries. Paraplegia occurs in around 9% of operative repairs (Fabian *et al.* 1997).

Conclusion

The treatment of chest trauma requires an assessment of problems that may potentially cause death. A high index of suspicion should be maintained in all high-velocity accidents for internal chest injuries.

Algorithms based on available evidence should be developed in individual institutions to improve outcomes for patients with chest trauma.

References

Barie P, Oswanski M, Spain D (1998) Prophylactic antibiotic usage in trauma. In: Luchette FA (ed) *EAST practice parameter guideline work group for tube thoracostomy*. www.east.org.

Demetriades D, Gomez H, Velmahos GC, Asensio JA, Murray J, Cornwell ER *et al.* (1998) Routine helical computed tomographic evaluation of the mediastinum in high-risk blunt trauma patients. *Archives of Surgery* 133: 1084–1088.

Fabian TC, Richardson JD, Croce MA *et al.* (1997) Prospective study of blunt aortic injury: multicenter trial of the American Association for the Surgery of Trauma. *Journal of Trauma* 42: 374–380.

Fabian TC, Davis KA, Gavant ML *et al.* (1998) Prospective study of blunt aortic injury: helical CT is diagnostic and antihypertensive therapy reduces rupture. *Annals of Surgery* 227: 676–677.

Pasquale M, Fabian TC (1998) Practice management guidelines for trauma from the Eastern Association for the Surgery of Trauma—blunt aortic injury. *Journal of Trauma* 44: 956–957.

Pasquale MD, Nagy K, Clarke J (1998) Practice guidelines for screening of blunt cardiac injury. In: *EAST practice parameter guideline work group for screening of blunt cardiac injury*. www.east.org.

Pate JW, Gavant ML, Weiman DS, Fabian TC (1999) Traumatic rupture of the aortic isthmus: program of selective management. *World Journal of Surgery* 23: 59–63.

RACS (1997) *Early management of severe trauma*. Course handbook. Royal Australasian College of Surgeons, Melbourne.

Further reading

Mattox KL (1996) In: Feliciano D, Moore EE, Mattox KL (eds) *Trauma*, 3rd edn. Appleton Lange Stamford, CT.

12

CHAPTER 12

Abdominal injuries

PETER BARRY, ANTHONY J SHAKESHAFT, AND RODNEY STUDD

CHAPTER 12
Abdominal injuries

PETER BARRY, ANTHONY J SHAKESHAFT, AND RODNEY STUDD

Abdominal trauma accounts for up to 20% of trauma-related operations. Geography largely determines the distribution of blunt and penetrating injury, the latter being more common in urban areas. Although the enforcement of the wearing of seatbelts has seen a reduction in the incidence of head, chest, and solid visceral injury, their use is associated with pancreatic, intestinal, and mesenteric injury as a result of compression against the lumbar spine.

Key points

- Earlier diagnosis and management of abdominal trauma reduces morbidity and mortality.
- Maintain a high level of suspicion based on history of trauma and related injuries.
- Always manage trauma in accordance with the principles and protocols of ATLS/EMST.

General surgeons have an essential role in the immediate resuscitation and decision-making process for multiply injured patients. The abdomen is potentially responsible for major morbidity and death from early haemorrhage and late sepsis. Diagnosis may be obscured by multiple injuries rendering clinical signs inaccurate. Nevertheless several indications for laparotomy exist including:

- penetrating trauma to the abdomen (with breach of the peritoneum)
- hypotension in the face of obvious abdominal trauma, obvious peritonitis, or evisceration through a wound (excluding omentum)
- gastrointestinal haemorrhage following abdominal trauma.

In most instances, however, these conditions are not present and clinical assessment aided by investigations must be judiciously used to select those patients who require laparotomy.

Although an aggressive laparotomy policy will enable the existence of intra-abdominal injury to be confirmed, an unnecessary operation confers a finite risk to all patients, including hypothermia, and—of more concern—may divert attention away from injuries deserving higher priority for management. However, needless over-investigation and delay where a laparotomy is needed may also result in greater harm to the patient. The importance of clinical reassessment to re-evaluate abdominal signs as well as the response to fluid challenge cannot be overemphasized.

The extent of the abdominal cavity is usually underestimated. It extends from the level of the nipple (fourth intercostal space) to the perineum. It may be conceptually divided into three compartments—the retroperitoneum, the peritoneum, and the pelvis—which are subject to differing patterns of injury and clinical signs. Interpretation of clinical signs pertaining to the abdomen may be rendered inaccurate as a result of a number of general factors (e.g. alcohol, head injury) and local factors such as thoracic, abdominal wall, and bony pelvic injuries.

Clues to abdominal injury begin with the history. The force of impact in a motor vehicle accident indicates the energy transferred to intra-abdominal viscera. The mechanism of injury is also important. Examination of the abdominally injured patient is in many cases the most important part of the assessment. It should be thorough, including a rectal examination, and should be targeted towards the mechanism of injury and any obvious external signs of injury. These may include bruising by seatbelt, tyre marks, or hoofmarks at the site of impact. For penetrating injuries the entry and exit sites must be carefully evaluated and trajectories must be carefully analysed, especially where exit wounds are not found.

Investigations

When laparotomy is not absolutely indicated yet doubt as to the possibility of abdominal trauma still exists, several means of further investigation are available: ultrasound, CT scan, diagnostic peritoneal lavage (DPL), laparoscopy, and laparotomy.

Ultrasound

Ultrasound provides a means of simple, rapid assessment in the resuscitation bay. Its main advantages over CT are that it is cheap, safe, and mobile; rapid evaluation may be carried out at the bedside, and repeated. Its limitations include operator dependence (expertise in this technique is essential), an inability to assess the extent of visceral damage, and a significant rate of missed injury, up to 10% in the best centres. The best results are obtained by centres experienced in trauma and personnel trained in the technique. Most importantly, reproducibility is maximized by using ultrasound as a screening technique where the end point is the presence of free fluid within the abdominal cavity. Its greatest value lies in demonstrating a positive finding in a stable patient. An additional advantage is assessing fetal viability in the pregnant patient.

Computed tomography

Many units have had excellent results from CT scanning in terms of sensitivity and specificity for particular findings, but it has not been a uniform experience and several variables will influence a particular unit's choice of investigation.

Findings which are reliably detected are:

- free blood or fluid in the peritoneal cavity
- solid visceral injury, especially to liver, spleen, pancreas, and kidneys
- free gas
- small pneumothoraces which may have been missed on supine chest radiographs.

Although most retroperitoneal injuries will be detected, gastrointestinal perforations may be missed. The absence of free fluid or gas does not exclude a hollow visceral injury, and use of enteric contrast may improve sensitivity of detection. CT does not give information about the rate of continued blood loss.

The main limitations of CT scanning include the need to transport the patient to the scanner, relative inaccessibility of the patient during scanning, and the risk of a patient becoming haemodynamically unstable during transport or scanning. Haemodynamic compromise remains an absolute contraindication to CT scanning. The more widespread use of helical CT scanning has substantially reduced the time taken for the investigation.

Diagnostic peritoneal lavage

Despite advances in the above imaging modalities, DPL is an important indicator of intra-abdominal injury. Overall accuracy is reported at >97%. The only absolute contraindication is an established indication for laparotomy. DPL does not indicate the source or volume of haemorrhage, nor whether the haemorrhage is ongoing. It will not give information about retroperitoneal injuries and pelvic fractures with haematoma tracking up into the DPL wound site may give a false-positive result. A positive result is an indication for laparotomy.

Technique

1 Insert nasogastric/orogastric tube to decompress the stomach.

2 Insert urinary catheter to empty bladder.

3 Prepare skin around and below umbilicus.

4 Local anaesthesia—lignocaine (lidocaine) 1% with adrenaline.
5 Midline incision just below the umbilicus.
6 Vertical incision through linea alba commencing at the umbilical cicatrix.
7 Apply clips to the peritoneum before incision.
8 Insert a purse-string suture through the peritoneum and linea alba.
9 Insert peritoneal dialysis catheter towards pelvis (if indicated—see below).
10 Rapid infuse 20 mL/kg of warmed normal saline (usually 1000 mL in adults).
11 Roll the patient from side to side, 30 seconds for each side.
12 Lower fluid bag and siphon fluid from the abdominal cavity.
13 Remove catheter and close wound.

Placement of the incision may need modification where there are pre-existent scars or pelvic fracture, or if pregnancy is suspected. Surgical trainees may be taught the technique, which is similar to that used for elective laparoscopic procedures, increasing the chance that the procedure is safely and rapidly conducted during the trauma assessment.

The criteria for a positive test include the withdrawal of free blood or enteric contents on opening the peritoneum, the lavage of blood, inability to read typewritten print behind the lavage tubing due to the colour of the haemoserous fluid, or a laboratory red cell count of >100 000/mL or a white cell count >500/mL. Microscopy for organisms or enteric content should be performed. The white cell count may not be elevated if <3 hours has elapsed from the time of injury. DPL may lead to a non-therapeutic laparotomy in up to 25% of cases. A greatly elevated amylase may be found in the presence of pancreatic injury of upper gastrointestinal perforation.

Laparoscopy

Increasing use and familiarity of laparoscopic techniques in elective general surgery has lead to their widespread availability and use in emergency assessment of trauma to minimize the need for unnecessary laparotomy. General anaesthesia is required and preparation for a trauma laparotomy must be made. Laparoscopy should only be used in the haemodynamically stable patient. Advantages and uses include confirmation of peritoneal penetration of a stab wound and damage to nearby structures, diaphragmatic injury, and ongoing haemorrhage from solid viscera. Examining the entire small bowel and retroperitoneal structures is difficult, but it is nevertheless possible and may be increasingly utilized in centres with extensive experience in elective advanced laparoscopic procedures.

Exploratory laparotomy

In certain situations this remains the most effective way of assessing and dealing with intra-abdominal injuries. The main indications in blunt trauma are peritonitis and hypovolaemia/shock.

Peritonitis

Peritonitis is usually due to rupture of a hollow viscus such as the duodenum, intestine, bladder, or gallbladder. Free intraperitoneal blood from solid viscus injury or mesenteric vascular injury may also cause significant peritoneal irritation without ongoing haemodynamic compromise.

Hypovolaemia/shock

Exploratory laparotomy is useful in cases of hypovolaemia/shock where no other obvious source of blood loss exists. A plain chest radiograph is required to exclude significant haemothorax, and a pelvic radiograph will exclude fractures which may give rise to significant bleeding. Other sources of ongoing blood loss such as major limb fractures and scalp lacerations can usually be controlled. Further haemodynamic compromise after short period of initial resuscitation should alert the clinician to the probability of an intra-abdominal source.

Key points

- Safe assessment of abdominal trauma involves:
  - adequate history from patient (if possible), available witnesses, and paramedical staff

- repeated measurement of vital signs: heart rate, blood pressure, or saturation
- complete physical examination including rectal examination
- prompt and correct use of diagnostic investigation
- repeated examinations to detect progressive physical signs

◆ All the above investigations must be utilized in conjunction with, not as a substitute for, regular and careful clinical evaluation.

Penetrating and blast injuries

In the UK, penetrating and blast injuries account for up to 20% of abdominal injuries. Stab wounds are the commonest, but even where the peritoneum has been breached they will cause significant damage in only 50% of cases. The stabbing victim who is haemodynamically unstable, exhibits peritonism, gastrointestinal bleeding or evisceration (excepting omental evisceration alone) or continuing external haemorrhage is best dealt within the operating theatre and will require laparotomy. In the absence of these findings patients may be assessed in the resuscitation room under local anaesthesia to determine direction and depth of penetration of the wound by exploration. Blind probing of wounds should be avoided. Whether the peritoneum has been breached needs to be determined, and if this is not possible then laparoscopy may be employed. Where no peritoneal entry is found, wound care is effected and if appropriate, retroperitoneal structures may be assessed by CT scanning using gastrograffin enema contrast as well as intravenous contrast to assess the presence of injury to the renal tract as well as the ascending or descending colon. When the peritoneum is found to be breached, DPL may select those patients who do not otherwise exhibit a clear indication for immediate laparotomy. Just as effective is frequent, careful serial physical examination to reduce the need for a non-therapeutic laparotomy. Weapons and other objects *in situ* at assessment should not be removed until the patient is in the operating theatre. Abdominal gunshot wounds and other missile injuries necessitate exploratory laparotomy as visceral damage is almost a certainty (>90%). A missile will cause tissue damage along the track it makes in its path traversing the tissues. The amount of damage sustained outside the track depends on the amount of excess energy transferred by the missile. High-velocity bullets such as those from rifles and machine guns may cause cavitation. A temporary cavity within the tissue destroyed is formed, and debris may be sucked into it. Secondary bone fragments may cause further, more extensive damage. The actual damage sustained is related to a number of variables; it is important to treat the wound, not the weapon. Explosions may cause injury by several mechanisms including blast waves, burns, missile fragments, and throwing of victims into the air.

The principles of surgical management include careful, extensive exploration, debridement of devitalized tissues, removal of foreign bodies where access to them does not impart further risk of tissue damage or morbidity, lavage, and open management of wounds. Repeated exploration may be required where tissue necrosis may extend and demarcate more clearly, and delayed primary closure or healing by secondary intention is usually required. Without careful adherence to these principles wound sepsis is likely to ensue, with its attendant mortality and morbidity.

Specific abdominal injuries: evaluation and treatment

Careful evaluation of the patient with potential intra-abdominal injury begins with a detailed history to elucidate the mechanism of injury, e.g. seatbelt-related, deceleration, direction of impact, speed of impact. Repeated clinical examination supplemented as indicated by the above investigations will lead to detection of the injuries and prevent missed injury resulting in disaster. Particular patterns of injury will direct enquiry towards specific organs:

◆ Right-sided lower rib fracture suggests possible liver injury.

- Left-sided rib fracture may be associated with splenic or left renal injury.
- Fracture of the upper lumbar spine (Chance fracture) may be associated with duodenal injury and pancreatic neck/body injury with disruption of the main pancreatic duct.
- A deceleration injury with a seatbelt sign may indicate duodenal transection, mesenteric vascular injury, and laceration of small bowel at junctions of fixity/mobility such the duodenojejunal flexure, and terminal ileum as well as hepatic or splenic damage.
- Pelvic fracture may have associated bladder, urethral, or rectal injury as well as significant vessel injury.
- Associated limb, chest, or head injury may give clues as to the likely site of abdominal trauma, even if signs are not obvious, especially in the unconscious patient.

Before the insertion of a nasogastric tube or urethral catheter, signs which may signify a base of skull fracture or partial urethral injury must be excluded. These include periorbital haematoma; epistaxis; clear dishcarge indicating cerebrospinal fluid from nostril; perineal haematoma; and blood at the urethral meatus and a high-riding prostate on rectal examination. Rectal examination is also essential to rule out potential spinal cord injury. The presence or otherwise of bowel sounds and assessment of abdominal girth are useless in the evaluation of trauma.

Key point

- The nature of trauma indicates a likely pattern of injury: stabbing, low-velocity gunshot, high-velocity gunshot, blunt impact, or deceleration.

Principles of the trauma laparotomy

Operating theatre staff should be informed about a multiply injured patient and preparation for major vascular and gastrointestinal procedures as well as suction, red cell recycling devices, and packs. The surgical team must be prepared for unexpected findings. The patient is positioned supine. A subcostal retraction device (e.g. Goligher or Wynn Jones frame) should be placed and if pelvic trauma is suspected, the legs should be placed in stirrups (Lloyd-Davies or Allen) to allow perineal access and assistant placement. Preparation is from the nipples to midthighs. A generous midline incision should allow exposure of all abdominal viscera. Blood is first aspirated and the four quadrants of the abdomen as well as the pelvis are packed carefully. A wide Deaver retractor held by an assistant over a pack placed on the visceral surface of the liver can retract this organ against the diaphragm to compress the organ firmly but gently. A systematic search can be made for specific sites of haemorrhage by removing individual packs sequentially. The liver should be examined finally, allowing adequate delay for non-significant haemorrhage to abate. Almost all haemorrhage can be controlled by direct pressure, either digitally or with packs. Torrential haemorrhage can be controlled by direct supra-coeliac aortic compression (manually or with an aortic compressor) or cross-clamping. Internal control can also be obtained by a distal aortotomy and retrograde passage of a large (e.g. 26G) Foley urinary catheter, inflating the balloon proximally. Once haemorrhage is temporarily controlled, blood and blood products may be infused by the anaesthetic team before the definitive repair of specific injuries. Once the life-threatening injuries have been dealt with, all other abdominal viscera must be exposed and examined to exclude occult injury. Manoeuvres to attain exposure include opening the lesser sac; Kocherization of the duodenum (after mobilization of the hepatic flexure of the colon) to expose the right renal hilum, inferior vena cava, and head of the pancreas; mobilization of the fourth part of the duodenum to expose the aorta; and, if indicated, mobilization of the left colon to expose the left renal vascular pedicle. Haematomas associated with pelvic fractures be left intact and controlled by packing, fractures stabilized by fixation, and endovascular embolization carried out following angiography if haemorrhage continues.

Key points

- Principles of trauma laparotomy.
  - control bleeding
  - control sepsis
  - definitive surgical management may be delayed 1–2 days if patient has gross metabolic derangement
  - seek further specialist assistance as necessary, e.g. liver, vascular, urology.

Damage control surgery

The concept of damage control surgery has arisen by observation of problems which ensue in the multiple injured patient where delay to definitive surgery or prolonged surgery results in hypothermia, acidosis and coagulopathy, and multiple organ failure. Rapid control of haemorrhage by packing and stapling of bowel injuries to prevent further peritoneal contamination is all that is effected during the first laparotomy. Stabilization of the patient in the intensive care unit then allows planning of definitive surgery 24–48 hours later. Emergency control of haemorrhage may still be required in up to 20% of patients managed in this way, and abdominal compartment syndrome may also be one of the sequelae. This is characterized by rising intra-abdominal pressure leading to anuric renal failure, increasing ventilatory requirements with a rise in airway pressures and eventually carbon dioxide, as well as impediment to venous return from the lower limbs.

Trauma in pregnancy

See Chapter 37, 'The injured pregnant woman'.

Abdominal wall injury

Blunt injury may give rise to significant abdominal wall injury. Significant bruising or soft tissue damage to the abdominal wall may indicate intra-abdominal injury, but may also simulate the diagnosis of peritonitis and render exclusion of intra-abdominal trauma difficult if not impossible. Pedestrians may be run over by heavy vehicles with resultant shearing of the subcutaneous tissues, devitalizing the overlying skin. Judicious use of early debridement is necessary to prevent the onset of serious necrotizing infection. Debridement includes removal of all visible foreign material and devitalized tissue. Copious lavage with saline should follow. Dressings and repeated debridement may be necessary before definitive reconstruction, which may involve delayed primary closure, skin grafting or even myocutaneous flaps and synthetic (polypropylene) mesh for significant abdominal wall defects.

Spleen

The spleen is the most commonly injured organ after blunt abdominal trauma, principally after motor vehicle accidents. It is a highly vascular but friable organ. A pathologically enlarged spleen is more likely to be injured with lesser degrees of trauma. The extent of injury ranges (Table 12.1) from subcapsular (contained) haematoma, through

Table 12.1 Severity of splenic injury

Type	Description
I	Subcapsular or intraparenchymal haematoma with an intact capsule
II	Open parenchymal tears of fractures which do not reach the hilum
III	Large open fractures which extend into the hilum
IV	Shattered or pulpified spleen with hilar disruption or avulsed fragments

parenchymal fractures which may extend to the hilum, to actual avulsion from the vascular pedicle. The spleen is susceptible to deceleration injury because of its relative mobility between all of its neighbouring attachments. It is at the junction of the attachments that capsular tears occur. Fractures may be caused by contact of the convex diaphragmatic surface against the ninth to eleventh ribs. Clues to the presence of splenic injury include a history of deceleration, usually involving an motor vehicle accident or a direct blow to the left lower ribs or left upper quadrant of the abdomen. There may be transient hypotension before resuscitation, and signs of peritoneal irritation maximal in the left upper quadrant of the abdomen may be present. Referred pain to the left shoulder tip due to left hemidiaphragmatic irritation may be a feature. Plain chest radiographs may reveal fractures of the left ninth to eleventh ribs, an elevated left hemidiaphragm, and medial displacement of the gastric bubble before nasogastric tube insertion. CT scanning remains the mainstay of diagnosis and non-operative assessment of splenic injury. Lacerations appear as low-density irregular bands within the parenchyma. Subcapsular haematomas appear as peripheral low density lesions which flatten the convex contour of the splenic surface.

The risk of overwhelming post-splenectomy infection (OPSI) following splenectomy and the success of several spleen-conserving techniques has meant a reduction in the rate of splenectomy in adult blunt trauma. Conservative management may be non-operative or operative conservation of the spleen (or part thereof). The phenomenon of delayed rupture occurs in up to 5% of non-operatively managed splenic injuries. Three-quarters of such ruptures occur within 2 weeks of the initial trauma, but delayed rupture has been reported years later. Its mechanism is thought to involve liquefaction of a contained haematoma leading to an influx of fluid due to its hyperosmolality. The cavity pressure rises and expands the capsule, resulting in rupture and secondary haemorrhage. Splenic cysts which may be symptomatic or be found incidentally on imaging may be associated a history of trauma to the spleen managed non-operatively. Selection of patients for non-operative management (up to 25% of adult splenic trauma) is made in the setting of blunt trauma where splenic injury is an isolated injury, or associated injuries do not require operative intervention. Haemodynamic stability persists despite no more than 2 units of blood transfused within the first 24 hours. Non-operative management of splenic injury as seen by CT scanning in the haemodynamically stable patient requires careful selection and monitoring of patients. Patients should be observed closely in a high dependency unit or surgical intensive care ward. CT scanning is useful to monitor morphological changes in the observation period. If laparotomy is being performed, it should proceed as previously indicated. Once blood and clots have been removed from the peritoneal cavity, the left upper quadrant should be carefully inspected. If clot but no active bleeding is seen, this should be gently removed to display the splenic surface. Omental and other congenital adhesions should be divided to 'defuse' the spleen, preventing iatrogenic injury. Capsular tears or adherent clots may be visualized and the spleen should be carefully palpated to detect other injuries. If no other injuries are seen, the spleen may be left in place with a dry pack next to it. After attending to other sites within the abdomen, the pack can be removed and the spleen inspected for ongoing haemorrhage. If active bleeding is present, mobilization of the spleen is mandatory. This must be done with care not to cause further injury. The splenocolic and lienorenal ligaments and lateral adhesions are divided while medial countertraction over a moistened pack is applied over the convex surface of the spleen by the surgeon. The apical short gastric vessels will need to be ligated and divided to achieve full mobility. If the exact site of hilar haemorrhage is hidden by the short gastric vessels, then these may all be ligated and divided. Although splenectomy may remain the safest option in cases of major disruption of the splenic substance, approximately 50–75% of spleens can be repaired once laparotomy has been indicated. Techniques include partial resection (suturing or stapling), ligation of feeding vessels, and compressing the splenic substance within an absorbable (Dexon) mesh. Once haemostasis has been obtained the risk, of further haemorrhage from the spleen is minuscule (<2%). Haemostatic agents such as topical thrombin or surgicel (oxidized cellulose), fibrin glue, and argon-beam coagulation are also effective in stopping surface haemorrhage. It is important to completely mobilize the spleen and have access to the vascular pedicle before attempting repair. The death rate from isolated splenic injury should be well under 10%. Patients who have undergone splenectomy, especially children, are at risk of developing OPSI principally with encapsulated organisms. This is a result of reduced clearance of organisms from the blood during episodes of bacteraemia, reduced levels of IgM antibodies, and reduction in opsonization of encapsulated organisms due to absence of the opsonic factor tuftsin. After splenectomy the patient must be immunized against *Pneumococcus*, *Meningococcus*, and *Haemophilus influenzae* B.

Liver

Liver injuries are common in blunt trauma. Commonly (up to 70%), hepatic injury is discovered on CT scanning and many cases will be managed non-operatively in specialized units where the surgical team is prepared should sudden potentially life-threatening haemorrhage take place. Injuries associated with haemorrhage rendering laparotomy necessary may often appropriately be managed by perihepatic packing and, once stabilized, the patient should be transferred to a specialist hepatobiliary centre for definitive management. This is usually the safest approach when massive blood loss and delays have already resulted. Liver injuries may be graded on the basis of the depth of laceration, the extent of haemorrhage, and the presence of major hepatic venous injury (Table 12.2). Penetrating wounds usually cause abdominal bleeding with minimal tissue destruction, whereas high-velocity missiles may cause extensive parenchymal damage.

Table 12.1 Liver injury scale[a]

Grade	Description
I	Haematoma: subcapsular, non-expanding, <10% surface area Laceration: capsular tear, non-bleeding with <1 cm depth parenchymal disruption
II	Haematoma: subcapsular, non-expanding, 10–50% ; intraparenchymal, non-expanding, <2 cm diameter Laceration: <3 cm parenchymal depth, <10 cm length
III	Haematoma: subcapsular, <50% surface area or expanding; ruptured subcapsular haematoma with active bleeding; intraparenchymal haematoma <2 cm Laceration: <3 cm parenchymal depth
IV	Haematoma: ruptured central haematoma Laceration: parenchymal destruction involving 25–75% of hepatic lobe
V	Laceration: parenchymal destruction <75% of hepatic lobe Vascular: juxtahepatic venous injuries (major hepatic veins/retrohepatic cava)
VI	Vascular: hepatic avulsion

[a] When two or more injuries exist, the grade should be increased. The grading is based on the best available evidence such as CT scanning, laparotomy, or autopsy.

Blunt trauma to the upper abdomen or lower right-sided rib cage tends to produce explosive bursts or linear lacerations of the liver surface (Fig. 12.1). Again, significant parenchymal damage often results. Stellate bursts tend to affect the posterior superior segment of the right lobe (Couinaud segment VII) due to its vulnerable location, convex surface, relative fixity, and concentration of hepatic mass. Associated shearing forces due to deceleration may cause tearing of the major hepatic veins at their junction with the liver.

The main surgical aims are to control bleeding and debride devitalized tissue. Bleeding from grade I injuries usually subsides spontaneously and does not require operative management. It may be responsible for a positive DPL. Ongoing haemorrhage from grade II injuries will either respond to packing or will require suture ligation of individual vessels and bile radicles. Grade III injuries may need perihepatic packing while the portal triad is controlled and prepared for cross-clamping (the Pringle manoeuvre) which can usually safely be maintained for up to 30 minutes. Once this has been achieved, a hepatotomy (tractotomy) may be performed to assist in identifying the source of continued bleeding (usually hepatic veins) which can be suture or clip ligated. Grade IV injuries will eventually require lobar or segmental resection, but it may be appropriate to delay formal resection until the patient has been stabilized with interim packing and debridement. Hepatic resection after acute injury should be minimized, and performed only as a life-saving last resort. Bile leaks should be actively sought and repaired; the Pringle manoeuvre may assist in their localization by increasing upstream pressure within the bile duct. Techniques such as omental plugging of hepatic cavities or raw surfaces and drainage are a useful adjunct. After control of significant vessels, raw surfaces can often be controlled with the use of argon-beam coagulation which is now available to most hepatobiliary units. Perihepatic packing will usually suffice to control all but the severest forms of hepatic bleeding (grades I–IV), allow the patient to be stabilized in the intensive care unit and to be and transferred to a specialized hepatobiliary unit while coagulopathy and hypothermia are corrected. Re-exploration to remove packing and effect definitive treatment can be carried out 24–48 hours later.

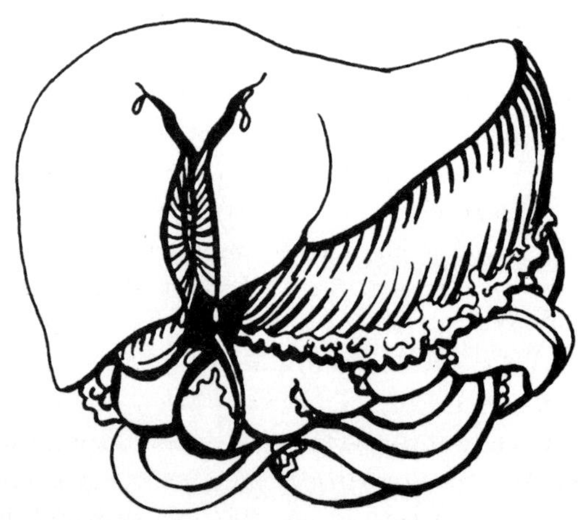

Figure 12.1 Laceration of the liver.

Grade V injuries with injury to the retrohepatic cava or major hepatic veins may not respond to packing and will then require either insertion of an atriocaval shunt or total vascular isolation by controlling the infra- and suprahepatic inferior vena cava after a Pringle manoeuvre. Re-bleeding from the liver after initial suture ligation will require re-exploration and usually lobectomy. Angiography may provide a useful preoperative adjunct. The latter procedure is the procedure of choice in the event of haemobilia. Selective angiography may be followed by embolization of the feeding vessel. Mortality following liver trauma depends on associated injuries as well as the extent of hepatic injury. Shock at the time of admission is associated with a 30% mortality rate. The death rate after penetrating trauma is around 1%, contrasting with 20% mortality from blunt trauma.

Bile duct and gallbladder

Minor lacerations to the gallbladder may be repaired, but in most instances a cholecystectomy will be required. Injuries to the common bile duct

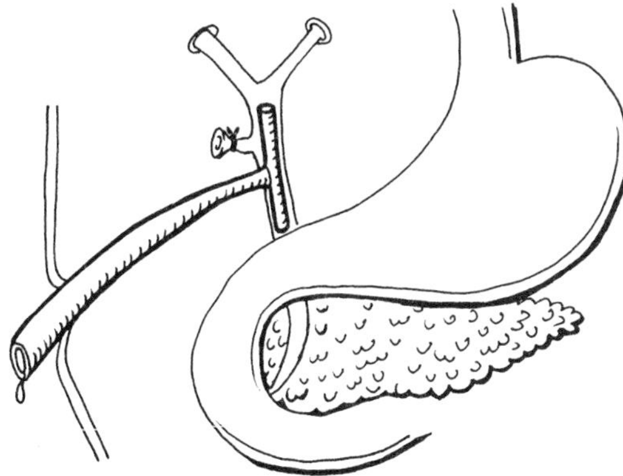

Figure 12.2 T-tube.

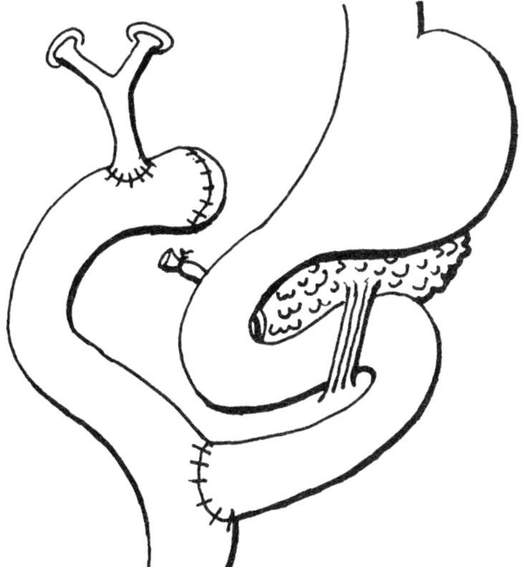

Figure 12.3 Roux-en-Y choledochojejunostomy.

or hepatic duct can be closed primarily and decompressed with a T-tube (Fig. 12.2). Transection or avulsion of the common bile duct will require Roux-en-Y choledochojejunostomy (Fig. 12.3).

Stomach

Gastric injuries are more likely to occur as a result of blunt injury in the presence of a distended stomach. This results in a blowout rupture. Gastric injuries as a result of penetrating trauma must be searched for carefully, with special attention to the posterior surface and the margins of the lesser and greater curvatures where omentum may conceal an injury, clues to which may only be a small haematoma. An exit wound indicating a through and through laceration must be assumed to exist until proven otherwise. These sites must be exposed by opening the lesser sac, aided by the use of dye instilled in the nasogastric tube (e.g. methylene blue) as well as distal clamping across the pylorus and instillation of air down the nasogastric tube to distend the organ to accentuate small leaks, allowing easier recognition and immediate repair. Management of such an injury may require debridement, and suture in one or two layers with a continuous, haemostatic suture will usually suffice. Decompression postoperatively by nasogastric tube is a necessity. Extensive damage to the stomach from a blast injury may require subtotal or total gastrectomy. Stress ulcers are common in the multiply injured patient postoperatively, and antisecretory agents should be considered.

Duodenum and pancreas

The commonest mode of blunt trauma is sudden deceleration in the presence of a seatbelt restraint. These retroperitoneal, immobile organs are compressed against the lumbar vertebrae during spinal flexion. Duodenal rupture should be suspected from aspiration of blood from the nasogatric tube, retroperitoneal gas, or loss of the psoas shadow on plain radiograph. A CT scan with fine cuts through the duodenum and nasogastric gastrograffin contrast may aid in diagnosis where laparotomy is not otherwise indicated. Isolated duodenal injury is rare and partial lacerations with minimal devitalization may be repaired. Nasogastric and external drainage is recommended.

Pancreatic injury may be suspected from elevations in serum amylase and DPL amylase level as well as CT scanning. Assessment of damage to the main pancreatic duct will dictate definitive management. This is usually difficult to assess in the acute setting as either endoscopic retrograde cholangiopancreatography (ERCP) or magnetic radiologic cholangiogram (MRCP) is required. In the absence of major duct injury, suture ligation to control bleeding, omental plugging, and drainage are the main management techniques. Where transection of the pancreas (anterior to the lumbar vertebra) has occurred, resection of the tail with or without splenic preservation and Roux-en-Y loop drainage of the injured surface of the pancreas and main duct as well as external drainage is required. External drainage alone may suffice in the acute setting (see 'Damage control surgery'). Additional techniques include diversion of the enteric stream away from the duodenum by performance of a duodenal 'diverticulization' or pyloric exclusion with a gastrojejunostomy or triple tube diversion via a gastrostomy, retrograde drainage of the duodenum after primary repair via a jejunostomy and a distal feeding jejunostomy. Upper gastrointestinal injuries including liver injury may be also supported by the use of enteric feeding by tube jejunostomy.

Small intestine

Small-intestinal injury is usually amenable to simple suture repair. Where devitalization of small intestine has occurred, resection and primary anastomosis (if appropriate) may be effected. Perforation may be concealed along the mesenteric border and areas may be devascularized as a result of concomitant mesenteric shearing injuries. Preservation of as much small-bowel length as possible is the main surgical principle. Expanding haematomas within the mesentery should be explored. They may be otherwise treated conservatively.

Colonic injuries

The general condition of the patient is paramount in deciding on major issues in colonic injuries. The questions raised are whether a diverting stoma should be created, and should primary repair or resection with or without a primary anastomosis be performed. A randomized controlled trial (Sasaki *et al.* 1995) has reported primary repair or resection with anastomosis in penetrating colonic injuries as the treatment of choice. Primary repair may be considered safe in a stable patient with a wound involving less than one-third of the colonic circumference, located around the antimesenteric surface if there is no compromise in the vascular supply. If there is gross contamination, peritonitis, a post-injury delay of greater than 8 hours, or the patient is shocked, primary repair is to be avoided. Blunt colonic injuries may generally be managed by resection and immediate anastomosis if the patient is otherwise stable. A loop ileostomy or double-barrelled stoma may be indicated and will facilitate operative closure.

Rectal injury

Injuries of the intraperitoneal rectum may be treated as described for colonic injuries. Injuries involving the extraperitoneal rectum need to be carefully assessed before surgical treatment. A gastrograffin enema and careful examination under anaesthesia are highly advantageous to planning treatment. The usual causes are pelvic fracture, foreign body, and knife or gunshot wounds. The management principles are usually a defunctioning proximal stoma, debridement, and drainage of the wound. The rectal stump may be irrigated to minimize contamination. Direct primary repair is difficult and rarely justified. Sphincter injuries should be managed by a specialist in this field, but will usually require defunctioning, debridement and perhaps repair, either immediate or delayed. Broad-spectrum antibiotics are necessary in rectal injury.

Renal injury

Blunt trauma to the kidneys is common and usually minor, requiring no active surgical intervention in 85% of cases. It is usually suspected by the site of injury or presence of associated injuries. Macroscopic haematuria is indicative until proven otherwise. Microscopic haematuria does not require further investigation if it resolves on repeat testing. Haematuria may be absent with severe renal trauma such as avulsion of the vascular pedicle. Usually hypotension and loin tenderness will be present. CT scanning with intravenous contrast is now the investigation of choice and will give anatomical and functional information about both kidneys. Indication for operative exploration include persistent retroperitoneal bleeding, extensive urinary extravasation, or non-viable renal parenchyma needing debridement.

The operative approach should commence with vascular control via a midline laparotomy before opening Gerota's fascia. Perinephric haematomas found at the time of laparotomy should only be explored if they are expanding or pulsatile, or preoperative CT demonstrates urinary extravasation. Injuries not requiring emergency intervention are best dealt with by specialist urological units.

Bladder

Rupture of the bladder is liable to occur in blunt injury when the bladder is full. Intra- or extraperitoneal rupture may occur (the latter in 75% of cases) and may be clinically silent initially. Preoperative diagnosis is by cystography and repair is followed by at least 10 days of decompression by an indwelling catheter. The anterior wall can be accessed through a midline laparotomy and a posterior wall defect may need to be sutured from within the bladder via an anterior cystotomy. A cystogram (trans-catheter) is performed to exclude a leak prior to catheter removal.

Urethra

When signs of urethral injury are present (blood at the meatus, perineal haematoma, and a high-riding prostate on rectal examination) a urethrogram should be obtained and specialist urological opinion sought before catheter insertion. A suprapubic catheter may need to be inserted but bladder fullness should be confirmed by ultrasound if not obviously palpable, to avoid iatrogenic injury to nearby structures.

Pelvic fractures usually cause disruption at the membranous urethra with a high-riding prostate. Suprapubic drainage is the initial management with definitive reconstruction (urethroplasty) usually delayed for 2–3 months. The bulbous or penile urethra may be injured by a direct blow to the perineum. Again, suprapubic diversion of urine is all that is required initially. A voiding cystourethrogram can be performed to assess the injury radiologically prior to consideration of any definitive intervention.

Male genitalia

Skin loss and testicular rupture with haematoma are the commonest forms of injury. The penis and penile urethra are usually spared. Skin loss can be managed with debridement and skin grafting. An exposed testis can be debrided and protected temporarily in the subcutaneous tissues of the upper thigh. Testicular haematomas are usually managed conservatively, unless expanding.

Uterine injury

Injury to the uterus is usually in combination with associated rectal or urinary tract injury (e.g. bladder) and is infrequent. Injury to the fundus can usually be directly repaired. In extensive injuries a hysterectomy may be necessary.

The vaginal cuff may be left open to provide drainage, especially if associated injuries are present. Direct trauma to the gravid uterus usually results in fetal death. Haemorrhage from the uterus in late stages of pregnancy may be massive, and hysterectomy is usually required after caesarean section.

Pelvic fractures

See Chapter 20, 'Pelvic injuries'.

Conclusion

Abdominal trauma is one component in the multiply injured patient, and priorities for resuscitation and treatment must be developed. Rapid control of intra-abdominal haemorrhage may be required immediately after assessment and stabilization of the airway and breathing components of the initial (primary) survey. Close co-operation between specialties is essential, and co-ordination is best carried out by personnel who understand the priorities in treatment as well as the principles of surgical repair of the injuries. All possible significant injuries must be excluded and meticulous secondary survey must minimize chances of missing less immediately life-threatening injuries which may have delayed adverse consequences on the patient's outcome. All specialists involved in trauma care should use the EMST/ATLS system of trauma care as a basis for streamlined management of all trauma patients.

References

Sasaki LS, Allaben RD, Golwala R *et al.* (1995) Primary repair of colon injuries: A prospective randomized study. *Journal of Trauma* 39: 895–901.

Further reading

EAST Evaluation of blunt abdominal trauma, www.east.org

13

CHAPTER 13

Urogenital injuries

SIMON V BARIOL AND HOWARD LAU

CHAPTER 13
Urogenital injuries

SIMON V BARIOL AND HOWARD LAU

Isolated trauma to the genitourinary system is rare. Urological injuries are more often seen in the patient with multiple trauma. Injury to the urinary tract occurs in up to 10% of patients suffering from blunt or penetrating abdominal trauma. The aetiology of urological trauma varies between trauma centres, but the majority are due to blunt force.

It is important to establish priorities in the trauma patient and develop a consistent, systematic method of clinical assessment. Trauma to the urinary tract is rarely life-threatening, but can cause significant long-term morbidity, especially when diagnosis is delayed. In the case of patients with suspected urological trauma, the priorities are the same as for all patients: establishing and maintaining an airway; ensuring adequate ventilation; cervical spine control; and providing adequate organ perfusion.

This chapter outlines the classification of genitourinary trauma, and important steps in diagnosis and management of these injuries. The wide availability of CT scanning has improved diagnostic accuracy of upper urinary tract injuries and reduced the requirement for operative exploration in stable patients, in favour of a more conservative approach.

Most urological injuries may be managed non-operatively, but outcome depends on prompt recognition of injury and minimizing potential complications. The goal is always patient safety and preservation of kidney function. To this end, we will discuss clinical indications and guidelines for appropriate radiological evaluation. Management decisions are based on a combination of clinical and radiographic information.

Key points

- Isolated trauma to the genitourinary system is rare.
- Most urological trauma may be managed non-operatively.

Renal injury

Renal trauma is traditionally classified in broad terms as major or minor. Major renal trauma includes large lacerations of the renal parenchyma with or without injury to the collecting system or the renovascular pedicle. Minor trauma includes simple laceration, renal contusion, and subcapsular haematoma (Fig. 13.1).

Minor trauma accounts for approximately 70% of renal injuries overall. Of the remaining major injuries, almost half involve the renovascular pedicle. Minor injuries are usually managed non-operatively, but there is widespread debate over the appropriate management of major renal injuries.

It may be more informative to classify renal trauma as blunt or penetrating, as this is more relevant for management. Penetrating injuries should be explored, with few exceptions. Most penetrating injuries to the kidney have other associated intra-abdominal injuries, especially in the case of gunshot wounds. In contrast, the majority of blunt renal injuries may be managed by conservative measures; associated injuries are less common and usually less severe. In the Parkland Memorial Hospital series, all cases of blunt renal trauma which required surgery had associated non-renal injuries (Feagins 1994a,b).

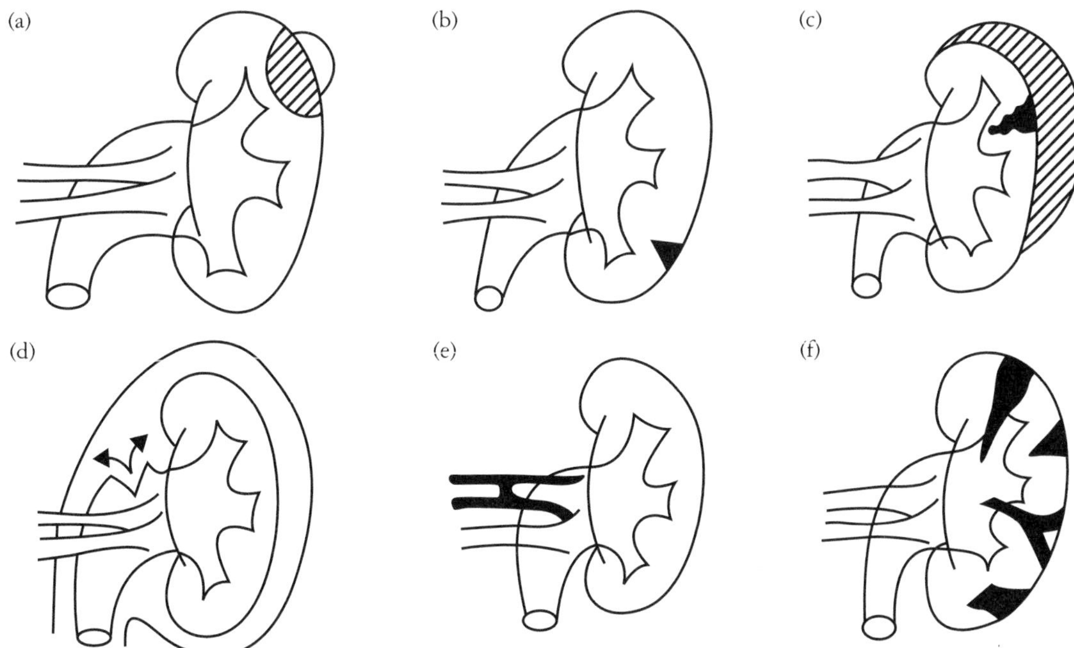

Figure 13.1 Major and minor renal injuries: (a) renal contusion and subcapsular haematoma; (b) simple laceration; (c) laceration and perirenal haematoma; (d) ruptured renal pelvis and urinoma; (e) renal artery intimal tear; (f) renal rupture/explosive injury.

The diagnosis of renal trauma is based on history, physical examination, and radiographic evidence. A history of blunt or penetrating injury to the abdomen, back, or flank, or sudden deceleration accidents, should all raise suspicion to the possibility of a renal injury. The patient may complain of flank pain or renal colic associated with clot haematuria. The patient's haemodynamic appearance depends on the degree of renal injury and any associated injuries; there may be flank bruising and tenderness, and gross or microscopic haematuria. The passing of clots is particularly suggestive of large bleeding from the upper urinary tract.

All patients with gross haematuria warrant further investigation. Patients with microscopic haematuria warrant further investigation only in the following settings:

- penetrating injury
- blunt injury with shock including transient hypotension
- high-impact trauma.

CT is the preferred method of evaluating renal trauma (Fig. 13.2). Although a normal intravenous pyelogram (IVP) almost excludes serious renal injury, an abnormal study is inadequate to define the degree of renal trauma. CT gives accurate staging information on renal trauma and has the added advantage of assisting with the diagnosis of any other intraabdominal injuries. It detects extravasation of contrast from the urinary tract with great sensitivity, and gives a more precise demonstration of blood flow to the renal parenchyma. The role of angiography in renal trauma is controversial. Selective renal angiography defines any areas of ischaemia, and will diagnose injuries to the renal

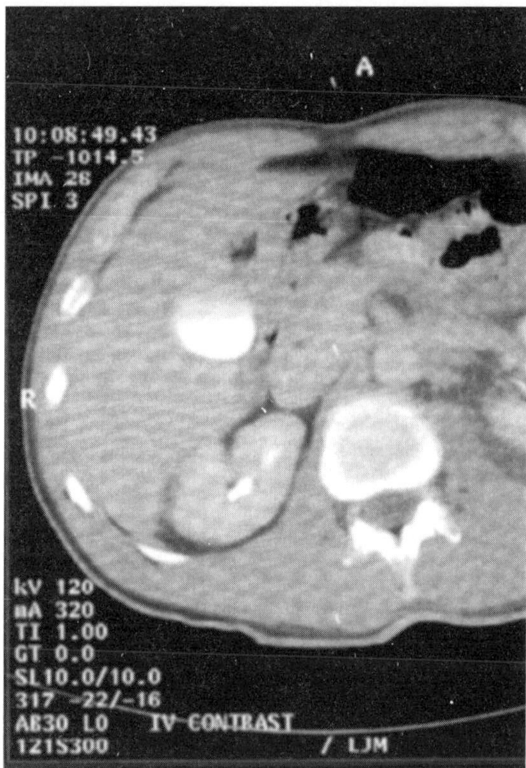

Figure 13.2 CT scan showing left perirenal haematoma. Note vicarious excretion of contrast in the gallbladder. (Courtesy Dr Rick Usher, Sutherland Hospital, Sydney.)

artery and its main branches. Therapeutic embolization can be carried out at the time of angiogram to stop bleeding arteries or arteriovenous fistula. Angiography should only be considered in an adequately stabilized patient; otherwise, laparotomy and open exploration of the injured kidney is more appropriate.

Management may be operative or expectant. The presence and condition of contra-lateral kidney is important and can be easily assessed on IVP or CT scan. The ultimate goal of treatment should be patient safety and preservation of renal function, with the lowest complication rate. In the stable patient with a 'minor' renal injury on CT scan and no associated non-renal injuries, it is safe to manage conservatively. This applies to 80–85% of all patients with renal trauma. Conservative management includes strict bed rest, with gradual mobilization if the patient remains stable and when macroscopic haematuria has cleared. The patient should be observed for haemodynamic changes and the abdomen examined regularly. If an expanding mass is observed or the patient becomes compromised, exploration should be undertaken. CT surveillance, coupled with percutaneous or endoscopic interventions when appropriate (e.g. drainage of fluid collections) allows selected patients with major renal injuries to be managed non-operatively, with less morbidity and a lower rate of nephrectomy (Mansi and Alkhudair 1997). Blood pressure surveillance every 3–6 months should continue for 5 years, as up to 10% of patients will develop hypertension after renal trauma.

Indications for urgent exploration are penetrating injuries or haemodynamic instability; a patient undergoing laparotomy for another reason may warrant exploration of the retroperitoneum if a pulsatile or expanding haematoma is observed. Blunt renal injuries should be explored if there is disruption with a significant devascularized segment, major urinary extravasation, or in the case of renal pedicle injuries. Associated injuries should not affect the decision about management of the renal injury; reconstruction or repair is safe in the face of colonic or pancreatic injury (Rosen and McAnich 1994, Wessels and McAnich 1996).

Surgical exploration is best preformed via a midline approach, which enables complete examination of all abdominal organs including the kidneys. The renal vessels should be controlled before approaching the kidney in case bleeding should occur upon release of the fascial covering of the kidney. This can be achieved by exposing the aorta with an incision of the retroperitoneum between the inferior mesenteric vein and duodenojejunal flexure. Simple lacerations may be repaired with absorbable suture after debridement, and should be drained. Exposed defects in the collecting system or parenchymal vessels should also be oversewn with fine absorbable suture before reflecting the capsule over bare parenchyma. If closure of the capsule is not possible, the area may be covered with free peritoneum, omentum, or a piece of synthetic mesh. Drainage should be provided with a closed suction drain, and broad-spectrum antibiotic prophylaxis commenced. Nephrectomy should be reserved for unstable patients with persistent bleeding or severe injuries to the vascular pedicle.

Renal injuries in children

In children, the kidney is far more prone to injury from blunt trauma because of its intra-abdominal location. Indeed, the kidney is the most frequently injured abdominal organ in children. Radiological evaluation should not be reserved for unstable patients, and the degree of haematuria is an unreliable predictor of renal injury (Abou-Jaoude *et al.* 1996). Therefore all patients with haematuria (including microscopic haematuria) or deceleration injuries should have further radiographic assessment, with either CT or renal tract ultrasound. The indications for operative and conservative management are the same as for adults.

Key points

- There is widespread debate over the appropriate management of major renal injuries.
- CT scan is the preferred method of evaluating renal trauma.

Ureteric injury

Isolated trauma to the ureter is uncommon because of its retroperitoneal location and its mobility. There are three major types of injury:

- penetrating
- blunt
- iatrogenic.

Penetrating injuries and surgical mishaps are by far the most common cause of injury to the ureter. Blunt injuries are extremely rare, but may occur in association with a pelvic fracture. The incidence of iatrogenic ureteric injuries following gynaecological surgical procedures is estimated at 2.5%, with a much higher incidence in abdominal approaches than vaginal (Mariotti *et al.* 1997). Colorectal operations, as well as vascular and endourological surgery, can also result in ureteric injuries.

Clinical presentation varies with aetiology. In the trauma setting, penetrating injuries to the flank with or without haematuria may herald a ureteric injury. Alternatively the patient with an iatrogenic ureteric injury which was not recognized intraoperatively will have a delayed presentation of flank pain, fever, and leukocytosis. In either scenario imaging of the urinary tract with either CT or IVP should assist in making the diagnosis.

A number of factors determine appropriate management of a ureteric injury:

- the site of the injury (i.e. proximal, middle, or distal third)
- co-existing injuries and illnesses
- time taken for the injury to be recognized
- mechanism of injury
- presence of normal contralateral kidney
- bladder mobility.

More than 90% of penetrating ureteric injuries are associated with other abdominal injuries. Simultaneous colonic injury is associated with a poor outcome in patients undergoing ureteric anastomosis for penetrating trauma (Velmahos *et al.* 1996). Early recognition of iatrogenic ureteric injury has been shown to improve outcome. Primary repair is not possible if there has been a delay in diagnosis and secondary infection or ureteric necrosis has occurred.

Management is aimed at providing an anastomosis which is tension-free and viable. Urinary drainage with ureteric stent or bladder catheter should be continued for at least 3 weeks. Urinary diversion by nephrostomy and delayed repair is indicated when the patient is haemodynamically unstable, in patients with multiple injuries (especially bowel), or in the presence of sepsis.

Distal injuries should be managed with ureteroneocystotomy. Mid-ureteric injuries should be considered for primary repair or ureteroureterostomy if the diagnosis has been made promptly. After debridement the ureteric ends are spatulated and then repaired. Care must be taken to preserve the blood supply to the anastomosis. A double-J stent should be placed across the repair and adequate drainage permitted outside the ureter.

In the case of destruction of a segment of ureter, a few options are available. Mobilization of the kidney or bladder (e.g. the Boari flap) may allow sufficient length for a primary repair. Secondly, a delayed reconstruction with an interposed segment of ileum has been employed with good results. Transverse ureteroureterostomy has a high complication rate, and nephrectomy should be only be considered if there is a normal contralateral kidney. Autotransplant can be considered if expertise is available.

Key point

- Penetrating injuries and surgical mishaps are by far the most common cause of ureteric injury.

Bladder trauma

Bladder injuries are classified into four major groups:

- bladder contusion
- extraperitoneal bladder rupture
- intraperitoneal bladder rupture
- combined intra- and extraperitoneal bladder rupture.

The distinguishing feature of bladder contusion is that there is no urinary extravasation. Intraperitoneal rupture may be caused by a blunt or penetrating injury, including a motor vehicle accident, an abdominal blow, gunshot, or stab wound. A history of alcohol consumption before injury should raise clinical suspicion. A bladder injury should always be considered in the hotel or bar patron who has been assaulted and presents with abdominal pain and voiding difficulty. The diuretic effect of alcohol increases bladder volume and gives it a more abdominal position, where it is less protected by the bony pelvis. On the other hand, extraperitoneal rupture is normally associated with pelvic fractures with a sharp fragment penetrating the bladder wall.

Gross haematuria is the most important finding in patients with a bladder rupture; in addition, most patients will complain of suprapubic pain; some patients complain of voiding difficulty. Examination reveals tenderness in the lower abdomen. It is important to examine the bony pelvis for instability or tenderness, and the genitalia and perineum for any associated injuries.

Urgent cystogram should be performed to confirm the diagnosis. Particular attention should be paid to whether the contrast tracks into the peritoneal cavity (Fig. 13.3). The contrast material is best delivered by gravity and small leakage often seen only after the contrast has drained. More than 250 mL of contrast material is recommended to distend the bladder sufficiently to demonstrate a perforation.

Management depends largely on whether the rupture has occurred intra- or extraperitoneally, and the presence of any associated abdominal or pelvic

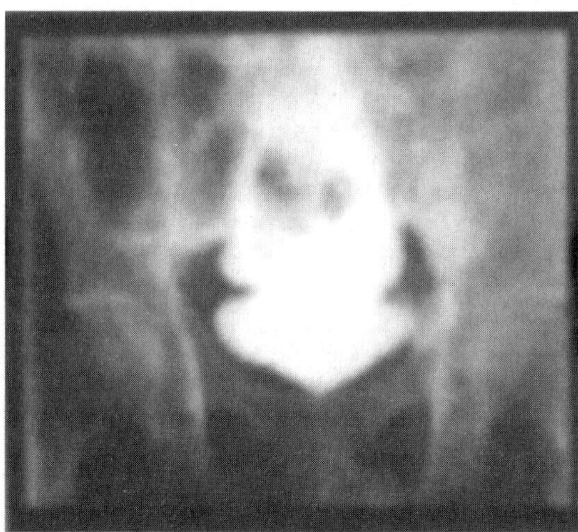

Figure 13.3 Cystogram showing intraperitoneal bladder rupture. (Courtesy Dr Peter Maher, Concord Hospital, Sydney.)

injuries. All patients should be on appropriate broad-spectrum antibiotic cover to prevent septic complications.

Extraperitoneal rupture may be managed by catheter drainage for a minimum of 2 weeks, then a follow-up cystogram. Continuous unobstructed bladder drainage by either indwelling urethral catheter or superpubic catheter is absolutely essential, and if this cannot be achieved the patient should undergo exploration, repair, and formal tube drainage.

Intraperitoneal or combined intra- and extraperitoneal ruptures should be explored through a laparotomy, with primary repair of the bladder, suprapubic tube cystostomy and drainage. The suprapubic catheter is removed at 2 weeks if the patient is voiding well and repeat cystogram is normal. Similarly, if a patient requires laparotomy for any other reason, the bladder should be repaired at that time.

Urethral trauma

Traumatic injuries to the urethra are traditionally classified anatomically as anterior or posterior. Colapinto and McCallum (1977) devised a classification system based on the findings of retrograde urethrography, and a modified system has been proposed by Goldman *et al.* (1997) (Table 13.1).

Although urethral injuries are much less common in women than men, they can occur in association with pelvic fractures. The short length of the female urethra and its lack of attachment to the pubis makes it less prone to injury.

Posterior urethral disruption

The posterior urethra is the segment proximal to and including the area of the external urinary sphincter. Disruption of the posterior urethra is a devastating injury which carries a high morbidity rate. Trauma to the posterior urethra is normally associated with extreme blunt trauma to the lower abdomen and pelvis, along with fractures to the pelvis (especially fractures through the ilium or pubic rami). Lower urinary tract injuries occur in up to 25% of patients with pelvic ring disruptions.

Blood at the external urethral meatus is the cardinal sign of urethral injury. Blood may also be present at the urethral meatus of females with urethral trauma, but is often mistaken for vaginal bleeding. Rectal examination of the male patient with a posterior urethral injury may reveal a high-riding prostate. Voiding may be difficult or impossible, but the patient who voids is not necessarily clear of

Table 13.1 Classification of urethral injuries

Description of injury	Classification		
	Anatomical	Colapinto and McCallum (1977)	Goldman *et al.* (1997)
Posterior urethra intact but stretched	Posterior	Type I	Type I
Partial or complete tear of membranous urethra above urogenital diaphragm	Posterior	Type II	Type II
Partial or complete combined posterior/anterior urethral injury with disruption of urogenital diaphragm	?	Type III	Type III
Bladder neck injury with extension into urethra	—	—	Type IV
Base of bladder injury with periurethral extravasation	—	—	Type IVA
Partial or complete pure anterior urethral injury	Anterior	—	Type V

urethral injury. Indeed, it is impossible to exclude posterior urethral injury on the basis of clinical findings alone. A patient who is suspected of having a urethral injury should not be catheterized until such an injury has been excluded by urethrogram, otherwise there is a high risk of converting a partial tear into a more complex injury or introducing infection into a periurethral haematoma.

Radiologic evaluation of urethral injuries consists of retrograde urethrography, performed by injecting 50 mL of water-soluble contrast through a catheter-tip syringe with screening radiography. If a urethral catheter has already been passed and is working, the study is performed through a smaller catheter introduced alongside the Foley catheter. Extravasation of contrast material reveals the level of the injury (Fig. 13.4).

Management of posterior urethral injuries is somewhat controversial. Although there has been renewed interest in early repair (endoscopically assisted), most authors favour delayed urethroplasty at least 3–6 months after the injury, when the haematoma and inflammation has resolved. At the time of the injury a large-bore suprapubic catheter is inserted operatively and antibiotic prophylaxis commenced. Stricture formation occurs in 95% of these patients, but this is corrected at the time of reconstruction. Realignment of the urethra and careful positioning of a urethral catheter at the time of injury will reduce the rate of stricture formation and may make delayed repair an easier undertaking. The other major long-term complications are urinary incontinence, which occurs in 10–15% of patients, and impotence, occurring in up to 50%. Although primary realignment does not improve the complication rate, it has the advantage of earlier removal of the suprapubic catheter.

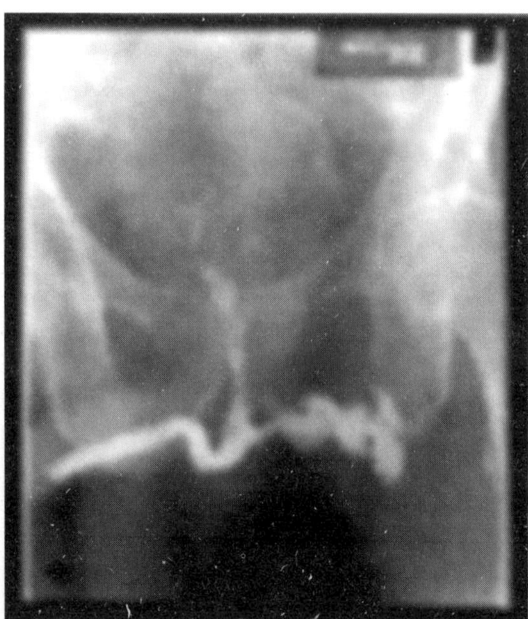

Figure 13.4 Urethrogram showing posterior urethral rupture, resulting from improper catheter insertion after transurethral prostate resection. (Courtesy Dr Peter Maher, Concord Hospital, Sydney.)

Key point

- Blood at the external urethral meatus is the cardinal sign of urethral injury.

Anterior urethral rupture

Trauma to the anterior urethra is more common than posterior urethral trauma, and most often result from straddle-type injuries to the perineum. Anterior urethral injury may also occur in association with a penetrating injury to the penis. Clinical features of voiding difficulty and blood at the urethral meatus are still present, but in addition there may be evidence of urinary extravasation. The extent of extravasation depends on the integrity of Buck's fascia; if this is disrupted, urine and blood may track along Collie's and Scarpa's fascia into the perineum ('butterfly haematoma') and abdominal wall, limited only by its fusion with the fascia lata of the thigh and the coracoclavicular fascia in the neck.

Retrograde urethrography confirms the diagnosis. Blunt injuries are best managed with suprapubic catheterization and delayed reconstruction. Early exploration and debridement is indicated for penetrating injuries; depending on the severity of the injury, primary repair over a Silastic catheter may be possible. The catheter is maintained for 2–3 weeks after primary repair, and voiding cystourethrogram is performed after removal.

Iatrogenic injury

Traumatic catheterizations are an unfortunately common occurrence in the hospital setting, resulting from either improper technique, anatomical difficulties (e.g. prostatic hyperplasia), or a combination of these. The use of urethral catheter introducers and suprapubic catheters should be reserved for experienced medical staff only. The use of portable bladder ultrasound to measure bladder residuals provides a non-invasive alternative to urethral catheterization.

Key points

- Traumatic catheterizations are an unfortunately a common occurrence in the hospital setting.

Genital injuries

Penile trauma

Degloving injuries

A degloving injury of the penis usually follows an accident with farming or industrial machinery. Careful examination of the penis under anaesthetic reveals the extent of skin which has been avulsed, and its viability. Injuries are classified as complete or partial avulsions.

It is important to remove any clothing or other foreign material which may contaminate the wound. Any remaining distal penile skin in a partial avulsion should be debrided as far as the coronal sulcus prior to skin graft. Depending on the degree of contamination delayed grafting with split-thickness skin (to allow expansion during erection) is ideal.

Amputation

Amputation of the penis is usually a self-inflicted injury by a psychotic patient, or less commonly the result of an assault by a jilted lover. Principles of storage of the severed part are the same as for any amputation; it should be cleaned with sterile saline, wrapped and kept cool (not on ice). Bleeding from the penile stump should be controlled with direct pressure rather than a tourniquet. The patient should be transferred to an appropriate centre with a microsurgical team; if such a facility is unavailable, reapproximation of the corpora and urethra frequently results in a successful outcome. The most important factor in survival of the penis is re-establishment of venous drainage. Most patients recover with reasonable erectile function and sensation.

Key point

- Amputation of the penis is usually a self-inflicted injury by a psychotic patient.

Penile fracture

Fracture of the penis is a rare injury, usually caused by vigorous intercourse with the partner in the dominant position. The patient gives a history of sudden forceful bending of the erect penis during coitus, accompanied by pain and loss of erection. The patient will occasionally hear a loud 'crack'. Urethral injury occurs in about 20% of cases. Examination reveals a swollen and bruised organ with deviation away from the injured side. In patients whose presentation is delayed, the amount of swelling and bruising is such that the organ is said to resemble an aubergine.

Management consists of early primary repair of the disrupted corpus, to maximize chance of maintaining erectile function, and the urethral injury if present. Repeated subclinical penile fracturing is one of many theories for the pathogenesis of Peyronie's disease.

Scrotal trauma

Penetrating scrotal injury may be associated with a degloving injury to the penis or occur as an isolated event. Management varies with the depth of trauma and the surface area involved. Lacerations which breach the dartos layer should be explored to exclude underlying testicular injury.

Degloving injury where testes are on view requires subcutaneous placement of the testes in the thigh temporarily, or coverage with perineal flaps or skin graft. In contaminated wounds it is advisable to dress the testes with wet dressings initially until an area of granulation tissue has formed, before embarking on a definitive procedure. Orchiectomy is avoided if possible.

Key point

- Lacerations which breach the dartos layer should be explored to exclude underlying testicular injury.

Testicular trauma

Penetrating injuries are normally associated with significant scrotal injury, and will be discovered during operative exploration. Laceration through the tunica albuginea is managed by thorough debridement, irrigation, and drainage; the tunica albuginea may be closed primarily.

Blunt trauma to the testis should be assessed with ultrasound, but exploration is often necessary if this is non-contributory and clinical suspicion of testicular rupture is high. This will enable the surgeon to exclude testicular torsion as a cause of pain. If an haematocoele is evacuated a Penrose drain should be placed and the scrotum closed primarily. A supportive dressing or jockstrap prevents haematoma formation and reduces pain.

Female genital injuries

Urologic and rectal injury should be considered in all female patients presenting with blunt or penetrating trauma to the perineum. The incidence of associated injury to the urinary tract has been reported as up to 30% (Goldman *et al.* 1998). Minor cutaneous injuries may be treated locally with primary repair but larger wounds may require grafting. Temporary faecal or urinary diversion should be considered to prevent wound contamination.

Clinical examination of traumatic injuries to the female external genitalia in children is notoriously inaccurate. A study comparing the findings on preoperative evaluation with those on examination under anaesthetic found that over 70% of patients had more serious injuries than had been appreciated preoperatively (Lynch *et al.* 1995). Assault must always be considered as a cause for genital injury and appropriate referrals made.

Key point

- Urological and rectal injury should be considered in all female patients presenting with blunt or penetrating trauma to the perineum.

References

Abou-Jaoude WA, Sugarman JM, Fallat ME, Casale AJ (1996) Indicators of genitourinary tract injury or anomaly in cases of pediatric blunt trauma. *Journal of Pediatric Surgery* 31(1): 86–89.

Colapinto V, McCallum RW (1977) Injury to the male posterior urethra in the fractured pelvis: A new classification. *Journal of Urology* 118: 575–580.

Feagins B (1994a) Urogenital trauma. In: Lopez-Viego MA (ed) *Parkland Memorial Hospital: The Parkland trauma handbook*. Mosby, St. Louis, Mo., pp 309–317.

Feagins B (1994b) Ureteric trauma. In: Lopez-Viego MA (ed) *Parkland Memorial Hospital: The Parkland trauma handbook*. Mosby, St. Louis, Mo., pp 319–323.

Goldman SM, Sandler CM, Corriere JN Jr, McGuire EJ (1997) Blunt urethral trauma: a unified, anatomical mechanical classification. *Journal of Urology* 157: 85–89.

Goldman HB, Idom CB Jr, Dmochowski RR (1998) Traumatic injuries of the female external genitalia and their association with urological injuries. *Journal of Urology* 159(3): 956–959.

Lynch JM, Gardner MJ, Albanese CT (1995) Blunt urogenital trauma in prepubescent female patients: more than meets the eye. *Pediatric Emergency Care* 11(6): 372–375.

Manzi MK, Alkhudair WK (1997) Conservative management with percutaneous intervention of major blunt renal injuries. *American Journal of Emergency Medicine* 15(7): 633–367.

Mariotti G, Natale F, Trucchi A, Cristini C, Furbetta A (1997) Ureteric injuries during gynecologic procedures. *Minerva Urologica e Nefrologica* 49(2): 95–98.

Rosen MA, McAnich JW (1994) Management of combined renal and pancreatic trauma. *Journal of Urology* 152: 22–25.

Velmahos GC, Degianis E, Wells M, Souter I (1996) Penetrating ureteric injuries: the impact of associated injuries on management. *American Surgeon* 62(6): 461–468.

Wessels H, McAnich JW (1996) Effect of colon injury on the management of simultaneous renal trauma. *Journal of Urology* 155(6): 1852–1856.

14

CHAPTER 14

Skin injuries and burns

NICHOLAS LOTZ, PETER G HAYWARD, AND NHI NGUYEN

CHAPTER 14
Skin injuries and burns

NICHOLAS LOTZ, PETER G HAYWARD, AND NHI NGUYEN

Skin injuries

The skin (Fig. 14.1) is the largest organ of the body and is inevitably involved in most trauma. This chapter provides an overview of soft tissue injuries, concentrating on skin damage and loss. Penetrating wounds to the hand and to vessels and nerves in other areas are reviewed in other chapters.

Initial (ABC) management of the patient with soft tissue injuries is identical for all trauma victims. For patients with extensive soft tissue injuries, care should be exercised in assessing shock. It is uncommon for soft tissue injuries alone to lead to shock. Although major lacerations can produce significant haemorrhage, underlying visceral or chest injuries should not be overlooked or discounted if systemic shock is present. The search for associated injuries should not be halted by the drama of a disfiguring soft tissue injury.

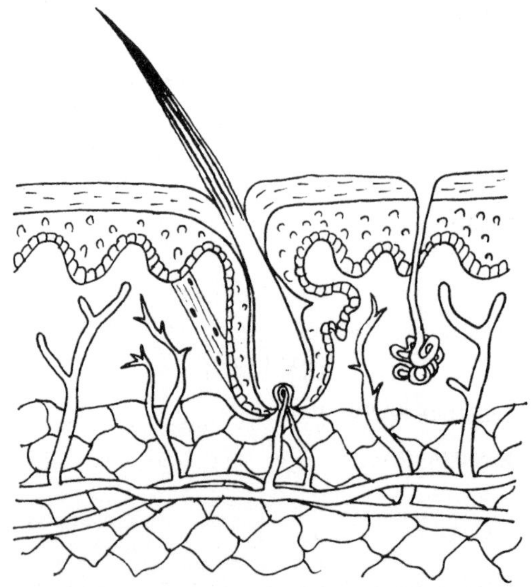

Figure 14.1 Anatomy of skin.

Attention to treatment of soft tissue injuries is often difficult in the acute phase. Assessment of the damage needs a supine patient and a good light. Blood and debris should be cleaned away with saline to allow an adequate inspection of the wounds, which should be probed with the gloved finger. Desiccation is the enemy of any exposed organ and so wet saline packs should be used as temporary or transit dressings to protect exposed structures. Undue time and resources can be wasted in the emergency treatment areas in trying to control bleeding from soft tissue injuries. In the main, haemorrhage from soft tissue can be controlled by pressure dressings. Vain efforts to control scalp bleeding with haemostats in the emergency department serve as an example. As a general principle, significant soft tissue injuries and associated haemorrhage should be treated in the operating theatre.

In any injury that involves a limb, neurovascular function of the limb needs to be assessed. Feeling for all peripheral pulses distal to the site of injury, checking the capillary return and comparing the warmth and colour of the distal parts of the limb with the other side all help to exclude any vascular injury resulting from the trauma. Sensation needs to be tested to exclude underlying nerve damage. It should be noted that most patients with traumatic nerve injuries will report paraesthesia, not anaesthesia. Commonly, the patient will say that the affected area feels different and will frequently compare the effect to that experienced after administration of local anaesthetic. Motor function of the distal limb and digits should be tested to exclude motor or tendon damage. Movement should be tested not only actively and passively, but also against resistance. This is important, since partial tendon injuries may reveal a normal range of motion but pain will occur at the site of injury when movement is resisted.

Radiography should be performed whenever there is a possibility of bony injury or radio-opaque foreign bodies. On occasion ultrasound will resolve the presence of foreign bodies better than conventional radiographs. Urgent angiography should be performed in any patient who has circulatory compromise to a limb where the extent and site of damage is not readily determined. These patients need to be prioritized for operative intervention. Muscle necrosis occurs after a few hours of warm ischaemia, and the viability of the limb will be threatened unless circulation is restored.

Specific locations create specific problems in wound repair. Blunt trauma to trilaminar structures such as the lip, nose, or ear is often much more complex to repair when finally confronted in theatre. The initial appearance of these wounds can be deceptive. When examination is carried out under anaesthesia, the need for a multilayered repair becomes obvious. Staff involved in the triage of soft tissue injuries have to liaise with reconstructive surgeons. The observation that tissue is missing is a critical one. The mechanism of injury dictates the pattern of injuries and often the ultimate amount of primary and secondary tissue loss. The history of the injuring force is important in this regard. Blunt trauma does not remove tissue. Swelling, haematoma, and muscle spasm will often conspire to give rise to an apparent soft tissue defect. Subsequent debridement and repair may show no real tissue loss. The difference between the real and apparent deficit can be great. History is also important by virtue of the destructive power of different tools and missiles. The aphorism 'glass cuts to the bone' is particularly true of penetrating trauma. Particularly in the upper limb, shards of glass have an exquisite ability to find and lacerate tendons and nerve trunks leaving rather small and innocuous entry wounds.

Key points

- The skin is the largest organ of the body and is inevitably involved in most trauma.
- Assess for shock in initial ABC management.
- Control soft tissue haemorrhage with pressure dressings and, if significant, treat definitively in operating theatre.
- Assess neurovascular function.
- Useful imaging includes radiograph, ultrasound, and angiography.

Anaesthesia

Most skin wounds can be closed with local anaesthetic. Making this as non-traumatic as possible enhances patient confidence and satisfaction. Plain lignocaine (lidocaine) 1% should be used. A small-bore needle and syringe should be used, with infiltration through the edges of the wound if possible. Slow infiltration reduces pain, as does having the local anaesthetic at body temperature and buffered with bicarbonate (8.4%, 1 mL per 9 mL of lignocaine). In children topical anaesthesia of small open wounds can be helpful before infiltration, and a number of topical mixtures including cocaine have been advocated.

Typical patterns of wounding are seen in the skin. Greater, more directed force correlates with more tissue damage or loss. Each typical wound presentation has specific management issues that are reviewed below.

Key point

- Most skin wounds can be closed with local anaesthetic (plain lignocaine [lidocaine] 1%).

Haematoma

Haematoma is a *sine qua non* of trauma to all tissues. Small haematomas absorb, but larger collections of blood are often worth draining on their own merits. If there are no problems with tissue viability or compartment pressures then haematomas can be left for 10 days to liquefy. Drainage of liquefied haematoma can then be carried out with a large-bore needle or even under ultrasound control if desired. Because of other injuries, haematomas are often ignored. In the face large haematomas that can be drained, should be drained. Large, organizing haematomas in the face can be disfiguring and difficult to treat later. Large haematomas under traumatic flaps in the limbs tend to act as foci for infection. Secondary pressure and chemical effects of these collections can threaten flap viability. Accordingly, such haematomas should be drained at the time of initial wound debridement.

Abrasion and tattoos

The management of a small abrasion is elementary first aid. Large abrasions associated with major trauma can lead to skin contamination and superficial sepsis which can complicate future treatment such as internal fixation of fractures. Skin denuded of surface epithelium will heal, but will do so best in a moist environment. Desiccation is the enemy of all exposed soft issues, particularly of the exposed dermis. There is an interminable array of moist wound dressings available, but there is little evidence to show that the traditional Vaseline gauze or xeroform dressings are inferior management. Extensive abrasions of the face can be managed exposed liberally coated in antibiotic ointment that is reapplied at regular intervals.

Where dirt, gunpowder, or industrial grime has been ground into the dermis, producing a traumatic tattoo, the wound should be surgically scrubbed with a topical antiseptic with some detergent properties. Savlon or betadine will suffice. In these situations a scrubbing brush is often more effective and cheaper than pulsatile lavage. Subsequent 'wet to dry' saline gauze dressings for a few days will often lift surface particle still adherent to the wound. Permanent, disfiguring tattooing will need to be treated secondarily by dermabrasion or laser ablation.

Key point

- The management of a small abrasion is elementary first aid with moist wound dressings, Vaseline gauze, or xeroform dressings.

Foreign body

In deciding to remove a foreign body, always weigh the risks versus the benefits. Removing a subcutaneous foreign bodies can be either a simple procedure, or a frustrating and time-consuming exercise. Where a decision is made to remove a foreign body surgically, the procedure should be carried out in an operating theatre in a bloodless field. Metallic foreign bodies should be removed with the ready availability of image intensification. Delegating junior staff in the emergency department to dissect aimlessly in the soft tissues for foreign bodies should be avoided.

Puncture wounds

In essence, puncture wounds are those which are small but deep, where the penetrating object is likely to have caused division of vital structures. The management of penetrating wounds of the chest and abdomen is covered elsewhere. In this section it is pertinent to look at puncture wounds of the face and upper limb.

In the face, deep penetrating wounds may create full thickness penetration of the conjunctiva, nasal passages, and mouth. Intraoral examination is particularly important with major facial lacerations. Every attempt should be made to assess whether the globe is intact. The facial nerve and the parotid duct can be divided with wounds to the cheeks. Both of these injuries can be occult. Parotid duct injuries are confirmed only by exploration and probing in theatre. Assessment of the facial nerve can be very difficult in a grossly swollen face. For triage purposes, lacerations anterior to a vertical line dropped from the lateral canthus are unlikely to have cut a major branch of the facial nerve. More correctly, the facial nerve beyond this line tends to function as a plexus and division of minor branches can leave little discernible facial asymmetry. This does not apply to truncal injuries or those to named branches posterior to the above-mentioned line. These injuries should be repaired primarily, as secondary dissection of the facial nerve is particularly tedious in the face of established scarring.

Penetrating trauma to the hands also deserves special mention. As noted above, the adage 'glass cuts to the bone' applies particularly to hand and wrist wounds. All significant wounds to the hand and forearm should be repaired in theatre. Because of the compact anatomy it is uncommon to find a significant puncture wound to the hand which has not injured an important structure. Assessing staff should realize that physical examination often underestimates the surgical findings in relation to hand trauma. Not only is a physical finding rarely in error, but the actual damage in the hand and forearm will usually exceed the acute assessment. Nowhere is this more so than in nerve trauma. The initial symptoms of nerve injury are usually not anaesthesia but rather paraesthesia. This should not be assumed to represent an in-continuity lesion if there is an associated penetrating wound. In these cases the nerve should always be explored acutely. Acute repair is technically simpler, and delay in repair of truncal nerves often creates gapping, requiring nerve grafts to achieve a tension-free repair.

Key points

- Intraoral examination is important with major facial lacerations.
- All significant wounds to the hand and forearm should be repaired in theatre.

Lacerations

Large disfiguring lacerations are closed in the same manner as smaller wounds. The key to closure of large soft tissue lacerations is minimal, 'inside out' debridement and closure of key anatomic points such as crease lines. The remainder of the wound is then closed using halving sutures to avoid 'dog ear' formation. The urge to carry out complicated flaps and Z-plasties at the time of initial repair should be avoided. Apart from accurate restoration of anatomy, no scar revision procedures should be carried out in the acute phase since the results are much better and more predictable when carried out 6–12 months later. Where a layered structure has been divided it should be repaired in layers. The cosmetic result of a full-thickness laceration to the nose is enhanced if mucosa, cartilage, and skin are closed in that order, so that the structural anatomy is accurately reconstructed beneath the overlying skin.

Experience in the Vietnam era (1960s–1970s) led to a penchant for delayed primary closure of wounds which had been caused by high-velocity weapons and were often heavily contaminated. In a civilian setting with lower-velocity injuries, there are fewer indications for this approach. Many low-velocity trauma wounds can be debrided and closed acutely. Delayed closure may be undertaken to accommodate the need for serial debridement where the full extent of necrosis becomes apparent with time. However, in the face for instance, delayed closure is less satisfactory as secondary oedema makes the accurate repair of cosmetic units more difficult.

Key point

- Low-velocity trauma wounds should be managed with debridement and closed acutely rather than with delayed primary closure.

Traumatic soft tissue flaps

A flap is a piece of tissue with its own blood supply. Surgically created flaps are crafted to maximize blood flow to the area being sculpted. Traumatic flaps are rarely this precise. Judging whether a traumatic skin flap will survive is often difficult. The greater the force involved during the injury, the less likely any tissue, including a skin flap, is to survive. In the limbs the geometry of flaps is key to survival. Proximally based flaps rely on orthograde arterial flow and so run with the anatomic 'grain' of the vascular tree in the limb. Distally based flaps rely on retrograde blood flow. Since the force raising a distally based flap is likely to have damaged proximal vessels, the ultimate survival of traumatic, distally based flaps in the lower limb is often poor. The key to management of traumatic flaps is judicious debridement and gentle handling. Acute appearances of inflamed tissue make it difficult to decide which tissue segments need to be removed. A second look may well be required to judge the final degree of debridement necessary. Fluoroscein and a Wood's lamp can be used to assess viability, but the passage of 72 hours usually allows visual inspection to predict tissue survival reliably. Tight closure of wounds accelerates tissue pressure rises associated with secondary oedema. This interstitial pressure rise leads to venous occlusion which is the forerunner to flap loss. Accordingly, limbs bearing traumatic flaps should be elevated and flaps should only be tacked into place with a few loose sutures.

Fat necrosis is often invisible at initial assessment. Because the fascial and dermal vascular arcades run parallel, the intervening fat is nourished by vascular arcades coursing between the two systems. If the fat is elevated with a flap then it becomes parasitic on the flap blood supply. Characteristically the skin survives but the fat necroses. If secondary infection intervenes, the skin wound will dehisce. An appreciation of the fascial vascular plexus is needed to understand the plane at which tissue cleaves in a limb. If a fasciocutaneous flap is being surgically raised the fascia is included so that the skin fat and fascia are raised as an anatomic unit with an intact vascular tree. In traumatic degloving the skin and fat is forcibly torn off the fascia, which is left covering the muscle. This traumatic plane creates a much less viable flap. This vascular mechanism explains why the ultimate survival of avulsed traumatic flaps in the limbs is often much less than initially predicted.

Key points

- A flap is a piece of tissue with its own blood supply.
- Judging whether a traumatic skin flap will survive is often difficult.
- The key to management of traumatic flaps is judicious debridement and gentle handling.

Management of tissue deficits

Providing skin cover to a traumatic defect involves techniques of varying complexity. When confronted by a defect requiring closure there are always four choices to be considered (in order):

- dressings allowing healing by secondary intention
- suturing or primary closure
- grafting with either split or full-thickness skin grafts
- flap repair using tissue from elsewhere incorporating its own blood supply.

Skin grafts and skin flaps

A skin graft is a parasite. It is a piece of skin shaved or cut from one area (the donor site) and placed into the defect, where it 'takes'. Clearly, the piece of freshly cut skin has no blood supply and is doomed to necrose. New blood vessels need to grow into the graft and connect to its existing vasculature to allow the graft to take. Such neovascular ingrowth comes from the 'bed' or recipient site. Grafting assumes the traumatic defect can generate a new blood supply for a graft. This is a key judgment. In general, if an area can produce granulation tissue it can be grafted. Certain tissues are notorious for not being able to generate granulation tissue, including bare bone, bare cartilage, and bare tendon. These structures normally have investing layers, periosteum for instance, which can generate granulation and can be grafted. However, in traumatic wounds these structures are usually denuded 'bare' and are not suitable for skin grafting.

Where skin grafting is not an option, flap repair will be required. A flap is a piece of tissue with its own blood supply. It can fill a defect that cannot generate granulation tissue and can even revascularize injured tissue it covers (like the tibia in a compound injury). Flaps can be composed of any tissue combination that can be linked together on a single blood supply; they may contain skin, muscle, fat, bone, nerves, etc. in limitless variety. Flaps can be described by their predominant movement in space—rotation, transposition, or advancement. Alternatively, they can be designated by predominant tissue type can also be used—skin flap, muscle flap, etc. A flap can be dissected free of the body and its pedicle vessels anastomosed to recipient vessels near the defect—the microsurgical 'free' flap.

Key points

- A skin graft is a piece of skin, without its own blood supply, harvested from one area and placed into another area where it 'takes'.
- Certain tissues do not generate granulation tissue and are not sites for grafting (bare bone, bare cartilage, bare tendon).
- Where skin grafting is not an option, flap (piece of tissue with its own blood supply) repair will be required.

Open limb fractures

The management of soft tissue injuries exposing injured bone can be exceedingly complex. The advantages of rigid internal fixation have meant that lower limb wounds require an intact integument to cover fixation devices. The ever-present risk of osteomyelitis is multifactorial. Clearly debridement, soft tissue closure, fixation, and antibiotics have a role to play. The difficult question is often deciding what needs to be debrided and then, when is the wound safe to close. Stratifying patients according to risk is important. The Gustilo classification (Table 14.1) of lower limb trauma takes into account the amount of skin loss and the bony injury as well as the presence or absence of neural and vascular injuries.

Table 14.1 Gustilo classification of open fractures

Type	Wound size	Soft tissue, bone, other factors	Incidence of infection (%)
I	<1 cm long	Little soft-tissue injury No crush injury Simple fracture with little comminution Moderately clean	0–2
II	>1 cm long	No extensive soft-tissue damage, flap or avulsion Slight or moderate crush injury Moderate comminution of fracture Moderate contamination	2–7
III	Extensive	Extensive soft tissue damage to muscle, skin, neurovascular structures Extensive comminution and instability Extensive contamination	10–25 (III overall)
Subdivided			
IIIA		Adequate soft tissue coverage	7
IIIB		Extensive injury to or loss of soft-tissue Periosteal stripping Exposure of bone	10–50
IIIC		Fractures associated with arterial injury which must be repaired	25–50 (amputation rate >50%)

From Gustilo *et al.* (1990).

High-speed trauma generating large forces on the lower limb produces not only complex fractures but also soft tissue wounds with a damaged vascular tree. Where these wounds are left open for prolonged periods, infection may supervene. The pioneering work of the microsurgeon Marko Godina showed that sepsis rate was reduced by early closure of the soft tissues over the bony damage. This principle remains undisputed, but the definition of early closure varies in units around the world. Most authorities would prefer such lower limb wounds closed in the first week after injury. Because the degree of tissue necrosis evolves over time, it is not always possible to complete closure at the first debridement. More commonly a second or third debridement is necessary. The advantage of conservative serial debridement is that tissue is preserved and the microvasculature has time to stabilize after the acute injury. Where major flap repair is to be carried out after serial debridement this will usually mean that definitive closure will occur at around 72 hours after injury.

Many flap options for the coverage of the lower limb are available, and they are beyond the scope of this chapter. Defects exposing bone below the knee are closed with local fasciocutaneous flaps, muscle flaps or free flaps. Fasciocutaneous flaps rely on the anatomy of skin blood supply which relies on perforators that run in the fascial plane. As noted above, this fascial plane is really the surgical dissecting plane cleaving fascia from the underlying muscle. Although these fasciocutaneous flaps have simplified much soft tissue management in the lower limb, they have limited application in the management of high-velocity limb trauma. The 'field of injury' concept holds that the vascular damage associated with bony trauma is widespread, extending above and below the level of fracture. This means that local vascular anastomoses and venous drainage patterns may become non-functional following the oedema and endothelial damage created adjacent to the fracture. Since fasciocutaneous flaps rely on an intact fascial perforator system they become unreliable where there has been extensive soft tissue injury involving muscle compartments. In the main such flaps are reserved for covering small areas of uninjured bone in low-velocity injuries. Muscle flaps such as the gastrocnemius flap are essentially more robust and rely on the well-demarcated vascular supply of some lower limb muscles. However, the vascular anatomy of muscle is such that flaps can only be reliably moved distal to proximal. This geometric consideration means that a gastrocnemius muscle can be detached from its insertion and translated superiorly to cover a defect over the knee. The same muscle does not have a range of movement that allows it to cover tibial defects below the upper third of the tibia. It is in these low tibial wounds that free flaps come into their own. Often these are high-force wounds and the microvascular field of injury is proportionately large. Unfortunately the lower third of the leg is also a watershed in terms of its blood supply, with relatively few accessible truncal arteries for anastomosis. Free flap reconstruction in the lower tibial area has a number of advantages. Distant flaps such as the latissimus dorsi muscle can bring large amounts of uninjured tissue to an area. In this way fractures and hardware can be covered with minimal dead space. The pedicle of the dissected flap can be quite long and allow vascular anastomoses outside the affected area avoiding vascular compromise. As a secondary benefit, free flap coverage provides adequate soft tissue coverage in case secondary bone grafting is required. The logistics of free flap coverage need to be considered by the team treating the patient. These microvascular procedures are lengthy and require close observation postoperatively. Postoperative use of anticoagulants after microsurgery has declined in popularity, but many units use anticoagulation temporarily. For these reasons, all other surgical procedures required by the patient should be completed before major flap coverage is undertaken. In particular, the patient should be stabilized after the acute trauma and residual anaemia should have been corrected. Often the patient will have been transferred to a care area skilled in the management of microsurgical cases.

Key points

- The Gustilo classification stratifies patients with lower limb trauma by taking account of the amount of skin loss and the bony injury.
- Complex fractures and soft tissue wounds left open for prolonged periods are at risk of infection.

Associated burn management

Some brief observations on the management of burn injuries have been included here (see below for detailed management). Commonly, however, burns will be part of a multiple trauma presentation and the comments here are directed at triage and first aid management of these cases. The triage officer has to distinguish burns which will be self-healing from those require admission to a burn unit for grafting or specialized dressings. Depth and area of the burn are critical assessments. Emergency physicians are familiar with Lund and Bowder charts that simplify surface area measurement. When looking at a burn, consider what is erythema and what is real burn. Patients seen immediately after burn injury demonstrate inflammatory erythema around a burn which will resolve within hours. If this erythema is included in the burn area assessment, over-resuscitation will occur. Depth estimation is more difficult. Separating full- from partial-thickness burns can be easy where the full-thickness injury is grey/white and insensate. Where there are blisters, there is life. A blister is caused by the fluid cleavage of layers of skin between the living and the dead. A blistered wound is by definition a partial-thickness injury. Blisters should not be acutely debrided—they are hindering dressings. The need for escharotomy in full thickness, circumferential burns of the extremities is an essential assessment. Where there is doubt, little harm is done by an escharotomy. This resembles fasciotomy in that if an assessor considers it may be necessary, then it should be carried out. In approaching a burn, take a history. Note the mechanism of burn injury. Boiling water really does burn like fire, and the temperature of the liquid in question is important. Was the victim clothed? Clothing may protect the victim, but can also retain heat on the body surface, exacerbating the injury. Respiratory injury is commonest from smoke inhalation. It often occurs when the victim is trapped in an enclosed space. Finally, make a record of the type and time of first aid given. Prolonged cooling of a burn immediately after injury reduces necrosis. The commonest error in the community is to apply cooling for too short a period of time.

With respect to dressings, if the patient is to be transferred to a specialist burn facility then the burn should be covered with saline packs instead of silver sulfadiazine (SSD). Because all burn units will reassess on admission, a laborious SSD dressing applied in the emergency room will be removed as soon as the patient arrives in the new facility. Care should be take to avoid hypothermia after burn injury, as thermoregulatory function of the injured skin will be lost.

A specific burn injury, which creates assessment problems, is electrical burns (see Chapter 24, 'Electrical injuries'. These come in many forms including arc burns, contact burns, exit wounds, and high-tension injures. They require very careful assessment. Loss of a limb from such an injury usually requires high electrical tension (>1000 V). The history of what type of electrical contact was made is very important. With high-tension injuries there can be extensive myonecrosis with skin preservation. Judging the level of amputation and the extent of ultimate debridement can be difficult. MRI can be very useful in defining necrosis in these cases.

Reconstructive aftermath

An integral part of triage of soft tissue wounds is documentation. In major multiple trauma cases the documentation of relatively minor soft tissue wounds may be overlooked. Patients emerging from the ravages of multiple trauma and the subsequent rehabilitation are faced with a variety of problems. Many struggle to make sense of why a given catastrophe occurred to them. Increasingly, litigation and the search for compensation have become part of the process of bringing finality to the trauma. Documentation of injuries is becoming a large part of the bureaucracy of post-trauma care. Physicians who have had to attend these legal matters will agree that a lack of clear, cogent records of all the injuries sustained frustrates this reporting process, which may take place years after the patient's injury. Patients may fixate on their external scarring as their main complaint late after injury. Their scars are what they can see, and what others around them identify as being trauma related. Relatives cannot see the results of a splenectomy or of internal fixation, but they can identify facial scarring or asymmetry. For these reasons soft tissue repair at the time of trauma surgery should be as accurately carried out as possible. This not only improves outcomes but also reduces the need for secondary scar revision. As noted above, scar revision, where required, is usually undertaken 6–12 months after injury when the collagen in the scar has matured and remodelled. At the time of initial assessment, issues of scarring should be properly canvassed. It is inappropriate to suggest to patients and their relatives that visible signs of their injuries can be made to disappear. The reality of scar revision is that it generally improves the quality of some (but not all) scars. Realism should be gently introduced at an early stage, so that the patient does not emerge from the process later with the belief that the visible signs of trauma can be totally erased.

Burns

Burns are relatively common injuries. Although the majority of burn injuries are minor and can be managed in an outpatient setting, a significant number require admission to hospital or a burns unit. The management of major burns requires a multidisciplinary team, and recovery can be a long process. The mortality and morbidity of burn injuries is dependent on early assessment and management of the burn and appropriate wound care in the recovery period.

Types of burns

Scalds

Scalds are thermal injuries caused by boiling water or steam. The depth of the burn is dependent on the duration of contact and the first aid measures taken immediately after the injury.

Flame

The tissue injury results from the direct effect of burning gases on the skin. Such burns are usually deep and involve high temperatures. Concomitant inhalational injury may be sustained. Prognosis depends on the extent of the area burned.

Contact

Direct contact of skin and a hot surface can cause contact burns. Rapid withdrawal reflexes mean that the contact is usually brief. However, in cases where there is a loss of consciousness or occupational mechanical injury, contact burns may be very deep.

Friction burns

These burns often involve large areas of abrasions leading to the generation of heat. Friction burns may occur in pedestrian–vehicle accidents when the person is dragged along the road.

Electrical burns

Resistance of tissues, voltage, and amperage determine the severity of the burn. Electrical energy is transformed into thermal injury, resulting in small but deep burns. The body becomes part of an electrical circuit. The most serious of the wounds occur at the point of entry.

Chemical burns

The chemical causing burns may be acid or alkali. The extent of the burn depends on the concentration of the chemical and the duration of the contact. Acid burns tend to be more superficial, and are limited by neutralization from the proteins in the areas affected. Alkali burns such as those caused by caustic soda penetrate deeply. First aid management of these burns should involve continuous irrigation with water.

Key points

- Types of burns:
  - scalds
  - flame
  - contact
  - friction
  - electrical
  - chemical.

Depth of burn

The depth of the burn needs to be assessed, as this affects the clinical outcome. Traditionally, burns have been classified as first, second, or third degree depending on the estimated depth of the burn. A more clinically significant classification may be that of partial-thickness burns, which heal spontaneously, or full-thickness burns which require skin grafting (see Table 14.2).

First-degree burns

The most common cause of first-degree burns is brief scalding and sunburn. The epidermis is involved, with erythema and localized pain being the associated features. There are only minor microscopic changes and the skin barrier remains in tact. Pain lasts for 48–72 hours, and healing is uneventful with no residual scarring.

Second-degree burns

Second-degree burns are deeper, and involve all of the epidermis and some of the dermis. The depth of dermis involved reflects the degree of systemic manifestations and the amount of undamaged dermis is directly related to the quality of healing. More superficial burns form blisters which can continue to enlarge due to the osmotic forces which draw water into the blister. Healing occurs over 10–14 days, with few complications and no scarring. Deeper partial-thickness burns have a more reddish appearance, and a layer of non-viable dermis may be evident as a white layer of tissue adherent to the underlying unaffected tissue. The remaining dermis gives rise to the healing epithelium. Without skin grafting, deep burns can give rise to hypertrophic scarring.

Third degree burns

Third-degree burns are full-thickness burns that have a white waxy appearance. The burn may be brown, dark red, or black if the underlying fat and

Table 14.2 Characteristics of burns

	First-degree burns	Second-degree burns	Third-degree burns
Causes	Exposure to sunlight	Limited exposure to hot liquid, flame, or chemical agent	Prolonged exposure to flame or hot object or chemical agent Contact with high-voltage electricity
Color	Red	Pink or mottled red	Pearly white, charred, translucent or parchment like deeply tanned in strong acid burns Dark red in young children
Surface	Dry, blanches with pressure	Bullae or moist weeping surface, blanches with pressure	Dry with thrombosis of superficial vessels Focal tissue loss in high-voltage electric injury
Sensation	Painful	Painful	Insensate surface
Healing	3–6 days	10–21 days for superficial >21 days for deep	Requires grafting

subcutaneous layer has been affected. There is no potential for healing, as all the layers have been destroyed. The skin lacks sensation and there is no capillary refill.

Key points

- Burn injury are classified according to depth of burn:
  - first-degree burns are superficial burns involving the epidermis. Common causes are scalds and sunburn
  - second-degree burns are partial thickness burns and involve the epidermis and some of the dermis
  - third-degree burns are full thickness burns which have no potential for healing hence needs grafting.

Pathophysiology of thermal injury

Thermal injury causes distinct changes to the affected tissues. Principally there is coagulation necrosis. The depth to which this extends depends on the temperature and duration of exposure to the noxious stimulus. Three zones are associated with the burned area.

- The first is the zone of coagulation, with irreversible vessel damage and no capillary flow.
- A zone of stasis surrounds this central zone. There is a moderate degree of vascular damage that causes a decrease in tissue perfusion. The release of local mediators can convert this zone of stasis to a partial-thickness or full-thickness injury. Appropriate management can help prevent the extension of the burn to involve this area.
- The third zone is the area of reactive hyperaemia.

The direct effect of heat as well, as the release of vasoactive mediators from the damaged tissue, results in increased capillary permeability and hence a rapid loss of fluid and protein from the intravascular into the extravascular compartment. The magnitude of the fluid shift and the resultant shock reflect the extent of the burn. It is important to assess the burn size accurately in order to estimate the amount of fluid loss and hence the amount which needs to be replaced. There is also an associated decrease in cardiac output and increased peripheral vascular resistance. The development of tissue oedema is greatest in the period immediately after the burn, volume loss being greatest in the first 6–8 hours. Haemodynamic stability begins at approximately 24 hours.

The diminished blood volume and cardiac output causes a decrease in renal blood flow and glomerular filtration rate. Oliguria may progress to acute renal failure if left untreated.

The body responds to a thermal injury the same way it responds to other injuries: there is an increase in the release of catecholamines, cortisol, and glucagon. The body is in a catabolic state, and there is a tendency to retain sodium and water and excrete potassium. The metabolic rate is greatly increased in the period of the burn, up to 150% above the basal rate. These patients have increased energy and protein requirements, which need to be met, in order to ensure adequate wound healing and increase resistance to infections. Early enteral feeding should be considered.

Immunological factors in burns

The loss of skin integrity in itself predisposes the patient to infections. Thermal injury also affects the cells and function of the immune system further increasing the risk of sepsis. There are decreased serum levels of IgA, IgM, and IgG, and leukocytes from burn patients have also been found to exhibit decreased chemotactic activity.

Initial hypovolaemia may result in rapid shallow respirations in those patients whose injuries do not include the thorax or airways. In the period of hypermetabolism following resuscitation, the patient may develop a mild respiratory alkalosis due to hyperventilation. With wound healing, there is typically a corresponding decrease in the degree of hyperventilation.

Key points

- There are three distinct zones in the injured tissue.
- Physiological response to thermal injury:
  - increased release of vasoactive mediators
  - increased capillary permeability results in rapid fluid loss from the intravascular space
  - decreased cardiac output and increased peripheral vascular resistance
  - decreased renal blood flow and glomerular filtration rate
  - increased basal metabolic rate.

Management

The initial management of burn patients involves the removal of the patient from the source of any ongoing injury. Where possible, first aid measures should be implemented. The affected area should be placed under cold running water for as long a period as possible. Major burns requires stabilization at the site and immediate retrieval to the nearest hospital facility. The definitive management of burns requires the accurate assessment of the nature and depth of the burn.

Superficial burns

Minor burns includes those which are full thickness but less than 1% of surface area, or partial-thickness burns less than 15% of body surface area. These burns can be managed in an outpatient setting. In minor burns or scalds, the initial management is to irrigate the wound immediately with cold running water. In most cases this would have been done at the initial site of injury. The area should be cleaned with saline or antiseptic. Appropriate analgesia should be given. The wound can be dressed with an absorbent layer of cotton wool and gauze covered by a crepe bandage. The patient can be allowed to go home with a follow-up appointment in 2 days. The area should be pain free and kept clean. Repeat dressings can be done every 5 days until the wound heals. Once there is evidence of epithelization, the wound can be covered dry or left exposed. There should be adequate healing by 10–12 days. If not, these patients should be referred to a specialist team for assessment of the need for skin grafting.

Major burns

First and foremost, the management of major burns must start with the basic ABC procedure. Assessment of the airways is particularly important in burns involving the face, as well as burns caused by fires, because inhalation of smoke causes intense inflammation of the airways. The airway may swell quickly, causing stridor followed by complete blockage, so the need for intubation must be initially assessed. Blood should be collected for carboxyhaemoglobin levels to confirm exposure to carbon monoxide, and 100% oxygen should be administered. Arterial blood gases should be tested and ECG and oxygen saturation should be monitored. At this time, examination for concomitant trauma is appropriate.

Fluid loss from the intravascular space can lead to shock, so adequate fluid resuscitation is crucial to the management of burns. The amount of fluid loss can be estimated from an accurate assessment of the amount of area burned. Here, the 'rule of nines' can be applied: 9% is allocated to the head and neck, 9% each to the back and front trunk, 9% to each arm, and 18% to each leg, with the remaining 1% accounted for by the genital area. The main goal of fluid resuscitation is to support the patient through the first 24–48 hours where there can be profound hypovolaemia due to sequestration of fluid following burn injury. There are numerous formulae to determine the appropriate amount of fluid to be given, depending on the degree of injury. Either crystalloids or colloids can be used. Typical formulas are, per percentage point of body surface burned, 2–4 ml/kg of crystalloids or 0.5 ml/kg of colloids. Children (<15 years) require more fluid as they have a greater ratio of surface area to body mass. Half of the calculated fluid needs for the first 24 hours should be given in the first 8 hours after the burn, with the remaining half infused over the next 16 hours. All formulae should be seen as guidelines only, and the adequacy of resuscitation must be monitored constantly. The insertion of a urinary catheter and measurement of hourly urine output is a good clinical indicator of adequate perfusion. Urine output should be of the order of 0.5–1.0 ml/kg per hour. The fluid infusion rate should be adjusted accordingly if the hourly urinary output exceeds or is less than the desired amount by 30% for 2–3 hours. The patient should be weighed daily as a clinical indicator of fluid balance.

Wound care

The key to wound care is the prevention of infection, as this delays healing. Superficial burns do not require topical antibiotics. The use of occlusive dressings will aid in healing by decreasing exposure to the air, and will decrease pain. If there is no infection then the burn will heal spontaneously. The goals of management for third-degree burns involve not only the prevention of wound sepsis but also the removal of dead tissue and covering the wound with skin as soon as possible.

A full-thickness burns is relatively avascular and if it becomes infected the avascular tissue forms a barrier against host defences and systemic antibiotics. Current therapy hence involves topical therapy, which penetrates the wound. Topical antibiotics should be used when there is a high risk of infection, such as in second- and third-degree burns. SSD is the most widely used agent, others being mafenide, silver nitrate, povidone-iodine, and gentamicin ointment. SSD is effective against gram-negative organisms. If used in large areas, it may cause a transient leukopaenia secondary to bone marrow suppression. Mafenide is more effective in that it is able to penetrate the wound but causes pain on application in many patients. This agent is used as a second line agent if the use of sulfadiazine has failed.

There are several modalities of management. The burn area can be exposed to air, dressed, or excised early and grafted. The decision as to which modality should be used depends on the size of the burn and the nature of the injury.

In partial-thickness and mixed-thickness wounds, exposure of the wound to the surface can promote the formation of an eschar over 2–3 days. Exposure to air keeps the wound dry and hence discourages bacterial growth. The eschar consists of protein exudate and necrosed tissue, which lifts off as the burn heals. The eschar lifts off early to reveal the re-epithelized surface. After 2 weeks, any remaining eschar should be removed as the risk of bacterial colonization and infection increases. During this therapy, if there are signs of infection or there is difficulty in keeping the wound dry, then the wound should be promptly dressed as moist surfaces encourage the growth of gram-negative bacteria such as *Pseudomonas aeruginosa*.

Dressing the wound minimizes contamination and provides the appropriate environment to encourage epithelization. Most dressings contain a topical antiseptic, hence limit bacterial colonization. Dressings should have a medicated, non-adherent layer in contact with the wound surface with several layers of cotton gauze to absorb any exudate as well as a layer of cotton wool underneath a firm crepe bandage. Bacterial colonization is difficult to prevent, but the frequent changing of dressings helps prevent sepsis. If infection of the wound occurs, then the dressing should be changed twice a day. Infected wounds should be assessed for the need of excision and grafting. If there is no evidence of infection, then the wounds should be dressed every few days, as frequent dressings will further expose the skin and increases the risk of infection.

Escharotomy

An aggressive approach to burn wound excision is now the accepted modality in severe burns. Early excision and closure in large burns of >30% total body surface area has been shown to decrease mortality. Skin in full-thickness burns loses its elastic properties. With the tissue oedema following fluid resuscitation of these burns, particularly circumferential burns of the limbs, there is a significant risk of decreased peripheral blood flow, hence compromising tissue perfusion distal to the burn injury. The clinical signs that signify a problem include decreased capillary refill and weak peripheral pulses that are most accurately assessed by Doppler studies. If vascular impairment is present, there should be an immediate decision to proceed to escharotomy. Escharotomy can be performed in the ward setting or the operating theatre. It involves making an incision through the full depth of the eschar and extending the cut down the length of the limb, thus relieving the underlying pressure. Third-degree burns are painless; hence these incisions can be done without anaesthetic. Any bleeding vessels can be controlled by cautery or stitching.

Wounds produced by excisions must be closed by autografting. This may be difficult with extensive burns, and in these cases biological dressing or a skin substitute is required. The patient should have successive excisions and debridement until all non-viable tissue is removed. The surface should be firm and red, with granulation tissue formation indicating a graftable wound bed.

Wound closure

Functional areas such as hands, neck, elbows, knees, and feet should be attended to first. Early healing of the hands, for instance, gives the patient some independence. The availability of donor sites depends on the extent of the burn. Usual donor sites are the thighs, calves, and buttocks. The scalp is a good donor site as it heals rapidly and can be used several times. The risk of alopecia at scalp donor sites has been reported.

Skin grafts may be applied as sheets, strips, or mesh. Meshed skin grafts are commonly used in unexposed areas. The skin can expand several times and the holes in the graft allow for the drainage of blood, serum, and pus. This enhances the graft take and accelerates wound closure. Split skin grafts should be taken thinly to allow for the donor site to heal rapidly. A hand-held dermatome is most commonly used to harvest the grafts.

The graft site should be dressed with Vaseline impregnated gauze and several layers of cotton gauze covered by a firm bandage. Dressings should be changed after 5 days, leaving the Vaseline gauze unless there are signs of infection, in which case the dressings should be changed more frequently.

Key points

- The management of burns requires the assessment of the depth of the burn.

Considerations include:

- minor burns
  - full thickness <1% of surface area or partial thickness of <15%
  - complete healing without complications is expected within 10–12 days.
- major burns
  - ABCs
  - adequate fluid resuscitation
  - use of topical antibiotics
  - exposure or closed method of dressing the wound
  - escharotomy and excision
  - skin grafting.

Complications

Infection

Infection is the principle complication leading to mortality in the period after the burn. Within 24 hours of the injury, the burn is colonized by flora from the patient as well as the environment. The problem arises when the organisms are present in sufficient numbers to invade normal healthy tissue. With poor blood flow and host defences, this may lead to invasive sepsis, septicaemia, and death. Common organisms include *Staphylococcus aureus* and haemolytic streptococci as well as opportunistic organisms *Pseudomonas aeruginosa* and *Streptococcus faecalis*.

Clinical signs of burn wound infection include focal dark brown or black discoloration of the wound, erythematous wound margin, conversion of second-degree burn to full-thickness necrosis, and haemorrhagic discoloration of subeschar fat.

To minimize infection risk, aseptic measures should be taken at all times when dealing with the wound. Those attending to the wound should wear gowns, masks, and gloves. Loose tissue should be removed and the burn cleaned with an antiseptic solution. If the wound is exposed to the air, it should be kept dry, as a moist surface would encourage the growth of bacteria. As noted earlier, if there are signs of infection such as early cellulitis the wound should be cleaned and covered and antibiotic therapy given. If the wound is to be dressed, the dressing should provide a barrier to contamination. In this case, antibacterial prophylaxis can be administered in the form of topical creams. The wounds should be regularly monitored for bacterial growth and sensitivity such that if the need arises appropriate antibiotic therapy can be given.

If an infection has established, these dressings are not adequate to control infection. An infected wound should be cleaned frequently. It is the actual cleaning and removing of contaminated dressings which can prevent the progression to sepsis, and not the antibiotic therapy *per se*.

Specific topical antibacterials are of limited use as they are not able to penetrate the eschar adequately. More heavily infected and necrotic tissue should be excised down to fascia and covered with viable skin. The patient should have high-dose broad-spectrum antibiotic cover, and supportive measures should also be undertaken for fluid and blood loss.

Septicaemia

Typically gram-negative sepsis has a slow and insidious onset, with falls in temperature, white cells, and platelet counts. Abdominal distension and ileus may follow it. Clinically the most important sign is the fall in urinary output and agitation or delirium. Gram-positive septicaemia results in a rapid rise in temperature, raised white cell count, and severe confusion. Blood cultures may be negative in both instances. The treatment hence is directed primarily towards basic support, that is rapid transfusion of blood, infusion of plasma expanders to improve tissue perfusion, and oxygen therapy. High doses of the appropriate antibiotics should be given intravenously.

Pneumonia

Pneumonia is a common cause of death in burn patients. The pneumonia can be of two types, haematogenous (i.e. from a septic focus elsewhere) or airborne. Airborne or bronchopneumonia is more common. The burn patient is an immunocompromized host, so the causative organism is often *S. aureus* or gram-negative opportunistic organisms. The patient often has evidence of atelectasis on chest radiograph and increased secretions, which should be cultured for potential pathogens and sensitivities. The first sign of haematogenous pneumonia may be a solitary rounded infiltrate. The source of the infection is often the burn wound, but other sources need to be explored. Haematogenous pneumonia is associated with a higher mortality.

Marjolin's ulcer (burn scar carcinoma)

Marjolin's ulcer is a rare complication of burn injury. Typically the scar is unstable, continually breaking down and healing. The latent period for malignant change can be many years. The carcinomas are usually squamous cell and are highly invasive. All ulcerated lesions in burn scars should be aggressively investigated with excision and adequate margins.

Gastrointestinal ulcers

Gastric and duodenal ulcers as a complication of major complication of major burns were first described by Curling in 1842. These ulcers were previously responsible for significant blood loss in the recovery period. The incidence of gastrointestinal complications has decreased since the early administration of antacids and nutritional therapy as well as decreased rates of sepsis.

Key points

- Complications of burn injury include:
  - local infection
  - sepsis
  - pneumonia
  - Marjolin's ulcer
  - Curling's ulcers.

Long-term therapy and rehabilitation

After the healing of grafts, therapy is directed at maximal restoration of function. Burn scars contract, and this results in decreased function and limited range of movements. Intensive physiotherapy during the recovery period involves passive and active movements of limbs and joints, to build muscle strength. Early splinting of scars across joints helps to limit contractures as the wound heals. The use of pressure garments can decrease the formation of hypertrophic scars and keloids. Splints and pressure garments should be worn at all times except for dressing changes, exercises, baths, and meals. The splints should be worn until the force of contractures has decreased such that they could be overcome by active stretching and muscle strength.

Rehabilitation after burn injury is a long process involving many disciplines.

References and further reading

Clarke JA (1992) *A colour atlas of burn injuries*. Chapman & Hall Medical, London.

Davey RB (1999) The changing face of burn care: The Adelaide Children's Hospital Burn Unit: 1960–1996. *Burns* 25: 62–68.

Gustilo RB, Merkow RL, Templeman D (1990) Current concept review: the management of open fractures. *Journal of Bone and Joint Surgery* 72A: 299–303.

Monafo WW (1996) Current concepts: initial management of burns. *New England Journal of Medicine* 335(21): 1581–1586.

Nguyen TT, Gilpin DA, Meyer NA, Herdon DN (1996) Current treatment of severely burned patients. *Annals of Surgery* 223: 14–25.

Rose JK, Herndon DN (1997) Advances in the treatment of burn patients. *Burns* 23 (Suppl 1): S19–S26.

Sabiston D (1997) *Textbook of surgery*, 15th edn. W.B. Saunders, Philadelphia, Pa.

Sparkes BG (1997) Immunogical responses to thermal injury. *Burns* 23: 106–113.

15

CHAPTER 15

Vascular injuries

ALEXANDRE K H CHAO AND JOHN P FLETCHER

CHAPTER 15
Vascular injuries

ALEXANDRE K H CHAO AND JOHN P FLETCHER

Epidemiology

Although vascular injuries constitute only between 0.25% and 3.7% of all trauma, civilian and military (Caps 1998), morbidity from the resultant limb-threatening ischaemia and life-threatening haemorrhage is high. Mortality rates range from 13% to 25% and in one series was more than twice that of patients without vascular injuries (Oller *et al.* 1992). Patients also tend to have higher injury severity scores and longer hospital stays, and incur a greater economic burden.

Penetrating vascular injuries account for 50–90% of all vascular trauma (Frykberg 1995). The majority of penetrating civilian vascular injuries are caused by low-velocity weapons (handguns, knives, picks). High-velocity missile penetration results in injuries of greater severity, largely due to the cavitation effect (Holt and Kostohryz 1983). This pattern is commonly seen on the battlefield, although the increasing use of military weapons in the civilian sector has resulted in the rising incidence of such injuries seen in civilian hospitals.

Blunt vascular trauma is frequently associated with more severe injuries and higher kinetic forces. There is a higher incidence of blunt vascular trauma in a civilian setting, mainly due to the higher incidence of motor vehicle accidents and falls from heights. Certain orthopaedic injuries, e.g. joint dislocations and pelvic fractures, are also associated with a higher incidence of blunt vascular injury. For instance, 23% of patients with knee dislocation have been found on angiography to have blunt popliteal artery injury (Trieman *et al.* 1992). Vascular injuries resulting from blunt trauma also have poorer outcomes because of the greater extent of associated injury to surrounding tissue. The spectrum of vascular injuries is shown in Fig. 15.1.

Iatrogenic vascular trauma is on the rise as a result of the increasing number of invasive diagnostic, monitoring, and therapeutic procedures being performed (Nehler *et al.* 1998). Also becoming more common are vascular injuries in intravenous drug abusers, which range from arterial and venous thromboembolism, through false and mycotic aneurysms, to arteriovenous fistulae (Yellin *et al.* 1995).

Initial assessment

History

In major trauma, the history is often not available or is given by a witness or emergency medical technician. However, the mechanism of injury gives valuable clues to the extent and pattern of trauma and has important prognostic implications. Shear forces from deceleration can result in significant lacerations of major visceral vessels. The energy dissipated by a projectile is proportional to its velocity and therefore one can expect extensive tissue damage with high-velocity missiles. Because of the effects of cavitation, injuries may be produced in a remote site. In contrast, most of the damage caused by low-velocity injuries is confined to the tract of the weapon.

The time of injury should be noted, as the incidence of limb loss has been shown to be related to the duration of ischaemia. The classic experiment conducted by Miller and Welch (1949) where they ligated the femoral artery in dogs and restored perfusion at different time intervals, showed the limb

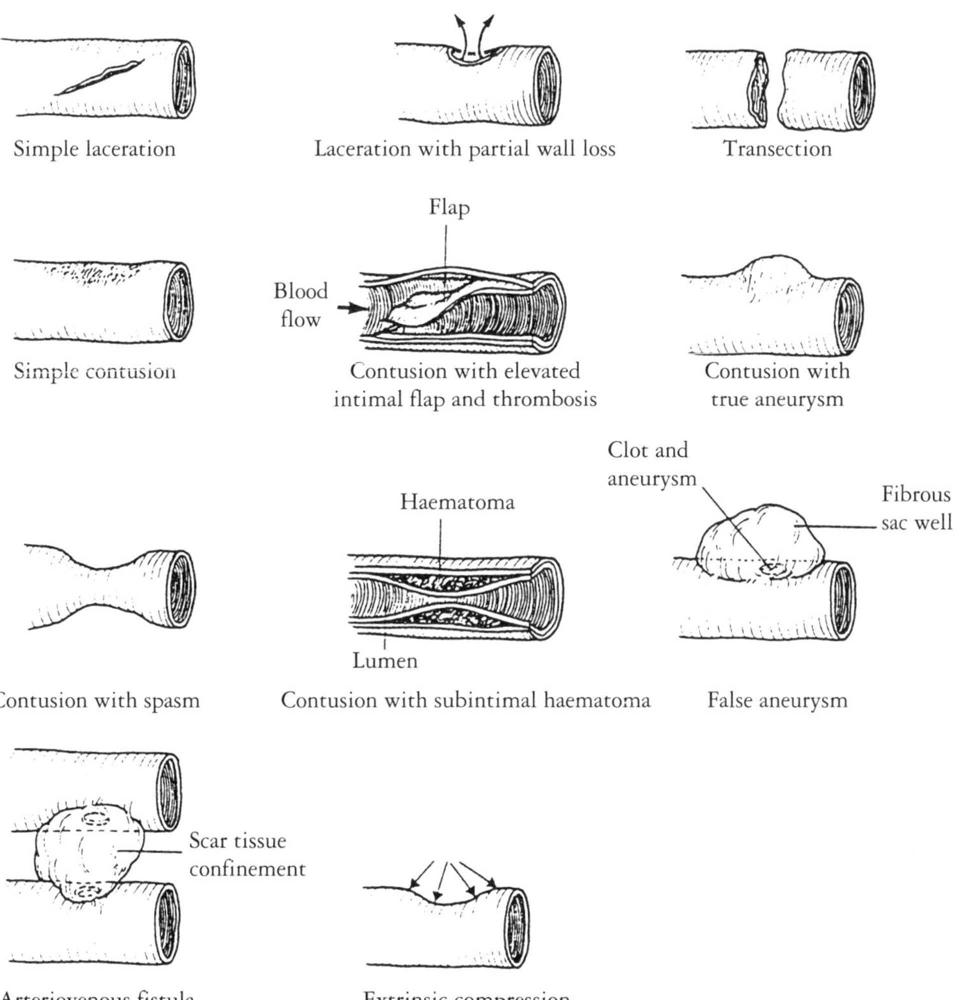

Figure15.1 Types of vascular injuries. (Reproduced with permission from Frykberg E. vascular trauma in vascular surgery: Theory & Practice (Callow AE & Ernst CB editors) 1995.)

salvage rate to be 90% with an ischaemic time of less than 6 hours, 50% from 12–18 hours, and only 20% when circulation was interrupted for more than 24 hours. Debakey and Simeone (1946) also showed a rising amputation rate with delays in definitive treatment of vascular injuries beyond 10 hours sustained by casualties during World War II. These and other empirical observations indicate that the critical period of limb ischaemia from vascular injury should not exceed 6–8 hours for the results of revascularization to be optimal (Fletcher 1992).

It should also be noted that some vascular injuries may not present immediately and may be delayed for anything from a few days to months. False aneurysms may present months or even years later, and it is prudent to inform the patient suspected of sustaining vascular trauma of this possibility.

Physical examination

A good clinical examination is still paramount in the diagnosis of vascular injuries. One study of 2674 patients evaluated a year after the initial trauma

Table 15.1 Physical signs of arterial injury

'Hard' signs	'Soft' signs
Distal ischaemia	History of haemorrhage
Pulse deficit	Small, stable haematoma
Pulsatile mass	Neurological deficit (sensory, motor)
Active bleeding	Hypotension
Expanding haematoma	Extensive bruising
Bruit/thrill	Proximity injury
	Decreased capillary refill

showed that physical examination yielding hard signs of vascular injury (Table 15.1) had a positive predictive value of nearly 100% of penetrating vascular trauma requiring surgery, with a false negative rate of 0.7% missing only two vascular injuries (Frykberg *et al.* 1991).

During the secondary survey, the extent of the vascular injury should be carefully documented. Dressings and bandages controlling actively haemorrhaging wounds should only be taken down in the operating theatre. In missile injuries, the entry point and exit wound should be examined and the path of the missile determined if any major vascular structures are at risk of being traversed. Bear in mind that possible ricochet effects and shrapnel can also result in vascular injury in sites outside the trajectory of the missile.

Pulses should be ascertained, but the presence of a pulse does not exclude vascular injury. In one study, 64% of patients with proximal thoracic vascular injuries had palpable peripheral pulses (Calhoon *et al.* 1992). Capillary refill and skin temperature are unreliable signs, as patients may be vasoconstricted from shock or exposure to cold. An expanding haematoma and the presence of a pulsatile mass are hard signs of vascular injury (see Table 15.1) (Frykberg *et al.* 1991).

Auscultation may reveal a bruit—a systolic bruit suggests a false aneurysm, and a continuous bruit suggests an arteriovenous fistula.

A neurological examination is important not only to document associated peripheral neural injury, but also because it may reveal signs suggestive of compartment syndrome (paraesthesia, paralysis). It is especially important in evaluating injuries to the head and neck region where blunt carotid artery trauma may result in hemiparesis or even hemiplegia.

Where a joint dislocation has occurred, the dislocated joint should first be reduced as far as possible and the arterial circulation re-assessed. If a pulse deficit still persists, then the patient should proceed to further diagnostic imaging. It should be noted that vasospasm may take several hours to resolve after reduction of a dislocated joint, and it may therefore be prudent to re-assess the patient for distal pulses later, especially if other hard signs of vascular injury are not present (Fig. 15.2).

In some patients, assessment of the pulses may be difficult because of tissue swelling. The highest systolic pressure in the pedal arteries should be obtained and its ratio to the brachial pressure, called the ankle–brachial index (ABI), calculated. It should be remembered that the mere presence of a pulse on Doppler does not exclude vascular injury.

Investigations

Angiography has been the gold standard in the evaluation of patients suspected of possible traumatic vascular injury. However, angiography is not without its attendant risks, increases the cost of trauma care, and may also delay definitive treatment. Careful selection of patients for angiography is needed. In the absence of objective clinical findings, angiography for 'proximity' wounds reveals arterial injury in $<10\%$ of patients (Weaver *et al.* 1990).

Non-invasive vascular testing has been found to be reliable in excluding occult extremity arterial trauma. Johansen *et al.* (1991) found that an ABI of <0.9 had a sensitivity and specificity of detecting

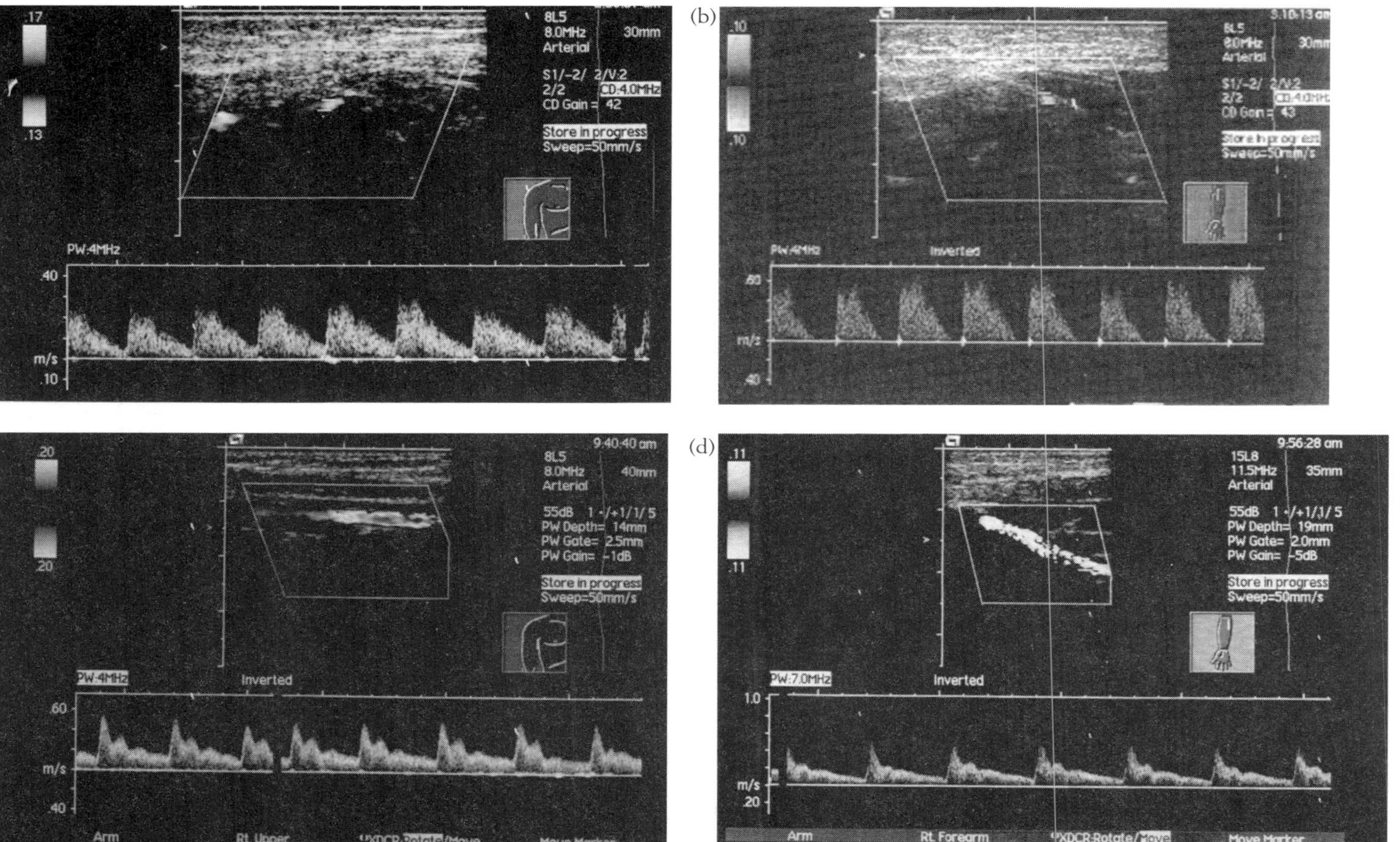

Figure 15.2 Posterior dislocation of the elbow in a 6 year old boy. Radial and ulnar pulses were absent before and after successful reduction of the elbow. Capillary refill was prolonged but the extremity was not threatened. Duplex ultrasound was performed 1 hour after reduction, showing a vasospastic segment of brachial artery over the elbow joint (a, b) and 4 hours later, with restoration of flow (c) and palpable radial and ulnar pulses (d). Note the turbulent flow and spectral broadening on pulsed Doppler in (b), compared to the normal triphasic waveform in (c). (Courtesy of Department of Radiology, New Children's Hospital, Westmead.)

major arterial trauma of 95% and 97%, respectively. Conversely, the negative predictive value of an ABI >0.9 was 99% in excluding major vascular injury.

Hood *et al.* (1998) have proposed an algorithm (Fig. 15.3) based on the use of the ABI to stratify patients according to their risk of vascular injury. In their analysis of 514 patients who had penetrating extremity trauma, patients with hard signs of vascular injury (Table 15.1) proceeded to operative repair and on-table angiography. Those with 'soft' or no signs of vascular injury were classified as either of intermediate risk (ABI <1.0 or pulse deficit) or low risk (ABI> 1.0, no pulse deficit).

Those at low risk of injury were managed by close observation and did not develop further signs of vascular injury in the first 24 hours of observation and on follow-up. The intermediate risk group proceeded to angiography, and the sensitivity of an ABI of <1.0 in predicting major arterial injury was 96%. The negative predictive value of an ABI >1.0 was 99%. The authors concluded that patients who have a normal pulse and an ABI >1.0 do not require angiographic evaluation. All clinically occult injuries requiring intervention were found in extremities with a distal pulse deficit or an ABI <1.0 or both.

Duplex ultrasound has emerged as a useful modality for screening and follow-up of patients with vascular injury. Indeed, definitive diagnosis is often possible in the vessels of the extremity and the

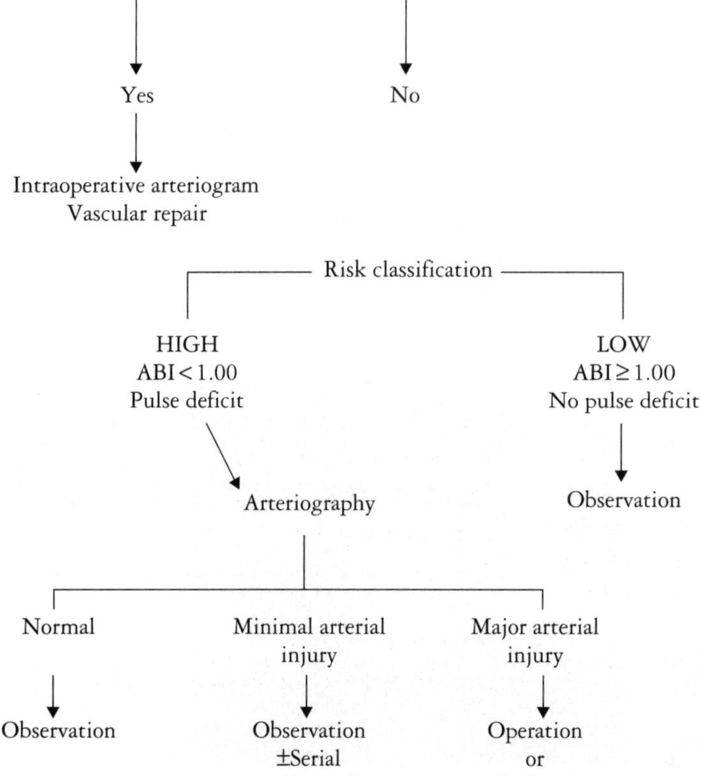

Figure 15.3 Algorithm for managing vascular injuries. (Reproduced with permission from Hood DB, Weaver FA, Yellin AE (1998) Changing perspectives in the diagnosis of peripheral vascular trauma. *Seminars in Vascular Surgery* 11(4): 255–260.)

neck region. Several studies have correlated its accuracy with angiography and operative findings, yielding sensitivities of between 90–100% and specificities of 98–100% (Bynoe *et al.* 1991, Fry *et al.* 1993, Kuzniec *et al.* 1998). It is particularly useful for distinguishing pseudoaneurysms from haematomas (Jargiello *et al.* 1998). Intimal flaps and arteriovenous fistulae can be identified on B-mode and colour-flow duplex. Arterial occlusion gives a characteristic 'thump' on pulsed wave Doppler. Associated venous thrombosis and isolated venous injuries can also be detected (Gagne *et al.* 1995). Some centres are now utilizing duplex ultrasound as the primary modality of imaging for detecting vascular injuries, which has the advantage of lower cost as well as virtually no procedural complications (Fry *et al.* 1993).

Key points

- Note duration of ischaemia.
- Reduce fractures/dislocations first before assessment.
- Check peripheral pulses of all limbs.
- Look for 'soft' and 'hard' signs.
- Obtain ankle (or wrist)–brachial systolic pressure index.
- Vasospasm may occur in blunt injury—reassess later if limb not threatened.

General principles of management

The principles of resuscitation must be upheld—securing the airway is a priority. Providing supplementary oxygen via face mask or nasal prongs ensures optimal oxygenation of blood in both haemorrhage and ischaemia.

Active haemorrhage should be controlled by direct pressure and packing. The use of tourniquets and blind arterial clamping should be avoided. Appropriate fluid resuscitation should be administered according to the severity of the injury.

The stable patient suspected of arterial injury should be managed according to the algorithm above (Fig. 15.3). Not all vascular injuries require surgical intervention; some can be observed (Table 15.2) (Stain *et al.* 1989). If a non-operative strategy is adopted, close monitoring of vital signs and the affected extremity, with repeat assessment of the injury for progression by angiography or duplex ultrasound, is mandatory.

The haemodynamically unstable patient should be brought to the operating theatre without delay. Undue delays in obtaining angiography should be avoided, as this can be performed on the operating table if necessary (Fletcher and Little 1981).

The management plan and priorities in treatment for the patient must be decided and agreed upon in the presence of all the various teams involved. The patient should be positioned to allow both vascular and orthopaedic surgical approaches. A radiolucent operating table should be utilized as far as possible to facilitate imaging. Autotransfusion devices (e.g. Cell-Saver) and a full range of vascular instruments (Fogarty balloon catheters, arterial clamps, shunts, etc.) should be available. The uninjured lower limb should also be prepared for saphenous vein harvesting if required.

The preferred surgical incision in the extremity would be along the injured vessel's anatomical course, as in an elective procedure. Existing open wounds may be extended in the line of the vessel.

Table 15.2 **Criteria for conservative management of vascular injuries**
Transient pulse deficit
Blunt injury/proximity injury with intact distal circulation
No active haemorrhage
Asymptomatic intimal defects on angiography
Pseudoaneurysms <5 mm
Small intimal flaps directed downstream

Care should be taken to preserve as many collateral vessels as possible during dissection. The injured vessel is explored to expose a normal segment proximally and distally. It should be remembered that thrombosis can and usually will extend well proximal to the point of injury, and every attempt should be made to expose healthy artery distally.

Systemic heparinization may increase the risk of bleeding in multiple trauma patients and should be used cautiously. It is generally best avoided except in isolated penetrating injuries. Most patients with significant haemorrhage are already in a mild coagulopathic state, and local administration of heparinized saline usually suffices.

Vasospasm is common in trauma, but may also mask underlying intimal damage. A segment in spasm can be treated with topical papaverine and flow reassessed. An embolectomy catheter should be used to gently retrieve any clot from the distal arteries until good backflow is seen.

The intima of the injured vessel should be inspected carefully, preferably with the aid of magnifying loupes. Any segment of artery with damaged intima should be resected, other than a simple flap, which can be successfully tacked. End-to-end anastomosis of transected vessels should only be attempted if they are tension-free with adjacent joints in full extension.

Where an interposition graft is required, autogenous saphenous vein is the conduit of choice. Size discrepancy is usually well tolerated and is not an issue in vessels of the extremity. The ends are spatulated, stay sutures may be used for approximation, and either continuous or interrupted polypropylene sutures are used for the anastomosis. In children, interrupted sutures are used to permit radial growth of the vessel. The proximal end is best constructed first to allow an accurate estimation of the length when the vein graft is distended with arterial inflow. When vein is not available, prosthetic material has been used with good results and low infection rates. Soft tissue cover is desirable to protect the anastomoses regardless of the material used.

Postoperative monitoring of the peripheral circulation is mandatory. Early thrombosis is usually technical and should be re-explored. The use of anticoagulation or rheologic agents should only be used as an adjunct in carefully selected cases. The early signs of compartment syndrome (see 'Reperfusion syndromes,' below) should be recognized and fasciotomy undertaken if any concern arises.

Management of concomitant orthopaedic injuries

The question of whether concomitant orthopaedic injuries should be stabilized first or vascular repair proceeded with initially remains controversial. In broad terms, the vascular injury takes priority because of ongoing limb ischaemia or haemorrhage. But where there is an unstable fracture, e.g. an open-book fracture of the pelvis, this should be stabilized first. A dislocated joint should also be first reduced before arterial injuries are assessed and managed. With all other stable orthopaedic fractures without gross deformity, the vascular injuries should be repaired first to minimize ischaemic time. The fear of disrupting an initial vascular repair by orthopaedic manipulation is largely unfounded (Winkelaar and Taylor 1998).

An exception may be made if the degree of limb ischaemia is mild. For instance, in patients with vascular injuries of upper limb, where the collateral circulation is usually adequate, it may be expedient to stabilize any associated orthopaedic injury first. The patient shown in Fig. 15.4 sustained open humeral and radial/ulnar fractures, resulting in a 'floating' elbow, following a motor vehicle accident. He had lost his distal arterial pulses and angiography was performed. The bony injuries were fixed first and the brachial artery explored and repaired with an interposition vein graft. The postoperative angiogram (Fig. 15.4c,d) demonstrates good restoration of perfusion to the distal forearm and hand, preserving limb viability.

Where the collateral circulation is deemed inadequate or where limb viability is threatened, and orthopaedic stabilization is imperative, the use of temporary plastic or silastic shunts (e.g. Javid) may be employed to re-establish perfusion to the distal

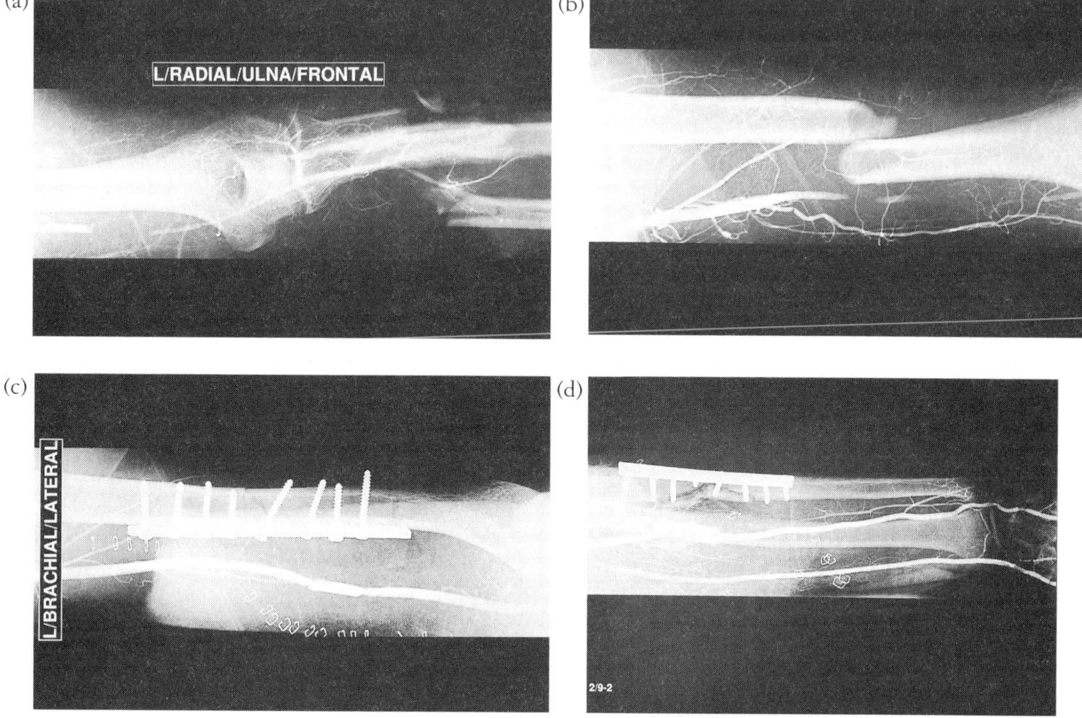

Figure 15.4 The patient shown in the figure sustained open humeral and radial/ulnar fractures, resulting in a 'floating' elbow, following a motor vehicle accident (a). He had lost his distal arterial pulses and angiography was performed (b). The bony injuries were fixed first and the brachial artery explored and repaired with an interposition vein graft. The postoperative angiogram (c, d) demonstrates good restoration of perfusion to the distal forearm and hand, preserving limb viability.

extremity. Definitive vascular repair can then be safely undertaken later once the orthopaedic injury has been fixed.

Key points

- Control active haemorrhage with direct pressure.
- Do not apply a tourniquet.
- Supplemental oxygen by face mask.
- Unstable fractures usually stabilised first.
- Surgical approach to expose healthy artery proximally and distally.
- Defects >2 cm should be repaired with interposition vein grafts.
- Assess for compartment and reperfusion syndromes.

Specific vascular injuries

Cervicothoracic vascular injuries

Monson and Freeark (1969) divide the neck into three anatomical zones for managing penetrating cervical trauma. Zone I extends from the sternal notch to 1 cm above the clavicular head, zone II from this point to the angle of the mandible, and zone III from the angle of the mandible to the base of the skull. They proposed that stable patients with injuries in zone I and III should be evaluated with angiography, a view which is generally held today. Controversy surrounds the management of zone II injuries, which Monson and Freeark propose warrant mandatory exploration. However, several series of mandatory exploration yielded a negative rate of 40–60% (Byrne 1995), and one study showed that physical examination alone is a good predictor of arterial injury (Beitsch *et al.* 1994). The use of duplex ultrasound has also made it possible to accurately diagnose zone II vascular injuries without the risk of angiography.

High cervical (zone III) injuries of the internal carotid artery, if stable, should be managed conservatively or with angiographic embolization (with either coils or detachable balloons) (Ditmars *et al.* 1997). Surgery is reserved for patients who are actively bleeding, or require surgical exploration for associated injuries.

Surgical exposure of zone II injuries is best achieved with an oblique incision along the anterior border of the sternomastoid, and if a high carotid injury is suspected, adjunctive measures such as nasotracheal intubation, division of the posterior belly of the digastric muscle, and jaw subluxation may be necessary for access. A Fogarty balloon catheter may be useful in controlling bleeding from the distal internal carotid arteries. Primary repair may be attempted but seldom achieved. Patch angioplasty or interposition graft using autogenous saphenous vein is usually necessary. The branches of the external carotid may be ligated with impunity.

Blunt carotid trauma constitutes 3–10% of all carotid artery injuries (McIntyre and Ballard 1998). It can arise from a direct blow to the neck, hyperextension injury, intraoral trauma (in children), or base of skull fractures (Beitsch *et al.* 1994). There is a high association with other injuries. More than half of these patients may develop neurological signs ranging from transient ischaemic attack to dense hemiplegia. There is usually a characteristic delay in the onset of symptoms. The usual arterial lesion is a dissection or intimal flap resulting in thrombosis. The prognosis is generally poor and in this situation conservative management is recommended. Surgical thrombectomy has not resulted in improved outcomes in patients who have neurological deficits compared with anticoagulation alone (Teehan *et al.* 1997, Englund *et al.* 1988). Patients are anticoagulated for 3–6 months. Some thrombosed arteries are found to have recanalized on follow-up.

Management of arterial injuries at the root of the neck and thoracic outlet (zone I) involving the subclavian, common carotid, and innominate arteries presents a major challenge to the surgeon. These arteries are well protected within the thoracic cavity and their injury reflects the magnitude of the incident forces. Claviculectomy, median sternotomy, and trapdoor incisions may be required for proximal vascular control and repair. Outcomes are generally poor owing to the high incidence of associated head and major truncal and soft tissue injury (Fletcher 1988).

Injuries of the thoracic aorta are dealt with in Chapter 11, Chest injuries.

Abdominal vascular injuries

Whether retroperitoneal haematomas should be explored depends on the mechanism of injury. As a rule, all penetrating injuries should be explored as the extent of vascular disruption is usually limited and amenable to direct repair. The exception would be with stable perinephric haematoma, where preoperative CT evaluation has excluded major pedicle injury or extravasation of urine, it would be permissible to follow up the patient with serial imaging (see section on renal trauma in Chapter 12).

Injuries of the abdominal aorta may present as a central retroperitoneal haematoma. Depending on the level of injury, a left medial visceral rotation may be necessary to obtain full exposure of the aorta. This will also expose the coeliac axis, proximal superior mesenteric artery, and left renal artery. Isolated lacerations of the aorta may be repaired primarily. More extensive injuries may require the use of prosthetic graft material. To minimize the risk of prosthetic graft infection in the presence of concurrent bowel injury, rifampicin-soaked gelatin-sealed grafts may be used together with meticulous debridement of all devitalized tissue and copious irrigation of the peritoneal cavity. In extreme contamination, aortic ligation below the renals with axillobifemoral bypass may be performed.

Exploration of haematomas associated with pelvic fractures should be avoided, unless the patient is exsanguinating. The pelvic fracture should be stabilized before assessment of ongoing haemorrhage is made. Bleeding is best controlled via angiographic embolization.

Injuries of the inferior vena cava may also produce a central retroperitoneal haematoma. Exposure is obtained by a right medial visceral rotation (Kocher manoeuvre). Control is best obtained by the use of sponge sticks or using a side-biting Satinsky clamp. Up to 50% reduction in the diameter of the cava following repair is well tolerated.

Wherever possible, the splanchnic vessels should be repaired. The superior mesenteric artery should be reconstituted if injured in its proximal segment, because of the high incidence of bowel necrosis with ligation. The coeliac and inferior mesenteric arteries can be ligated if necessary as long as the superior mesenteric artery is intact, as the collateral supply through the gastroduodenal or marginal arteries is usually adequate. Injuries to the liver, hepatic vasculature, and retrohepatic cava are dealt with elsewhere in this book.

It may be necessary to monitor the intraabdominal pressure postoperatively to detect abdominal compartment syndrome. This is characterized by a tense abdomen, oliguria/anuria, increased airway pressure and ventilatory requirements, and decreased cardiac output (Schien *et al.* 1995). Prompt reversal of these manifestations are obtained with decompression. An intraabdominal pressure of >30–35 mmHg mandates surgical re-exploration (Kron *et al.* 1994).

Venous injuries

Venous injuries constitute about 35–63% of all extremity vascular trauma (Frykberg 1995), the majority of which are associated with major arterial injury (Rich 1992). The management of venous injury has been embroiled in controversy over the past few decades. Ligation used to be favoured over repair because of the high incidence of thrombosis of such repairs and the fear of thromboembolism, which is probably unfounded. The impetus for venous repair is derived from experimental and clinical studies showing that ligation is associated with increased morbidity from high venous pressures following venous ligation leading to oedema, compartment syndrome, and even impaired arterial inflow threatening limb viability (Rich 1992). However, venous repair is associated with a high rate of thrombosis, which does not appear to affect limb salvage. Recanalization may subsequently occur in these thrombosed segments (Nypaver *et al.* 1992). Recent clinical data now suggests that adverse long-term sequelae from extremity venous ligation are minimal, and most complications that arise are transient, and often manageable with conservative measures such as limb elevation and compression (Meyer *et al.* 1992).

Major proximal extremity venous injuries should only be repaired if the patient is stable, and can be performed primarily with lateral suture or end-to-end anastomosis. In unstable patients with multiple injuries or in venous injury in the distal extremity, ligation should be performed. Where major arterial and venous injuries coexist, it is recommended that venous repair be performed first to facilitate venous outflow upon revascularization, avoiding severe limb oedema. A temporary shunt can be used to restore arterial perfusion in the interim.

Reperfusion syndromes

Much of the morbidity from vascular injury occurs with re-establishment of flow to ischaemic tissue. *Compartment syndrome* is the term given to the pathophysiological effects of elevated tissue pressure. The muscle compartments most susceptible to damage are those in the calf and the forearm. Following successful revascularization, if prophylactic fasciotomy has not already been done, monitoring of compartmental tissue pressure by clinical observation is mandatory looking out for pain and pain on passive stretching of the muscles within the compartment. The tissues most sensitive to tissue hypoxia are the type C sensory fibres carrying fine touch. A later symptom of compartment syndrome is the development of previously undocumented paraesthesia.

Where compartment syndrome is suspected, intracompartmental pressures may be obtained using a simple manometric device shown in Fig. 15.5. Normal tissue compartmental pressure should be <8 mmHg (Whitesides *et al.* 1975). Fasciotomy is clinically indicated when the tissue compartment pressure is >30 mmHg. Other experimental means of detecting the clinicopathological effects of raised intracompartmental pressure include the detection of abnormal venous haemodynamics on duplex ultrasound (Ombrellaro *et al.* 1996), and diminished somatosensory evoked potentials (Present *et al.* 1993). The clinical findings of compartment syndrome are summarized in Table 15.3.

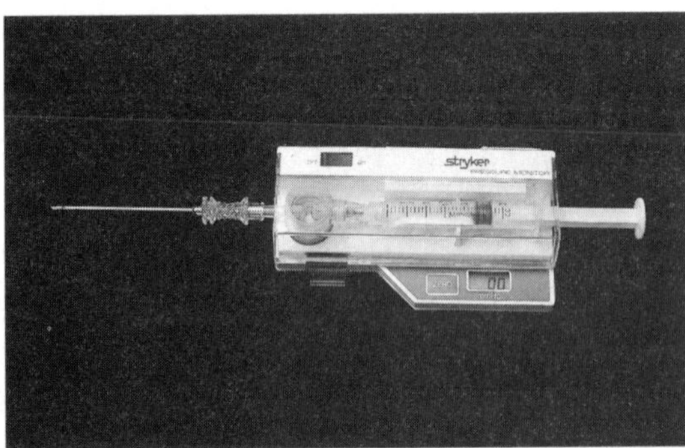

Figure 15.5 Compartment manometer.

Table 15.3 Clinical findings of compartment syndrome

More pain than expected
Pain on stretching of the muscles within the compartment by passive flexing and/or extending the toes
Later
Paraesthesia
Late
Loss of sensation Muscle paralysis Absent peripheral pulses

Complete fasciotomy in the leg consists of release of all four compartments: the anterior, lateral (peroneal), superficial, and deep posterior compartments. This can be achieved through either a single lateral incision or, more commonly, through two separately placed skin incisions (Gulli and Templeman 1994). (Fig. 15.6) The incisions made laterally should extend from the fibular head to the malleolus. Access to the deep posterior (soleal) compartment may be difficult and the best strategy is to start at the distal tendinous portion of the gastrocnemial–soleal muscle complex. If there is any doubt, a complete decompression of the deep compartment can be achieved with a middle third fibulectomy.

Closure of fasciotomy may be performed once tissue swelling subsides, usually within 7–14 days. The problem of skin retraction can be countered by

(a)

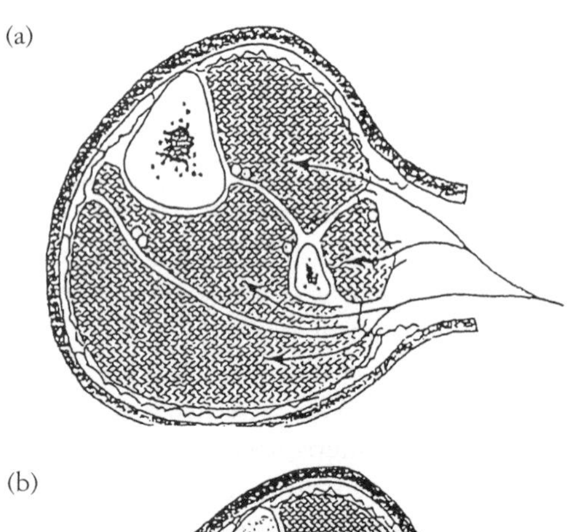

(b)

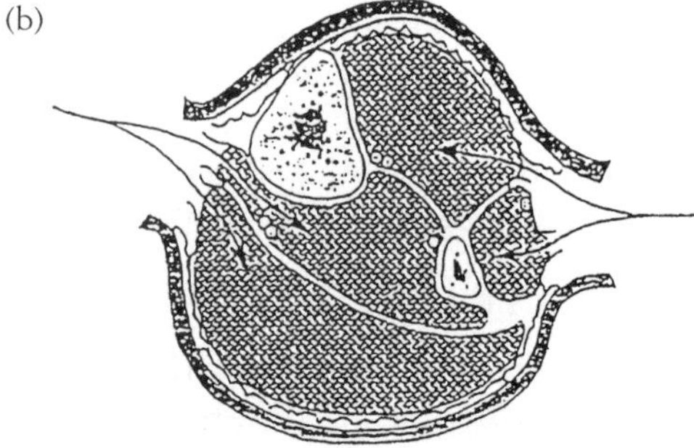

Figure 15.6 Fasciotomy incisions in the lower limb: (a) a single anterolateral incision (b) anterolateral and medial incisions. (Reproduced with permission from Gulli B, Templeman D (1994) Compartment syndrome of the lower extremity. *Orthopedic Clinics of North America* 25: 677–684.)

threading a soft vessel loop through strategically placed skin staples in a 'shoelace' fashion and tightened daily (Berman *et al.* 1994). Commercial devices are also available to facilitate skin apposition. If two incisions are made, one can be closed primarily and the other grafted with a split-skin graft.

Other compartments that may be affected include the forearm, where decompression of both compartments may be achieved through a single incision on the volar aspect of the forearm starting from the elbow down to the wrist, including the carpal tunnel. The muscles of the foot may sometimes be affected, characterized by pain and swelling in the plantar region following revascularization, and may have to be decompressed as well with incisions over the dorsum and over the medial plantar aspects of the foot.

The other consequence of revascularization of ischaemic skeletal muscle tissue is the *myonephropathic syndrome* (Haimovici 1973). The breakdown of a large mass of ischaemic muscle tissue leads to metabolic abnormalities such as hyperkalemia, metabolic acidosis, elevated creatine kinase, lactate dehydrogenase, and myoglobinuria. Myoglobin precipitation within the tubules may result in acute tubular necrosis and renal failure. In severe cases the adult respiratory distress syndrome and even cardiac arrest may ensue. Recent evidence suggest that mannitol, besides its diuretic effect, also acts as a scavenger of oxygen free radicals generated during ischaemia, which have been implicated in the pathogenesis of reperfusion syndrome (Shah *et al.* 1996). Alkalinization of the urine is beneficial, and diuretics such as frusemide (furosemide) which acidify the urine should be avoided. Patients should also be adequately hydrated to replace the diuretic loss. Metabolic acidosis and other electrolyte derangements should be treated aggressively.

Endovascular treatment

Angiographic intervention in the treatment of vascular injuries is not new, but its indications are expanding. Major pelvic bleeding is often difficult to control surgically and has traditionally been treated by embolization, particularly in the unstable patient.

Injuries of arteries not surgically accessible (e.g. distal internal carotid artery and carotid-cavernous fistulae) may also be treated by embolization with coils or detachable balloons.

There are reports of successful obliteration of false aneurysms of the aorta using stents covered with vein, polytetrafluoroethylene, or polyester (White *et al.* 1997, Scharrer *et al.* 1998, Parodi *et al.* 1999). Traumatic arteriovenous fistulae may also be treated in the same way. Initial results have been good, but the long-term patency and function of these stent-grafts remain to be evaluated (Parodi *et al.* 1999).

An endovascular approach to the treatment of vascular injuries has the advantage of being minimally invasive and is able to treat vessels which are difficult to access through conventional surgery.

References

Beitsch P, Weigelt JA, Flynn E *et al.* (1994) Physical examination and arteriography in patient with penetrating zone II neck injuries. *Archives of Surgery* 129(6): 577–581.

Berman SS, Schilling J, McIntrye KE (1994) Shoelace technique for delayed primary closure of fasciotomies. *American Journal of Surgery* 167: 435–436.

Bynoe RP, Miles WS, Bell RM *et al.* (1991) Non-invasive diagnosis of vascular trauma by duplex ultrasonography. *Journal of Vascular Surgery* 14(3): 346–352.

Byrne MP (1995) Penetrating and blunt extracranial carotid artery injuries. In: Ernst CB, Stanley JC (eds) *Current therapy in vascular surgery*. Mosby, St. Louis, Mo., pp. 598–603.

Calhoon JH, Grover FL, Trinkle JT (1992) Chest trauma: approach and management. *Clinical Chest Medicine* 13: 55–67.

Caps MT (1998) The epidemiology of vascular trauma. *Seminars in Vascular Surgery* 11(4): 227–231.

DeBakey ME, Simeone FA (1946) Battle injuries of the arteries in World War II. An analysis of 2471 cases. *Annals of Surgery.* 123: 534.

Ditmars ML, Klein SR, Bongard FS (1997) Diagnosis and management of zone III carotid injuries. *Injury* 28(8): 515–520.

Englund R, Harris JP, May J (1988) Blunt trauma to the internal carotid artery. *Annals of Vascular Surgery* 2(4): 362–6.

Fletcher JP, Little JM (1988) Injuries to the branches of the aortic arch. *Australian and New Zealand Journal of Surgery* 58(3): 217–9.

Fletcher JP (1992) Vascular trauma. *Annals of the Academy of Medicine, Singapore* 21(2): 294–296.

Fletcher JP, Little JM (1981) Vascular trauma. *Australian and New Zealand Journal of Surgery* 51(4): 333–336.

Fry WR, Smith RS, Sayers DV *et al.* (1993) The success of duplex ultrasonographic scanning in diagnosis of extremity vascular proximity trauma. *Archives of Surgery* 128(12): 1368–72.

Frykberg ER (1995) Vascular trauma: history, general principles and extremity injuries. In: Callow A, Ernst C (eds) *Vascular surgery, theory and practice.* Appleton and Lange, Norwalk, CT, pp. 1001–1006.

Frykberg ER, Dennis JW, Bishop K (1991) The reliability of physical examination in the evaluation of penetrating extremity trauma for vascular injury: results at one year. *Journal of Trauma* 31(4): 502–511.

Gagne PJ, Cone JB, Macfarland D *et al.* (1995) Proximity penetrating extremity trauma: the role of duplex ultrasound in the detection of occult vascular injuries. *Journal of Trauma* 39(6): 1157–1163.

Gulli B, Templeman D (1994) Compartment syndrome of the lower extremity. *Orthopedic Clinics of North America* 25: 677–684.

Haimovici H (1973) Myopathic-nephrotic-metabolic syndrome associated with massive arterial occlusions. *Journal of Cardiovascular Surgery* 14: 58–600.

Holt GR, Kostohryz G Jr (1983) Wound ballistics of gunshot injuries to the head and neck. *Archives of Otolaryngology* 109: 313–318.

Hood DB, Weaver FA, Yellin AE (1998) Changing perspectives in the diagnosis of peripheral vascular trauma. *Seminars in Vascular Surgery* 11(4): 255–260.

Jargiello T, Zubilewicz T, Janczarek M *et al.* (1998) Pulsating mass after accidental arterial trauma: diagnosis with duplex ultrasound and the role of arteriography. *Vasa* 27(2): 111–117.

Johansen K, Lynch K, Paun M *et al.* (1991) Non-invasive vascular tests reliably exclude occult arterial trauma in injured extremities. *Journal of Trauma* 31(4): 515–519.

Kron IL, Harman PK, Nolan SP (1984) The measurement of intra-abdominal pressure as a criterion for abdominal re-exploration. *Annals of Surgery* 199: 28–30.

Kuzniec S, Kauffman P, Molnar LJ *et al.* (1998) Diagnosis of limbs and neck arterial trauma using duplex ultrasonography. *Cardiovascular Surgery* 6(4): 358–366.

McIntyre WB, Ballard JL (1998) Cervicothoracic vascular injuries. *Seminars in Vascular Surgery* 11(4): 232–242.

Meyer JP, Schuler JJ, Flanigan DP (1992) Management of peripheral venous injuries. In: Flanigan DP (ed) *Civilian vascular Trauma.* Lea & Febiger, Philadelphia, Pa., pp. 373–383.

Miller HH, Welch CS (1949) Quantitative studies on the time factor in arterial injuries. *Annals of Surgery* 130: 428–438.

Monson DO, Saletta JD, Freeark RJ (1969) Carotid vertebral trauma. *Journal of Trauma* 9: 987–999.

Nehler MR, Taylor LR, Porter JM (1998) Iatrogenic vascular trauma. *Seminars in Vascular Surgery* 11(4): 283–293.

Nypaver TJ, Schuller JJ, McDonnell P (1992) Long term results of venous reconstruction after vascular trauma in civilian practice. *Journal of Vascular Surgery* 16: 762–768.

Oller DW, Rutledge R, Clancey T (1992) Vascular injuries in a rural state: A review of 978 patients from a state trauma registry. *Journal of Trauma* 32: 740–745.

Ombrellaro MP, Stevens SL, Freeman MB (1996) Ultrasound characteristics of lower extremity venous flow for the early diagnosis of compartment syndrome: an experimental study. *Journal of Vascular Technology* 20: 71–75.

Parodi JC, Schonholz C, Bergan J (1999) Endovascular stent-graft treatment of traumatic arterial lesions. *Annals of Vascular Surgery* 13(2): 121–129.

Present DA, Nainzedeh NK, Ben-Yishay A (1993) The evaluation of compartmental syndromes using somatosensory evoked potentials in monkeys. *Clinical Orthopedics* 287: 276–285.

Rich NM (1992) Principles and indications for primary venous repair. *Surgery* 91: 492–496.

Rich NM, Hughes CW, Baugh JH (1970) The management of venous injuries. *Annals of Surgery* 171: 724–730.

Scharrer-Palmer R, Gorich J, Orend KH (1998) Emergent endoluminal repair of delayed abdominal aortic rupture after blunt trauma. *Journal of Endovascular Surgery* 5: 134–137.

Schien M, Wittmann DH, Aprahamian CC (1995) The abdominal compartment syndrome: the physiological and clinical consequences of elevated intra-abdominal pressure. *Journal of the American College of Surgeons* 180: 745–753.

Shah DM, Bock DE, Darling RC III (1996) Beneficial effects of hypertonic mannitol in acute ischaemia-reperfusion injuries in humans. *Cardiovascular Surgery* 4: 97–100.

Stain SC, Yellin AE, Weaver FA *et al.* (1989) Selective management of nonocclusive arterial injuries. *Archives of Surgery* 124: 1136–1141.

Teehan EP, Padberg FT Jr, Hobson RWII (1997) Carotid arterial trauma: assessment with the Glasgow Coma Scale as a guide to management. *Cardiovascular Surgery* 5(2): 196–200.

Trieman GS, Yellin AE, Weaver FA (1992) Evaluation of the patient with a knee dislocation: The case for selective arteriography. *Archives of Surgery* 127: 1056–1063.

Weaver FA, Yellin AE, Bauer M (1990) Is arterial proximity a valid indication for arteriography in penetrating extremity trauma? *Archives of Surgery* 125: 1256–1260.

White RA, Donayre CE, Walot I (1997) Endograft repair of an aortic pseudoaneurysm following gunshot wound injury: Impact of imaging on diagnosis and planning of intervention. *Journal of Endovascular Surgery* 4: 344–351.

Whitesides TE Jr, Haney TC, Morimoto K *et al.* (1975) Tissue pressure measurements as a determinant for the need of fasciotomy. *Clinical Orthopedics* 112: 43–51.

Winkelaar GB, Taylor DC (1998) Vascular trauma associated with fractures and dislocations. *Seminars in Vascular Surgery* 11(4): 261–273.

Yellin AE, Frankhouse JH, Weaver FA (1995) Vascular injury secondary to drug abuse. In: Ernst CB, Stanley JC (eds) *Current therapy in vascular surgery*, 3rd edn. Mosby, St. Louis, Mo., pp. 637–644.

16

CHAPTER 16

Introduction to musculoskeletal injuries

EUGENE SHERRY AND BELLA VAN DALEN

CHAPTER 16
Introduction to musculoskeletal injuries

EUGENE SHERRY AND BELLA VAN DALEN

Musculoskeletal injuries comprise over one-third of all trauma. That is why orthopaedic injuries occupy a sizeable part of this text.

Fractures are described according to (Fig. 16.1):

- which *bone*
- which *part* of that bone (proximal, middle, distal)
- fracture *pattern or direction* (oblique/spiral, transverse (pathological), segmental, or comminuted)
- then *displacement or alignment* of the position of distal fragment as *tilt* (angulation), *shift* (percentage of end-to-end contact), or *twist* (rotation—may be hard to assess but often important)
- whether *nearby joint involved*
- *associated factors* (dislocation, open fractures, etc.).

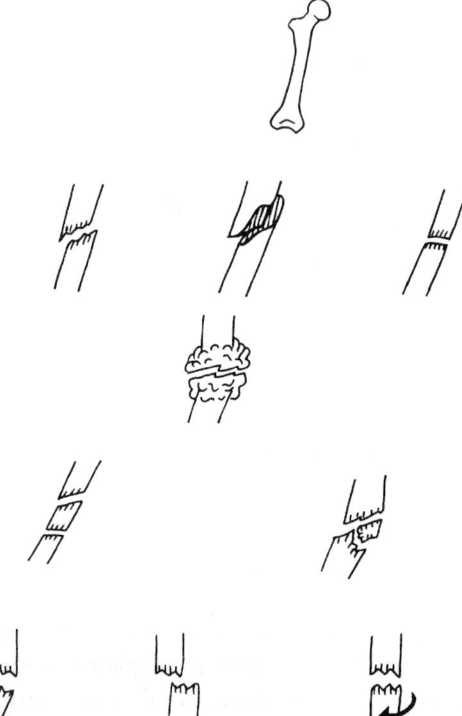

Figure 16.1 Description of fractures. See text for details.

It is useful to know the mechanism of injury to help assess the *personality* of the fracture and thus its treatment (e.g. compression forces result in angulated or T-type fractures; rotational forces in spiral fractures; traction injuries in avulsion fractures).

Open fractures

Open fractures communicate with the skin, and should be handled with extreme care as contamination and soft tissue disruption may result in disaster. Formal, thorough debridement with irrigation (normal saline), preferably pulsed, should be performed within 8 hours of injury, otherwise serious infection may result.

The basic steps to the management of open fractures are:

- debride the soft tissues and debride the bone
- stabilize the soft tissues and stabilize the bone
- reconstruct the soft tissues and reconstruct the bone.

First- or second-generation cephalosporin and an aminoglycoside should be given for 48 hours. Use of penicillin should be considered for farmyard or clostridial infections; also appropriate immobilization and fixation is required.

Gunshot wounds are open fractures (see Chapter 3). The resultant soft tissue disturbance and bone destruction is usually based on the velocity of the bullet. The relatively low velocity of handguns causes the least soft tissue destruction, and treatment usually consists of debridement of entry and exit wounds. The high velocity of military rifle bullets causes massive soft tissue destruction, which requires stage II debridement of the entire missile track. Intra-articular bullets should be removed, as they may cause lead intoxication. Beware of arterial injury: signs of this include diminished pulses and haematoma. An arteriogram should be sought.

Life-threatening conditions

Advanced Trauma Life Support (ATLS) guidelines should be followed. Where these guidelines are applied, preventable death has decreased markedly—from 14% to 3% (see Chapter 2).

Concept of the golden hour

The causes of adult trauma include gunshot wounds, motor vehicle accidents, stabbings, industrial accidents, sport, recreational and domestic accidents. The concept of the 'golden hour' is explained in Chapter 1.

First stabilize—'life before limb'. Do not delay surgery, but make sure everything is ready and optimal (metabolic and cardiopulmonary status, the team is available, equipment, and your plan). Then assess the associated bone trauma once the patient is stabilized.

Orthopaedic procedures

Radiographs are important to assess bony and soft tissue trauma. Obtain standard AP and lateral views with joints above and below the fracture. For periarticular fractures, oblique views are useful. Tomograms (a cross-section 'slice') are helpful. MRI provides excellent three-dimensional images but is expensive and is best reserved for spinal work. CT scans are useful for most injuries except those to the spine, pelvis, and calcaneus. Bone scans will 'find' injuries, including stress fractures, and are also useful in screening for child abuse.

Reduction of fractures

The inexperienced often agonize over which fractures to reduce, how to reduce them, in what position to hold them, and how to hold them. In principle, a displaced fracture often needs to be reduced. The best position is the original anatomical position (if possible), and the best way to hold the reduction is the simplest method (usually plaster of Paris).

Having said that,

- there are a lot of *difficult fractures* (multiple, pathological, open, comminuted, into joint or involving growth plates)
- under *difficult circumstances* (war or simply no proper equipment, hospital, staff)
- with *difficult patients* (obese, unwell, unreliable, drug addicts).

Closed reduction

The treatment of a Colles' fracture may be taken as an example of the closed reduction technique (Fig 16.2):

1. Use a suitable anaesthetic: a general anaesthetic may be required.
2. Apply traction (traction reduces most fractures).
3. Manipulate the distal radius with the thenar eminence of non-dominant hand.
4. Use fluoroscopy, otherwise palpate bony landmarks (tip of radial styloid 1 cm longer than ulnar head).
5. Get out to length. Gently flex wrist 10° and 10° ulnar deviation (probably just as stable in neutral position).
6. Apply plaster of Paris as assistant holds arm in this position. Never apply full plaster of Paris to a new injury—there is a risk of compartment syndrome, which is irreversible, unlike loss of position, which can be re-manipulated.

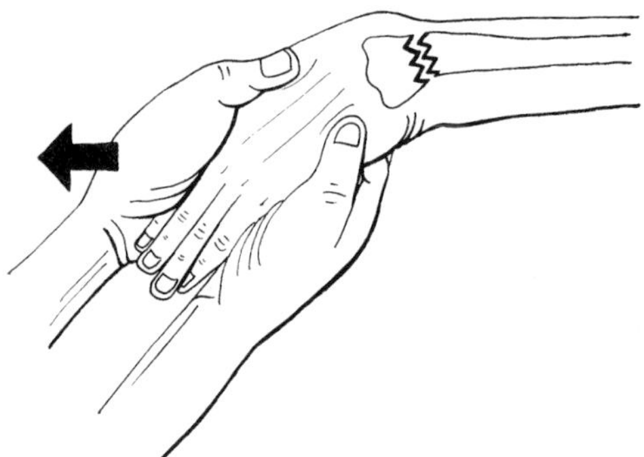

Figure 16.2 Reduction of Colles' fracture. See text for details.

7 Apply back slab on dorsum: below elbow for adults, above for children.

8 Put on soft underlayer, then shaped plaster slab (about six layers; use thicker layers for more difficult patients).

9 In 48 hours complete plaster of Paris or apply fibreglass (plaster of Paris is simpler to use).

10 Give instructions regarding plaster of Paris checks. Follow-up at 1 week and then 6 weeks (more frequent if necessary).

Functional bracing

An excellent way of treating selected fractures of the tibia (or humerus or ulna), which allows nearby joints to move, has been developed by Sarmiento (1999). Functional bracing is suitable for:

- low-energy closed transverse fractures which are not displaced, or have been reduced and remain axially stable
- low-energy closed axially unstable fractures (oblique, spiral, comminuted with <12 mm shortening)
- closed asegmental fractures with minimal displacement and <12 mm shortening
- grade 1 open fractures which meet the above criteria
- as above, provided angulation is <5° after reduction and application of initial or corrective above-the-knee cast
- isolated tibial or fibular fractures which meet the above criteria in patients who do not have other fractures that preclude ambulation with aid.

Relative contraindications are:

- selected diaphyseal tibial fracture with an intact fibula
- multiple trauma patients who cannot use an aid to walk
- axially unstable fractures with initial shortening >12 mm where length has been restored by traction, unless patients are kept from weight-bearing for a period of time to allow stability to develop.

Humeral shaft fracture

- *For:* closed diaphyseal fractures without marked distraction between fragments; closed fracture associated with radial nerve palsy similar to above; open fractures without significant soft-tissue injury.
- *Relative contraindications:* bilateral humeral fractures; multiple trauma where the patient is unable to ambulate with support.

Isolated ulnar fracture

- *For:* isolated shaft fracture without displacement; type I and II open fracture as above; no dislocation of proximal radius; bilateral closed ulnar fracture without multiple trauma.
- *Relative contraindications:* open fractures with a lot of soft tissue injury; dislocation of radial head.

Technique used to apply traction

Reduction may be *closed* (manipulate/apply traction) or *open*, usually with internal fixation (open reduction with internal fixation, ORIF). Both types can be held externally with plaster of Paris, a functional brace, a splint, or an external fixator, or internally with plates, screws, or nails. Joint surface involvement demands a very close reduction

(<2 mm). Consider the age and state of the wound and pre-injury function.

See Appendix E.

Immobilization

Immobilization decreases movement at the fracture, prevents displacement, and relieves pain. It may be achieved by traction, internal or external fixation, splinting, functional bracing, casting, or orthotics.

Preservation of function

The ultimate goal is rehabilitation (see Chapter 42).

Orthopaedic complications

- Complications may result from the injury or other organ systems. They include bone healing problems usually due to limited healing potential from limited or disturbed blood supply.
- They may be caused by infection or inadequate fixation, inadequate blood supply, excessive space between fracture fragments, too much or too little motion at the fracture site, soft tissue interposition, *delayed union* (free movement of bone ends >4 months after injury or beginning of treatment), or *non-union* (free movement >6 months).
- They are classified as *hypervascular* (hypertrophic) or *avascular* (atrophic) on the basis of their biological reaction.
- Treatment includes injection of bone marrow or other osteo-stimulating materials, more secure internal fixation, excision of gap tissue, applying compression across the gap, bone graft, electrical stimulation, or prosthetic replacement.

Malunion

Malunion, i.e. healing in a 'crooked' position, may result from a management problem or may be unavoidable. It causes shortening where there is overlap. Treatment means correction by osteotomy. Shortening can also result from bone loss or growth plate injuries.

Avascular necrosis

Bone death or avascular necrosis (AVN) is seen in intra-articular fractures, especially of the femoral head and neck, femoral condyles, proximal scaphoid, talar neck, and proximal humerus. It results from disruption of the blood supply. AVN causes non-union, and may lead to osteoarthritis and collapse.

Infection

Infection is always a possible complication of open fractures. Immediate and adequate debridement of all open fractures is essential—both initially, and again if infection becomes apparent. Watch for 'fight bites' and the bites of cats or dogs. The symptoms of infection are persistent pain; stiffness; and progressive, concentric joint space narrowing. It may result in severe pain or systemic disturbance, and may become life-threatening.

Beware of *tetanus* caused by *Clostridium tetani* which flourishes in dead tissue (the micro-organism secretes an exotoxin which passes to the central nervous system). It can be avoided by early toxoid boosters and extreme care. Signs and symptoms are contractions (jaw and facial muscles, then diaphragm and intercostals leading to asphyxia). Treatment includes intravenous antitoxin and heavy sedation with a muscle relaxant or tracheal intubation, if necessary.

Gas gangrene

Gas gangene is a life-threatening condition due to *Clostridium* species or, in rare cases, a group G streptococcal infection. Severe symptoms within 24 hours include a foul-smelling, serosanguinous brown discharge; oedema; progressive pain; ultimate toxaemia; and coma.

Treatment includes penicillin G (20 million units per day in adults), clindamycin, hyperbaric oxygen, and amputation in advanced cases.

Toxic shock syndrome

Toxic shock syndrome is caused by gram-positive bacteria. Superinfection results from toxaemia, not septicaemia. Symptoms (severe) are fever, hypotension, an erythematous macular rash, systemic disturbance, and serous exudate (gram-positive cocci). Treatment requires incision and drainage as a matter of urgency, plus intravenous antibiotics and fluid.

Necrotizing fasciitis

Necrotizing fasciitis is an aggressive, life-threatening fascial infection usually with an underlying vascular disease (e.g. diabetes). It is often associated with streptococcal gangrene, and polymicrobial (with both aerobes and anaerobes). Treatment is wide surgical incision and drainage and intravenous antibiotics.

Acute osteomyelitis

Acute osteomyelitis may develop into chronic disease. It occurs in the metaphyses or epiphyses of long bones, and *Staphylococcus aureus* is the most common organism. Symptoms include pain, loss of function, soft tissue abscess with soft tissue swelling, demineralization, sequestra and—in the latter stages—involucrum. Treatment is to identify the organism, select and give appropriate antibiotics, and halt tissue destruction.

Soft tissue injuries

There may be direct or indirect injuries to nerves, vessels, or other soft tissue.

- *Arterial injuries* are rare but devastating; they may be seen with shoulder dislocations, knee dislocations, and supracondylar elbow fractures. Repair, if necessary, within 6 hours. Fasciotomy may be required.
- *Nerve injuries* are uncommon; most are neuropraxias from stretch (>70% heal within 6 weeks).
- *Compartment syndrome*: Increasing pressure can lead to serious sequelae. There is a further increase of risk with the use of antishock garments. Symptoms include pain (increasing with active and passive movement of muscle involved), paraesthesia, and much later (too late) pallor, paralysis, and pulselessness. Treatment includes fasciotomy within 48 hours (to avoid muscle necrosis) and judicious muscle debridement for any ischaemic muscle lacking the capacity to bleed or contract.

Key point

- Compartment syndrome is most common following serious injury to the forearm or leg.

Pulmonary complications

- *Pulmonary embolism* is the most common pulmonary complication. It requires intermittent pneumatic compression, low-molecular-weight heparin, and warfarin.
- *Adult respiratory distress syndrome (ARDS)* results from aspiration and inhalation or from shock and sepsis. The hallmark is pulmonary oedema and decreased pulmonary function, made worse by prolonged hypovolaemia and decreased left ventricular function. Measurement of arterial blood gases (ABG) is useful. Treatment is with ventilation with postive end-expiratory pressure (PEEP).
- *Fat embolism* is a form of ARDS. which usually follows cases of multiple fractures, mostly of the long bones. It results in changes in chylomicron stability and conversion to free fatty acids in the lung tissue. Symptoms, within 72 hours, are tachycardia, hyperthermia, tachypnoea, hypoxea, and change in mental state (confusion). Treatment includes stabilization of the bony injury (the earlier the better, especially for pelvic fractures) and pulmonary support (steroids may help).

Bleeding disorders

Excessive bleeding can cause disseminated intravascular coagulation (DIC) and hypovolemic shock.

Shock is the manifestation of decreased tissue perfusion); it causes pale and cool extremities, oliguria, and tachycardia.

The diagnosis of DIC is made by noting decreased levels of antithrombin III and fibrinogen and increased values of prothromin time (PT) or partial thromplastin time (PTT) and fibrin split products. Treatment includes immediate whole blood, intravenous fluids, and dextran solutions. It is important to treating the underlying cause. Heparin, platelets, and deamino-D-arginine vasopressin (DDAVP) should be used cautiously, as excessive anticoagulation can lead to bleeding into the soft tissues. The use of albumin should be avoided.

Gastrointestinal complications

Gastrointestinal complications may be either the result of trauma or a complication. They include stress ulcers and *cast syndrome*, which is sometimes seen with spine fractures in plaster of Paris. It results from compression of the second part of the duodenum by the superior mesenteric artery, with small-bowel obstruction and projectile vomiting. Treatment is to remove the cast and place a nasogastric tube.

Reflex sympathetic dystrophy

Reflex sympathetic dystrophy (also known as complex regional pain syndrome type 1, formerly called causalgia; Topper 2000) is a neurological disorder after trauma, surgery, or immobilization. There is intense pain, a vasomotor disturbance, increased sweating, slow recovery, dryness, swelling, osteopaenia, and skin changes. It is said to be caused by a sustained efferent sympathetic activity locked into a reflex loop. Lankford and Evans have described three stages (Lankford 1988):

- *Acute:* onset within 3 months, there is pain, swelling, redness, decreased range of movement, and sweating. Radiograph is normal; three-phase bone scan is positive.
- *Subacute:* onset 3–12 months. Increased pain, blueness, dryness, increased stiffness, skin atrophy, osteopenia.
- *Chronic:* >12 months. There is decreased pain, fibrosis, dry and cool skin, stiff joints, and extreme osteopenia.

Diagnosis

The diagnosis is made on four main signs (severe pain, swelling, stiffness, and discolouration). Thermography, radiography, and bone scan are required. An early diagnosis is important for treatment.

Treatment

Physiotherapy (range of movement exercises, hydrotherapy, TENS) is helpful. Pain can be controlled by sympathetic nerve blocks: chemical (four of the stellate ganglion) or surgical, if the chemical blocks are unsuccessful (after >6 months). Analgesics (e.g. NSAIDs) and psychological help are also important.

Late complications

- *Myosotis ossificans* may occurs where there are large haematomas, as late as 6 months after injury.
- *Post-traumatic osteoarthritis* commonly follows intra-articular fractures (if not anatomically reduced). Treatment is adult reconstruction.
- *Immobilization hypercalcaemia* is rare. It is seen after childbirth and in Paget's disease. Symptoms are nausea, vomiting, severe abdominal pain, and acute personality changes.
- *Heterotopic ossification* is seen after acetabular fracture surgery and in head injuries. Treatment is with indomethacin and irradiation.

Key point

- The essential long-term goal of all orthopaedic trauma care is to avoid or minimize the development of secondary osteoarthritis.

Soft tissue trauma

Soft tissue trauma is important; it may be severe or life threatening. It occurs with initial bone trauma and then with subsequent care.

- Thermal burns, freezing injuries, electrical shocks, chemical burns, chemotherapeutic extravasation (see also Chapter 14): Treatment is symptomatic; avoid infection. Amputation is sometimes necessary (especially with electrical injury).
- High-pressure injection injuries: From accidental injections (paint or grease guns) with resultant tissue necrosis or fibrosis. Treatment is intravenous antibiotics, incision and drainage, plus steroids.
- Snake bites may produce extensive soft tissue destruction, often leading to compartment syndrome (see Chapter 27).

Principles of open reduction and internal fixation

Surgical details of ORIF are not included here. Some cases, such as anterior acetabular fractures, should probably only be treated by an experienced pelvic surgeon.

The principles of ORIF have been worked out by the AO (Arbeitsgemeinschaft für Osteosynthesefragen), a non-profit organization dedicated to improving the care of patients with musculoskeletal injuries and their sequelae, through research, development, education and quality assurance in the principles, practice, and result of fracture treatment. Their account of the principles of fracture management (Ruedi and Murphy 2001) is essential reading.

Key points

- Fractures almost always treated by ORIF:
  - pathological (especially tumours)
  - femoral in adults and femoral neck in children
  - multiple trauma
  - where there are nursing diffculties (elderly, multiple injuries).
- Fractures almost never treated by ORIF:
  - most children's fractures
  - tibial shaft non-displaced
  - those of unreliable or disturbed patients.

Fixation devices

Commonly used fixation devices are shown in Fig 16.3. Preoperative planning is essential, as well as a thorough knowledge of the local anatomy, mechanical demands, and injury characteristics. See Appendix D for surgical approaches.

Plates and screws

Lag screws are often used with compression plates (the basis for the AO technique). Compression of the fracture is achieved by overdrilling the proximal cortex.

Compression plate

A compression plate (DCP) is used on the tension side of transverse or short oblique fractures. It provide stability and acts as a load-sharing device.

Contoured plates

These are plates pre-contoured to the shape of the bone and make ORIF a lot easier and more accurate.

Reconstructive plates

Reconstructive plates are useful for pelvic and distal humerus fractures. They are pliable, and allow positioning for use as neutralization platea.

Intramedullary fixation

The use of intramedullary (IM) nails is an old technique, but still a commonly used and successful method of fixation for lower-limb diaphyseal fractures.

- Allows early weight-bearing.
- Nails can be placed using a closed technique.
- Allows good axial alignment (but canal diameter can limit size of nail used).

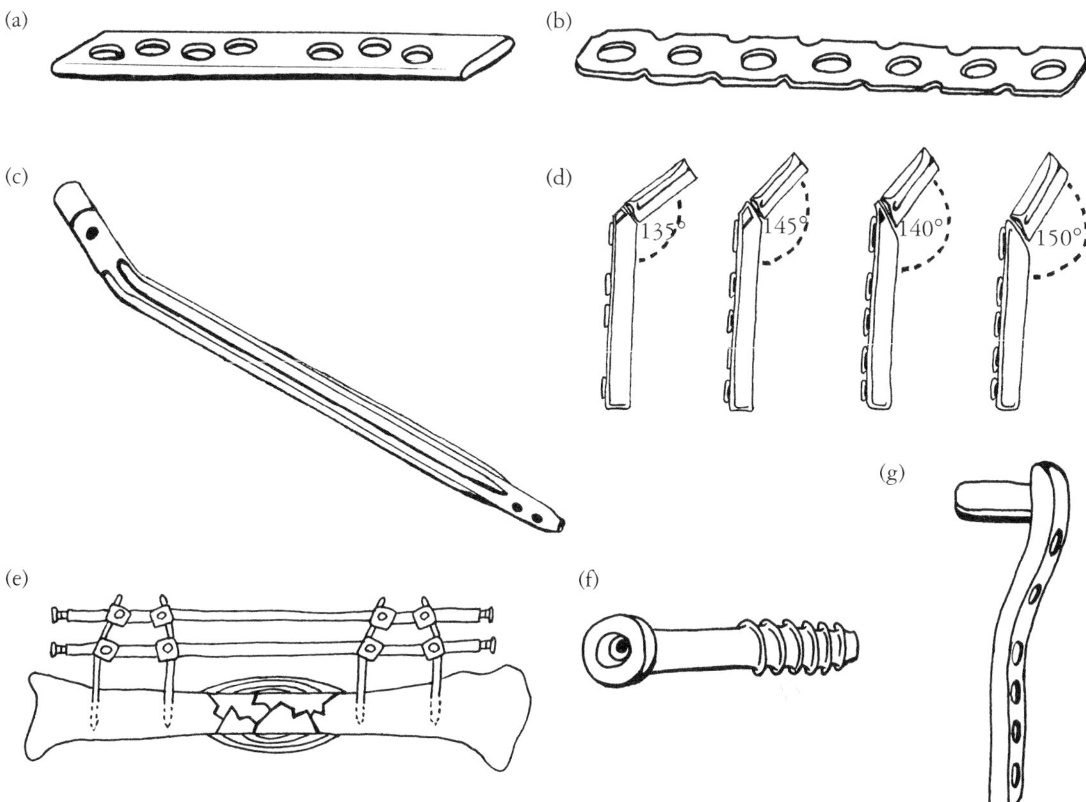

Figure 16.3 Fixation devices: (a) dynamic compression (AO) plate, (b) reconstructive plate, (c) IM nail, (d) dynamic hip screw, (e) external fixator, (f) cannulated screw, (g) dynamic condylar screw sideplate.

- Disrupts endosteal blood supply (may cause embolism).
- May need to lock to achieve rotational control. Modern designs (e.g. the SWEL nail) do not require cross-locking.
- Remove after 12 months.

For IM nails, reaming may not be required. They may also be used in children (e.g. the Nancy Nail from Landos).

External fixation

External fixation is useful for grade III open tibial fractures where there is too great a risk of infection for ORIF. It allows access to the wound. This technique is also useful for anterior disruption of the pelvis or distal radial fractures.

Special devices

Many special devices are available. Among the most useful are most useful are the following.

- *Dynamic hip screw:* A load-sharing device allowing screw insertion at various angles, most useful for femoral neck fractures.
- *Cannulated screws:* Very useful for a variety of fractures, especially femoral neck fractures (use guide wires).
- *DC screw sideplates:* Useful for unstable subtrochanteric fractures and distal femur fractures.
- *Tension band wiring:* Allows fixation on the tension side and so relies on motion to promote union on the compression side; parallel

Kirschner wires placed close to the outer cortex with cerclage wire under these before being tightened to apply compression. Useful for patella and olecranon fractures.

References

ATLS American College of Surgeons Chicago, Illinois. www.facs.org/dept/trauma/atls/index.html

Lankford LL (1988) Reflex sympathetic dystrophy. In: Green dp (ed.), *Operative hand surgery*, 2nd edn. Churchill Livingstone, New York, pp. 633–663.

Ruedi TP, Murphy WM (2001) *AO Principles of Fracture Management.* Thieme Verlag, Stuttgart.

Sarmiento A (1999) Functional fracture bracing. *Journal of the American Academy of Orthopaedic Surgeons* 7: 66–75.

Topper SM (2000) Hand and microsurgery. In: Miller MD (ed.) *Miller's review of orthopaedics*, 3rd edn. W.B. Saunders, Philadelphia, p. 321

Further reading

Hotchkiss RN (1999) *Problems of the wrist and hand.* Orthopaedic Review Course, Anaheim.

McRae R (1999) *Pocketbook of Orthopaedics and Trauma.* Churchill Livingstone. Edinburgh.

Wheeless' Textbook of Orthopaedics. www.medmedia.com

17

CHAPTER 17

Shoulder injuries

EUGENE SHERRY AND NICHOLAS NEAL

CHAPTER 17
Shoulder injuries

EUGENE SHERRY AND NICHOLAS NEAL

The unconstrained nature of the shoulder joint allows great and unique axial and rotational mobility (and makes it vulnerable to injury and dislocation). This joint is required to provide a large range of movement with speed and force, so it is not surprising that is prone to injuries from the stresses applied.

Anatomy and biomechanics

The scapula, humerus, and clavicle are connected by a complex web of 18 muscular origins and insertions, which suspend the humerus from the scapula and the shoulder girdle from the spine and rib cage (Miller and Miller 1996). The shoulder function depends on four separate joints: the glenohumeral, acromioclavicular, sternoclavicular, and scapulothoracic articulations.

- The *glenohumeral joint* is a ball and socket joint with the humeral head comprising almost one-third of a sphere. The articular surface has a medial angulation of 45° to the shaft and is retroverted about 30°. The glenoid fossa is pear shaped with a radius of curvature equal to half that of the humeral head and a small area of bony contact. The glenoid labrum increases the depth of the fossa and increases the contact area of the humeral head and the glenoid. Ligamentous stability is provided by the superior, middle, and inferior glenohumeral ligaments and the capsule. Further stability arises from a negative intra-articular joint pressure, the rotator cuff muscles, and the coracohumeral ligament.

Material drawn, with permission, from Sherry E (1998) Shoulder. Chapter 8 in Sherry E, Wilson SF (ed.) *Oxford Handbook of Sports Medicine*, Oxford University Press, Oxford.

- The *acromioclavicular joint* is a diarthrodial joint, which links the arm to the axial skeleton. There is little inherent bony stability. It has a variable fibrocartilaginous disc or meniscus. The capsule and the superior acromioclavicular ligaments, along with the coracoclavicular ligaments, the conoid, and trapezoid, stabilize the joint at physiological loads.
- The *sternoclavicular joint* has two incongruent articular surfaces with fibrocartilaginous disc forming two independent joints, which is stabilized by the interclavicular, anterior, and posterior sternoclavicular ligaments and the costoclavicular ligament. The joint has three planes of motion, the fulcrum being the costoclavicular ligament.
- At the *scapulothoracic articulation* the scapula glides on the posterior thoracic wall. Upward rotation is provided by trapezius and serrratus anterior; downward rotation by the rhomboids and levator scapulae. It is prone to grating, bursitis and dissociation.

Despite the low weight of the arm (5% of body weight, i.e. around 3.6 kg in a 70 kg man), high torque forces are generated by a long lever. The rotator cuff and other shoulder muscles generate movement and provide glenohumeral control. When throwing, all the muscles of the trunk and upper limb work in a synchronized manner to propel an object forward. Imbalance, fatigue, or damage to these structures may result in pain and instability. With ageing, the medullary canal expands, the humeral cortex thins and the trabecular bone density diminishes, so making the proximal humerus prone to fracture.

The blood supply of the humeral head is from the anterior humeral circumflex artery and its intraosseous continuation, the arcuate artery. An abundant intraosseous anastamosis of the postero-medial metaphyseal vessels can maintain perfusion in four-part fractures if these soft tissue attachments are maintained (Brooks *et al.* 1993). The major muscle attachments of the humeral shaft determine the displacement of fracture fragments.

Injuries of the shoulder girdle

Fractures of the scapula

Scapular fractures are said to be a rare injury, but not so when a cause is sought for periscapular pain after high-velocity injury.

The fractures may be classified anatomically (Miller and Ada 1992; Fig. 17.1). Most are of the body then the neck and in 96% of cases they are associated with rib fractures, pulmonary injury, head injury, clavicle fractures and acromioclavicular injury.

Radiological investigation

Anteroposterior and lateral Y views should be used. If there is nothing to be seen on the radiograph the injury is probably not important. Some use CT, especially when deciding on the approach to the glenoid.

Treatment

Most well non-surgically, with low non-union rate. Displaced neck fractures may be symptomatic (abductor weakness and pain). Many of the symptoms (especially type III, intraarticular and some spine injuries) are related to an associated rotator cuff problem ('pseudorupture' of the rotator cuff is thought to be from haemorrhage into the cuff muscles with paralysis) (Neviaser 1956). Treatment is aimed at restoring this rotator function.

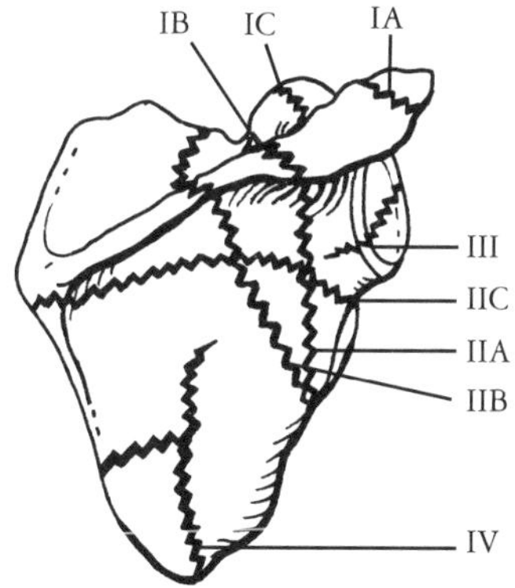

Figure 17.1 Classification of scapular fractures. I, acromion (A, acromion; B, base; C, coracoid); II, neck (A, lateral to base of acromion; B, extending to base or to spine; C, transverse); III, glenoid (intra-articular); IV, body. (Reproduced with permission from Miller and Ada 1992.)

Currently the following injuries are recommended for ORIF (Miller and Ada 1992):

- IA
- 1B >5–8 mm displacement
- IIA, B, C. 40° angular displacement in transverse or coronal planes and >1cm displacement of glenoid surface
- III with >3–5 mm step-off.

Key point

- Majority do well non-surgically with low non-union rate.

Authors' preferred technique

Non-surgical management of most scapular fractures with ORIF where significant glenoid step-off (>3–5 mm) and marked angulation of neck (>40°) or spine. Leave most body fractures alone. If proceeding to surgery then: for anterior rim fractures approach anteriorly and conversely (transverse glenoid fractures reduced through the anterior approach and fixed percutaneously through the deltoid).

Anteriorly use the deltopectoral approach, may need to osteotomize the coracoid and later re-attach.

For posterior approach (fractures of posterior glenoid and lateral scapular margin): prone or lateral position with the arm supported; curved skin incision starts at lateral prominence of acromion, courses medially along scapular spine and caudally to inferior angle of scapula, detach deltoid from scapular spine and retract laterally; extend approach through interval between- infraspinatus and teres minor. Use pointed reduction forceps.

Scapulothoracic dislocation

Scapulothoracic dislocation injuries are high-velocity injuries associated with other complex multisystem problems. It is most important to direct attention to associated disruption of subclavian vessels and brachial plexus from the severe traction applied to the upper limb. The injury may be intrathoracic (inferior angle of scapula lodged between two ribs) or lateral. For an intrathoracic dislocation the arm should be abducted and direct manipulated. A lateral dislocation is ominous; it is the equivalent of a partial, closed amputation. It can be seen on a centred chest radiograph with laterally displaced scapula. Arteriography should be performed and vascular repair considered.

Fractures of the clavicle

Unlike scapular fractures, clavicular fractures are common; they may result from direct trauma or a fall on to an outstretched hand, probably from a posteriorly directed force applied to the shoulder over the fulcrum of the first rib.

Classification

Fractures occur in the mid third, medial and distal thirds of the clavicle. Those in the distal third are subdivided into:

- *type I:* lateral to coracoclavicular complex and stable.
- *type II:* distal clavicle intact but oblique fracture which separates the clavicle from underlying coracoclavicular ligament, and bony avulsion of coracoclavicular ligament.
- *type III:* intra-articular fracture of AC joint/ distal clavicle, may lead to osteoarthritis.

Evaluation

There is pain, swelling and deformity over the site of the fracture. Neurological lesions are rare (brachial plexus), as are vascular injuries.

Treatment

Mid third of clavicle

Treat with figure-of-eight or sling (with swathe). ORIF is indicated

- if the fracture remains grossly displaced
- for an open injury with associated neurovascular injury
- if there is tenting of skin and lack of normal proprioception
- if a high-performance athlete insists upon it for early return to sport.

Medial third

Special radiographic views may be needed (anteroposterior 30° cephalic tilt). Otherwise as for mid third fracture.

Distal clavicle

If non-displaced, treat with a sling. If displaced, consider ORIF if there are no signs of union after 4–6 weeks. Some aggressively use ORIF for type II injuries (with Krischner-wires across the acroclavicular join into clavicle, or suture loop clavicle to coracoid).

Non-union of clavicle

The non-union rate is 0.1–23%. Delayed surgery is as good as immediate surgery. There is usually a painful hypertrophic non-union with decreased range of movement. Treatment is ORIF with intramedullary pins or plate (3.5 mm reconstructive/DCP plate) and bone graft. Care must be taken not to shorten the clavicle. A sculptured bicortical interposition bone graft may be considered. The wound may heal with hypertrophic scar.

Authors' preferred technique

Treat most clavicle fractures with a sling and delayed ORIF when necessary. Special cases (e.g. a patient concerned about deformity) may subject themselves to aggressive closed reduction, figure-of-eight or aggressive closed reduction.

If there is non-union, place the patient in the barber's chair position, make the incision in deltoid-trapezius interval, expose non-union site and freshen. If the gap is small (hypertrophic), then use intramedullary technique. Drill, retrograde, with (6.5 mm) Steinmann pin from site laterally to exit posterior border of clavicle, reduce and then antegrade pin across site. Place a 6.5 mm short-threaded cannulated screw over pin guide. If the gap is large or atrophic then use a low-profile 3.5 mm reconstructive plate and intercalary bone graft.

A plate is better than an intramedullary screw for a distal fracture.

Key points

- Most unite without problem with a sling.
- Special cases may require ORIF, but it is fraught with problems.

Acromioclavicular joint injuries

Injuries of he acromioclavicular joint occur from a fall on to the point of the shoulder and are either chondral or meniscal. Severe injuries may result in subluxation or dislocation of the joint. Treatment remains controversial.

Classification

There is a range of injuries, from a sprain to a markedly displaced dislocation. The classification in Rockwood and Matsen (1999) is useful (Fig. 17.2).

Examination

There is localized tenderness and swelling. In dislocations the outer clavicle appears to be superiorly displaced (really the shoulder sags below the clavicle). Forced cross-body adduction will cause pain.

Radiological investigations

Radiographs should include the clavicle shaft with standing weighted views of the joint (with the weights applied to the wrists of the patient).

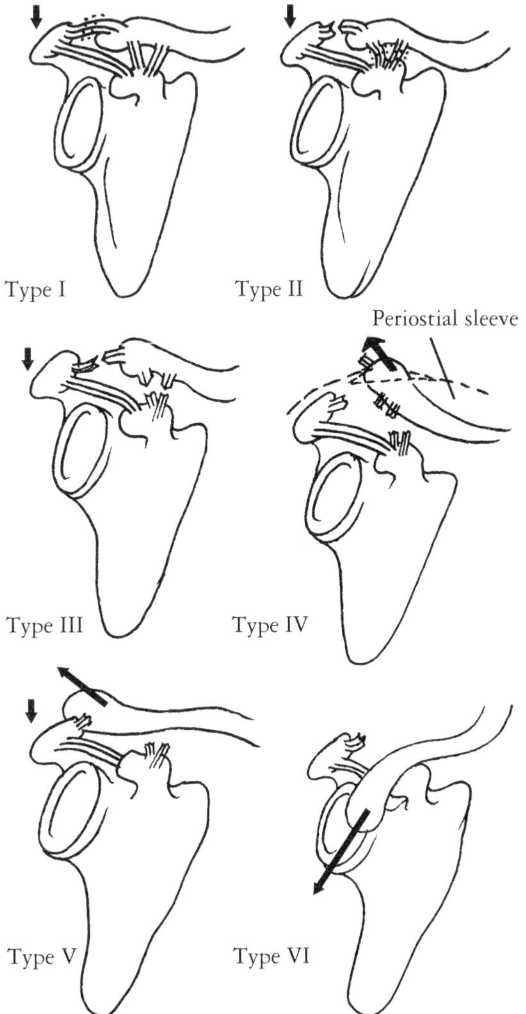

Figure 17.2 Classification of acromioclavicular injuries (separations). (Reproduced with permission from Rockwood 1988.)

Treatment

Treatment is controversial, but we suggest

- For *undisplaced injuries (types I, II, III):* Ice, rest and then gradual return to activity over a 2–6 week period (seemingly minor acromioclavicular injuries may give rise to grumbling discomfort for up to 6 months).
- For *type III in manual workers* (and in athletes if their dominant arm is involved and they participate in upper limb sports): Surgical repair is advisable.
- *Major dislocations (types IV–VI):* These injuries usually require surgical stabilization. They may be associated with a fracture of the coracoid process.

The surgical technique is controversial. Options include transfixing wires of acromioclavicular joint (high pull-out rate) with tension band wiring and coracoclavicular fixation (screw, woven Dacron loop, Mitek bone anchor).

Late treatment

Only a few untreated acromioclavicular injuries are chosen for later fixation. For a painful acromioclavicular joint (arthritis), resection of the distal clavicle usually suffices. This may be done arthroscopically, but is very easy with a small incision over the acromioclavicular joint). For neglected type II–VI injuries the coracoclavicular ligament complex (along with resection of distal clavicle) can be reconstructed using the Weaver–Dunn (1972) technique.

> **Authors' preferred technique**
>
> We treat most acromioclavicular separations nonsurgically except where demanded by significant displacement or patient dictates (manual worker or overarm athlete). We use the Weaver–Dunn technique for both acute and late cases.
>
> The patient is placed in the barber's chair position and the distal clavicle is resected (<1 cm). The coracoacromial ligament is mobilized from the acromion and attached to the hollow of distal clavicle via drill holes. It is left loose until the clavicle is reduced and anchored to the coracoid by a Mitek bone anchor to the knuckle of the coracoid (or use a coracoclavicular screw) and the free end fixed by further drill holes to the distal clavicle. The coracoacromial ligament is then secured to the distal clavicle. Treat with a sling for 6 weeks.

Key point

- Most do well non-surgically. Do not rush to fix surgically.

Sternoclavicular dislocation

Dislocation of the sternoclavicular joint is rare. In the <25 age group it may occur as a growth plate fracture-dislocation. Mechanism of injury is a direct blow or fall on to the side.

Classification

These injuries are classified as either anterior or posterior. Anterior are usually obvious from the painful medial prominence of the clavicle. Abduction/external rotation will be painful. A CT scan may be needed to confirm whether the injury is anterior or posterior as radiographs of this area are difficult to interpret.

Treatment

Many surgeons prefer to leave the dislocation and treat the patient symptomatically, as the clavicle is said to contribute little to activities of daily living. In the acute situation the dislocation should be reduced closed. The arm should be abducted with a sandbag under the spine (as fulcrum) and direct pressure applied. A Velpeau bandage is used for 3 weeks, then exercises. If it remains unstable, the deformity must be accepted, or the medial clavicle resected or stabilized.

Posterior dislocation may cause pressure on vital structures in the neck with dysphagia, dyspnoea, or compression of the great vessels. This is a surgical emergency. Posterior dislocations should be reduced urgently if there is compromise of the thoracic outlet mediastinal structures. A bolster is placed between the shoulder blades and posterior pressure applied to the shoulders. If the clavicle does not reduce, a sterile surgical towel clip can be hooked around the clavicle and pulled forwards.

Key point

- A posterior dislocation should be reduced urgently if it is causing pressure on vital structures in the neck.

Fractures of the proximal humerus

Fractures of the proximal humerus are increasing as the population ages. Although our treatment is becoming more aggressive, it is less invasive. The proximal humerus is a common site of metastases.

Classification

Neer's four-part classification (Neer 1970b) remains the gold standard (Fig. 17.3).

The AO classification is based on the blood supply of the humeral head and describes three categories based on the severity of the injury:

- Type A is the least severe. It is extracapsular and presents as two main fragments, such that avascular necrosis is unlikely.
- In the type B fracture, which is partially intracapsular, there is a low risk of avascular necrosis and two or three fragments are seen radiologically.
- Type C fractures are most severe and are intracapsular with complete isolation of the

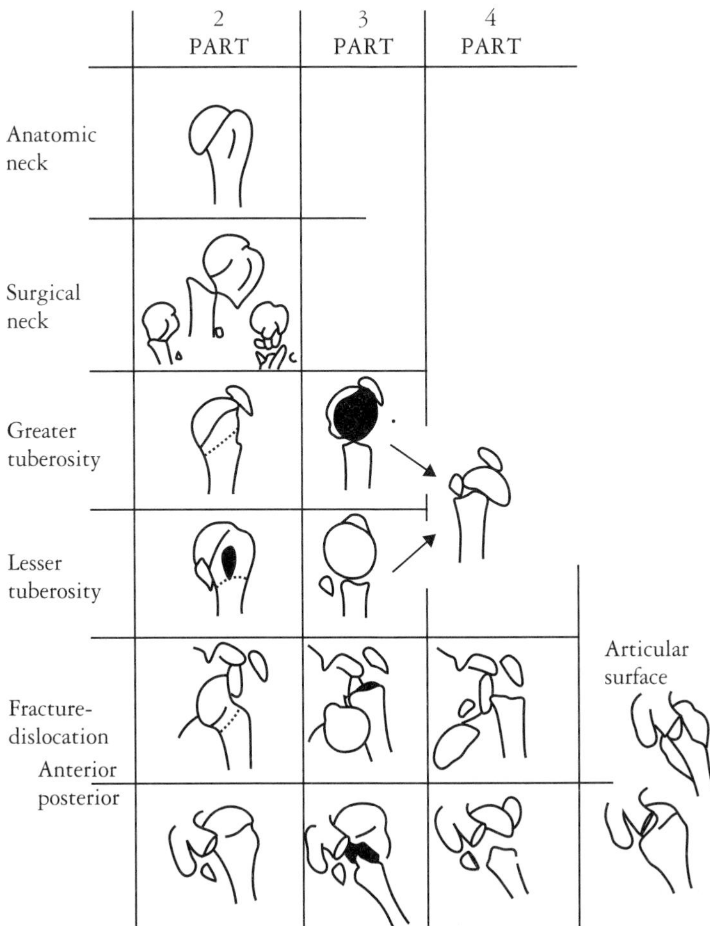

Figure 17.3 Neer's four-part classification of fractures of the proximal humerus. (Reproduced with permission from Neer CS II (1970) Displaced proximal fractures: Part I. Classification. *Journal of Bone and Joint Surgery* 52A: 1077–1089.)

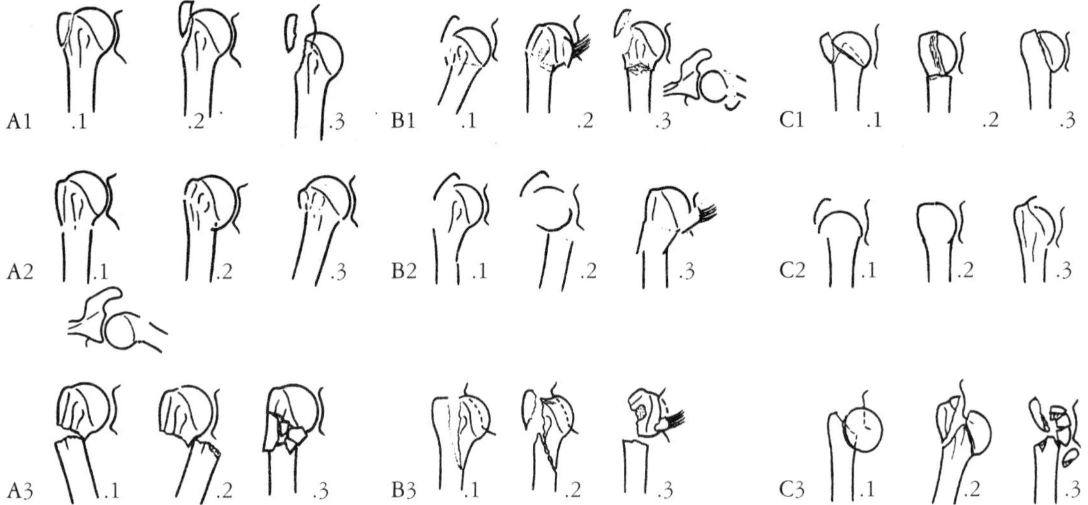

Figure 17.4 AO classification: A (extracapsular); B (partial intracapsular); C (complete intracapsular). Each further subdivided into nine types. (Reproduced with permission from Müller *et al.* 1990).

articular segments, producing a high risk of avascular necrosis. Radiologically, they may have two, three or four fragments. There is further subdivision into nine parts for each group (Fig. 17.4).

ORIF may produce poor results in elderly osteoporotic patients.

Key points

- The proximal humerus is a common site of neoplasms (benign and malignant; including metastases) and tumour-like conditions (Paget's, tumoral calcinosis).
- There may be a need for prophylactic fixation or ORIF of pathological fractures with adjuvant chemotherapy/radiotherapy and surgical excision and reconstruction/amputation. Cement (PMMA) is often used to augment bony deficiencies.
- An appropriate text on bone tumours should be consulted (e.g. Lewis 1992).

Treatment

Non-displaced and impacted fractures, which constitute over 80% of these injuries, should be treated with a sling and mobilized when the pain settles (3–4 weeks).

For displaced fractures (>45° or >1.5 cm):

- two part lesser tuberosity (usually seen with posterior dislocations); if large fragments then ORIF is indicated.
- two-part greater tuberosity (AO classification A1): associated with rotator cuff tear and so should use ORIF when >1 cm displacement or fragment >2 cm. Use Tension band wiring over a screw or Kirschner wires should be used (Fig. 17.5a).
- two- or three-part displaced/unstable fractures (A3, B1, B2, B3): should be reduced (closed or open) and fixed internally. Retrograde intramedullary fixation should be considered. A prosthesis should be considered in a three-part fracture in osteoporotic bone.

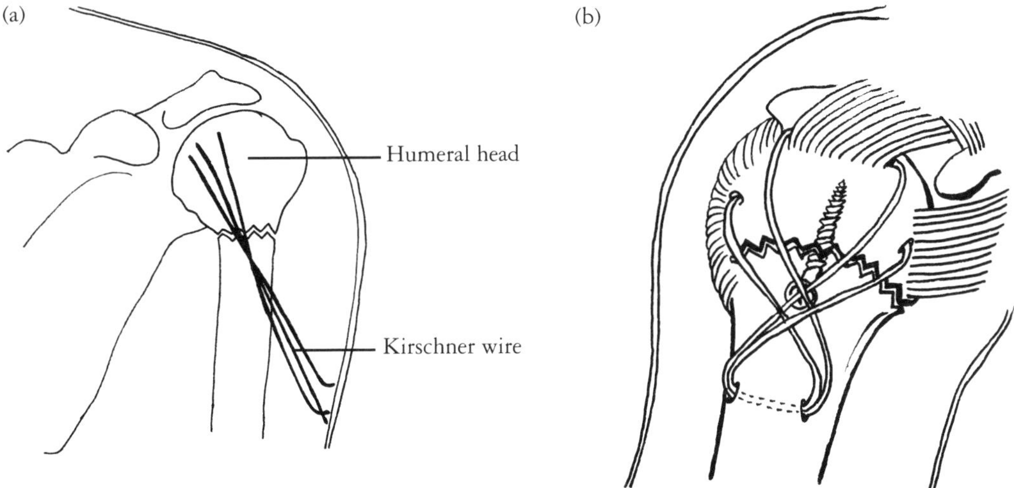

Figure 17.5 (a) Kirschner wire in humerus. (b) TBW technique over a screw for a two-part proximal fracture (wires should not entrap long head of biceps).

Authors' preferred technique

For two-part or three-part fractures, where the greater tuberosity is not much displaced, we perform closed reduction (by applying traction and abducting) under intensive imaging control. Then:

- *Either* use two percutaneous 2.5 mm Schanz pins (or large Kirschner wires). Jupiter (1995) advises a minimum of four pins (at least two from proximal shaft to head and one from greater tuberosity to medial shaft). If closed reduction is unsuccessful then open and use the tension band wiring technque, with the patients in the barber's chair position. The deltopectoral incision/interval is used. The long head biceps is a critical landmark. The superior portion of the pectoralis major may be released. Mobilize with an osteotome. Stay sutures to major fragments. Transverse drill holes distal and proximal fragments. Then use two figure-of-eight tension band wires. A #5 Dacron suture can be used instead of wire, and a screw may be added (Fig. 17.5b). Close the subscapularis–supraspinatus gap.
- *Or* place an intramedullary nail from the top. There is a high risk of avascularity and often poor results from non-surgical treatment (Neer 1970).
- We suggest (hemi-) prosthetic replacement (the patient will become pain free but remain stiff) for: head-splitting, fracture-dislocations, where severe osteoporosis and in anatomical neck fractures in patients >50 *but* ORIF (with multiple pins) in younger patients where young or valgus-impacted fracture (AO classification C2) where soft-tissue attachments to posteromedial neck and some circulation to the head are intact.
- *Humeral prosthetic technique:* Barber's chair position, deltopectoral incision. Identify long head of biceps. May release superior portion pectoralis major. Mobilize fragments. Tag greater and lesser tuberosities. Remove head. Shaft preparation: drill holes to distal shaft to re-attach tuberosities to both shaft and prosthesis. Retrovert prosthesis 25–40°. Trial reduction to check length restoration (monitor tension of long head biceps) tension. Tuberosities should be under head. There is often postoperative stiffness.

Fractures of the humeral shaft

In the past most fractures of the humeral shaft were treated non-surgically with hanging casts or moulded thermoplastic splints. Now ORIF (with plates and intramedullary nails is more likely to be used.

Classification

The AO classification is standard and useful (Fig. 17.6). The fracture may be pathological.

Evaluation

Pathological fracture, or a young athlete on steroids, must be excluded. The radial nerve may be involved.

Treatment

Most humeral shaft fractures can be treated non-surgically with careful follow-up. The arm will tolerate up to 20° anterior angulation, 30° of varus, and 3 cm of shortening.

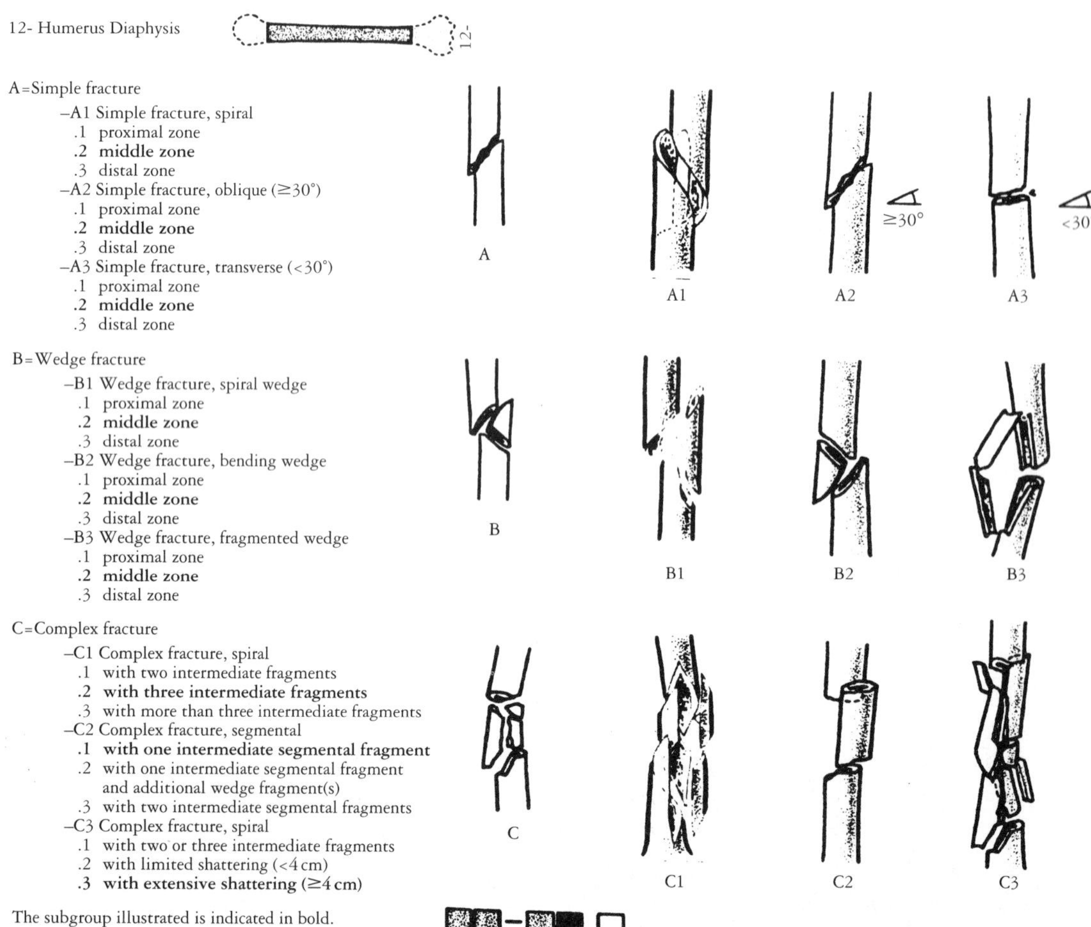

Figure 17.6 AO classification of humeral shaft fractures: A (simple); B (wedge); C (complex). Each subdivided into three types. (Reproduced with permission from Müller ME, Allgöwer M, Schneider R *et al.* (ed.) (1991) *Manual of internal fixation, 3rd edn*. Springer-Verlag, Berlin, pp. 118–150. © Springer-Verlag 1991.)

A hanging arm cast (Fig. 17.7) may be used initially to help maintain alignment. This is cheap but awkward. A moulded thermoplastic splint (functional brace) is better and can be applied at 7–10 days when the swelling and pain are subsiding (Sarmiento *et al.* 1977).

ORIF (Lange 1996) is used for failed treatment of closed fractures, some open fractures, or fractures with vascular or neurological compromise. This type of fixation can also be used if there is a floating elbow, segmental fractures, multiple fractures, pathological fractures, fractures associated with brachial plexus injuries, or if the patient has Parkinson's disease.

In general terms, IM nail fixation is used to stabilize pathological fractures and fractures in patients with multiple injuries. Short, rigid nails are particularly useful to control proximal simple fracture patterns, such as AO type A. The retrograde method of insertion is preferred to avoid violation of the rotator cuff and subsequent shoulder pain. With this approach, care must be taken to ensure that the entry point does not creep proximally to encroach upon the fracture. Locked IM nails are particularly useful to support comminuted segmental, unstable fractures, where shortening and malrotation may be a problem. IM devices cannot provide adequate fixation when the fracture is close to either end of the bone.

When plating humeral shaft fractures, 4.5 mm dynamic compression plates are recommended, with the aim of obtaining six cortices of fixation proximally and distally. The anterolateral approach provides access to much of the humerus. The posterior approach should be used when dealing with distal, especially intra-articular fractures and fractures associated with radial nerve palsy.

External fixators are particularly useful to maintain bony stability in the more severe, open injuries, particularly when there is vascular injury.

Complications

- *Associated radial nerve problems:* Occur in up to 20% of humeral shaft fractures, usually a contusion of the nerve with neuropraxia which recovers in >70% cases in about 3 months. Immediate surgical exploration of the nerve is indicated where palsy associated with open fractures, Holstein–Lewis distal-one third spiral fracture and secondary palsy following closed reduction (little solid data for last two indications). Rockwood and Matsen (1999) advise exploration if 'nerve injury occurs after manipulation'.

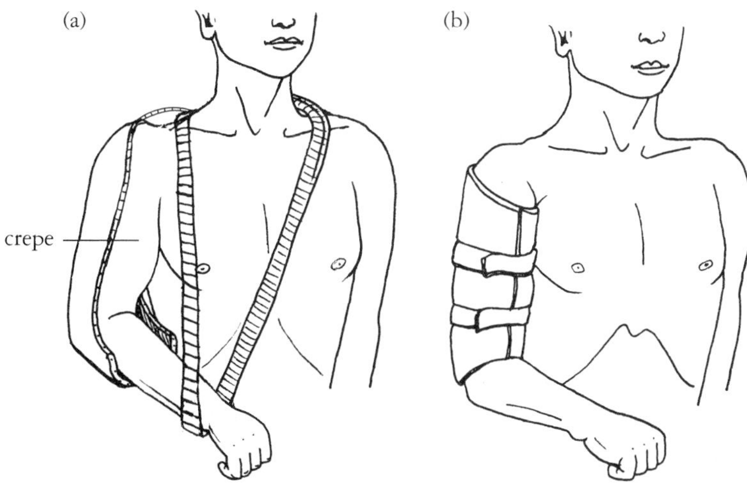

Figure 17.7 (a) Hanging cast; connect the neck collar-and-cuff to the hanging cast. (b) Functional brace.

Key points

Immediate exploration of radial nerve injury: in open fractures and when it occurs after manipulation.

- *Non-surgical treatment problems:* Non-union (usually from big gap, most require ORIF with bone graft except in elderly people with osteopaenia and little pain), malunion, radial nerve palsy, shoulder stiffness.
- *Surgical treatment problems:* All the above plus infection, implant problems, and nerve injury.

Authors' preferred technique

We use a functional brace whenever possible, but follow closely with radiographs and are prepared to remanipulate. For simple fracture patterns (AO type A) intramedullary nails are easy to insert and lock. For complex fractures (AO types B and C) we use a 4.5 mm plate via an anterolataral approach.

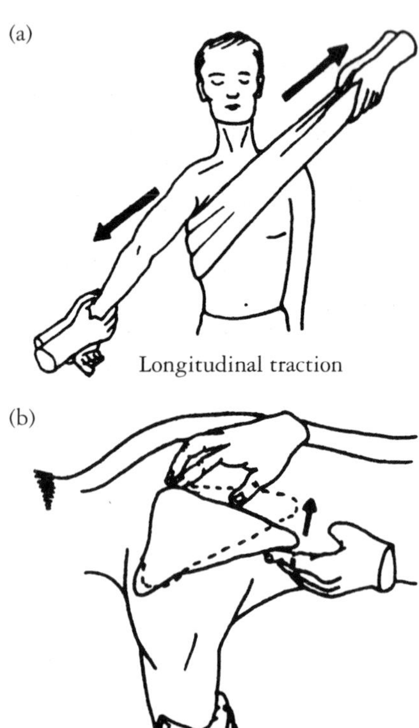

Figure 17.8 Shoulder reduction techniques for reduction of anterior shoulder dislocation. (Reproduced with permission from Sherry and Wilson 1998.)

Shoulder instability

Shoulder instability is common. There is a wide range of symptoms from a (frank) dislocation to variable degrees of slipping of the shoulder.

With *anterior dislocation* (the most common) (Fig. 17.8), the anterior capsule, labrum, and rotator cuff may be torn or avulsed, the glenoid rim fractured, and the (posterolateral) humeral head indented (Hill–Sachs lesion). Avulsion of the rotator cuff is seen in older patients after dislocation where they cannot abduct the shoulder.

A *subluxation* is a partial dislocation. It is not an insignificant injury, as joint damage may occur from 'instability events'. Almost all (95%) of shoulder instability is anterior/anteroinferior direction; others include posterior and multidirectional.

Anterior instability is seen with abduction/external rotation when an anterior force is applied to the shoulder.

In chronic instability there may be no obvious traumatic event.Overhead sports (such as baseball or tennis) cause a gradual stretch of the anterior capsule and subsequent symptoms of the slipping of the shoulder.

Note the hierarchy of support mechanisms controlling glenohumeral stability and so the cascade of injury.

Evaluation

Symptoms of instability include frank dislocation; slipping; pain with the arm in abduction or external rotation, apprehension when using the arm overhead, or a 'dead arm' feeling with overhead movement. The examiner should heck the range of motion, strength and whether there is increased anteroposterior translation of the humeral head (by holding the acromion and with the other hand testing if the humeral head moves anteriorly or posteriorly) (Fig. 17.9), apprehension (Fig. 17.10) and relocation signs,. Coincident tendinitis, labral tears or signs of ligament laxity (hyperextended knee, elbow and metacarpophalangeal joints of the hand with flexion of the wrist so hand touches forearm) should also be looked for.

The natural history of the first acute anterior shoulder instability is known (Hovelius 1987). Recurrence in young patient (<22 years of age) is 62% (for a participant in contact sports repeat instability is over 90%). In older patients (30–40 years) the recurrence rate is 25%. Over a 10 year period there is a 12% chance of a contralateral instability and a 20% incidence of arthritic changes on radiography (9% moderate or severe).

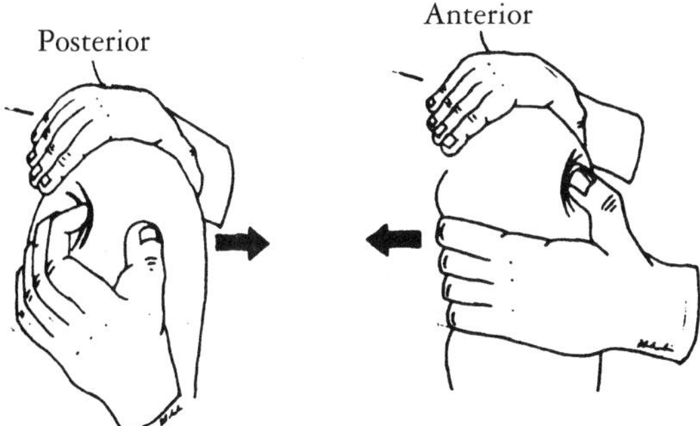

Figure 17.9 Checking instability of the shoulder, whether anterior or posterior. (Reproduced with permission from Sherry and Wilson 1998.)

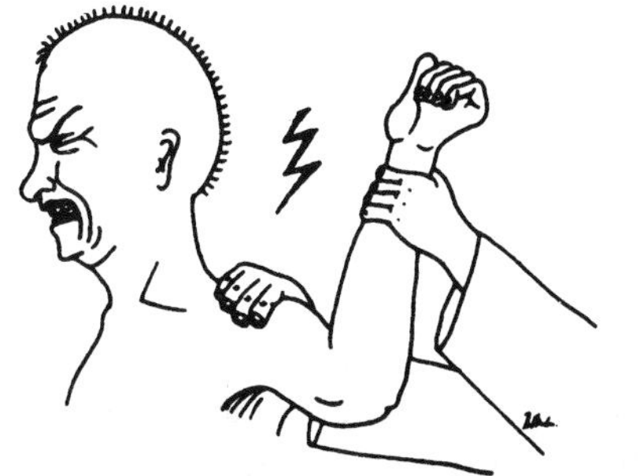

Figure 17.10 Apprehension test for anterior instability of the shoulder. (Reproduced with permission from Sherry and Wilson 1998.)

Key point

- Shoulder dislocation recurrence rate in young patients is high.

Treatment

Acute dislocation

It is important to check for vascular or nerve injury (10% incidence of axillary nerve palsy; up to 60% for luxatio erectae). The shoulder should be radiographed (anteroposterior and lateral view in plane of scapula). Closed reduction can be performed outside the operating theatre using either pethidine (50–100 mg intravenous infusion), diazepam (5 mg intravenous infusion), or nitrous oxide (Sherry *et al.* 1989), or with an intra-articular injection of lignocaine (lidocaine) 1% (5 mL). General anaesthesia may be required if there is excessive muscle spasm (as in a young man with a huge shoulder muscle girdle). Techniques for closed reduction of the dislocated shoulder are listed in Table 17.1.

Thereafter the arm should be placed in a sling and physiotherapy organized after 1–3 weeks. Younger patients have a high risk of recurrence; so for special sporting requirements consider an acute arthroscopic assessment and capsular/labral repair.

Recurrent dislocation

If *recurrent* instability becomes a problem, options include: avoidance of the precipitation event, a rehabilitation programme to strengthen the shoulder; or surgical reconstruction of the shoulder. Several surgical techniques are used, either correcting the pathology or tightening or using bone blocks to avoid dislocation (Table 17.2)

Correction of the pathology includes repairing the avulsed inferior glenohumeral ligament (*Bankart lesion*) and correcting any associated capsular redundancy (*capsular shift*). This is the preferred option

Table 17.1 Techniques for closed reduction of the shoulder joint

Technique	Details/comment
Scapular rotation	Patient lies prone on table with injured arm hanging over the edge of the table. The scapula is manipulated to open the front aspect of the joint to restore congruence of the humeral head and the glenoid, i.e. push the inferior tip of the scapula towards the spine
Longitudinal traction	Patient lies supine and the affected arm is slightly abducted and traction applied with the operator's foot (minus shoe) placed in the axilla or sheet around chest to apply counter traction (an old technique, which is often effective but may cause a traction injury to the brachial plexus)
Stimson's technique	Patient lies prone and weight is applied to the arm with the affected shoulder hanging off the edge of a table
Kocher manoeuvre	Patient lies supine. With the elbow flexed, longitudinal traction is applied to the arm, which is slowly externally rotated. While maintaining traction, the arm is adducted across the front of the chest and finally the upper limb is rotated internally
Forward elevation manoeuvre	Patient lies supine. The arm is gently elevated in the plane of the scapula up to about 160°. Traction is applied in elevation with outward pressure on the humeral head

From Sherry and Wilson (1998), with permission.

Table 17.2 Types of shoulder reconstruction

Type	Surgical details
Anatomical	
Bankart repair	The anterior detached capsule and labrum are repaired back onto the glenoid neck
Capsulorraphy	Plication of stretched or redundant capsule
Inferior capsular shift	Similar with inferior extension
Non-anatomical	
Putti-plan	The anterior capsule and subscapularis muscles are divided, overlapped and tightened. Decreases external rotation of the arm
Bristow's procedure	The coracoid process is transferred
Magnusen–Stack procedure	The subscapularis, capsule and a portion of the lesser tuberosity is detached fixed more laterally on the humeral; head. This tightens the anterior should structures decreasing external rotation

From Sherry and Wilson (1998), with permission.

in surgical management of the unstable shoulder. The success rate for surgery is 95%. Non-anatomical reconstructions restrict external rotation and so restrict athletes.

Multidirectional instability

Most shoulders show a variable degree of laxity (and are normal); however ,where there is marked laxity this may become a problem. It may be insidious in onset or related to trauma. It is important to differentiate laxity from instability. *Laxity* is a physical finding, whereas *instability* is the combination of symptoms and signs.

Diagnosis

There is instability in are least two directions (inferior plus either anterior or posterior or both). There is pain and weakness.

For a small subgroup of MDI patients there is a habitual or voluntary aspect to the problem. Associated psychological problems and potential secondary gains should be evaluated. Surgical procedures will fail in this group.

Treatment

Treatment is focused on rehabilitation to strengthen the rotator cuff and scapula stabilizers; proprioceptive/biofeedback techniques can be used and activities should be modified.

If necessary, surgery will include an inferior capsular shift with closure of the rotator capsular interval and tightening of the superior glenohumeral ligament. The results of surgery are 80–90% good.

Posterior instability

Posterior dislocation is uncommon (<5% in most series). It may occur from a fall, electrocution, or a grand mal convulsion. The diagnosis is often delayed or missed. There is pain and the arm is locked in internal rotation. The (anteroposterior) radiograph may appear 'normal' (actually it has a symmetrical or ice-cream cone appearance), so check the axillary view (which is diagnostic) should be checked. If there is any doubt then a CT scan should be performed.

Key points

- Posterior dislocations are often missed.
- If radiograph appears 'normal' then do axillary view or CT scan.

Associated problems

Tendinopathy and impingement

The supraspinatus tendon is vulnerable to degeneration and susceptible to inflammation as it passes under the coracoacromial arch in the relatively combined space between it and the greater tuberosity. Tendon damage can occur from overload of the cuff tendons or fatigue of their muscles. The acromion may be shaped so as to reduce the space available for the cuff tendons, so predisposing to impingement. Tendinitis may occur in patients with very lax shoulders (the muscles are overworked to stabilize the humeral head). Beware of tendinitis in younger patients (<25 years) as this may be secondary to subtle/unrecognized instability.

Typically there is pain over the anterior aspect of the shoulder with radiation into the deltoid (minimal at rest and rarely radiates down the arm or into the neck; aggravated with overhead and rotation activities). Night pain with waking indicates a severe case.

Rotator cuff tendinopathy is typically diagnosed with a history of pain on the anterior aspect of the shoulder, which radiates towards the insertion of the deltoid. The pain rarely extends further down the arm or up into the neck. It is aggravated by shoulder abduction, over head and rotational activities. In severe cases, sleep may be disturbed.

Examination

There is tenderness over the greater tuberosity and positive impingement signs (Fig. 17.11).

- *Speed's test* (Rockwood and Matsen 1999) is positive when pain is localized in the bicipital groove when the shoulder is flexed against resistance with the elbow extended and the forearm supinated.
- *Yergason's sign* (Yergason 1931) is elicited when there is pain on the anterior aspect of the

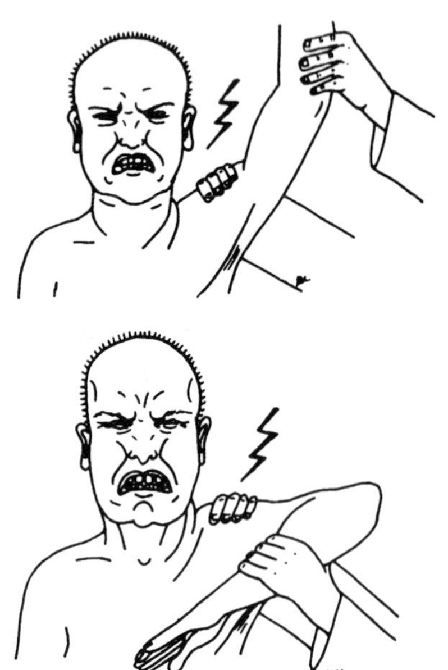

Figure 17.11 Impingement tests. (Reproduced with permission from Sherry and Wilson 1998.)

shoulder in the region of the bicipial groove when, with the elbow flexed, the forearm is supinated against resistance.

Wasting is seen early. Neck pathology must be excluded.

Diagnosis

The diagnosis is clinical. A plain tadiograph is useful (including a supraspinatus outlet view) as is the *impingement test*: 5–10 mL of lignocaine (lidocaine) is injected into the subacromial bursa, after 5 minutes there is then a significant decrease in pain on forward elevation of the arm to perform the impingement sign (Fig. 17.11). Ultrasound (in good hands) is accurate.

Treatment

Initially, the treatment of these lesions requires non-steroidal anti-inflammatory drugs (NSAIDs), modification of activities, and physiotherapy. Persistent symptoms may be helped with subacromial injection of local anaesthetic and steroid. Initially, the local anaesthetic is injected alone and then the shoulder manipulated with flexion and abduction to confirm the diagnosis before the steroid is infiltrated. If still painful after 6 months, then an open or arthroscopic acromioplasty should be considered.

Rotator cuff tears

In young people a violent force is required to tear the retotaor cuff, but in older people it may be a result of underlying degeneration.

Examination

The symptoms are very similar to those of tendinopathy, but with large tears,there will be a reduced range of movement. In the chronic situation, plain radiographs may be of use as they will show narrowing of the acromiohumeral gap when the tear is large. The diagnosis is usually confirmed with arthrogram, ultrasound, or an MRI scan.

Treatment

In patients <50 years of age treatment with rotator cuff repair and an acromioplasty is required, as there is a risk of increase in tear size and deterioration of shoulder function. In older patients a short trial of activity modification, NSAIDs, physiotherapy, and corticosteroid injection is reasonable and surgery may be performed later.

Internal derangements within the glenohumeral joint

Labral tears and SLAP (superior labral antero/posterior) lesions Snyder *et al.* (1990) can result from trauma and instability. The labrum tears in the upper shoulder and extends into the biceps anchor. Loose bodies result from trauma or synovial disease (synovial chondrometaplasia).

Outer clavicular osteolysis

Outer clavicular osteolysis (Scarenius and Iverson 1992) is a condition most commonly seen in who work out in the gymnasium on overhead machines, or take part in overhead sports. Radiographs of the acromioclaviucular joint show irregularity of the outer clavicle with osteolysis ('sucked candy' appearance). A bone scan (not always necessary) will be 'hot'. Treatment is with rest, activity modification, NSAIDs, or surgical excision.

Medical clavicular sclerosis (osteitis condensans)

Clavicular sclerosis is a rare disorder where there is osteosclerosis of the medial end of the clavicle.

Muscle and tendon ruptures

Muscle ruptures

Muscle ruptures about the shoulder include pectoralis major; long head of biceps, and subscapularis.

- The torn pectoralis major bunches on contraction.
- Long head of biceps rupture may be associated with rotator cuff disease.
- Subscapularis rupture presents weakness on the posterior lift-off test (see box Benson 1979).

Biceps tendon injuries

The biceps may be injured with anterior instability or inflamed with impingement and rotator cuff tears. In 95% of cases biceps tendonitis is secondary.

Lift-off test

The patient places the dorsum of the hand on the affected side on the small of their back so that the palm faces backward and then the strength of subscapularis is tested by lifting the hand backward away from the small of the back against resistance.

Nerve injuries

Nerves involved include the axillary, suprascapular, musculocutaneous, long thoracic, and radial nerve. Brachial plexus injuries follow high-velocity trauma such as motorcycle accidents and, if complete and associated with nerve root avulsion, have a devastating effect. Transient lesions described as 'burners' or 'stingers' may occur when the shoulder is traumatized during sporting activities such as rugby or American football.

Thoracic outlet syndrome describes a variety of clinical features caused by compression of neurovascular structures passing from the neck to the upper limb through the gap between the scalene muscle and across the top of the first rib. Causes include cervical ribs, abnormally long transverse processes at C7, callus from fractures of the clavicle restricting the gap between this bone and the first rib, abnormalities of the scalene muscles—indeed, any pathology around the shoulder girdle that modifies the position of the scapula. On examination, the Wright manoeuvre is particularly useful to confirm the diagnosis. This involves abducting and externally rotating the shoulder and turning the head away, while feeling the radial pulse. The test is positive when the pulse is weak or absent and there is reproduction of the patient's sensory symptoms.

Usually the injury is a neuropraxia and will recover. Electromyography is useful. If the lesion does not recover within 6 months it should be explored and repaired.

References

Benson BL (1979) Surgical repair of the pectoralis major rupture in an athlete. *American Journal of Sports Medicine* 7: 348–351.

Bokor D (1997) Shoulder injuries. In: *Manual of Sports Medicine*. GMMs, London, pp. 125–144.

Brooks CH, Revell WJ, Heatley FW (1993) Vascularity of the humeral head after proximal humeral fractures: An anatomical study. *Journal of Bone and Joint Surgery* 75B: 132–136.

Hovelius L (1987) Anterior dislocation of the shoulder in teenagers and young adults: five year prognosis. *Journal of Bone and Joint Surgery* 69A: 393–399.

Jupiter JB (1995) Open reduction and internal fixation of displaced fractures and nonunions of the proximal humerus. In: Craig EV (ed.) *The Shoulder. Master Techniques in Orthopaedic Surgery*. Raven Press, New York.

Kyle RF, Schmidt AH (1995) Open reduction and internal fixation of fractures and nonunions. In: Craig EV (ed.), *The Shoulder.* Master Techniques in Orthopaedic Surgery. Raven Press, New York, Chapter 9, p. 183.

Lange RH (1996) Fractures of the humeral shaft. In: Levine AM (ed.) *Orthopedic Knowledge Update: Trauma*. AAOS, Rosemont, Illinois.

Lewis MM (1992) *Musculoskeletal Oncology: A Multidisciplinary Approach*. Saunders, Philadelphia.

Miller EM, Ada JR (1992) Injuries to the shoulder girdle. In: Browner BD *et al.* (ed.) *Skeletal Trauma*, Vol. 2. Saunders, Philadelphia, pp. 1291–1310.

Miller EM, Miller CE (1996) Injuries to the shoulder girdle: fractures of the scapula, clavicle, acromioclavicular joint, and sternoclavicular joint. In: Levine AM (ed.) *Orthopedic Knowledge Update: Trauma*. AAOS, Rosemont, Illinois.

Müller ME, Nazarian S, Kock P *et al.* (ed.) (1990) *The Comprehensive Classification of Fractures of Long Bones*. Springer-Verlag, Berlin.

Müller ME, Allgöwer M, Schneider R *et al.* (ed.) (1991) *Manual of Internal Fixation*, 3rd edn. Springer-Verlag, Berlin, pp. 118–150.

Neviaser JS (1956) Injuries in and about the shoulder joint. In: Raney RB (ed.) *AAOS ICL* XIII 187–216.

Neer CS II (1970a) Displaced proximal fractures: Part I. Classification. *Journal of Bone and Joint Surgery* 52A: 1077–1089.

Neer CS II (1970b) Displaced proximal humerus fractures: Part II. Treatment of three-part and four-part displacement. *Journal of Bone and Joint Surgery* 52A: 1090–1103.

Rockwood CA Jr (1988) Subluxations and dislocations about the shoulder. In: Rockwood CA Jr, Green DP (ed.) *Fractures in adults*. Lippincott, Philadelphia PA, pp. 722–985.

Rockwood CA, Matsen FA (1999) *Orthopaedic Review Course*. AAOS Annual Meeting, Anaheim, CA.

Sarmiento A, Kinman PB, Galvin EG, Schmitt RH, Phillips JG (1977) Functional bracing of fractures of the shaft of the humerus. *Journal of Bone and Joint Surgery* 59A: 596–601.

Scarenius M, Iverson BF (1992) Non traumatic clavicular osteolysis in weight lifters. *American Journal of Sports Medicine* 29: 463–467.

Sherry E, Wilson SF (ed.) (1998) *Oxford Handbook of Sports Medicine*. Oxford University Press, Oxford.

Sherry E, Henderson A, Cotton J (1989) Comparison of midazolam and diazepam for the reduction of shoulder dislocations and Colles' fractures in skiers on an outpatient basis. *Australian Journal of Science and Medicine in Sport* 5: 5–6.

Snyder SJ, Karzel RP, Del Pizzow *et al.* (1990) SLAP lesions of the shoulder. *Arthroscopy* 6: 274.

Weaver JK, Dunn HK (1972) Treatment of acromioclavicular injuries, especially complete acromioclavicular separations. *Journal of Bone and Joint Surgery* 54A: 1187–1194.

Yergason RM (1931) Rupture of biceps. *Journal of Bone and Joint Surgery* 13: 160.

18

CHAPTER 18

Elbow injuries

PETER THOMAS, GAWEL KULISIEWICZ, SIMON R HUTABARAT, JOHN ROONEY, AND EUGENE SHERRY

CHAPTER 18
Elbow injuries

PETER THOMAS, GAWEL KULISIEWICZ, SIMON R HUTABARAT, JOHN ROONEY, AND EUGENE SHERRY

The elbow joint is frequently injured and often difficult to treat. Elbow injuries account for about 10% of all fractures in childhood (see Chapter 18). The injuries are commonly the result of a fall, typically on an outstretched hand. The prominence of the olecranon and epicondyles predisposes the elbow to direct trauma.

Anatomy

The elbow is a diarthrodial joint at the meeting of three bones forming three separate articulations. This arrangement allows rotational movement in two axes. One axis passes through the centre of capitellum and trochlea, allowing flexion and extension. The second axis passes through the radial head in line with the radius and allows pronation and supination.

The distal articular surface of the humerus comprises the trochlea, which articulates with the proximal ulna, and the capitellum, which articulates with the radial head. The *trochlea–ulnar articulation* is effectively a hinge joint with very little lateral movement due to the prominent medial and lateral trochlear ridges that house the articular surface of the proximal ulna. The carrying angle is 7° of valgus in men and 13° in women.

Movements at the proximal *radioulnar joint* allow pronation and supination of the forearm. For this movement the cylindrical radial head rotates in the radial notch of the proximal ulna. The normal range of movement is 140° of flexion from the straight and 180° pronation from full supination. The functional range of movement is less; 30–130° of flexion with 50° of supination and pronation. Loss of the last 30° of extension is only obvious as a deformity when both arms are held out with the hands palm-up. The elbow is prevented from falling into valgus by the *radiocapitellar articulation* and the medial collateral ligament, composed of the anterior, posterior, and transverse bundles. The most important part is the anterior, which can be distinguished from the capsule. The lateral collateral ligament consists of four parts: the annular, radial, ulna, and accessory collateral ligaments. It stabilizes the elbow during varus loading. The biceps, brachialis, and triceps muscles provide dynamic stability. The annular ligament wraps around the radial neck stabilizing the proximal radioulnar joint.

The *ulnar nerve* is wrapped closely around the posterior aspect of the medial epicondyle. It may be damaged by direct trauma or stretched by an acute extreme valgus deformity. If a cubitus valgus deformity develops slowly as a result of asymmetrical growth around the elbow or malunion of a fracture, the ulnar nerve may be progressively damaged producing a tardy ulnar palsy. The *radial nerve* is more commonly affected by more proximal fractures of the humerus. The *median nerve* passes through the antecubital fossa with the brachial artery where the two structures can be affected together. They are particularly at risk in a severely displaced supracondylar fracture of the humerus in a child.

Clinical evaluation

It is important to determine the mechanism of injury. This will give useful clues as to the severity and pattern of injury. Information about the patient's work and hobbies may guide the surgeon when deciding on the most appropriate treatment.

Localize the areas of tenderness. An effusion is most easily detected posterolaterally. The stability of the joint and the range of motion should be compared to the normal opposite elbow. The tips of the epicondyles and the tip of the olecranon normally form an equilateral triangle. An abnormality in this relationship may be used to distinguish between intra-articular fractures, dislocations and supracondylar fractures. If the patient is toxic or the swelling and pain are out of proportion to the injury, consider infection or an inflammatory arthropathy. It is especially important to exclude infection in a child who is febrile with a swollen painful joint and a high erythrocyte sedimentation rate (ESR).

Neurovascular status should be assessed and recorded both before and after treatment. Remember that muscle ischaemia and compartment syndrome can be developing despite the presence of a distal arterial pulse. Prompt treatment should prevent the disaster of Volkmann's ischaemic contracture. Pain on passive stretching is the most sensitive clinical test for muscle ischaemia, but in the unconscious patient one must rely on the monitoring of muscle compartment pressures.

Key points

- Exclude infection as a cause of pain in a child's elbow.
- If unsure of reading a child's radiograph with growth plates, compare with normal side.
- Consider compartment syndrome where there is increasing pain (despite reasonable analgesia), pain on passive stretching of flexors or extensors and dysaesthesia. Absent pulse and paralysis are very late signs. Mechanical or electronic compartment pressure readings may be wrong: never let such measurements over-ride your clinical judgment.

Radiological findings

The anteroposterior view is useful for determining displacement or deformity. This view may not always be possible because of pain to the patient. A comprise is made by taking a film that is perpendicular to the humerus but through the flexed forearm (Jones' view). This view should be compared with the normal side (especially in children).

An important sign on the lateral radiograph is the *fat pad sign*. This is a sign of intrarticular effusion and may suggest an intra-articular fracture. Occasionally an arthrogram may be useful in defining the articular surface in the child. CT and MRI scans are occasionally useful where there is an occult fracture or where more information is required.

Fractures of the distal humerus account for 2% of all adult fractures but have a bad reputation for poor outcomes, especially in the elderly, from a high-energy injury, or when they are intra-articular (Asprinio and Helfet 1996, Trigg 1997). Two factors determine the eventual outcome: stable anatomical reduction and early restoration of joint movement. In displaced fractures, and especially in those which extend into the articular surfaces, open reduction and internal fixation (ORIF) is usually required to hold the fragments in a good position while the elbow is subsequently mobilized. The goal of treatment is restoration of anatomy and full functional recovery.

When considering ORIF, think of the distal humerus as consisting of medial and lateral osseous columns which diverge to support an intervening 'spool-shaped' trochlea and spherical capitellar articular surface. This forms a triangular construct (Fig. 18.1).

The goal of surgery is to restore this triangle and to place screws, if possible, in the strong columns.

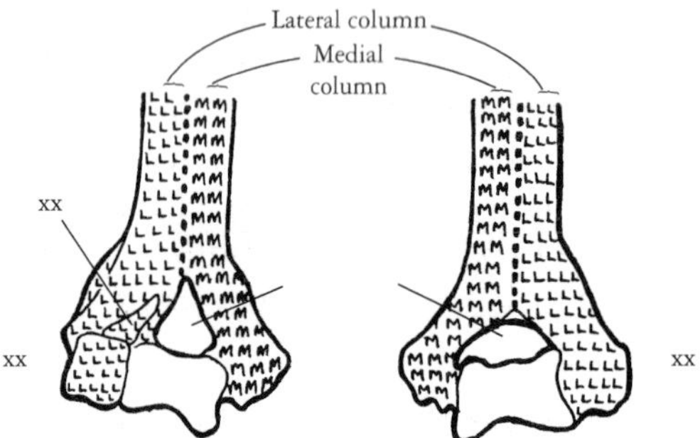

Figure 18.1 The medial (M) and lateral (L) osseous columns of the distal humerus diverge to support an intervening 'spool-shaped' trochlea articular surface (a triangular construct).

Key points

- Think of the distal humerus as a triangular construct.
- Of the several classification systems available, including Riseborough and Radin (1969), the AO classification is probably most useful (Fig 18.2).

Clinical evaluation

Often there is marked swelling and deformity. Examine the function of the three main peripheral nerves which cross the elbow. Examine for the vascularity of the forearm and hand.

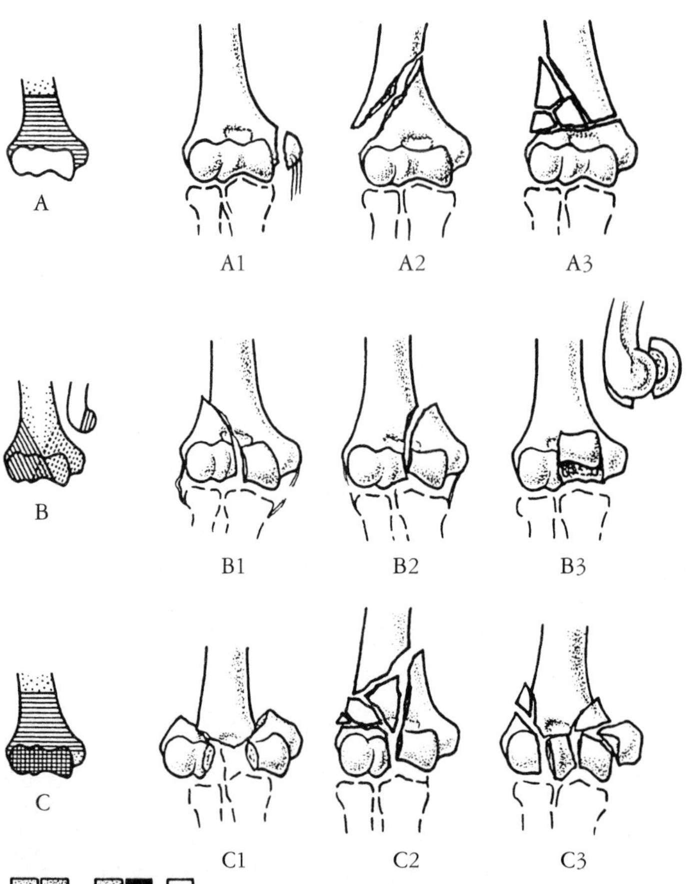

Figure 18.2 The AO provide a comprehensive classification (extra/periarticular, partial articular, complete articular and subdivided) of fractures of the distal humerus. (Reproduced with permissionfrom Müller *et al.* 1990.)

Investigations

Usually the two standard views previously described are adequate. The *radial head–capitellar view* is useful if a fracture of the capitellum or radial head is suspected. CT can be helpful in planning the operative reconstruction of a complex fracture. Three-dimensional reconstruction views from the CT scans can be more useful than the simple CT cuts. An intraoperative arthrogram can be performed by injecting radio-opaque dye into the elbow joint. This technique can show the extent of damage to cartilage in intra-articular fractures in children, in whom a significant fracture may be missed on a plane radiograph which shows only the calcified parts of bones.

Treatment

Displaced intra-articular fractures

Nearly all displaced intra-articular fractures require ORIF. Unstable fractures close to the elbow joint usually require fixation if movement of the elbow is likely to cause the fracture to heal in a displaced position. Fractures nearer the midshaft of the humerus may be treated without operative fixation. The judgement about which fractures to treat conservatively requires experience. Whichever method of treatment is used, it must allow early movement of the elbow and the other joints of the arm. The worse the fracture, the stiffer it will become if immobilized. After surgery it is safe, and kinder, to immobilize the elbow for a week in a plaster of Paris splint before beginning supervised movement under the auspices of a physiotherapist. For the first few weeks the arm should be rested between treatments in a cloth-covered foam collar-and-cuff sling, which is discarded after about 6 weeks or so when the fracture has healed.

Extra-articular fractures

Widely displaced avulsed fragments from the epicondyles usually require internal fixation. Distal shaft fractures may be managed conservatively, provided early movement of the elbow will not cause an unacceptable degree of displacement. A collar-and-cuff sling allows the weight of the forearm to help to reduce the fracture while allowing active movement of the elbow. Various designs of brace have been used to maintain reduction of the fracture while allowing movement of the elbow. If the distal shaft fracture is too displaced or unstable, it will need to be fixed with interfragmentary screws and a plate.

Predominantly intra-articular fractures

Intra-articular fractures are often difficult to fix internally. However, the results from successful internal fixation are much better than those from conservative treatment. The exposure of the damaged joint surfaces is crucial. It must be adequate to allow proper visualization of all the fracture fragments so that they can be reconstructed. The patient is positioned on one side with the affected arm on a gutter support, the upper arm horizontal and the forearm hanging vertical. A tourniquet is essential. Some surgeons approach the elbow joint through an osteotomy of the olecranon, lifting the whole of the triceps insertion up with it. This approach gives an excellent view, but the olecranon osteotomy can cause problems later, due to incongruency of the articular surface or non-union. A triceps splitting approach gives as good a view. A long distally based triangle is cut in the triceps and hinged down distally on its olecranon insertion. Each fracture tends to be unique, but it is usually best to begin by putting the articular fragments back together before re-attaching the reconstructed articular portion to the shaft of the humerus. It is often necessary to place a plate up each supracondylar ridge. The preoperative CT scan with three-dimensional reconstruction will help in the planning of the operation.

Complications

Loss of fixation can occur. Non-union (1–11%), including that of an olecranon osteotomy, can be difficult to treat and usually requires re-fixation with bone graft. Infection is a risk with any internal fixation. The ulnar nerve may be stretched at the time of surgery. This is why it is important to record any preoperative neurological deficit. Heterotopic ossification causes increasing stiffness over the first few months after the injury and is often difficult to treat. Some degree of stiffness, or reduction in the range of movement, is inevitable after intra-articular fractures. Patients must be warned of this at the outset to avoid the treatment being blamed for the inevitable poor result of a serious injury.

Supracondylar fractures in children

Supracondylar fracture is a common injury in children, and can result in significant complications if not treated properly. It is dealt with Chapter 29.

Fractures of the olecranon

Olecranon fractures are produced by as direct blow to the point of the elbow, often the result of a fall. In direct injuries the fragments are often comminuted and there is more significant overlying soft tissue damage. Indirect injuries produce transverse or oblique fracture patterns, often with the two fragments separated by the pull of the triceps. A combination of a direct force and flexion will produce a displaced and comminuted fracture. If the force is severe there may be an additional fracture of the radial head with or without dislocation of the elbow joint.

Clinical evaluation

There is pain around the elbow and usually swelling. The fracture gap can sometimes be felt. It is usually difficult or impossible for the patient to extend the elbow against resistance.

Radiological findings

The fracture is best seen in the lateral view. More complex imaging techniques are usually unnecessary.

Treatment

Undisplaced fractures are treated by external immobilization using a splint or split cast with the elbow in 45° of flexion. After 1 month supervised passive motion is started, and after 6 weeks active movement is encouraged. Displaced fractures require ORIF.

Several techniques are available; the best known is tension band wiring (TBW). A compression screw can also be used with TBW. The TBW AO technique converts distractive forces into compressive by placing the wires dorsal to mid-axis ulna; some say the transverse hole in the ulna should be anterior so as not to distract the fracture, but this is controversial. In avulsion-type fractures where the proximal fragment is small, it may be excised and the triceps tendon reattached distally with non-absorbable sutures.

Treatment of comminuted fractures depends largely on the extent of the injury. If confined to the olecranon, the fragments may be excised and the triceps tendon reattached. If, however, part of the ulnar shaft is affected an attempt at fixation may be made with plates (applied to dorsal or tension side), screws, and pins. It is important to achieve fixation and prevent recurrent dislocation from developing in such fractures. (It is worth remembering that in children olecranon fractures may be associated with injuries to the radial head and the epicondyles.)

Complications

- Loss of range of movement is less common than with the other intra-articular elbow fractures.
- Non-union can occur especially if fixation fails.
- Osteoarthritis may result from poor reduction, but it is an uncommon complication in comparison to the other intra-articular fractures of the elbow joint.
- Nerve damage should be rare, as the closest nerve—the ulnar—is still well clear of the tissues which are cut in the posterior approach.

Radial head fracture

Fractures of the radial head are usually caused by a fall onto the outstretched hand. Pain is felt around the lateral side of the elbow and is often aggravated

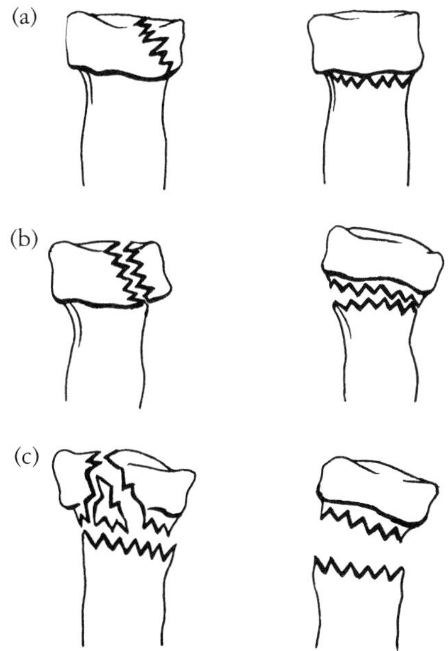

Figure 18.3 Fractures of the radial head: (a) type I; (b) type II; (c) type III.

by rotation of the forearm. Four types have been described in adults (Mason 1954) (Fig. 18.3):

- *type I:* undisplaced
- *type II:* displaced
- *type III:* comminuted
- *type IV:* fracture of radial head with an associated elbow dislocation.

In children, a fracture of the radial head usually involves angulation or separation of the entire head, with the fracture line running transversely through the physeal plate or the metaphysis.

Investigations

Plain radiographs are adequate to show the nature and extent of the fracture.

Treatment

Type I fractures (undisplaced)

The haemarthrosis should be aspirated and replaced with 5 mL of a long-lasting local anaesthetic agent, such as bupivacaine. This will produce an instant and gratifying relief of pain which will allow the patient to begin to mobilize the elbow, resting it between exercises in a collar-and-cuff sling. Although the residual pain should settle over the first 4 weeks or so, the patient should be warned that they will probably lose the last 10° of extension in the elbow, and that this loss of movement will be permanent.

Type II fractures (displaced)

Shear or marginal fractures with angulation of >30°, >3 mm of articular step, or a fragment greater than one-third of the diameter of the head need ORIF. This is done with small interfragmentary screws.

Type III fractures (comminuted)

The haemarthrosis is replaced with bupivocaine and a trial of mobilization is started. If pain and movement are not improving steadily after 3 weeks, the radial head fragments are excised. If the movement continues to improve, the radial head fragments are left in place. If there is an increase in pain later, the radial head fragments are excised then.

Type IV fractures (associated with an elbow dislocation)

These must be reduced and internally fixed if possible. However, most radial head fractures in this situation are too comminuted to be reconstructed and must be replaced with a prosthetic radial head to restore stability to the elbow joint. The lateral collateral ligament should also be reconstructed if the elbow is unstable into varus.

Fractures with associated dislocations

Monteggia fracture

Because the forearm contains two parallel bones linked at each end by joints, wide displacement of one part necessitates displacement at another. In 1814 Monteggia described the fracture now named after him when he realized, too late, the reason for the continuing pain and deformity in the forearm of a young woman whose radial head remained dislocated due to a malunion of a fracture of the ulna.

The radial head most commonly dislocates anteriorly and less commonly posteriorly or laterally. The concomitant fracture of the ulna must be internally fixed when the radial head is reduced.

Essex-Lopresti fracture

The opposite of the Monteggia fracture is that described by Galeazzi in 1934. It is a fracture of the radial shaft associated with disruption of the distal radioulnar joint. Although this fracture does not involve the elbow, another fracture of similar mechanism does. A fracture of the radial head may be associated with disruption of the distal radioulnar joint. Two cases were described by Essex-Lopresti in 1951. If the radial head fracture cannot be reconstructed, replacement with a prosthetic radial head will reduce the risk of later subluxation of the distal radioulnar joint. When the radial head is fixed or replaced, the distal radioulnar joint must also be reconstructed or stabilized. Supinating the forearm may keep the distal radioulnar joint reduced, but sometimes it must be explored and repaired.

Fractures of the capitellum

Fractures of the capitellum are rare injuries which are associated with a fall on an outstretched hand. They are classified as type I (large trochlea piece, Hahn–Steinthal), type II (minimal subchondral fragment, Kocher–Lorenze), and type III (comminuted).

Treatment

Splint if undisplaced for 2–3 weeks. ORIF if displaced, excise if fragmented.

Complications

There is usually a loss of the last 10° of extension in the elbow.

Fractures of the coronoid process

The coronoid process is fractured in 10% elbow dislocations. For type I (avulsion of the tip) and type II (fragment less than 50% of the articular surface) the treatment is early mobilization. For type III fractures, involving greater than 50% of the articular surface, ORIF is necessary.

Dislocation

Dislocation of the elbow is usually caused by a fall onto an outstretched hand. It is exceedingly painful, and is often associated with a temporary ulnar nerve palsy.

Classification

Posterior dislocation is the commonest: medial, lateral, and anterior dislocation are rare. Very rarely, the proximal radius and ulna are divergent.

Associated injuries are often overlooked and may account for difficulties in achieving reduction:

- 50% of cases have radial head or neck fractures.
- 10% have an avulsion fracture of lateral or medial epicondyles.
- 10% have a coronoid fracture while 10% have another intra-articular fracture.
- Damage to the median or ulna nerves occurs in about 20% cases. This is usually a neurapraxia, but may be an axonotmesis or neurotmesis.

Treatment

The elbow dislocation should be reduced as soon as possible to avoid further damage to nerves, and because it is so painful and distressing for the patient. A closed reduction is usually possible under sedation or general anaesthetic. In the posterior dislocation, the commonest, the elbow is extended to allow an easy and atraumatic reduction. It is important to remember that articular cartilage can be damaged by reduction which is not gentle.

Complications

Injury to the ulnar nerve usually recovers. Late instability of the elbow is surprisingly uncommon, occurring in only 1% of dislocations. It can be treated by repair of the lateral collateral ligament.

References

Asprinio D, Helfet DL (1996) Fractures of the distal humerus. In: Levine AM (ed.) *Orthopedic Knowledge Update: Trauma*. AAOS, Rosemont, Illinois.

Mason ML (1954) Some observations on fractures of the radial head: a review of 88 cases and the analysis of the indications for excision of the radial head and non-operative treatment. *Journal of Bone and Joint Surgery* 42: 123–132.

Müller ME, Nazarian S, Kock P *et al.* (ed.) (1990) *The Comprehensive Classification of Fractures of Long Bones*. Springer-Verlag, Berlin.

Riseborough EJ, Radin EL (1969) Intercondylar T fractures of the humerus in the adult: a comparison of operative and non-operative treatment in 29 cases. *Journal of Bone and Joint Surgery* 51A: 130–141.

Trigg SD (1997) Fractures of the adult distal humerus. Complex Fracture Management Course Trauma Update. Vail Colorado.

19

CHAPTER 19

Hand, wrist, and forearm injuries

CHARLES EATON

CHAPTER 19

Hand, wrist, and forearm injuries

CHARLES EATON

Incidence

Upper extremity trauma accounts for one-third of injuries treated by physicians (Kelsey *et al.* 1980). Hand injuries account for about one out of five injuries treated by physicians.

Management priorities

Evaluation

History

Severe upper extremity injuries are frequently dramatic and attended by emotional factors. Because of this, it is usually best to obtain a history in a deliberate, orderly way. If possible, after hearing the story, the examiner should physically demonstrate the scenario of injury back to the patient to confirm an understanding of the details, including the position of the extremity at the time of injury. Were the fingers in a fist or opened straight when the palm was cut? Did the patient land on their palm with their wrist extended or on the dorsum of their wrist? Was the patient able to pull their hand out, or was it trapped, requiring extrication? If an injury involves machinery unfamiliar to the examiner, it should be described well enough to be visualized, in simple mechanical terms.

Key point

- Severe upper extremity injuries are frequently dramatic and attended by emotional factors.

Examination

A working knowledge of anatomy usually allows much of the examination for an acute injury to be performed without touching the actual site of injury. *Posture* of the fingers can indicate specific tendon injuries. Even under anaesthesia, if the tendons and phalanges are intact, the fingers should assume a position of progressively more flexion of both proximal and distal interphalangeal joints proceeding from the index to the little finger. *Colour* of the skin and nail beds compared to the opposite side can indicate arterial or venous insufficiency, and *bruising* at a site away from an area of impact strongly suggests an underlying skeletal injury even with normal radiographic appearance. Sensory, motor, and vascular examination *distal to the injury* can provide clues as to the status of more proximal wounds. Active unresisted motion may be limited, but even so can provide information regarding tendon and nerve status. Allen's test for patency of the radial and ulnar arteries can be performed by applying pressure to the palm without requiring the patient to make a fist. This gentle approach is clearly preferable to attempting to define the injury by instrumenting the wound itself in the emergency department.

Evaluation of an acute injury commences with triage: brief history ('the door closed on my hand'), brief examination (wounds? deformity?), and then a more directed and detailed history, radiographs and detailed examination.

Key points

- Check posture, colour, bruising, motor/sensory and vascular function, Allen's test, active unresisted movement.
- Be gentle.

Closed injuries

Phalangeal fractures

Classification

Except for fractures involving tendon avulsion from the base of the distal phalanx, phalangeal fractures are generally classified by both exact and interpretive description. Exact descriptions include mention of the *bone* (thumb, index, middle, ring, small; proximal, middle, distal phalanx), *location* (head, neck, shaft, base, condyle, tuft, epiphysis), *pattern* (transverse, oblique, spiral, unicondylar, comminuted), *displacement* (non-displaced, minimally displaced, impacted, displaced), and *soft tissue status* (open, closed). Interpretive descriptions include mention of the energy of injury (high energy, low energy) and the stability of the fracture complex (stable, unstable).

General treatment principles

The most common problem following phalanx fractures is stiffness, and the best way to prevent this is early protected motion. Many factors contribute to stiffness. The internal wound from a proximal or middle phalanx fracture always breaches both flexor and extensor tendon surfaces, and tendon adhesions of both systems are the rule—even in non-displaced fractures. The combination of swelling and immobility alone frequently results in flexion contractures of the proximal interphalangeal joint and extension contractures of the metacarpophalangeal joint. These joints are always sprained or injured to some extent by the forces that produced the adjacent fracture. The proximal and distal interphalangeal joints may remain stiff, painful, and swollen for as long as a year after a closed injury—even without a fracture. Additionally, the finger extensor mechanism easily unbalanced by relatively small changes in phalangeal length from either shortening or angulation, leading to secondary joint contractures distal to the fracture. The precision cascade of motion of the fingers may be grossly disrupted by minor degrees of phalangeal malunion, much more so than for other fractures. For these and other reasons, it is best to achieve anatomical reduction and stable fixation, and begin early motion. A variety of external, percutaneous, and open fixation techniques may be used. Plate and screw fixation systems for phalangeal fractures have become increasingly refined and popular, but adhesions produced by the necessary surgical exposure for open reduction may compound the tendency for stiffness. Fortunately, tubular hand bones heal rapidly, and in most cases fixation is required for no more than a month, allowing many fractures to be treated with percutaneous fixation. If gentle stress on the fracture site is painless, healing is probably strong enough to withstand unresisted active motion without fixation. For metacarpal and phalangeal fractures, this clinical evaluation is more important than radiographic evidence of healing. In general, patients must begin moving their fingers before solid bone bridging is visible on the radiograph. For every finger fracture non-union, you will see a hundred stiff fingers.

Most patients are critically uninformed about problems with stiffness and about the frequently lengthy recovery period associated with phalangeal fractures ('it's just a finger'). During the initial interview, a blunt discussion by the examiner—demonstrating with their own hand what they mean by 'stiffness' by making a fist and then straightening the other fingers while holding one finger fixed in partial flexion—is time well spent.

The management of hand fractures as with fractures elsewhere can be broken down into a simple decision tree, based on the injury, technically possible goals, and patient participation (Fig. 19.1).

Key points

- The most common problem following phalanx fractures is stiffness.
- Percutaneous fixation is often effective.

Common and special types

Distal phalanx tuft fractures

A distal phalanx tuft fracture is a common injury which should be suspected whenever a patient has a subungual hematoma in the proximal half of the

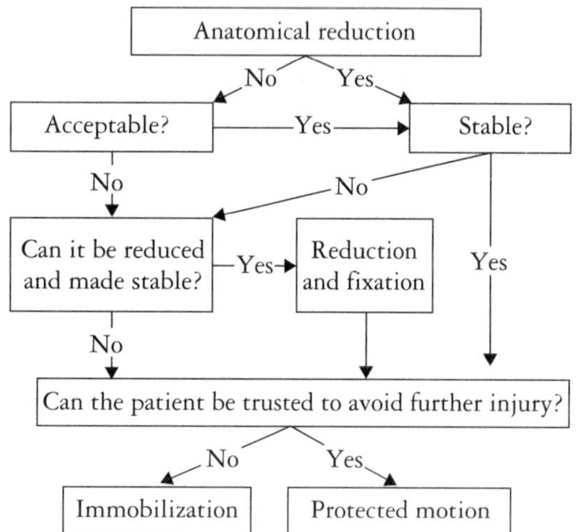

Figure 19.1 Generic hand fracture protocol.

nail bed. In most closed tuft fractures, the nail plate acts as a splint and healing is uneventful. Some patients may benefit from a small splint, but this should only span the distal phalanx, not crossing the distal interphalangeal joint—otherwise, it may transfer of the force of the profundus tendon to the fracture site and either delay or prevent union.

Middle phalanx base fractures

The most common type of middle phalanx base fracture is a small *volar plate avulsion fracture*, which commonly accompanies a sprain or dislocation of the proximal interphalangeal joint. This usually heals with a painless fibrous union. This injury requires no specific treatment other than what is indicated for the associated joint injury. Less common but much more troublesome are *fracture-dislocations of the proximal interphalangeal joint.* If the fracture line extends through the proper collateral ligament, the joint will become unstable, and the middle phalanx will displace with subluxation. Dorsal fracture-dislocations with a large palmar fragment are more common than volar fracture-dislocations. Either can be complicated by central articular impaction. Treatment is controversial, with advocates for internal or external fixation using a variety of techniques, but common principles include correction of subluxation, bone graft to correct impaction, and early motion.

Unicondylar phalanx head fractures

Following an oblique longitudinal impaction, unicondylar phalanx head fractures may involve either proximal or middle phalanx. Typically, the fracture line extends from the intercondylar notch to the junction of the phalangeal head and neck. These usually require open reduction, and are particularly suited to the use of small (1.0–1.3 mm) screws. Because the fragment is small, a helpful technique is to achieve provisional fixation using two Kirschner wires, and then remove the wires one at a time, and place screws in the wire drill holes. These fractures are frequently neglected, but if the finger has not been immobilized properly, healing is delayed, and it is usually possible to achieve satisfactory open reduction even several weeks after injury.

Proximal phalanx shaft fractures

Fractures of the proximal phalanx shaft typically result in dorsal angulation (apex volar) because of the palmar force of the intrinsic muscles on the proximal fragment and the dorsal force of the extensor mechanism on the distal fragment. These are generally unstable unless the force of the intrinsic muscles can be counteracted. They are commonly treated either by reduction and percutaneous fixation with longitudinal intramedullary Kirschner wires, open reduction with intraosseous wires and Kirschner wires, or open reduction and fixation (ORIF) with miniplates and screws. In either case, early motion of the proximal and distal interphalangeal joints is needed to prevent stiffness.

Intra-articular proximal phalanx base fractures

Often high-energy injuries, intra-articular proximal phalanx base fractures are frequently comminuted, impacted, and may displace in the same fashion as proximal phalanx shaft fractures. Because the metaphyseal bone is soft, it is more difficult to achieve adequate percutaneous fixation, and open reduction is required more often than for proximal phalanx shaft fractures.

Very comminuted phalangeal fractures

Fingers are at risk for severe crushing and other high-force mechanisms, which result in many small fracture fragments. Treatment requires ingenuity, judgment, patience, and luck to achieve a satisfactory result. In addition to the usual treatment options, these fractures may require treatment with immediate bone grafting or external fixation. Unfortunately, after a high-energy phalangeal fracture, many fingers are doomed to stiffness regardless of surgical efforts (Duncan *et al.* 1993).

Key point

- Treatment requires ingenuity, judgment, patience and luck to achieve a satisfactory result.

Paediatric fractures

As elsewhere, *Salter II* fractures (Salter and Harris 1963) predominate . In the young child, after fingertip injury, the most common hand fracture is a *fracture of the proximal phalanx base* with ulnar or radial angulation. If seen within the first 2 days, the fracture usually can be reduced with a local block, using a pencil or the examiner's finger in the web space as a fulcrum. A less common pattern is the paediatric *mallet fracture,* in which a portion or the entire growth plate is translated dorsal relative to the remainder of the distal phalanx. This fracture is unstable, and temporary Kirschner wire fixation is reasonable. In the older male pre-adolescent, *boxer's fracture* becomes more common. This may be Salter II, but more often is metaphyseal, and in either case is treated as an adult boxer's fracture.

Mallet fracture and profundus avulsion fractures are discussed in the section below covering closed tendon ruptures.

Key point

- Salter II fractures predominate.

Metacarpal fractures

Classification

Except for fractures with an associated eponym, metacarpal fractures are generally classified according to the same guidelines described above for phalangeal fractures.

Common and special types

Metacarpal neck fractures

Boxer's fracture is a displaced fracture of the little finger metacarpal neck, typically with palmar angulation (apex dorsal). These are usually not stable and often present late after injury. Considerable angulation may be tolerable because of compensation through the mobile little finger metacarpophalangeal joint and the little finger carpometacarpal joint. It is not possible to reliably secure and maintain reduction with a cast alone, although a number of authors have recommended this. Residual angulation will result in a cosmetic loss of dorsal prominence of the little finger metacarpal head and prominence of the metacarpal head in the palm, neither of which routinely justifies surgery. However, if the patient has more angulation than can be compensated for by their joint motion, extensor tendon imbalance will result and patient will develop a secondary flexion contracture of the proximal interphalangeal joint. Reduction and fixation is indicated when the patient can not fully straighten the proximal interphalangeal joint of their little finger, rather than by a radiographic classification of the fracture itself. Percutaneous reduction may be achieved using longitudinal Kirschner wires driven from distal to proximal, or open reduction with tension band or plate and screw technique may be used. Open boxer's fractures should be suspected for possible *clenched-fist bite wound injury*, discussed below.

Key point

- Considerable angulation may be tolerable.

Intra-articular metacarpal base fractures

Bennett's fracture (Fig. 19.2a) is an oblique volar coronal fracture through the thumb metacarpal base, with the smaller fracture fragment remaining attached to the volar carpometacarpal ligament. The unresisted force of the abductor pollicis longus tendon results in proximal and radial subluxation of the larger metacarpal fragment, carrying the entire thumb with it. *Reversed Bennett's fracture* (Fig. 19.2b) is a similar fracture-dislocation of the little finger metacarpal base. In analogous fashion, the force of the extensor carpi ulnaris attached to the larger fracture fragment produces instability requiring fixation. In either of these variations, closed reduction and percutaneous fixation of the metacarpal base to the proximal carpal bone is straightforward and satisfactory. The ring and small metacarpal bases may sustain a combined fracture-dislocation injury associated with a *dorsal hamate fracture*, also usually amenable to percutaneous fixation. *Rolando's fracture* is a comminuted intraarticular fracture of the thumb metacarpal base. Unlike Bennett's fracture, the additional comminution makes percutaneous fixation much less satisfactory. Although technically difficult, ORIF gives the best chance of restoring a working joint surface.

Key point

- Bennett's fracture is usually amenable to percutaneous fixation.

Carpal fractures

Classification

Except for scaphoid fractures, carpal fractures are classified simply by description of the fracture location (tubercle, body), pattern (coronal, comminuted, etc.), soft tissue status (open, closed), and associated ligament injuries (e.g. transscaphoid perilunate fracture dislocation). In a severe high-energy injury, any of the carpal bones may be fractured in patterns that defy neat categorization. In low-energy injuries, by contrast, the scaphoid and hamate represent the majority of carpal fractures sustained.

Common and special types

Scaphoid fractures

The scaphoid fracture is well known for several reasons. It is the most common carpal fracture sustained in a fall. The scaphoid acts as the primary mechanical link between the proximal and distal

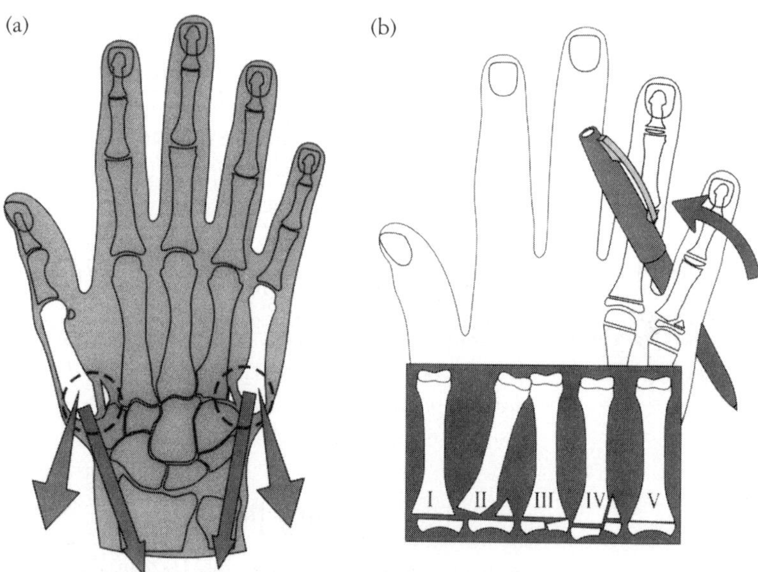

Figure 19.2 (a) Bennett's fracture; (b) Reversed Bennett's fracture.

carpal rows. Differential forces on these rows serve both to produce fracture and then to maintain motion and instability at the fracture site despite external immobilization (Fig. 19.3). Scaphoid fractures are not always obvious on initial radiographs. Patients with wrist pain and tenderness in the anatomic snuffbox after a wrist hyperextension injury should be assumed to have a scaphoid fracture even if initial radiographs are normal. They are best treated in a cast for 2 weeks and then re-evaluated with repeat films. As little as 2 mm of displacement can indicate gross instability and high risk for non-union. Many patients believe that they have sprained their wrist when in fact they have fractured their scaphoid, and may have intermittent symptoms for years before seeking medical attention. Scaphoid fractures are prone to non-union because the proximal pole of the scaphoid is entirely articular and the blood supply to the proximal pole of the scaphoid is largely from the distal pole, which is disrupted by fracture. Avascular necrosis of the proximal pole can occur, changing the alignment of the other carpal bones and over years resulting in degenerative arthritis of the radioscaphoid joint, the midcarpal joint and ultimately the remaining wrist joints, referred to as scapholunate advanced collapse (SLAC) wrist (Fig. 19.3). Some believe that even asymptomatic scaphoid fractures should be treated to prevent this late problem. Although the role of vascular supply to the proximal pole has received much attention in the experimental study of scaphoid non-union, since the introduction of the Herbert screw, adequate bone fixation has been recognized to be at least as important. There has been a trend away from the extreme of conservative management (4–8 months of immobilization in an above-elbow-to-fingertip cast) to earlier surgical intervention. Herbert has classified scaphoid fractures (Krimmer *et al.* 2000), and this classification can be used as a basis for treatment recommendations (Fig. 19.4). Indications for open reduction of acute scaphoid fractures currently include displaced fractures, perilunate fracture dislocations, and selected minimally displaced fractures to reduce recovery time. A volar surgical exposure is used for fractures involving the middle or distal third, and a dorsal surgical exposure is best for proximal fractures or those associated with perilunate injuries.

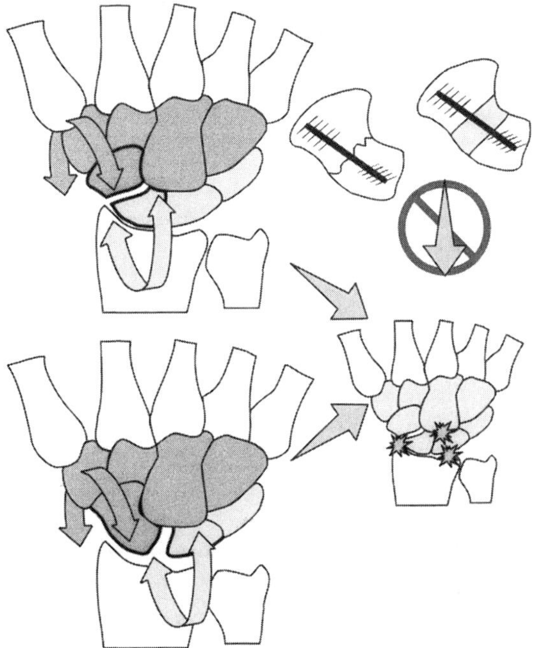

Figure 19.3 Scaphoid fractures.

Key points

- Scaphoid fractures are not always obvious on initial radiographs.
- Patients with wrist pain and tenderness in the anatomic snuffbox after a wrist hyperextension injury should be assumed to have a scaphoid fracture even if initial radiographs are normal.

Hamate fractures

Fractures of the hook of the hamate may be sustained in a fall, but more often occur in sports such as tennis, baseball, and golf, in which a handle sharply impacts the proximal hypothenar palm. As with the scaphoid, these fractures are frequently missed initially, and may not be visible on standard

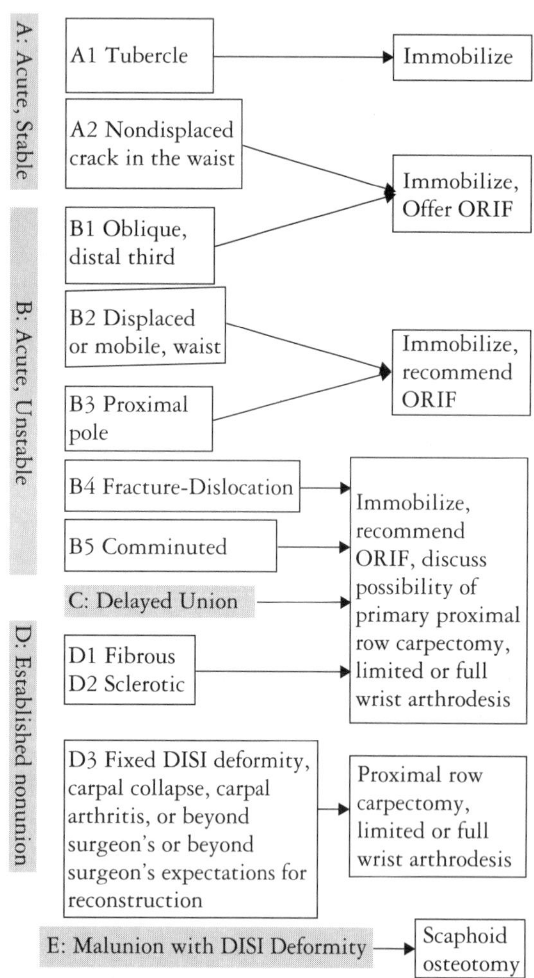

Figure 19.4 Modified Herbert classification of scaphoid fractures.

radiographs. Also similar to the scaphoid, they are prone to non-union and may result in secondary complications. The hook of the hamate is the point of attachment for hypothenar muscles, and when fractured through the base, these muscles alternately stress the fracture in different directions, predisposing to non-union. The hook also functions as a trochlea for the flexor tendons of the little finger and surface irregularities or chronic local inflammation can result in flexor tendon rupture, ulnar neuritis, and ulnar artery occlusion in Guyon's canal. Confirmation of this diagnosis may require special radiograph views of the hamate, including carpal tunnel view and 20° supinated oblique views, bone scan, or CT scan. Standard treatment is excision of the hook fragment and smoothing the base to prevent future tendon chafing.

Forearm fractures

Classification

Forearm fractures are generally classified as distal radius fractures (with or without distal ulna fractures), single bone forearm fractures, and forearm fracture-dislocations.

Common and special types

Distal radius fractures

Fractures of the distal radius account for about one out of every six fractures seen in the accident ward, and three out of four forearm fractures. Distal radius fractures are difficult to classify, as evidenced by the fact that there are over 20 different published classification systems for them, based on mechanism of injury, on fracture geometry, and on relative treatment indications. The simplest classification describes these fractures as being non-displaced, displaced extra-articular, and displaced intra-articular. The most simple subclassification of intraarticular distal radius fractures identifies the number of fracture fragments: two-part, three-part, four-part and comminuted. Many operative and non-operative treatment options exist, and many of them appear to give comparable results. Optimum treatment is controversial because alignment documented on late radiographs does not correlate well with the extent of late symptoms. Recent publications reflect an increasing awareness of the unpredictability of repeated closed reductions and a trend toward a more aggressive primary operative approach for these fractures. There is a need to restore articular congruity especially in younger patients. Operative treatment options include external fixation, percutaneous pinning, open reduction with or without bone grafting, and any combination of these. Poor final outcome is more likely when the fracture is initially very displaced, when the distal radioulnar joint is involved, and when the radiocarpal joint is comminuted. Progressive loss of reduction is more common in the elderly patient who depends more on upper-extremity weight bearing. Reflex sympathetic dystrophy, finger stiffness, and ulnar styloid non-union are common complications. Carpal tunnel syndrome, posttraumatic arthritis, tendon rupture, and carpal instability are also associated complications. Prolonged (6–12 months) symptomatic recovery is typical, as are long-term subjective symptoms, such as pain, fatigability, and loss of grip strength. Despite this, at least three out of four patients on the average have a satisfactory functional result following distal radius fracture.

Key points

- The simplest classification describes these fractures as being non-displaced, displaced extra-articular, and displaced intra-articular.
- Optimum treatment is controversial because alignment documented on late radiographs does not correlate well with the extent of late symptoms.

Isolated ulna fractures

Nightstick fracture of the ulna is the second most common single bone forearm fracture, generally resulting from blunt forearm trauma. The junction of the middle and distal thirds of the ulna is mechanically the most susceptible to fracture because of its cross-sectional geometry at that point (Hsu *et al.* 1993). Because this is usually a low-energy injury, it may be treated in a cast with close observation, reserving plate or intramedullary fixation for displaced fractures or those failing closed treatment. Isolated radial shaft fractures are less common, more often presenting as a Galeazzi fracture-dislocation.

Both-bone forearm fractures

Fractures of both forearm bones are relatively more common in children than adults because of differences in diaphyseal bone mechanics. Because of this, both-bone forearm fractures in adults are more likely than those seen in children to be high-energy open fractures. Traditionally, both-bone forearm fractures in children are treated closed much more often than both-bone forearm fractures in adults. In general, complications are more common and prognosis is worse for displaced fractures and for open fractures. On the average, non-displaced fractures take 6–8 weeks to heal, and displaced fractures take 3–5 months. Satisfactory functional end results may be expected in about 8 out of 10 patients with non-displaced fractures and about one-half of those with displaced fractures. Function may be most obviously affected with loss of pronation or supination, and as many as half of patients with both-bone forearm fractures will have obvious loss of forearm pronation, which may or may not be functionally significant. Loss of forearm rotation is most likely when fractures occur in the middle third of the forearm. Synostosis between the radius and ulna is much more common in proximal than in distal forearm fractures, occurring in about 1 out of 15 patients with proximal fractures. Synostosis is also more likely in children, with open fractures, with single incision access to both forearm bones, and following high-energy injuries. Non-union occurs in as many as 1 out of 10 patients. Early protected motion appears to improve the odds of satisfactory final motion. Internal or external fixation is usually indicated for open or very unstable fractures, accepting the risk that postsurgical infection may occur in as many as 1 out of 20 patients.

Key point

- Loss of forearm rotation is most likely when fractures occur in the middle third of the forearm.

Combined forearm fractures

Combined fractures include three special combinations of injury:

- *Galeazzi fracture-dislocation* is a fracture of the shaft of the radius associated with dislocation of the distal radioulnar joint.

- *Monteggia fracture-dislocation* is fracture of the ulna with dislocation of the radial head. Each of these fracture-dislocation patterns is best treated with open fracture reduction and closed treatment of the dislocation.
- *Essex–Lopresti lesion* is longitudinal disruption of the radioulnar interosseous membrane and proximal migration of the radius associated with fractures involving the proximal radioulnar joint, the distal radioulnar joint, or both sites. The most common presentation of Essex–Lopresti is associated with radial head excision for fracture, resulting in ulnocarpal impingement syndrome. Treatment is controversial. When diagnosed acutely in the context of an unreconstructable radial head fracture, Essex–Lopresti justifies use of a temporary radial head implant. Late surgical options include ulnar shortening osteotomy or the developing technique of ligament reconstruction with a tendon graft.

Tendon and ligament avulsion fractures are discussed in the next sections.

Key point

- Treatment of combined forearm fractures is controversial.

Dislocations

Classification

Classification of dislocations is descriptive and exact, referring to the joint involved, the direction of displacement of the distal bone (volar, dorsal, lateral, dorsolateral, etc.), soft tissue status (open, closed), association with fractures (simple dislocation, fracture-dislocation), and interposition of soft tissue which prevents closed reduction (simple or complex/irreducible).

Key point

- Interposition of soft tissue may make closed reduction impossible.

General treatment principles

Patients may reduce their own finger dislocations, or the emergency department physician may easily reduce a dislocation, which may give the impression that the injury was inconsequential. However, the mechanics of the very large ratio of surface area to volume in small joints makes them much more slow and difficult to recover than might be expected. The first thing to explain to the patient is that in terms of recovery, there is no such thing as a 'simple dislocation': it is common for a patient who has sustained a proximal interphalangeal joint dislocation to have swelling, stiffness, and some pain with use for 6–12 months after injury. This should be explained to the patient at the first possible opportunity.

Key points

- There is no such thing as a 'simple dislocation'.
- It is common to have swelling, stiffness, and some pain with use for 6–12 months after injury.

Common and special types

Simple dorsal phalangeal dislocations

Dorsal dislocations of the metacarpophalangeal, proximal interphalangeal, or distal interphalangeal joints follow a hyperextension injury, and are 'simple' only because reduction is usually straightforward: block anaesthesia; irrigate and cleanse any open injuries; obtain radiographs; stress the joint in the direction which produced the injury to open the internal path for relocation; apply gentle progressive pressure on the base of the dislocated bone; 'pop'—the joint is reduced; obtain confirmatory radiographs. This is a typical scenario, and most often involves the proximal interphalangeal joint. Not all dislocations are easily reduced. If an attempt at closed reduction under anaesthesia is unsuccessful, the patient should be considered a candidate for open reduction rather than aggravating the injury with repeated attempts at closed reduction.

Complex dislocations

Irreducible or complex digital dislocations are those in which local structures pass in or around the joint space in a way which prevents closed reduction. This often is associated with a 'buttonhole' anatomy for which attempts at closed reduction simply tighten a soft tissue noose around the head of the proximal bone. Complex dislocations most often involve the border digit metacarpophalangeal joints, and are more common in joints which have associated sesamoid bones. They are much less common than simple dislocations, but carry the risk of digital nerve injury during the course of open reduction, as digital nerves may be stretched over the protruding surface of the proximal bone head. Complex dislocation should be strongly suspected when there is dimpling of the skin or when radiographs show sesamoid bone interposition in the joint space.

Key point

- A 'buttonhole' anatomy may result in attempts at closed reduction simply tightening a soft tissue noose around the head of the proximal bone.

Perilunate injuries

Lunate dislocations and perilunate fracture dislocations represent a spectrum of injuries involving the ligamentous attachments of the lunate bone. In a wrist hyperextension injury, mechanical failure frequently begins at the proximal radial wrist, either as a scaphoid fracture or as a scapholunate ligament disruption. Depending on the energy of injury, this initial location of injury will progress from radial to ulnar around the lunate. The path of injury may be entirely through ligaments, progressively disrupting the scapholunate, midcarpal, and lunotriquetral joints, resulting in a *lunate dislocation* (Fig. 19.5), or may pass through the radius, scaphoid, or capitate, or involve less common patterns of *perilunate fracture-dislocation* (Fig. 19.5). Many perilunate dislocations can be reduced closed, but all should have open ligament repair, often requiring a combined dorsal and palmar approach.

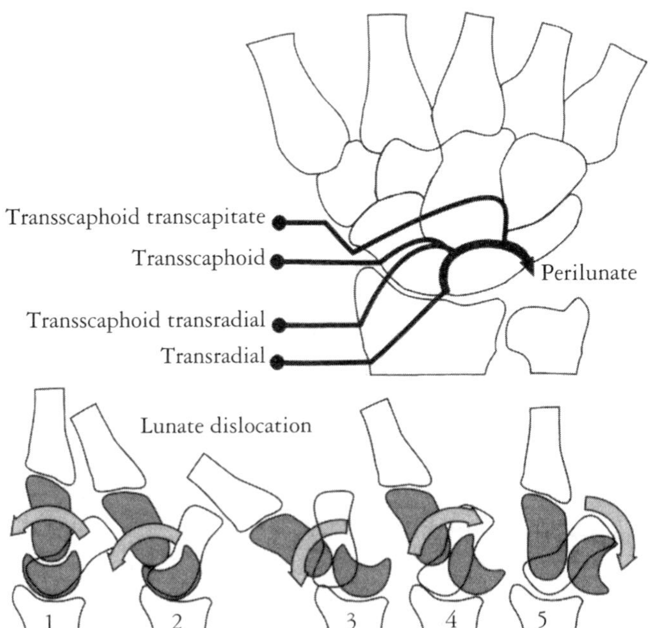

Figure 19.5 Perilunate injuries.

Key point

- Lunate dislocations often missed.

Ligament injuries

Classification

Other than gamekeeper's thumb, classification of hand and forearm ligament injuries is descriptive, referring to the joint involved, the ligament involved, soft tissue status (open, closed), associated avulsion fractures, and assessment of stability or extent of the lesion (partial, complete).

General treatment principles

A partial closed ligament injury is treated in the same fashion as a non-displaced stable fracture: early protected motion in the reliable patient, immobilization in the unreliable patient. The treatment of complete closed ligament disruptions depends on the joint involved, as described below.

Common and special types

Interphalangeal joint ligament injuries

If radiographs show no translation or subluxation, complete ligament tears involving the proximal or distal interphalangeal joints are usually stable and may be treated with buddy taping during waking hours and static extension splinting during hours of sleep. Otherwise, open ligament repair is indicated. Small proximal interphalangeal joint volar plate avulsion fractures are very common with hyperextension injuries, and usually heal as a painless non-union, unlike fractures involving either the central articular surface or the lateral cortex the base of the middle phalanx. This latter finding should prompt consideration for reduction and fixation. Lateral angulation of the finger must be assessed with radiographs. Angulation may not be obvious clinically because of swelling and stiffness in the acute setting. However, if allowed to heal, almost any radial or ulnar angulation will be obvious and difficult to correct later on.

Gamekeeper's thumb (also known as skier's thumb)

An acute radial stress on the thumb metacarpophalangeal joint may disrupt its ulnar support. Tissue failure is usually rupture of the ulnar collateral ligament from its insertion at the base of the proximal phalanx. Injury can occur in the form of an avulsion fracture, less commonly as a combined fracture and ligament tear, or as a ligament rupture through the central or proximal ligament. The historical eponym refers to the gamekeeper who repeatedly dispatched small animals by pushing forcefully with a thumb to on the back of the animal's head, breaking its neck. The injury may result in an irreducible displacement of the end of the ligament. For irreducible ligament displacement, the following events must occur: at the time of maximum displacement, the extensor mechanism overlying the ligament tears, allowing the torn ligament end to protrude through a buttonhole, where it becomes trapped in a subcutaneous position. This specific scenario is referred to as the *Stener lesion* and is important because spontaneous ligament healing is prevented by interposition of the thumb extensor mechanism, requiring surgery to prevent chronic instability. The Stener lesion occurs in a sizable minority of thumb ulnar collateral ligament injuries, and should be suspected when the metacarpophalangeal joint is grossly unstable, or when there is a persistent firm mass on the ulnar aspect of the thumb metacarpal head. In most cases, ligament reinsertion is possible months or even years after injury, and should be considered to stabilize the thumb and prevent early degenerative changes from persistent subluxation.

Treatment: For incomplete ulnar collateral ligament/metacarpophalangeal joint injuries (>30° of radial deviation on stress testing) place in a S-Thumb splint (Johnson & Johnson Medical), For complete tears (painless deviation >30°) surgical repair is necessary and then 6 weeks postoperatively in an S-Thumb splint.

Key points

- Incomplete injuries (>30° of radial deviation on stress testing) place in an S-Thumb splint.

- Complete tears (painless deviation >30°) surgical repair is necessary and then 6 weeks in an S-Thumb splint.

Scapholunate ligament injuries

The scapholunate ligament maintains the proximal pole of the scaphoid adjacent to the lunate (scapholunate gap) and stabilizes the palmar rotation force of the scaphoid against the dorsal rotation force of the lunate (scapholunate angle). This structure is injured when the wrist hyperextension mechanism that might result in a scaphoid fracture instead disrupts the adjacent scapholunate ligament. This may occur as a partial tear with pain but no instability, best treated by arthroscopic debridement. More complete injuries may result in dynamic scapholunate instability, with normal plain radiographs, but pain with use and increase in the scapholunate gap with wrist in ulnar deviation with a strongly clenched fist. Complete disruption of the scapholunate ligament results in an instability pattern visible on plain radiographs with widening of the scapholunate gap, palmar flexion of the scaphoid and dorsiflexion of the lunate—referred to as *scapholunate dissociation with DISI* (dorsal intercalary segment instability). Acute repair of scapholunate injuries associated with instability may be possible, and many surgeons augment this with some form of wrist capsulodesis. Results of repair are unpredictable and often disappointing if delayed months after the initial injury. Over time, the abnormal position of the scaphoid and lunate result in degenerative changes at the radioscaphoid, midcarpal, and then radiolunate joints and, referred to as scapholunate advanced collapse or SLAC wrist (see Fig. 19.3). Salvage procedures include, among others, proximal row carpectomy, scaphoid excision with midcarpal fusion, and full wrist fusion.

Key point

- Complete injuries may result in dynamic scapholunate instability (plain radiographs are normal).

Triangular fibrocartilage injuries

The triangular fibrocartilage complex (TFCC) provides an articular surface between the ulna and the ulnar carpal bones and provides stability to the distal radioulnar joint while allowing pronation and supination. This structure may be torn in a hyperextension/pronation mechanism, or associated with a distal radius fracture. Palmer (1989) has classified traumatic TFCC injuries as follows:

A central perforation

B ulnar avulsion with or without distal ulnar fracture

C distal avulsion

D radial avulsion with or without sigmoid notch fracture.

Additionally, acute injuries of the triangular fibrocartilage complex may be described as non-destabilizing, destabilizing, or associated with fractures of the distal radius and/or ulnar styloid. Non-destabilizing injuries, such as a central perforation, are usually treated with several months of immobilization before considering arthroscopic debridement. Destabilizing injuries, such as disruption of the radial attachment with instability of the distal radioulnar joint, may be technically difficult to repair, requiring a combination of arthroscopic and open techniques. Injuries associated with distal radius fractures are underdiagnosed, and account for residual ulnar pain and distal radioulnar instability following fracture. Hopefully, more aggressive arthroscopic management of these lesions will reduce the incidence of long-term symptoms.

Key point

- Injuries associated with distal radius fractures are underdiagnosed.

Closed tendon rupture

Classification

Acute traumatic tendon ruptures nearly always occur at the point of tendon insertion. Mallet finger, boutonnière finger, and profundus avulsion injuries account for the great majority of tendon ruptures. These may occur as pure soft tissue injuries or may be associated with avulsion fractures. Attritional ruptures may occur at sites where tendons pass over fracture lines, and interestingly are more common in non-displaced than displaced fractures. The most common post-traumatic attritional ruptures are extensor pollicis longus rupture after a distal radius fracture and little finger flexor digitorum profundus rupture after a hook of hamate fracture.

Key point

- Mallet finger, boutonnière finger, and profundus avulsion injuries account for the great majority of tendon ruptures.

General treatment principles

Treatment is individualized for each of these injuries. Some residual deformity is to be expected in any of the acute traumatic injuries. Post-traumatic attritional ruptures are treated in the same fashion as non-traumatic attritional ruptures, with either tendon transfer or intercalated tendon graft rather than primary repair.

Key point

- Some residual deformity is to be expected in any of the acute traumatic injuries.

Common and special types

Mallet finger

In the adult, mallet injury commonly occurs as either a soft tissue injury, less often associated with a dorsal avulsion fracture. It arises from the combination of an external flexion force on the distal interphalangeal joint at the same time as attempted extension of this joint, with tissue failure occurring at the extensor tendon insertion. Soft tissue mallet injuries may occur after a relatively trivial event, such as using the fingertips to push folds out of a bedspread, a painless event with no bruising. Soft tissue mallet injuries are best treated with continuous extension splinting for 6–8 weeks. Splinting may be helpful even if the initial treatment is delayed as long as 3 months. If the patient can not tolerate a continuous splinting programme, the distal interphalangeal joint may be pinned in slight hyperextension for 6 weeks. Mallet fractures more often result from obvious trauma, such as being struck on the fingertip while trying to catch a ball: *'baseball finger'*. In the majority of adult mallet fractures, the distal phalanx articulation remains congruent and the fracture fragment involves less than one-third of the joint surface. These injuries are best treated with extension splinting for 1 month. Residual deformity is more likely with delayed treatment, with an associated hyperextension posture of the proximal interphalangeal joint, and in mallet fractures with a large avulsion fragment or with palmar subluxation of the distal phalanx. Recognizing both the technical difficulty and known complications of open treatment, these latter two fractures are probably best treated with a percutaneous indirect reduction using extension block pinning (Darder-Prats *et al.* 1998). The majority of *paediatric mallet injuries* are fractures involving the growth plate—usually Salter I, less often Salter III.

Key point

- Soft tissue mallet injuries are best treated with continuous extension splinting for 6–8 weeks.

Boutonnière finger

A closed boutonnière finger results from a mechanism similar to that of a mallet injury in that there is a tear of the insertion of the extensor mechanism to the dorsal base of the phalanx. However, unlike the mallet, the extensor mechanism continues past the proximal interphalangeal joint, and a tear in the tendon mechanism at this point resembles a buttonhole ('boutonnière'), with the protruding head of the proximal phalanx forming the 'button'. This alters the normal distribution of tension over the extensor mechanism sheet, allowing the force of proximal pull on the mechanism to bypass the proximal interphalangeal joint, leaving it flexed and diverting it to the distal joint, which becomes hyperextended. Acutely, these injuries are best treated closed with 4–6 weeks of 'four-point' finger splinting to maintain the proximal interphalangeal joint in extension and slightly flex the distal interphalangeal joint, allowing flexion of the distal interphalangeal joint. Residual deformity is often more of a cosmetic than functional problem. Typically, the injury is a pure soft tissue mechanism. Boutonnière associated with a dorsal avulsion fracture should be considered a volar fracture dislocation and may be associated with palmar subluxation of the middle phalanx.

Key point

- Boutonnière finger injuries are best treated closed with 4–6 weeks of 'four-point' finger splinting to maintain the proximal interphalangeal joint in extension and slightly flex the distal interphalangeal joint, allowing flexion of the distal interphalangeal joint.

Profundus avulsion

Avulsion of the profundus tendon insertion usually occurs when something strongly grasped is suddenly pulled away (*'rugby jersey finger'*), either tearing the tendon from the bone, producing a volar avulsion fracture, or both. The injury is compounded to a variable degree by devascularization of the tendon from disruption the attachments of the vincula. For example, in the soft tissue variety of injury, the tendon usually retracts into the palm, tearing away the attachments of both the long and short vincula. If treatment is delayed (which often is the case), at the time of exploration, the distal tendon segment found in the palm is either necrotic or firm and contracted to such a degree that it is unsuitable for reattachment. If the injury is associated with an avulsion fracture, the end of the tendon is usually trapped at either the base of the distal phalanx, the A4 pulley (mid-middle phalanx) or the A2 pulley (mid-proximal phalanx) with avulsion fracture fragments of diminishing size, respectively. Obviously, the greater distance the tendon retracts, the more brief the window of opportunity for primary repair. If the end of the tendon is trapped at or distal to the proximal interphalangeal joint, only the short vinculum is disrupted. More proximal retraction results in disruption of both the long and short vincula, with unavoidable tendon devascularization. Minimally displaced avulsion fractures may be repaired many weeks after injury, but in this instance, the examiner should have the patient demonstrate some active flexion of the distal interphalangeal joint to confirm that this is not the combined injury of avulsion fracture and complete soft tissue tendon avulsion. If primary reinsertion is not possible, either distal interphalangeal joint capsulodesis or arthrodesis is less complicated than staged flexor tendon reconstruction with a temporary silastic rod.

Key point

- 'rugby jersey finger'.

Closed vascular injuries

Ulnar artery aneurysm, thrombosis-related ischaemia, or emboli of the fingers may occur from repeated blunt trauma to the hypothenar palm injuring the ulnar artery in Guyon's canal, referred to as *'hypothenar hammer syndrome'* or *'hypothenar hammer hand'*. Often, symptoms of ulnar neuritis predominate. This is more common in smokers, may occur in young men, and may be confused with Buerger's disease. Treatment includes preoperative evaluation for possible hook of hamate fracture, and then excision of the diseased section of artery. If the artery is occluded, the patient is a smoker, and the remaining circulation is normal, simple excision and ligation is adequate. Otherwise, or based on the surgeon's preference, the segment may be repaired primarily or with a small vein graft.

Hand–arm vibration syndrome or *vibration-induced white finger* is a poorly understood syndrome in which patients exposed to vibrating hand-operated tools develop activity- or cold-related finger vasospasm. The most productive intervention for this appears to be avoidance of further hand vibration

(Bovenzi *et al.* 1998). Digital artery thrombosis associated with closed ring avulsion injury (discussed below) has been reported, but is rare.

Open injuries

Open injuries of the hand and forearm are common both because we use our hands to manipulate dangerous objects such as knives and moving machinery, and because our protective reflexes instinctively place our hands in harm's way when we are confronted with a fall, a flying object, or a fight.

Classification

Open injuries are described as for closed injuries, and in addition are classified by description of the mechanism of injury (sharp, crush, avulsion, pressure injection, abrasion, burn, ballistic, etc.), the type of wound (puncture, simple laceration, burst, stellate, distally based flap, amputation, etc.), contamination of the wound (clean, contaminated, heavily contaminated with debris, etc.), and vascularity of the wound area (viable, devascularized, indeterminate viability).

General treatment principles

Management of deep open upper extremity wounds is rarely as simple as repairing the mechanical disruption. Treatment must be undertaken with the long-term outcome in mind at all times. The two main priorities are healing and function.

- *Healing goals* are adequate blood supply, stable skeleton, and mobile soft tissue cover.
- *Functional goals* are nerve function, passive range of motion, and active range of motion.

Along with these goals, the orderly sequence of procedures must be carefully considered.

Healing

Blood supply

The surgeon must ensure adequate blood supply with debridement, revascularization, or both. Vascular injuries, and particularly those associated with muscle devascularization, place severe time constraints on the surgeon. Although revascularization may be the most important step of the operation, it should not be the first step taken. An orderly planned approach is needed to give the best chance for limb salvage. Debridement is critical: postoperative infection is evidence of inadequate debridement. It must include tissues that are devascularized and those that can not be revascularized. Debridement should be approached in the same fashion as tumour surgery: removal, not rinsing; surgical excision, not scrubbing. It is best done under tourniquet control and before vascular repairs, which reduces intraoperative blood loss and allows for the most accurate evaluation of injury. Pulsatile irrigation should be withheld until after sharp debridement, for it may blur evidence of the zone of injury. Muscle ischaemia time should be limited to 4 hours, but definitive vascular repairs should be deferred until after debridement, skeletal fixation, and repair of muscular tenderness structures adjacent to the site of vascular or repair. This requires planning and a deliberate stepwise approach, and may involve provisional revascularization with a shunt. A common pitfall in the management of large wounds involving transection of artery and muscles is to have a vascular surgeon perform vascular repair using a vein graft, as the first step. Then, after adjacent muscles are repaired, the original ends of the vessel are indirectly approximated to the extent that the vein graft becomes redundant, kinks, and must be removed. Carrying out debridement and muscle repair before vessel repair helps to avoid this scenario. If grafts are needed, vein grafts are generally satisfactory for forearm vessels, but in the palm and fingers, branches and small diameter may be difficult to match with vein grafts. In some circumstances, a branched arterial graft from the thoracordorsal system may provide a solution.

Key point

- Debridement is critical: postoperative infection is evidence of inadequate debridement.

Stable skeleton

The principles of skeletal fixation discussed above also apply in open wounds. In addition, optimum management of open fractures includes immediate intravenous broad-spectrum antibiotics and definitive fracture cleansing within 4 hours of injury. The extent of soft tissue injury in open phalangeal fractures has profound influence on expected outcome. Duncan *et al.* (1993) evaluated open phalangeal fractures along the lines of the Gustilo classification as follows:

- I tidy laceration <1 cm in length, no soiling, no soft tissue loss or crush; basically a puncture wound from within or without
- II tidy laceration <2 cm in length, from outside in, no soiling, no soft tissue crush or loss; partial muscle laceration
- IIIA laceration >2 cm, penetrating or puncturing projectile wound; any frankly soiled wound
- IIIB same as IIIA + any periosteal elevation or stripping, either by injury or by surgeon
- IIIC same as IIIB + neurovascular injury.

Using the criteria of total active motion for evaluation of outcome, Duncan *et al.* (1993) found that three-quarters of patients with a grade I injury and half of patients with a grade II injury had a good or excellent result. In contrast, almost all patients with a grade IIIB or IIIC injury had a poor result with >50% normal range of motion. For phalangeal fractures, periosteal stripping—either by injury or by the treating surgeon—contributes strongly to a poor result.

Mobile soft tissue cover

A stable, well-vascularized, supple soft tissue cover is a prerequisite to functional recovery. This requires adequate debridement and, if needed, flap cover. If a flap is required, and particularly if a free flap is required, timing is critical. The risk of osteomyelitis and wound healing problems, as well as the length and cost of hospital care, are directly related to the interval of time between injury and flap cover. Definitive wound closure with a free flap has the lowest complication rate if performed within 3 days of injury, and the highest complication rate if performed during the 'subacute' phase, after granulation tissue has formed (Godina 1986). This timing relationship goes against traditional teachings of delayed primary closure, possibly because of differences arising from the use or the need for a flap. As elsewhere, the 'reconstructive ladder' of wound closure is as follows, and the surgeon should begin at the bottom and consider each rung before advancing to the next:

- free flap
- distant flap
- regional flap
- local flap
- skin graft
- delayed primary closure
- primary closure
- spontaneous healing.

Local and regional flaps from the hand and adjacent fingers are commonly used for finger and thumb tip amputations, and are discussed below. Commonly used larger regional flaps from the forearm include to the radial forearm flap and the posterior interosseous (dorsal forearm) flap. These and other available flaps make free flap reconstruction less frequently indicated for upper-extremity reconstruction than for lower-extremity reconstruction. When available, single-stage flap reconstruction is preferred. Compared to staged reconstruction such as that involving a pedicled groin flap, single-stage flaps require less immobilization and allow better elevation of the hand. Every effort should be made to achieve healing as soon as possible. In the hand, stiffness, difficulty with use, and ultimate disability are directly related to the length of time required for wound healing.

Key points

- A stable, well-vascularized, supple soft tissue cover is a prerequisite to functional recovery.

- Stiffness, difficulty with use and ultimate disability is directly related to the length of time required for wound healing.

Function

Nerve function

Nerve injuries should be approached aggressively in open injuries, as there is never a better time to evaluate and to perform repairs. In the context of an adjacent open wound, nerve dysfunction should be considered an open nerve injury until proven otherwise. Partial nerve lacerations are clearly best treated by early repair. If untreated, the nerve heals with a large neuroma, and partial function returns. If such an injury is explored late, it may be impossible to distinguish neuroma from scarred nerve fibres in continuity, and the surgeon may face the no-win choice of either leaving things as they are or performing a segmental complete nerve excision and grafting, possibly leaving the patient worse off than they were before surgery.

If a nerve appears injured, but is not explored, nerve studies may not be helpful in distinguishing neuropraxia from more severe nerve injury for several weeks. At that point, conditions may not be favourable for nerve exploration, and it may be reasonable to wait for nerve recovery, assuming that the nerve is injured but in continuity. How long is it reasonable to wait before expecting to see signs of muscle recovery following an in continuity injury? This can be calculated, making a few assumptions:

- Muscle recovery is poor if motor point reinnervation is delayed past 12 months, and unlikely if delayed past 18 months.
- After repair, axon growth proceeds at an average of 30 mm per month.
- The probable site of the nerve injury is known.
- There is no other evidence contrary to the diagnosis of a closed stretch injury.

If these assumptions apply, it should be 'safe' to wait for distal muscle to show signs of reinnervation for a period of 12 months minus the distance in millimetres (d) from injury to motor end point divided by 30 mm per month, or $12-(d/30)$ months. Within that time frame, recovery could still be anticipated even if delayed excision and repair is performed. So, for example, in an ulnar nerve injury, if the distance from a forearm injury to the first dorsal interosseous muscle along the course of the ulnar nerve is 180 mm, it would be 'safe' to wait up to $(12-180/30)=6$ months before the window of opportunity for surgical success begins to close.

Key point

- If a partial nerve laceration is explored late, it may be impossible to distinguish neuroma from scarred nerve fibres in continuity.

Passive range of motion

As mentioned above, the injured hand tends to become stiff in a characteristic position due to the anatomy and soft tissue constraints of each joint. After a period of swelling and immobility, it is common to be faced with flexion contractures of the interphalangeal joints, extension contractures of the metacarpophalangeal joints, and pronation contracture of the forearm. Less frequently recognized, but equally common and important, are intrinsic muscle contractures of the hand and adduction contracture of the first web space. These structures should be specifically stretched and length maintained as much as possible during recovery. Stable skeletal fixation, anatomic joint reconstruction, early wound healing, and early range of motion are key to preserving the potential motion of all moving structures. As elsewhere, early range of motion after injury promotes synovial surface healing, reduces the tethering effects of adhesions and maintains the necessary dimensions of the joint capsule.

Key point

- Stable skeletal fixation, anatomic joint reconstruction, early wound healing, and early range of motion are key to preserving the potential motion of all moving structures.

Active range of motion

Strong active range of motion is built on the foundation of the goals just described, with the prerequisite of painless, stable, passive range of motion and the most powerful tool of early active motion. Secondary salvage with tenolysis, joint releases, tendon transfers, and in rare cases free functional muscle transfers may be indicated, but are unlikely to achieve the potential made possible with primary healing and early active motion. Such procedures are contraindicated for patients who have persistent local pain or who have developed a strong pattern of disuse of the hand.

Common and special types of open injuries

Complex open wounds

The dramatic presentation of severe upper extremity wounds may create problems independent of the specific details of injury. When confronted with the gruesome wounds, bleeding, and amputated parts as well as the immediate demands of the patient and family ('you *can* save it, can't you?'), one must maintain perspective and look for potentially missed injuries such as blunt abdominal trauma, proximal skeletal injuries, brachial plexus injuries, and compartment syndrome.

Key point

- Maintain perspective and look for potentially missed injuries.

Iatrogenic injuries

One must avoid iatrogenic injuries which, in the emergency department, are usually related to efforts to control bleeding. Fortunately, even major arterial upper extremity haemorrhage can be controlled with elevation of the arm and direct pressure. Attempts to control bleeding in the emergency depatment with either arterial clamps or a proximal pneumatic tourniquet are dangerous and inappropriate for anyone other than the surgeon who will be performing the definitive repairs.

Subtotal amputation

One of the most difficult complications of a severe open upper extremity injury is the failure to amputate. If amputation is a consideration, the best time to amputate is at the first operation. Faced with a mangled upper extremity, many patients are pessimistic about salvage, but when they return from the operating theatre and see that their hand is 'still there', they are given hope that may be entirely unfounded. Once started on this road of reconstruction, many patients are unable to consent to amputation later, even after many operations, chronic pain and an extremity that is more a burden than an asset. Faced with a mangled upper extremity, it may be helpful to ask yourself: 'If this were a complete amputation, would it be worth the effort to replant?' or 'If this survives, will the final result be better than a prosthesis?' If the answer is no, primary amputation should be strongly considered. In complex wounds with poor wound definition, mixed viability, and those for which the source of distal vascular supply is uncertain but for which the final outcome is likely to be better than a prosthesis, a conservative approach is reasonable. Wound healing is unpredictable in these indeterminate wounds, and efforts at radical debridement and complex reconstruction are more likely to fail or have serious complications. A conservative approach gives wounds the opportunity to heal while minimizing additional risk to the patient. Principles of conservative management include minimal debridement, no additional incisions, percutaneous fracture reduction, early active and passive motion, repeated debridement, and skin grafts. Obviously, expectations are less: such an approach gives greater likelihood for stiffness and poor function but also lessens the chances for major iatrogenic complications. Conservative management should be considered when the anticipated margins of radical debridement are not clear or if debridement itself may precipitate an unsalvageable situation.

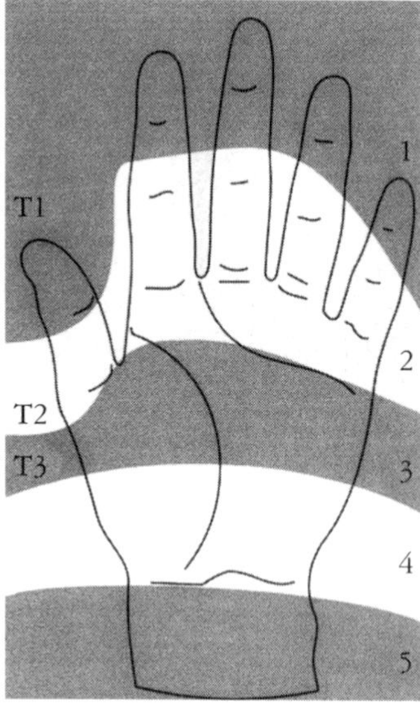

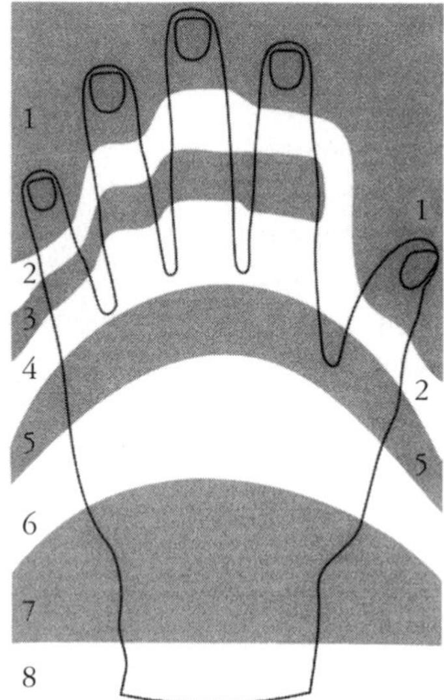

Figure 19.6 Zones of flexor tendon injuries.

Key point

- One of the most difficult complications of a severe open upper extremity injury is the failure to amputate.

Flexor tendon injuries

Open flexor tendon injuries are very common, and the source of considerable disability. Prognosis is strongly influenced by the location of tendon injury (Fig. 19.6), with worst results anticipated for injuries in zone 2. In this zone, the profundus and superficialis tendons are tightly constrained within the flexor tendon sheath from the metacarpophalangeal joint to the mid-middle phalanx. As noted above, outcome is also markedly worse when tendon injury is associated with fracture or nerve injury. Tendon repairs require special suture technique, generally a combination of a central 'core' suture or sutures and a peripheral epitendinous suture (Fig. 19.7). Suture technique is critical, and there is a strong ongoing trend to increase the number of core sutures such that four, six, or more suture strands cross the tendon repair site. This trend is matched by a trend in postoperative management away from immobilization, currently using early controlled motion, but moving toward early active motion. Noting this, current postoperative management would involve (for the unreliable patient) immobilization in wrist and metacarpophalangeal joint flexion or (for the co-operative patient) beginning early controlled motion with elastic traction to passively flex the fingers while allowing active extension against resistance.

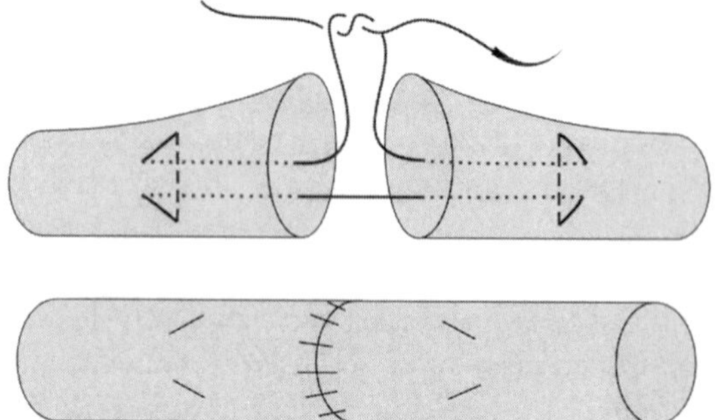

Figure 19.7 Suture technique for tendon repair.

Extensor tendon injuries

Open extensor tendon injuries are classified according to location on the hand and wrist (Fig. 19.7) relative to adjacent joints. By this system, the odd-numbered zones—1, 3, 5, 7—are difficult management problems because they usually correspond to open mallet injury, open boutonnière injury, clenched-fist bite wounds, and multiple tendon injuries, respectively. Clean open mallet or boutonnière injuries are treated by primary tendon repair (absorbable sutures are preferred because they extrude less frequently than non-absorbable ones) and then a splinting programme appropriate for a similar but closed injury. Along the same lines, clean tendon lacerations over the dorsum of the hand or wrist may be repaired primarily and then splinted with the wrist and metacarpophalangeal joints in comfortable extension for 4–6 weeks. Clenched-fist bite wounds are different, and are discussed below.

Amputations

Fingertip, finger, and thumb amputations are unfortunately common. Replantation of amputations at any level from shoulder to fingertip pulp is technically possible and has been performed for years. Replantation is a considerable undertaking, more so for the patient than for the surgeon, because it usually involves a prolonged recovery period, often multiple operations, intensive therapy, and, when complete, it is realistic to expect only partial recovery of range of motion and sensation. If replantation is a consideration, a regional centre performing replantation surgery should be contacted to confirm with the receiving surgeon that referral for replantation is appropriate and that such services will be available. Replantation obviously does not take precedence over potentially life-threatening injuries, and particularly in a blunt trauma scenario such as a motor vehicle accident, the drama of the amputation should not be allowed to curtail thorough evaluation for other more dangerous injuries.

If replantation is not performed, amputation wounds may require skeletal shortening for simple primary closure. Skeletal shortening should be avoided in the digits if possible, because a relatively small loss of length may critically change the functional outcome of the digit. Fingertip amputation is the most common situation to test the knowledge and ingenuity of the surgeon. Pure soft tissue fingertip defects 1 cm or less in diameter may be treated with dressing changes, allowing the wound to heal by secondary intent. If the defect extends to the distal nail bed, the scar will come to lie beneath the fingernail and may not be visible. Larger defects or those in which bone is exposed require flap cover. Many flaps have been described for fingertip cover. The three most common and useful regional flaps for fingertip cover are the central V–Y palmar advancement flap, the thenar flap, and the dorsal cross-finger flap (Fig. 19.8). The three most common and useful regional flaps for thumb tip cover are the Moberg palmar advancement flap, dorsal cross finger flap from the index finger, and neurovascular island flap.

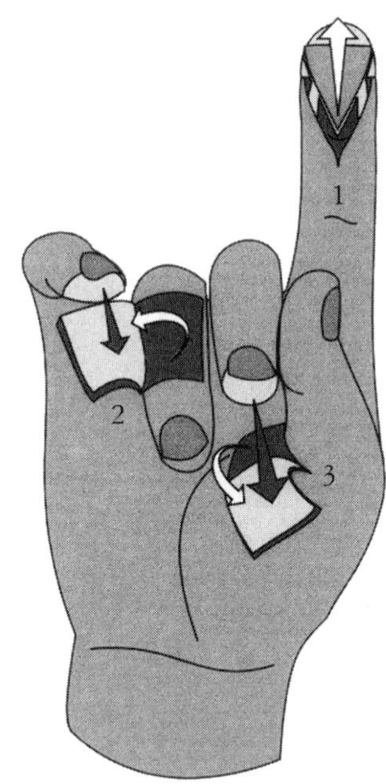

Figure 19.8 Flaps for fingertip cover.

Key point

- Replantation is a considerable undertaking, more so for the patient than for the surgeon, because it usually involves a prolonged recovery period.

Ring avulsion injuries

Patients may catch their wedding band or other finger ring on moving machinery or on a protrusion from a surface as they jump or move away from it. The sudden pull on the ring may result in a small wound, a circumferential wound, or an amputation. These injuries have been classified most recently (Kay *et al.* 1989) as follows:

I circulation adequate

II circulation inadequate

IIA digital arteries injured only

IIB digital arteries + skeletal injury

IIC digital veins injured only

III complete amputation.

With this mechanism, the actual extent of injury is always much greater than it appears. High-speed photography of the injury in a cadaver model has shown that relatively little force is required to momentarily turn the entire soft tissue envelope of the finger inside out. Because the external wound may be small and motion maintained through the intact flexor and extensor tendons, the extent of injury may not be appreciated initially and the patient may be discharged, only develop signs of progressive ischaemia. Arterial thrombosis along the length of the finger may prevent successful revascularization even with grafts, and the possibility of a proximal or even ray amputation should be discussed with the patient at the time of initial evaluation.

Injection injuries

High-pressure injection injuries of paint, sand, lubricating fluid, and other materials are uncommon, but important because they are also on the list of injuries missed in the accident ward. Typically, the patient has briefly placed their hand or fingertip over a pressure spray nozzle, sustaining an injection of material into the soft tissues. Under pressure, this material tracks up tissue planes next to flexor tendons, nerves, and arteries, and through the named bursae and compartments of the hand and arm. Debris may be driven from the fingertip to the chest wall. The examiner may be misled by a small visible wound and (depending on the material injected) relatively few physical findings, and the patient may be discharged only to return within 24 hours because of worsening symptoms. Radiographs may show air, particulate debris, or pigment from certain types of paint in the soft tissues. Treatment is emergency radical debridement. The pressure-injected material tends to track through the loose areolar tissue along longitudinal structures, and careful debridement may allow preservation of all vital structures. In contrast, late surgical treatment may require *en bloc* tumour-like excision of contaminated zones.

Key point

- High-pressure injection injuries of paint, sand, lubricating fluid, and other materials are uncommon but important.

Clenched-fist bite injuries

When someone strikes another person's face with their fist, they may cut the dorsal surface of their proximal phalanx or distal metacarpal head on the victim's tooth, usually involving the middle or ring finger. This extremely contaminated bite wound equivalent may divide the extensor mechanism and contaminate the metacarpal head joint surface. Because such injuries frequently occur while the patient is intoxicated, initial medical evaluation is often delayed, and the patient may not present until they have progressive infection. Neglected injuries may require ray amputation. All suspicious injuries in this area should be taken very seriously. Because the wound is made while the hand is in a fist, inspection of the wound with the fingers straight does not usually reveal the true extent of the injury. Standard radiograph views may be normal even if the patient has sustained an osteochondral fracture. There are two components of this injury. The first and most important is a septic open joint injury. Once this mechanism is suspected, patients immediately should be given intravenous broad-spectrum antibiotics appropriate for oral and skin organisms and be brought to the operating room at the earliest opportunity for a formal joint inspection and debridement. Documented joint surface injuries should be re-inspected in the operating theatre 24–48 hours after the initial procedure. The second component is the extensor tendon injury. In the presence of infection, the extensor mechanism should not be repaired. If the injury involves the middle or ring finger, the injured metacarpophalangeal joint should be supported in a splint which maintains the joint at greater extension than that of the adjacent fingers. Because of the action on the tendinous junctures, splinting in this position results in approximation of the divided tendon ends and may provide a satisfactory result without further surgery.

Key point

- Initial medical evaluation is often delayed.

References

Bovenzi M, Alessandrini B, Mancini R, Cannava MG, Centi L (1998) A prospective study of the cold response of digital vessels in forestry workers exposed to saw vibration. *International Archives of Occupational and Environmental Health* 71(7): 493–498.

Darder-Prats A, Fernandez-Garcia E, Fernandez-Garbada R, Darder-Garcia A (1998) Treatment of mallet finger fractures by the extension-block K-wire technique. *Journal of Hand Surgery* 23B(6): 802–805.

Duncan RW, Freeland AE, Jabaley ME, Meydrech EF (1993) Open hand fractures: an analysis of the recovery of active motion and of complications. *Journal of Hand Surgery* 18A(3): 387–394.

Godina M (1986) Early microsurgical reconstruction of complex trauma of the extremities. *Plastic and Reconstructive Surgery* 78(3): 285–292.

Hsu ES, Patwardhan AG, Meade KP, Light TR, Martin WR (1993) Cross-sectional geometrical properties and bone mineral contents of the human radius and ulna. *Journal of Biomechanics* 26(11): 1307–1318.

Kay S, Werntz J, Wolff TW (1989) Ring avulsion injuries: classification and prognosis. *Journal of Hand Surgery* 14A(2 Pt 1): 204–213.

Kelsey JL, Pastides H, Krieger M, Harris C, Chernow RA (1980) *Upper extremity disorders: a survey of their frequency and cost in the United States*. C V Mosby, St Louis.

Krimmer H, Schmitt R, Herbert T (2000) Scaphoid fractures—diagnosis, classification and therapy. *Unfallchirurg* 103(10): 812–819. In German.

Palmer AK (1989) Triangular fibrocartilage complex lesions: a classification. *Journal of Hand Surgery* 14A: 594–606.

Salter RB, Harris WR (1963) Injuries involving the epiphyseal plate. *Journal of Bone and Joint Surgery* 45: 587–632.

Further information

e-Hand (www.eatonhand.com)

20

CHAPTER 20

Pelvic injuries

EUGENE SHERRY, DAVID STANTON, KE HUANG, DANIEL RAHME, AND PATRICK H WARNKE

CHAPTER 20
Pelvic injuries

EUGENE SHERRY, DAVID STANTON, KE HUANG, DANIEL RAHME, AND PATRICK H WARNKE

Pelvic fractures

Fractures of the pelvic ring represent a unique and potentially devastating problem. They often result in serious long-term functional disability, pain, and death. Soft tissue injuries associated with the fractures add to short-term and medium-term morbidity, and mortality.

Thanks to the improved Advanced Trauma Life Support protocol and landmark papers by a number of leaders in the field (Tile 1996b), the management of pelvic ring fractures is now more logical and comprehensive, with a markedly decreased morbidity and mortality. The classification system used recognizes that diagnosis and treatment may be improved when force vector analysis and fracture patterns are studied.

The classification systems used in treatment of pelvic fractures consider the following:

- understanding of the relevant anatomy
- re-creation and understanding of mechanisms and forces involved in injury
- knowledge of the diagnostic options and the relevant investigations that may be performed
- understanding of the associated soft tissue injuries
- familiarity with the various treatment options
- experience with potential complications and the need for rehabilitation and other interactions.

Key points

- In pelvic fractures, it is the complexities of fracture and soft tissue injury, combined with the potential for mortality, that make these fractures such a specialized field.
- A good surgical text for this material is Wiss (1998).

Surgical anatomy

Bony pelvis

The *pelvic ring* is composed of two innominate bones and the sacrum, joined at the anterior and posterior iliac joints. The innominate bones are joined at the pubic symphysis.

The *hip bone* itself is formed from three bones that fuse in a Y-shaped epiphysis involving the acetabulum. The pubis and ischium form an incomplete wall for the pelvic cavity. The ilium forms the brim between the acetabulum and the sacrum (McMinn 1994).

It is important to note the correct anatomical position of the bone. The pubic tubercle and anterior superior iliac spines lie in the same vertical plane, whereas the upper borders of symphysis pubis and ischial spines lie in the same horizontal plane. Thus the position of the whole sacrum is often described as oblique.

The *cavity* of the bony pelvis is divided into two subcavities by the arcuate lines of the sacrum posteriorly and the upper part of pubis bone anteriorly—this is known as the *brim* of the pelvis. The true pelvis below the brim houses the pelvic viscera; the false pelvis above the brim forms part of the abdominal cavity.

The *weight-bearing arches* are columns of thick bones within the innominate bones. These transfer weight from the L5 vertebra to the upper three pieces of sacrum, then to the sacroiliac joint. Weight is then transferred to the thick, weight-bearing pieces of ilium, thence to the roof of the acetabulum or the ischial tuberosity, depending upon whether the person is standing or sitting. It can thus be stated that the ilium is the primary transference element in transmission of weight forces from the spine to the lower extremities when standing, whereas the ischium serves as the terminal point of weight transmission within the sitting position.

The *pubic body* forms the anterior border of the true pelvis and forms part of the origin for the adductor muscles.

The *sacrum* is a part of the pelvic ring in that not only does it have the sacral nerves from the pelvic plexus, but it also is involved in the transmission of weight to the acetabulum from the spine.

Pelvic joints and ligaments

Sacroiliac complex

The stability of the bony pelvis is dependent upon the posterior sacroiliac joint complex. This consists of

- interosseous sacroiliac ligaments (sacrospinous and sacrotuberous)
- iliolumbar ligaments
- anterior and posterior transverse sacroiliac ligaments.

The effect of these ligaments is to prevent superior and anterior displacement of the complex, and includes some of the strongest ligaments in the body. It is also important to note that the anterior sacroiliac joint helps to prevent external rotation.

Pubic symphysis

This joint complex is covered with hyaline cartilage and composed of the superior pubic ligament above and arcuate pubic ligament below.

Soft tissues of the pelvis

It is beyond the scope of this chapter to describe in detail the contents of the true pelvis, but it is vitally important to recognize and quantify the types of injury to soft tissues when interpreting a radiograph of an acute fracture. Consider the bladder and rectum.

It is possible to estimate clinically the amount of vascular damage to the vessels of the pelvis via the type of fracture. Force-vector analysis of the fracture pattern has been shown to be predictive of the patient population at high risk for massive haemorrhage. Note that approximately 50–70% of those with unstable pelvic fractures will require 4 units of blood or more and 30–40% will require 10 units or more (Levine 1996).

Mechanism of injury

The recognition and analysis of direction and intensity of force involved is important in order to determine possible outcomes in trauma management. The details of force may be recovered from various sources—patient, witnesses, scene investigators, and paramedics, as well as intuitive analysis.

Pelvic fractures can be classified into two major types:

- *low energy:* for the most part resulting in isolated bony fracture
- *high energy:* most likely to lead to pelvic ring disruption.

As a part of this analysis, two other factors must be considered:

- impact versus crush injury
- direction of forces involved.

Low-energy fracture

Low-energy pelvic fractures usually result from domestic falls and avulsion injuries of the muscular apophyses in skeletally immature patients.

About one-third of all pelvic fractures are fractures of a single element of the pelvic ring. Recently, with the aid of better imaging and analysis, it has been shown that if the pelvic ring is fractured in one area it must also be broken in another (the only exception is a greenstick injury). It is extremely important to recognize this in initial trauma assessment. Pubic ramus fractures are often associated with ipsilateral ramus fracture and posterior ring injury; sacral fractures with pelvic ring fracture; and iliac injury with abdominal and thoracic injuries.

High-energy fracture

High-energy forces result in more severe injury to the pelvic ring, associated soft tissues, and viscera. Pelvic fractures vary in the degree of stability, and this is related to the direction of the injurious force. This can be classified as an external rotation force, an internal rotation forces, or a shearing force.

External rotation forces

An external rotation forces acts through either an intact femur or the anterior or posterior iliac spines, via anteroposterior compression forces. External rotation forces through the pelvic ring, in order of decreasing severity of injury, tend to:

- cause 'open-book' fractures of the pelvis via disruption of the symphysis pubis or fracture of rami
- rupture the pelvic floor
- tear the anterior sacroiliac ligaments
- cause rotation of the pelvis unilaterally or bilaterally, but with the pelvic ring remaining stable by virtue of an intact posterior sacroiliac joint complex.

Lateral or internal rotational forces

The first injury caused by a lateral rotational force is often fracture of the anterior rami, with pelvis rotating internally. The next injury depends on the strength of the posterior ligament versus the sacrum: there may be fracture of the sacrum if the ligaments are stronger or, if the sacrum is stronger, then the ligaments may tear. In both scenarios the pelvic floor and its ligaments remain intact, and thus major posterior and vertical translation is impossible. However, these forces are more likely to cause puncture wounds to viscera.

Shearing forces

Shearing forces are generally perpendicular to soft tissue structures and bony trabeculae, so these forces may overcome the sacroiliac joint complex and result in an unstable hemipelvis. Note that external rotation and shearing forces disrupt the ligaments more commonly than lateral compression forces and are more likely to cause visceral, nerve, and vascular injuries.

Evaluation

Use EMST/ATLS principles (see Chapter 2). Evaluation in the emergency department consists of the ABCs of trauma management. A primary survey of the patient is performed, along with baseline observations, and insertion of monitoring and resuscitative devices.

Physical examination includes:

- inspection for fresh blood from rectum or anus, and penis or vagina
- gentle palpation at the anterior superior iliac spine (ASIS), looking for instability in internal or external rotation, and instability with superior or inferior distraction, compression or springing
- digital rectal examination and perineal examination (note position of prostate). *Destot's sign* is blood above inguinal ligament or in scrotum; *Roux's sign* is decrease distance from greater trochanter to pubic tubercle and *Earle's sign* is tender swelling found on rectal examination. Depending upon the result of the rectal examination, further examination with placement of an indwelling catheter (perhaps with urethrogram), or proctoscopic inspection may be necessary.
- Detailed neurological and vascular examination. Note there is a 50% incidence of plexus injuries in the patient with unstable pelvic fracture or fractures that involve sacral ala or foramina (Tile 1996a).

In the unstable patient, bleeding into the intra-abdominal space must be ruled out either by CT if the patient is haemodynamically normal, or by diagnostic peritoneal lavage (DPL) if haemodynamically unstable. If DPL is to be used the entry point must be placed supraumbilically to prevent decompression of tamponade haematoma.

Key points

- Early haemorrhage must be ruled out
- Fluid resuscitation
- Open wounds—use sterile dressing.

Radiology

An anteroposterior (AP) radiograph is standard and should be taken in all patients with blunt trauma; special care should be taken with possible sacral fractures that are easily missed. If this is abnormal, then:

- inlet views (40° caudad) are best for sacral fractures or displacement of posterior elements
- outlet views (40° cephalad) are best for vertical displacement/assessment of pelvic ring.

CT scan

This helps clinicians to further interpret fracture patterns and indeed helps in diagnosis of posterior element fracture, especially sacral fracture. CT scanning helps with sub-classification of fracture with reference to various classification systems. MRI is not routinely used in the acute setting.

Key points

- AP radiograph of pelvis
- 40° caudad
- 40° cephalad
- CT scan
- MRI is not routinely used in the acute setting.

Classification

Burgess *et al.* (1990), Tile (1996a) and the AO group have produced a classification system which incorporates the vector forces involved, stability, and fracture configuration (Table 20.1) (Wiss 1999).

The aim of any classification system is to quantify and standardize treatment and decision-making in the management and subsequent follow-up of patients. However, all fractures must be considered individually in terms of soft tissue injury, compound injury, and associated non-pelvic injury.

Key point

- All fractures must be considered individually in terms of soft tissue injury, compound injury, and associated non-pelvic injury.

Table 20.1 Pelvic fracture classification system

Type	Description	Subtypes
A	Stable (posterior arch intact)	A1: Avulsion injury (ring not involved) A2: Minimally displaced ring fracture (iliac wing, anterior arch ,transverse sacrococcygeal fracture)
B	Rotationally unstable-vertically stable (partially stable; incomplete disruption of posterior arch)	B1: Open book injury (external rotation) B2: Lateral compression injury (internal rotation); ipsilateral B3: Lateral compression-contralateral
C	Rotationally and vertically unstable (complete disruption of posterior arch)	C1: Rotationally and vertically unstable C2: Bilateral C3: Associated acetabular fracture

- Stress fractures of the pubis/pubic rami are not uncommon in osteoporotic patients.
- Type A fractures do not fracture through the pelvic ring.
- Type B fractures are partially stable, and no posterior or vertical displacement is possible. This is often difficult to determine on the initial radiograph, and other imaging modalities may be required in order to fully visualize this area.
- Type C fractures are inherently unstable because of posterior disruption, leading to the possibility of posterior or vertical movement. These are generally high-energy injuries, with gaps of the posterior elements of greater than one centimetre on initial views, associated with severe disruption of the anterior elements, leading to an unstable hemipelvis.

The radiographic signs of pelvic instability (Fig. 20.1) include:

- displacement of the posterior sacroiliac complex >5 mm in any plane
- fracture gap posteriorly
- presence of a fracture (avulsion) of the transverse process of L5 (where iliolumbar and lateral lumbosacral legs attached and so indicates vertical instability); ischial spine (attachment of the sacrospinous ligament; resists external rotation of hemipelvis); or ischial tuberosity (attachment of sacrotuberous lig; resists sagittal rotation).

(a)

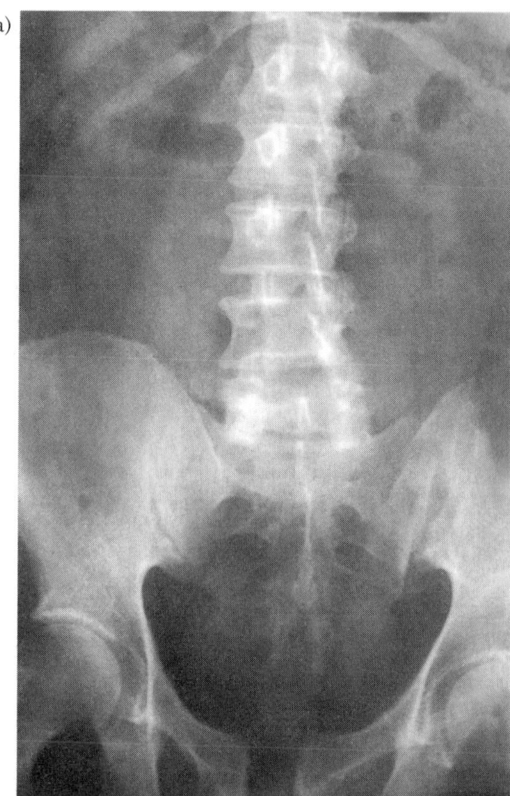

(b)

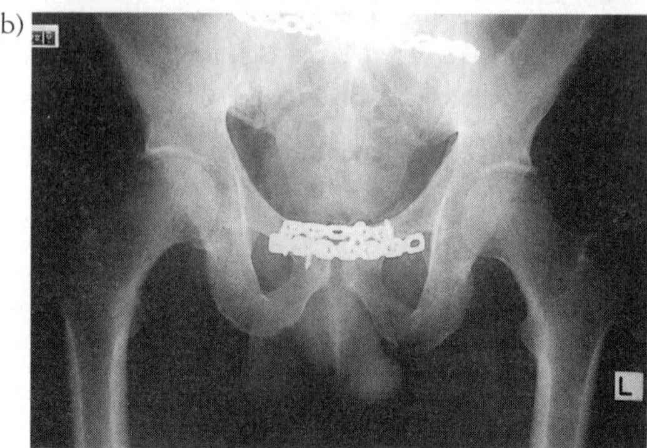

Figure 20.1 (a) Pre- and (b) postoperative radiographs of type C1 pelvic fracture (also L5 fracture).

Key point

- Most fractures are type A or B.

Treatment

Early management

Immediate resuscitation must proceed along EMST/ATLS guidelines. The multiple-trauma patient may have other life-threatening injuries apart from the pelvic fracture.

In the patient in which pelvic fracture is the leading injury, initial assessment must address notable associations:

- retroperitoneal haemorrhage
- pelvic ring instability

- soft tissue injury (especially lower bowel and genitourinary)
- open fracture.

Haemorrhage has been shown to be the leading cause of death in the patient with a pelvic fracture (approximately 60%). Most of the blood loss is from fracture site or retroperitoneal veins, not arterial injury (Levine 1996). The unstable patient has a tenfold increased chance of dying. The chest and abdomen should also be excluded as sites of bleeding.

Open wounds require aggressive incision and drainage. Any communication with the gastrointestinal tract should be removed; a diverting colostomy should be considered for rectal or vaginal injuries. Temporary external fixation should be carried out.

Closed degloving injuries (Morel–Lavalle lesion), where skin and subcutaneous tissue are separated from fascia, create a huge potential space, and surgical exposure may compromise flaps.

Genitourinary disruption requires primary bladder and urethral repair via a Pfannenstiehl incision. The urologist works via the anterior pelvic disruption. A Foley catheter is needed for 6 weeks after a urethral tear. A suprapubic catheter should not be used. Open reduction and internal fixation (ORIF) should be carried out as required.

A positive peritoneal aspirate in the face of pelvic fracture warrants laparotomy to assess the extent of abdominal injury. Provisional stabilization of the pelvic fracture prior to laparotomy can be obtained by application of an external fixator, pelvic clamp, or MAST suit (easy and safe to apply; it should be deflated slowly in the emergency department after large-bore intravenous lines have been placed).

Key point

- The multiple-trauma patient may have other life-threatening injuries apart from the pelvic fracture.

External fixators

- *Advantages:* May be life saving; decreases pelvic volume; temporary simple frames available.
- *Disadvantages:* Not suitable for all fractures; pin tract problems; limits abdominal access; does not control posterior pathology.

Authors' preferred technique

Pelvic (Ganz) clamp (Fig. 20.2)

The entry point is 3–4 finger breadths anterolateral to the posterior superior iliac spine (PSIS), along a line from PSIS to the anterior superior iliac spine (ASIS). An assistant holds the clamp, and the operator then slides Steinmann pins on to the outer cortex of the ilium, and drives them in 1 cm. The sidearms are pushed centrally and threaded bolts advanced with a wrench to engage and compress the fracture diastasis.

External fixator

Two pins per cut are placed in the iliac crest, on both sides: one at ASIS, one at the iliac tubercle, at about 45° to each other. The complete frame is an anterior rectangle.

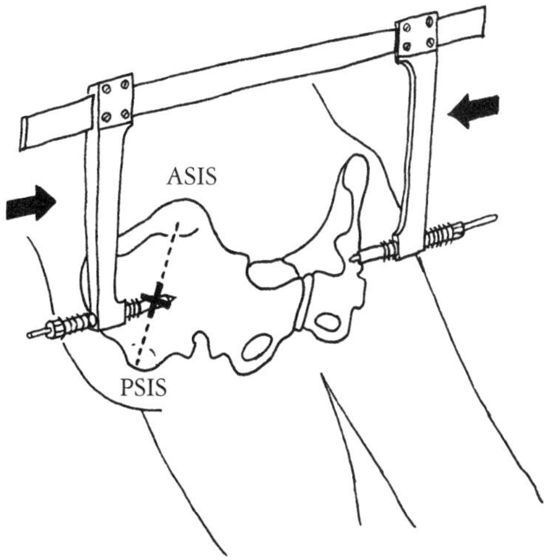

Figure 20.2 Pelvic C-clamp can be applied in the emergency department to stabilize (tamponade) haemodynamically unstable displaced pelvic fracture (probably not of use for non-displaced pelvic fracture and may open type C, posterior pelvic fracture).

The orthopaedic team must be present at the time of laparotomy to aid in assessment and management of fracture. Opening the abdomen may decompress the tamponaded pelvic haematoma and allow expansion and a further hypotensive episode, making closure of the abdomen impossible.

An interventional radiologist and an angiography suite should be on stand-by in case urgent embolectomy is required. If the haemorrhage is uncontrollable, then temporary cross-clamping of the aorta may be necessary to allow for packing of the retroperitoneal space or for transport to the angiography suite.

The orthopaedic team may also decide to continue with definitive stabilization of the fracture after the laparotomy is performed. The aims of management in this case are to decrease haematoma by decreasing pelvic volume (due to stabilization of the fracture) and thus causing a retroperitoneal tamponade, as the strong pelvic fascia limits the rupture of blood into the peritoneal cavity.

Key points

- Control venous bleeding.
- Give fluid and blood replacement.
- Use simple external fixator.
- Apply pelvic C-clamp.
- May need angiographic embolization.
- Consider early/urgent internal fixation under these circumstances:
  - at time of exploratory laparatomy
  - urethral realignment or bladder repair
  - ongoing haemorrhage
  - open wounds
  - loss of nerve function
  - patient under general anaesthetic for other orthopaedic injuries.

Definitive management

In the haemodynamically normal patient, definitive stabilization should be attempted (Tile 1988) (Fig. 20.3). The timing of this procedure is critical in determining the outcome, and must be individualized.

Type A fracture

The need for definitive fixation in type A fractures is small, apart from the displaced iliac wing fracture, with or without involvement of the greater sciatic notch area. Angiographic evaluation of blood supply is required before open reduction of these fractures.

The iliac wing approach is performed via an external or internal iliac exposure; use lag screws and plates.

Type B fractures

ORIF is often needed.

Type B1

- Anterior symphyseal disruption <2.5 cm results in a good functional outcome without operative intervention.
- Anterior symphyseal disruption >2.5 cm is best treated with anterior fixation via plate and screws. This is generally done through a Pfannensteil incision and two 4.5 mm reconstructive plates, one anteriorly, the other along the superior border, each with 4–6 holes. An alternative is external fixation for at least 8–12 weeks.

Types B2 and B3 A type B2 or B3 fracture is usually treated with rest and symptomatic care unless there is concern about leg length discrepancy. In this case, application of external fixation may be considered in order to rotate the pelvis externally and restore leg length.

The so-called *locked symphysis* may occur in this type of injury, and is usually reduced by closed means. Most patients can tolerate some internal rotation of the hemipelvis.

Type C

A type C fracture is in essence a sacral fracture (or fractures) either with or without sacroiliac dislocation. Treatment is difficult. Definitive

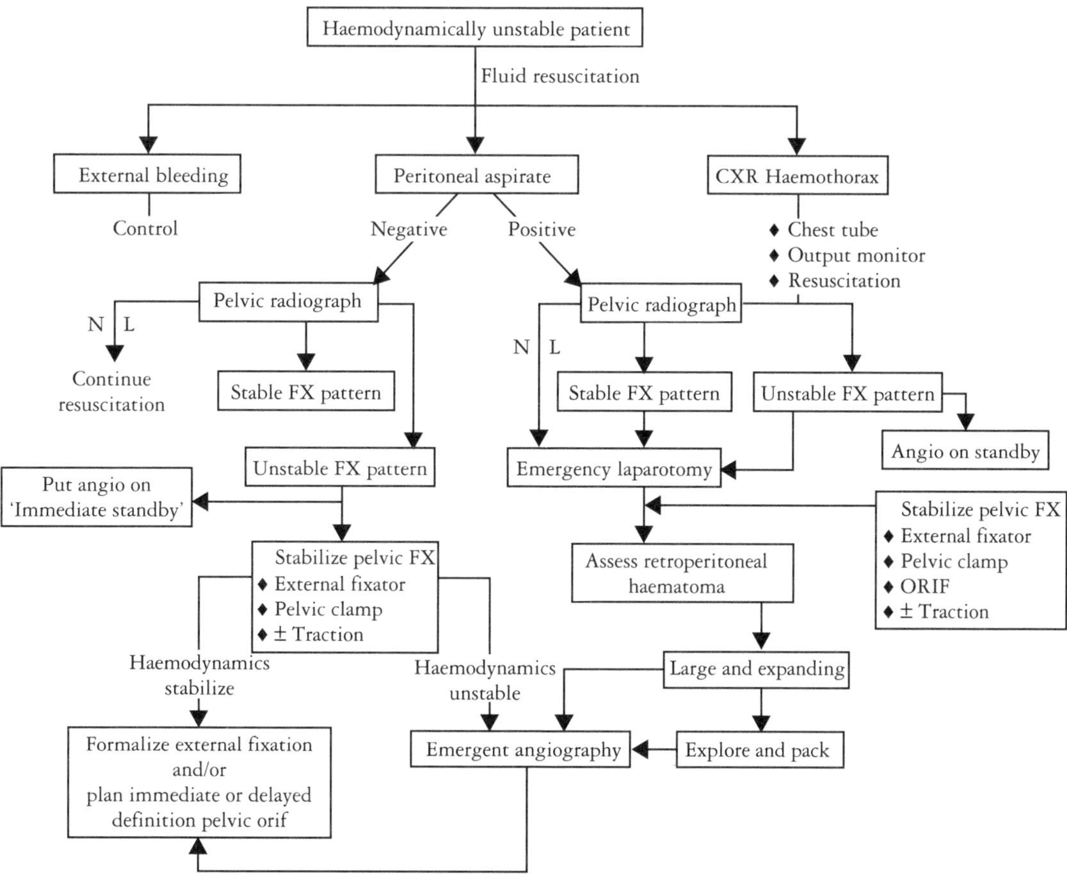

Figure 20.3 Stabilization algorithm.

stabilization of these unstable injuries is required, in other words both anterior and posterior fixation.

Key points

- Posterior fixation.
- Operate usually within the first 5–7 days.
- Provide antibiotic cover and haemodynamic monitoring with or without a cell saver.
- Consider somatosensory evoked potentials (SSEP) or neurological monitoring.
- The type of approach is dependent on soft tissue injury.
- Use image intensification (fluoroscopy).

For sacral fractures, surgical options include iliosacral screws, posterior spanning plate, and transiliac screws or rods (sacral bars). For sacroiliac dislocation, anterior stabilization with dynamic compression plate (DCP) is easy but puts the L5 nerve root at risk. The other option is posterior stabilization with iliosacral screws and transiliac rods or plates (details in box). Rods and screws must not be over-tightened, especially if there are sacral fractures.

Fixation of sacroiliac dislocation

Posterior approach

Two 6.5 mm cannulated screws are required. These should be passed from the ilium to the sacral ala at the junction of the lower and middle thirds. The operator's index finger should be kept in the incisura ischium to aim the drill. Under fluroscopic control (a lateral sacral image is required) the guide wire is passed through the ilium and into the sacroiliac body, avoiding the sacral foramina, spinal canal, and great vessels. A percutaneous technique may be considered (Matta *et al.* 1989).

Anterior approach

The iliac muscle is stripped from the inner wall of the ilium to expose the sacroiliac, which is fixed with two short DCPs. Only one of these screws into the sacrum, to avoid the L5 nerve.

Transiliac rods (Harrington) are easy to put in: two rods are used. The prominence of the rod ends and subsequent wound breakdown are a problem. A plate on the end of the rod, contoured on to the posterior ilium, may help. A 4.5 mm reconstruction plate across the iliac crests (through windows) and contoured on to the posterior ilium may also be used.

Key point

- Iliosacral screws require good knowledge of spatial anatomy and are ideally left to an expert in pelvic fractures. Transiliac rods (sacral bars) and plates are not so difficult.

Postoperative care

The patient requires standard wound care with antibiotics and no weight bearing for 8–12 weeks, or on the less affected side for transfers. This period can be reduced to 3–6 weeks for a stable configuration, or increased for a disrupted posterior element.

Postoperative radiographs should be done weekly for 4 weeks, then monthly for 3 months, then 3-monthly for a further year.

Prognosis

The prognosis of pelvic fractures is directly related to the degree of injury. Severe fractures lead to worse postoperative pain, inability to return to pre-fracture work, and altered sexual function. Mortality is 5–20%, up to 42% for open fractures (this worsens with age; at >70 years it is >50%). Pedestrians have 50% mortality, and in pregnancy there is 33% fetal loss (20–40% of women subsequently need a caesarean section).

Complications

Complications are:

- infection (0–25%, especially where there is bowel injury)
- nerve palsy (usually peroneal component of sciatic nerve) in 11.2% (20.4% of posterior fractures)
- thromboembolism (versus risk of early haemorrhage): use compression stockings or calf

Authors' preferred technique

Anterior pelvic (open book) fracture

Two reconstruction plates should be used, via a Pfannenstiel incision. The linea alba is exposed in midline, then divided. The two heads of the rectus abdominus are retracted laterally to reveal the pubic bone. Pointed retractors or Matta's two-screw technique are used to reduce the fracture.

Posterior pelvic fracture

ORIF with vertical displacement is preferred. Skeletal traction (up to 40 kg) shoud be applied for 2–3 days to bring the hemipelvis down. For surgery, the patient is placed prone and two vertical lateral parailiac incisions are made (off the prominence). Skeletal traction is kept on. A reconstruction plate (3.5 or 4.5 mm) is passed from the window in one posterior iliac crest across the posterior of the sacrum to the window in the other posterior iliac crest, contoured on to the posterior ilium, and fixed.

compression devices, anticoagulation, possibly an inferior vena cava filter
- malunion: this can be devastating and cause low back pain, sitting problems, and limb length differences with gait problems
- non-union (rare but crippling): tends to occur in younger patients and may require bone grafting
- ectopic bone formation occurs in about 20%: use indomethacin and consider possible carcinogenic effect of radiation in young people.
- post-traumatic osteoarthritis, seen in 4–15%: depends on quality of reduction.

Almost one-third of unstable fractures (13% overall), have a urethral injury, so a retrograde urethrogram is required before an indwelling catheter is inserted, with a cystogram and intravenous pyelogram (IVP) if indicated. Bladder rupture is usually extraperitoneal and may form vesicocolic and vesical fistulas. Erectile dysfunction is evident in about 40%.

Conclusion

The diagnosis and management of pelvic fractures has improved markedly over recent decades, but future directions such as percutaneous pin fixation with image intensification, and the development of guidance systems for pin fixation, make this one of the most exciting areas in trauma management.

Acetabular fractures

Fractures of the acetabulum are a major challenge to the orthopaedic surgeon. Many important matters remain to be resolved in their management, including:

- decision-making (i.e. whether to operate in the acute setting or at a planned later stage)
- details of surgical technique
- avoidance of complications.

Articular fractures, especially in weight-bearing joints of the lower extremity, require anatomical reduction, either closed or open, for good long-term function. The complicated anatomy of the acetabulum makes exposure of the fracture difficult, and severe comminution is often part of the personality of the fracture, making reduction and fixation difficult. Also, fractures of the acetabulum frequently occur in multiple-trauma patients with major associated injuries and have a high morbidity and disability rate no matter what the treatment. Anatomical reduction may not be possible even in the best circumstances. In a young patient, the benefits of ORIF are worth the risks (Matta *et al.* 1994), but in an older patient other forms of operative care, such as early total hip arthroplasty, may be preferable.

Surgical anatomy

When viewed from the side the acetabulum forms an inverted Y, one limb forming the anterior column and one the posterior column.

- The anterior column extends from the iliac crest to the symphysis pubis and includes the anterior wall of the acetabulum.
- The posterior column begins at the superior gluteal notch and descends through the acetabulum, obturator foramen, and inferior pubic ramus and includes the posterior wall of the acetabulum and the ischial tuberosity. The superior weight-bearing area, which includes a portion of both the anterior and posterior columns, has been called the acetabular dome or roof.

The pathoanatomy of any acetabular fracture depends on the position of the femoral head at the moment of impact. The femoral head acts like a hammer, shattering the acetabulum on impact. Fractures of the posterior column are produced when the femoral head is rotated internally, and those of the anterior column are produced when the head is rotated externally. If the femoral head is adducted, the superior aspect of the dome is involved; and if it is abducted, the inferior aspect is involved. The actual fracture or fracture-dislocation produced depends on the magnitude of the force causing it, as well as on the strength of the bone. High-energy injuries from motor vehicle or motor cycle accidents may occur at any age and produce fractures of any anatomical variety, depending on the force direction. Comminution with articular impaction fractures is common. Older patients with osteopenia may fracture the acetabulum with relatively low forces, such as simple falls.

High-energy injuries have a high incidence of major associated injuries, whereas low-energy injuries are usually isolated.

Key points

- Complex fractures of major weight-bearing joint.
- Anatomy and surgery are difficult.
- Often require ORIF.
- Sub-specialist help often needed.

Evaluation

After initial resuscitation, a complete physical examination is required to determine the associated injuries. The extremity should be examined for soft tissue injury, which may give insight into the mechanism of injury. Especially important are local bruises in the area of the greater trochanter and areas of massive subcutaneous haemorrhage. The ipsilateral knee must be carefully examined for posterior instability and patellar fracture, both common in posterior-type patterns. Because nerve injury is relatively common, careful documentation of any neurological deficit is essential. Sciatic nerve involvement may be present in up to 40% of posterior types. Femoral nerve involvement with anterior column fractures is rare but not unknown. Also, vascular examination of the limb is mandatory to rule out penetrating injuries to the femoral artery by the anterior column.

Patient factors

The general medical fitness of the patient, and the type of trauma involved, affect the choice of management. Anatomical open reduction and stable fixation is important in young, fit patients. Choices are not so clear in older patients. If there is a strong indication for ORIF and the surgery is relatively straightforward (such as a posterior wall fracture in isolation or with a transverse or column fracture), then go to open reduction. However, with severe comminution in osteoporotic bone, especially if secondary congruence can be achieved by traction in a both-column fracture (type C), non-operative care with traction is the preferred option. Good outcomes can be expected in some cases. If not, a total hip replacement should be carried out (Duwelius *et al.* 1998).

If surgery is not planned then traction should be continued until healing has occurred, usually at 8–12 weeks. If the pain has diminished at that time, the patient should be rehabilitated. A reconstructive procedure such as arthroplasty or arthrodesis can be performed at this time or later, as directed by patient's symptoms. In older patients with fractures that clearly would be difficult to fix and maintain anatomically, early arthroplasty may be the best choice especially if a fracture of the femoral head or neck is present.

Radiology

Radiographs are often hard to read. Standard and special views are needed, as well as a CT scan. The ability to interpret radiographs and CT scans of the pelvis and acetabulum is essential for decision-making.

Standard views

Anteroposterior inlet and outlet views will determine whether the pelvic ring is involved in the acetabular fracture.

Special views

To the standard anteroposterior view of the hip joint have been added a 45° internal rotation view (obturator oblique view obtained by rotating patient 45° on to the unaffected side) and a 45° external rotation view (iliac oblique view; rotate; 45° on to the side of the fracture) (Judet *et al.* 1964) (Fig. 20.4). By examining these three views, two of which are at 90° to each other, the clinician can determine the overall pattern of the fracture.

Another useful view is roof angle—a measurement of how much dome is intact. On the anteroposterior

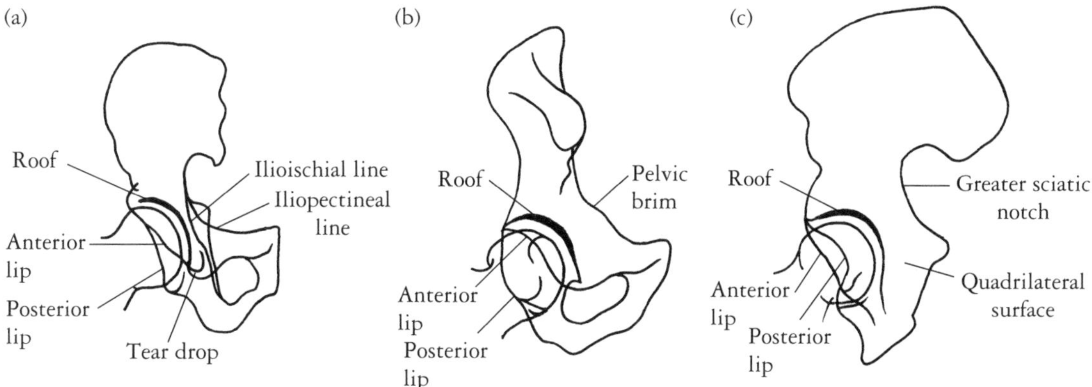

Figure 20.4 (a) Anteroposterior, (b) obturator, and (c) iliac oblique views/landmarks of acetabulum.

view, draw a line vertically from the acetabulum roof to the centre of the femoral head, and a second line from the edge of the fracture to the centre of the head. The roof angle is below these lines. If the roof angle is >45°, operative treatment is rarely needed.

CT scan

CT is useful for showing the fine detail in the acetabular fracture, but not for viewing the overall pattern. It shows with great precision fragments of the anterior or posterior wall, marginal impaction, retained bone fragments in the joint, comminution, the presence or absence of a dislocation, and sacro-iliac pathology. Three-dimensional reconstruction looks good, though it does not always add much, and will assist in understanding acetabular comminution (subtract the femoral head to see the interior of the acetabulum).

Classification

Judet *et al.* (1964) published the first comprehensive classification, dividing all the fractures into elementary/simple and associated/complex types. All further attempts to classify these fractures stem from their efforts.

- *simple fractures:* anterior wall, anterior column, posterior wall, posterior column, transverse
- *complex fractures:* posterior column–posterior wall, transverse–posterior wall, T-shaped, anterior column–posterior hemitransverse, both columns.

The current classification is based on the AO comprehensive fracture classification, which groups all fractures into A, B, and C types (in order of increasing severity) (Fig. 20.5). The types are anatomical, based on the Letournel–Judet classification, and modifiers are added in Table 20.2 to denote prognostic indicators (with Greek letters).

Key point

- Each injury is different, and each fracture has its own personality.

Treatment

Primary treatment is urgent closed reduction for all fracture-dislocations (with sedation/muscle relaxant). Then assess stability:

- For posterior fracture-dislocations cautiously flex and slightly adduct hip whilst checking for subluxation; for anterior injuries, extend and abduct.
- If the femoral head dislocates the fracture is unstable and surgery is required.
- Monitor sciatic nerve function.
- Check the adequacy of reduction with radiography.

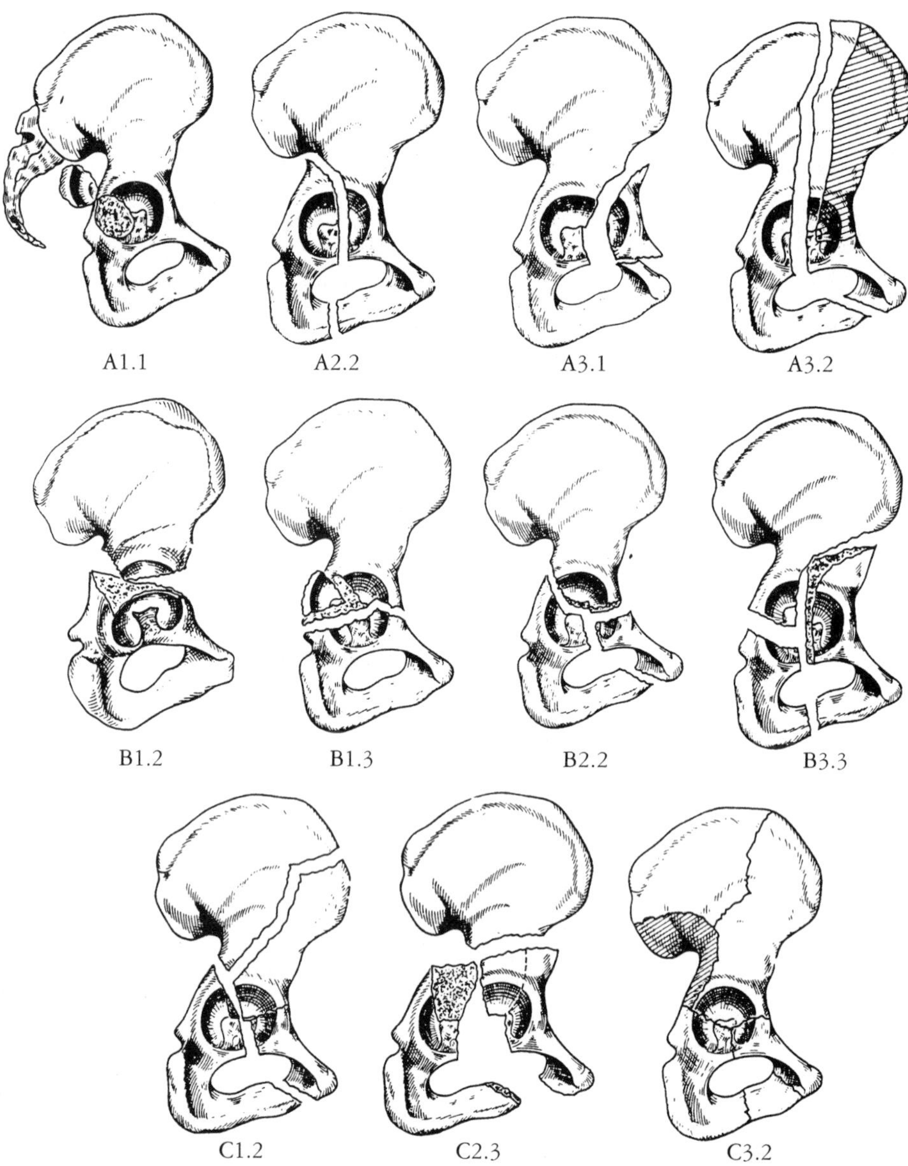

Figure 20.5 AO classification of acetabular fractures. (Reproduced with permission from Müller ME, Allgöwer M, Schnieder P *et al.* (1990) *AO Manual of Internal Fixation*, 3rd edn. Springer-Verlag, Heidelberg. © Springer-Verlag 1990.)

Non-operative management

Non-operative management may be indicated for injuries where congruity of the hip joint is maintained. These include:

- displacement of <2–5 mm in the dome, depending on the location of the fracture and patient factors
- distal anterior column fractures
- distal transverse fractures (infratectal) in which congruity of the hip is maintained by the large remaining medial buttress

Table 20.2 Classification (after Letournel) of acetabular fractures. Modifiers are added to denote prognostic indicators (Greek letters)

Type	Description	Comments	Subtypes
A	Partial articular one-column fracture		A1: Posterior wall A2: Posterior column A3: Anterior wall and/or anterior column
B	Partial articular transverse oriented fracture	Transverse types with portion of the roof attached to intact ilium	B1: Transverse + posterior wall B2: T types B3: Anterior with posterior hemitransverse
C	Complete articular, both-column fracture	Both columns are fractured and all articular segments, including the roof, are detached from the remaining segment of the intact ilium, the 'floating acetabulum'	C1: Both column: anterior column fracture extends to the iliac crest (high variety) C2: Both column: anterior column fracture extends to the anterior border of the ilium (low variety) C3: Both column : anterior fracture enters the sacroiliac joint

Qualifiers: Additional information can be documented concerning the condition of the articular surfaces to further define the prognosis of the injury. The information should be, as additional qualifiers, identified by Greek letters: α1, femoral head subluxation, anterior; α2, femoral head subluxation, medial; α3, femoral head subluxation, posterior; β1, femoral head dislocation, anterior; β2, femoral head dislocation, medial; β3, femoral head dislocation, posterior; γ1, acetabluar surface, chondral lesion; γ2, acetabular surface, impacted; δ1, femoral head, chondral lesion; δ2, femoral head, impacted; δ3, femoral head, osteochondral fracture; ε1, intra-articular fragment requiring surgical removal; φ1, non-displaced fracture of the acetabulum.

- both-column fractures with secondary congruence without major posterior column displacement
- $<$20% posterior wall involved.

Surgery

Indications for surgery are:

- deteriorating sciatic nerve function after closed reduction
- incarcerated fragment preventing congruent reduction
- failure to achieve closed reduction
- presence of femoral neck fracture
- associated vascular injury
- open injury
- roof arc measurements $<$45°
- fracture displacement $>$3 mm
- unstable hip.

Operative treatment is generally indicated for the unstable or incongruous joint. Emergency surgery is rarely indicated because these procedures are difficult and must be done under optimal conditions.

Unstable hip

Posterior instability: Fractures of the posterior wall of the acetabulum are the most common acetabular fracture (50%). They are often thought to be easy to treat, but poor outcomes are not unusual (up to 80% of those treated non-operatively) (Baumgaertner 1999). The usually occur in motor vehicle accidents from indirect force applied to the knee from impact with the dashboard (up to 22% may have associated knee injury and sciatic nerve injury). Any acetabular fracture containing a posterior wall fragment large enough (generally accepted to involve >50% of posterior wall; <20% are stable) to cause instability of the joint in the normal resting position must be operated on to stabilize the hip.

Central instability: This may occur when the quadrilateral plate fracture is large enough to allow the femoral head to sublux medially. In such cases some form of medial buttress with a spring plate or cerclage wire is required to restore stability.

Anterior instability: Large anterior wall fragments either in isolation with an associated anterior dislocation or as part of an anterior type with posterior hemitransverse pattern (type B3) may be large enough to allow anterior hip instability and therefore require operative fixation.

Prepare for ORIF within the first 7 days. Surgery is difficult and ideally undertaken by experienced surgeons. Strive for anatomical reduction of all fractures and stable fixation, so as to allow early motion.

Postoperative mobilization depends on the quality of the bone, adequacy of reduction, and stability of the internally fixed fracture. In general, postoperative traction is for 7 days with continuous passive motion (CPM). If stability is good and the bone adequate, the traction may be removed and the patient allowed out of bed. Weight-bearing is not started until signs of union are present, usually 6–8 weeks after surgery.

If there is concern about the quality of the bone, or gross comminution is present, maintain traction for 6–8 weeks until the fragments have healed. Then ambulate, followed by progressive weight bearing at about 12 weeks.

Surgical approaches are varied, and too specialized to describe here.

Posterior wall fractures (Levine 1996)

Blood loss is usually >700 mL, so consider the use of blood cell savers. The need for SSEP monitoring is controversial, and we do not use it. An operating table that allows fluoroscopic imaging should be used. The patient is placed on one side or prone, and skeletal traction is maintained. The Kocher–Langenbeck posterior approach is used, and the incision is centred at the posterosuperior corner of the greater trochanter. The gluteus maximus is split proximally until the first crossing branches of the inferior gluteal nerve are reached (otherwise it is denervated). The deep lower half of gluteus maximus is then released from femur. The sciatic nerve should be identified under haematoma. The quadratus femoris should be preserved: it carries the medial circumflex artery which supplies the femoral head. The piriformis and obturator internus tendons should be dissected from the capsule and divided mid substance. The gluteus minimus is elevated from the ilium (taking care near the sciatic notch to avoid damage to superior gluteal artery, vein, and nerve). The joint should be examined, and distracted with a Schanz screw in trochanter. Any free cartilaginous bits should be removed. The concentrically reduced femoral head should be used as a template to guide replacement of fragments (including the marginally impacted fragments), and gaps filled with cancellous bone graft. Slight abduction and external rotation relieves capsule tension to allow reduction. A buttress reconstructive plate (6–9 mm from rim) is usually used as well as lag screws to hold reduction (3–5 lag screws are seldom enough). The plate (slightly underbent to aid reduction) may be place down to the ischium. The screws should be directed away from the joint (i.e. parallel or posterior to the coronal plane). Fluoroscopy should be used for a final check. Post-operative prophylaxis for deep venous thrombosis (DVT) is required.

Key points

- Posterior wall/column fixation:
  - Kocher-Langenbeck approach
  - prone or lateral
  - neutralize with plate.

Anterior wall fractures

This approach also accesses the iliac wing, anterior sacroiliac joint, and pubic symphysis (Helfet 1997). The ilioinguinal approach is used, with the patient supine on a fluoroscopic table. The incision is made from the mid iliac crest to the ASIS, parallel to the inguinal ligament, to end 2 cm above the symphysis pubis. The lateral aspect of the external oblique is released, then subperiosteal dissection is required to expose the internal iliac fossa. The external oblique aponeurosis is incised 5 mm from its insertion into the inguinal ligament. The ilioinguinal nerve and contents of the inguinal canal must be protected. The conjoint tendon is incised from the inguinal ligament, protecting the lateral femoral cutaneous nerve. The rectus abdominis is released from pubic tuberososity to the symphysis pubis (the bladder and the space of Retzius can now be seen). The iliopsoas muscle and the femoral nerve are mobilized with a Penrose drain. The iliopectineal fascia is isolated and dissected off the pelvic brim (from the pectineal eminence to the sacroiliac joint). Ligate the corona mortis artery if it is present. Place the Penrose drain around the femoral vessels, lymphatics and the conjoint tendon. Access to the acetabulum has now been created via three windows (medial, middle, and lateral). Now via the medial and middle windows, perform stepwise reduction of the fracture from the margin of the fracture. A Schanz screw in the lateral femoral head allows distraction. Flex the hip to improve access. Remove loose fragments. Start at the iliac crest.

Restore the normal concavity to the internal iliac fossa. You will require reduction clamps, lag screws, 3.5 mm (carefully moulded) reconstruction plates. Stabilize the iliac crest and reduce the anterior wall/column to the intact iliac wing. Check with fluroscopy. Place drains into the space of Retzius, re-attach the rectus abdominis to the symphysis pubis. Repair the floor and roof of the inguinal canal. Re-attach the external oblique to the inguinal ligament. Further detail on Wheeless' Textbook of Orthopaedics (http://www.media.com/004/149.htm accessed July 1, 2002)

Other acetabular fractures are specialized and beyond many surgeons; details are not within the scope of this text. For more detail access Ortho Search at www. orthosearch. com or see Matta (1998).

Prognosis and complications

Prognosis

The prognosis for an acetabular fracture depends on both the fracture and the treatment (Letournel and Judet 1993). The major factors are:

- degree of violence: high energy versus low energy
- location: superior roof of the acetabulum or the posterior wall or column, allowing instability
- degree of articular comminution on both the femoral head and acetabulum, including osteochondral fractures, chondral fractures, and marginally impacted fragments
- degree of displacement
- presence of joint dislocation: anterior, central, or posterior
- associated injuries in the patient and the limb.

Key point

- Quality of the reduction restoring both congruity and stability to the joint is the most important factor in the prognosis.

Complications

Complications associated with acetabular fractures are not uncommon. Those influencing prognosis are:

- thromboembolic disease
- infection
- nerve injury
- heterotophic ossification
- avascular necrosis (necrosis of the femoral head gives rise to acetabular fragments)
- chondrolysis.

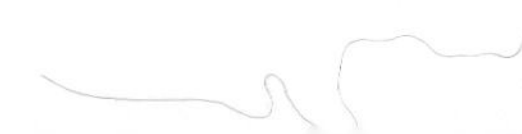

Nerve injury

- The *sciatic nerve* may be injured at the time of trauma or during surgery. The reported incidence is 16–33%.
- Rarely, the spike of the anterior column or during surgery injures the *femoral nerve*.
- The *superior gluteal nerve* is vulnerable in the greater sciatic notch, where it may be injured during trauma or during surgery, resulting in paralysis of the hip abductors. Paralysis of the hip abductor mechanism is a major disability.
- Other nerves can be injured. The *pudendal nerve* can be compressed on the traction table, but it usually recovers. Also, the *lateral femoral cutaneous nerve* of the thigh is commonly stretched or cut during anterior approaches. The patient usually tolerates sensory loss in the lateral aspect of the thigh.

Heterotopic ossification

Heterotopic ossification is one of the major unsolved problems in acetabular surgery (incidence 3–69%).

Avascular necrosis

Avascular necrosis of the femoral head is a devastating complication. Avascular necrosis of the acetabular segment may also occur, causing collapse of the joint.

Chrondrolysis

Chrondrolysis after acetabular trauma can occur with or without surgical intervention; it may lead to early osteoarthritis. After ORIF, the surgeon must suspect infection or metal in the joint. Occasionally, avascular necrosis of acetabular fragments causes early collapse and chondrolysis may ensue. Causative factors are:

- injury related (the amount of articular damage to the femoral head or acetabulum, the development of avascular necrosis, or the onset of other complications)
- surgeon related (whether reduction is adequate and iatrogenic complications exist).

Fractures with hip instability or significant incongruity, especially posterior types, high transverse or T types involving the dome, or fractures with a triangular dome fragment, require accurate open reduction and stable internal fixation allowing early motion. If anatomical reduction is achieved and complications are avoided, good to excellent results can be expected.

References

Baumgaertner MR (1999) Fractures of the posterior wall of the acetabulum. *Journal of the American Academy of Orthopedic Surgeons* 7(1): 54–65.

Burgess AR, Eastridge BJ, Young JW *et al.* (1990) Pelvic ring disruptions: Effective classification system and treatment protocols. *Journal of Trauma* 30: 848–856.

Duwelius PJ, Moed BR, Olson SA. Templeman DC (1998) *Surgical approach to acetabular fractures.* Instructional Course Lecture 463, American Academy of Orthopaedic Surgeons, New Orleans.

Helfet DL (1997) Acetabular fractures: surgical approaches and technique. In: Sledge CB (ed.) *The Hip. Master techniques in orthopedic surgery*. Lippincott-Raven, Philadelphia, Pa., pp. 73–91.

Judet R, Judet J, Letournel E (1964) Fractures of the acetabulum: classification and surgical approaches for open reduction. *Journal of Bone and Joint Surgery* 46A: 1615–1646.

Letournel E, Judet R (ed.) (1993) *Fractures of the acetabulum*. Springer-Verlag, Berlin.

Levine A (1996) *Orthopedic knowledge update: Trauma*. AAOS, Rosemont, Illinois, pp. 241–251.

Matta JM, Mehne DF, Roffi R (1994) Operative management of acetabular fractures through the ilioinguinal approach: a 10 year prospective. *Clinical Orthopedics* 305: 10–19.

McMinn RMH (1994) *Last's Anatomy, Regional and Applied*, 9th edn. Churchill Livingstone, Edinburgh, UK, pp. 413–420.

Müller ME, Allgöwer M, Schnieder P *et al.* (1990) *AO Manual of Internal Fixation*, 3rd edn. Springer-Verlag, Heidelberg.

Tile M (1988) Pelvic ring fractures :should they be fixed? *Journal of Bone and Joint Surgery* 70B: 1–12.

Tile M (1996a) Acute pelvic fracture—causation and classification. *Journal of the American Academy of Orthopedic Surgeons* 4: 143–151.

Tile M (1996b) Acute pelvic fracture—principles of management. *Journal of the American Academy of Orthopedic Surgeons* 4: 152–161.

Wiss DA (ed.) (1998) *Fractures. Master Techniques in Orthopaedic Surgery*, Chapters 35–42. Lippincott-Raven, Philadelphia.

Wiss DA (1999) Trauma: orthopaedic review course. *AAOS 66th Annual Meeting*, Anaheim, California, pp. 1–2.

21

CHAPTER 21

Hip and femur fractures

EUGENE SHERRY AND
KEVIN SMITH

CHAPTER 21
Hip and femur fractures

EUGENE SHERRY AND KEVIN SMITH

Fractures of the femur are relatively common, with diaphyseal injuries occurring in the younger age group and fractures of the hip and distal metaphysis predominating in elderly people. Fortunately, most of the bone has a good blood supply and most fractures are amenable to surgical fixation.

Fractures of the proximal femur (hip)

Broadly speaking, there are two types of fractures—intracapsular and extracapsular. Their incidence is increasing with the increase in the elderly population, and is predominately due to age-related osteopenia and increased susceptibility to falls. The risk may be reduced by exercise, quitting smoking, avoiding sedatives, reducing caffeine intake, treating impaired vision, maintaining bone density (postmenopausal women should consider hormonal replacement and calcium supplements), and reducing home hazards (Cauley *et al.* 1995, Cummings *et al.* 1995).

Intracapsular hip fractures

The anatomy is important. The proximal femoral epiphysis fuses at age 16 (skeletal maturity). The neck shaft angle is $130 \pm 7°$, anteversion $10 \pm 7°$ (Turen 1996). The calcar is the posteromedial portion of the upper femur and critical for the mechanical stability of this region. The blood supply of the femoral head is critical and vulnerable, accounting for the complications of fractures in this region as a result of avascular necrosis (AVN) and non-union. The femoral head is principally supplied by the medial and lateral femoral circumflex arteries, with a contribution from the gluteal arteries, forming an extracapsular arterial ring at the base of the neck. The major branch of this arterial ring is the lateral epiphyseal artery, which runs in the posterior retinaculum and to a large extent supplies the femoral head.

A fracture of the femoral neck disrupts this blood supply to the head to a varying extent depending upon the degree of displacement. In marked displacement there is a tear of the posterior retinaculum, but if the displacement is less, the expanding haematoma may cause a problem because of tamponade.

Evaluation

Symptoms may be mild, especially in the older patient, if there is impaction or incomplete displacement. Otherwise there is hip or groin pain with shortening and external rotation of the leg. The multiple trauma patient must be carefully evaluated for such injuries.

Radiography

Standard anteroposterior hip and a cross-table lateral radiographs are required, to adequately assess both the injury and degree of displacement. Sometimes the fracture is not obvious and a bone scan, CT, or MRI is required.

Classification

Garden's classification remains the gold standard (Fig. 21.1). Types I and II are non-displaced with a low rate of subsequent AVN, with the converse being true for types III and IV. Pauwel's system is based on the angle between the fracture line and the horizontal after reduction, and reflects stability, not displacement.

Treatment

The aim of treatment is restoration of function. This should entail reduction and fixation of fractures in patients who are relatively fit with a reasonable life

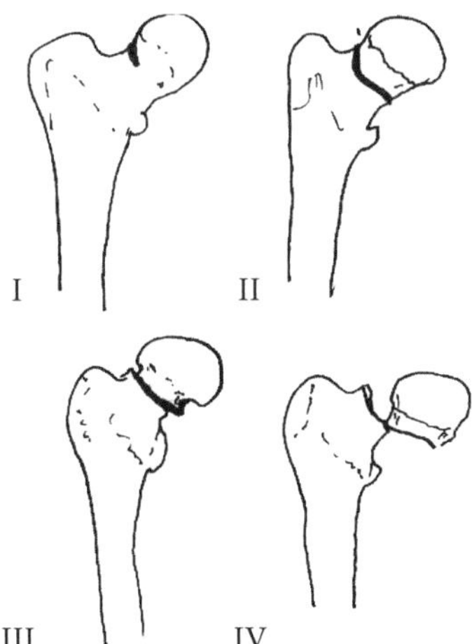

Figure 21.1 Garden's classification of intracapsular hip fractures: type I, incomplete; type II, complete, non-displaced; type III, displaced but <50%; type IV, complete and >50%.

expectancy. Elderly or infirm patients with displaced fractures are usually treated by hemiarthroplasty using an uncemented prosthesis (e.g. Austin-Moore), though undisplaced fractures may still be fixed.

Non-displaced or minimally displaced fractures have a lower risk of AVN and non-union than displaced fractures. These risks are higher in younger patients with displaced fractures, reflecting the magnitude of the injury.

It is important to achieve a good reduction to avoid failure of fixation and subsequent AVN.

Key point

- The adequacy of reduction and the density of the head and neck are the key features determining stability after fixation.

Methods available for reduction and fixation include gentle manipulation under image intensifier (II) control, followed by fixation with either three parallel cannulated screws or a compression screw plate device, placing a large compression screw in middle of the head on both anteroposterior and lateral views, supplemented with a 4.5 mm screw in the superior head for rotational control.

If the decision is made not to reduce and fix, then a hemiarthroplasty can be performed, usually in a Garden III or IV fracture in an elderly unfit patient.

Total hip replacement should be reserved for cases of delayed treatment in patients otherwise suitable for reduction and fixation, and in cases where there is significant pre-existing degenerative change in the hip joint. This is relatively rare. It may also be the treatment of choice when there is rheumatoid arthritis, renal failure, or metastatic disease.

Key point

- If the decision is made to reduce and fix the fracture, this should be done as soon as possible (Swiontkowski 1994).

Ipsilateral hip and femoral shaft fractures

In this special situation, use an intramedullary (IM) nail with provision for oblique screws to be placed up the femoral neck (reconstruction nail) or consider an IM nail with cannulated cancellous screws placed in front of and behind the nail.

Authors' preferred technique

- *Garden I and II fractures:* Proceed to three parallel cannulated screws using a percutaneous technique. Consider performing an anterior capsulotomy to decompress the haemarthrosis.
- *Garden III and IV fractures:* If the patient is fit, reduce and fix as above. If unfit or demented, perform an hemiarthroplasty.
- In young patients, preserve the femoral head at all costs. This will entail an emergency reduction and fixation.
- In patients who are demented and non-ambulatory with a valgus impaction fracture, consider non-operative management, though there is a risk of subsequent displacement.

Complications

- AVN may occur in a significant proportion of cases and may ultimately require prosthetic replacement if symptomatic degenerative changes develops.
- Non-union can be treated by either refixation or grafting or prosthetic replacement.
- Other complications include infection, dislocation, and deep vein thrombosis (DVT).

Key point

- Early adequate reduction is the key to reducing the risk of AVN.

Femoral head fractures

Fractures of the femoral head usually occur in high-energy injuries in the younger patient, often associated with a dislocation of the hip joint. Loss of congruency of the femoral head may result in premature degenerative change. CT is the most useful imaging modality.

Classification

Pipkin (1957) devised the following classification for fractures associated with posterior dislocations:

- *type 1:* fracture caudad to fovea centralis
- *type 2:* fracture cephalad to fovea centralis
- *type 3:* type 1 or 2 with associated femoral neck fracture
- *type 4:* type 1,2 or 3 with associated acetabular fracture.

Treatment

Treatment of these fractures is dictated by their type:

- *Type 1:* Primary closed reduction followed by 6 weeks in traction with range of motion exercises. If the fragment blocks reduction of the hip joint it must be excised via a small arthrotomy.
- *Type 2:* Primary closed reduction of the joint followed by CT scan to determine adequacy of reduction of the fragment. If inadequate, open reduction and internal fixation (ORIF) should be performed although this is a complex undertaking even for experienced hip surgeons.
- *Type 3:* In younger patients the femoral neck fracture should be fixed and the head fracture dealt with by either fixation or excision depending on its size. In elderly patients, consider primary prosthetic replacement.
- *Type 4:* Primary consideration is given to the acetabular fracture, with the femoral head fracture being dealt with subsequently as previously described.

Key points

- In young patients where there is a fracture of the femoral head and neck, urgent ORIF is required.
- All patients should have post-reduction CT to assess adequacy of reduction.

Extracapsular (intertrochanteric) hip fractures

Most extracapsular hip fractures require ORIF (Koval 1998). Stability must be obtained, ideally by restoring the posteromedial buttress. Unstable fracture patterns are seen where there is loss of this buttress, subtrochanteric extension of the fracture, or a reverse oblique fracture pattern.

Evaluation

Patients may present in severe pain with shortening and external rotation of the leg, but this may be absent if there is minimal displacement.

Radiographs

Standard anteroposterior hip and cross-table lateral radiographs are required, sometimes augmented with a 15° internal rotation view.

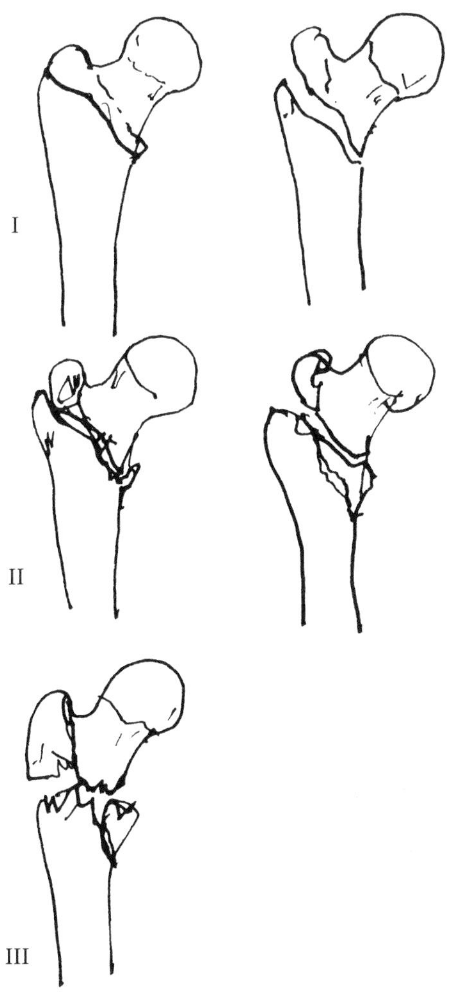

Figure 21.2 Evans–Jensen classification of intertrochanteric fractures: type I, stable, two-part; type II, unstable, three-part; type III, very unstable, four-part.

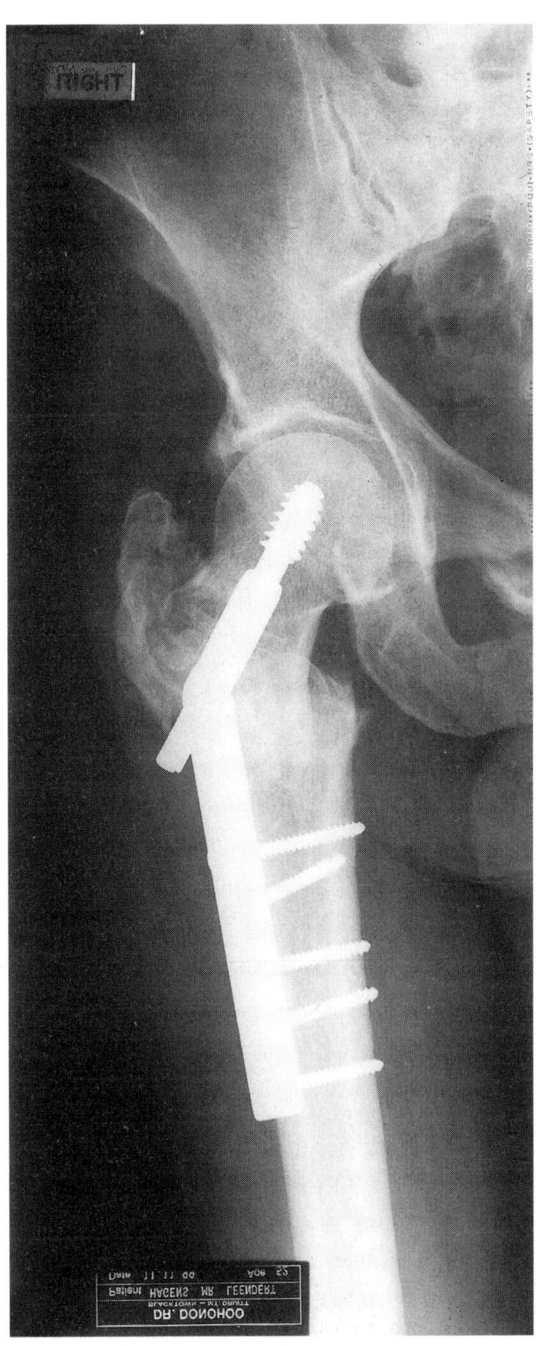

Figure 21.3 Sliding hip screw in 56 year old man.

Classification

The Evans–Jensen system (Evans 1949, Jensen 1980) is the best one to use (Fig. 21.2).

Treatment

The surgical options are either an IM device such as the Gamma nail, or a sliding hip screw system such as the dynamic hip screw (DHS) (Fig. 21.3).

Authors' preferred technique: sliding hip screw

Place the patient on fracture table and achieve reduction by applying traction with the leg internally rotated. Check the reduction in two orthogonal planes using II. The fracture may require additional manipulation to obtain reduction.

Access to the proximal femur is gained via a straight lateral approach, through the iliotibial band, splitting vastus lateralis and ligating the perforating branches of the femoral artery. Using a 135° jig, a guide wire is introduced into the middle of the femoral head, stopping 5 mm from the subchondral bone in both AP and lateral views using II. A second parallel wire should be introduced superiorly to prevent rotation during reaming, tapping and screw insertion. The appropriate length screw is selected. A reamer is used to create the appropriate shaped hole and the screw is introduced after tapping. A 135° plate is then applied over the screw (short barrel if screw <80 mm). This plate is then loosely clamped to the femoral shaft, traction is released to allow some impaction, and the plate fixed using cortical screws. A compression set screw may be added to initiate compression but should be removed.

Key point

- Do not place a screw in the anterosuperior part of the femoral head.

Other situations

- In unstable fracture patterns, in a younger patient, one may consider reduction of the posteromedial fragment with a lag screw, to prevent excessive screw-barrel slide and consequent limb shortening.
- Basicervical fractures, with fracture lines proximal to or at the intertrochanteric line, may require a supplementary cancellous antirotation screw, parallel to the lag screw.
- Subtrochanteric extension of the fracture requires the use of a longer plate or a 95° sliding screw plate.
- A displaced greater trochanter may be reattached using either a cerclage wire or trochanteric capture plate.

Postoperative treatment

Postoperative weight-bearing is dictated by the stability of the fixation, but protected as pain allows is the norm. Prophylaxis against DVT may be used, with a recent multinational study suggesting that aspirin is a suitably efficacious agent. Mortality in the first year after hip fracture may be as high as 40%. If the fixation fails it may be revised or replaced by a 95° sliding screw device and bone grafting.

Subtrochanteric femoral fractures

Subtrochanteric fractures are potentially problematic as this region is subject to large bending stresses. The presence of cortical rather than cancellous, metaphyseal bone may also mean that fractures take longer to unite. Fixation is more technically demanding than for intertrochanteric fractures. The initial evaluation, however, is the same as stated above.

Key points

- Subtrochanteric fractures are problematic because of high bending stresses in this region and the presence of cortical bone (slow to heal).
- Aim for anatomical alignment, not anatomical reduction (Wiss 1999).

Classification

These fractures are described regarding their position relative to the lesser trochanter, their degree of comminution and their displacement. A commonly used classification is that of Russell-Taylor (Garden 1974):

- 1A: lesser trochanter intact.
- 1B: lesser trochanter involved.

- 2A: fracture extends from lesser trochanter towards the isthmus, with a secondary extension into the piriformis fossa.
- 2B: fracture extending to the greater trochanter, with comminution of the medial cortex.

Treatment

Fractures at or above the lesser trochanter can be fixed using either a 95° dynamic compression screw (DCS) plate (a two-piece screw/plate system easier to use than the 95° blade plate), or a second-generation reconstruction IM nail.

A standard interlocking nail can be used if the fracture is below the level of the lesser trochanter, but this does place the implant at a mechanical disadvantage.

Complications

Delayed union, malunion, non-union, infection, and fixation failure are seen. Related factors are inadequate ORIF, involvement of posteromedial cortex, inappropriate weight-bearing, and extension into the intertrochanteric region.

Femoral shaft fractures

It is generally accepted that fractures of the femoral diaphysis are best treated by a reamed locked IM nail.

Evaluation

Obvious shortening, rotation, or angulation of the femur may be present. These are usually high-energy injuries so the patient should be managed along ATLS guidelines to exclude life-threatening and pelvic or hip injuries, especially hip dislocation. Thorough neurovascular assessment is required, as is haemodynamic monitoring as even closed injuries may account for a loss of 2–3 units of blood.

Authors' preferred technique

- Consider ORIF using a 95° DCS plate in cases where the fracture is subtrochanteric but above the lesser trochanter, where there is marked comminution or where there is reverse obliquity of fracture. Note that it can be difficult to place an IM nail after adducting the leg on the traction table with the patient supine. (Fig 21.4). Preoperative planning is useful with three-dimensional reconstruction CT. The entry point landmark is lateral and proximal to the most prominent part of greater trochanter, allowing placement of the lag screw in inferior half of the head. The patient should be supine on the fracture table. II is required. Using the direct lateral approach, as described above, place the guide wires using the 95° jig. After appropriate reaming, insert the lag screw, apply the plate to shaft and reduce shaft fragments onto plate. Final fixation to plate is achieved using cortical screws: 8–10 cortices are recommended below the fracture. Autogenous bone grafting to the area of the medial buttress may be considered. Weight-bearing should be protected until callus is visible.
- Second-generation reconstruction nail (Smith & Nephew) (Russell 1998): This device is recommended for fractures involving the lesser trochanter but not the greater trochanter, as the latter may compromise the proximal locking device. The patient is placed supine on traction and the leg adducted. The distal leg is rotated to realign with the upper femur (15° anteversion, up to 30° in Asians). A direct lateral approach is used. The entry point is 3 mm anterior to piriformis fossa. Use a guide-pin, overream the guide pin, then insert a bent-tip, 3.2 mm guide wire to gain access to the femoral canal. Adjust the leg position to reduce the fracture. Advance the guide wire across the fracture and then ream over the guide wire. Insert the nail with the jig attached. Align the proximal locking holes with the femoral head in the correct anteversion. Distal locking is obligatory and best done by a freehand technique. Protected weight-bearing is recommended until evidence of union is apparent, in an effort to minimize implant failure.

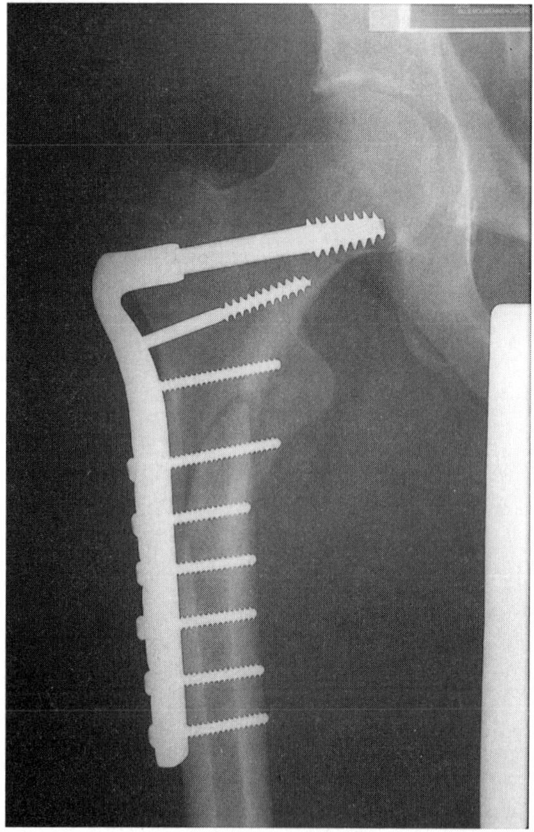

Figure 21.4 ORIF with 95° DCS plate for subtrochanteric fracture with reverse obliquity (type III, three part).

Key point

- Exclude life-threatening and pelvic/hip injuries (especially hip dislocation).

Classification

The standard classification is that of Winquist and Hansen (1984) (Fig. 21.5).

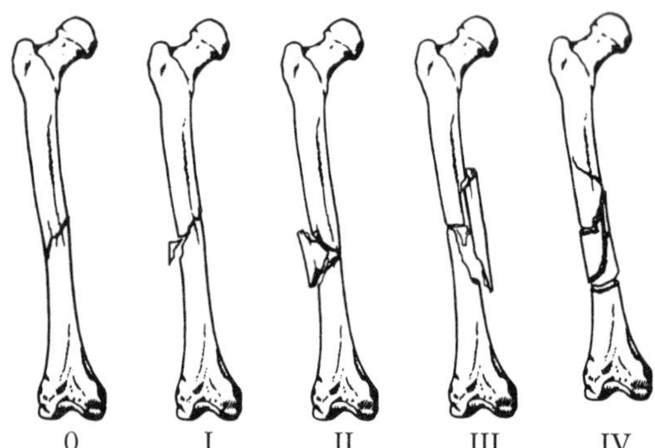

Figure 21.5 Winquist classification of femoral shaft fractures: type I, transverse <25% butterfly; type II, transverse 25–50% butterfly; type III, >50% comminution, unstable; type IV, extensive comminution, no cortical contact, unstable; V, segmental bone loss, unstable. Types I and II are stable; III and IV are comminuted and unstable. (Reproduced with permission from Poss R (ed.) (1990) *Orthopedic Knowledge Update 3*. AAOS, Park Ridge, Illinois, pp. 513–527.)

Treatment

Traction

Although traction is still safe and predictable, a prolonged stay in hospital is required. This is expensive, and also exposes the patient to the risks of prolonged recumbency. It is best reserved for those not suitable for ORIF, or where the equipment or expertise to fix is not available. Use skeletal traction with later cast-brace. There are associated problems of shortening, malrotation, and knee stiffness.

External fixation

External fixation is rarely indicated. It is used mainly in cases where ORIF is not feasible or if there is a severe open fracture. Pin tract problems are frequent.

Plating

Plating is now seldom performed, but may be useful when IM nailing is not possible. It may be suitable in children to stabilize the femur in the presence of associated vascular, pelvic, or hip injuries. Use a direct lateral approach.

Intramedullary nail

The use of an IM nail is regarded as the best technique, allowing early mobilization, thus avoiding prolonged hospitalization and knee or hip stiffness. Most shaft fractures are best nailed using a closed, reamed, statically locked system. The nail will only need to be dynamized if evidence occurs of delayed union. The operation should be carried out within 24 hours once critical conditions such as head or chest injuries have been optimized. The most commonly used method uses an antegrade approach with the patient supine on a traction table. Image intensification is mandatory. Some use the femoral distractor to both reduce and hold the femur during nailing.

- Unreamed nails are slower to heal, although offering a reduced surgical time. They may also be prone to implant failure.
- In adolescents, one may consider using flexible retrograde nails, inserted proximal to the distal femoral growth plate.
- There may be an increased incidence of infection if nailing is performed after external fixation.
- Open fractures require urgent debridement and intravenous antibiotics and stabilization by insertion of a reamed nail.
- Expanding nails (eg the SWEL nail) which do not require cross-locking screws, will be the way of the future to reduce operating time and so radiation exposure.

Special situations

Ipsilateral neck and shaft fractures

The neck fracture should be stabilized with screws then nailed, or a second-generation (reconstruction) nail used. This is a difficult technique.

Gunshot wounds

The wounds should be aggressively debrided and stabilized using a locked nail. Sequential debridement may be required. Stabilizing the skeleton affords the best environment for soft tissue healing.

Adolescents

The use of a plate, external fixation, or retrograde flexible nailing should be considered. If a standard IM nailing technique is used, care should be taken to avoid the proximal and distal growth plates. A direct lateral approach should be used.

Vascular injuries

The aim is to stabilize the fracture, ideally with a nail or plate, and then perform the vascular repair. Some vascular surgeons would advocate initial vascular shunting to reduce ischaemic time.

Authors' preferred technique

- Patient supine or lateral decubitus.
- Measure the appropriate length from either the other limb or a standardized radiograph. Use of the fracture table is recommended.
- Reduce fracture using traction and a reduction device, such as the F-bar, if necessary.
- The incision should be gently curved posteriorly as it progresses proximally from the greater trochanter, to account for the anterior femoral bow when introducing the guidewire, reamers, and the nail.
- Entry point is centred on canal in both projections (use a curved awl). Then pass T-shaped awl.
- Insert guide wire, check with image intensification in two planes to make sure it is in distal shaft, ream, and exchange with straight wire via a plastic sheath for insertion of nail.
- Lock proximally. This will be either transversely or diagonally, depending upon the system used.
- Freehand distal lock (Kirschner wire centred on hole, indent, then drill).

Complications

Fat emboli and adult respiratory distress syndrome (ARDS) can be associated with reaming, but one can still proceed with an immediate reamed nail in the presence of a chest injury, in order to stabilize the fracture and reduce the risk of further pulmonary complications.

Infection

Infection is unusual after IM nailing, with rates ideally <1%. If it occurs, it may be treated by debridement, antibiotics, and exchange nailing, with over- reaming of the medullary canal to clear infected granulation and fibrous tissue. A larger-diameter nail is usually then inserted to maintain stability.

Non-union

There is an incidence of <1%. Initial treatment is by exchange nailing.

Malunion

Malunion can either be corrected early or by a corrective osteotomy later. Newer alternatives include the use of circular frames and callotasis.

Other complications

Compartment syndrome in the thigh is rare, as is nerve injury from traction or positioning on the table. Heterotopic ossification may occur adjacent to the entry point.

Supracondylar femoral fractures (fractures of the distal metaphysis)

Supracondylar femoral fractures are either high-energy fractures in the distal 9 cm of the femur in young adults, or the result of relatively minor trauma in elderly people. There may be shortening with varus or posterior angulation.

Anatomy

The medial condyle is larger in the anteroposterior plane than the lateral and extends further distally. The condylar block is trapezoidal (the posterior aspect is wider than the anterior aspect). The shaft joins with the anterior half of the condyles. The anatomic axis is 9°and the mechanical is 3°. It is important to be aware the close relationship of the popliteal neurovascular bundle, and always to check for associated injuries.

Classification

In the AO classification this is area 3.3. It is further subdivided into A (extraarticular), B (unicondylar), and C (bicondylar). These groups can again be further subdivided into smaller subsections.

Treatment

These fractures usually require reduction and fixation, with non-operative management reserved for impacted or undisplaced fractures in the elderly, which may be treated in a plaster cast. The newer IM devices can be used in elderly patients where osteopenia would have previously precluded internal fixation.

Key point

- Surgery must not be delayed in open injuries and should be immediate if there is associated vascular compromise or compartment syndrome.

Author's preferred technique: dynamic compression screw

- The DCS system is still preferred for most cases.
- At least 4 cm of intact medial femoral condyle is needed for the 6.5 mm cancellous screw.
- A straight lateral approach should be used, on a radiolucent table.
- The knee joint is opened, and guide wires placed along distal and anterior condylar surfaces as guides.
- The condylar articular fragments are reduced first and fixed with cancellous lag screws and the condylar segment then reduced to the shaft.
- Using the 95° plate as a guide, the lag screw is inserted parallel to the articular surface and the plate then applied and fixed.
- Protected weight-bearing should be observed for 8 weeks.

Open reduction and internal fixation

- ORIF can be difficult surgery (Wiss 1999).
- The aim is to restore anatomy and joint congruency if there is an intra-articular component to the fracture.

The techniques recommended are a 95° DCS plate, augmented with bone graft where necessary, or a retrograde IM locked nail (supracondylar nail).

Retrograde IM locked nail

The retrograde IM locked nail (supracondylar nail) is a good technique (Seligson 1998) (Fig. 21.6). It is not as difficult as might be expected, though not so useful if there is distal articular comminution as in a type C fracture, unless one is prepared to perform open reduction of joint surfaces. The fracture can usually be reduced by manual traction with the knee flexed over a bolster. II is required, so a radiolucent table should be used. The portal of entry is the intercondylar notch, which is approached via a 3 cm vertical skin incision over the patellar tendon, which is either split in the line of its fibres or retracted

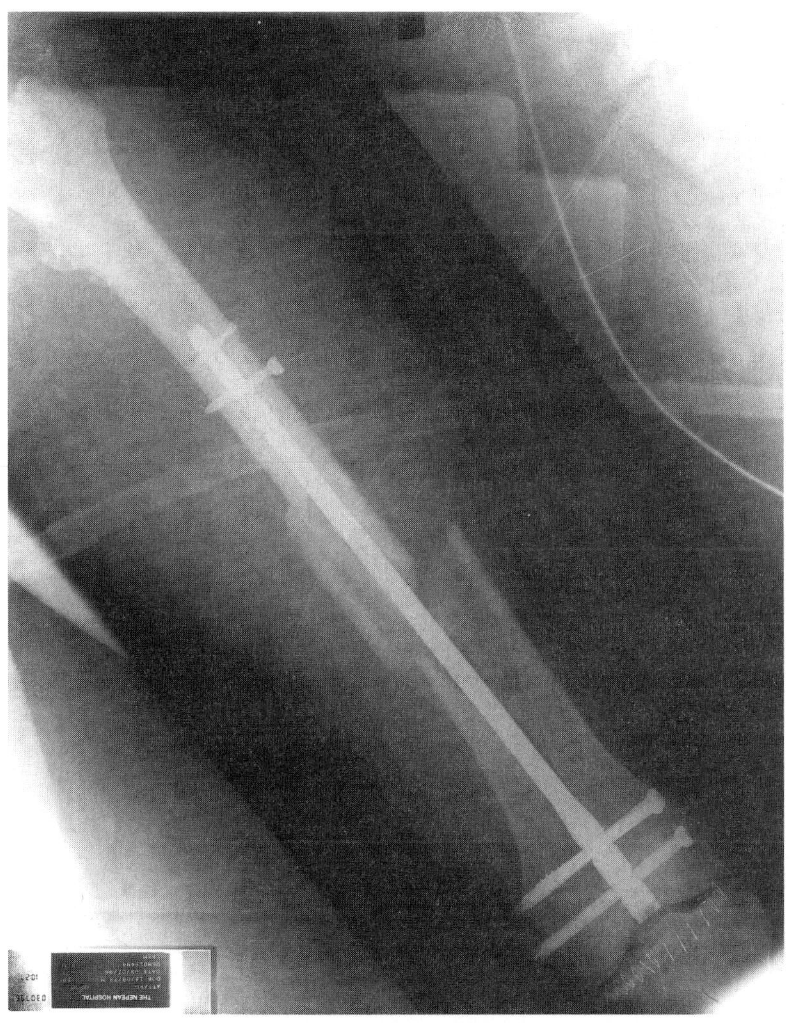

Figure 21.6 Retrograde IM locked nail (supracondylar nail).

laterally. An awl is used to gain access to the canal, then the guide wire is passed across the fracture. After minimal reaming the nail is gently inserted. Proximal and distal locking is accomplished using the jig provided.

Complications

Complications include infection and non-union rates of up to 6% with a lower incidence of malunion and implant failure. Postoperative knee stiffness may be prolonged, but usually responds to physiotherapy.

References

Cauley JA, Seeley DG, Ensrud K *et al.* (1995) Estrogen replacement therapy and fractures in older women. *Annals of Internal Medicine* 122: 9–16.

Cummings SR, Black DM, Nevitt MC *et al.* (1995) Risk factors for hip fracture in white women. *New England Journal of Medicine* 332: 767–773.

Evans EM (1949) The treatment of trochanteric fractures of the femur. *Journal of Bone and Joint Surgery* 31B: 190.

Garden RS (1974) Reduction and fixation of the subcapital fractures of the femur. *Orthopedic Clinics of North America* 5: 683–712.

Jensen JS (1980) Classification of trochanteric fractures. *Acta Orthopaedica Scandinavica* 51: 803.

Koval KJ (1998) Intertrochanteric hip fractures: sliding hip screw. In: Wiss DA (ed.) *Fractures. Master Techniques in Orthopedic Surgery*. Lippincott-Raven, Philadelphia, pp. 223–241.

Pipkin G (1957) Treatment of grade IV fracture dislocation of the hip. A review. *Journal of Bone and Joint Surgery* 39A: 1027–1042.

Poss R (ed.) (1990) *Orthopedic Knowledge Update 3*. AAOS, Park Ridge, Illinois, pp. 513–527.

Russell TA (1998) Subtrochanteric femur fractures: reconstruction nailing. In: Wiss DA (ed.) *Fractures. Master Techniques in Orthopaedic Surgery*. Lippincott-Raven, Philadelphia, pp. 255–272.

Seligson D (1998) Supracondylar femur fractures: IM nailing. In: Wiss DA (ed.) *Fractures. Master Techniques in Orthopaedic Surgery*. Lippincott-Raven, Philadelphia, pp. 321–334.

Swiontkowski MF (1994) Intracapsular fractures of the hip. *Journal of Bone and Joint Surgery* 76: 129–138.

Turen CH (1996) Intracapsular hip fractures. In: Levine AM (ed.) *Orthopedic knowledge update: Trauma*. AAOS, Rosemont, Illinois, pp. 113–119.

Winquist RA, Hansen ST, Clawson DK (1984) Close IM nailing of femoral fractures: a report of 520 fractures. *Journal of Bone and Joint Surgery* 66A(4).

Wiss DA (1999) Trauma: orthopaedic review course. *AAOS 66th Annual Meeting*, Anaheim, California, pp. 1–2.

22

CHAPTER 22

Knee and tibial injuries

RHIDIAN MORGAN-JONES, JAYNATH SUNDAR SAMPATH, AND BALAKRISHNAN ILANGO

CHAPTER 22

Knee and tibial injuries

RHIDIAN MORGAN-JONES, JAYNATH SUNDAR SAMPATH, AND BALAKRISHNAN ILANGO

Bony injuries

Fractures of the patella

Fractures of the patella constitute 1% of all skeletal injuries and occur mostly between 20 and 50 years of age (Bostrom 1972). The functional significance of the patella was poorly understood in the past, leading to wide variations in the management of patellar fractures.

Anatomy

The patella is the largest sesamoid bone in the body and lies within the quadriceps tendon. It is triangular in shape, with a broad proximal pole. The quadriceps muscle and most of the aponeurosis insert into the superior aspect of the patella. The narrow distal pole gives origin to the patellar tendon. The blood supply to the patella is through an anastomotic ring of vessels that enter the bone through the middle and distal pole. With displaced transverse fractures, the proximal pole is at risk of avascular necrosis. The medial and lateral extensor retinacula are extensions of the quadriceps on either side of the patella.

Biomechanics

The patella improves the mechanical advantage of the extensor mechanism by elevating it from the axis of knee motion. It helps nourish the anterior articular cartilage of the femur and protects it from direct injury.

Key point

- The patella improves the mechanical advantage of the extensor mechanism.

Mechanism of injury

Patellar fractures may be caused by direct or indirect forces. Direct injuries include a fall on the knee or a direct blow to the anterior surface and commonly cause undisplaced, comminuted fractures. In contrast, displaced transverse fractures are caused by strong eccentric contraction of the quadriceps in a partly flexed knee during a fall; the patella failing in tension. Transverse fractures are associated with rupture of the medial and lateral quadriceps expansions.

Signs and symptoms

The patient collapses on to the knee and is unable to bear weight on the affected side. There is painful swelling of the knee and a defect may be palpable anteriorly. Active extension of the knee against gravity is restricted or abolished. In direct injuries that result in undisplaced fractures, the retinacula are frequently intact, and active straight leg-raising is possible. Patellar fractures are associated with a painful haemarthrosis that may require aspiration.

Classification

Fractures of the patella can be transverse, comminuted, displaced, undisplaced, polar, or vertical. Osteochondral fractures involving the medial facet of the patella can occur following lateral dislocation of the patella (Hammerle and Jocob

1980). Transverse fractures are the most common type and account for 50–80% of fractures. Vertical or marginal fractures result from direct injuries.

Key point

- Classification—transverse, comminuted, displaced, undisplaced, polar, or vertical.

Investigations

Anteroposterior and lateral radiographs of the knee are sufficient for most fractures. Skyline views may be obtained to demonstrate vertical fractures. The accessory ossification centre in the superolateral pole of the patella occasionally fails to unite with the rest of the bone. This is called a *bipartite patella*, which may be mistaken for a vertical fracture.

Key point

- Note the accessory ossification centre in the superolateral pole of the patella.

Management

The goals of treatment are to restore continuity of the extensor mechanism of the knee and preserve the function of the patella.

Non-operative treatment

Undisplaced fractures with preserved extensor mechanism function are treated non-operatively (Braun *et al.* 1993). A tense haemarthrosis can cause considerable discomfort, and is aspirated under sterile conditions (Carpenter *et al.* 1993). A cylinder cast or extension brace is applied and the patient is allowed to bear full weight as tolerated, with crutches for support. Cast immobilization is maintained for 4–6 weeks. Early quadriceps exercises and straight-leg raises are essential for an optimal functional result.

Operative treatment

Open reduction with internal fixation (ORIF) is required in displaced fractures (Bostman *et al.* 1981). Partial patellectomy is performed if there is significant comminution and a portion of the patella is sacrificed to restore articular continuity (Hugh *et al.* 1993). Total patellectomy is reserved for highly displaced comminuted fractures (Jakobsen *et al.* 1985), but should be avoided if at all possible. Surgery is recommended if the displacement is >2–3 mm in transverse fractures. Osteochondral fragments require anatomic reduction and internal fixation.

The universally accepted operative technique is tension band wiring that incorporates an anterior tension band with cerclage wiring (Curtis 1990). Two Kirschner wires placed across the fracture site provides rotational stability. This may be supplemented by 4 mm AO cancellous lag screws. The construct converts tension forces into compressive forces, dynamically closing the fracture site with knee flexion (Thakur 1997). Transverse and distal pole fractures are ideally suited for this method. In comminuted fractures, small fragments may be removed to restore articular continuity.

Authors' recommended treatment

We prefer tension band wiring for displaced fractures and cast immobilization for undisplaced fractures. The wire is inserted in a figure-of-eight configuration with double loops on either side of the fracture for equal compression.

Postoperative care

Early rehabilitation with partial weight-bearing is recommended after stable internal fixation, and this is continued for at least 6 weeks.

Complications

Complications associated frequently with patellar fractures are persistent anterior knee pain and loss of motion in the patellofemoral joint. This leads to early arthritis in the patellofemoral compartment and non-unions (in 'neglected' fractures or failure of fixation following surgery).

Acute dislocation of the patella

Acute dislocation of the patella is a relatively rare injury and usually occurs in the lateral direction. The mechanism of injury is internal rotation of the femur on an externally rotated tibia, in a weight-bearing partially flexed knee. The medial retinaculum ruptures and the patella is forced over the edge of the lateral femoral condyle (Morscher 1971).

On examination, an obvious mass is seen over the lateral aspect of the knee and an associated haemarthrosis. The patient complains of pain over the medial retinaculum and cannot flex the knee. The patella is relocated under intravenous anaesthesia or nitrous oxide and oxygen analgesia. The haemarthrosis is aspirated, carefully looking for fat globules on the surface of the aspirate. The presence of lipohaemarthrosis should raise a strong suspicion of an osteochondral fracture. If the patella has relocated spontaneously before the patient presents to hospital, the clinical picture is limited to medial pain and a haemarthrosis. In late presentations, there may be a history of locking and buckling of the knee due to an osteochondral loose body within the joint. Radiographs of the knee must include tangential and tunnel views to exclude associated osteochondral fractures of the lateral femoral condyle or the medial facet of the patella.

The knee is placed in a cylinder cast or extension brace for 3–4 weeks, and quadriceps strengthening exercises are started (Cofield and Bryan 1977). Full restoration of flexion can be expected by 6 weeks. If an osteochondral fragment is present, immediate arthroscopic evaluation must be carried out. Depending on size and location, an excision or operative repair is carried out. Operative repair of the medial retinaculum or arthroscopic release of the lateral retinaculum is required only in cases that progress to recurrent patellar subluxation.

Key point

- The patella is relocated under intravenous anaesthesia or nitrous oxide and oxygen analgesia.
- History of dislocations.

Tibial plateau fractures

Fractures of the tibial plateau account for 1% of all fractures, rising to 8% in the elderly population. Reported series show that the great majority of these injuries affect the lateral tibial plateau (55–70%) (Wiss and Tracy Watson 1996). Isolated injuries to medial plateau account for 10–20% and fractures that involve both condyles (bicondylar fractures) are, fortunately, less frequent. These fractures cover a broad spectrum of injuries, ranging from low-energy patterns in elderly people that respond well with non-operative treatment to high-energy trauma in young adults that merits aggressive management (Blokker *et al.* 1984).

Anatomy and biomechanics

The tibia is the major weight-bearing bone in the leg. The tibial shaft expands in its proximal portion into the medial and lateral tibial condyles or plateaux. The proximal fibula acts as a buttress to the lateral tibial condyle and the fibular shaft merely provides attachment to the muscles in the leg. The tibial condyles are lined with articular cartilage and covered in their periphery by the menisci. The proximal tibia and fibula provide attachment to the collateral and cruciate ligaments of the knee, thus playing a crucial role in ensuring knee stability. Any injury to the proximal tibia is therefore likely to affect the stability and function of the knee joint.

Mechanism of injury

Fractures of the tibial plateau occur as a result of a large valgus or varus force combined with axial loading (Kennedy and Bailey 1968). The femoral condyle is driven into the tibial plateau by compressive and shear forces. This results in a split fracture, a depressed articular fragment, or both. Split fractures are common in young adults and depressed fractures are seen in elderly people. This is related to the quality of the cancellous bone in the proximal tibia (Koval and Helfet 1995). Common mechanisms include fall from a height, motor vehicle accidents, and sports injuries.

Classification

The Schatzker classification is the most widely used (Fig. 22.1). All fractures are grouped into six types

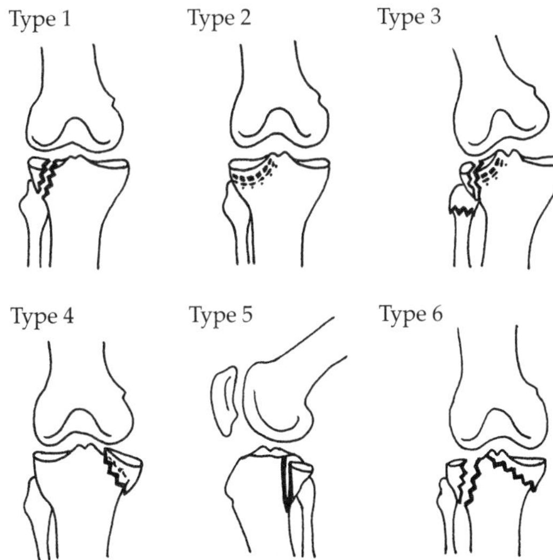

Figure 22.1 Schatzker classification of tibial plateau fracture (see text for details).

in increasing order of severity (Schatzker *et al.* 1979, Schatzker 1987):

Type 1: A split fracture of the lateral tibial plateau, without articular depression. If the fragment is displaced, there may be associated soft tissue disruption such as a lateral meniscal tear.

Type 2: A split-depressed fracture of the lateral tibial plateau. It occurs in a slightly older age-group than the split fractures.

Type 3: A pure depression of the lateral tibial plateau. The depressed fragment is usually central. Lateral and posterior depressions are associated with a greater degree of instability at the knee joint. All of the above patterns are caused by valgus forces.

Type 4: A fracture of the medial tibial plateau. It results from a varus force acting on an axially loaded knee.

Type 5: Bicondylar fractures of the tibia are the result of high-energy trauma with significant disruption of soft tissues around the affected knee. This renders early operative intervention risky and technically difficult. The usual pattern is a split fracture of the medial tibial plateau combined with a type 1 or 2 injury.

Type 6: A bicondylar fracture of the tibia with metaphyseal-diaphyseal dissociation. It usually results from high-energy injuries and has been described as an 'explosive' fracture.

The neurovascular status of the limb has to be closely monitored as there is a high risk of compartment syndrome with this pattern.

Key point

- The Schatzker classification (types 1–6) is the most widely used.

Signs and symptoms

The patient presents with a painful swollen knee and is unable to bear full weight on the affected leg.

Investigations

In general, routine anteroposterior and lateral radiographs will show tibial plateau fractures. Oblique radiographs in two planes may be obtained to define the fracture pattern in three dimensions. Whenever there is uncertainty about the degree of comminution or the location and extent of the articular depression, additional imaging studies are required.

- *CT* is useful. CT imaging with three-dimensional reconstruction is often used.
- *MRI* is a relatively new diagnostic tool for tibial plateau fractures, and is useful for preoperative evaluation (Barrow *et al.* 1994).
- *Arteriography* is occasionally used in Schatzker types 4–6 to rule out disruptions and intimal tears of the popliteal artery (Wiss and Tracy Watson 1996). A high index of suspicion in high-energy injuries and the clinical findings will help in deciding the need for an arteriogram.

Key point

- CT imaging with three-dimensional reconstruction is used routinely.

Management

The goals in treatment of tibial plateau fractures are to obtain a stable, well-aligned, congruous, and painless knee joint with a good range of motion. In order to determine the optimal treatment plan, the 'personality' of the fracture has to be determined (Table 22.1).

Non-operative treatment

Undisplaced or minimally displaced lateral tibial plateau fractures are suitable for non-operative treatment (DeCoster *et al.* 1988). The haemarthrosis is aspirated and the knee joint is examined under anaesthesia for instability. If the knee is stable, a hinged cast-brace locked in full extension is applied. Close clinical and radiographic follow-up is required initially at weekly intervals to prevent loss of reduction and to allow adjustment of the brace. Progressive range of motion is permitted (90° flexion at 4 weeks). The brace is worn for up to 12 weeks, until union is achieved. Weight-bearing is initially restricted until adequate callus formation is seen. Patients with coexisting medical conditions, osteoporotic patients, and those with severe open fractures may also be considered for non-operative management.

Key point

- Undisplaced or minimally displaced lateral tibial plateau fractures are suitable for non-operative treatment.

Indications for operative management

Long-term clinical studies and cadaver experiments have helped determine the factors associated with poor clinical outcomes (Brown *et al.* 1988, Delamarter and Hohl 1989). The presence of neurovascular impairment or compartment syndrome is an absolute indication for surgery. Lateral plateau fractures with joint instability, and most medial tibial plateau and bicondylar fractures, are commonly managed using closed or open reduction techniques with internal or external fixation. Varus or valgus instability >5–10° at any point from 0–90° of flexion, >7° of malalignment in the frontal plane, displacement of the tibial plateau rim fragment with condylar widening, and articular surface depression >3 mm are generally considered indications for operative intervention in fit and healthy patients.

Table 22.1 Personality of a fracture (factors to consider in the treatment of a fracture)

Patient factors	Disease factors	Treatment factors
Age	Knee stability	Experience and training of surgeon
General medical problems	Degree of displacement	Availability of equipment
Osteoporosis	Presence of comminution	Physiotherapy staff
Presence of multiple trauma	Fracture location	Expert nursing care
Skin condition	Associated injuries	Financial constraints
Level of activity	Neurovascular damage	
	Open fractures	

Key point

- The presence of neurovascular impairment or compartment syndrome is an absolute indication for surgery.

Operative technique: Preoperative planning is essential and details of the approach, choice of metalwork, and reduction techniques are worked out beforehand. In the presence of severe soft tissue contusion, surgery is best delayed for a few days. The patient is placed supine and a thigh tourniquet is applied. A straight midline or a medial or lateral parapatellar incision may be used. Image intensification is used during the procedure to confirm restoration of the articular congruity and joint stability.

- *Displaced type 1:* fractures are reduced indirectly and fixed using percutaneous 6.5 mm cannulated cancellous screws. An arthroscopy of the knee is carried out at the same time to address meniscal tears.
- *Type 2: fractures (split-depressed):* The depressed articular fragment is elevated and cancellous bone graft harvested from the iliac crest is used to fill the defect in the tibial metaphysis. An AO buttress plate (T- or L-shaped plate) is then applied to the lateral cortex.
- *Type 3: fractures:* A cortical window is made in the lateral cortex of the tibia and the depressed fragment is elevated using a punch. The defect is filled with bone graft and supported by percutaneous cancellous screws inserted just below and parallel to the articular surface. A buttress plate is applied over the site of the cortical window. Arthroscopy of the knee is used to confirm anatomical restoration of the articular surface.
- *Type 4: fractures:* require ORIF with buttress plating over the proximal anteromedial tibial metaphysis, deep to the pes anserinus.
- *Types 5 and 6 fractures:* are high-energy injuries with severe soft tissue compromise. The previously advocated methods of open reduction and dual buttress plating are associated with high rates of wound dehiscence and infection. Therefore, surgical dissection is kept to a bare minimum using indirect reduction techniques. Femoral distractors are used to align the condyles by ligamentotaxis, and limited internal fixation of the articular fragments is carried out through small incisions. Hybrid external fixation is emerging as an alternative technique with numerous advantages. The articular fragments are reduced indirectly and held with highly tensioned wires. A circular frame is applied proximally and connected to half-pins applied to the tibial diaphysis. Any deformities noted after the fixator is applied can be corrected by adjusting the construct and hybrid fixators allow early joint motion, thereby preventing knee stiffness.

Key point

- Surgery is difficult and best undertaken by an expert in this area.

Postoperative care

Range of movement in the knee is encouraged with the help of continuous passive motion (CPM) machines. Weight-bearing is delayed until 6–8 weeks after surgery, gradually progressing to full weight-bearing at about 12 weeks.

Management of open tibial plateau fracture

Open tibial plateau fractures represent an emergency situation, requiring immediate treatment. The principles closely mirror management of open fractures elsewhere in the body (see 'Open tibial shaft fractures'). Primary internal fixation is advised only when facilities exist for immediate, definitive soft tissue cover. Delayed minimal internal fixation with hybrid external fixation can be carried out when the soft tissues allow, at the first available opportunity. 'Joint-bridging' external fixators that span the knee joint may be used instead of skeletal traction, to facilitate recovery of the soft tissue envelope whilst maintaining length and alignment.

The management of these injuries is fraught with difficulty, and early referral to specialist trauma centres is the safest option.

Key point

- An open tibial plateau fracture represents an emergency.

Complications

Tibial plateau fractures are the source of numerous complications that may result from the injury itself or as a consequence of surgical management of the fracture. Deep infection is treated by early aggressive debridement, removal of all metalwork, high-dose intravenous antibiotics based on bacterial sensitivity, and early soft tissue cover. Vascular injury is mostly seen in Schatzker 5 and 6 fractures. Rapid, temporary skeletal stabilization using an external fixator is performed before arterial repair, in order to protect the vascular anastomosis. Compartment syndrome may occur immediately after the injury or in the postoperative period. If the compartment is tense, fasciotomy may be performed after internal fixation. Knee stiffness is also a common problem, especially in elderly people. Post-traumatic osteoarthritis results from the initial insult to the articular cartilage. Incongruity of the articular surface and knee instability after surgery accelerate the onset of arthritis. Non-union is rare after tibial plateau fractures, thanks to the abundance of cancellous bone in the proximal tibia. The treatment of any serious complication must be tailored to each individual case and is best dealt with by an experienced surgeon.

Key point

- Complications are numerous.

Tibial shaft fractures

The tibial diaphysis is the most commonly fractured long bone. The average age of patients is 37 years and about 25% of all tibial fractures are open injuries (Court-Brown and McBirnie 1995).

Anatomy

The tibia is subcutaneous along its entire anteromedial surface. The lack of protection from overlying muscles makes it susceptible to high-energy injuries. In addition, most of the blood supply to the adult tibia is from the intramedullary circulation, with a minor contribution from periosteal vessels (Nelson *et al.* 1964). This has obvious implications for fracture and soft tissue healing, especially after open fractures. The tibial shaft is enclosed on its lateral and posterior aspects by three muscle compartments. The anterior compartment contains the dorsiflexors of the ankle, supplied by the anterior tibial nerve. The lateral compartment containing the peroneal muscles is responsible for eversion at the subtalar joint. The posterior compartment is divided into superficial and deep compartments, comprising the plantar flexors of the ankle and foot; they are supplied by the posterior tibial nerve.

Key point

- Most of the blood supply to the adult tibia is from the intramedullary circulation, with a minor contribution from periosteal vessels; this has obvious implications for fracture and soft tissue healing.

Mechanism of injury

Tibial shaft fractures constitute a spectrum of injuries ranging from stable undisplaced low-energy fractures to high-energy trauma associated with neurovascular compromise, soft tissue disruption, and bone loss. Tibial fractures are caused by torsion, bending, or direct violence. *Torsional (twisting) forces*, commonly seen in skiing and contact sports such as football, produce spiral fracture patterns. Short oblique and transverse fractures are caused by *three- or four-point bending forces.* A *direct blow* to the subcutaneous surface of the tibia results in considerable soft tissue disruption and comminution at the fracture site. The tibia is frequently involved in pedestrian accidents (car bumper), motorcycle accidents, dashboard injuries, and crushing farming accidents.

Signs and symptoms

Pain, inability to move the affected leg, and deformity are almost always present. The degree of deformity is a rough clinical guide to the fracture pattern, whether stable or unstable. The entire leg is carefully inspected for soft tissue swelling and bruising, fracture blisters, or obvious crush injuries (Table 22.2). Any open wound is inspected for its shape, size, contamination, arterial bleeding, and communication with the fracture site. The dorsalis pedis and posterior tibial pulses are checked clinically. If they are absent, a Doppler probe is used. The posterior tibial artery is usually patent even in severe injuries. Therefore, local soft tissue flaps using the calf muscles (based on the posterior tibial artery) can be fashioned in the management of open fractures. The presence or absence of normal sensation is noted and motor function is tested in all muscle groups. Close monitoring of pain level and neurovascular status of the limb is mandatory in all tibial fractures irrespective of severity, due to the ever-present danger of compartment syndrome.

Table 22.2 Tscherne classification of soft tissue injury with closed tibial shaft fractures

Grade	Description
0	Negligible soft tissue injury
1	Superficial abrasion or contusion caused by fragment pressure from within
2	Deep, contaminated contusion associated with skin or muscle contusion (also, impending compartment syndrome)
3	Extensively contused or crushed skin and possibly severe muscle damage (also, overt compartment syndrome and vascular injury)

From Tscherne and Gotzen (1984).

Key point

- For open fractures use the Gustilo and Anderson (1976) classification (see Table 14.1).

Associated injuries

In a major trauma situation tibial fractures are seen in association with fractures of hip, knee, foot, spine, and upper limb. These injuries are carefully documented during the secondary survey. Early operative treatment of tibial fractures in the multiple trauma victim reduces the incidence of pulmonary and systemic complications (Bone *et al.* 1989).

Classification

Fractures of the tibia may be closed or open. Numerous classifications of tibial fractures have been developed. The system presented by Johner and Wruhs (1983) in association with the AO/ASIF group is widely used (Fig. 22.2). Four factors are considered in classifying tibial fractures: mechanism of injury, degree of comminution, associated soft tissue injury, and initial and final displacement.

- Group A fractures include all simple fractures with no comminution.
- Group B involves a butterfly fragment in which one cortex is broken once and the other cortices are broken several times.
- Group C includes fractures with all cortices broken more than once and all segmental fractures.

Key points

- Four factors are considered in classifying tibial fractures:
  - mechanism of injury
  - degree of comminution
  - associated soft tissue injury
  - initial and final displacement.

Investigations

Anteroposterior and lateral radiographs are sufficient for the evaluation of most tibial fractures. The entire leg including knee and ankle joints must be

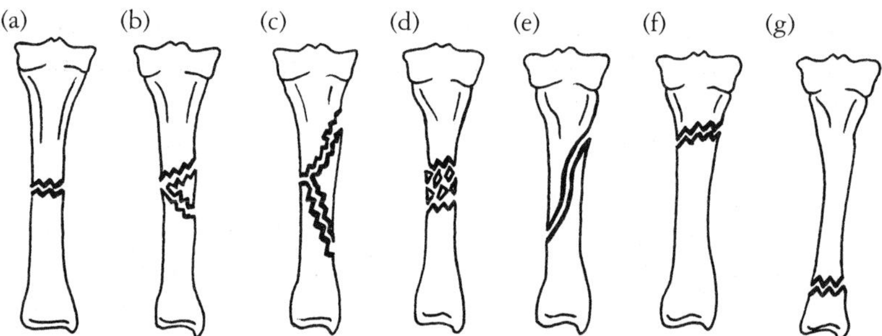

Figure 22.2 Types of tibial shaft fractures: (a) transverse; (b) small butterfly; (c) large butterfly; (d) segmental; (e) spiral; (f) proximal; (g) distal.

seen on the same film in order to assess rotational deformities. Oblique radiographs in two planes are sometimes obtained to assess malunion.

Management

The ultimate goal of any treatment is to restore the structural continuity and the mechanical axis of the tibia. The current guidelines for acceptable reduction are 5° for varus or valgus angulation, 10° for anteroposterior alignment (Nicoll 1964), up to 10° for rotation, and 1 cm of shortening. Comparison with the uninjured extremity establishes the baseline for the individual patient. Distraction of the fragments delays healing time considerably (Ellis 1958). Any displacement is corrected to enhance fracture stability (at least 50% cortical contact at the fracture site). These criteria are designed to ensure bony union and early restoration of normal gait. In practice, the surgeon may modify these criteria on the basis of the patient's age and functional status.

Key points

- The goal of treatment is to restore the structural continuity and the mechanical axis of the tibia.
- The current guidelines for acceptable reduction are 5° for varus or valgus angulation, 10° for anteroposterior alignment, up to 10° for rotation, and 1 cm of shortening.

Options

The main treatment modalities are closed reduction with cast or brace immobilization, ORIF, external fixation, and intramedullary (IM) nailing. In severe injuries, the indications for limb salvage are not yet clearly defined and the decision to amputate requires considerable judgement.

Key point

- The main treatment is closed reduction with cast.

Closed treatment

Isolated, low-energy, stable tibial fractures are treated initially by immobilization in a full leg cast (Sarmiento *et al.* 1989). Closed reduction under intravenous sedation or general anaesthesia may be necessary. The patient is positioned with the leg hanging off the edge of the table. Using an image intensifier, the fracture is manipulated and a well-padded plaster cast applied from inches below the greater trochanter to the toes with the knee in 5° flexion and the ankle in neutral position. The cast is moulded over the ankle and the subcutaneous surface of the tibia. The patient is kept non-weight-bearing for 4 weeks.

Clinical and radiographic examination is performed every week. The full leg cast is then replaced with a moulded brace or a Sarmiento patellar-tendon bearing cast (Sarmiento 1967). Full weight-bearing is allowed at this stage. Loss of reduction $<10°$ can be corrected by wedging the cast. The patient is reviewed until clinical and radiographic union. With closed treatment, the reported rate of union is up to 97.5%. Malunion rates in any direction are in the region of 20–30% and 90% of fractures have healed by 26 weeks (Sarmiento *et al.* 1995). Ankle stiffness is a common problem (Oni *et al.* 1988) and long-term functional loss can be significant. An intensive rehabilitation programme instituted early can help prevent some of these problems.

Internal fixation with plates and screws

The current indications for ORIF with compression plates and screws are tibial shaft fractures involving the metaphyseal region of the tibia, associated with displaced intra-articular fractures of the knee or ankle (Whittle 1998). Plating is sometimes performed for short oblique and transverse fractures, and in treating non-unions.

Ilizarov technique

The Ilizarov technique is a highly technical but effective method for severe soft tissue and bony injuries. A description of this technique is beyond the scope of this text but can be found using the search engine google (www.google.com) and in Aronson 1997 and Shertsav 1997. Also, note that the Ilizarov is not the only external fixateur used and is possibly the least commonly used.

Intramedullary nailing

IM nailing is ideally suited for unstable tibial fractures located at least 7 cm below the knee and 4 cm above the ankle joint (Bradford Henley 1989). The principal advantages are simple technique, good rotational control of the fracture, preservation of the soft-tissue envelope, and the possibility of early weight-bearing. Earlier designs such as flexible pins and centromedullary nails have lost favour because they gave poor rotational control, and the interlocking nail is now the implant of choice.

Nails are usually inserted using a closed technique, and may be locked in static or dynamic modes. Static locking results in better control of unstable tibial fractures. Reaming the medullary canal allows larger diameter nails to be inserted with greater stability, and the reamings act as bone graft at the fracture site. The main disadvantages of reaming are damage to the endosteal circulation and fat embolism. Unreamed nails can be inserted with less blood loss, shorter operating times, and fewer pulmonary complications from fat embolism. This is particularly relevant in major trauma where rapid skeletal stabilization improves overall survival rates. Unreamed nails are mechanically less stable than reamed nails.

Key point

- IM nailing is ideally suited for unstable tibial fractures located at least 7 cm below the knee and 4 cm above the ankle joint.

Operative technique: Preoperative planning is essential. The patient is positioned supine on the fracture table with traction applied through a calcaneal pin. A tourniquet is used and the lower thigh is supported on a padded bolster. The hip and knee are flexed to allow horizontal orientation of the tibia. The fracture is reduced using image intensification. Failure to reduce the fracture requires open exploration. A 5 cm incision is made medial to the patellar tendon. The tendon is retracted laterally and the insertion point is identified. The canal is opened with a curved bone awl. A curved-tip guide wire is inserted across the fracture. The canal is reamed initially with a 9 mm reamer inserted over the guide wire, and then in 0.5 mm increments until the diameter of the endosteal canal at the isthmus is reached. For unreamed tibial nails, the proximal tibial metaphysis is expanded to 12 mm with the awl and the diameter of nail determined using sounds. The nail length is measured and the guide wire exchanged. The tibial nail is then driven into the medullary canal until the proximal end is countersunk firmly into the entry portal. Proximal and distal interlocking screws are inserted using a radiolucent power drill and image intensification. The wounds are closed and a crepe bandage is applied.

Postoperative care: The patient is mobilized from the second postoperative day, weight-bearing with crutches as tolerated. Knee and ankle exercises are started in hospital and continued until functional restoration. The fracture is radiographed at frequent intervals for signs of callus formation. Full weight-bearing is usually possible at 6 weeks. Depending on the amount of callus and fracture consolidation, additional procedures such as exchange reamed nailing, dynamization, or autogenous bone grafting may be required. *Dynamization* is a process by which micromovement at the fracture site is produced, in order to provide mechanical stimulus for callus formation and accelerated fracture healing. This can be accomplished by removal of the proximal or distal interlocking screw.

External fixation

External fixators are primarily used in the initial management of open tibial fractures and for comminuted fractures with bone loss. These indications are expanding to include definitive treatment of closed fractures and secondary reconstruction for bone loss, non-union, and malunion. The two basic types of constructs are pin and ring fixators. The two methods can be combined to form 'hybrid' fixators. Pin fixators can provide stability in one or more planes depending upon the fracture pattern. Ring fixators consist of rings that are connected to the bone using highly tensioned wires, producing a 'trampoline' effect (Whittle 1998). With the help of hinges and interconnecting rods, ring fixators can be configured to correct angulation, translation, and rotational deformities. The advantages of external fixation are minimum interference with blood supply, rapid application in multiple-trauma victims, and ease of access for soft tissue procedures such as vascular flaps. External fixators can be 'dynamized' by sequential disassembly of the construct to provide mechanical stimulus for callus formation. Drawbacks of external fixation include pin-track infection, pin loosening, loss of frame stability and the need for secondary definitive fixation once the soft-tissues have healed.

Key point

- External fixators are often used in the initial management of open tibial fractures and for comminuted fractures with bone loss.

Operative technique: A number of different external fixators are available for stabilizing tibial fractures.

Post-operative management:

Pin-site care begins after the first postoperative dressing change. Partial weight-bearing with crutches is allowed at 3–6 weeks. The fixator is dynamized at 6 weeks and removed when the fracture has consolidated clinically and radiologically. Bone grafting, via a posterolateral apporach to the tibia, may be required at 6– 8 weeks.

Treatment of open tibial fractures

All open fractures require urgent orthopaedic intervention. Wounds should be covered with antiseptic dressings in the emergency department. Polaroid photographs may be taken to prevent repeated uncovering of wounds during examination. High-dose broad-spectrum antibiotics are administered intravenously and tetanus prophylaxis is given. The first operation should be undertaken within 6 hours from the time of the injury. Plastic surgical input at the initial assessment allows early decision-making regarding soft tissue cover and improves the outcome (Fischer *et al.* 1991).

At operation, the wound is fully assessed for degree of contamination, tissue necrosis, periosteal stripping, and bone loss. The skin is scrubbed clean and the wound irrigated using pulsed lavage with 3–6 L of warm normal saline solution. All necrotic tissue must be excised using sharp dissection, and unattached bone fragments are removed (Burgess *et al.* 1987b). Skin incisions for the debridement should be planned with the plastic surgeon in order not to compromise any future reconstructive flap designs. The wounds are left open. The fracture is stabilized after debridement. An external fixator is usually applied but primary IM nailing combined with early soft tissue cover is associated with lower malunion rates (Tornetta *et al.* 1994). Skeletal stabilization must avoid any further devascularization of the remaining bone fragments. External fixators can be extended to include the foot, since this rests the muscles of the leg and helps soft tissue healing. If bone loss is present, autologous grafting and bone transport procedures may be needed.

Scheduled repeat wound inspection in theatre is done at 48 hours. Further debridement is performed if required at this stage. Soft tissue cover must be obtained within 4–7 days with whatever plastic procedure (delayed closure, skin grafts, local flaps, or microvascular tissue transfer) will provide optimal conditions for healing. Intravenous antibiotics are continued postoperatively.

The degree of callus formation is monitored closely over the next 6 weeks. Preemptive bone grafting for grade 3 open fractures has resulted in decreased time to healing and increased rates of union (Burgess *et al.* 1987a). With careful attention to detail, 90% of severely injured tibiae can be returned to useful function.

Key point

- All open fractures require urgent orthopaedic intervention.

Prognosis

The average time to union for low-energy closed fractures is 12–15 weeks, for high-energy closed fractures 12–28 weeks. Grade 3A and 3B open fractures require 30–50 weeks for union. Long-term function depends on restoring knee and ankle motion. Younger patients do uniformly better than older people with poor bone quality. In the absence of complications, return to former employment can be expected.

Complications

Infected non-union and osteomyelitis are the worst complications after tibial fracture. Treatment includes radical debridement of all infected bone and soft tissues, stable fixation, soft tissue coverage, and antibiotics based on bacterial culture and sensitivity results (Koval *et al.* 1991). In severe cases, vascularized autograft, allograft, or bone transport is required to restore limb length.

Delayed union and non-union are more common in high-energy injuries. The important causes are infection, poor fixation, and patient-related factors. Treatment is aimed at modifying mechanical factors (revising external fixators to plate osteosynthesis, exchange nailing, supplementary fixation) or biological factors (bone grafting, Ilizarov distraction histogenesis, reaming). Malunion causing significant functional limitation or deformity is best treated by osteotomy and external fixation. Refracture, secondary osteoarthritis, ankle stiffness, and reflex sympathetic dystrophy are also encountered. Anterior knee pain is unique to IM nailing and requires removal of the nail in affected patients (Court-Brown *et al.* 1997).

Acute compartment syndrome

Acute compartment syndrome is a condition in which the circulation within a closed osseofascial compartment is compromised by an increase in the pressure within it, leading to necrosis of the muscles and nerves and in extreme cases, the skin surrounding the compartment. Any muscle or muscle group bound by inelastic deep fascia can be affected by compartment syndrome, the muscles in the leg being the most commonly affected.

Key point

- Acute compartment syndrome is a medical emergency.

Aetiology

Acute compartment syndrome is usually the result of bleeding from a fracture into the compartment leading to increased interstitial pressure. Fractures of the tibial shaft, both closed and open, are the commonest cause of compartment syndrome in normal clinical practice. Acute compartment syndrome can also result from muscle contusions, crush injuries, bomb blasts, snake bites, bleeding diatheses, and reperfusion following acute limb ischaemia.

Pathophysiology

According to Matsen (1989), the increased pressure within the compartment leads to a corresponding rise in the pressure within the intracompartmental veins. This reduces the arteriovenous gradient and with it, the local blood flow. When local blood flow is unable to sustain tissue metabolic demands, the tissue loses function and viability. As the intracompartmental pressure is less than the arterial pressure, the distal arterial blood flow and pulses are intact. Because the capillary bed of the toes drains into extracompartmental veins, the digital arteriovenous gradient and the digital blood flow are preserved. Thus, peripheral pulses and digital circulation are poor indicators of blood flow within the compartment.

Clinical features

The most important sign is pain out of proportion to that expected from the injury. The involved compartment feels tense on palpation, the muscles are tender, and frequently there is pain on passive stretching of the muscle groups. Paraesthesia and hypoaesthesia in the sensory distribution of nerves running through the compartment is an early sign of raised pressure. Motor weakness and vascular insufficiency occur late, when irreversible muscle necrosis is likely. These classical features are blunted or absent in patients with multiple injuries or altered consciousness, and in children. Continuous monitoring of compartment pressure may therefore be useful in these patients (McQueen *et al.* 1996).

Key points

- The most important sign is pain out of proportion to that expected from the injury; others include:
  - tense compartment on palpation
  - pain on passive or active movement of the muscles of concern
  - paraesthesia and hypoaesthesia.
- Motor weakness and absent pulse are (too) late signs.

Investigations

In the acute situation, intracompartmental pressures are measured as a matter of urgency. A Stryker hand-held monitor can be used for single measurements and continuous monitoring. This device provides accurate and reliable results with minimal training and experience. Under aseptic conditions, the side-ported needle is introduced into the compartment. The needle is connected to the monitor through a syringe and tubing filled with normal saline. About 0.3 mL of saline is injected slowly into the compartment, to allow equalization with the interstitial pressure. The monitor is placed at the same level as the leg and the pressure is measured. A compartment pressure >30 mmHg in the presence of clinical signs indicates the need for urgent decompression. Studies have shown that the difference between the diastolic blood pressure and the compartment pressure is more reliable than the compartment pressure alone. A differential pressure <30 mm Hg is considered significant (McQueen and Court-Brown 1996).

Management

A simple measures such as splitting the cast and underlying padding down to the skin decreases pressures significantly. The affected leg is positioned at the same level as the heart. High elevation of the extremity decreases arterial perfusion and worsens the problem. These measures are instituted in conjunction with pressure readings. If there is any doubt, the compartment is decompressed. For fasciotomy following tibial fractures, we use the 'double incision fasciotomy'.

Key points

- Split the cast to the skin but not including the skin.
- Position the affected leg is at the same level as the heart.
- These measures are instituted in conjunction with pressure readings.
- If there is any doubt, the compartment must be decompressed (fasciotomy).

Operative technique

A 20–25 cm skin incision is made over the anterior compartment, centred halfway between the crest of the tibia and the fibular shaft. The incision is widened by generous subcutaneous dissection, anteriorly and posteriorly. The lateral intermuscular septum is exposed and the superficial peroneal nerve is identified just posterior to the septum. The anterior compartment is released along its entire course, in line with the tibialis anterior and the lateral compartment is decompressed, in line with the fibular shaft. A second longitudinal skin incision is made 2 cm posterior to the posterior margin of the tibia. The saphenous vein and nerve are retracted anteriorly. A transverse incision is made to identify the septum between the superficial and deep posterior compartments. The gastrocsoleus compartment is decompressed first. Through a separate incision over the flexor digitorum longus muscle, the deep posterior compartment is released. The wound is lightly packed and the patient is taken back to theatre at 48–72 hours. If the swelling has subsided, the wound is closed. Any unviable muscle can be debrided at the second-look procedure. Split skin grafts may be required on occasion, for soft tissue cover.

Prognosis

Decompression performed within 24 hours of the onset of compartment syndrome carries a good prognosis. There is no benefit from decompression beyond this critical period. Thanks to early recognition and prompt treatment, contracture from neglected compartment syndrome is fortunately rare in modern orthopaedics.

Soft tissue and ligament injuries

Studies into the functional anatomy of the knee have established that the supporting structures around the knee work in perfect synchrony. It seems unlikely that isolated injuries to knee ligaments (e.g. isolated rupture of the anterior cruciate ligament) can occur without some degree of damage to other related structures. There are three principal mechanisms of injury to the knee (Miller 1998).

- *Abduction, flexion, and internal rotation of the femur* on the tibia is the commonest, seen when the weight-bearing leg is subjected to a deceleration force from the lateral side. This causes serial disruption of the medial collateral ligament, the anterior cruciate ligament (ACL) and the medial meniscus (the 'unhappy triad' of O'Donoghue).
- *Adduction, flexion, and external rotation of the femur* causes disruption of the fibular collateral ligament, the lateral capsule, the arcuate ligament complex, the popliteus, the iliotibial band, the biceps femoris, and the lateral popliteal nerve.
- *Hyperextension and anteroposterior displacement* cause disruption of the cruciate ligaments. The flexed knee striking the dashboard leading to a posterior cruciate ligament (PCL) rupture is a classic example of this mechanism.

Key point

- Abduction, flexion, and internal rotation of the femur on the tibia is the commonest mechanism of injury.

Classification

Instability arising from acute injuries to the knee has been classified by the American Orthopaedic Society of Sports Medicine. The tibia is taken as the reference point and any abnormal movement of the tibia in relation to the femur on stress testing is noted. Instability can be one-plane, rotary or combined. The system helps correlate clinical findings with structural defects. For example, one-plane medial instability in full extension indicates rupture of the medial collateral ligament and the ACL, whereas one-plane instability detected at 30° flexion suggests tear of the medial structures only. Rotary and combined instabilities result from major disruptions of the collateral and cruciate ligaments.

Key point

- *For assessing instability:* the tibia is taken as the reference point and any abnormal movement of the tibia in relation to the femur on stress testing is noted.
- Consider the ACL as providing the stable platform for the qaudriceps to work from; and the converse for the PCL and the hamstrings.

Presentation

History

A careful and detailed history will help localize and grade the severity of most acute injuries to knee ligaments. The history of the mechanism of injury should include position of the knee, magnitude and location of the forces applied to the knee, exact activity involved during the impact, and position of the leg after the injury. Inability to bear full weight immediately afterwards is significant. The patient's description of the experience will give valuable clues; an audible 'pop' and knee buckling are characteristic of cruciate ligament tears. The onset and timing of pain and swelling of the knee and freedom of active movement help distinguish cruciate and meniscal pathology. Swelling within 2 hours of injury suggests haemarthrosis, and an effusion occurring overnight indicates an acute traumatic synovitis. Any previous injuries or instability should be noted.

Physical examination

A precise and systematic examination carried out as soon as possible after the injury will minimize problems due to a tense effusion and reflex muscle spasm, as these tend to blur physical signs. The normal knee is first examined to establish the baseline for the individual patient. Quadriceps wasting is invariably seen after any significant knee injury.

Collateral ligament injuries

Injuries to the collateral ligaments commonly occur during sporting activities. They can occur as isolated ligament injuries or in combination with cruciate ligament tears.

Anatomy

According to Warren and Marshall (1979), the stabilizing structures on the medial and lateral aspects of the knee are arranged in three basic layers. On the medial side, the superficial layer is the investing deep fascia that encloses the entire medial aspect of the knee. The second layer is composed of the parallel fibres of the superficial medial collateral ligament. The true capsule of the knee joint and the deep medial collateral ligament constitute the deepest layer. The tendon of semimembranosus and its investing sheath merge with the two deeper layers. Active contraction of the semimembranosus tenses the posterior oblique ligament (a thickened portion of the posteromedial capsule), providing added dynamic stability on the medial side during knee flexion.

The lateral collateral ligament is a tendinous structure extending from the lateral femoral epicondyle to the fibular head. The iliotibial band, the popliteus, and the lateral collateral ligament cross each other during flexion and provide additional stability against varus stress. Seebacher *et al.* (1982) identified three distinct anatomic layers in the posterolateral corner of the knee. Layer 1 is formed by the iliotibial band and the biceps femoris insertion, layer 2 by the patellofemoral ligaments, and layer 3 by the lateral capsular ligament. The arcuate ligament is a Y-shaped structure extending from the fibular head to the oblique popliteal ligament, on the posterior aspect of the femur. More recently, Maynard *et al.* (1996) have identified a distinct structure called the popliteofibular ligament that connects the fibula to the femur through the popliteus. The arcuate ligament complex is a functional musculotendinous unit on the lateral aspect of the knee composed of the arcuate ligament, the lateral collateral ligament, the popliteus, and the lateral head of gastrocnemius (Baker *et al.* 1983). A detailed knowledge of the functional anatomy of each structure is essential when repairing acute tears of the lateral ligament complex (Veltri and Warren 1994).

Investigations

Standard anteroposterior and lateral radiographs may show an avulsion of the bony attachments of the collateral ligaments. In chronic cases, the origin of the medial collateral ligament (MCL) may be calcified (Pellegrini–Steida disease). Stress radiographs are useful in younger patients to differentiate ligamentous laxity from abnormal movement at the growth plates due to physeal injury. MRI is highly sensitive for detecting MCL ruptures, especially the superficial lamina which is not visualized on arthroscopy (Rasenberg *et al.* 1995).

Management

Conservative

Isolated grade I and II collateral ligament injuries should be managed conservatively (Hastings 1980). There is some controversy in the management of isolated grade III collateral ligament tears, but prospective studies have shown conservative treatment to be superior to surgical repair (Simonsen *et al.* 1984). Before deciding on any treatment regimen, the integrity of the cruciate ligaments must be determined clinically and by arthroscopy or MRI.

Initial management aims to control pain and swelling by rest, elevation, ice massage, and anti-inflammatory drugs. Quadriceps-strengthening exercises are started once the inflammation subsides. The knee should be protected in a hinged knee brace and return to functional activities is gradually encouraged. The patient can resume running and contact sports once the knee is stable on stress testing, and range of movement is normal.

Key point

- Isolated grade I, II, and III medial collateral ligament injuries should be managed conservatively.

Operative treatment

The decision to operate depends on the degree of joint laxity and the presence of associated pathology. If a meniscal tear is present, the meniscus is excised or repaired. Surgical repair of collateral ligaments is usually reserved for selected patients with combined collateral and cruciate ligament injuries.

Operative technique—(medial collateral ligament) (Miller 1998): With the patient in the supine operative position and the knee flexed to 60°, the side of the knee is approached through a midmedial incision extending from above the adductor tubercle to 5 cm below the joint line. The great saphenous vein and the sartorial branch of the saphenous nerve are protected. The tibial attachment of the medial collateral ligament is exposed by retracting the pes anserinus. The rest of the ligament is exposed by dissecting the patellar retinaculum off the medial capsule. The knee joint is exposed through a parapatellar capsulotomy. The medial and lateral menisci, the cruciates and the articular surface are inspected for damage. The integrity of the posteromedial capsule and the posterior oblique ligament must be checked. A midsubtance tear is repaired by multiple interrupted absorbable sutures with tension sutures to protect the repair. If the ligaments are avulsed off bone, they can be reattached using transosseous sutures, suture anchors, or AO screws with a ligament washer. Alternatively, they may be buried under a flap of bone and secured with a table staple. The isometric point on the bone has to be chosen and marked before reattachment. The arthrotomy is closed first and the ligament repair performed in 60° flexion. The knee is immobilized in a long leg cast or a hinged knee brace with the knee in 45° flexion and mild internal rotation.

Anterior cruciate ligament injuries

The reported incidence of ruptures of the ACL following acute traumatic haemarthrosis of the knee, in the absence of a fracture, is between 40% and 70% (Simonsen *et al.* 1984, Johannsen and Fruensgaard 1988). ACL ruptures are a significant cause of disability, and ACL-deficient knees are at risk of developing early degenerative joint disease and secondary meniscal tears (Hawkins *et al.* 1986). There is considerable debate about the natural history of an ACL rupture and its treatment, many key issues remaining unresolved (Daniels and Fithian 1994).

Key point

- ACL-deficient knees are at risk of developing early degenerative joint disease and secondary meniscal tears.

Anatomy and biomechanics

The ACL extends from the medial aspect of the lateral femoral condyle to its tibial attachment in front of the anterior tibial spine. It is composed of anteromedial, posterolateral, and intermediate bundles. Blood vessels enter the ligament through its femoral attachment and the anterior synovial covering. The ACL is classically described as 'intra-articular' but 'extrasynovial'. The anteromedial bundle is tight in flexion and the posterolateral band is tight in extension (Sakane *et al.* 1997). As a result, partial tears of the ACL involving one bundle may be missed on clinical examination (Lintner *et al.* 1995).

Key point

- The ACL is classically described as 'intra-articular' but 'extra-synovial'.

Mechanism of injury

The ACL is torn by non-weighted twisting (skiing injuries) or in contact sports. It is forced against the posterior cruciate ligament (PCL) in external rotation and against the lateral femoral condyle during internal rotation (Feagin and Lambert 1985). The dimensions of the intercondylar notch is an important aetiological factor in ACL ruptures (narrow notch, higher risk) (Souryal and Freeman 1993, LaPrade and Burnett 1994).

Examination findings

A thorough examination of the knee confirms associated ligament and meniscal pathology. The following are common clinical tests for anterior instability.

- The *anterior drawer test* is performed with the patient supine, the hip flexed to 45° and the knee to 90° (Marshall *et al.* 1975). Sit on the dorsum of the patient's foot and feel behind the knee with both hands for relaxation of the hamstrings. Gently pull and push the proximal part of the leg, noting the movement of the tibia on the femur. The test is performed with the knee in internal, external and neutral rotation. A difference of 6–8 mm or more, when compared to the opposite side, indicates a torn ACL.
- The *Lachman test* is more sensitive and useful in the acutely injured knee (Kim and Kim 1995). The knee is placed in 15–30° flexion and slight external rotation. The femur and tibia are held firmly and any anterior translation is noted on attempting to lift the proximal tibia.
- *The pivot–shift test:* Lift the foot with the knee extended, internally rotate the leg, and apply a valgus force to the knee. The knee is gradually flexed and the tibia subluxes anteriorly due to the deficient ACL. When the knee is past the 30° mark, the tibia reduces back on to the lateral femoral condyle with a 'clunk' (Fetto and Marshall 1979).

Various rotary tests such as the *flexion rotation drawer test* and the *reverse pivot shift test* are described that attempt to diagnose complex instabilities (Heron and Calvert 1992). The *dynamic extension test* is useful in the acutely injured knee. The patient lies supine with the knee flexed 30° over the examiner's arm and asked to lift the foot off the bed. The tibia subluxes forward, as the platform is no longer stable.

Key point

- At first presentation, the knee with an ACL rupture is swollen and full of blood.
- The Lachman test is most accurate for diagnosis.
- The dynamic extension test is useful in the acutely injured knee.

Diagnostic techniques

Arthroscopy is the best method of confirming a ruptured ACL. MRI has a sensitivity of up to 96% and specificity of up to 98% for diagnosing ACL tears (Vellet *et al.* 1989, Friedman and Jackson 1996). The use of non-orthogonal cuts (knee placed in 15° of external rotation) has improved the sensitivity of MRI scans (Jomha *et al.* 1999). It has the added benefit of diagnosing associated soft tissue and bony lesions in acute knee injuries. Examination under anaesthesia is a valuable adjunct to arthroscopy for the assessment of knee instability.

Management

The management of ACL ruptures can be broadly divided into non-operative and operative methods. There are no uniform criteria for inclusion into either group. The decision to operate depends on a number of factors: activity level, nature of sports, frequency and severity of symptoms (mainly 'giving way'), patient's expectation, and the degree of instability on objective measurement (Daniels and Fithian 1994). Recent long-term studies have indicated less radiological evidence of osteoarthritis in patients who have undergone ACL reconstruction (Jomha *et al.* 1999). When considering the need for surgery, a positive pivot-shift test is considered specially significant.

Key point

- The decision to operate depends on: activity level, nature of sports, frequency and severity of symptoms mainly 'giving way', patient's expectation, and the degree of instability on objective measurement.

Conservative treatment

Knee braces are usually used in the period immediately after the injury (Barrack *et al.* 1990). They help improve the patient's confidence in undertaking light sporting activities and may be useful in protecting partial tears from further injury. In addition, an intensive rehabilitation programme involving quadriceps and hamstring sets, pedal biking, and closed-chain kinetic exercises are useful in regaining movement and function in the affected knee. Full extension of the knee is avoided in order to reduce stress transmission through the ACL.

Operative treatment

Acute repair of the ruptured ACL is controversial, though some authors have claimed good results when a patellar tendon graft is used to augment the repair (Fruensgaard *et al.* 1992, Cross *et al.* 1993). ACL reconstruction is usually advocated for patients who have failed a trial of conservative management or in professional athletes with greater functional demands. The developments in ACL surgery have closely mirrored the improved understanding of knee biomechanics (Woo *et al.* 1997). Reconstruction of the ACL is performed with autografts (bone–patellar tendon–bone or quadruple hamstring graft), allografts, or synthetic ligament combinations (Miller and Harner 1993, Ochi *et al.* 1993, Shelton *et al.* 1997). Arthroscopic surgery has minimized the morbidity associated with these procedures (Bray and Dandy 1987).

Key point

- Acute repair of the ruptured ACL is controversial.

Posterior cruciate ligament injuries

Injuries to the PCL are less common and less well understood than ACL injuries. The incidence of PCL injuries is between 3% and 20% of all knee injuries (Clendenin *et al.* 1980). The most common mechanism is a direct blow to the anterior aspect of the knee (Cooper *et al.* 1991). The PCL originates from the lateral aspect of the medial femoral condyle and inserts on the posterior aspect of the intercondylar area of the tibia. The PCL accounts for 95% of the restraining force against posterior displacement of the tibia on the femur (Rubenstein *et al.* 1994).

Diagnosis is made on the basis of mechanism of injury, presence of haemarthrosis, and clinical findings. There is an obvious posterior sag of the tibia when the knee is viewed from the side. The posterior drawer test is performed with the knee flexed to 90° and any abnormal posterior displacement of the tibia on the femur is noted (Rubenstein *et al.* 1994). Injuries to the PCL are frequently associated with disruption to the posterolateral structures of the knee and the clinical picture is complicated (Fleming *et al.* 1981). An avulsion fracture of the posterior tibial spine may be seen on a lateral radiograph of the knee. MRI is highly sensitive and specific for PCL disruption, best demonstrated on sagittal images (Sonin *et al.* 1994, Sonin *et al.* 1995). Any diagnostic doubt must prompt an examination under anaesthesia and arthroscopy of the knee.

Treatment of PCL injuries depends on the magnitude of the tear and an understanding of the natural history of the disease. After an injury to the PCL, there is increased posterior sagging of the tibia leading to higher joint contact forces in the tibiofemoral and patellofemoral joints (Skyhar *et al.* 1993, MacDonald *et al.* 1996). This leads to premature degenerative joint disease. Complex algorithms have been developed for managing PCL injuries, but reconstruction is generally indicated when the posterior displacement is >8–10 mm (Veltri and Warren 1993). An avulsion fracture of the tibial spine is treated by ORIF with 4.0 mm cancellous lag screws. Rehabilitation and physical therapy focus on strengthening the quadriceps by closed- and open-chain kinetic exercises (Wilk 1994).

The prognosis after PCL injuries is variable (Hughston *et al.* 1980). Progressive degenerative changes have been noted in spite of surgical reconstruction, though many studies report superior results in terms of symptoms and activity level following surgery in selected patients (Clancy and Pandya 1994, Kim *et al.* 1999).

Key point

- The most common mechanism is a direct blow to the anterior aspect of the knee.
- The dynamic flexion test is useful in diagnosis. The patient is supine with knee flexed 30° and asked to lift and drag heel backwards. The tibia subluxes backward as the platform is no longer stable (converse of ACL test).

Meniscal injuries

General principles

Injuries to the semilunar cartilages are common after knee injuries. They are frequently seen in association with tears of the collateral and cruciate ligaments (Maffulli *et al.* 1993).

Key point

- Semilunar cartilages injuries are common after knee injuries.

Anatomy

The medial meniscus is a C-shaped structure with a larger radius of curvature than the lateral meniscus. The peripheral border of the medial meniscus is attached to the capsule and the lateral meniscus is anchored to the popliteus tendon and the meniscofemoral ligaments. The lateral meniscus covers the tibial articular surface to a larger extent than the medial meniscus.

Ultrastructure and biomechanics

The menisci act as a joint filler, increasing the contact surface area between the femur and tibia. This directly decreases the contact stresses generated in the articular cartilage and prevents mechanical damage to the chondrocytes. They also play a role in load transmission, shock transmission, and joint lubrication (Shrive *et al.* 1978). They act as secondary stabilizers of the knee joint in all directions, especially in rotational planes and when the primary stabilizers such as the cruciate ligaments are absent (Shoemaker and Markolf 1986). The meniscus is composed of dense, tightly woven type I collagen fibres that are predominantly circumferential in orientation. 'This highly oriented collagen ultrastructure of the menisci makes the tissue anisotropic in tension, compression and shear and appears to dominate its behaviour under all loading conditions' (Fithian *et al.* 1990).

Key point

- The menisci act as a joint filler.

Mechanism of injury

A meniscus is usually torn by a rotational force in a partially flexed joint. Forcible internal rotation of the flexed knee pushes the medial meniscus posteriorly. The meniscus is caught between the femur and tibia when the joint is extended from this position. This results in a classic *bucket-handle tear.* The lateral meniscus, by virtue of its shape and attachment to popliteus and to the femur through the meniscofemoral ligaments, can get 'pulled out of the way', rendering it is much less susçeptible to injury (McMinn 1994).

Key point

- A meniscus is usually torn by a rotational force in a partially flexed joint.

Presentation

There is a history of a twisting injury to the weight-bearing knee and effusion that develops a few hours after the injury Two distinct syndromes are associated with meniscal tears. The classic 'locked' knee denotes an inability to extend the injured knee fully compared to the normal side. In the chronic tear, joint line discomfort after activity is associated with recurrent 'giving-way' episodes and swelling.

Key point

- Meniscal tears present as 'locked' knee, or in the chronic tear: joint line pain and recurrent 'giving-way' episodes with swelling.

Diagnostic tests

Numerous manipulative tests for meniscal integrity are described. The *McMurray test* and the *Apley Grinding test* are commonly used. In the McMurray test, the knee is fully flexed with the patient lying supine. The examiner's hand is placed over the joint line. The integrity of the medial meniscus is tested by gradually extending the knee with the foot in external rotation. For the lateral meniscus, the test is repeated with the foot in external rotation. If a meniscal tear is present, a click may be felt over the medial joint line or the symptoms may be reproduced (Kim *et al.* 1996).

Classification

The most useful classification system is based on findings at operation. Types of tears include (1) bucket-handle, (2) flap, (3) horizontal cleavage, (4) radial, (5) degenerative, and (6) tears of discoid menisci. The bucket-handle tear is a vertical longitudinal cleavage that occurs frequently with ACL ruptures.

Key point

- Types of tears include (1) bucket-handle, (2) flap, (3) horizontal cleavage, (4) radial, (5) degenerative and (6) tears of discoid menisci.

Investigations

Routine anteroposterior and lateral radiographs must be obtained to rule out bony lesions. Tunnel views may be requested to rule out loose bodies or chondral fractures in the intercondylar area that may mimic meniscal pathology. MRI is non-invasive, and 98% accuracy for medial meniscal tears has been reported (Polly *et al.* 1988). It has the additional advantage of diagnosing tears of the collateral and cruciate ligaments.

Management

There is an increasing trend towards a selective approach to treating meniscal tears. Several factors such as length of the tear, vascularity, and the presence of associated ACL rupture are considered in the decision-making process (DeHaven 1990). Diagnostic arthroscopy represents the gold standard for the suspected acute meniscal tear, although MRI is superior to arthroscopy in diagnosing intrasubstance meniscal tears and pathology within discoid lateral menisci (Biedert 1993).

Initial

The knee is immobilized in a bandage or splint for 2–4 weeks until the acute pain and swelling settle. The knee is re-examined at this stage and further management is based on the clinical findings. If the knee is locked, diagnostic arthroscopy may be indicated. A program of rehabilitation consisting principally of isometric quadriceps and hamstring exercises is instituted. MRI scans are obtained at this stage if in doubt and where facilities are available.

Operative treatment

The management of meniscal injuries is technically demanding and requires considerable clinical judgement.

Traumatic dislocation of the knee

Knee dislocation is extremely rare (Fig. 22.3). In general, both cruciate ligaments and at least one of the collateral ligaments have to be disrupted for the knee to dislocate (Bratt and Newman 1993).

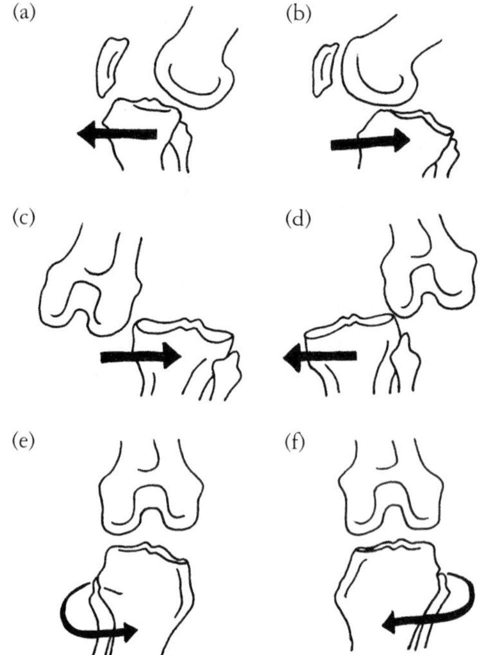

Figure 22.3 Knee dislocations: (a) anterior, (b) posterior; (c) lateral; (d) medial; (e) anteromedial; (f) anterolateral.

The popliteal artery and vein traverse the posterior aspect of the knee joint bounded proximally and distally by fibro-osseous tunnels. The popliteal vessels are thus particularly vulnerable to disruption and the presence of vascular insufficiency is a major factor in the planning the management of these complex injuries (Kaufman and Martin 1992).

Dislocations of the knee may be classified as open or closed dislocations, and reducible or irreducible. The tibia may be displaced anteriorly, posteriorly or in the mediolateral plane (Hill and Rana 1981). Spontaneous reduction can occur, resulting in occult dislocations that can be missed on clinical examination. The diagnosis is apparent on inspection. There is a high incidence of arterial injury, and the distal neurovascular status should be carefully assessed. The popliteal artery and the peroneal nerve are commonly affected. Radiographs must be obtained only after the knee is manually relocated. Clinical examination will usually reveal gross multi-plane instability due to extensive soft tissue damage (Yu *et al.* 1995). Arterial injury can occur with normal distal pulses and an angiogram is always obtained (Gable *et al.* 1997).

Treatment depends on the severity of the injury. Early vascular consultation is mandatory. If there is popliteal artery injury, primary repair with a vein graft is performed (Walker *et al.* 1994). If the ischaemic time is >6 hours, a prophylactic fasciotomy is done at the same time. Injuries to the peroneal nerve are repaired primarily using an operating microscope. The treatment of ligamentous injuries is more controversial. Studies comparing operative treatment with conservative management indicate better long-term function and less stiffness with early, primary operative repair (Shapiro and Freedman 1995). If the femur has buttonholed through the soft tissues, urgent open reduction may be necessary (Nystrom *et al.* 1992). Postoperative management is aimed at restoring early range of movement in the first 6 weeks, followed by strengthening exercises. The prognosis after knee dislocations is satisfactory (>80% excellent to good results) (Noyes and Barber-Westin 1997) if modern techniques of vascular, nerve, and ligament repair combined with an aggressive rehabilitation programme are adopted.

Key point

- Knee dislocation is extremely rare and an emergency.

Extensor mechanism injuries

Rupture of the quadriceps tendon

Ruptures of the extensor mechanism of the knee occur in old age from direct sharp or blunt trauma. Repeated microtrauma or collagen diseases increase the likelihood of tendon ruptures (Miskew *et al.* 1980). The quadriceps usually ruptures within 2 cm of the superior pole of the patella (Siwek and Rao 1978). The patient presents with pain over the superior aspect of the patella, swelling of the knee, and inability to bear weight on the affected side. Not infrequently, the symptoms are minimal and the diagnosis is missed in the acute period.

Patients with chronic or neglected ruptures (history >2 weeks) will complain of repeated 'giving way' episodes, especially on ascending stairs (Ramsey and Muller 1970).

Physical examination will reveal a palpable defect in the quadriceps tendon and an inability to actively extend the knee. There may be an associated effusion within the knee joint. Lateral radiographs of the knee joint may show the patella to be in a low position (patella baja). In case of diagnostic difficulty, an ultrasound or MRI scan can be obtained.

Key point

- Not infrequently, the symptoms of quadriceps tendon rupture are minimal and the diagnosis is missed in the acute period.

Management

Acute ruptures: If the quadriceps tendon is not repaired in the acute period, it may ride proximally on the femur and adhere to the surrounding soft tissues. Most authors agree that early, end-to-end repair offers the best chance of a good outcome from these injuries (Siwek and Rao 1981). The torn edges of the tendon are freshened and repaired with interrupted non-absorbable sutures. The edges of the tendon should overlap slightly to relieve any tension. The repair is protected by a local reinforcement flap, as advocated by Scuderi (1958). In this technique, a distally based partial thickness flap of the quadriceps tendon in the shape of an isosceles triangle is turned down over the suture line and secured with tacking stitches. The primary repair may be protected by means of a dacron graft or the middle third of the patellar tendon. The knee is immobilized in a cylinder cast for 6 weeks. Partial ruptures of the quadriceps tendon can be treated conservatively.

Key point

- Early, end-to-end repair offers the best chance of a good outcome.

Chronic ruptures: The popular technique for chronic ruptures is the Codivilla V–Y lengthening.

Ruptures of the patellar tendon

Acute ruptures of the patellar tendon are rare injuries. They usually result from forceful contraction of the quadriceps muscle on a partially flexed knee. These injuries occur commonly in middle age and there may be a history of patellar tendinitis or steroid injections into the tendon.

The patient presents with severe pain in the region of the patellar tendon and inability to bear weight. On examination, there is significant swelling and subcutaneous ecchymosis associated with a palpable defect over the patellar tendon. The patient cannot actively extend the knee or straight leg-raise in the supine or sitting positions. Lateral knee radiographs are helpful in determining patellar height. Gradient-echo or T2 weighted MRI may be employed in difficult or chronic cases.

Key point

- Note history of patellar tendinitis or steroid injections into the tendon.

Management

Direct end-to-end repair at the earliest opportunity offers the best results (Larsen and Lund 1986). The tendon is approached through a midline longitudinal incision. The ends are identified, freshened and repaired using no. 2 non-absorbable sutures. Various techniques have been used to augment and protect the repair. In uncomplicated cases, a 1.0–2.0 mm wire is passed around the edges of the patella and anchored distally by means of a drill hole through the tibial tubercle, in a figure-of-eight pattern. This protects the repair by acting as a tension band across the patellar tendon. In order to augment the repair, the semitendinosus and gracilis tendons can be harvested, passed through transverse drill holes in the patella and sutured in an end-to-end manner. Whatever the technique employed, it is vitally important to restore normal patellar tracking, height, and rotation. At the end of the procedure, the knee is flexed to 90° in order to ensure normal tracking and adequate strength of the repair. Intraoperative lateral radiographs of the knee confirm patellar height. In the presence of significant retraction of the tendon, Z-plasty of the quadriceps tendon is used to restore length. The knee is closed in the routine manner and a cylinder cast applied with the knee in full extension. Chronic ruptures can be reconstructed using hamstring grafts or achilles tendon allograft (Ecker 1979).

Postoperative management and rehabilitation

The principles of rehabilitation of all injuries to the extensor mechanism are similar in most aspects. The knee is immobilized in a cylinder cast for 6 weeks. The patient can be allowed to bear weight fully as tolerated. Once the cast is removed, a control-dial hinged knee brace is applied. Progressive flexion is allowed in increments of 10–20° each week. Isometric quadriceps exercises and active assisted straight-leg raises are commenced in this period. Knee flexion should be fully restored at 3 months from the operation. The brace can be discarded once 90° of flexion is obtained. Strengthening exercises help functional recovery and return to normal activities can be expected at 6 months. The results following reconstruction of chronic and neglected ruptures are less consistent than with acute repairs.

Dislocation of the superior tibiofibular joint

Acute dislocation of the superior tibiofibular joint is a rare injury. It may be the result of direct or indirect trauma. The normal superior tibiofibular joint has two major anatomical variants: horizontal and vertical. According to Ogden (1974), the more vertically oriented joints have a higher risk of dislocation. The tibiofibular articulation also has a role in rotation at the ankle joint, by relieving rotational stresses.

The patient presents with pain, tenderness, and local swelling over the upper, lateral aspect of the leg. There may be associated signs of peroneal nerve involvement. True anteroposterior and lateral radiographs of the tibiofibular joint are difficult to obtain. Therefore, the diagnosis is made by comparison with radiographs of the normal extremity taken in roughly the same orientation.

There are four main patterns of tibiofibular dislocations.

- *Subluxation:* This is due to generalized ligamentous laxity (Ehler–Danlos syndrome) and may cause peroneal nerve dysfunction. If the symptoms and nerve palsy do not respond to a brief period of cast immobilization, the fibular head may have to be resected.
- *Anterolateral dislocation:* This results from indirect forces transmitted from a violent twisting injury to the ankle joint. Due to the presence of more severe associated injuries such as compound dislocations of the ankle joint, it is frequently missed on clinical examination. There is an obvious prominence of the fibular head and an abnormal anteriorly curving course of the biceps tendon (Falkenberg and Nygaard 1983). Treatment is by closed reduction. The knee is flexed to relax the collateral ligament, and the foot is pronated, dorsiflexed and externally rotated. Direct pressure over the fibular head reduces it back into its sulcus in the proximal tibia (Sharma and Daffner 1986).
- *Posteromedial dislocation:* This is caused by direct high-energy trauma. It may be associated with injuries to the lateral supporting structures of the knee joint. Treatment is by closed reduction, failing which open reduction and ligamentous repair is advocated.
- *Superior dislocation:* These injuries are the result of a displaced tibial shaft fracture with an intact fibula (Brana *et al.* 1983). Stabilization of the tibial fracture usually reduces the dislocation. If this is unsuccessful, closed or open reduction may be necessary. The reduction may be held with Kirschner wires, until the supporting ligaments heal.

Key points

- Dislocation of the superior tibiofibular joint is rare.
- There maybe associated signs of peroneal nerve involvement.

Postoperative management

Most authors recommend immobilization in a cast for 3–6 weeks, followed by active exercises. Weight-bearing is restricted only in the first 2 weeks following the injury. Full functional restoration can be expected within 3 months. The presence of persistent symptoms is an indication for fibular head resection or open reduction and internal fixation of the joint. Arthrodesis of the joint interferes with the rotation at the ankle joint and is no longer recommended.

References

Aronson J (1997) Limb strengthening, skeletal reconstruction and bone transport with the Ilizarov method. *Journal of Bone and Joint Surgery* 79(8): 1243–1258.

Baker C, Norwood L, Hughston J (1983) Acute posterolateral instability of the knee. *Journal of Bone and Joint Surgery* 65A: 614.

Baratz ME, Fu FH, Mengato R (1986) Meniscal tears: the effect of meniscectomy and of repair on intra articular contact areas and stress in the human knee. A preliminary report. *American Journal of Sports Medicine* 14(4): 270–275.

Barrack RL, Bruckner JD, Kneisl J, Inman WS, Alexander AH (1990) The outcome of nonoperatively treated complete tears of the anterior cruciate ligament in active young adults. *Clinical Orthopedics* 259: 192–199.

Barrett GR, Field MH, Treacy SH, Ruff CG (1998) Clinical results of meniscus repair in patients 40 years and older. *Arthroscopy* 14(8): 824–829.

Barrow BA, Fajman WA, Parker LM *et al.* (1994) Tibial plateau fractures: evaluation with MR imaging. *Radiographics* 15: 553.

Bennett WF, Browner B (1994) Tibial plateau fractures: a study of associated soft-tissue injuries. *J Orthop Trauma* 8: 183.

Biedert RM (1993) Intrasubstance meniscal tears. Clinical aspects and the role of MRI. *Archives of Orthopaedic and Trauma Surgery* 112(3): 142–147.

Blokker CP, Rorabeck CH, Bourne RB (1984) Tibial plateau fractures and analysis of treatment in 60 patients. *Clinical Orthopedics* 182: 193.

Bone LB, Johnson KD, Weigelt J, Scheinberg R (1989) Early versus delayed stabilisation of fractures: a prospective randomized study. *Journal of Bone and Joint Surgery* 71A: 336–340.

Bostman A, Kiviluoto O, Nirhamo J (1981) Comminuted displaced fractures of the patella. *Injury* 13: 196–202.

Bostrom A (1972) Fractures of the patella : A study of 422 patellar fractures. *Acta Orthopaedica Scandinavica* 143 (Suppl): 1–80.

Bradford Henley M (1989) Intramedullary devices for tibial fracture stabilisation. *Clinical Orthopedics* 240: 87–96.

Brana VA, Mieres BP, Montes MS (1983) Traumatic luxation of the proximal tibiofibular joint: superior variety. A case report. *Acta Orthopaedica Belgica* 49: 479–482.

Bratt HD, Newman AP (1993) Complete dislocation of the knee without disruption of both cruciate ligaments. *Journal of Trauma* 34(3): 383–389.

Braun W, Weidemann M, Ruter A, Kundel K, Kolbinger S (1993) Indications and results of nonoperative treatment of patellar fractures. *Clinical Orthopedics* 289: 197–201.

Bray RC, Dandy DJ (1987) Comparison of arthroscopic and open techniques in carbon fibre reconstruction of the anterior cruciate ligament: long-term follow-up after 5 years. *Arthroscopy* 3(2): 106–110.

Brown TD, Anderson DD, Nepola JV *et al.* (1988) Contact stress aberrations following imprecise reduction of simple tibial plateau fracture. *Journal of Orthopaedic Research* 6: 851.

Burgess AR, Poka A, Brumback RJ, Bosse MJ (1987a) Management of open grade III tibial fractures. *Orthopedic Clinics of North America* 18: 85–93.

Burgess AR, Poka A, Brumback RJ *et al.* (1987b) Pedestrian tibial injuries. *Journal of Trauma* 27: 596–601.

Carpenter JE, Kasman R, Matthews LS (1993) Fractures of the patella. *Journal of Bone and Joint Surgery* 75A: 1550–1561.

Clancy WG Jr, Pandya RD (1994) Posterior cruciate ligament reconstruction with patellar tendon autograft. *Clinics in Sports Medicine* 13(3): 561–570.

Clendenin MB, DeLee JC, Heckman JD (1980) Interstitial tears of the PCL of the knee. *Orthopedics* 3: 764–772.

Cofield RH, Bryan RS (1977) Acute dislocation of the patella: results of conservative treatment. *Journal of Trauma* 17(7): 526–531.

Cooper DE, Warren RF, Warner JJP (1991) The posterior cruciate ligament and the posterolateral structures of the knee: anatomy, function, and patterns of injury. *Instructional Course Lectures* 40: 249–270.

Court-Brown CM, McBirnie J (1995) The epidemiology of tibial fractures. *Journal of Bone and Joint Surgery* 77B: 417–421.

Court-Brown CM, Gustilo T, Shaw AD (1997) Knee pain after intramedullary nailing: its incidence, aetiology, and outcome. *Journal of Orthopaedic Trauma* 11(2): 103–105.

Cross MJ, Wootton JR, Bokor DJ, Sorrenti SJ (1993) Acute repair of injury to the anterior cruciate ligament. A long-term follow up. *American Journal of Sports Medicine* 21(1): 128–31.

Curtis MJ (1990) Internal fixation of fracture of the patella: a comparison of two methods. *Journal of Bone and Joint Surgery* 72B: 280–282.

Daniels DM, Fithian DC (1994) Indications for ACL surgery. *Arthroscopy* 10(4): 434–440.

DeCoster TA, Nepola JV, El-Khoury GY (1988) Cast brace treatment of proximal tibial fractures. A ten-year follow-up study. *Clinical Orthopedics* 231: 196–204.

DeHaven KE (1990) Decision-making factors in the treatment of meniscus lesions. *Clinical Orthopedics* 252: 49–54.

Delamarter R, Hohl M (1989) The cast brace and tibial plateau fractures. *Clinical Orthopedics* 242: 26–31.

Ecker ML, Lotre PA, Glazer RM (1979) Late reconstruction of the patella tendon. *Journal of Bone and Joint Surgery* 61A: 884.

Ellis H (1958) The speed of healing after fracture of the tibial shaft. *Journal of Bone and Joint Surgery* 40B: 42–46.

Falkenberg P, Nygaard H (1983) Isolated anterior dislocation of the proximal tibiofibular joint. *Journal of Bone and Joint Surgery* 65B: 310–311.

Feagin JA Jr, Lambert KL (1985) Mechanism of injury and pathology of anterior cruciate ligament injuries. *Orthopedic Clinics of North America* 16(1): 41–45.

Fetto JF, Marshall JL (1979) Injury to the anterior cruciate ligament producing the pivot-shift sign. *Journal of Bone and Joint Surgery* 61A(5): 710–714.

Fischer MD, Gustilo RB, Varecka TF (1991) The timing of flap coverage, bone-grafting, and intramedullary nailing in patients who have a fracture of the tibial shaft with extensive soft-tissue injury. *Journal of Bone and Joint Surgery* 73A: 1316–1322.

Fithian DC, Kelly MA, Mow VC (1990) Material properties and structure–function relationships in the menisci. *Clinical Orthopedics* 252: 19–31.

Fleming R, Blatz D, McCarroll J (1981) Posterior problems in the knee: posterior cruciate insufficiency and posterolateral rotatory insufficiency. *American Journal of Sports Medicine* 9: 107.

Friedman RL, Jackson DW (1996) Magnetic resonance imaging of the anterior cruciate ligament: current concepts. *Orthopedics* 19(6): 525–532.

Fruensgaard S, Kroner K, Riis J (1992) Suture of the torn anterior cruciate ligament. 5-year follow-up of 60 cases using an instrumental stability test. *Acta Orthopaedica Scandinavica* 63(3): 323–325.

Gable DR, Allen JW, Richardson JD (1997) Blunt popliteal artery injury: is physical examination alone enough for evaluation? *Journal of Trauma* 43(3): 541–544.

Gustilo RB, Anderson JT (1976) Prevention of infection in the treatment of 1025 open fractures of long bones: retrospective and prospective analysis. *Journal of Bone and Joint Surgery* 58A: 453–458.

Hammerle CP, Jocob RP (1980) Chondral and osteochondral fractures after luxation of the patella and their treatment. *Archives of Orthopaedic and Trauma Surgery* 97: 207–211.

Hastings DE (1980) The nonoperative management of collateral ligament injuries of the knee joint. *Clinical Orthopedics* 147: 22–28.

Hawkins RJ, Misamore GW, Merritt TR (1986) Followup of the acute nonoperated isolated anterior cruciate ligament tear. *American Journal of Sports Medicine* 14(3): 205–210.

Henning CE, Lynch MA, Yearout KM *et al.* (1990) Arthroscopic meniscal repair using an exogenous fibrin clot. *Clinical Orthopedics* 252: 64–72.

Heron CW, Calvert PT (1992) Three-dimensional gradient-echo MR imaging of the knee: comparison with arthroscopy in 100 patients. *Radiology* 183(3): 839–844.

Hill JA, Rana NA (1981) Complications of posterolateral dislocation of the knee: case report and literature review. *Clinical Orthopedics* 154: 212–215.

Honkonen SE, Jarvinen MJ (1992) Classification of fractures of the tibial condyles. *Journal of Bone and Joint Surgery* 74B: 840.

Hugh LK, Lee SY, Leung KS, Chan KM, Nicholl LA (1993) Partial patellectomy for patellar fracture: tension band wiring and early mobilization. *Journal of Orthopaedic Trauma* 7: 252–260.

Hughston JC, Bowden JA, Andrews JR, Norwood LA (1980) Acute tears of the posterior cruciate ligament. Results of operative treatment. *Journal of Bone and Joint Surgery* 62A(3): 438–450.

Jakobsen J, Christensen KS, Rasmussen OS (1985) Patellectomy—a 20-year follow-up. *Acta Orthopaedica Scandinavica* 56: 430–432.

Johannsen HV, Fruensgaard S (1988) Arthroscopy in the diagnosis of acute injuries to the knee joint. *International Orthopaedics* 12(4): 283–286.

Johner R, Wruhs O (1983) Classification of tibial shaft fractures and correlation with results after rigid internal fixation. *Clinical Orthopedics* 178: 7–23.

Johnson DL, Bealle D (1999) Meniscal allograft transplantation. *Clinics in Sports Medicine* 18(1): 93–108.

Jomha NM, Borton DC, Clingeleffer AJ, Pinczewski LA (1999) Long-term osteoarthritic changes in anterior cruciate ligament reconstructed knees. *Clinical Orthopedics* 358: 188–93.

Kaufman SL, Martin LG (1992) Arterial injuries associated with complete dislocation of the knee. *Radiology* 184(1): 153–155.

Kennedy JC, Bailey WH (1968) Experimental tibial plateau fractures. *Journal of Bone and Joint Surgery* 50A: 1522.

Kim SJ, Kim HK (1995) Reliability of the anterior drawer test, the pivot shift test, and the Lachman test. *Clinical Orthopedics* 317: 237–242.

Kim SJ, Min BH, Han DY (1996) Paradoxical phenomena of the McMurray test. An arthroscopic investigation. *American Journal of Sports Medicine* 24(1): 83–87.

Kim SJ, Kim HK, Kim HJ (1999) Arthroscopic posterior cruciate ligament reconstruction using a one-incision technique. *Clinical Orthopedics* 359: 156–166.

Koval KJ, Helfet DL (1995) Tibial plateau fractures: evaluation and treatment. *Journal of the American Academy of Orthopedic Surgeons* 3(2): 86–93.

Koval KJ, Clapper MK, Brumback RJ *et al.* (1991) Complications of reamed intramedullary nailing of the tibia. *Journal of Orthopaedic Trauma* 5(2): 184–189.

LaPrade RF, Burnett QM II (1994) Femoral intercondylar notch stenosis and correlation to anterior cruciate ligament injuries. A prospective study. *American Journal of Sports Medicine* 22(2): 198–203.

Larsen E, Lund PM (1986) Ruptures of the extensor mechanism of the knee joint. *Clinical Orthopedics* 213: 150–153.

Lintner DM, Kamaric E, Moseley JB, Noble PC (1995) Partial tears of the anterior cruciate ligament. Are they clinically detectable? *American Journal of Sports Medicine* 23(1): 111–118.

MacDonald P, Miniaci A, Fowler P, Marks P, Finlay B (1996) A biomechanical analysis of joint contact forces in the posterior cruciate deficient knee. *Knee Surgery, Sports Traumatology, Arthroscopy* 3(4): 252–255.

Maffulli N, Binfield PM, King JB, Good CJ (1993) Acute haemarthrosis of the knee in athletes. A prospective study of 106 cases. *Journal of Bone and Joint Surgery* 75B(6): 945–949.

Marshall JL, Wang JB, Furman W, Girgis FG, Warren R (1975) The anterior drawer sign: what is it? *J Sports Med* 3(4): 152–158.

Matsen FA III (1989) Compartment syndromes: Part A. Pathophysiology of compartment syndromes. *Instructional Course Lectures*, 43: 463.

Maynard MJ, Deng X, Wickiewicz TL, Warren RF (1996) The popliteofibular ligament. Rediscovery of a key element in posterolateral stability. *American Journal of Sports Medicine* 24(3): 311–316.

McMinn RMH (1994) Lower limb. In: McMinn RMH (ed.) *Last's Anatomy, Regional and Applied*, 9th edn. Churchill-Livingstone, Edinburgh, UK.

McQueen MM, Court-Brown CM (1996) Compartment monitoring in tibial fractures: the threshold for decompression. *Journal of Bone and Joint Surgery* 78B(1): 99–104.

McQueen MM, Court-Brown CM, Christie J (1996) Acute compartment syndrome in tibial diaphyseal fractures. *Journal of Bone and Joint Surgery* 78B(1): 95–98.

Miller MD, Harner CD (1993) The use of allograft. Techniques and results. *Clinics in Sports Medicine* 12(4): 757–770.

Miller RH (1998) Acute traumatic lesions of ligaments. In: Terry Canale S (ed.) *Campbell's Operative Orthopaedics*, Vol. 2. Mosby, St. Louis, Mo., pp 1113–1299.

Miskew DBW, Pearson RL, Pankovich AM (1980) Mersilene strip suture in repair of disruptions of the quadriceps and patellar tendons. *Journal of Trauma* 20(10): 867–872.

Morscher E (1971) Cartilage–bone lesions of the knee joint following injury. *Reconstruction Surgery and Traumatology* 12: 2–26.

Nelson GE, Kelly PJ, Peterson F, Janes J (1964) Blood supply of the human tibia. *Journal of Bone and Joint Surgery* 42A: 625–635.

Nicoll EA (1964) Fractures of the tibial shaft: a survey of 705 cases. *Journal of Bone and Joint Surgery* 46B: 373–387.

Noyes FR, Barber-Westin SD (1997) Reconstruction of the anterior and posterior cruciate ligaments after knee dislocation. Use of early protected postoperative motion to decrease arthrofibrosis. *American Journal of Sports Medicine* 25(6): 769–778.

Nystrom M, Samimi S, Ha'Eri GB (1992) Two cases of irreducible knee dislocation occurring simultaneously in two patients and a review of the literature. *Clinical Orthopedics* 277: 197–200.

Ochi M, Yamanaka T, Sumen Y, Ikuta Y (1993) Arthroscopic and histologic evaluation of anterior cruciate ligaments reconstructed with the Leeds–Keio ligament. *Arthroscopy* 9(4): 387–393.

Ogden JA (1974) Subluxation and dislocation of the proximal tibiofibular joint. *Journal of Bone and Joint Surgery* 56A: 145–154.

Oni OO, Hui A, Gregg PJ (1988) The healing of closed tibial fractures: the natural history of union with closed treatment. *Journal of Bone and Joint Surgery* 70A(5): 787–790.

Polly DW Jr, Callaghan JJ, Sikes RA *et al.* (1988) The accuracy of selective magnetic resonance imaging compared with the findings of arthroscopy of the knee. *Journal of Bone and Joint Surgery* 70A(2): 192–198.

Ramsey RH, Muller GE (1970) Quadriceps tendon rupture: a diagnostic trap. *Clinical Orthopedics* 70: 161–164.

Rasenberg EI, Lemmens JA, Van Kampen A *et al.* (1995) Grading medial collateral ligament injury: comparison of MR Imaging and Instrumented valgus–varus laxity test-device. A prospective double-blind study. *European Journal of Radiology* 21(1): 18–24.

Rubenstein RA Jr, Shelbourne KD, McCarroll JR, VanMeter CD, Rettig AC (1994) The accuracy of the clinical examination in the setting of posterior cruciate ligament injuries. *American Journal of Sports Medicine* 22(4): 550–557.

Sakane M, Fox RJ, Woo SL *et al.* (1997) In situ forces in the anterior cruciate ligament and its bundles in response to anterior tibial loads. *Journal of Orthopaedic Research* 15(2): 285–293.

Sarmiento A (1967) A Functional below-the-knee cast for tibial fractures. *Journal of Bone and Joint Surgery* 49A: 855–875.

Sarmiento A, Gersten LM, Sobol PA, ShankwilerJA, Vangsness CT (1989) Tibial shaft fractures treated with functional braces. *Journal of Bone and Joint Surgery* 71B: 602–609.

Sarmiento A, Sharpe FE, Ebramzadeh E, Normand P, Shankwiler JA (1995) Factors influencing the outcome of closed tibial fractures treated with functional bracing. *Clinical Orthopedics* 315: 8–24.

Schatzker J (1987) Fractures of the tibial plateau. In: Schatzker J, Tile M (eds) *Rationale of Operative Fracture Care*. Springer-Verlag, New York, N.Y.

Schatzker J, McBroom R, Bruce D (1979) Tibial plateau fractures: the Toronto experience 1968–1975. *Clinical Orthopedics* 138: 94.

Scuderi C (1958) Ruptures of the quadriceps tendon. *American Journal of Surgery* 95: 626–635.

Seebacher JR, Inglis AE, Marshall JL, Warren RF (1982) The structure of the postero-lateral aspect of the knee. *Journal of Bone and Joint Surgery* 64A: 536–541.

Shapiro MS, Freedman EL (1995) Allograft reconstruction of the anterior and posterior cruciate ligaments after traumatic knee dislocation. *American Journal of Sports Medicine* 23(5): 580–587.

Sharma P, Daffner RH (1986) Idiopathic, anterolateral dislocation of the fibula at the proximal tibiofibular joint. *Skeletal Radiology* 15: 505–506.

Shelton WR, Papendick L, Dukes AD (1997) Autograft versus allograft anterior cruciate ligament reconstruction. *Arthroscopy* 13(4): 446–449.

Shertsov VI (1997) Professor GA Ilizarov's contribution to the method of transosseous osteosynthesis. *Bulletin Hospital Joint Disorders* 56(1): 11–15.

Shoemaker SC, Markolf KL (1986) The role of the meniscus in the anterior-posterior stability of the loaded anterior cruciate-deficient knee. Effects of partial versus total excision. *Journal of Bone and Joint Surgery* 68A(1): 71–79.

Shrive NG, O'Connor JJ, Goodfellow JW (1978) Load-bearing in the knee joint. *Clinical Orthopedics* 131: 279–287.

Simonsen O, Jensen J, Mouritsen P, Lauritzen J (1984) The accuracy of clinical examination of injury of the knee joint. *Injury* 16(2): 96–101.

Siwek KW, Rao JP (1978) Bilateral simultaneous rupture of the quadriceps tendon. *Clinical Orthopedics* 131: 252–254.

Siwek KW, Rao JP (1981) Ruptures of the extensor mechanism of the knee joint. *Journal of Bone and Joint Surgery* 63A(3): 351–356.

Skyhar MJ, Warren RF, Ortiz GJ, Schwartz E, Otis JC (1993) The effects of sectioning of the posterior cruciate ligament and the posterolateral complex on the articular contact pressures within the knee. *Journal of Bone and Joint Surgery* 75A(5): 694–649.

Sonin AH, Fitzgerald SW, Friedman H *et al.* (1994) Posterior cruciate ligament injury: MR imaging diagnosis and patterns of injury. *Radiology* 190(2): 455–458.

Sonin AH, Fitzgerald SW, Hoff FL, Friedman H, Bresler ME (1995) MR imaging of the posterior cruciate ligament: normal, abnormal, and associated injury patterns. *Radiographics* 15(3): 551–561.

Souryal TO, Freeman TR (1993) Intercondylar notch size and anterior cruciate ligament injuries in athletes. A prospective study. *American Journal of Sports Medicine* 21(4): 535–539.

Stone KR (1996) Meniscus replacement. *Clinics in Sports Medicine* 15(3): 557–571.

Thakur AJ (1997) *The elements of fracture fixation*, Chapter 2. Churchill Livingstone, London.

Tornetta PI, Bergman M, Watnik N, Berkowitz G, Steuer J (1994) A prospective randomised comparison of external fixation and non-reamed locked nailing. *Journal of Bone and Joint Surgery* 76B(1): 13–19.

Tscherne H, Gotzen L (1984) *Fractures with soft tissue injuries*. Springer-Verlag, Berlin.

Vander Schilden JL (1990) Improvements in rehabilitation of the postmenisectomized or meniscal-repaired patient. *Clinical Orthopedics* 252: 73–79.

Vellet AD, Marks P, Fowler P, Munro T (1989) Accuracy of nonorthogonal magnetic resonance imaging in acute disruption of the anterior cruciate ligament. *Arthroscopy* 5(4): 287–293.

Veltri DM, Warren RF (1993) Isolated and combined PCL injuries. *Journal of the American Academy of Orthopedic Surgeons* 1(2): 67–75.

Veltri DM, Warren RF (1994) Operative treatment of posterolateral instability of the knee. *Clinics in Sports Medicine* 13(3): 615–627.

Walker DN, Rogers W, Schenck RC Jr (1994) Immediate vascular and ligamentous repair in a closed knee dislocation: case report. *Journal of Trauma* 36(6): 898–900.

Warren LF, Marshall JL (1979) The supporting structures and layers on the medial side of the knee. *Journal of Bone and Joint Surgery* 61A: 56–62.

Warren RF (1990) Menisectomy and repair in the anterior cruciate ligament-deficient patient. *Clinical Orthopedics* 252: 55–63.

Whittle AP (1998) Fractures of the lower extremity: tibial shaft. In: Terry Canale S (ed.) *Campbell's operative orthopaedics,* Vol. 3. Mosby, St. Louis, p 3.

Wilk KE (1994) Rehabilitation of isolated and combined posterior cruciate ligament injuries. *Clinics in Sports Medicine* 13(3): 649–677.

Wiss DA, Tracy Watson J (1996) Fractures of the proximal tibia and fibula. In: Rockwood C, Green D, Bucholz R (eds) *Fractures in adults*, 4th edn. Lippincot-Raven, Philadelphia.

Woo SL, Chan SS, Yamaji T (1997) Biomechanics of knee ligament healing, repair and reconstruction. *Journal of Biomechanics* 30(5): 431–439.

Yu JS, Goodwin D, Salonen D *et al.* (1995) Complete dislocation of the knee: spectrum of associated soft-tissue injuries depicted by MR imaging. *American Journal of Roentgenology* 164(1): 135–139.

23

CHAPTER 23

Foot and ankle injuries

LORETTA B CHOU AND NICOLA MAFFULLI

CHAPTER 23
Foot and ankle injuries

LORETTA B CHOU AND NICOLA MAFFULLI

Ankle sprains

General principles

Ankle sprains are very common. Inversion injuries cause about 85% of all ankle injuries, with the lateral collateral ligamentous complex as the most frequently injured structure (Cardone *et al.* 1993). A recent study showed that at the United States Military Academy during a 2 month period, there were 104 ankle injuries, which was 23% of all injuries seen. Of these, there were 96 ankle sprains (Gerber *et al.* 1998).

Key point

- Ankle sprains, especially of the lateral collateral ligamentous complex, are one of the most common musculoskeletal injuries.

Anatomy and biomechanics

The ankle joint is a mortice joint that is made of the distal tibia and fibula and the talus. The lateral collateral ligamentous structure consists of the anterior talofibular (ATF), calcaneofibular (CF), and posterior talofibular (PTF) ligaments. The medial collateral ligament is made of the superficial and deep portions of the deltoid ligament.

Mechanism of injury

The ATF ligament is taut in plantar flexion, and it is the most commonly injured ligament. The mechanism of injury is inversion while the foot is plantar flexed. The CF ligament is taut in dorsiflexion, and can be injured with the ATF ligament. Less commonly injured is the deltoid ligament. Jumping and cutting increase the risk of an ankle sprain while participating in sports such as basketball, tennis, and soccer.

Key point

- The ATF ligament is taut in plantar flexion, and it is the most commonly injured ligament.

Presentation

Signs and symptoms

The most common complaint is acute onset of pain after an injury. Associated symptoms are swelling, difficulty with weight-bearing, and instability.

Classification of injury

Sprains of the ankle can be classified by the degree of injury to the lateral collateral ligamentous structures. A grade I injury is stretching of the ATF without laxity, grade II injury is partial tear of the ATF ligament and CF ligament with mild laxity, and grade III injury is a complete rupture of the ATF, CF, and PTF ligaments with gross laxity. In the study by Gerber *et al.* (1998) the vast majority of sprains were classified grade I or grade II. By 6 weeks after injury, 95% of the patients had returned to full activity in the military academy.

Key points

- Sprains of the ankle classified (by the degree of the lateral collateral ligamentous structures) are:
  - grade I injury: stretching of the ATF without laxity

- grade II: partial tear of the ATF ligament and CF ligament with mild laxity
- grade III: complete tear of the ATF, CF, and PTF ligaments with gross laxity.

Possible associated injuries

Radiography will help with the diagnosis of other injuries which may occur with ankle sprains, which include talar dome fractures, avulsion fractures of the lateral or medial malleolus, and other bony injuries.

Diagnosis

Examination findings

The examination of a patient with an ankle injury should begin with the patient uncovering both legs from the knee. The skin is checked for lacerations or abrasions, swelling, and blisters. Generally, the patient will have point tenderness at the area of injury, over the lateral and medial ankle. The anterior drawer test may be positive with an injury to the ATF ligament, and an increased talar tilt indicates an injury to the CF ligament.

Key points

- There is point tenderness at the area of injury (over the lateral and medial ankle).
- The anterior drawer test may be positive with an injury to the ATF ligament.
- An increased talar tilt indicates an injury to the CF ligament.

Diagnostic techniques

Radiographs are an essential component of the evaluation of the injured patient to exclude fractures. After the clinical examination, three views of the foot or ankle are obtained. Stress views can be obtained to evaluate the extent of the injury, and these may be taken in the chronic case. Acute injuries are usually too painful to manipulate for these views. MRI is a sensitive study to show tears that are acute or chronic. Generally, this exam is not required for diagnosis. Cardone *et al.* showed good correlation between MRI and surgical findings (Chrisman and Snook 1969). MRI demonstrated ATF and CF ligament injuries in a study of 43 patients with ankle sprains. It was also helpful in demonstrating soft tissue and osseous injury.

Key point

- MRI is a sensitive study to show tears that are acute or chronic, but is not generally required for diagnosis.

Ottawa ankle rules (Stiell *et al.* 1995)

1. An ankle radiograph series is needed if there is any pain in medial and/or lateral malleolus and bony tenderness over the medial or lateral malleolus, and inability to bear weight both immediately after the injury and in the emergency department.
2. A foot radiograph series is needed if there is any pain in the midfoot and bone tenderness over the base of the fifth metatarsal or the navicular, and inability to bear weight both immediately after the injury and in the emergency department.

Management

Initial

Acute injuries are treated with rest, ice, compression, and elevation (the RICE regimen). In moderate to severe injuries, a short course of immobilization (up to 5 days) in a splint or cast with the ankle in neutral position is helpful to allow the symptoms to improve, and in bearing weight. Once the pain and swelling decrease, active and passive range of motion exercises can be initiated. Physical therapy is helpful for recovery of strength and motion, particularly peroneal strength. An ankle stirrup may be used for additional support until strength is regained and symptoms are resolved.

Key point

- Acute injuries are treated with rest, ice, compression, and elevation (the RICE regimen).
- Moderate to severe injuries require a short course of immobilization in a splint or cast in neutral.

Surgical indications

The majority of ankle sprains are treated non-operatively. In cases of chronic recurrent injuries with failure of non-operative management and recurrent ankle injuries or instability, surgical reconstruction can be considered.

Key point

- The majority of ankle sprains are treated non-operatively.

Surgical techniques available

Over 80 surgical techniques have been described for the reconstruction of the lateral collateral ligaments. These procedures involve anatomical repair of the torn ligaments or reconstructive procedures with tendon transfers, such as with use of the peroneus brevis tendon. The most commonly used techniques include the modified Brostrom repair and the Chrisman–Snook procedure. The Brostrom repair is an anatomical repair of the torn ATF ligament, whereas the Chrisman–Snook procedure incorporates half of the peroneus brevis tendon to reconstruct the ATF and CF ligaments (Chrisman and Snook 1969). The Evans repair also uses the peroneus brevis tendon, but in this procedure half of the tendon is brought through a drill hole through the fibula and then inserted into the base of the fifth metatarsal (Rosenbaum *et al.* 1997). Non-anatomical repairs can lead to reduced mobility of the subtalar joint and cause impaired eversion, with the possibility of increased development of arthrosis of the subtalar joint.

Authors' preferred technique

The Brostrom procedure with the Gould modification consists of a repair of the ATF ligament (Brostrom 1966, Hamilton *et al.* 1993).

Use a curvilinear incision just distal to the lateral malleolus, taking care to identify and protect the lateral branch of the superficial peroneal nerve (the intermediate dorsal cutaneous nerve) and the sural nerve. the lateral aspect of the extensor retinaculum is mobilized and then the capsule is incised while identifying the scarred ATF ligament. The CF ligament is also identified. The ATF and CF are repaired with the 'vest over pants' technique or with drill holes into the fibula. The extensor retinaculum is then repaired with absorbable suture with the ankle held in neutral.

Key point

- An anatomical repair of the torn ATF is the surgical technique of choice.

Postoperative care

The patient is immobilized in a short leg cast for 6 weeks, with the initial 3 weeks non-weight-bearing. Gentle range of motion exercises can be initiated once the patient is weight-bearing.

Complications and management

Complications from surgical repair include wound healing problems, surgical neuromas, continued instability, and stiffness. Taking care to protect the sensory nerves and gentle handling of soft tissue will help to avoid these complications. Physical therapy may be used to treat persistent instability or stiffness.

Prognosis

Patients have good relief of pain and instability in most cases, although up to 40% of patients may continue to experience ankle dysfunction (Gerber *et al.* 1998).

Following a modified Brostrom procedure, there were 26 excellent results, 1 good, and 1 fair in 28 ankles in 27 patients (Hamilton *et al.* 1993). There were no failures, stretch-outs, re-dos, or complications. This procedure is an excellent choice for dancers, athletes, or non-athletes alike.

Achilles tendon tears

General principles

Rupture of the Achilles tendon is a common injury in the men, usually in the 4th–5th decade. Acute ruptures are usually associated with low grade symptoms from underlying tendinosis (Novacheck 1998). This is known as the 'weekend warrior' injury, with acute stress placed on an already abnormal tendon.

Anatomy and biomechanics

The Achilles tendon is made up of the gastrocnemius–soleus complex, the largest muscle in the leg. It spans two joints, contracts eccentrically and concentrically, and twists 90° in its course from its origin to its insertion. The area of hypovascularity, 4–6 cm from the insertion (Saltzman and Tearse 1998) is where most of the acute subcutaneous tears take place. Advanced intratendinous degeneration is a feature of acute ruptures (Maffulli *et al.* 2000).

Mechanism of injury

The aetiology of a rupture is usually multifactorial, and the most common cause is training errors, such as increase in intensity, duration, or overuse. The patient is usually engaged in an acceleration–deceleration sport, which causes the rupture.

Key point

- Most patients sustain a tear when engaged in an acceleration–deceleration sport.

Presentation

Patients complain of sudden onset of pain in the posterior aspect of the lower leg. Frequently, they describe that they felt a 'kick' in the affected ankle. They may not be able to bear weight, and may find it difficult to walk. There is associated swelling and bruising.

Diagnosis

The diagnosis can reliably be made by history and physical examination (Maffulli 1998).

Examination findings

The patient has localized swelling of the involved foot and ankle, and cannot plantar flex the foot. The area of rupture has a palpable defect.

Key point

- The Thompson test is performed with the patient prone: absence of plantar flexion of the foot when the calf is squeezed indicates a complete rupture of the Achilles tendon, and constitutes a positive Thompson test.

Imaging

An MRI scan may be used to help confirm the diagnosis. This is especially useful with a false-positive Thompson test or with a partial tear. Ultrasonography may be more accurate and less costly than an MRI scan, but this is dependent on the ultrasonographer's experience.

Management

Initial

The patient should be treated with ice, elevation, splinting, and crutches. These measures will help with the acute symptom of pain and inability to bear weight.

Options

With a complete rupture, the patient can be treated with a course of immobilization, with a short leg cast in equinus for approximately 3 months, gradually decreasing the amount of equinus.

Surgical indications

For the healthy, active patient, most surgeons recommend surgery. Although there are definite surgical risks, the risk of re-rupture is approximately one-tenth of that of conservative management, and return to sport is faster and more predictable.

Key point

- For the healthy, active patient, most surgeons recommend surgical treatment.

Surgical techniques available

Direct repair of the tendon is commonly used, and a large non-absorbable suture is incorporated for the repair. There is a method of percutaneous repair, but the results are variable, and there can be complications with nerve entrapment.

> **Authors' preferred technique**
>
> The Achilles tendon is exposed through a longitudinal incision just medial to the midline, to avoid a scar directly over the tendon and the sural nerve. The ends of the tendon are debrided if necessary and then re-approximated with a non-absorbable suture in a modified Kessler technique. Next, an absorbable suture, such as 3-0 plain gut, is used as a tidying stitch. The paratenon is repaired with absorbable suture, followed by the subcutaneous tissue and skin. The foot and ankle are maintained in 30° of equinus. A bulky compression dressing and splints are applied to protect the repair.

Postoperative care

The patient is instructed to use crutches and not bear weight on the extremity. The sutures are removed 2 weeks after surgery. A cast is placed with the foot held in equinus. The cast is changed every 2–3 weeks, gradually decreasing the amount of equinus. Once 10° is attained, the patient may begin toe-touch weight-bearing. The final cast is at neutral, and the patient may bear weight as tolerated. At 10–12 weeks from the time of the repair, the cast is removed and the patient may ambulate with a 2.5 cm (1 inch) heel.

Complications and management

Complications of surgical repair include wound infection, skin healing problems, sural nerve injury or neuroma, re-rupture, and weakness.

Prognosis

The prognosis following surgical repair is good, and usually the maximum strength is achieved 8–12 months after the procedure. There may be residual swelling and weakness.

Ankle fractures

General principles

Fractures of the ankle are common. Most fractures are displaced and require treatment with open reduction and internal fixation (ORIF).

Key point

- If fractures are displaced, and require ORIF.

Anatomy and biomechanics

The ankle joint consists of the distal tibia and fibula and the talus, which are held together with ligaments. The tibiofibular syndesmosis is made of the anterior tibiofibular ligament, posterior tibiofibular ligament, transverse tibiofibular ligament, and the interosseous membrane. Approximately 70% of dorsiflexion and plantar flexion takes place at the ankle joint. With displacement in a fracture, the weight-bearing portion of the talus can change dramatically. Therefore, anatomical reduction is crucial for regaining function and prevention of early secondary osteoarthritis.

Key point

- Anatomic reduction is necessary for regaining function.

Mechanism of injury

Frequently, an ankle fracture occurs from a fall, with an inversion and rotation injury, or is associated with a sports activity. The mechanism determines involvement of the lateral, medial, or posterior malleolus of the ankle joint.

Presentation

As with other ankle injuries, patients present with acute onset of pain and inability to bear weight. Swelling usually develops rapidly.

Signs and symptoms

Most patients will have moderate to severe pain. There can be a deformity of the ankle with a displaced fracture. The swelling is localized to the foot and ankle, and in severe cases, fracture blisters can develop. The patient may have difficulty with motion because of pain and swelling. There is localized tenderness at the fracture site.

Classification of injury

The most common classification is the Danis–Weber scheme (Harper 1992). It describes the position of the fracture of the lateral malleolus. A type A injury is a fracture of the lateral malleolus below the syndesmosis, a type B fracture is at the level of the syndesmosis, and a type C fracture is above the syndesmosis. This is a simple classification, is reproducible, and allows for determination of management.

The other well known classification is that of Lauge-Hansen (1950), the first to be based on the mechanism of injury. It was determined from the results of a cadaver study. The first term indicates the position of the foot and the second term describes the direction of the deforming force. There are four types: supination–adduction injury, supination–external rotation injury, pronation– abduction injury and pronation–external rotation injury. Each type has stages of the mechanism of injury.

Key point

- The most commonly used classification is the Danis–Weber scheme.

Possible associated injuries

The syndesmosis may be injured with an ankle fracture. Fixation with a syndesmosis screw is necessary if the fracture lies 3–4.5 cm proximal to the mortice (Boden *et al.* 1989).

Diagnosis

The diagnosis of an ankle fracture can be made with history of the mechanism of injury, physical examination, and radiographic examination.

Examination findings

The skin is examined for lacerations, abrasions, swelling, and fracture blisters. Gentle palpation of the malleoli, medial and lateral collateral ligaments, syndesmosis, and proximal fibula will help determine the structures involved. Tenderness of the deltoid ligament indicates a deltoid tear, and this may require treatment if there is an associated displaced lateral malleolus fracture.

Diagnostic techniques

After history taking and physical examination, radiographs are taken (anteroposterior, lateral, and mortice views of the ankle joint). Further diagnostic studies are generally not required unless there is a suspicion of a stress fracture or occult injury, in which case a bone scan may be helpful.

Management

Initial

The initial treatment for a displaced fracture is immediate reduction. Adequate reduction is then confirmed by radiography. Generally, any ankle fracture is to be immobilized, preferably with a splint. Ice and elevation should be used to control the swelling, and help with pain control.

Options

Cast immobilization may be used once the swelling has diminished. Non-surgical treatment is used with undisplaced fractures or minimally displaced isolated medial or lateral malleolus fractures. Also, patients with significant co-morbidities and limited activity level may be candidates for non-operative treatment.

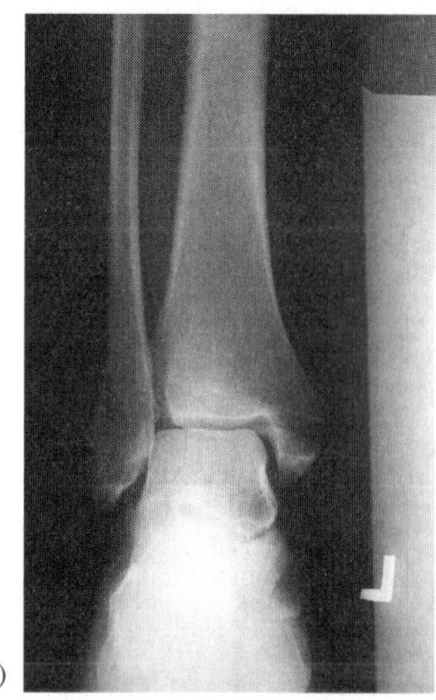

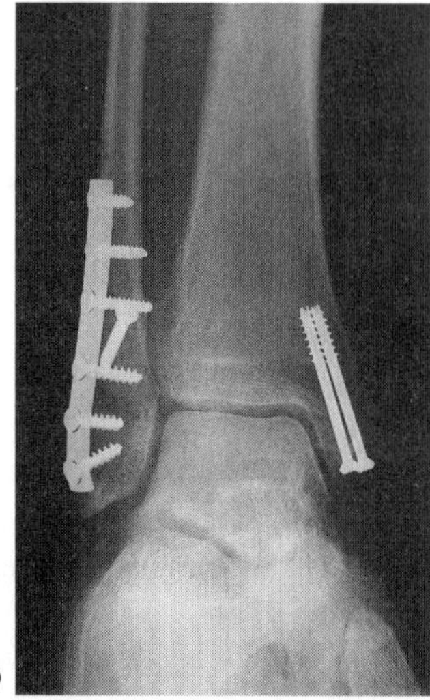

Figure 23.1 (a) Preoperative mortice radiograph demonstrating a displaced bimalleolar ankle fracture in a 43° year old man following an inversion injury while playing softball. (b) Postoperative mortice radiograph shows anatomical reduction with internal fixation.

Key point

- The initial treatment for a displaced fracture is immediate reduction.

Surgical indications

ORIF of ankle fractures is indicated in bimalleolar fractures (Fig. 23.1) or displaced isolated medial or lateral malleolus fractures. Generally, >2 mm of displacement significantly affects the function of the ankle joint and the development of post-traumatic arthritis.

Key point

- >2 mm of displacement significantly affects the function of the ankle joint.

Surgical techniques available

The lateral malleolus is anatomically reduced to ensure normal function of the ankle joint, and lag screws may be used if the fracture pattern is a spiral or long oblique. Frequently, a one-third semi-tubular is placed on the lateral aspect of the lateral malleolus, especially if the fracture has a short oblique configuration or if comminution is present. The medial malleolus is treated with 1–2 malleolar screws. If the fragment is too small to accommodate two screws, then a Kirschner wire may be used to help control rotation.

Fractures that have injury of the syndesmosis (Danis–Weber type C or a Lauge-Hansen pronation external rotation injury), should be evaluated for the need of a syndesmosis screw.

The posterior malleolus requires reduction and internal fixation if it involves >25% of the articular surface. This fragment is reduced through a posterolateral incision, and the screws penetrate the anterior cortex to gain compression at the fracture site.

> **Authors' preferred technique**
>
> All surgery is performed without tourniquet. For the syndesmosis screw, we prefer to use a 3.5 or 4.5 mm cortical screw, placed approximately 2 cm above the plafond. We include only three cortices, and the foot is held in maximum dorsiflexion while the screw is inserted at a 25–30° angle from posterolateral to anteromedial. The screw is removed 12 weeks after surgery, and the patient is informed that there is a possibility of screw breakage.
>
> If the posterior malleolus fragment is >25% of the articular surface, it should be anatomically reduced. This is achieved using a posterolateral incision that will also allow access to the lateral malleolus. The posterior fragment is reduced and the guide wire of the 4.0 mm cannulated screw provides initial fixation. Intraoperative image intensification is used to confirm reduction, and then the screw is placed from posterior to anterior, approximately 1–1.5 cm from the joint. Two screws can be used, but one is often sufficient.

Postoperative care

The patient is placed in a bulky compression dressing with splints as the ankle is kept in neutral. The sutures are removed 2 weeks after surgery, and a short leg cast is applied. The leg is kept non-weight-bearing for 4 weeks, and then the patient is allowed to bear weight in a walking cast for an additional month. The time of protected weight-bearing is increased when there is severe comminution.

Complications and management

Infection and wound healing problems are rare in healthy patients, but surgical neuromas, stiffness, and post-traumatic arthritis are seen more frequently. Fracture-dislocations are associated with many more complications, especially when there is a delay in surgical treatment. Fracture blisters are seen more frequently with fracture-dislocations, because of the greater extent of soft tissue injury. Immediate reduction, even before radiographs are taken, is recommended and surgical fixation will decrease the severity of this occurrence. Once blisters occur, it is generally recommended to wait until they resolve before proceeding with open reduction.

Special considerations

Patients treated with a syndesmosis screw should maintain protected weight-bearing until the screw has been removed. This may be difficult to achieve if the surgeon elects to maintain the screw for 12 weeks. Physical activities should be avoided during this time. With highly comminuted fibular fractures, the syndesmosis screw should be maintained until there is evidence of healing of the fracture (Ebraheim *et al.* 1997).

Prognosis

With anatomical reduction and stable fixation, the patient has a good chance of returning to most pre-injury activities. Post-traumatic arthritis may result from an ankle fracture, is more commonly seen with displaced bimalleolar fractures, and usually occurs within the first 2 years after the injury (Ebraheim *et al.* 1997).

Key points

- Post-traumatic arthritis:
  - may result from an ankle fracture
  - is more commonly seen with displaced bimalleolar fractures
  - usually occurs within the first 2 years after the injury.

Osteochondral defects of the talus

General principles

These lesions of the talus are also known as osteochondral fractures and osteochondral lesions. The diagnosis may be difficult to make, and it is not uncommon for the injury to be misdiagnosed as an ankle sprain.

Key point

- The diagnosis of osteochondral defects may be difficult to make.

Anatomy and biomechanics

The area of involvement is the chondral surface of the talar dome. On the lateral aspect, the anterior portion is usually involved. The posterior aspect is affected with a medial injury.

Mechanism of injury

The most common mode of injury is inversion of the ankle. Other mechanisms include motor vehicle accidents or falling from a height.

Presentation

The patient complains of pain of the ankle, and can have difficulty with weight-bearing and associated swelling. If the diagnosis is not made initially, the patient may develop chronic pain, swelling, instability, stiffness, and possibly locking with a loose fragment.

Signs and symptoms

Clinical examination may show localized tenderness over the lesion. There may be swelling and decreased motion compared to the uninjured ankle. Attempted motion of the ankle may reproduce symptoms.

Classification of injury

Osteochondral injuries of the talus are classified according to the system of Berndt and Harty (1959). Stage I is a compression lesion, stage II is a fragment that is still attached to the talus, stage III is a fragment without attachment but undisplaced, and stage IV is a displaced fragment.

Possible associated injuries

Other injuries that can be concurrent include lateral collateral ligament injury, peroneal tendon injury, and fracture of the ankle.

Diagnosis

Most lesions can be seen on radiographs of the ankle, anteroposterior, mortice, and lateral views (Fig. 23.2). An MRI scan will reveal lesions not found on plain radiographs. This study will also delineate associated injuries, especially of the surrounding soft tissues.

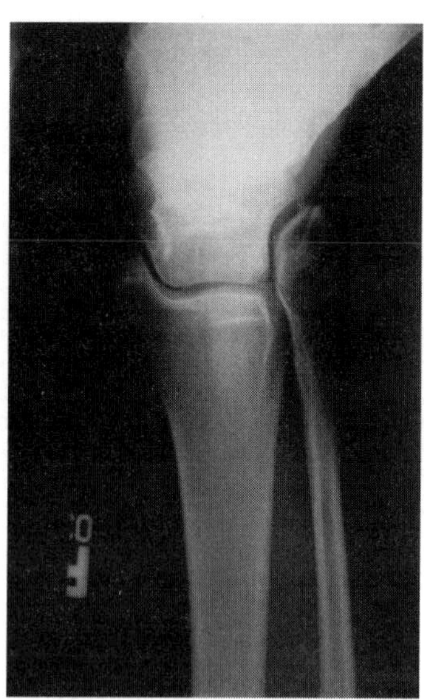

Figure 23.2 Mortice radiograph of a 26 year old woman who fell and twisted her right ankle. A small osteochondral defect is seen in the lateral talar dome.

Key point

- An MRI scan will reveal lesions not found on plain radiographs.

Management

Initial

In stage I, II, and III injuries, it is important to immobilize and initiate protected weight-bearing to help prevent detachment or displacement of the lesion. Splinting and use of crutches can be used until the fragment begins to heal, at about 4–6 weeks. At that time, gentle range of motion can be included in the treatment. This is followed by a short leg weight-bearing cast for an additional month.

Surgical indications

The most important indication for surgical treatment is a displaced fragment (stage IV). Occasionally, a stage III lesion will not heal with immobilization, and then surgical treatment is warranted.

Key point

- If the fragment is displaced, surgery is indicated.

Surgical techniques available

These lesions can be treated with arthroscopic or open techniques.

Authors' preferred technique

Our preference is to treat unhealed stage III lesions and stage IV lesions arthroscopically. Large fragments should be fixed with mini or small fragment screws, absorbable pins, or Herbert screws. Smaller fragments may be removed and the osteochondral base drilled. Some posterior fragments may require an osteotomy of the medial malleolus to gain access for fixation or debridement. There is a technique in which the drill is brought through the medial malleolus, into the joint, and then to the medial talar dome. Intraoperative image intensification is required to confirm positioning of the drill.

Key point

- Consider treating stage III and stage IV lesions arthroscopically.

Postoperative care

After arthroscopic debridement, the patient is placed in a short leg splint and crutches until the sutures are removed. If the lesion is large, non-weight-bearing is continued for about 6 weeks to allow for fibrocartilage ingrowth. This treatment plan is used for fragments that are repaired. After healing is seen on postoperative radiographs, the patient can progress to weight-bearing in a removable cast. Range of motion exercises can also be performed.

Complications and management

The most common complication is the development of secondary arthritis, usually determined by the extent of the initial injury. Other complications include non-union, malunion, symptoms from the fixation means used, and surgical neuroma. Non-union and malunion of the fragment should be treated surgically if the patient is symptomatic. Removal of hardware might help decrease some symptoms. Surgical neuromas can be treated symptomatically. Exploration and resection is sometimes warranted.

Prognosis

Undisplaced lesions generally heal with little consequence. Displaced and stage III non-unions may result in post-traumatic arthritis, and progress with time. These patients should be followed, and treatment may include bracing, or possibly ankle fusion in the severe cases.

Fractures of the talus

Anatomy and biomechanics

The talus is an important structure of the foot and ankle. It articulates with the distal tibia and fibula, forming the ankle joint. It also articulates with the calcaneus in the subtalar joint, and with the navicular in the talonavicular joint. Injury to the talus may involve one or more of these joints, and may affect motion of the foot or the ankle.

Mechanism of injury

Common causes of talus fractures include sports injuries, such as inversion or eversion injuries. Other causes include motor vehicle accidents or falling from a height.

Presentation

Signs and symptoms

Generally, patients with a fracture of the talus will present with acute onset of pain and swelling. They will have difficulty with weight-bearing.

Classification of injury

Hawkins (1970) classified talar neck fractures. Type 1 fractures are non-displaced, type 2 are displaced with subtalar joint subluxation or dislocation, and type 3 are displaced and involve the subtalar and ankle joint with subluxation or dislocation. A type 4 fracture has been added to the system to include subluxation or dislocation of the talonavicular joint.

Key point

- The classification system developed by Hawkins (1970) is still commonly used.

Diagnosis

Examination findings

There is diffuse swelling around the ankle and foot. There is also significant tenderness to gentle palpation. Vascular and neurological examination should always be included, as these systems can be injured with displacement or dislocations.

Diagnostic techniques

The diagnosis is made with plain radiographs of the foot and ankle. The displacement and dislocation is obvious. Sometimes, a CT scan may be helpful to define the nature of the fracture if there is significant comminution.

Management

Initial

The patient should be placed in a splint and prompted to partial weight-bearing. Ice and elevation will help with swelling and pain. A subluxation or dislocation requires immediate reduction and splinting. If reduction is not achieved, then emergency open reduction is indicated.

Options

Type 1 injuries do not require surgical treatment. The patient is placed in a non-weight-bearing cast for 6 weeks, followed by radiographic examination. If fracture consolidation is seen, weight-bearing may be allowed in a short leg cast. Range of motion exercises may be initiated once the swelling and pain allow.

Surgical indications

Displaced types 2 and 3 fractures of the talar neck require open reduction and internal fixation to try and prevent avascular necrosis (AVN).

Authors' preferred technique

A dorsomedial incision is used. Once the fracture is reduced, the guide wire from the cannulated 4.0 mm screw system is used to maintain the reduction while the screw is introduced. Intraoperative image intensification and intraoperative plain radiographs are used to check positioning.

Key points

- Displaced types 2 and 3 fractures of the talar neck require ORIF to try and prevent AVN.
- Surgery is undertaken through a dorsomedial incision, and partially threaded screws are used.

Postoperative care

After surgery, the patient is placed in a bulky compression dressing with splints. The sutures are removed at 2 weeks, and a short leg cast is placed. Non-weight-bearing is continued until 6 weeks after surgery, at which time radiographs are taken. If there is evidence of healing, the patient may begin weight-bearing in a short leg walking cast. This may be removed for range of motion exercises.

Complications and management

The most important complication is AVN, which can be seen by 6 weeks after the injury. *Hawkins' sign* is a radiolucency of the talar dome from hypervascularization of the fracture, and absence of this indicates AVN. AVN is managed by prolonged non-weight-bearing in a cast until there is evidence of revascularization. MRI can be used to monitor the healing process.

Other complications include malunion and non-union. Malunion can be avoided by obtaining anatomical reduction at surgery.

Key points

- The most important complication is AVN. This can be seen by 6 weeks after the injury.

- Hawkins' sign is a radiolucency of the talar dome from hypervascularization of the fracture.

Prognosis

The prognosis depends on the severity of the initial injury. Type I injuries heal without complications and return of function occurs. Patients with type II or III injuries usually have residual pain, stiffness, and swelling.

Fractures of the calcaneus

General principles

The calcaneus is the most commonly fractured tarsal bone. A fracture of the calcaneus may be intra-articular or extra-articular. Most extra-articular injuries can be treated non-operatively, whereas intra-articular fractures frequently may require ORIF.

Key point

- Most extra-articular injuries can be treated non-operatively.

Anatomy and biomechanics

The calcaneus is an important component of the gait cycle, especially with heel strike, foot flat, and toe off. The subtalar joint allows inversion and eversion, both necessary for walking on uneven surfaces. Restoration of the anatomy of the calcaneus is important to maintain the lever arm of the triceps mechanism.

Mechanism of injury

Most intra-articular fractures occur from axial loading following a fall from a height or motor vehicle accident.

Presentation

Most patients with calcaneus fractures will have severe pain and swelling, causing difficulty with weight-bearing. Usually, the associated swelling is moderate to severe.

Signs and symptoms

On physical examination, the patient will have obvious swelling and bruising, possibly with fracture blisters. The foot and ankle may be diffusely tender, with most of the tenderness at the heel.

Possible associated injuries

Depending on the mechanism of injury, a calcaneal fracture may be associated with other skeletal injuries, including a fracture of the contralateral calcaneus, of the pelvis, or of the lumbar spine. Therefore, a careful clinical examination is necessary, and radiographs of the other areas should be obtained if clinical examination warrants them.

Key point

- A calcaneal fracture may have associated skeletal injuries, including fracture of the contralateral calcaneus, the pelvis, or the lumbar spine.

Classification of injury

Extra-articular fractures can involve the body, posterior tuberosity, anterior process, medial process, and lateral process. Intra-articular fractures are classified by a primary and secondary fracture lines. The primary fracture line is a constant finding in displaced calcaneal fractures, caused by the talus wedging into the calcaneus. The sustentaculum tali fragment maintains its attachment to the talus by the interosseous ligament. A secondary fracture line usually occurs, producing a tongue-type or joint depression fracture. The tongue-type fracture is produced when the fracture line continues to the posterior facet and then completes through the posterior tuberosity. In the joint-depression type fracture, the fracture line continues into the posterior facet only.

Sanders' classification is based on CT coronal views of the comminution involvement of the posterior facet (Sanders *et al.* 1993). Type I injury is undisplaced or extra-articular, type II is one fracture line with displacement, type III has two fracture lines, and type IV has three fracture lines or more, creating four or more fragments. Type IV is associated with poor results.

Diagnosis

Examination findings

Moderate to severe swelling is usually seen. With severe injuries, fracture blisters may develop. Also, bruising and loss of motion are commonly found. Paraesthesia may develop in conjunction with swelling.

Key point

- With severe injuries, fracture blisters may develop.

Diagnostic techniques

Plain radiographs will reveal the fracture. If there is intra-articular extension, then Broden's views will help visualize the posterior facet. These views are obtained by placing the foot in internal rotation, 45°, and angling the beam from cephalad from 10° to 40°.

If operative management is planned, then a CT scan with coronal views of the posterior facet is helpful in planning the surgical reconstruction.

Key point

- A CT scan with coronal views of the posterior facet is helpful in planning the surgical reconstruction.

Management

Initial

As with other fractures of the foot and ankle, immediate splinting, elevation, and use of ice will help decrease further swelling and possibly soft-tissue damage. A foot pump can be used to treat the significant swelling that occurs with calcaneal fractures. Patient tolerance for a foot pump is variable; some patients require analgesics while the pump is operating.

Key point

- A foot pump can be used in an attempt to reduce the marked swelling that occurs with calcaneal fractures.

Options

The spectrum of treatment options for calcaneal fractures remains broad, and includes elevation, compression dressing, early motion, closed manipulation, placement of a percutaneous pin, ORIF, and primary subtalar fusion.

Extra-articular fractures that are minimally displaced can be treated with a non-weight-bearing cast for 4–6 weeks, followed by a weight-bearing cast for an additional 4–6 weeks. Fractures that involve the articular surface can be treated non-operatively provided they have little displacement (<2 mm).

Key point

- The spectrum of treatment options for calcaneal fractures remains broad.

Surgical indications

Any extra-articular fracture with significant displacement or causes subluxation of the subtalar or calcaneocuboid joint, or an intra-articular fracture with >2 mm of incongruity warrants open reduction (Fig. 23.3). Other important considerations are widening of the calcaneus or loss of calcaneal height.

Surgical techniques available

Open reduction can be achieved through medial or lateral incisions. The medial incision allows for exposure of the sustentaculum tali, but visualization of the posterior facet requires a lateral exposure. Generally, the medial fragment can be reduced indirectly through the lateral exposure.

(a)

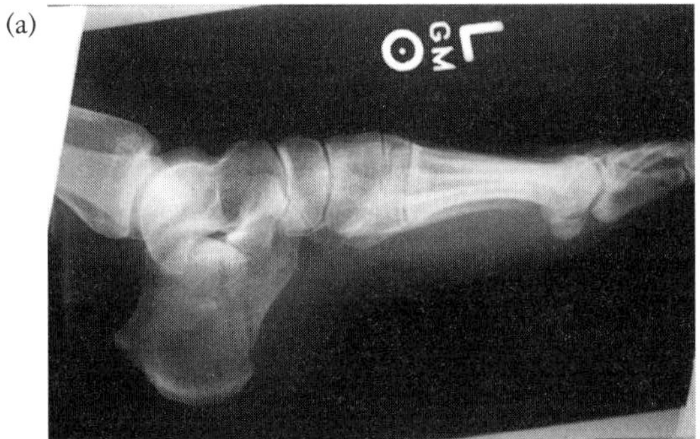

(b)

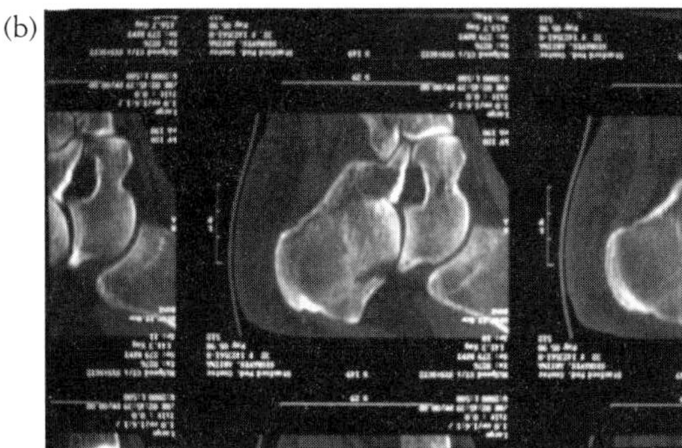

(c)

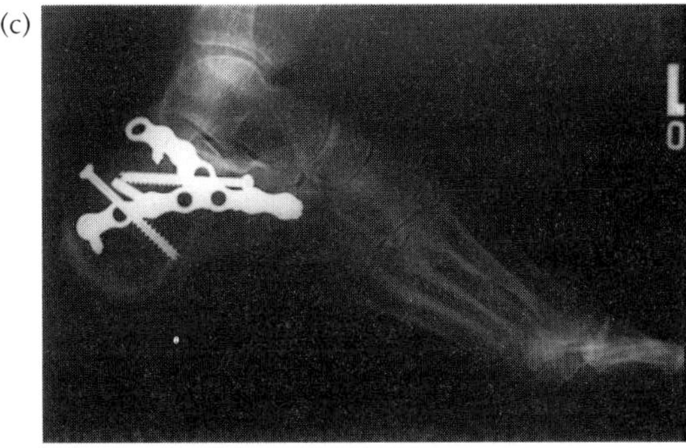

Figure 23.3 (a) Preoperative lateral radiograph of a 33 year old woman who jumped off a 4 m (12 foot) cliff and sustained an intra-articular calcaneus fracture. (b) Preoperative CT scan demonstrates a large depressed fragment of the posterior facet. (c) Postoperative lateral radiograph shows anatomical restoration of the posterior facet joint surface.

Key point

- An extended lateral approach is preferred for operative management of most calcaneal fractures.

Authors' preferred technique

We prefer an extended lateral approach. The patient is placed supine with a sandbag under the hip of the injured side, and the table is tilted to the contralateral side. A tourniquet is used, and a L-shaped incision is made just posterior to the peroneal tendons and sural nerve. A full thickness soft-tissue flap is raised, and two Kirschner wires are placed into the talus for retraction. The lateral wall is removed, and the posterior facet fragments are reduced through the exposure. The sustentaculum tali is reduced with the guide wire of a 4.0 mm cannulated system. Kirschner wires may be used for provisional fixation, then the lateral wall is replaced. Bone graft can be placed if the cancellous defect is large. A Y- or H-shaped calcaneal plate is contoured to the lateral surface of the calcaneus, and then the screw holes are filled with 3.5 mm cortical screws. Image intensification is used to confirm the reduction and screw placement, and plain radiographs should be obtained before completion of the procedure. A drain is placed for 24–48 hours. A bulky compression dressing is placed with splints. The patient is maintained on elevation and ice until discharge, approximately 2–3 days after surgery.

Postoperative care

The sutures are removed after 3 weeks. No weight is placed on the foot for 3 months. Radiographs are obtained to determine the extent of healing. Once consolidation is satisfactory, then partial weight-bearing can be initiated, in a walking cast. Range of motion exercises can be started once the sutures have been removed.

Complications and management

The most common complication is residual pain, swelling, and stiffness. Post-traumatic arthritis is common, and is dependent on the amount of comminution of the posterior facet. Therefore, anatomical reduction is important to help restore as much function as possible. Another important complication is wound healing problems, occurring in about 10% of patients (Macey *et al.* 1994). This can be minimized by waiting for the swelling to resolve, and by not using a tourniquet. If a wound dehiscence or infection occurs, it can usually be treated with oral antibiotics and local wound care. Approximately 20% of patients develop peroneal tendinopathy that requires removal of the hardware (Macey *et al.* 1994).

Special considerations

Although operative versus non-operative treatment remains controversial, the general trend is for open reduction, as this allows for restoration of calcaneal height, width, and joint surface. In the case of a severely comminuted fracture, operative management may not provide a better outcome. Primary subtalar fusion should be considered, as it yields good relief of pain without the need for a secondary procedure.

Key point

- Operative versus nonoperative treatment remains controversial, but the general trend is for open reduction, as this allows for superior restoration of calcaneal height, width, and joint surface.

Prognosis

The prognosis for an intra-articular fracture depends on the amount of comminution of the joint surface and the restoration of congruity. Most patients can return to weight-bearing activities with some limitations. They may also may be limited to wearing wide, flat shoes. Macey *et al.* (1994) reported preliminary results of surgical treatment of calcaneal fractures in over 100 displaced intra-articular calcaneal fractures. In that study 65% of patients were limited only in their ability to participate in vigorous activities and sports, and 70% of patients were completely satisfied with their surgical outcome.

Key point

- The prognosis for an intra-articular fracture depends on the amount of comminution of joint surface and the restoration of congruity.

Lisfranc fracture-dislocations

General principles

Injuries involving the tarsometatarsal articulation, or Lisfranc joint, can be misdiagnosed as a foot or ankle sprain, with potentially disastrous consequences.

A Lisfranc fracture-dislocation is usually misdiagnosed and frequently appropriate management is instituted late. It is important to suspect the injury, and confirm its presence by radiographs.

Key point

- A Lisfranc fracture-dislocation can be misdiagnosed as a foot or ankle sprain.

Anatomy and biomechanics

The Lisfranc ligament is a strong structure spanning the medial cuneiform to the base of the second metatarsal base. Injury to this ligament can allow for subluxation of the Lisfranc joint. Since the tarsometatarsal joint is an important component of the arch of the foot, disruption of the ligaments can lead to collapse of the arch and post-traumatic arthritis.

Mechanism of injury

The mechanism of injury is direct trauma to the Lisfranc joint, or axial force on to a plantar flexed foot, such as in a sports activity or motor vehicle accident.

Presentation

Signs and symptoms

The patient will present with pain around the midfoot. There can be mild to marked swelling, depending on the extent of the injury. Neurovascular examination is usually normal, but the possibility of a compartment syndrome of the foot should be kept in mind.

Key point

- The presenting complaint after a Lisfranc joint injury may be pain, which may be diffuse about the midfoot.

Possible associated injuries

Frequently, a fracture of a metatarsal can be associated with a dislocation. The most common such fracture is at the medial aspect of the base of the second metatarsal from an avulsion injury of the Lisfranc ligament. Other metatarsals can be involved, with fracture patterns involving the base or the diaphysis.

Classification of injury

A classification system was described by Quenu and Kuss (see Perez Blanco *et al.* 1998) that describes the displaced components. Type 1 is ipsilateral direction of displacement, type 2 is isolated with only one or two of the metatarsals displaced, and type 3 is divergent, where there is displacement of all of the metatarsals and separation between the first and second metatarsals.

Diagnosis

Examination findings

Patients have swelling, tenderness, and bruising of the foot. The swelling is generally diffuse, and can be moderate to severe. With severe injuries, there is a risk of compartment syndrome.

Diagnostic techniques

Most diagnoses can be made with plain radiograph. Anteroposterior views may show disruption of the medial border of the second metatarsal in relation to the medial border of the middle cuneiform. An oblique view may show loss of congruity of the medial border of the fourth metatarsal to that of the cuboid. A true lateral radiograph can show loss of the normal curvature of the arch of the midfoot, particularly when in a weight-bearing position. A CT scan is helpful in subtle injuries. Widening will be seen between the first and second metatar-sal bases as compared to the uninjured foot. Also, a bone scan will show increase uptake at the involved joint.

Key point

- Plain radiography is usually sufficient to diagnose an injury to the Lisfranc joint.

Management

Initial

After clinical and radiographic examination, the patient should be placed in a splint and kept non-weight-bearing until surgery is undertaken.

Surgical indications

Previously, closed reduction and percutaneous pinning was the most common surgical treatment, but loss of reduction can occur once the pins are removed and weight-bearing is permitted. ORIF is the current recommended treatment for these potentially devastating injuries. Open reduction allows for anatomical restoration of the alignment of the Lisfranc joint, if closed reduction is not possible because of haematoma or scar formation.

Key point

- ORIF is the current recommended treatment for these potentially devastating injuries.

Surgical techniques available

The procedure is performed through multiple longitudinal incisions, depending on the metatarsals involved. The first tarsometatarsal joint is exposed through a dorsal incision. The second and third are approached through a second intermetatarsal incision, and the fourth and fifth through a fourth intermetatarsal incision. Pins or screws can be used for fixation (Fig. 23.4).

Authors' preferred technique

Once reduction is achieved with a guide wire, we prefer to use cannulated 4.0 mm screws. The screw pattern and number depends on the type of injury. One screw is usually placed from the medial cuneiform into the base of the second metatarsal, to stabilize the Lisfranc ligament. An additional screw can be placed between the bases of the first and second metatarsals. The other metatarsals can be fixed with longitudinal screws.

(a)

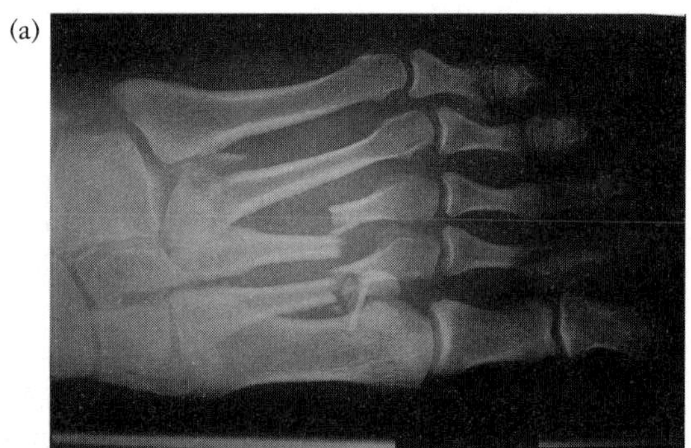

(b)

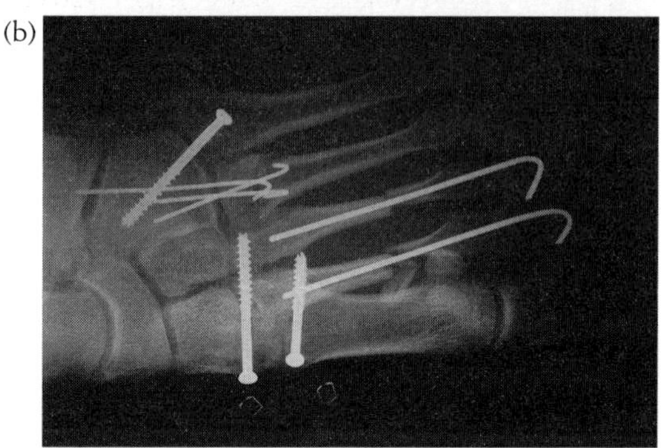

Figure 23.4 (a) Preoperative oblique radiograph of a 26 year old man who sustained an open left Lisfranc fracture dislocation. (b) Postoperative oblique radiograph demonstrates satisfactory alignment after internal fixation.

Postoperative care

The limb is placed in a bulky dressing with splints. Non-weight-bearing and elevation are continued. The staples are removed after 2 weeks, at which time range of motion exercises can be commenced in a removable cast. After 4–6 weeks, partial weight-bearing is begun and then progressed to full weight-bearing in a cast. The screws are maintained for 3–6 months.

Complications and management

Patients usually experience prolonged stiffness and swelling with limitation of their weight-bearing activities. The long-term complication is post-traumatic arthritis, which is determined by the initial injury and the adequacy of reduction. Some patients benefit from an arch support, orthotic device, or possibly tarsometatarsal arthrodesis for severe arthritis.

Prognosis

The patient should be advised of the possibility of developing arthritis of the Lisfranc joint, as most patients will suffer some form of this. Most patients can return to many pre-injury activities, but the rehabilitation may be prolonged and footwear may be limited to wide, flat shoes.

Jones fractures

General principles

The importance of the Jones fracture is that a delayed union, non-union, or re-fracture may occur. Correct diagnosis is critical in proper treatment of a Jones fracture: it should be differentiated from an avulsion fracture of the base of the fifth metatarsal.

Key point

- The importance of the Jones fracture is that a delayed union, non-union, or re-fracture may occur.

Anatomy and biomechanics

There is an area of hypovascularity between the diaphysis and the tuberosity, exactly in the region where Jones fractures occur. This lack of blood supply affects healing potential.

Mechanism of injury

The cause of this fracture is usually an inversion injury. It can also be caused by a direct blow or result from overuse, as in a stress fracture.

Presentation

Signs and symptoms

The patient has complaints of lateral forefoot pain. There may be associated swelling and a limp. With stress fractures, the complaints may be minimal.

Classification of injury

The fracture involves the junction of the metaphysis and diaphysis of the fifth metatarsal, unlike the avulsion fracture which is caused by an avulsion of the insertion of the peroneus brevis tendon.

Diagnosis

Examination findings

Physical examination reveals localized tenderness at the base of the fifth metatarsal. In an acute injury, there is usually swelling and bruising.

Diagnostic techniques

The diagnosis is made with plain radiographs of the foot (Fig. 23.5). If a stress fracture is suspected but not seen on the radiograph, a bone scan may be obtained.

Management

Initial

A Jones fracture should be treated with immediate immobilization in a non-weight-bearing cast (Torg *et al.* 1984) for 6–8 weeks until there is evidence of radiographic healing. This is followed by a short leg walking cast for an additional 4 weeks.

Key point

- A Jones fracture should be treated with immediate immobilization and non-weight-bearing for 6–8 weeks until there is evidence of radiographic healing

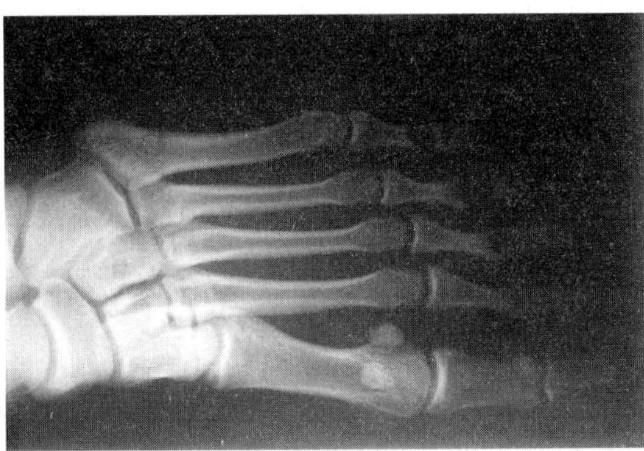

Figure 23.5 Oblique radiograph of a 21 year old man demonstrates an undisplaced Jones fracture.

Surgical indications

Most Jones fractures can be treated non-operatively, but intramedullary fixation is recommended for an athlete or in a delayed or non-union (Torg *et al.* 1994).

Surgical techniques available

An intramedullary screw is placed percutaneously through a small dorsolateral incision, using a 4.5 mm AO/ASIF malleolar screw with protected weight-bearing until radiographic union is evident (Torg *et al.* 1984).

Postoperative care

After internal fixation, the patient is treated with immobilization, as for non-operative treatment.

Complications and management

A delayed union can be diagnosed by the radiographic finding of intramedullary sclerosis and absence of callus with widening of the fracture line. A nonunion has the appearance of a widened fracture line with sclerosis. If these develop, then surgical treatment is recommended.

Even after surgical treatment, failures can occur. Glasgow *et al.* (1996) reported surgical failures in 11 patients who were treated with intramedullary screw fixation or inlaid corticocancellous bone graft. These included delayed union in 3 patients, re-fracture in 7 patients, and non-union in 1 patient.

Prognosis

The prognosis for surgical treatment is good so that an athlete can return to sports activities once the fracture has healed.

Compartment syndrome of the foot

General principles

With fractures or crush injuries, swelling and haematoma can ensue and compromise the vascularity of the foot.

Anatomy and biomechanics

Nine compartments have been identified in the foot by gelatin dye injection studies: medial, superficial, lateral, adductor, four interossei, and calcaneal compartments (Manoli and Weber 1990, Shereff 1990). Each is contained in a fibro-osseous space and must be released individually.

Presentation

Signs and symptoms

The patient will complain of severe pain of the foot, with inability to bear weight or move the foot and ankle.

Possible associated injuries

Frequently, fractures are associated with this syndrome. Most common are multiple metatarsal fractures, and fractures of the calcaneus or talus. A severe crush injury to the foot can also result in a compartment syndrome even without a fracture.

Diagnosis

Examination findings

The foot has significantly swollen compartments and is diffusely tender. The pulses may or may not be palpable. The most important factor in making the diagnosis of a compartment syndrome of the foot is clinical suspicion. If this syndrome is suspected, then compartment pressure should be measured and plans made for surgical release.

Diagnostic techniques

Most trauma centres have compartment pressure monitors. The clinician should be familiar with the anatomy of the compartments, so that they can be measured accurately. If the pressure is >30 mmHg, or <30 mmHg below the diastolic blood pressure, then the diagnosis is confirmed.

Management

Initial

The injured foot should be splinted and closely monitored. Elevation should not be above the heart level, as this may further diminish blood flow to the extremity.

Surgical indications

Once the diagnosis is made, it is a surgical emergency to release all of the compartments of the foot.

Surgical techniques available

There are two common approaches to release. The medial approach utilizes one incision, and the dorsal approach has two incisions. The dorsal incisions are generally used when fixation of metatarsal fractures is performed.

Authors' preferred technique

Our preferred approach is through two dorsal incisions. All the compartments can be released, and then the wounds can be repaired with split thickness skin grafts 5–7 days later. Occasionally, the wounds can be closed without skin graft.

Key points

- The foot is diffusely tender and the swelling may not be marked.
- Peripheral pulses may or may not be palpable.
- The most important factor in making the diagnosis of a compartment syndrome of the foot is clinical suspicion.
- Once the diagnosis is made, it is a surgical emergency to release all of the compartments of the foot.

Postoperative care

The patient can be treated in a splint to protect the associated fractures. If there are no fractures, then weight-bearing may begin once the soft-tissues have healed.

Complications and management

Prompt treatment of compartment syndrome of the foot will usually prevent complications. If there is a delay in diagnosis and treatment, a claw foot deformity may result. It is important to release the calcaneal compartment, as this can be associated with calcaneal fractures.

Prognosis

If the syndrome is treated promptly, there should be little residual deficit.

References

Berndt AL, Harty M (1959) Transchondral fractures (osteochondritis dissecans) of the talus. *Journal of Bone and Joint Surgery* 41A: 988–1020.

Boden SD, Labropoulos PA, McCowin P *et al.* (1989) Mechanical considerations for the syndesmosis screw: a cadaver study. *Journal of Bone and Joint Surgery* 71A: 1548–1555.

Brostrom L (1966) Sprained ankle. *Acta Chirurgica Scandinavica* 132: 551–565.

Cardone BW, Erickson SC, Hartog BD Den, Carrera GF (1993) MRI of injury to the lateral collateral ligamentous complex of the ankle. *Journal of Computer Assisted Tomography* 17: 102–107.

Chrisman OD, Snook GA (1969) Reconstruction of lateral ligament tears of the ankle: an experimental study and clinical evaluation of seven patients treated by a new modification of the Elmslie procedure. *Journal of Bone and Joint Surgery* 51A: 904–912.

Ebraheim NA, Mekhail AO, Gargasz SS (1997) Ankle fractures involving the fibula proximal to the distal tibiofibular syndesmosis. *Foot and Ankle International* 18: 513–521.

Frost SC, Amendola A (1999) Is stress radiography necessary in the diagnosis of acute or chronic ankle instability? *Clinical Journal of Sport Medicine* 9: 40–45.

Gerber JP, Williams GN, Scoville CR, Arciero RA, Taylor DC (1998) Persistent disability associated with ankle sprains: a prospective examination of an athletic population. *Foot and Ankle International* 19: 653–660.

Glasgow MT, Naranja RJ, Glasgow SG, Torg JS (1996) Analysis of failed surgical management of fractures of the base of the fifth metatarsal distal to the tuberosity: the Jones fracture. *Foot and Ankle International* 17: 449–457.

Hamilton WG, Thompson FM, Snow SW (1993) The modified Brostrom procedure for lateral ankle instability. *Foot and Ankle* 14: 1–7.

Harper MC (1992) Ankle fracture classification systems: a case for integration of the Lauge-Hansen and AO–Danis–Weber schemes (review). *Foot and Ankle* 13(7): 404–407.

Hawkins LF (1970) Fractures of the neck of the talus. *Journal of Bone and Joint Surgery* 52A: 991–1002.

Lauge-Hansen N (1950) Fractures of the ankle, II. Combined experimental-surgical and experimental roentgenologic investigations. *Archives of Surgery* 60: 957–985.

Macey LR, Benirschke SK, Sangeorzan BJ, Hansen ST (1994) Acute calcaneal fractures: treatment options and results. *Journal of the American Academy of Orthopaedic Surgeons* 2: 36–43.

Maffulli N (1998) The clinical diagnosis of subcutaneous tear of the Achilles tendon. A prospective study in 174 patients. *American Journal of Sports Medicine* 26: 266–270.

Maffulli N, Barrass V, Ewen SW (2000) Light microscopic histology of achilles tendon ruptures. A comparison with unruptured tendons. *American Journal of Sports Medicine* 28: 857–863.

Manoli AII, Weber TG (1990) Fasciotomy of the foot: An anatomical study with special reference to release of the calcaneal compartment. *Foot and Ankle* 10: 267–275.

Novacheck TF (1998) Running injuries: a biomechanical approach. *Journal of Bone and Joint Surgery* 80A: 1220–1233.

Perez Blanco R, Rodriguez Merchan C, Canosa Sevillano R, Munuera Martinez L (1988) Tarsometatarsal fractures and dislocations. *Journal of Orthopedic Trauma* 2(3): 188–194.

Rosenbaum D, Becker J, Sterk J, Gerngross H, Claes L (1997) Functional evaluation of the 10-year outcome after modified Evans repair for chronic ankle instability. *Foot and Ankle International* 18: 765–771.

Saltzman CL, Tearse DS (1998) Achilles tendon injuries. *Journal of the American Academy of Orthopaedic Surgeons* 6: 316–325.

Sanders R, Fortin P, Dipasquale T *et al.* (1993) Operative treatment in 120 displaced intra-articular calcaneal fractures: results using a prognostic computed tomography scan classification. *Clinical Orthopaedics* 290: 87–95.

Shereff MJ (1990) Compartment syndromes of the foot. In: Greene WB (ed.) *Instructional Course Lectures* 39. American Academy of Orthopaedic Surgeons, Rosemont, Ill., pp. 127–132.

Stiell I, Wells G, Laupacis A *et al.* (1995) Multicentre trial to introduce the Ottawa ankle rules for use of radiography in acute ankle injuries. *BMJ* 311: 594–597.

Torg JS, Balduini FC, Zelko RR *et al.* (1984) Fractures of the base of the fifth metatarsal distal to the tuberosity: Classification and guidelines for non-surgical and surgical management. *Journal of Bone and Joint Surgery* 66A: 209–214.

24

CHAPTER 24

Electrical injuries

JOSEPH DUC HUY TRIEU, GARY YEE, KOUROSH TAVAKOLI, AND MARK KOHOUT

CHAPTER 24
Electrical injuries

JOSEPH DUC HUY TRIEU, GARY YEE, KOUROSH TAVAKOLI, AND MARK KOHOUT

'Electricity' comes from the Greek *electron*, the word for amber. The ancient Greeks observed that amber, when rubbed, acquired the ability to attract objects such as straw. However, William Gilbert, the physician to Queen Elizabeth who wrote the book *De magnete* in 1600, was the first to use the term electricity. The incandescent lightbulb was introduced in 1879, by which time concepts of electricity were already well established by 1880. In 1800, Alessandro Volta announced that electricity could be drawn from a pile of alternating zinc and silver discs stacked one on the other. Michael Faraday, in 1821, discovered that a current carrying conductor would rotate about a magnetic pole and that a magnetized needle would rotate about a wire carrying an electric current (Meyer 1971). In 1879, Edison introduced the incandescent electric light. This single application fuelled a tremendous growth in the use of electricity and electrical equipment and the consequent inevitable emergence of electrical injury from manufactured sources. The first fatality due to electricity was recorded in France in 1879, when a stage carpenter was killed by an alternating current of 250 V (Harvey-Sutton *et al.* 1992) Before 1880, electrical injury to humans came primarily from lightning (Bernstein 1994).

Comprehensive literature pertaining to electric injury statistics or of the costs involved is surprisingly lacking (Lutton 1994). Collection of data about injury and death due to electricity is difficult due to inconsistencies in injury definitions, data reporting, and record maintenance.

From information that is available, the national rates for fatal electrical accidents per million inhabitants in 1967 ranged from 1.3 (Northern Ireland) to 7.6 (Italy) (Kieback 1998). The victims of electrical injury are most likely to be workers in the electric utility and construction industries (Loomis *et al.* 1999). Electrocution is the fifth leading cause of fatal occupational injury in the USA (Statistics BoL 1997), where from 1980 to 1992, 5348 workers died from contact with electrical energy (an average of 411 deaths per year) (Stout 1998). The mortality from electrical injuries ranges from 3% to 15% (Lee 1997), and 3–4% of admissions to a hospital burn unit are related to electrical injuries (DiVincenti *et al.* 1969, Saffle *et al.* 1995).

The costs of electrical injury are high, and continue long after the initial injury. Many of those injured are young and become permanently disabled. Costs can therefore persist for decades. In addition to the direct costs of the injury, indirect costs include lost employment time; productivity loss; equipment damage; replacement employee hiring and training; fire loss; accident investigation; and overhead costs associated with running a self-insurance programme. It is estimated that it takes fewer than 650 cases worldwide to cost US$ 1billion (Wyzga and Lindroos 1999).

Away from the workplace, most injuries are due to lightning strikes or to domestic low-voltage (<1000 V) electrical contact. Lightning strikes account for several hundred deaths each year in the USA, with mortality approaching 30% (NSC 1983). The rate of disability is high because of neurological effects (Andrews *et al.* 1991). Domestic low-voltage power frequency electrical shocks commonly involve small children in and around the home (Hunt 1992).

Physical concepts

- *Electricity* is the movement of electrical charge along a material.
- *Current* (I) is a measure of the rate of flow of electrical charge that is flowing. It is measured in amperes (A). Electrical current flow requires the presence of an electric potential difference between two points. By convention, electrical current flow occurs in the direction opposite to the flow of electrons between the two points.
- *Voltage* (V) is a measure of the electrical force that is driving the flow of current. It is measured in volts (V).
- *Resistance* (R) is the degree to which a material opposes the flow of current through it. It is measured in ohms (Ω).

  If an analogy were drawn between an electrical circuit and water flowing through a hose, current would be the rate at which water is flowing through the hose and voltage would be the water pressure driving the flow of water. There are also two equations in the physics of electricity that are relevant to electrical injuries.
- *Ohm's law* relates voltage, current and resistance:

  $$V = I \times R.$$

  This means that for any given voltage level, the amount of current flow will increase as resistance to flow decreases.
- *Joule's law* quantities the amount of heat generated in a conductor:

  $$\text{Heat} = I^2 \times R \times \text{time} = V^2/R \times \text{time}$$
- The *electric field strength* is the rate of change of potential difference per unit distance (V/m) or the gradient of the potential difference with respect to distance.
- The *field frequency* is the rate of change of the field strength.
- *DC* (direct current) indicates a field frequency of zero. *AC* (alternating current) indicates change of polarity of the field with time.
- *Capacitative coupling* refers to the phenomenon whereby an alternating electric field can transfer energy to charged molecules in the field (without actual physical transfer of charge) and cause them to rotate so as to align with the direction of the alternating electric field. The efficiency of capacitative coupling is very dependent on the frequency of the field (Lee 1997). However, as the frequency of the field increases, energy absorption occurs at an atomic level. At frequencies $>10^{15}$ Hz, electrons in the outer orbits may become unpaired leading to the formation of free radicals. Electric fields of this frequency are termed *ionizing fields* and mediate cellular damage via the free radicals (Harm 1980).
- *Arc contact* or *dielectric breakdown* occurs when the electric field strength in a conducting medium is of such magnitude that atoms are pulled apart and a hot gas of ions called 'plasma' (a very good conductor of electricity) is created. Consequently, in a strong electric field created by a high-voltage power source, an arc can mediate direct electrical contact and allow passage of current along its length before mechanical contact is established with the victim. For example, the breakdown strength of air is approximately 2×10^6 V/m. Arcing can occur when the forearm of a grounded victim is 3–4 mm away from a 7500 V power line source. The threshold for arc initiation depends on the geometry of the arcing surfaces. Arcing can occur across greater distances when, for example, an outstretched finger or a pointed object held in the hand approaches the power source. The threshold also depends on the weather. Humidity decreases the threshold. At <300 V, arcing cannot be initiated through normal air and direct mechanical contact must precede electrical contact (Lee 1997).
- A *thermoacoustic blast* arises from the sudden (sub-second) thermal expansion of air due to the high temperatures (5000°C or higher) within electric arcs (Capelli-Schellpfeffer *et al.* 1999).

Such a blast may propel the victim away from the electric source. Barotrauma from the blast include perforated eardrums, blast lung, abdominal blast injury and secondary acceleration/deceleration injuries from impact, and impact from shrapnel.

Electrophysiological interactions

Electrochemical reactions at the skin

Low-frequency current produces ions on direct contact with the body surface. These alter the tissue oxygen level and pH. Such electrochemical reactions at the interface with the skin do not occur when contact is made through an aqueous electrolyte solution or during capacitative and magnetic coupling of electrical power into the body across the tissue interface (Lee 1997).

Resistance of the epidermis

The epidermis forms a barrier to ion transport and contributes 95–99% of skin resistance to passage of DC current. On the palms and soles, the epidermis is 2–3 times thicker and therefore has 2–3 times greater resistance (Freiberger 1934).

Epidermal resistance is dependent on three factors:

1. *Current frequency*: alternating currents can capacititatively couple across epidermis and resistance is lower to AC currents than it is to DC current.

2. *Hydration*: resistance decreases with increased epidermal hydration.

3. *Voltage*: The resistance of the epidermis remains approximately constant until a breakdown voltage is approached and then it rapidly drops away with increasing voltage. The *breakdown voltage* is the voltage at which the epidermis undergoes structural destruction and electrical conducting channels in the epidermis are formed. The breakdown voltage is about 150 V in most areas and 400 V on the palms and soles. Complete epidermal destruction allows direct current passage to the dermis and subcutaneous tissues (Freiberger 1934, Prausnitz *et al.* 1993).

Current

Muscle and nerve cells use ion currents for intra- and extracellular communication. Action potentials are generated by sufficiently large transmembrane electric fields, which produce neurological responses and muscle contraction. Neuromuscular responses to electric currents are dependent on frequency. Alternating currents at frequencies $\geqslant$50 Hz pass through nerve and muscle membranes capacitatively without altering the transmembrane potential enough to generate an action potential.

- The threshold of human perception for current passing through a finger is 1 mA (Dalziel 1960). At 16 mA, at what is known as the 'let-go threshold' (Dalziel 1943), the forearm muscles contract involuntarily, resulting in a clenched fist because the flexor muscles are stronger than the extensors. The fist position cannot be released unless the current stops.
- Respiratory muscle spasm occurs at a transthoracic current threshold of 20 mA to produce respiratory arrest (Dalziel and Lee 1969).
- Atrial or ventricular fibrillation can result if there is passage of non-physiological current of 60 mA during the repolarization phase of the cardiac cycle. The vulnerable period is at the end of ventricular systole and correlates with the early T wave component of the ECG (Wiggers and Wegria 1939).

Tables 24.1 and 24.2 summarize thresholds for electrophysiological responses.

Distribution of current within tissues

The current distribution is dependent on the relative conductivity of the various tissues and the frequency of the current. The tissues behave like a volume conductor with the conductivity of normal saline solution because the difference in conductivity of most tissues is small. Current density is highest at contact points (Sances *et al.* 1981, Daniel *et al.* 1988).

Table 24.1 Correlation between current and injury

Current (mA)	Effect
>5000	Thermal burn Cardiorespiratory failure
60	Ventricular fibrillation
30	Respiratory muscle tetanus
15	Skeletal muscle tetanus
5	Pain

From Monafo and Freedman (1987).

Table 24.2 Summary of current thresholds for electrophysiological responses

Response	Threshold current (mA)
Sensation of pain (fingertip contact)	1.0 (male) 0.5 (female)
The 'let go' threshold	16 (male) 11 (female)
Respiratory arrest	20
Cardiac: extrasystole	60
Cardiac: ventricular fibrillation	100
Permeabilization of nerve and muscle membranes	1500

Data from Dalziel (1943, 1960); Dalziel; and Lee (1969).

In the extremities, skeletal muscle carries the bulk of the current because it occupies a high proportion of the volume of the extremity, despite the higher conductivities and higher current densities within arteries and nerves. Cortical bone carries the least amount of current because of its high resistance and small cross-sectional dimensions (Sances *et al.* 1981).

The orientation of tissue planes also affects the magnitude of the electric field and current. If current passes parallel to the tissue planes, the electric field strength will be equal across the tissues but the current will be different in each tissue. If it passes perpendicular to the tissue planes, then magnitude of the current will be equal in the different tissues but the electric field will be different in each tissue, being maximal in the tissue of highest resistance (Lee and Kolodney 1987b).

Current mainly travels between cells because cell membranes are good insulators. Therefore, tissue resistance is proportional to cell density. Furthermore, the conductivity of muscle cells is higher in a plane parallel to the fibres than in a plane perpendicular to the fibres.

Axial position determines the relative volume fraction occupied by the various tissue types and therefore, the current distribution and total resistance. The high resistance of joints is due to the large proportion of the cross-sectional area occupied by skin and bone. For instance, 25% of total hand resistance is in the wrist and 30% of the foot resistance arises from the ankle (Freiberger 1934). When the epidermis is intact, the resistance between two points on a body surface is 100 000 Ω. On prolonged contact with a power source of >200 V, the resistance from one hand to foot falls to 1000 Ω, after epidermal breakdown (Kouwenhoven 1968). See Table 24.3.

Pathogenesis of tissue injury

Low-frequency, high-voltage electric fields produce acute tissue injury by:

- Joule heating of tissue (DiVincenti *et al.* 1969)
- permeabilization of cell membranes by *electroporation* (Lee and Kolodney 1987, Lee *et al.* 1988, Powell *et al.* 1989, Reilly 1994, Tung *et al.* 1994)
- cell membrane protein denaturation (Tsomg and Astumian 1987, 1988).

As frequency increases to the optical range and beyond, direct molecular absorption of electrical

Table 24.3 Tissue current density (J) in mA/cm^2 and resistivity r (ohm cm) in cross-section versus applied current from experiments using hogs' hind limbs

Total current (mA)	Approx. applied voltage (V)	Artery		Nerve		Muscle			Fat		Bone cortex	
		J	R	J	r	J	r_L[a]	r_T[b]	J	r	J	R
10	6	0.32	147	0.26	201	0.18	296	512	0.12	375	0.03	1828
30	15	1.18	145	0.86	209	0.50	282	525	0.43	360	0.09	1880
100	45	3.1	152	3.0	191	2.0	295	483	1.5	352	0.30	1832
300	135	9.8	140	8.7	197	7.0	287	501	4.9	377	0.85	1859
600	260	21.0	150	15.2	196	12.0	292	492	9.3	366	2.0	1876
1000	415	35.9	155	27.1	200	19.5	290	650	13.4	386	2.8	1836

[a] L, longitudinal; [b] T, transverse.
From Sances *et al.* (1981).

energy occurs, with consequent free radical mediated damage (Harm 1980). Cellular injury translates to tissue and organ dysfunction.

Thermal effects

- *Joule heating* refers to heat generated from the passage of ionic current.
- *Dielectric heating* refers to the heat generated from rotating molecular dipoles (e.g. water) in a high-frequency AC electric field. Rotation of molecular dipoles is resisted by viscous drag from interactions with neighbouring molecules. Small molecules such as water can oscillate at the frequency of the applied field up to the gigahertz range (Chou 1995). However, the frequency of oscillation of larger molecules, such as DNA and proteins, is highest at the radiofrequency range, giving rise to concern about the use of cellular telephones (Lee 1997).

The rate of tissue dielectric heating is dependent on (Lee 1997):

- the amplitude of the tissue electric field
- the density of the dipoles
- the frequency of the field.

Field frequency governs the relative contributions to the heat generated from an AC electric current.

Electrical effects

Pure electrical injury results from the direct action of electrical forces on electrically charged or electrically polarized cell components.

Electroporation

Transmembrane potentials of >300–400 mV lead to electroporation (Gowrishankar *et al.* 1999). This process involve the 'punching' of water molecules through molecular-sized pores in the cell membrane (Litster 1975) until the pore exceeds a critical size, beyond which the pore is energetically favoured to expand rather than close, disrupting the lipid bilayer of cell membranes (Taylor and Mitchell 1973). Structural membrane defects result in permeability to ions and molecules as large as DNA, leading to cellular dysfunction (Powell and Weaver 1986, Tsong 1991). Growth of the electropores is thought to be restricted by membrane proteins which comprise 30% of the total membrane mass. Although electropores can seal spontaneously (Bhatt *et al.* 1990, Canaday and Lee 1990,

Tropea and Lee 1992), a cell ceases to be viable if sufficient numbers of non-sealing pores form.

Electroconformational protein denaturation

Electroconformational protein denaturation refers to the denaturation of membrane proteins by the direct action of an electric field. Proteins are composed of amino acids which are electrical dipoles that collectively form a larger electric dipole (Tsong and Astumian 1988), and can be influenced by an electric field. Since the function of proteins is dependent on a precise three-dimensional structure, even minor distortions of configuration lead to protein dysfunction or even irreversible denaturation. An example of a protein susceptible to electroconformational damage is the potassium channel, one of the voltage-gated ion channels (Chen and Lee 1994, 1995).

Effects of AC frequency

The biological consequences of electrical injury are related to the frequency of the electric field producing the injury (Lee 1997) (Table 24.4). Most of the electrical injuries requiring medical attention arise from contact with electricity with the frequencies of commercial or domestic electricity supplies.

Microwave burns

Microwave-frequency electric burns are clinically different from low-frequency electric burns (Alexander *et al.* 1987, Nicholson *et al.* 1987, Sneed *et al.* 1992, van Rhoon *et al.* 1992). The epidermis forms a resistive barrier at low frequencies. In the microwave range, capacitative coupling permits passage of current with little dissipation of energy at the epidermis. Unless the epidermis has a high content of water, it may not even be burnt. The microwave field penetrates to a depth of 1 cm, characteristically heating up subepidermal tissue water.

Key point

- In a microwave injury the epidermis may not be burnt.

Clinical manifestations

Clinical presentations of electrical injury are variable, ranging from minor to severe multisystem injury (Taylor *et al.* 1962, DiVincenti *et al.* 1969, Rouge and Dimick 1978, Lee 1981, Halperin *et al.* 1983, Jensen *et al.* 1987, Capelli-Schellpfeffer

Table 24.4 Important frequency ranges of electrical injury

Frequency	Regimen	Applications	Harmful effects
DC-10 kHz	Low frequency	Commercial electrical power; soft tissue healing; transcutaneous electrical stimulation	Joule heating; destructive cell membrane potentials
100 kHz–100 MHz	Radiofrequency	Diathermy; electrocautery	Joule heating; dielectric heating of proteins
100 MHz–100 GHz	Microwave	Microwave ovens	Dielectric heating of water
10^{13}–10^{14} Hz	Infrared	Heating; CO_2 lasers	Dielectric heating of water
10^{14}–10^{15} Hz	Visible light	Optical lasers	Retinal injury; photochemical reactions
10^{15} Hz and higher	Ionizing	Radiotherapy; radiographic imaging; UV therapy	Generation of free radicals

From Lee (1997).

et al. 1995, Mann *et al.* 1996, Robinson and Chamberlain 1996).

The random nature of the circumstances in an accidental electric shock makes it impossible to formulate empirical guidelines for predicting the full extent of tissue damage. The variables include duration of contact, points of contact, frequency of current, electric field strength, magnitude of the thermoacoustic blast, radiant heat transport, associated falls, and fractures from involuntary muscle contraction (Lee 1981, Capelli-Schellpfeffer *et al.* 1995, 1999).

The consequences of contact with high-energy electrical sources are usually major and the upper extremity is almost always involved, but any or all systems may be affected. The clinical picture is dominated by primary electrical injuries to the skin, nerve, skeletal muscle, bone and cardiovascular system (Lee 1997). Secondary organ dysfunction often develops in the lung and kidney. An important concept is that *there is no correlation between the size of the contact skin wound and the actual total extent of all injuries*. The total extent of injury in high energy electrical shocks is almost always more extensive than is apparent at initial triage inspection.

Key points

- The consequences of contact with high-energy electrical sources are usually major.
- There is no correlation between the size of the contact skin wound and the actual total extent of all injuries.

Skin

There are always at least two points of skin contact. In low-voltage injuries, the current path is predictable. However, with high voltages, the current path is unpredictable as arcing may occur at multiple sites. The size and pattern of the skin wound is determined by the nature of contact with the power source in terms of area and topology (Lee 1997).

'Kissing wounds' occur when there is electrical breakdown of skin on opposite sides of a joint, most commonly at the axilla. The breakdown voltage for this occurrence is a hand–foot voltage difference of >1000 V (Lee 1997).

Electroplating of the skin in high-voltage arcing when metal contacts vaporize and deposit on the skin can manifest as a black metallic coating with sometimes only superficial thermal skin burns beneath. Thermal burns to the skin can also occur from ignition of clothing from electrical arcs (Lee 1997).

Skin necrosis may be full thickness or partial thickness.

Key point

- There are always at least two points of skin contact.

Heart

The cardiac sequelae of electrical injury are often transient, with resolution and complete recovery being the usual result. However, there is much evidence of delayed or permanent cardiac dysfunction after electrical injury (Jensen *et al.* 1987, Robinson and Chamberlain 1996). Ventricular fibrillation as a result of electrical injury has been reported to recur up to 6 months after electrical injury (Robinson and Chamberlain 1996). Experiments have shown AC to be more dangerous than DC. The injury produced by AC is dependent on frequency and voltage. Domestic frequencies carry the highest risk of inducing ventricular fibrillation. Very high frequencies (>1 kHz) are thought to be safe, producing only local tissue damage (Halperin *et al.* 1983). The incidence of ventricular fibrillation following AC injury is inversely proportional to voltage, whereas the incidence of atrial fibrillation and ventricular tachycardia is directly proportional to voltage (Lown *et al.* 1962).

Cardiac conducting tissue is primarily affected, particularly the sinoatrial and atrioventricular nodes. The reason for this predilection is unclear but may result from denaturation of ionic channels in the nodes or from ischaemia or infarction secondary to spasm of the right coronary artery, which is the coronary artery most commonly affected in electrical injury (James *et al.* 1990).

High-energy electrical injury can cause cardiac abnormalities ranging from sinus node dysfunction, atrial fibrillation, ventricular fibrillation, and asystole to myocardial infarction. Arrhythmias from electrical contact can be fatal, especially if there is a delay in resuscitation.

In the clinical setting, the incidence of cardiac abnormalities following electrical injury has been reported to range from 14% to 54%. The majority of these were arrhythmias and non-specific ECG changes, with only five cases of myocardial infarcts from 344 cases in one report (Arrowsmith *et al.* 1997). Patients who have a normal ECG within the first 24 hours rarely develop anomalies later (Fish 2000). Myocardial infarction following electrical injury has been well described (Kinney 1982), and often diagnosed solely on the basis of transient ST segment elevations or minor ECG changes. Q wave myocardial infarcts can occur without thrombus in the lumen or occlusion of the coronary arteries on angiography. Therefore, prolonged coronary artery spasm is proposed as the mechanism of injury.

Key points

- There is much evidence of delayed or permanent cardiac dysfunction after electrical injury.
- AC is more dangerous than DC.
- The right coronary artery is the coronary artery most commonly affected in electrical injury.
- Arrhythmias from electrical contact can be fatal, especially if there is a delay in resuscitation.
- Patients who have a normal ECG within the first 24 hours rarely develop anomalies later.

Skeletal muscle

Injury to skeletal muscle and its sequelae dominate the clinical picture immediately after electrical trauma. Fixed contracted skeletal muscle and myoglobinuria are amongst the clinical signs of electrical injury. The escape of intracellular proteins such as myoglobin and creatine phosphokinase into the circulation is the *sine qua non* of membrane permeabilization. Muscle dysfunction or death is characterized by the absence of twitching at surgical exploration. The systemic sequelae of the loss of these proteins into the circulation include renal failure from obstruction of the collecting systems by precipitated myoglobin and hyperkalaemia from cell lysis. Renal failure from myoglobin accumulation can have a mortality rate of 18% (Baxter 1970).

The nature of the 'progressive necrosis' of muscle seen at serial surgical explorations for debridement is currently uncertain. Initially, after World War II, it was thought that early surgical manipulation after electrical injury caused progressive necrosis of muscle. However, it is now postulated that the progressive recognition of initially already non-viable muscle has been misinterpreted as 'progressive necrosis' (Solem *et al.* 1997) Electrically injured muscle tissues lack the macroscopic appearances of necrosis at initial exploration but are already non-viable due to damage to their membranes from electroporation and electroconformational protein denaturation and only become visibly necrotic at later explorations (Artz 1967, Hammond and Ward 1994). However, it is likely that there are components of both progressive recognition and true progressive necrosis in electrically injured muscle (Lee 1997).

Skeletal system

Powerful tetanic skeletal muscle contractions secondary to electrical injury are often responsible for acute skeletal injuries such as long bone fractures, joint dislocations, and cervical spine fractures (Dalziel and Lee 1969, Oner *et al.* 1995).

Late skeletal complications include heterotopic ossification of soft tissues and disordered skeletal growth in adolescents. Heterotopic ossification can be found at joints, bursae, nerve sheaths, and ends of amputation stumps (Hunt *et al.* 1980, Oner *et al.* 1995).

Vascular system

Endothelial cells are susceptible to electroporation and electroconformational protein denaturation, because endothelial cells are electrically coupled through intercellular gap junctions (Cooper 1985, Reilly 1994). Injury to endothelial cells can result in activation of the clotting cascades and platelet adhesion. Platelet activation leading to vascular occlusion, can also result from thermal injury to blood macromolecules and thermal denaturation of elastin and collagen. Vessels >2–3 mm in diameter are rarely occluded in the acute post-electrical injury period.

In addition to intrinsic vascular injury, extrinsic compression from compartment syndromes due to soft tissue oedema may occlude vessels.

Delayed rupture of arteries is well described, especially in children after oral commissure injuries (the labial artery often ruptures at 10–14 days after injury).

Peripheral nerves

Literature on the clinical effects of electrical injury on peripheral nerves is limited. Symptoms include anaesthesia, paraesthesia, and dysaesthesia and are usually transient ('stunning'). Rarely, these may be permanent (Grube and Heimbach 1992). Paralysis is less common. Peripheral nerve lesions may develop immediately, but sometimes appear several weeks to 2 years after injury. Entrapment syndromes usually involve compression of nerves in areas where there is normally little room for swelling e.g. the median (carpal tunnel) and ulnar nerves (canal of Guyon), the peroneal nerve at the fibular head, and the anterior compartment of the lower leg (Fish 2000b). Transient autonomic disturbances, e.g. reflex sympathetic dystrophy and causalgia (see below), may also occur.

Often, neurological symptoms persist without any anomalies in electrophysiological studies. The degree of vulnerability, theoretically, is determined by a nerve axon's electrical space constant, which in turn depends on the diameter and degree of myelination of the axon. Since there are different functional types of axons in a peripheral nerve, the pattern of damage within a peripheral nerve is likely to be heterogeneous (Lee 1997).

Autonomic dysfunction associated with peripheral nerve injury is known as *causalgia.* Causalgia is not uncommon after high-voltage electrical injury, with possibly up to 33% of patients with major electrical injuries developing it (Baxter 1970). It typically presents in three stages (Cohen 1995):

- The *acute stage* occurs within hours or days of the injury and has a duration of weeks and consists of burning pain with hyperpathia, allodynia, hyperalgesia, hyperhydrosis, and oedema.
- The *dystrophic stage* occurs 3–6 months after injury and there is more oedema. Muscle atrophy, osteoporosis, nail and hair loss emerge.
- The *atrophic stage* sets in after 6–12 months. Pale and cool skin appears and pain subsides. Heterotopic calcification leads to stiffness and contractures.

The significant mechanism of injury to peripheral nerves from electricity is likely to be direct electrical effects, i.e. electroporation and electroconformational protein deformation, because computational simulations suggest it is unlikely for the peripheral nerve to reach substantially higher temperatures than the surrounding tissues (Lee 1967).

Central nervous system

A spectrum of transient or permanent central nervous system disabilities may manifest in victims of electrical shock, even though there may not have been direct physical contact of the conductor with the head (Triggs *et al.* 1994).

Pathological features of central nervous system injury include reactive gliosis, demyelinization, vacuolisation, and perivascular haemorrhage (Critchley 1934, Grube and Heimbach 1992). Alteration of brain function can be transient or permanent. Permanent changes are possible even without visible changes at the microscopic level.

There are various time courses of symptom development and regression including immediate and transient, immediate and prolonged or permanent, delayed, and often progressive.

Memory deficit is the most common neuropsychological complication. Others include acute and delayed behavioural changes (Critchley 1934, Christensen *et al.* 1980, Daniel *et al.* 1985, Mancusi-Ungaro *et al.* 1986, Hooshimand *et al.* 1989), and psychiatric changes including the development of phobias, anxiety, irritability, depression, somatoform disorders, and psychosis (Kelley *et al.* 1994). Symptoms can also result from traumatic brain injury secondary to falls or hypoxic brain injury secondary to cardiac or respiratory arrest.

Victims of electrical injury who were injured through mere peripheral contacts have been shown to have more prevalent somatic, cognitive, and emotional symptoms, as determined by a neuropsychological symptom checklist, than control individuals. They also underperform in attention and concentration, motor speed and dexterity, and memory especially visual memory. The symptoms were not related to the severity of the physical injury. No consistent relationship has been established between patient or injury-related characteristics and neuropsychological test performance (Pliskin *et al.* 1999).

There is often a delay in the onset of significant central nervous system dysfunction. Paralysis has been reported up to 5 years after injury without major intervening signs. Spinal cord nerve lesions are thought to be due to vascular thrombosis, haemorrhage, and resultant alteration in blood flow. The consequent ischaemia leads to later fibrosis of perineural structures. Spinal cord medullary lesions can resemble amyotrophic lateral sclerosis (including progressive development of spastic paralysis), transverse myelitis or ascending paralysis. Delayed nerve lesions are usually irreversible (Dendooven *et al.* 1990). The neuropsychological functions of post-acute (>3 months) injury victims were found to be worse than those of the acute victims (<3 months) (Pliskin *et al.* 1999).

Key points

- Memory deficit is the most common neuropsychological complication.
- There is often a delay in the onset of significant central nervous system dysfunction.

Cataracts

Cataracts induced by lightning are often bilateral (Fish 2000b). As with the central nervous system effects, cataracts have been formed in the absence of direct mechanical contact with the head. However, the patients at greatest risk of forming cataracts are those who have contact wounds on the head or neck and who have been exposed to voltages >1000 V (Saffle *et al.* 1985). The incidence of cataract formation is 5–20%. Most patients initially develop visual symptoms within 12 months of the injury. Although the morphological changes within the lenses are well described (Thomas and Hanna 1974), the exact pathophysiology of electrical cataracts remains obscure (Long 1962). Anterior subcapsular changes are most common. Most of the affected eyes respond well to surgery (Portellos *et al.* 1996).

Auditory system

Haemorrhage can occur in the tympanic membrane, middle ear, cochlea, cochlear duct, and vestibular apparatus, which may be complicated by infection producing mastoiditis, sinus thrombosis, meningitis, and cerebral abscess (Somogyi and Tedeschi 1977). The thermo-acoustic blast from lightning not uncommonly causes tympanic membrane rupture. Electrical injuries sustained from lightning though the telephone lines can cause tympanic membrane perforation, persistent tinnitus, sensorineural deafness, ataxia, vertigo, and nystagmus (Johnstone *et al.* 1986, Frayne and Gillligan 1987).

Clinical management principles

The clinical management of burn injuries are summarized in Table 24.5.

Field response

Extrication

It is essential to separate the patient from the energized conductor: turn off the power where possible.

Table 24.5 Summary of clinical management of electrical injuries

Field response	Separate patient from electrical source Immobilize cervical spine Support vital organ systems that may include cardiopulmonary resuscitation Fluid volume resuscitation Transport to trauma centre
Hospital initial	Assess other injuries Correct pH and other electrolyte imbalances Control cardiac arrhythmia Dilute and alkalinize myoglobin in urine Diagnostic imaging (X-ray, MRI and radionucleotide) Tetanus prophylaxis
Early	Transport to intensive care unit unit Decompress muscle and nerve compartments Surgical debridement Evaluate for cardiac muscle damage Second look procedures (48 h): biologic dressing or primary wound closure
Intermediate	Wound closure Begin surgical reconstruction Nutritional support Musculoskeletal splinting Neurophysiological evaluation Psychiatric consultation Coworker evaluation
Late	Rehabilitation (physical, psychological and occupational) Additional reconstructive measures as required Co-workers' and supervisors' education and follow-up

Once the victim is separated from the source, any electrical charge on the victim will dissipate within seconds.

Initial management should be in accordance with the Australian EMST guidelines or the American ATLS guidelines.

Cervical spine immobilization

The cervical spine should be immobilized in a hard collar until fractures are excluded. The patient should be on a resuscitation board should cardiopulmonary resuscitation (CPR) be required.

Resuscitation

Airway, breathing and circulation are assessed (ABC procedure).

The airway is cleared and oxygen is delivered via a mask in the breathing patient. The non-breathing patient is intubated. Intravenous access is obtained via an uninjured extremity. At least 2 large-bore intravenous cannulas should be inserted.

Arrhythmias should then be treated aggressively with appropriate drugs where possible. Ventricular arrhythmias are the most common and life threatening. Lightning and high-voltage electricity can cause cardiac asystole. The heart may restart spontaneously, but the associated respiratory arrest may last longer. If adequate ventilation is not established, a secondary cardiac arrest from hypoxia-induced ventricular fibrillation will ensue (Cooper 1995).

Intravenous fluid resuscitation should be free flowing, with concurrent and continuous monitoring of blood pressure, heart rate, and sensorium.

Retrieval

Victims of major electrical trauma should be transported to a tertiary trauma centre with an intensive care unit.

Initial evaluation

Primary survey and resuscitation

The victims of electrical injury often have associated thoracoabdominal and skeletal injuries due to falls or tetanic contractions. Therefore, the patient should be evaluated as for multisystem blunt trauma before concentrating solely on the electrical injuries.

Airway, breathing, circulation, and neurological status should be rapidly reassessed. Oxygen is delivered continuously. Venous access is checked and secured. An indwelling urinary catheter is inserted. Cardiac monitoring is commenced and arrhythmias are treated with appropriate drugs.

Intravenous fluid resuscitation is continued and titrated against blood pressure, urine output and heart rate. Urine output should be maintained at no less than 0.5 mL/kg per hour (25–50 mL/hour) unless dark urine suggests myoglobin/haemoglobin precipitation. Since there is no relationship between the size of the skin wounds and the extent of the subcutaneous tissue injury, it is impossible to produce a valid empirical formula for rate of initial fluid administration. However, despite this principle, various formulae based on contact wound area have been advocated ranging from 4 to 9 mL/kg percent of body surface area involved (Baxter 1970, Luce 2000).

If the urine is tea-coloured from myoglobin or haemoglobin, the urine output should be increased to 75–100 mL/hour to avoid acute tubular necrosis. Bicarbonate may be added to the resuscitation fluids to prevent intrarenal precipitation of myoglobin and haemoglobin. Arterial pH in preference to urinary pH should guide bicarbonate therapy. The arterial pH should be maintained >7.45 (AHA 1997). As soon as the urine colour clears, the rate of intravenous fluid administration should be reduced to produce a urine output of 30–50 mL/hour (or 1 mg/kg per hour in patients <30 kg). Sodium bicarbonate should also be ceased to reduce the sodium load.

A Swan–Ganz catheter should later be inserted if the ECG indicates cardiac injury or if there are large third-space losses or autonomic dysfunction leading to hypo- or hypertension.

A 12-lead ECG, a cross-table cervical spine radiograph and blood assays which include a full blood count, electrolytes, urea and creatinine, arterial blood gases, and creatine phosphokinase (CPK) levels should be obtained. Tetanus prophylaxis should be administered.

Secondary survey

A thorough history and examination should be performed, with attention to vascular and neurological systems. The distribution and extent of injury is determined. Skin contact points are located.

Peripheral pulses and arterial pressures are determined with a Doppler probe. Compartment syndrome and compression neuropathies are common manifestations of an electrical injury. Compartment pressure should be measured and documented, as clinical examination alone is not reliable. The classical clinical sign of pain on stretching may not be present, owing to associated nerve injury. The most common muscle compartments affected are the forearm and the leg, which have two and four compartments respectively. Repeat measurements of compartment pressure should be made at 8 and 24 hours after injury to exclude a compartment syndrome in evolution.

Monitoring of renal function by urine output and serum creatinine is continued.

Transfer to intensive care unit

Patients who are unable to maintain an airway or adequate ventilation (e.g. from quadriplegia) should be intubated and ventilated. A feeding tube should be inserted in all patients and enteral alimentation commenced within 6 hours of injury, unless there is suspicion of concurrent abdominal visceral injury. Electroencephalograms may be necessary to assess quality of seizure control in a paralysed patient. A 12-lead ECG should be performed daily for 3 days to detect evolving myocardial injury.

Diagnostic imaging

Cell membrane damage by thermal or electric forces is the hallmark of electrical injury. MRI can identify the inevitable oedema associated with cell membrane injury. Early MRI allows rapid localization of occult necrotic tissue, facilitating early debridement and wound closure to avoid later infection. MRI-detected oedema should guide attention to potential problem regions (Chen *et al.* 1994, Karczsmar *et al.* 1994). Nerves within oedematous fibro-osseous canals (e.g. carpal and tarsal tunnels, Guyon's canal) should be decompressed to prevent compression neuropathies. If imaging by MRI or CT is negative for oedema, it is unlikely that there has been significant muscle injury.

^{99m}Tc stannous pyrophosphate can be used as a marker of damaged muscle tissue (Hunt *et al.* 1979, Hammond and Ward 1994). It is useful in localizing non-viable muscle tissue, which may not become evident for 5–10 days. The isotope is administered intravenously and the scan performed 2 hours later. Scans are considered indicative of muscle injury by a region of hyperaemia. Muscle necrosis is seen as an area of lucency. Radionuclide scanning with ^{99m}Tc stannous pyrophosphate has been reported to have a positive predictive value of 100% (i.e. if the scan detects necrosis, there is true necrosis) and a sensitivity of 75% (i.e. the probability that the scan is positive if there is true necrosis) (Hammond and Ward 1994). However, use of the ^{99m}Tc pyrophosphate scan may not always translate into a reduction in hospital length of stay or the number of surgical procedures (Hammond and Ward 1994). Newer radioisotopes that may improve localization of necrosis include ^{99m}Tc methoxy isobutyl isonitrile, ^{201}Th thallous chloride and ^{99m}Tc DTPA.

Key points

- Cell membrane damage by thermal or electric forces is the hallmark of electrical injury.
- MRI can identify the inevitable oedema associated with cell membrane injury.
- Radionuclide scanning with ^{99m}Tc stannous pyrophosphate has been reported to have a positive predictive value of 100%.

Early surgical treatment

Decompression of muscle and nerve compartments

Compartment pressure >30 mmHg compromises fluid and gas exchange between blood and tissue and is an indication for fasciotomy. In smaller compartments such as the intrinsic muscles of the hand where measurement of pressure is technically difficult, fasciotomy should be performed empirically when these areas are involved. Fasciotomy should be performed under direct vision through adequate skin incisions.

Debridement

Damaged muscle often looks normal at initial exploration unless there has been severe heat denaturation. Due to the stunning effect of electric shock, intraoperative pinch and nerve stimulator tests of contractile response are unreliable indicators of muscle viability. Since the only current practical intraoperative indicators of muscle viability are colour, contractility, and bleeding, non-viable tissue will not be readily apparent at early surgical exploration.

Early debridement under histological guidance is accurate but protracted in duration (Quinby *et al.* 1978), which may increase morbidity due to prolonged general anaesthesia. The most commonly practised approach is to re-inspect the wound and debride obviously necrotic tissue every 48 hours. Between debridements, topical antibiotics such as silver sulfadiazine (SSD), furacin, or mafenide should be applied every 8 hours to marginal tissue. Allograft is applied to decompressed, exposed, and viable muscle.

Tertiary survey

Pain and anxiety should be treated pharmacologically initially. Persistent pain should be treated by transcutaneous electrical nerve stimulation (TENS).

A thorough neurological examination to localize and characterize any neuropathology should be performed. Paralysis and weakness should be managed with physiotherapy (to ensure that joint and tendon mobility is maintained), which may involve range of motion exercises in a warm environment. Physiotherapy is also useful in alleviating pain particularly in cases of causalgia. Non-narcotic analgesia, anti-inflammatory agents, and calcium channel blockers also attenuate any pain.

A spectral technique has been developed, which characterizes the conduction deficit of a nerve in terms of the distribution of the refractory periods of transmission (RPTs) of its constituent fibers. The RPT is a particularly sensitive index of conduction deficit and measures the ability of axons to conduct pairs of closely spaced impulses. The distribution of RPT in the nerve is used to determine the contribution of the various types of axons to the peripheral nerve; identifying normal from pathological fibres (Smith 1980, Smith and Hall 1980). The refractory transmission spectrum is a measure of the nerve fibre's ability to regenerate a transmembrane potential effectively, whereas the conventional compound action potential in nerve conduction studies describes the conduction velocity distribution within the nerve.

Investigations that should supplement a thorough sensory and motor neurological examination of the peripheral nerves include electromyography to assess motor nerve function. Nerve conduction velocity studies and refractory period spectral neurophysiological studies are required to completely evaluate the peripheral nerves.

Since any part of the entire neuraxis may be affected in high-energy electrical shock, an evaluation of the central nervous system is necessary. A structured psychiatric interview and a full neuropsychological assessment, (which includes cognitive, fine motor, sensory recognition, verbal and auditory memory, and the Minnesota Multiphasic Personality Inventory), should be performed.

Any blast injury (from thermoacoustic blast trauma) to the eyes and eardrums should be treated early.

Wound closure

The fundamental objective in wound closure is to remove all non-viable tissue and close the wound as soon as possible. Open wounds subject the nerve, muscle, and tendons to desiccation. Although it is imperative to remove all non-viable tissue before closure because bacterially contaminated muscle in a closed wound is a great risk for sepsis, not all the non-viable tissue is initially obvious. A second-look procedure at 48–72 hours should complete the debridement and provide closure in the majority of cases with skin grafts or fasciocutaneous local flaps. Management of electrically damaged bone follows the guidelines for other types of skeletal trauma. The basic tenets are also debridement and early cover with vascularized soft tissue. Progress in free microvascular tissue transfer has allowed salvage of extremities that would previously have required amputation and is useful to cover exposed nerve, cortical bone, and tendon.

Rehabilitation

Full functional rehabilitation involves the management of physical and neuropsychological problems. Neuropsychological evaluation, similar to that for mild to moderate head trauma, is necessary. Job retraining is also often required if the injury occurred at work, because the victim is unlikely to return to the same hazardous job. Residual disability such as impaired sensory and motor functions in extremities requires extensive physiotherapy and occupational therapy and may require further reconstructive surgery such as tendon transfers and nerve grafting.

The late development of medical sequelae following electrical injury is not uncommon, especially with ultra high-voltage or lightning injuries. Amongst these are neuromuscular problems (from muscle fibrosis and peripheral neuropathies coupled with joint stiffness and loss of tissue on debridements), sensory neuropathies, paraesthesia, dysaesthesia and reflex sympathetic dystrophy, cold intolerance, and complete spinal cord paralysis.

Growth disturbances can produce skeletal deformities that become long-term sequelae.

Cataracts tend to be bilateral and can occur in up to 5–20% of victims even when the current path does not involve the head or neck. However, vision can usually be improved with surgery e.g. cataract extraction and insertion of intraocular lens.

Post-traumatic stress disorder and phobias are also common in patients and witnesses.

The future

The major advances in the management of electrical injuries, in the future will stem from improved methods of rapidly imaging deep non viable tissue, restoring membrane integrity, restoring native conformation to damaged proteins, limiting systemic sequelae, and repairing nucleic acids (Lee 1997).

The development of cameras of higher resolution to quantify radioisotope uptake and identify and locate tissue with membrane damage more precisely, is currently under way and will aid early debridement of non-viable tissue.

It is known that electropore expansion can be limited by membrane proteins (Chang and Reese 1990). Naturally occurring proteins such as fusigenic proteins already induce sealing of porated cell membranes after exocytosis or fertilization. Furthermore, industrial surfactant polymers, called poloxamers, have been shown to seal electropermeabilized (Lee *et al.* 1994) and heat-permeabilized membranes (Padanilam *et al.* 1994). Antioxidants, such as ascorbate, have been shown to reduce wound oedema.

Lightning injuries

Lightning is the common term for dielectric breakdown. This occurs when the electric field strength in the air between clouds and other objects exceeds 2×10^6 V/m, producing an enormous current for a short time (10–100 ms). The current can exceed 30 000 A (Apfelberg *et al.* 1974, Andrews *et al.* 1992). The temperature in the arc can reach 30000 K, generating a high-pressure thermo-acoustic wave that expands and causes shock waves we know as thunder.

Approximately 400 people are struck by lightning annually in the USA. Of this number, fewer than 100 die.

A substantial voltage difference can occur between the feet of a person near a lightning strike. Voltage drops can reach 7500 V and currents up to 2–3 A can be induced to flow through the body between the legs (Lee 1997).

During direct contact with lightning, the body surface potential difference can reach several thousand volts, allowing current of several hundred amperes to flow for up to 10 sufficient to produce electroporation without substantial heating. Fortunately, membranes can spontaneously seal, possibly accounting for high survival rates amongst victims of lightning strikes (Lee 1967).

Large magnetic fields can be generated from the large currents in lightning. These magnetic fields can induce a current in conducting objects such as the body. Thermoacoustic blasts from lightning can be very destructive, strong enough to split trees and cause physical damage to the eardrums of victims or minor head injury.

Clinical manifestations

Although mortality from lightning accidents is high (25–32% in he US, according to source), significant number of victims survive. It is of paramount importance to be certain the victim is electrically discharged before providing aid immediately after a lightning strike.

The prime clinical feature observed in these patients is *keraunoparalysis*, or complete neurological and muscular stunning. The latter can be manifested by cardiorespiratory arrest. After this episode, victims can then suffer from amnesia, confusion, muscle ache, and visual disturbances for up to 7 days.

The severity of lightning injury is classified into mild, moderate and severe (Andrews *et al.* 1992):

- *Mild*: All symptoms are transient and recovery is complete. The clinical features vary from mild amnesia to temporary blindness and deafness.

- *Moderate*: Symptoms of keraunoparalysis and myocardial infarction. The victims tend to have superficial cutaneous thermal injury. If they survive, they can then suffer from chronic vascular spasm, and permanent neurophysiological disturbances such as lesions of peripheral motor and sensory nerves.
- *Severe*: Central nervous system (CNS) lesions, myocardial infarcts, or both (Cooper 1980), secondary to prolonged hypoxia from cardiorespiratory arrest. The rehabilitation potential is extremely poor.

Management

Initial resuscitation aims to establish airway, breathing, and circulation (ABC). Having been revived at the scene of the accident, the patient needs to be transferred to a major trauma and burns unit for further evaluation and treatment.

Obtaining a 12-lead ECG and baseline serum cardiac enzymes is imperative at the time of initial assessment. The patient will subsequently require continuous cardiac monitoring either in coronary care or in an intensive care unit. If there is substantial CNS or cardiac depression, there may be need for ventilatory support, until further assessment of severity of lightning injury has been made. Seizures, although uncommon, can occur and should be treated with anticonvulsant medication.

Thermal burns should be addressed early. It is imperative to establish the extent of cardiac and brain injury before surgical management. A co-ordinated plan should be constructed between the intensivists and the aesthetic team, for dressings and timing of any debridement, grafting, and reconstruction.

In the long term, lighting-strike patients need special trauma counselling. They may also suffer from CNS symptoms such as insomnia and regional pain disorders, which should be referred on to the chronic pain management team. Follow-up visits should therefore continue for several years.

References

AHA (1997) *Textbook of advanced cardiac life support*. American Heart Association, Dallas, pp. 11–17.

Alexander RC, Surrell JA, Cohle SD (1987) Microwave oven burns to children: an unusual manifestation of child abuse. *Pediatrics* 79: 255–260.

Andrews CJ, Cooper MA, Darveniza M, Mackerras D (1992) *Lightning injuries: electrical, medical and legal aspects*. CRC Press, Boca Raton, Fla.

Apfelberg DB, Masters FW, Robinson DW (1974) Pathophysiology of treatment of lightning injuries. *Journal of Trauma* 14: 453–460.

Arrowsmith J, Usgaocar RP, Dickson WA (1997) Electrical injury and the frequency of cardiac complications. *Burns* 23: 576–578.

Artz CP (1967) Electrical injury simulated crush injury. *Surgery, Gynecology and Obstetrics* 125: 1316–1317.

Baxter CR (1970) Present concepts in the management of major electrical injury. *Surgical Clinics of North America* 50: 1401–1418.

Bernstein T (1994) Electrical injury: Electrical engineer's perspective and an historical review. *Annals of the New York Academy of Sciences* 720: 1–10.

Bhatt DL, Gaylor DC, Lee RC (1990) Rhabdomyolysis due to pulsed electric fields. *Plastic and Reconstructive Surgery* 86: 1–11.

Canaday DJ, Lee RC (1990) Magnetism ion influx measurement in skeletal muscle cell electroporation. *Journal of Cell Biology* 111: 431a.

Capelli-Schellpfeffer M, Miller GH, Humilier M (1999) Thermoacoustic energy effects in electrical arcs. *Annals of the New York Academy of Sciences* 888: 19–32.

Capelli-Schellpfeffer MTM, Lee RC, Astumian RD (1995) Advances in the evaluation and treatment of electrical and thermal injury emergencies. *IEEE Transactions on Industry Applications* 31: 1147–1152.

Chang DC, Reese TS (1990) Changes in membrane structure induced by electroporation as revealed by rapid-freezing electron microscopy. *Biophysical Journal* 58: 1–12.

Chen CT, Aarsvold JN, Block TA *et al.* (1994) Radionuclide probes for tissue damage. *Annals of the New York Academy of Sciences* 720: 181–191.

Chen W, Lee RC (1994) Altered ion channel conductance and ionic selectivity induced by large imposed membrane potential pulse. *Biophysical Journal* 67: 603–612.

Chen W, Lee RC (1995) High intensity electric field-induced reduction of K^+ channel currents may result from electro-conformational changes in channel's voltage sensors: gating current reduction. *Biophysical Journal* 68: A354.

Chou CK (1995) Radiofrequency hyperthermia in cancer therapy. In: Bronzino JD (ed.) *The biomedical engineering handbook*. CRC Press, Boca Raton, Fla., pp. 1424–1430.

Christensen J, Sherman R, Balis G, Waunutt J (1980) Delayed neurologic injury secondary to high voltage current with recovery. *Journal of Trauma* 20: 166–168.

Cohen JJ (1995) Autonomic nervous system disorders and reflex sympathetic dystrophy in lightning and electrical injuries. *Seminars in Neurology* 15: 387–390.

Cooper MA (1980) Lightning injuries: prognostic signs for death. *Annals of Emergency Medicine* 9: 134–138.

Cooper MA (1995) Emergent care of lightning and electrical injuries. *Seminars in Neurology* 15: 268–278.

Cooper MS (1985) Electrical cable theory, transmembrane ion fluxes, and the motile responses of tissue cells to external electrical fields. *Frontiers of Engineering and Computing in Health Care 7th Annual Conference*, 1985, Chicago. IEEE/Engineering in Medicine and Biology Society.

Critchley M (1934) Neurologic effects of lightning and of electricity. *Lancet* i: 58–72.

Dalziel CF (1943) Effect of frequency on let go currents. *Transactions of the American Institute of Electrical Engineering* 62: 745–750.

Dalziel CF (1960) Threshold 60 cycle fibrillating currents. *Transactions of the American Institute of Electrical Engineers, III: Power Apparatus and Systems* 79: 667–673.

Dalziel CF, Lee WR (1969) Lethal electric currents. *IEEE Spectrum* 6: 44–50.

Daniel M, Haban GF, Hutcherson WL, Bolter J, Long C (1985) Neuropsychological and emotional consequences of accidental high voltage electrical shock. *International Journal of Clinical Neuropsychology* 7: 102–106.

Daniel RK, Ballard PA, P. H, Zelt RG, Howard CR. (1988) High voltage electrical injury. *Journal of Hand Surgery (Am)* 13: 44–49.

Dendooven AM, Lissens M, Bruyninckx F, Vanhecke J (1990) Electrical injuries to peripheral nerves. *Acta Belgica. Medica Physica* 13: 161–165.

DiVincenti FC, Moncrief JA, Pruitt Jr BA (1969) Electrical injuries: a review of 65 cases. *Journal of Trauma* 9: 497–507.

Fish RM (2000) Electric injury, part III: cardiac monitoring indications, the pregnant patient, and lightning. *Journal of Emergency Medicine* 18: 181–187.

Fish RM (2000b) Electric injury, Part II: Specific injuries. *Journal of Emergency Medicine* 18: 27–34.

Frayne JH, Gilligan BS (1987) Neurological sequelae of lightning stroke. *Clinical and Experimental Neurology* 24: 195–200.

Freiberger H (1934) *Der elektrische widerstand des menschlichen Korpers gegn technischen gleich und wechselstrom* [The electrical resistance of the human body to commercial direct and alternating currents]. Verlag Julius Springer, Berlin. Translated from German by Allen Translation Service, Maplewood, NJ, Item No. 9005.

Gowrishankar TR, Pliquett U, Lee RC (1999) Dynamics of membrane sealing in transient electropermeabilization of skeletal muscle membranes. *Annals of the New York Academy of Sciences* 888: 195–210.

Grube BJ, Heimbach DM (1992) Acute and delayed neurological sequelae of electrical injury. In: Lee RC, Carvalho EG, Burke JF (eds) *Electrical trauma: the pathophysiology, manifestations and clinical management*. Cambridge University Press, Cambridge, pp. 133–152.

Halperin DS, Oberhansli I, Rouge JC (1983) Cardiac and neurological impairments following electric shock in a young child. *Helvetica Paediatrica Acta* 38: 159–166.

Hammond J, Ward CG (1994) The use of technetium-99 pyrophosphate scanning in management of high voltage electrical injuries. *American Surgeon* 60: 886–888.

Harm W (1980) *Biological effects of ultraviolet radiation*. Cambridge University Press, Cambridge.

Harvey-Sutton PL, Driscoll TR, Frommer MS, Harrison JE (1992) Work-related electrical fatalities in Australia, 1982–1984. *Scandinavian Journal of Work and Environmental Health* 18: 293–297.

Hooshimand HF, Radfar F, Beckner E (1989) The neurophysiological aspects of electrical injuries. *Electroencephalography* 20: 111–120.

Hunt J, Lewis S, Parkey R, Baxter C (1979) The use of technetium-99m stannous pyrophosphate scintigraphy to identify muscle damage in acute electric burns. *Journal of Trauma* 19: 409–413.

Hunt JL (1992) Soft tissue patterns in acute electric burns. In: Lee RC, Cravalho EG, Burke JF (eds) *Electrical trauma: the pathophysiology, manifestations and clinical management*. Cambridge University Press, Cambridge, pp. 83–104.

Hunt JL, Sato RM, Baxter CR (1980) Acute electric burns: current diagnostic and therapeutic approaches to management. *Archives of Surgery* 115: 434–438.

James TN, Riddick L, Embry JH (1990) Cardiac abnormalities demonstrated postmortem in four cases of accidental electrocution and their potential significance relative to nonfatal electrical injuries of the heart. *American Heart Journal* 120: 143–157.

Jensen PJ, Thomsen PE, Bagger JP, Norgaard A, Baandrup U (1987) Electrical injury causing ventricular arrhythmias. *British Heart Journal* 57: 279–283.

Johnstone BR, Harding DL, Hocking B (1986) Telephone-related lightning injury. *Medical Journal of Australia* 144: 706–709.

Karczsmar GS, River LP, River J *et al.* (1994) Prospects for assessment of the effects of electrical injury by magnetic resonance. *Annals of the New York Academy of Sciences* 720: 176–180.

Kelley KM, Pliskin N, Meyer G, Lee RC (1994) The neuropsychiatric aspects of electrical injury: the nature of psychiatric disturbance. *Annals of the New York Academy of Sciences* 720: 213–218.

Kieback D (1988) International comparison of electrical accident statistics. *Journal of Occupational Accidents* 10: 95–105.

Kinney TJ (1982) Myocardial infarction following electrical injury. *Annals of Emergency Medicine* 11: 622–5.

Kouwenhoven WB (1968) Human safety and electric shock. Address to the Wilmington ISA Electrical Safety Course, Research Triangle Park, NC.

Lee RC (1997) Injury by electrical forces: pathophysiology, manifestations, and therapy. *Current Problems in Surgery* 34: 677–764.

Lee RC, Kolodney MS (1987a) Electrical injury mechanisms: dynamics of the thermal response. *Plastic and Reconstructive Surgery* 80: 663–671.

Lee RC, Kolodney MS (1987b) Electrical injury mechanisms: electrical breakdown of cell membranes. *Plastic and Reconstructive Surgery* 80: 672–679.

Lee RC, Gaylor DC, Bhatt D, Israel DA (1988) Role of cell membrane rupture in the pathogenesis of electrical trauma. *Journal of Surgical Research* 44: 709–719.

Lee RC, Myerov A, Maloney CP (1994) Promising therapy for cell membrane damage. *Annals of the New York Academy of Sciences* 720: 239–245.

Lee RH (1981) The other electrical hazard: electric arc blast burns. *IEEE Industry Applications Society Annual Meeting*, 1981.

Litster JD (1975) Stability of lipid bilayers and red cell membranes. *Physics Letters* 53A: 193–4.

Long JC (1962) A clinical and experimental study of electrical cataract. *Transactions of the American Ophthalmological Society* 60: 471–516.

Loomis D, Dufort V, Kleckner RC, Savitz DA (1999) Fatal occupational injuries among electric power company workers. *American Journal of Industrial Medicine* 35: 302–309.

Lown B, Neuman J, Amarsingham R, Berkovits BV (1962) Comparison of alternating current with direct current electroshock across the closed chest. *American Journal of Cardiology* 10: 223–233.

Luce EA (2000) Electrical burns. *Clinics in Plastic Surgery* 27: 133–143.

Lutton CE (1994) Economic impact of injuries associated with electrical events. *Annals of the New York Academy of Sciences* 720: 272–276.

Mancusi-Ungaro HR, Tarbox AR, Wainwright DJ (1986) Posttraumatic stress disorder in electric burn patients. *Journal of Burn Care and Rehabilitation* 7: 521–525.

Mann R, Gibran N, Engrav L, Heimbach D (1996) Is immediate decompression of high voltage electrical injuries to the upper extremity always necessary? *Journal of Trauma* 400: 584–587.

Meyer HW (1971) *A History of Electricity and Magnetism*. MIT Press, Cambridge, MA, p. 16.

Monafo WW, Freedman BM (1987) Electrical and lightning injury. In: Boswick JA (ed.) *The art and science of burn care*, Aspen, Rockville, pp. 241–253.

Nicholson CP, Grotting JC, Dimick AR (1987) Acute microwave injury to the hand. *Journal of Hand Surgery (Am)* 12: 446–449.

NSC (1983) *Accident facts*. National Safety Council, Chicago.

Oner N, Ozguzel H, Berker C, Gurtunka N, Kocabasoglu C (1995) Musculoskeletal system damage with electrical injury. *Fizik Tedavi Rehabilitasyon Dergisi* 19: 323–325.

Padanilam JT, Bischof JC, Lee RC *et al.* (1994) Effectiveness of poloxamer 188 in arresting calcein leakage from thermally damaged isolated skeletal muscle cells. *Annals of the New York Academy of Sciences* 720: 111–123.

Pliskin NH, Fink J, Malina A *et al.* (1999) The neuropsychological effects of electrical injury. New insights. *Annals of the New York Academy of Sciences* 888: 140–149.

Portellos M, Orlin SE, Kozart DM (1996) Electric cataracts. Arch Ophthalmol 114: 1022–1023.

Powell KT, Morganhelar AW, Weaver JC (1989) Tissue electroporation:observation of reversible breakdown in viable frog skin. *Biophysical Journal* 56: 1163–1171.

Powell KT, Weaver JC (1986) Transient aqueous pore in bilayer membranes: a statistical theory. *Bioelectrochemistry and Bioenergetics* 15: 211–227.

Prausnitz MR, B VG, Langer R, Weaver J C (1993) Electroporation of mammalian skin: a mechanism to enhance transdermal drug delivery. *Proceedings of the National Academy of Sciences of the USA* 90: 10504–10508.

Quinby WC, Burke JF, Trelstad RL, Caulfield J (1978) The use of microscopy as a guide to primary excision of high tension electrical burns *Journal of Trauma* 18: 423–429.

Reilly JP (1994) Scales of reaction to electric shock: thresholds and biophysical mechanisms. *Annals of the New York Academy of Sciences* 720: 21–37.

van Rhoon GC, van der Zee J, Broekmeyer-Reurink MP, Visser AG, Rheinhold HS (1992) Radiofrequency capacitative heating of deep-seated tumours using pre-cooling of the subcutaneous tissues: results on thermometry in Dutch patients. *International Journal of Hyperthermia* 8: 843–854.

Robinson NM, Chamberlain DA (1996) Electrical injury to the heart may cause long-term damage to conducting tissue: a hypothesis and review of the literature. *International Journal of Cardiology* 53: 273–277.

Rouge RG, Dimick AR (1978) The treatment of electrical injury compared to burn injury: a review of pathophysiology and comparison of patient management protocols. *Journal of Trauma* 18: 43–47.

Saffle JR, Crandall A, Warden GD (1985) Cataracts: a long-term complication of electrical injury. *Journal of Trauma* 25: 17–21.

Saffle JR, Davis B, Williams P (1995) Recent outcomes in the treatment of burn injury in the United States: a report from the American Burn Association Patient Registry. *Journal of Burn Care and Rehabilitation* 16: 219–232.

Sances A Jr, Myklebust JB, Larson SJ *et al.* (1981) Experimental electrical injury studies. *Journal of Trauma* 21: 589–597.

Smith KJ (1980) A sensitive method for the detection and quantification of conduction deficits in nerve. *Journal of the Neurological Sciences* 48: 191–199.

Smith KJ, Hall SM (1980) Nerve conduction during peripheral demyelination and remyelination. *Journal of the Neurological Sciences* 48: 201–219.

Sneed PK, Gutin PH, Stauffer PR *et al.* (1992) Thermoradiotherapy of recurrent malignant brain tumours. *International Journal of Radiation Oncology, Biology, Physics* 23: 853–861.

Solem L, Fischer RP, Strate RG (1977) The natural history of electrical injury. *Journal of Trauma* 17: 487–492.

Somogyi E, Tedeschi CG (1977) Injury by electric force. In: Tedeschi CG, Echert WG, Tedeschi LG (eds) *Forensic medicine, a study in trauma and environmental hazards*. W B Saunders, Philadelphia, pp. 661.

Statistics BoL (1997) *National census of fatal occupational injuries*. Statistics BoL, Washington, pp. 1996.

Stout NA (1998) *Worker deaths by electrocution*. National Institute for Occupational Safety and Health, Cincinnati.

Taylor GI, Michael DH (1973) On making holes in a sheets of fluid. *Journal of Fluid Mechanics* 58: 625–640.

Taylor PH, Pugsley LQ, Vogel EH (1962) The intriguing electrical burn: a review of thirty one electrical burn cases. *Journal of Trauma* 2: 309–324.

Thomas AH, Hanna C (1974) Electric cataracts. 3. Animal model. *Archives of Ophthalmology* 91: 469–473.

Triggs WJ, Owens J, Gilmore RL, Campbell K, Quisling R (1994) Central conduction abnormalities after electrical injury. *Muscle and Nerve* 17: 1068–1070.

Tropea BI, Lee RC (1992) Thermal injury kinetics in electrical trauma. *Journal of Biomechanical Engineering* 114: 241–250.

Tsong TY (1991) Electroporation of cell membranes. *Biophysical Journal* 60: 2977–306.

Tsong TY, Astumian RD (1987) Electroconformational coupling and membrane protein function. *Progress in Biophysics and Molecular Biology* 50: 1–45.

Tsong TY, Astumian RD (1988) Electroconformational coupling: how membrane-bound ATPase transduces energy from dynamic electric fields. *Annual Review of Physiology* 50: 273–290.

Tung LTO, Neunlist M, Jain S, O'Neill R (1994) Effects of strong electric shock on cardiac muscle tissue. *Annals of the New York Academy of Sciences* 720: 160–175.

Wiggers CJ, Wegria R (1939) Ventricular fibrillation due to single, localised induction and condenser shocks applied during the vulnerable phase of ventricular systole. *American Journal of Physiology* 128: 500–505.

Wyzga RE, Lindroos W (1999) Health implications of global electrification. *Annals of the New York Academy of Sciences* 888: 1–7.

Further reading

Baxter CR (1970) Present concepts in the management of major electrical injury. *Surgical Clinics of North America* 50: 1401–1418.

Demling RH, LaLonde C (1989) *Burn trauma*. Thieme Medical Publishers, New York, pp. 242–244.

Frank DH, Fisher JC (1984) Complications of electrical injury. In: Greenfield LJ (ed.) *Complications in surgery and trauma*. J B Lippincott, Philadelphia, pp. 50–59.

Kouwenhoven WB (1949) Effects of electricity on the human body. *Electrical Engineering* 68: 199–204.

Rudowski W, Nasilowski W, Zietkiewicz W, Zietkiewicz K (1976) *Burn therapy and research*, John Hopkins University Press, Baltimore, pp. 262–271.

25

CHAPTER 25

Radiation injuries

KERWYN FOO AND LEE COLLINS

CHAPTER 25
Radiation injuries

KERWYN FOO AND LEE COLLINS

General principles

Nuclear technology and the use of radiation have spread into fields from warfare to healthcare, and from space exploration to terrestrial transport. With this widespread use comes the possibility of accidents involving radiation, possibly combined with trauma.

Natural background radiation is the largest single source of radioactive exposure for most living things on earth. It is made up of cosmic radiation and radiation from naturally occurring radioactivity in the soil. Background radiation is weak and mostly unavoidable.

Other minor sources of small amounts of radiation abound in everyday life: building materials, televisions, smoke detectors, glaze in ceramics used in the home, even radon in the air we breathe. Occupational exposure can occur in nuclear power generation, industrial applications, medical and research facilities, and the disposal of nuclear waste.

Radiation injuries, like other trauma, have a scale of severity from minor incidental exposure to large-scale accidents such as Chernobyl and Goiania. The latter are medical, social, and ecological disasters, and thankfully are extremely rare. It is much more likely that the medical practitioner will encounter minor incidents, as a result of occupational or accidental public exposure. Radiation injuries are very uncommon, due in part to the fewer nuclear facilities compared to other industries, but also to the strict safeguards imposed by most authorities on the use, transport and disposal of radioactive material and products, as well as on the use of radiation-producing devices.

Key point

- Natural background radiation is the largest single source of radioactive exposure for most living things on earth.

Basic radiation science

Radiation damage is caused by transmission of energy from radiation sources to biological material. These sources may be radioactive materials which emit particles such as alpha- and beta-particles, neutrons, or gamma-rays (photons), or they may be artificial sources of radiation such as radiographic equipment.

Radioactive materials may in turn be sealed (where the source is encapsulated) or unsealed (where the source is a potential source of contamination).

Radiation can be measured in various ways:

- *Exposure*, measured in coulomb/kg, refers to the *ionization* produced in air by X-rays or gamma rays.
- *Absorbed dose*, measured in gray (Gy), refers to the *energy* absorbed per kilogram by a material such as an organ or tissue.
- *Equivalent dose*, measured in sievert (Sv) takes into account the differing effects that each type of radiation has on body tissue. For example, 1 Gy from alpha radiation has 20 times the effect on tissue that 1 Gy of gamma or X-radiation has.
- *Effective dose*, also measured in Sv, takes into account the differing sensitivity to radiation of various tissues. This allows assessment of severity of injury by converting separate tissue doses into a whole-body dose, which in turn can

be used to estimate the biological relevance of a person's radiation exposure. The effective dose is derived by adding the product of the equivalent dose and a tissue weighting factor for all exposed organs.

- The quantity of a radioactive material (radioisotopes or radionuclides) is called the *activity*, measured in becquerels (Bq). As the Bq is a very small amount, multiples such as kBq or MBq are common. Each radioisotope has different types and energies of emissions. For photon emitters a quantity sometimes called the *dose rate constant*, measured in Gy h^{-1} MBq^{-1} at 1 m, is used to describe the radiation intensity from a particular radioisotope.

Key point

- Radiation damage is caused by transmission of energy from radiation sources to biological material.

Types of radiation accidents

It is very important to understand the difference between *radiation exposure* and *contamination with radioactive materials*. Exposure from sources of X-rays and gamma rays does not itself create a radiation hazard to others. Internal or external contamination, even with low activities of radioisotopes, can create a significant radiation hazard to those treating the patient. In some cases the same radioisotope source can represent very different hazards, depending on whether the source is sealed or unsealed. For example, the amount of radium-226 once used in watches constitutes a low-level hazard while it remains contained, but can be quite toxic if incorporated into the body.

There are four types of radiation accidents:

- *Whole or partial body irradiation from external sources:* Examples of this type of accident are inadvertent exposure from industrial radiography sources, or from picking up a sealed radioactive source and carrying it in a pocket. These patients are not themselves radioactive, but may have received large localized or generalized absorbed doses, which may not have produced any symptoms at the time of presentation. They may be managed in the normal hospital environment quite safely once any sealed source is removed.
- *Internal contamination only:* The patient has ingested, inhaled, or otherwise incorporated an unsealed radioactive material into their body. These accidents may arise from industrial or medical incidents, or even (in bizarre cases) attempted suicides. The patient is radioactive, and is a potential source of contamination. If the contamination is totally internal, the patient may be treated in the emergency department, but all body fluids must be assumed to be contaminated until proven otherwise.
- *External contamination with or without internal contamination:* Typical accidents are those arising from transport or handling unsealed radioactive materials. They are a potentially significant source of contamination, and special precautions may be needed to prevent the spread of contamination to the local environment and staff, and to prevent internal contamination of the patient. Patients may need concurrent treatment of injuries, and in most cases, the urgent treatment of injuries should take precedence over decontamination. Use of universal precautions will minimize the risk of contamination in this phase. Once the patient is stabilized, the contamination should be dealt with.
- *Radioactive sources embedded within the patient:* This is an unusual situation, usually arising from explosive accidents, but some patients who are being treated with implanted radioactive material and discharged could conceivably be an emergency admission due to other causes. The embedded source may be of low activity and hazard, or may be a significant source of radiation.

Many accidents involving the whole body can cause multisystem problems that result in systemic symptoms, where more limited exposure will only manifest as local effects. It is therefore important in radiation injuries to assess not only the patient, but also the incident, and determine the type and dose of radiation. An accident history should be compiled as soon as possible to allow proper assessment of treatment and risks.

Key points

- Understand the difference between radiation exposure and contamination with radioactive materials.
- Many accidents involving the whole body can cause multisystem problems that result in systemic symptoms, whereas more limited exposure will only manifest as local effects.
- In most cases, the urgent treatment of injuries should take precedence over decontamination.

Effects of radiation exposure

The injuries that result from radiation exposure depend on several factors, including:

- dose
- type of radiation
- source of radiation
- body part exposed
- length and intensity of exposure
- whether contamination is present.

Radiation effects are divided into two categories, stochastic and deterministic:

- *Stochastic effects* are those where there is assumed to be a probability of the effect occurring at any dose, with the probability increasing with dose (the linear, no threshold hypothesis). Stochastic effects include carcinogenesis and leukaemogenesis. The period between the radiation exposure and the manifestation of the effect may be many years—longer for solid tumours than for leukaemia. The overall population lifetime probability of fatal cancer radiation for low doses at low dose rates is assumed to be 5%/Sv.
- *Deterministic effects* are those where there is a threshold dose, below which the effect does not occur. Above the threshold, the severity of the effect increases with dose. Examples are epilation, radiation sickness, erythema, radiation cataract, and sterilization. The thresholds vary markedly. Acute radiation effects are basically a severe form of deterministic effects.

There is a relatively long latent period between the radiation exposure and the clinical manifestation of stochastic effects—up to decades for solid tumours. For deterministic effects, the latent period is very short—hours to days in many cases.

Key point

- Radiation effects are divided into two categories, stochastic and deterministic.

Acute radiation syndrome

Acute high-level (usually >1 Gy) whole-body irradiation by penetrating radiation such as photons (gamma or X-rays) may result in damage to multiple organ systems—a complex clinical entity called acute radiation syndrome (ARS). Such radiation exposure can occur in reactor accidents or industrial accidents involving unprotected individuals, or from the use of nuclear weapons. Fortunately such exposures are rare, but they call for an immediate and careful response. In over 80% of fatal radiation accidents, it is the whole-body radiation exposure that has been the cause of death.

Organ systems damaged include:

- *Haematopoietic:* Bone marrow suppression occurs, resulting in neutropenia and thrombocytopenia. An initial reactive rise in neutrophils is followed by a decline that occurs 1–21 days after radiation exposure. Recovery of cell numbers starts about 30 days after exposure. A brief rise in neutrophils may occur earlier but is not usually sustained. Serial lymphocyte counts can give a prognosis: if the trough count is $>1.2 \times 10^9$/L then there will probably be a benign course. Treatment will be required below this. Troughs $<0.5 \times 10^9$/L indicate severe illness, and near total lymphopenia in the first 6 hours is usually quickly fatal.

- *Gastrointestinal:* The effects are related to the loss of gastrointestinal epithelium. Initial symptoms are nausea, vomiting, and diarrhoea. A dose of >12 Gy precludes mucosal regeneration. The damage to the mucosa results in decreased gut motility, absorption, and secretion. Diarrhoea, malabsorbtive syndromes, and gastrointestinal infections result. Bloody diarrhoea indicates a very poor prognosis.
- *Cardiovascular:* High-dose radiation of about 15 Gy causes tissue oedema and cytokine release which manifests as hypotension, fever, and vomiting. Oedema of specific organs has its own consequences, e.g. cerebral oedema. Extreme doses (50 Gy) can affect cell membranes directly to cause neurological impairment before death.

For convenience, the temporal sequence of events following exposure is somewhat arbitrarily divided into four periods (Table 25.1):

1. The *prodromal period* occurs in the few hours after exposure, and is when transitory symptoms are apparent. The type, timing, and severity of these depend on dose.
2. The *latent period* is the time before the development of the symptoms of bone marrow, gastrointestinal, or neurovascular abnormalities.
3. A period of *manifest illness* then occurs which consists of the organ system damage effects described above.
4. The course of illness is completed by *recovery* over months or *death* if the organ damage was too high. Death can occur at any stage.

The approximate timing of some of the symptoms of ARS is shown in Table 25.2.

Key point

- Acute high-level (usually >1 Gy) whole-body irradiation by penetrating radiation such as photons (gamma- and X-rays) may result in damage to multiple organ systems—a complex clinical entity called acute radiation syndrome.

Table 25.1 Temporal stages in the acute radiation syndrome

Prodromal	Latent (asymptomatic)	Illness
Anorexia, nausea, vomiting, diarrhoea, abdominal pain	Leukopenia	Gastrointestinal: nausea/vomiting, diarrhoea, abdominal pain, jaundice
Fatigue, disorientation, fever	Thrombocytopenia	Skin: erythema, hair loss
Shock, oliguria Changes in sensation		Neurological: sensation changes, ataxia, confusion, loss of consciousness
Erythema, conjunctivitis		Haematological: infection, fever, purpura

Table 25.2 Timing of some clinical features of the acute radiation syndrome

Dose rage (Gy)	Likely clinical effects	Typical time interval	Prognosis
0.25–2.5	Nausea Fatigue Vomiting Fever	3–20 h 3 h–6 weeks 6–24 h 2 days– 5weeks	Very good
2.5–7.5	Nausea Fatigue Vomiting Fever Haematological damage	1–72 h 1 h–6 weeks 3–24 h 1–5 weeks 2–21 days	Good
>7.5	Nausea Fatigue Vomiting Fever Haematological damage	1–72 h 1 h–2 weeks 1–48 h 10–14 days 1–5 days	Guarded to poor
>50	CNS Cardiovascular	Hours Hours	Death certain

Local injury effects

In any radiation exposure accident there is usually a variation in absorbed dose along the exposed region of the body. If the trunk dose is not high enough to cause ARS, but there has been a high dose to a limited area, it is usually referred to as *local radiation injury*. Such exposure can occur when body parts or skin are exposed to small radioactive sources outside their normal containment, or when exposed to direct X-ray beams in industrial or medical settings. High-dose radiotherapy can have the same effects. The local effects depend on the tissue affected and the depth of penetration of the radiation. The type of radiation is therefore important, given that photons (gamma and X-rays) penetrate much further than beta-particles, which give a high dose to superficial tissue. It is important to realize that, even if the exposure was very localized, ARS may still co-exist with local effects.

Skin reactions are the main effect of local exposure since skin (most often the hand) generally receives the highest dose in these cases. The effects may be erythema with or without oedema, loss of hair, flaking of skin, blisters, and dry or moist desquamation with subsequent tissue necrosis. Time frames and duration vary, as shown in Fig. 25.1. When radiation damages cutaneous and subcutaneous tissue, subsequent disease may be related to the loss of sweat glands, nerve tissue, hair follicles, and blood vessels, with some damage occurring similar to burns. Radiation damage may persist long after the

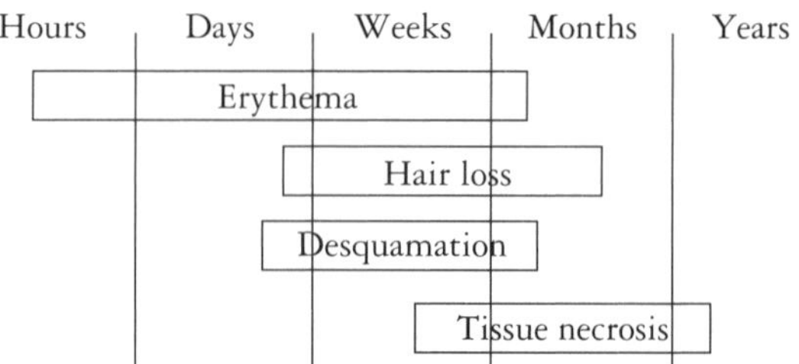

Figure 25.1 Timing of skin changes in response to radiation injury.

corresponding physical trauma and become manifest years later as necrosis or tissue breakdown.

Key point

- Skin reactions are the main effect of local exposure.

Long-term effects

Local long-term effects from radiation include fibrosis, tissue atrophy, necrosis, and chronic skin conditions. Both skin and underlying tissue, such as lung, gut, or muscle can be affected, long after the other injuries from exposure have resolved. For example, lung fibrosis can follow years after chest exposure to high-energy photons during breast radiotherapy. Specific disorders include joint stiffening and decreased range of movement due to tendon and synovial thickening or breakdown, changes to sensation of exposed skin, and the development of cataracts in the eyes.

The sequelae of whole-body exposure depend on the complications from the acute radiation syndrome. Infection and damage to haematopoietic and other systems will dictate the course of illness and recovery. Exposure of the whole body will produce similar late effects to exposed areas as from local exposure if the skin dose was sufficiently high.

Radiation has the potential to transform genetic material. Radiation exposure to the fetus can result in mental retardation of the infant and an increased risk of the future development of leukaemia and other childhood cancers years after the exposure, as well as organ maldevelopment. Although the doses needed to cause some of these effects are relatively high, fetal exposure may at times be a cause for concern.

Analysis of data after the atomic bombing of Hiroshima and Nagasaki, and later of major radiation accidents such as the reactor disaster at Chernobyl, has demonstrated increases in the incidence of cancer, supported by studies of people exposed to low-dose radiation by their occupation or environment. Cancers particularly associated with radiation are:

- *Skin cancers:* These result from larger doses, usually associated with radiodermatitis. The skin is more resistant to carcinogenesis by radiation than internal organs, but non-melanoma skin cancers can and do occur at higher doses.
- *Lung cancer*: This can be induced by inhalation of radioactive particles or gases (such as radon) or by exposure to external sources. Evidence of increased lung cancer has been found for both atomic bomb survivors and to early radiotherapy patients treated with high doses of X-rays to the chest.
- *Bone cancers*: e.g. osteosarcomas, have been induced especially by internalized sources such as radium, absorbed by the body by ingestion or contamination. Other radionuclides can have similar effects.
- *Thyroid cancer*: There is a confirmed link between thyroid cancer incidence and radiation exposure. This exposure includes direct exposure to external X-rays (e.g. medical equipment), ingestion of food products from a contaminated source, or from a radioiodine contaminated environment. The fetus is particularly at risk.
- *Leukaemias*: Even relatively small doses of radiation have been found to be associated with a rise in leukaemia incidence.
- *Breast cancer*: Modern mammographic techniques and equipment deliver very small doses to the breast.

Key point

- Local long-term effects from radiation include fibrosis, tissue atrophy, necrosis, and chronic skin conditions.

Management of radiation accident victims

Immediate management

Radiation accidents can involve trauma of more conventional nature. Burns, physical trauma, chemical effects, or inhalational injuries can be part of the accident and more acutely life threatening. Adequate resuscitation must take priority.

Particular care must be taken to ensure the safety of medical, paramedical, and emergency services staff attending an incident that has a possible radiation component. Hospitals near a nuclear site with potential for radiation accidents will normally have a disaster plan that incorporates procedures for dealing with accident victims.

In addition to resuscitation and treatment of acute conditions, the initial (hospital) management of the radiation accident victim should include:

- monitoring and decontamination: as above, with priority to remove any internal radioactive contamination
- serial blood and urine samples, to assess ingested radionuclide uptake and retention
- serial blood counts, for lymphocyte counts to help prognosis
- full history of any existing conditions or illnesses, especially incompletely treated infections or unhealed wounds, which may have an altered course as a result of the exposure.

In addition, the local radiation regulatory authorities must be informed, and radiation professionals such as medical physicists must be included in the treatment team at the earliest possible stage. This ensures appropriate procedures and equipment, such as the correct detectors for the particular radiation involved.

Information gathering about the event is vital. Much of the relevant history will be about the type of radiation, the period of exposure and the exposed body parts. The patient is unlikely to have this information, and it will have to be sought from the victim's employer, for example (see Table 25.3).

Key points

- Adequate resuscitation must take priority.
- Local radiation regulatory authorities must be informed, and radiation professionals such as medical physicists must be included into the treatment team at the earliest possible stage.

Decontamination

After identification of a radiation accident involving contamination, strict controls must be instituted to prevent further contamination outside those already affected. These include:

- Protective clothing and equipment for all rescue and treating staff.
- Establishment of a restricted and isolated zone incorporating the area of increased radioactivity. All personnel must be checked in and out and all equipment and contaminated clothing removed at the exit.
- Removal of patient's contaminated clothing, as soon as practicable given resuscitation needs and other injuries. Outer clothing should be cut off the patient. Outer surfaces should be folded inwards to prevent spread. Personal items can be kept safely but also in a controlled area until decontaminated.
- *Monitoring:* Use of detection devices to monitor what items are contaminated. Monitoring of all patients is required to separate those who are contaminated. Regular monitoring of staff is required to ensure their safety.
- Prevention of contamination or equipment. Place plastic sheets under equipment and casualties.
- If contamination could be spread to other areas of the hospital, for example with unstable patients, barriers and controlled areas should be set up within the hospital. There should be

Table 25.3 Basic information needed about a radiation accident victim

External source	Contamination with radioactive material	Other
Type and source of radiation	Radionuclide, activity and chemical form	Details of monitoring at the site
Exposed organ(s)	Amount and composition (liquid, size of particles)	Circumstances, time, and place of the exposure
Period of exposure	Method of contamination (inhalation, skin contact, ingestion), and what decontamination was performed	Other trauma or medical problems
Distance from source	What measurements have been made (smears, excreta, etc.)	Other persons involved

covered floors in the treatment area, and a covered route to and from the receiving area.

- There must be a system of collection and disposal of waste in labelled double bags to an appropriate facility.
- After clean-up, monitoring of the area is necessary to assess any persistent radiation.

Small numbers of contaminated particles on the skin can be removed at the scene. More extensive decontamination may need to take place at the hospital or disaster centre. Decontamination involves washing the skin many times with soap or detergent and monitoring between washes. Damage to the skin should be avoided. Covering of clean parts of the body while washing will reduce spread of contaminants. Wounds should be cleaned in the usual manner, but irrigated several times afterwards. Do not forget eyes, ears, mouth, and nose as possible areas of contamination. However, complete decontamination can rarely be achieved.

Inhaled, ingested, or absorbed contamination needs a more complex treatment, depending on the type of substance and route of contamination. Gastrointestinal clearance can be achieved by increasing transit speed, gastric lavage, and aspiration via nasogastric tube, and by manipulating the gut environment to reduce absorption of radioactive material.

In the case of absorbed radioactive iodine, the administration of stable iodine can saturate the thyroid gland to minimize further uptake of the radioisotope. Other substances can be diluted by administration of large amounts of non-radioactive isotopes to displace or increase excretion of the radioactive isotope. Chelating agents can also be used to bind radioisotopes. Examples are EDTA for transuranic elements, DTPA for transuranics and some rare earths, and desferrioxamine for plutonium.

More radical approaches for clearance of lungs, such as pulmonary lavage, are possible, but have significant associated morbidity.

In all cases, the effect of decontamination is assessed by monitoring the patient and the patient's urine and faeces to monitor absorption and clearance.

Key points

- Strict controls must be instituted to prevent further contamination.
- Small numbers of contaminated particles on the skin can be removed at the scene.
- More extensive decontamination may need to take place at the hospital or disaster centre.

Non-radiation trauma

In a disaster situation, it is likely that those affected will have physical or chemical trauma as well as the radiation effects. The treatment of these injuries may not be significantly affected by radiation exposure. There are some important factors to take into account:

- Radiation exposure can reduce healing. Radiation injury and other injuries will combine to give a longer recovery period and greater morbidity and mortality.
- Any surgical procedures necessary are best done in the *first 48 hours* before any fall in blood cell numbers occurs. Other surgery is best delayed by up to months to enable recovery from radiation syndromes.
- Infection control is of paramount importance.
- Haematology advice should be sought regarding transfusions, and platelet replacement before surgical procedures in the pancytopenic patient.
- The symptoms and signs of radiation illness are altered in the presence of other trauma. The patient may be assessed as having a higher dose of radiation due to thermal burns or gastrointestinal bleeding from physical trauma.

Key points

- Those affected will have physical or chemical trauma as well as the radiation effects.
- Infection control is of paramount importance.
- The symptoms and signs of radiation illness are altered in the presence of other trauma.

Treatment of specific conditions

Acute radiation syndrome

ARS is treated according to the dose received and severity of symptoms, and treatment is aimed at supporting the patient, treating the haematopoietic damage, and controlling opportunistic infection.

Supportive treatment aims to alleviate symptoms. Control of nausea is achieved using centrally and peripherally acting medications. $5HT_3$-receptor antagonists can be more effective in the control of radiation-induced emesis. Support in the form of fluids and adequate feeding is necessary to restore losses from diarrhoea and reduced absorption in the gastrointestinal system. The high turnover of cells also increases the body's requirements. A high-energy diet should be formulated that includes essential amino acids, vitamins A and E, and selenium. Specialist dietetic advice should be sought. Damage to the gastrointestinal system may require the use of antibiotic cover and parenteral feeds.

The treatment of the haematopoietic damage is aimed at supporting the patient while the system recovers. If the exposure leaves sufficient stem cells viable (about 10%), the patient will in time be able to regenerate the losses. Haematology review and supervision should be requested as the regime will be similar to that for haematology/oncology patients with neutro-, lympho- or thrombocytopenia. This may include colony stimulating factors, or even stem cell transplant if the patient has received a very high dose. Complications at this stage are bleeding and infection.

Control of infection starts when the patient is first assessed. All practical effort should be made to exclude or treat infection while the patient still has sufficient immune resources. If in hospital, isolation such as that for neutropenic oncology patients should be observed. Broad-spectrum antibiotic cover may be necessary for febrile patients, depending on specialist advice.

Key points

- Support the patient.
- Treat haematopoietic damage.
- Control opportunistic infection.

Local radiation effects

Care of superficial skin damage may be supportive, by keeping clean and excluding infection while the skin heals. Irritating methods and substances such as brushes and soaps should be avoided. Protection from sun exposure is required. For comfort, non-steroid creams can be applied.

More extensive skin damage involving deeper layers, pain, breaks in the skin, or tissue necrosis requires more active treatment. High doses of radiation result in skin that cannot be saved. Necrosis and ulceration occur and are treated on a symptomatic basis with adequate analgesia and prevention of infection. As in other extensive skin trauma, skin grafting may be required, particularly in larger areas of dead skin, radiodermatitis, or to improve function or appearance. In radiation trauma, there may be significant damage to underlying vascular tissue which may not be macroscopically apparent, and this can compromise graft survival. Late tissue necrosis may occur up to years after the dose, as well as skin cancers, tendon and joint degeneration.

Follow-up

Given the public sensitivity to radiation matters, and the potential for serious long-term effects, follow-up of radiation trauma patients is essential. As in other trauma, counselling is effective, but explanation of risks to expectant mothers, possible genetic risks, and the potential for future effects including cancer should all be addressed. For low-dose exposure, most patients will not require long-term follow-up. For more severe exposure, the patient should be made aware of the need to seek advice even at times far removed from the event.

Key point

- Follow-up of radiation trauma patients is essential.

Conclusion

Although it is unlikely that most hospitals will ever have to deal with radiation injury, it is important that plans are developed to seek the relevant advice should such an incident occur. Radiation safety officers or medical physicists are employed in many institutions using radiation equipment or radioactive materials, including hospitals. From accidental minor exposure in the workplace to large disasters, an awareness of the basic issues in radiation injury management will enable the trauma worker to identify when specialist help needs to be sought. With radiation a new technology but increasingly present in our lives, it behoves us to be ready to manage its potential dangers.

Acknowledgment

The authors wish to thank Dr Roland Yeghiaian-Alvandi, Staff Specialist, Department of Radiation Oncology, Westmead Hospital, Sydney, Australia for his assistance in the preparation of this chapter.

Further reading

Brown D, Weiss JF, MacVittie TJ, Pillai MV (1990) *Treatment of radiation injuries*. Plenum, New York.

Hendee WR, Edwards FM (1996) *Health effects of exposure to low-level ionizing radiation*. Institute of Physics Publishing, Philadelphia.

Mettler FA, Kelsey CA, Ricks RC (1990) *Medical management of radiation accidents*. CRC Press, Boca Raton, FL.

Swindon TN (1991) *Manual on the medical management of individuals involved in radiation accidents*. Commonwealth of Australia Department of Health for the Australian Radiation Laboratory.

26

CHAPTER 26

Drowning and diving accidents

ROBYN WALKER

CHAPTER 26
Drowning and diving accidents

ROBYN WALKER

Drowning

Epidemiology

Water sports are favourite recreational pursuits for many people and it is therefore unfortunate that so many, particularly the young, suffer injury through misadventure.

Drowning accidents are largely preventable and generally affect previously healthy individuals. Between 1992 and 1996 accidental drowning claimed the lives of some 1643 Australians and was the fifth most common 'external cause of death' behind suicide, motor traffic accidents, accidental falls and homicide (RLSSA 1997). The Royal Life Saving Society Australia also estimates there are approximately 90 000 'near misses' annually in Australia. The peak incidence of drowning is in the 0–4 year age group, followed by men in the 20–45 year age group. A combination of alcohol and risk-taking activity (boating, jet skis, surfing) occurs frequently. Hyperventilation before entering the water is known to increase breathhold time and prolong the time one may spend submerged. Hyperventilation lowers the arterial carbon dioxide level and hence removes the most potent respiratory stimulant. Hypoxia alone is a less powerful stimulant, and loss of consciousness and drowning may occur before the impulse to breath becomes apparent. Drowning may occur as the primary event or be secondary to, for example, a sudden cardiac event, epileptic seizure, or (in scuba divers) cerebral arterial gas embolism.

Key point

- Drowning accidents are largely preventable and generally affect previously healthy individuals.

Mechanism of injury

Whatever the cause, a drowning victim will initially hold their breath (voluntary apnoea) until they reach 'breaking point'. The levels of hypercarbia and hypoxia govern this breaking point. Once it is reached, inspiration of water occurs and this is usually followed by involuntary gasping. Significant volumes of water may also be swallowed. Progressive respiratory failure, metabolic acidosis, cardiac arrhythmias, and finally brain death ensue.

Key point

- A drowning victim will initially hold their breath (voluntary apnoea) until they reach 'breaking point'.

Classification of drowing accidents

The literature classifies the drowning syndromes in many ways. Drowning is defined as suffocation by submersion, especially in water (Modell 1993); *near drowning* is defined as survival, at least temporarily, after aspiration of fluid into the lungs (Golden *et al.* 1997). Classically the literature refers to 'wet' and 'dry' drowning and then further subdivides drowning according to whether fresh or salt water was involved.

Wet drowning (with aspiration of fluid into the lungs) is said to occur in 80–93% of cases. At least 85% of patients who survive near drowning are thought to aspirate 22 mL/kg of water or less (Modell 1993). The physiological basis of the hypoxia depends on the nature and the volume of the aspirated fluid. Most authors (Pearn 1985, Modell 1993, Mitchell and Gorman 1994, Weinstein and Krieger

1996, Golden *et al.* 1997, Reed 1998, Thanel 1998) refer to the theory of '*dry drowning*' and state that 7–20% of individuals who drown aspirate no fluid as a consequence of laryngeal spasm. It is stated a small volume of water enters the larynx or trachea and initiates laryngeal spasm, a vagally mediated reflex. In this case the progressive hypoxia occurs on a background of apnea. Edmonds (1998) questions the concept of dry drownings and states, 'dry drowning could well be an artifact of fluid absorption from the lungs or death from other causes'.

Key points

- Drowning is suffocation by submersion, especially in water whilst.
- Near drowning is survival, at least temporarily, after aspiration of fluid into the lungs.

Pathophysiology

Fresh water is hypotonic and rapidly absorbed into the pulmonary circulation, so the presence of the aspirate within the alveoli is not a problem. Although the fresh water is absorbed into the circulation and theoretically could cause hypervolaemia, electrolyte abnormalities, and red blood cell haemolysis, this is rarely seen in survivors. However, the fresh water denatures the alveolar surfactant, rendering the alveoli unstable and promoting alveolar collapse and ventilation–perfusion mismatching. Denaturization of the surfactant may continue even after rescue of the victim from the water, and damage to the alveolar epithelium results in a transudate into the alveoli and resulting pulmonary oedema. This transudate may be of such volume to render the survivor hypovolaemic on arrival at hospital.

Salt water is hypertonic and draws fluid from the intravascular space into the already fluid-filled alveoli. Ventilation–perfusion mismatching occurs and is compounded by the washing out of surfactant from the alveoli. This fluid shift again theoretically may result in haemoconcentration, hypovolemia, and electrolyte abnormalities, but this is rarely seen clinically.

No matter whether the fluid is salt or fresh water, the end result is pulmonary oedema and ventilation–perfusion mismatching with progressive respiratory distress, and the clinical management is identical for both groups. Consciousness is always lost within 3 minutes of involuntary submersion (Pearn 1985) and this is almost always due to cerebral hypoxia.

Initial management

The victim should be removed from the water without delay. Effective cardiopulmonary resuscitation (CPR) in water is not possible and although it is possible to perform mouth-to-mouth resuscitation in water, this must not delay retrieval to land. The focus of initial management is on restoring effective oxygenation and alleviating hypoxia. CPR should be instituted for the apnoeic and pulseless patient. The Heimlich manoeuvre (previously advocated to aid drainage of fluid from the lungs) should not be used unless obstruction of the airway from foreign body is strongly suspected (Weinstein and Krieger 1996). The patient should be transported promptly to a medical facility.

Key points

- Remove from water (effective CPR in water is not possible).
- Start CPR.
- Heimlich only for obstruction.
- Move to medical facility.

Definitive management

When the casualty arrives at the emergency department, medical staff should evaluate the airway and perform endotracheal intubation if indicated. Circulatory support with intravenous fluids should be initiated. For patients presenting pulseless and apnoeic, advanced clinical life support procedures should be continued until all hopes of achieving a salvageable patient are exhausted. Hypothermic patients must be rewarmed to a core temperature of 34°C before death is pronounced. A high index of suspicion should exist for cervical spine injury, particularly if there is any history of a diving or boating accident and cervical spine radiographs arranged.

Key points

- CPR.
- Where pulseless and apnoeic, continue advanced clinical life support procedures until all hope is gone.
- Warm hypothermic patients to a core temperature of 34°C.
- Check for cervical spine injury.

Patients with mild symptoms or no symptoms on arrival

All victims with a history of near drowning who arrive with minimal or no symptoms must be observed as secondary deterioration with the onset of pulmonary oedema may develop precipitously. As a minimum all patients should have a chest radiograph, arterial blood gases (ABGs), serum electrolytes, and ECG. Mild hypoxaemia should be managed with supplemental oxygen and ABGs on room air should have returned to normal before the patient is discharged.

Aspiration of water, particularly if contaminated, may result in pulmonary infection, but routine prophylactic use of antibiotics is not indicated. Antibiotics are indicated only if there is clinical signs of infection, and microbiological studies should be used to guide the choice.

Pulmonary oedema, if it occurs, will usually develop within several hours of aspiration and may be rapidly progressive. For this reason most authors suggest a minimum period of observation of 24 hours; however, for the subset of patients who are asymptomatic both clinically and biochemically at presentation, and remain so, discharge after 6 hours may be possible.

Key points

- Observe near drowning (with minimal or no symptoms) for at least 24 hours and do chest radiograph, ABGs, serum electrolytes, and ECG.
- May need antibiotics.

Patients with evidence of respiratory compromise

Patients with evidence of respiratory embarrassment require urgent intervention to correct the hypoxemia. The single treatment most effective in reversing hypoxemia, regardless of whether it is caused by aspiration of fresh water or seawater, is the application of continuous positive airway pressure (CPAP) (Modell 1993). CPAP may be used in both spontaneously breathing and mechanically ventilated patients and should be withdrawn gradually as the patient's ABGs and ventilation perfusion ratio normalizes. These patients require cardiac monitoring, serial ABGs, serum electrolytes, and chest radiographs. ABGs may vary between mild to severe hypoxemia with a widened alveolar-arterial gradient, and the PCO_2 may be low or high dependent on the level of alveolar ventilation. The chest radiograph may reveal patchy infiltrates suggestive of aspiration or frank pulmonary oedema. These patients may be significantly hypovolaemic as a consequence of pulmonary oedema (irrespective of the type of immersion) and a Swan–Ganz catheter may prove useful in monitoring their cardiovascular status. Consideration should be given to the insertion of a nasogastric tube to decompress the stomach.

Some centres in the past have recommended aggressive cerebral resuscitative techniques in near drowning victims in an attempt to maximize neurological salvage. The HYPER regime (Modell 1993) involved fluid restriction, hyperventilation, hypothermia, barbiturate coma, and invasive intracranial pressure monitoring, but these techniques have largely been abandoned due to lack of data supporting their use. Steroids have also been advocated in the past to in an attempt to reduce the lung injury, but again lack of supporting evidence for their benefit has seen a decline in use.

Animal studies (Waugh 1993) have suggested warm butyl alcohol vapour inspired in 100% oxygen may improve the hypoxaemia associated with aspiration of salt water. The entry of salt water into the lungs is associated with the production of foam bubbles that remain relatively stable due to the inclusion of surfactant from the alveolar lining. Waugh postulates the warm butyl alcohol vapour has a defoaming action within the small airways and may also act as a free radical scavenger to reduce the risk of oxygen toxicity. No human data is available at this time.

Key point

- Apply CPAP.

Outcome predictors

There are frequent newspaper reports of 'success' stories of drowning victims who have survived neurologically intact after prolonged periods of immersion, particularly in cold water, but the reported rates of survival with full neurological recovery vary. For patients presenting awake and alert, full neurological recovery is reported to be 100% (Modell 1993) and >90% of victims who arrive at the emergency department with a pulse survive neurologically intact (Reed 1998). For near-drowning victims who required admission to ICU, paediatric data reveals that 56% survived neurologically intact, 32% survived in a persistent vegetative state, and the remaining 32% died (Lavelle and Shaw 1993). Factors which are said to have an adverse effect on survival are prolonged submersion, delay in effective cardiopulmonary resuscitation, severe metabolic acidosis (pH <7.1), asystole on arrival at a medical facility, fixed dilated pupils, and a low Glasgow Coma Score (<5) (Modell 1993). However, survivors with intact neurological function have been reported after presenting with each of these factors. Hypothermia appears to be protective, but only if it occurs at the time of near drowning (Modell 1993); the basis of this appears to be the reduced cerebral oxygen requirements.

Key point

- Hypothermia appears to be protective, but only if it occurs at the time of near drowning.

Diving accidents

Recreational diving with self-contained underwater breathing apparatus (scuba diving) is a popular leisure activity. In Australia it is a growth industry. It is estimated that approximately 1.29 million scuba dives occur in Queensland waters each year, and the total value of the diving industry to Queensland in direct expenditure annually is approximately $100 million (Windsor 1996). In recent years there has also been a growing interest in the recreational community in mixed gas diving, i.e. diving on gas mixtures other than air, for example mixtures of nitrogen and oxygen (nitrox) and mixtures of helium and oxygen (heliox), and on closed circuit equipment, previously the realm of the military alone. Figures from Australian and New Zealand hyperbaric medicine units for the 1997/1998 financial year (HTNA 1998) reveal that some 398 divers required recompression therapy for a diving-related illness during this period. The most common injury in divers is middle ear barotrauma of descent, resulting from the non-equalization of the middle ear cavity with the ambient pressure, but the most serious injuries are those of decompression illness and pulmonary barotrauma with cerebral arterial gas embolism. It is these serious injuries that are dealt with in this chapter. Readers are referred to standard diving medicine texts for further information on the less serious forms of dysbaric illness.

Key point

- The most common injury in divers is middle ear barotrauma of descent.

Pulmonary barotrauma

Barotrauma is defined as the tissue damage resulting from the expansion or contraction of closed gas spaces, and is a direct effect of gas volume changes causing tissue damage (Edmonds *et al.* 1992). Pulmonary barotrauma of ascent or pulmonary overinflation syndrome is the tissue damage resulting from pressure changes acting on the lung when

Table 26.1 Depth-pressure relationship

Depth (msw)	Pressure (ATA)	Volume (L)
Surface	1	15
10	2	7.5
20	3	5
30	4	3.75
40	5	3
50	6	2.5

a diver ascends to the surface. Every time divers descend beneath the surface of the water, they subject their body to an increase in environmental pressure. This pressure relationship is illustrated in Table 26.1. Pascal's principle dictates that this pressure is distributed equally across all body tissues. Boyle's law states that if the temperature of a fixed mass of gas is kept constant, the relationship between the volume and the pressure will vary in such a way that the product of the pressure and the volume will remain constant (i.e. $P_1V_1 = P_2V_2$). It is important to recognize that the greatest pressure changes and therefore the greatest danger to a diver occurs at 0–10 m of sea water (msw), negating the popular myth that you cannot get into trouble if you only dive to shallow depths. Put simply this means if a diver fills his lungs with (5 L) gas at a depth of 20 msw or 3 atmospheres absolute (ATA) (101.325 kPa) and holds his breath until he reaches the surface, in accordance with Boyle's law the gas within his lungs will have expanded to 15 L. As the lungs cannot expand to accommodate this volume, pulmonary tissue damage is likely to occur. Pulmonary barotrauma occurs most commonly in novice and inexperienced divers and submarine escape training candidates who perform rapid ascents. Classically divers who suffer pulmonary barotrauma are seen to have an 'incident' at depth causing them to panic and then make a rapid uncontrolled ascent to the surface. A high-pitched scream may be heard as the diver breaks the surface of the water. This is said to be due to the exhalation of the expanding gas from the lungs.

Historically, individuals with a history of asthma or bullous lung disease, and therefore increased likelihood of gas trapping, have been excluded from diving owing to their theoretical increased risk of pulmonary barotrauma.

A transpulmonary pressure difference of as little as 70 mmHg in water near the surface (Edmonds *et al.* 1992) is enough to cause alveolar rupture and can result in pulmonary tissue damage, pneumothorax, pneumomediastinum/subcutaneous emphysema, and cerebral arterial gas embolism (CAGE). Although all four manifestations can occur simultaneously, this is uncommon and less than 10% of CAGE victims will have a detectable pneumothorax.

Key point

- Barotrauma is defined as the tissue damage resulting from the expansion or contraction of closed gas spaces, and is a direct effect of gas volume changes causing tissue damage.

Pulmonary tissue damage

Pulmonary tissue damage resulting in widespread alveolar rupture is rarely seen and is usually associated with a history of explosive decompression back to the surface. If the patient survives, first aid management includes ventilatory support with 100% oxygen.

Pneumothorax

Pneumothorax presents in the same way as a pneumothorax from non-diving causes. Clinically the diver may complain of sharp chest pain associated with shortness of breath with increased percussion note and decreased breath sounds. Resolution of the pneumothorax may be hastened by the breathing of 100% oxygen, needle aspiration, or the insertion of an intercostal drain.

Key point

- Clinically the diver may complain of sharp chest pain and shortness of breath.

Pneumomediastinum/ subcutaneous emphysema

Alveolar gas may also track through the interstitial pulmonary tissues and into the mediastinum (pneumomediastinum) and up into the subcutaneous tissues of the neck (subcutaneous or surgical emphysema, Fig. 26.1). The symptoms may occur immediately on exiting the water or take several hours to develop. The diver may complain of retrosternal chest pain, shortness of breath, a feeling of fullness in the throat, and changes in the character of the voice. On palpation of the neck region the 'crunching' sensation of subcutaneous emphysema may be felt. Radiologically, air may be seen tracking along the border of the heart and other mediastinal structures and along the major vessels in the neck region. Symptomatic relief will occur with the administration of 100% oxygen. Recompression is usually not indicated, although this will also provide symptomatic relief.

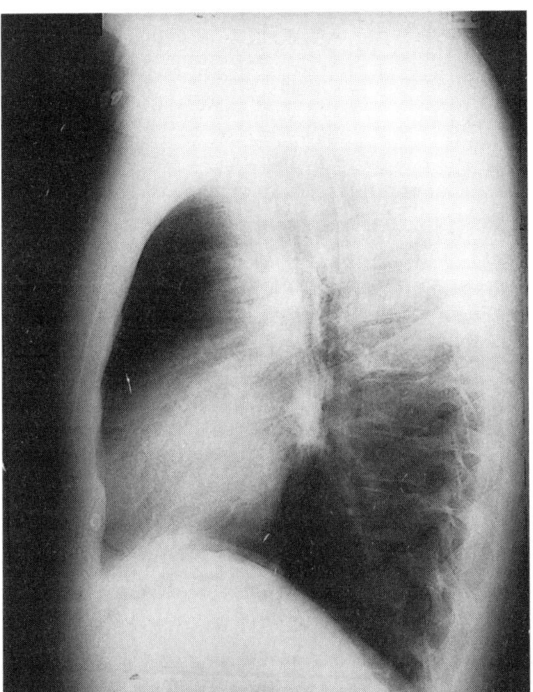

Figure 26.1 Chest radiograph showing surgical emphysema in the neck and superior mediastinum. There is no evidence of a pneumothorax.

Key point

- The diver may complain of retrosternal chest pain, shortness of breath, a fullness in the throat, and voice changes.

Cerebral arterial gas embolism

CAGE occurs when alveolar gas ruptures into the pulmonary veins and is then carried via the heart into the cerebral circulation. Typically the site of the alveolar rupture is not demonstrable even by sophisticated radiological techniques as rapid closure of the perforation site occurs. Bubbles reaching the arterial circulation distribute according to buoyancy in large blood vessels and according to flow in small blood vessels (Gorman *et al.* 1987) explaining why cerebral involvement is so common. Bubbles travelling to the brain can do one of three things:

- They may lodge permanently in the cerebral vasculature, typically in successive branching arterioles of 100 μm or less in diameter, resulting in an ischaemic infarct.
- They may lodge temporarily in the cerebral vasculature, and then redistribute, travelling back through the venous circulation to the lungs. This redistribution is a consequence of a reflex rise in arterial blood pressure, increased cerebral blood flow, and increased intracranial pressure resulting in the driving arterial pressure overcoming the surface tension of the bubble. The temporary arresting of blood flow secondary to lodgment of the bubble may cause clinical symptoms and signs, and bubbles also cause damage to the vascular endothelium as they pass through the cerebral vasculature

stripping the endothelium and activating inflammatory pathways. This process can result in progressive cerebral dysfunction via alterations in the blood–brain barrier and local cerebral blood flow even though the bubbles have long since passed.

- Most bubbles are not trapped within the cerebral vasculature and pass through into the venous system and back to the lungs. The bubbles again cause damage to vascular endothelium as they pass through. Accumulation of platelets and polymorphonuclear leukocytes at the site of injury and activation of inflammatory proteins such as kinins and complement pathways occurs. It is this inflammatory response which is believed to underlie many of the symptoms experienced by divers with decompression illness. The lungs are usually an effective bubble filter and the majority of bubbles will be trapped in the lungs (due to the low pulmonary pressures compared with the arterial circulation); the inert gas will then diffuse into the alveoli and be expired. This bubble filter may be overwhelmed in the presence of large numbers of bubbles, with bubbles again passing through into the arterial circulation and redistributing once more to the brain. This explains the presentation sometimes seen in divers who have collapse unconscious, recover, sit up (bubbles distributing with buoyancy), and then collapse once more. Bubbles may also reach the brain via abnormal arteriovenous channels within the lungs or through heart defects, e.g. a patent foramen ovale. Some 30% of the general population are said to have a probe-patent foramen ovale (Langton 1996) and reversal of flow across the defect can be seen in many with a Valsalva manoeuvre.

A diver presenting with acute neurological symptoms or signs either on surfacing or soon after a dive must be considered to have had a CAGE. CAGE may present as sudden death (typically with embolization of the brain stem), loss of consciousness, or with focal neurological abnormalities such as confusion, paralysis, convulsions, and variable sensory abnormalities. The first aid and definitive management of victims with CAGE is the same as for DCI and will be discussed below.

Key point

- A diver presenting with acute neurological symptoms or signs either on surfacing or soon after a dive must be considered to have had a CAGE

Classification of diving accidents

Conventionally serious diving accidents were classified as either decompression sickness type 1 or 2, or cerebral arterial gas embolism (CAGE). Type 1 decompression sickness was considered minor and involved the skin and joints; type 2 decompression sickness was considered serious and involved typically the neurological or respiratory systems. It has become apparent, however, that most divers presenting with decompression sickness have neurological involvement, which can be detected with careful neurological examination. In the past poor history taking and examination skills may have resulted in the overdiagnosis of type 1 disease. It is also difficult at times to differentiate between disease caused by pulmonary barotrauma with resultant CAGE and disease due to the arterialization of bubbles generated in the tissues. For this reason a new descriptive classification system encompassing all decompression illnesses has been introduced (Table 26.2). For example, a diver who makes a rapid uncontrolled ascent to the surface holding their breath, loses consciousness and then regains consciousness may be described as having acute resolving neurological DCI with evidence of pulmonary barotraumas, whereas a diver who presents with weakness of both lower limbs and who then develops urinary retention is described as having progressive neurological DCI with no evidence of pulmonary barotrauma.

Table 26.2 DCI classification

Evolutionary terminology	Progressive, static, spontaneously resolving, relapsing
Organ system terminology	Cutaneous, musculoskeletal, lymphatic, neurological, cardiorespiratory
Evidence of pulmonary barotraumas	

Decompression illness

Decompression illness (DCI) refers to the spectrum of diseases that result from decompression and the consequent lowering of pressure (Gorman 1993). When a diver descends below the surface of the water, the physical laws of Dalton and Henry explain why the diver's body absorbs an increased amount of inert gas (nitrogen, in most cases). Put simply, the partial pressure of nitrogen in the breathing mixture rises with the increase in ambient pressure, resulting in increased diffusion of nitrogen into the body tissues. While the diver remains at depth this increased nitrogen load is of no significance, but as the diver returns to the surface the inert gas must once more obey the laws of physics and one of two things may happen:

- The diver ascends at a rate which allows the dissolved inert gas to be carried back in solution to the lungs where it is expired.
- If the diver ascends at a rate that exceeds this capacity, bubbles will form in the tissues and venous blood.

These bubbles may then travel back to the lungs, which acts as a filter to trap the bubbles, and the bubbles may resolve through gas diffusion into the alveoli. Excessively large numbers of bubbles may overwhelm this filter, resulting in the passage of the bubbles into the arterial circulation. Bubbles formed in the tissues may also reach the arterial circulation via a patent foramen ovale or through pulmonary arteriovenous malformations.

Most divers will plan their dives using decompression tables or computers. These tables advise the diver as to how long they should stay at a particular depth and how to control their ascent. Unfortunately many of these decompression schedules have a failure rate varying between 0.5% and 5%, so the belief that staying within the tables excludes the possibility of developing DCI is wrong. Other factors which are said to increase the risk of DCI are dehydration, obesity, high levels of exertion during the dive, physical injury, multiple ascents, repetitive, and multiday diving exposures.

Key points

- DCI refers to the spectrum of diseases that result from decompression and the consequent lowering of pressure.
- Decompression tables or computers: advise the diver as to how long they should stay at a particular depth and how to control their ascent, but staying within the tables does not exclude the possibility of developing DCI.
- Other factors which are said to increase the risk of DCI are: dehydration, obesity, high levels of exertion during the dive, physical injury, multiple ascents, repetitive, and multiday diving exposures.

Effects of bubbles

Bubbles in the tissues cause direct mechanical damage, e.g. disrupting myelin sheaths in the spinal cord, cell rupture, and indirect damage through the activation of inflammatory pathways. Bubbles in the venous system damage the vascular endothelium, also activating inflammatory pathways. If bubbles are trapped in the lungs in sufficient quantity, the resultant back pressure on the venous drainage system can result in haemorrhagic infarction, particularly in the spinal cord. Bubbles in the arterial circulation will travel largely to the brain where they may lodge causing infarction or they may pass through into the venous circulation damaging the vascular endothelium as they pass. It is this damage, with the subsequent activation of the inflammatory cascade, that is thought to underlie many of the systemic symptoms of cerebral DCI.

Key point

- Bubbles in the tissues cause direct mechanical damage.

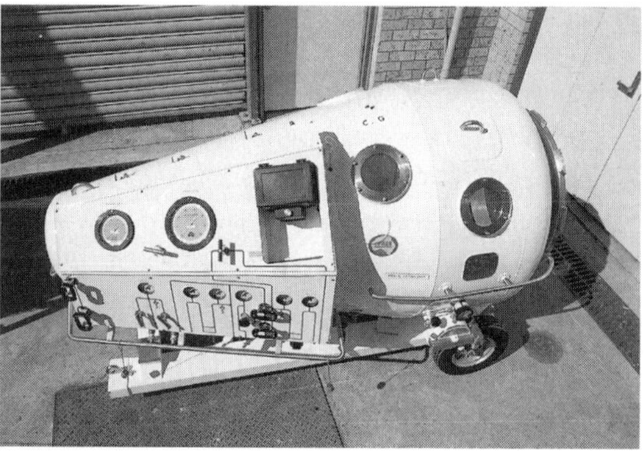

Figure 26.2 Portable recompression chamber.

Clinical presentation

DCI may affect all organ systems of the body. Most commonly divers present with constitutional symptoms which are believed to be secondary to activation of the inflammatory pathways. Patients complain of generalized malaise, fatigue, and headache. They often complain of profound tiredness despite a full night's sleep. Bubbles in and around a joint produce pain that can be severe and typically involves the knees, shoulders, elbows, and wrists. The pain is described as dull, throbbing, and gradual in onset, and is unaccompanied by effusion. The nervous system is almost always involved and cerebral involvement may present as difficulty in concentration or mentation, changes in personality, mild confusion, and impaired judgment to frank confusional states and loss of consciousness. Spinal cord involvement occurs frequently and presents with bladder, motor, and sensory disturbance. The presence of girdle pain should be taken seriously as it often progresses into serious spinal disease. Cutaneous involvement is often transient and varies from allergic type rashes, pruritus to purpura. Respiratory symptoms (breathlessness, increased respiratory rate, and chest pain) due to the overwhelming of the pulmonary bubble filter are uncommon, but indicate serious disease.

Management

The definitive treatment for a diver with DCI is recompression (Fig. 26.2), but not all patients will experience 100% resolution of their symptoms. Reported treatment failures vary from 32% to 54% (Drewry and Gorman 1992). Some evidence suggests that the earlier a patient is treated the better the prognosis. Early consultation with a specialist in diving medicine is encouraged.

Important history that should be obtained from the diver includes:

- depths/times of all recent dives
- the nature of the symptoms
- are the symptoms/signs stable, progressive, or resolving?
- were there any uncontrolled or multiple ascents during the dive?

A full examination including a detailed neurological evaluation with an assessment of mental state is essential and should be repeated as necessary to document any progression of the disease. The diagnosis of DCI is made on clinical findings and there are no specific laboratory investigations which will aid this decision process and which may in fact delay the time to definitive recompression. Specifically, a chest radiograph should not delay recompression if pulmonary barotrauma and CAGE is suspected.

First aid management includes the administration of 100% oxygen and intravenous fluids, and keeping the patient supine. In recent years divers were positioned in the head-down position in an attempt to prevent further embolization of the cerebral vasculature (bubbles distribute with buoyancy in large vessels), but this resulted in increasing cerebral oedema and is no longer recommended. A compromise is reached with lying the patient flat. Under no circumstances should a patient suspected of having a CAGE be allowed to stand. Fluid replacement using crystalloid (1 L immediately followed by 1 L over 4 hours, titrating to urinary output and haemodynamic status) is recommended, avoiding glucose solutions as they may contribute to cerebral oedema. Although pulmonary oxygen toxicity is possible with prolonged use of 100% oxygen, it is usual to apply it continuously unless advised differently by the consulting hyperbaric physician. A Hudson mask cannot deliver 100% oxygen and it is more appropriate to use a circuit made up of an anaesthetic mask, rebreather bag, and high-flow oxygen (Fig. 26.3). Alternatively a closed circuit rebreather system will conserve oxygen.

If aerial transfer to a recompression facility is required, consultation with the receiving unit is vital. Any ascent to altitude will result in an expansion of bubbles in both the tissue and the circulation, and may result in a further deterioration in their clinical state. Aerial transfer can be achieved safely in an aircraft capable of pressurizing the cabin to 1 ATA, or with rotary wing aircraft flying at an altitude <300 m. Similarly, if the patient is intubated the air in the endotracheal tube cuff will also expand with altitude and contract with recompression. For this reason it is advised that ventilated patients requiring recompression should have the air in the tube cuff replaced with water.

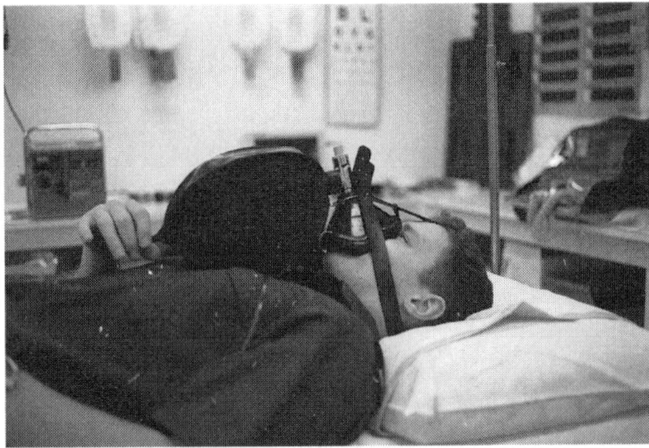

Figure 26.3 One method of delivering 100% oxygen. Requires a tight-fitting mask, rebreather bag, and oxygen flow rate of 12–15 L/min.

Key point

- The definitive treatment for a diver with DCI is recompression.

References

Drewry A, Gorman D (1992) A preliminary report on a prospective randomized, double-blind, controlled study of oxygen–helium in the treatment of air-diving. *SPUMS Journal* 22(3): 139–143.

Edmonds C (1998) Drowning syndromes: The mechanism. *SPUMS Journal* 28(1): 2–9.

Edmonds C, Lowry C, Pennefather J (1992) *Diving and subaquatic medicine*, 3rd edn. Butterworth-Heinemann, Oxford.

Golden F, St C, Tipton MJ, Scott R (1997) Immersion, near-drowning and drowning. *British Journal of Anaesthesia* 79: 214–225.

Gorman D (1993) *Diving and hyperbaric medicine*, 2nd edn. Course notes from the Royal New Zealand Navy and Royal Adelaide Hospital, p 10.1.

Gorman DF, Browning DM, Parsons DW, Traugott FM (1987) The distribution of arterial gas emboli in the pial circulation. *SPUMS Journal* 17(3): 101–116.

HTNA (1998) Hyperbaric Technicians and Nurses Association. Annual Report. HTNA, Sydney.

Langton P (1996) Patent foramen ovale in underwater medicine. *SPUMS Journal* 26(3): 186–191.

Lavelle JM, Shaw KN (1993) Near drowning: Is emergency department cardiopulmonary resuscitation or intensive care unit cerebral resuscitation indicated? *Critical Care Medicine* 21(3): 368–373.

Mitchell S, Gorman D (1994) Near drowning. *General Practitioner* 2(3): 8–9.

Modell JH (1993) Drowning. *New England Journal of Medicine* 328(4): 253–256.

Pearn J (1985) Pathophysiology of drowning. *Medical Journal of Australia* 142: 586–588.

Reed WJ (1998) Near drowning. *Physician and Sportsmedicine* 26(7): 31–36.

RLSSA (1997) *The national drowning report*. Edition 1. Royal Life Saving Society Australia, Sydney.

Thanel F (1998) Near drowning. *Postgraduate Medicine* 103(6): 141–153.

Waugh WH (1993) Potential use of warm butyl alcohol vapor as adjunct agent in the emergency treatment of sea water wet near-drowning. *American Journal of Emergency Medicine* 11(1): 20–27.

Weinstein MD, Krieger BP (1996) Near drowning: epidemiology, pathophysiology, and initial treatment. *Journal of Emergency Medicine* 14(4): 461–467.

Windsor D (1996) A study into the number of dives conducted on the Great Barrier Reef in 1994. *SPUMS Journal* 26(2): 72–74.

27

CHAPTER 27

Bites, stings, and venomous animals

JULIAN WHITE AND EUGENE SHERRY

CHAPTER 27

Bites, stings, and venomous animals

JULIAN WHITE AND EUGENE SHERRY

Bites and stings from animals, venomous and non-venomous, cause an unknown number of injuries per year, but statistics from a few key groups of venomous animals indicate that there are millions of cases annually, with at least 125 000 deaths worldwide. In most cases of venomous animal injury the primary problem is direct toxic effects of venom, but there may also be significant local tissue injury, and non-venomous animals will principally cause direct trauma. Because of the global magnitude of human injury, morbidity, and mortality from venomous animal bites and stings, this area will be dealt with in some detail, even though it encompasses more than just primary physical trauma.

Key point

- Bites and stings from animals, venomous and non-venomous, cause millions of injuries annually.

Venomous animals

Venomous animals are found in most groups or classes of the animal kingdom and in most habitats, terrestrial and marine, reflecting the selective advantage venom may bestow both in acquiring prey and in deterring predators. In this chapter, the types of animals, the types of venoms, clinical effects, and general comments on management will be covered. This is followed by a more detailed look at individual types of animals and their effects on humans.

Overview of venomous animals

Of the approximately 26 phyla of animals, at least 6 contain species that use venom or internal poison, as either pure defence, or for both offence and defence (Fig. 27.1). A few groups, however, account for the vast majority of cases of human envenoming or poisoning by animals:

- *venomous snakes:* >125 000 deaths/year
- *scorpions:* approximately 5 000 deaths/year
- *stinging insects:* hundreds of deaths/year due to anaphylactic reactions to venom
- *puffer fish:* several hundred deaths/year
- *jellyfish:* possibly scores of deaths/year
- *spiders:* perhaps 10–50 deaths/year
- *stinging fish:* perhaps 1–10 deaths/year
- *venomous molluscs:* perhaps 1–10 deaths/year.

Key point

- a few taxonomic groups account for the vast majority of cases of human envenoming or poisoning by animals

Taxonomy

A knowledge of the taxonomy of venomous animals is fundamental to the understanding of trauma from these animals; without a reliable way of identifying an animal, it will not be possible to accurately record cause and effect, which is essential in elucidating epidemiology, aetiology, pathophysiology, and clinical management. It is beyond the scope of this chapter to detail the taxonomy of all venomous animals, but a simplified scheme is outlined in Fig. 27.1.

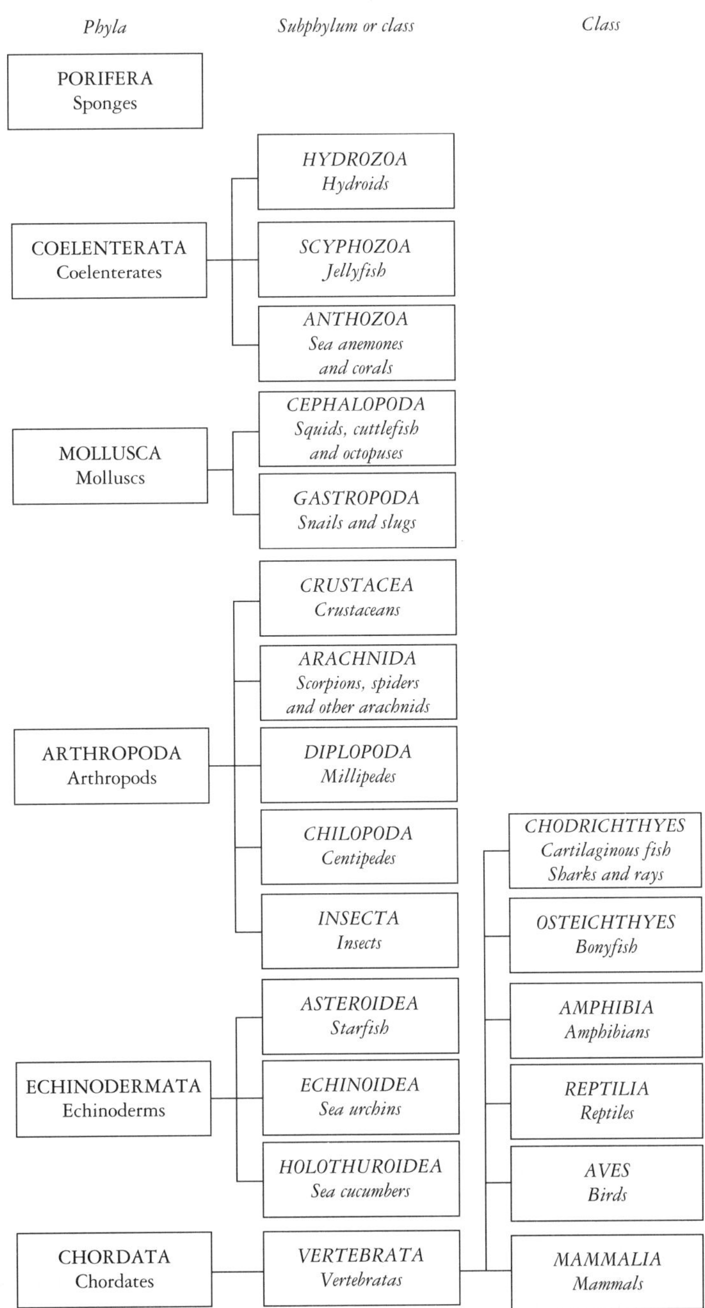

Figure 27.1 Some principal phyla containing venomous or poisonous animals, shown to class level.

Overview of venoms

Venoms are nearly always complex mixtures of varied biologically active substances (toxins) which may work independently or synergystically and each of which may have one or more quite distinct target sites and actions, resulting in a complex, multisystem disease process.

Venoms have evolved principally because they benefit the venomous animal, giving it some competitive advantage over related non-venomous species. In many species the venom has evolved from digestive juices, especially enzymes, the venom gland being a highly evolved digestive gland. It is not surprising, therefore, that many venomous animals use their venom principally to aid digestion, explaining many of the unpleasant effects on envenomed humans. At some point in evolution some venomous animals have evolved venom with rather different effects, designed

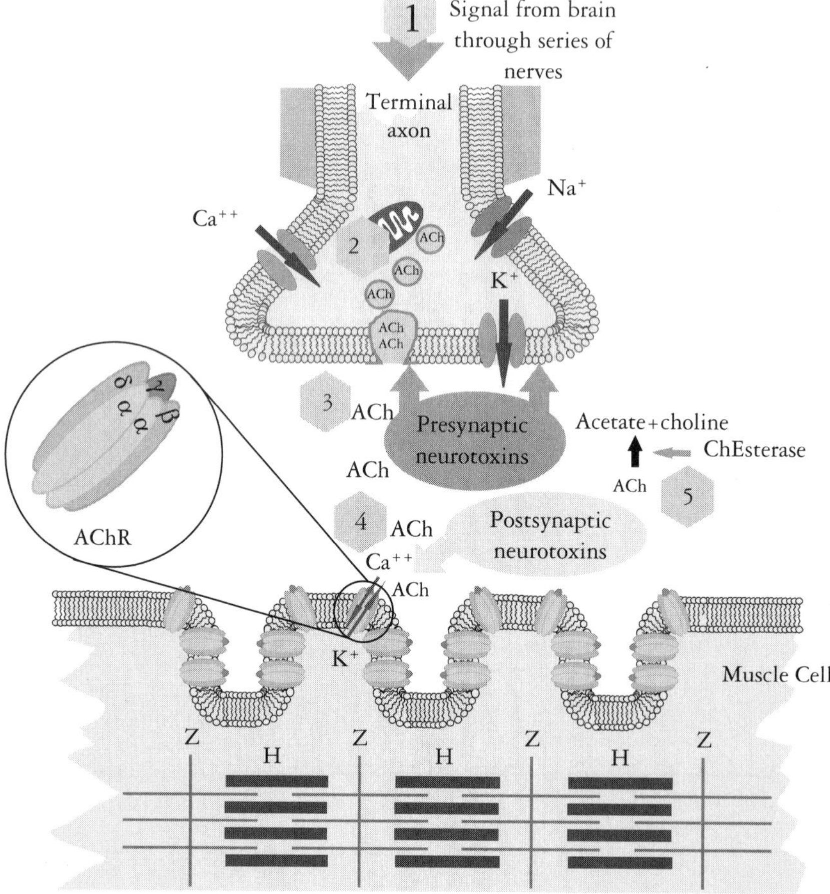

Figure 27.2 Mode of action of some principal types of paralysing neurotoxins active at the human neuromuscular junction: 1, Signal from brain arrives at nerve cell ending (terminal axon) through a series of nerves; 2, The neurotransmitter acetylcholine (ACh) is released from the terminal axon; 3, The ACh leaves the terminal axon and crosses the gap (synapse) to the muscle cell wall; 4, The ACh binds to receptors (AchR) on the muscle cell wall, causing changes in the cell that result is muscle contraction; 5, The ACh is released from the receptor and broken down by cholinesterase (ChEsterase). Illustration copyright Dr. Julian White.

to assist acquiring prey or as a defence against predators. Classic examples of this are the phospholipase A_2 (PLA_2) toxins that are so prominent in snake venoms and have evolved into potent toxins such as neurotoxins, myotoxins, procoagulants, anticoagulants, platelet-active toxins, and necrotoxins.

There are many methods of classifying venom components and types of toxins. The method used here is based on clinical effect. A single toxin may be active within several categories. The classification of clinical effects is as follows:

- neurotoxins
  - paralysing neurotoxins (Fig. 27.2)
  - presynaptic neuromuscular junction neurotoxins
  - postsynaptic neuromuscular junction neurotoxins
  - presynaptic and postsynaptic synergistic neuromuscular junction neurotoxins
  - sodium channel neurotoxins
  - potassium channel neurotoxins
  - excitatory neurotoxins
  - autonomic neurotoxins.
- myotoxins
- cardiotoxins
- coagulopathic toxins (Table 27.1 and Fig. 27.3)
- procoagulants
- anticoagulants (see Table 27.1)
- fibrinolytic agents
- platelet active agents
- haemorrhagins
- plasma serine protease inhibitors (SERPIN) inactivators
- nephrotoxins
- necrotoxins
- other venom components.

Table 27.1 Broad classification of types of action of snake coagulopathic and haemorrhagic toxins

	Specific activity
Procoagulants	Factor V activating Factor X activating Factor IX activating Prothrombin activating Fibrinogen clotting
Anticoagulant	Protein C activating Factor IX/X activating protein Thrombin inhibitor PLA2
Fibrinolytic	Fibrin(ogen) degradation Plasminogen activation
Vessel wall interactive	Haemorrhagins
Platelet activity	Platelet aggregation inducers Platelet aggregation inhibitors
Plasma protein activators	SERPIN inhibitors

Key point

- There are many methods of classifying venom components and types of toxins. The method used here is based on clinical effect.

Pharmacodynamics of envenoming

The way venoms are introduced by a bite or sting, the depth of injection, quantity involved, the size and action of venom components, size, age, pre-existing disease, and post-envenoming activity of the victim will all influence the rate of absorption,

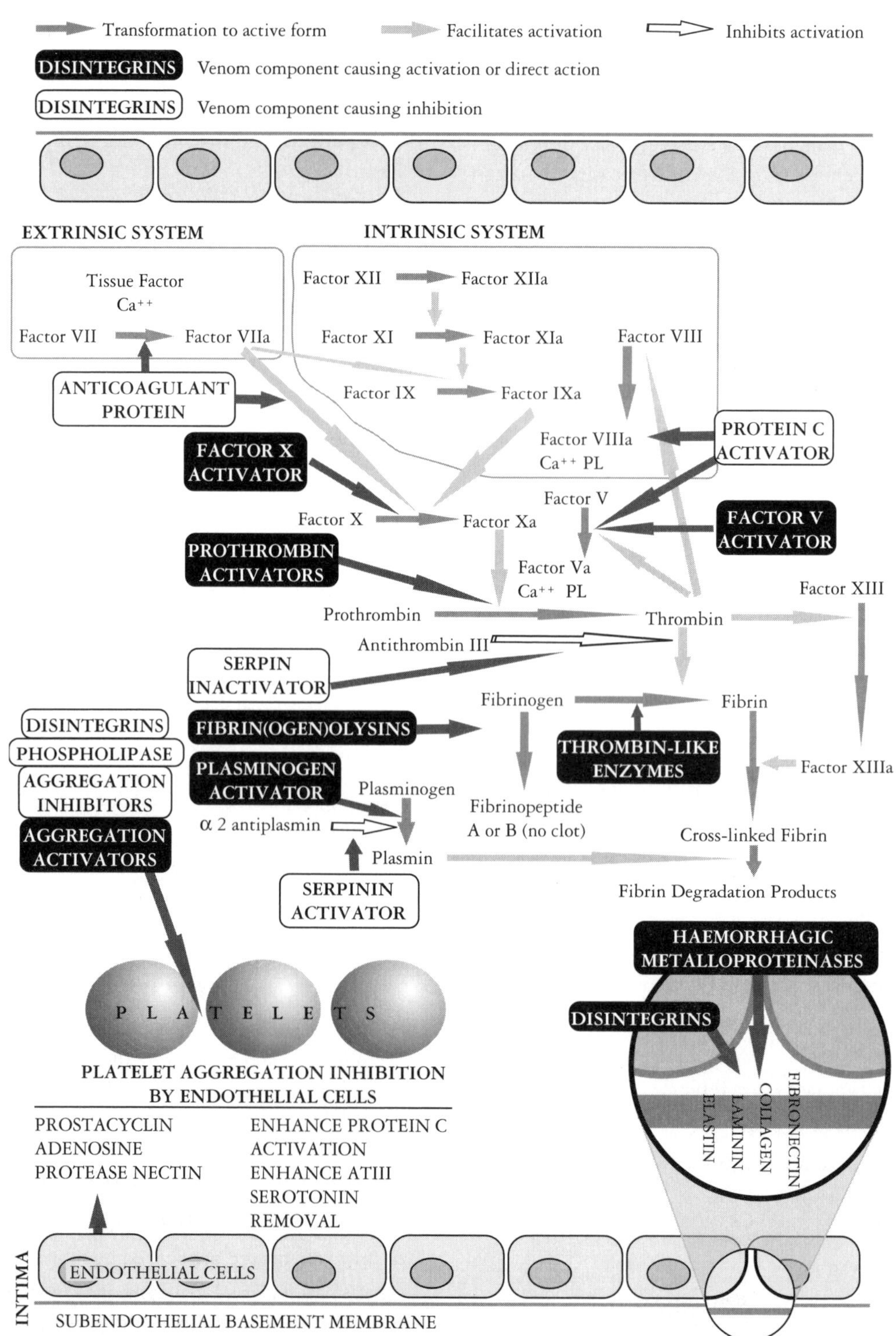

Figure 27.3 Sites of action of some principal snake coagulopathic and haemorrhagic toxins. Illustration copyright Dr. Julian White.

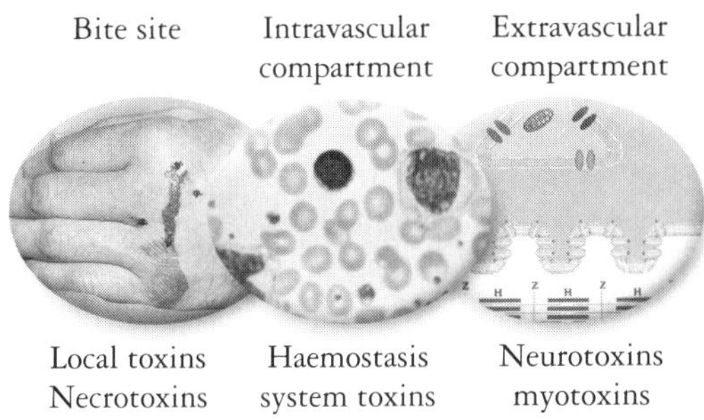

Figure 27.4 Distribution and sites of action of venom. Illustration copyright Dr. Julian White.

clinical effectiveness, and elimination of venom. With a range of quite different venom components all working at once, in different ways, understanding the pharmacodynamics of envenoming can be difficult. In general terms, however, the speed of onset of action of a particular component will be determined by its size and target tissue location. Thus necrotoxins and other locally active toxins may commence clinical effects almost immediately after the bite or sting, as they are already at their target site, while systemically active toxins must first reach the bloodstream (Fig. 27.4). Toxins active within the bloodstream will exert their effect rapidly, but toxins with extravascular targets, such as neurotoxins and myotoxins, will generally have a more delayed onset. The rapidity of effect will also be influenced by any latency period between time of binding to the target tissue and onset of detectable action. As an example, presynaptic neurotoxins may have a latency period of 60 minutes, whereas postsynaptic neurotoxins may have almost no latency period; these differences are reflected in the speed of onset of neurotoxic symptoms and signs. However, in real clinical circumstances, assessment is rarely so simple, for a single venom will contain a diverse array of toxins.

Key point

- In real clinical circumstances a single venom will contain a diverse array of toxins.

Clinical effects of venoms

With such a wide array of venomous animals and venom components, the range of clinical effects might be considered immense. However, a few major themes of venom action dominate, so that there are just a few major classes of clinical effect, with classic symptoms, signs, and laboratory findings. It must be remembered that venomous animals are not evolutionarily frozen; their venoms may still be evolving, so that effects may also evolve and change. This is clearly true for venomous snakes. Both the nature of venom components and the snakes' abundance, geographical range, and even diet are the subject of rapid change. It follows that whatever may presently be stated as the effects, range, habits, etc. for a given species of venomous animal must be continuously re-interpreted as the animals change, and the unexpected should always be looked for.

Key point

- There are just a few major classes of clinical effect, with classic symptoms, signs, and laboratory findings.

Neurotoxic paralysis

Neurotoxic paralysis is usually a result of neuromuscular junction pre- or postsynaptic neurotoxins which act systemically rather than locally, affecting voluntary and respiratory muscle. It is a classic effect of many snake venoms, but is also seen with envenoming by other animals such as paralysis ticks and a few marine animals, notably cone shells and blue ringed octopuses. Clinically symptoms involve progressive flaccid paralysis, often first seen in the cranial nerves, where it is easily missed if not sought by careful examination. Ptosis, partial then complete ophthalmoplegia, loss of facial tone, dysarthria and dysphagia are all common early signs of paralysis (Figs 27.5 and 27.6). The pupils may become dilated and unresponsive to light. Progressive weakness of limbs and bulbar function may follow, the latter often mandating intubation and ventilation to

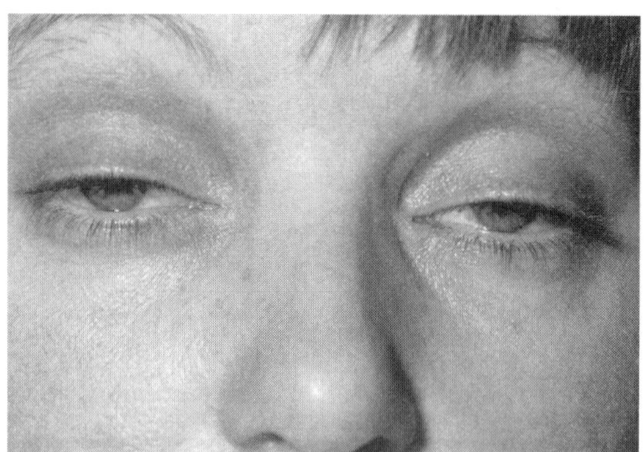

Figure 27.5 Early flaccid neurotoxic paralysis manifest as mild ptosis. Photo copyright Dr. Julian White.

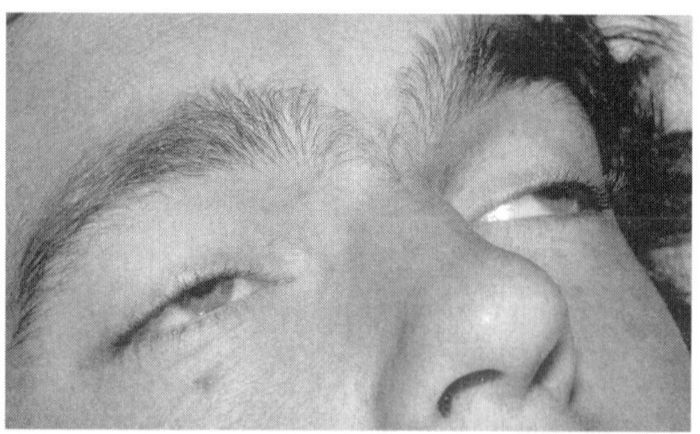

Figure 27.6 Early flaccid neurotoxic paralysis manifest as mild ptosis and partial ophthalmoplegia (divergent squint on lateral gaze due to selective sixth nerve paresis; Australian death adder bite). Photo copyright Dr. Julian White.

protect the airway. Accessory muscles of respiration may become prominent and the patient more agitated or drowsy as hypoxia develops. The diaphragm is often the last muscle to be paralysed and may not be fully affected for up to 24 hours after a neurotoxic snakebite. If the neurotoxin is extracellular, such as snake postsynaptic neurotoxins, tetrodotoxin, or conotoxins, then the paralytic effect may last only a few hours or may be reversible with treatment, such as antivenom or anticholinesterase, but presynaptic paralysis usually involves damage to the terminal axon, so reversal must await regeneration, which may take days, weeks, or months.

Exicitatory neurotoxin effects

Excitatory neurotoxins, as found in some arachnid (spider) and related arthropod (scorpion) venoms, usually cause very rapid onset of clinical effects, with potentially catastrophic effects possible within 10–30 minutes of a sting or bite. So rapidly are these toxins absorbed, transported, and bound to target tissues, that antivenom therapy is frequently administered too late to have optimal effect. The clinical effect will vary with species, but commonly includes local pain, rapid onset of anxiety, hypertension, tachycardia, and in some species, dyspnoea and pulmonary oedema (e.g. Australian funnel web spiders) or cardiac arrhythmias (e.g. some scorpions) or muscle fasciculation (some scorpions, spiders). There is often evidence of autonomic excitation, such as piloerection, priapism (banana spider), sweating, lachrymation, or hypersalivation, in addition to the cardiovascular manifestations.

Cardiotoxin effects

In many cases, cardiovascular effects are secondary to other venom actions, but direct cardiovascular effects, such as hyper- or hypotension, brady- or tachycardia, and cardiac arrhythmias can occur, particularly in scorpion venoms and a few jellyfish venoms (e.g. box jellyfish), as well as a few snake venoms (e.g. gaboon viper).

Myotoxin effects

Local myotoxins will cause local tissue damage, resulting in local effects such as pain and swelling and secondary effects such as compartment syndrome and hypovolaemic shock. Systemic myotoxins, such as those in some snake venoms, will cause progressive myolysis of skeletal muscle, resulting in muscle pain, tenderness, and weakness that may mimic paralysis, and secondary effects, notably myoglobinaemia, myoglobinuria (with potential secondary renal failure), hyperkalaemia (with potential secondary cardiac arrhythmia) and rise in serum enzymes, especially creatine kinase (CK), which may reach extraordinary levels. Myoglobinuria

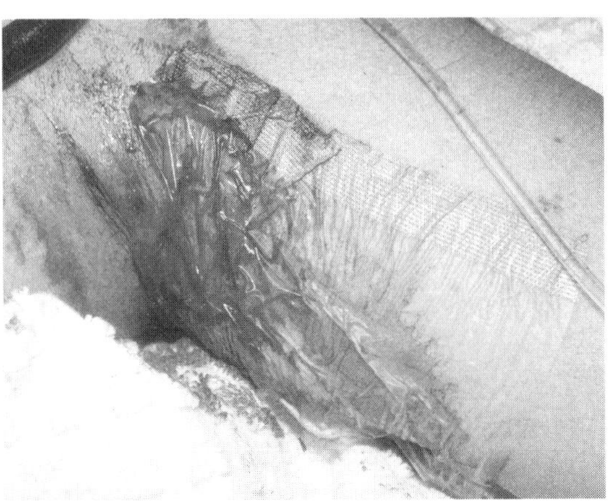

Figure 27.7 Persistent bleeding from a snake bite site, indicative of venom-induced coagulopathy (Australian inland taipan snake). Photo copyright Dr. Julian White.

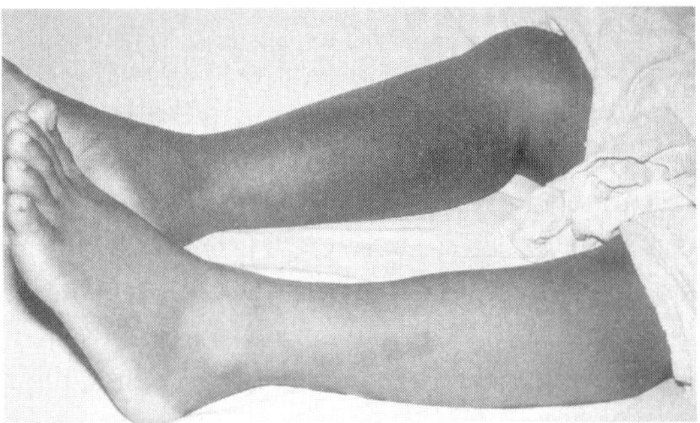

Figure 27.8 Severe bruising around a snake bite site secondary to venom induced coagulopathy and venom haemorrhagins (Thai green pit viper). Photo copyright Dr. Julian White.

gives the classic red to black urine that is positive to a dipstick test for blood.

Haemostasis effects

The wide variety of haemostatically active venom components, particularly present in many snake venoms, may give rise to a variety of clinical disorders of haemostasis, distinguishable by detailed coagulation and platelet function studies. However, just three basic syndromes are generally evident:

- incoagulable blood with bleeding tendency
- poorly coagulable or incoagulable blood without clinically apparent bleeding tendency
- thrombotic tendency.

The last of these is unusual, but is clearly present in envenoming by a few Central American vipers, where deep venous thrombosis (DVT) is a common sequela of envenoming. Those with bleeding tendency may exhibit no clinical signs other than persistent bleeding from the bite site (Fig. 27.7), but more commonly there is also bleeding from the

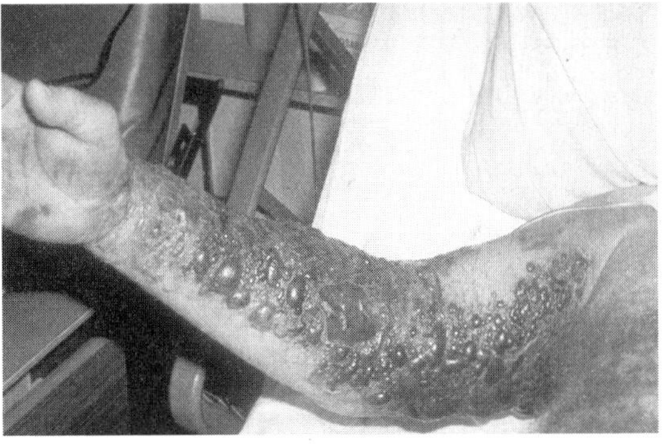

Figure 27.9 Severe local swelling. blistering, haemorrhage and developing necrosis after snakebite (North American rattlesnake bite). Photo copyright Dr. David Harvey.

gums, and gastrointestinal bleeding (manifest as haematemesis or malaena) and haematuria may also occur. Bleeding into a major organ or space (e.g. intracranial) will produce classic signs, but more localized bleeding, such as into the pituitary (Sheehan's syndrome following Burmese Russell's viper bite) may produce more subtle or delayed signs. Any artificial breach of vascular integrity, such as insertion of a cannula, may result in prolonged and significant bleeding. This has obvious management implications.

Haemorrhagin effects

The effects of haemorrhagins are similar to the more severe effect of haemostatically active toxins, in that they will produce clinically apparent bleeding. As the two groups of toxins are usually present together and are synergistic, bleeding can be major. There may be marked bleeding in the bitten area (Figs 27.8 and 27.9), as other venom components assist tissue breakdown and allow extravasation of blood from vessels damaged by haemorrhagins.

Nephrotoxin effects

Nephrotoxins, primary or secondary, will exert their effect somewhat silently at first, the first indication of problems often being a rapidly falling urine output, accompanied by rising creatinine and urea. In a case of envenoming where renal failure is possible, such as many snakebites, it is therefore advisable to carefully monitor fluid input and output and give an initial intravenous fluid load.

Other systemic effects

A variety of specific systemic effects may be induced by envenoming by certain species. Of particular note is haemolysis, seen with some snakebites and with severe envenoming by some spiders. Liver damage may also occur after bites or stings by many animals, but is rarely of major significance. Pancreatitis can be induced by some scorpion stings.

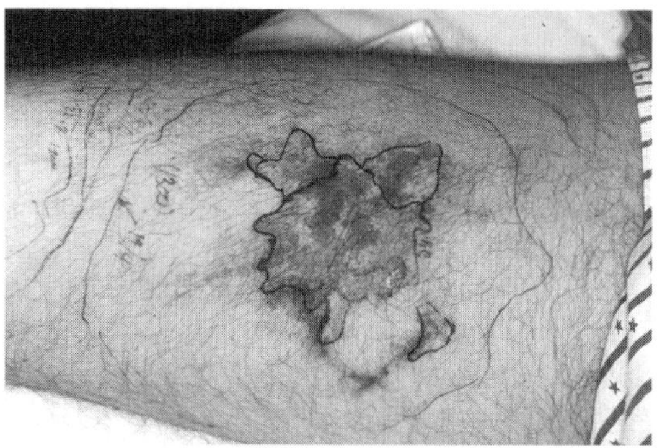

Figure 27.10 Local swelling, erythema, ecchymosis, and developing central necrosis following a recluse spider bite. Photo copyright Dr. Julian White.

Necrotoxin effects

The effects of necrotoxins may be rapidly evident, as is seen with some snakebites (e.g. many vipers, pit vipers, some cobras), as progressive swelling, blistering, ecchymosis, and darkening of skin, or liquefaction of skin (Fig. 27.9). Over 24–48 hours this may progress to clear skin necrosis, resulting in deep ulceration, sometimes involving muscle and other deeper tissues. Pain is present in most cases. Spider necrotoxins may cause more insidious effects, particularly those of recluse spiders. The bite may go unnoticed, frequently occurring at night while the victim is asleep. This is followed by local redness, sometimes but not always associated with local pain. Blisters may form after 12–48 hours, or areas of ecchymosis (Fig. 27.10), becoming darker and more clearly necrotic over the next 1–7 days, eventually developing a full-thickness skin ulcer or ulcers, which may occupy an area far greater than the original bite region. Jellyfish necrotoxins, such as those in box jellyfish venom, are associated with major envenoming. The sting is intensely painful, with wheal formation, with necrosis taking several days to become evident.

Other local effects

The local effects of envenoming, dependent on both species and dose, may include pain, swelling, blistering, ecchymosis, necrosis, persistent bleeding, blanching, wheal formation, or almost no visible effect at all, even in the presence of life-threatening systemic envenoming. Some elapid snakes and a variety of other animals can envenom sufficient to cause major systemic effects, yet leave little evidence locally, not even significant pain.

General systemic effects

The range of general systemic effects of envenoming is considerable and variable. Snakebite is often associated with headache, nausea, vomiting, and abdominal pain. Diarrhoea may also occur. Collapse and even convulsions may occur as early manifestations of major envenoming, especially in children.

First aid for envenoming

As a general rule immobilization of the bitten limb is a useful technique to reduce venom transport, as many venom components are of moderate to large molecular weight and lymphatic flow is important in their transport. The use of compression bandaging is more controversial, but is apparently beneficial for certain types of snake and spider bite and a few major marine toxins (cone shells, blue ringed octopus). Application of a cold pack to the wound area is a useful technique for many types of envenoming by marine invertebrates, especially jellyfish, and some terrestrial invertebrates, but is not applicable for envenoming by vertebrates (snakes, fish). For fish with venomous spines and for stingrays, immersion of the stung limb in hot water is effective in reducing local pain (be sure the water is not so hot that it may cause thermal injury).

There are some first aid methods which are known to be either of no value or potentially harmful and so should not be used. These include tourniquets, cutting and suction of the wound, application of chemicals such as Condy's crystals, use of cryotherapy, and electric shock to the bite site. All these methods are still used in various regions of the world, most commonly for snakebite, despite the evidence that they frequently cause harm without conferring benefit. Of these techniques, the use of medically supervised tourniquets has merit in certain circumstances, where the bite is from a lethal species and transport time to a hospital with appropriate antivenom is <30 minutes. The use of proprietary suction devices to remove venom is advocated by their manufacturers, but studies of efficacy do not inspire confidence in the technique, as even in optimal circumstances, at least 70% of the venom will be left in the victim. Cryotherapy has been clearly shown to be harmful. Electric shock for snakebite, though still promoted by manufacturers of these devices, has been shown to offer no benefit and its use may delay more appropriate first aid.

Key point

- Immobilization of the bitten limb is a useful technique.

Medical management of envenoming

Most doctors will see few cases of significant envenoming, so acquiring and maintaining skills in management is problematic. It is therefore advisable, when faced with a case of major envenoming, to seek expert advice at the earliest opportunity, either from a regional expert or from a regional poisons information centre, the staff of which may facilitate referral to an appropriate expert.

Diagnosis

Patients may present with a clear history of a bite or sting and either a good description of their assailant or the assailant itself. The latter may introduce further problems if it is still alive (such as an angry venomous snake!). In this situation, although the diagnosis may be clear, some expertise may be required to determine the true identity of the assailant, sometimes crucial in determining which type of antivenom to consider. Equally, the extent of envenoming may not be immediately apparent, and some major types of envenoming, such as paralysis, myolysis, coagulopathy, and renal damage may not be initially evident from examination, or require appropriate laboratory investigation.

Children may be unable to give a history of a bite or sting and may present with advanced envenoming, manifest as symptoms and signs that could point to a myriad of diagnoses. Beware the child with unexplained collapse and convulsions, which might be indicative of major envenoming by a snake, scorpion, or spider. Adults may also be unaware of being bitten, as some bites (e.g. by certain snakes, blue ringed octopuses, ticks) may be painless. They will later present with symptoms that might indicate a wide range of diagnoses and the lack of a noted bite may erroneously point the diagnostic process away from envenoming. Envenoming should be considered in otherwise unexplained collapse, convulsions, flaccid paralysis, autonomic stimulation, myolysis, coagulopathy, thrombosis (DVT), haemorrhage, renal failure, chest pain, abdominal pain, regional pain, muscle fasciculation, excessive sweating, nausea and vomiting, headache, local swelling, ecchymosis, blistering, ulceration, cardiac arrhythmias, and pulmonary oedema. This list covers only some of the more common effects of envenoming.

Key point

- Although the diagnosis may be clear, some expertise may be required to determine the true identity of the assailant.

History

The mix of the following points in history taking will be determined by the circumstances and the nature of the assailant.

- Precise date and time of the incident that might have involved a bite or sting.
- Geographic location at the time of the incident (to narrow down potential assailant fauna).
- A description of the assailant, if possible.
- A detailed description of how the bite or sting occurred, including how many bites or stings (multiple bites or stings are generally more severe), or the patient's activity at the time an unnoticed bite or sting might have occurred.
- What first aid, if any, was used, its timing after the bite or sting, and the patient's physical activity both before and after first aid applied (physical activity may decrease the effectiveness of first aid).
- A list of symptoms observed by the patient and their time of onset and cessation. Specifically ask for symptoms indicative of envenoming by likely assailant species.
- A list of any signs noted by those with the patient, including timing of onset and cessation.
- Relevant past medical history, including allergy, particularly to animals used to produce antivenom (e.g. horses, sheep, rabbits) and any medications used by the patient. Recent use of alcohol or recreational drugs that might affect symptoms or signs should also be queried.

Examination

It is easy to detect many signs of envenoming if looked for, but even easier to miss them if envenoming is not considered during examination. Envenoming frequently evolves over time, so repeated examination may be vital in detecting important signs. This is particularly true for systemic effects of envenoming (see Figs 27.5–10).

- The bite or sting site should be checked for evidence of bite or sting marks (is there a sting left behind, as in a honey bee sting), distance between bite marks (may indicate mouth size for snakebite), multiple bites or stings, local effects such as erythema, oedema, blistering, ecchymosis, necrosis, physical trauma (e.g. lacerations following sting ray injury).
- The regional lymph nodes should be checked for evidence of venom spread (swelling or tenderness).
- General systemic function should also be checked (blood pressure, pulse, respiration).
- Specific venom effects to look for are the following:
  - *Flaccid paralysis:* Ptosis, ophthalmoplegia (partial or complete), pupil dilation, loss of

facial tone, limited mouth opening or tongue extrusion, palatal paresis, drooling, limb weakness, gait disturbance, accessory respiratory muscle use, depressed or absent deep tendon reflexes, depressed or absent response to painful stimuli (note the patient still feels the pain, but cannot withdraw due to paralysis, so consideration for patient distress is important), cyanosis, signs of hypoxia, including confusion.

- *Excitatory neurotoxic effects:* Anxiety, restlessness, hyperreflexia, piloerection, increased sweating, salivation, lacchrymation, muscle fasciculation, confusion, hypoxia, pulmonary oedema, uncontrolled random limb movements (some scorpion stings).
- *Myotoxicity:* Muscle tenderness, pain on contraction against resistance, weakness (may mimic paralysis), muscle spasm, rarely compartment syndrome signs due to massive muscle swelling. ECG should be checked for evidence of hyperkalaemic effects.
- *Cardiotoxicity:* Cardiac arrhythmias, arrest, ECG abnormalities (various).
- *Coagulopathy and haemorrhagins:* Persistent ooze of blood from bite site, venepuncture sites, bleeding gums, bruising, occasionally signs consistent with a bleed into an internal organ or space (e.g. intracranial, etc.).
- *Nephrotoxicity:* Usually little to be found, but oliguria or anuria should be checked.

Key point

- It is easy to detect many signs of envenoming if they are looked for, but even easier to miss them if envenoming is not considered during examination.

Laboratory tests

Basic health facility

- *Urine output:* Haematuria or myoglobinuria should be checked (red or black urine; dipstick test positive for blood; simple microscopy for red cells).
- *Coagulopathy:* 20 minute whole blood clotting test (poor or absent clot indicates coagulopathy; requires only needle, syringe, and glass tube or container).
- *Venom detection (Australia only):* Simple commercial ELISA-based test for Australian snake venoms. The best sample is the bite site. If there is systemic envenoming, then urine could be tested, but blood is unreliable as a sample. A positive result indicates both that a snakebite has occurred and the most appropriate antivenom, but is not an indication to give antivenom, as venom can be present on the skin without significant systemic envenoming. A negative result does not exclude snakebite, so is of little diagnostic help.

Fully resourced hospital

- *Urine output:* Haematuria or myoglobinuria should be checked (red or black urine; dipstick test positive for blood; simple microscopy for red cells).
- *Blood tests:*
  - extended coagulation studies—(prothrombin time/International Normalized Ratio (standard of care for the management of anticoagulation [INR]); activated partial thromboplastin time (aPTT); fibrinogen level; fibrin(ogen) degradation products)
  - complete blood picture—raised white cell count suggestive of envenoming or infection; absolute lymphopenia suggestive of certain types of snake envenoming; haemoglobin level (evidence of haemolysis should be checked for); thrombocytopenia may indicate direct or indirect effect of some snake venoms or secondary disseminated intravascular coagulopathy (DIC)

- electrolytes and renal function—hyperkalaemia should be investigated if there is myolysis or renal failure
- CK—elevated, sometimes to extreme levels, in presence of myolysis
- liver function tests—enzyme levels may be elevated if there is myolysis.

◆ *Arterial blood gases:* Relevant only if advanced respiratory failure due to neurotoxic paralysis or pulmonary oedema.

◆ *Venom detection (Australia only):* As for basic health facility, above.

Critical care

The major requirement for intensive care is respiratory support for cases with advanced neurotoxic flaccid paralysis or severe pulmonary oedema. Respiratory support, including intubation and ventilation, may be needed only for a few hours, but for envenoming by some snake species, may be required for days, weeks, or months, until the neuromuscular junction regenerates. Tracheostomy should be avoided until there is complete resolution of any coagulopathy or haemorrhagic tendency (some snakebite cases); all invasive procedures with the potential to cause bleeding should be avoided for similar reasons.

In cases of cardiac arrest or severe dysfunction following envenoming by cardiotoxic species, notably the Australian box jellyfish, prolonged cardiac support may be required.

Key point

◆ The major requirement for intensive care is respiratory support.

Antivenoms

Antivenoms are the treatment of choice, where available, for most forms of major envenoming, particularly systemic envenoming. Old aphorisms suggesting that antivenom is more dangerous than envenoming are generally ill-founded and inappropriate. Nevertheless, antivenom therapy carries certain risks and should only be used when clearly indicated. However, for many venomous animals and in many less developed regions, antivenom is either unavailable or economically impractical.

Antivenoms are specific antidotes to venoms. Virtually all are whole or fractionated animal immunoglobulins raised against a target whole venom, not specific venom components. Antivenoms are polyclonal and may contain far more neutralizing activity against some venom components than others. To produce antivenoms, a source of venom for immunizing must be determined. The choice of venoms may strongly influence the clinical efficacy of an antivenom; if only a narrow range of species or species from a small part of a geographic range is used, then the antivenom may lack efficacy against bites from a wider range of species or against bites from the target species from other parts of its geographic range. The three major types of antivenom, based on the degree of fractionation, are whole IgG, $F(ab)^2$, and Fab (Fig. 27.11). Their individual characteristics are listed in Table 27.2.

Principles of antivenom therapy

The first principle of antivenom therapy is to tailor the dose to the individual situation. From this it follows that just as the degree of envenoming varies from nil ('dry bite') to severe systemic, so the amount of antivenom required will vary from none to potentially large quantities. The quantity required is therefore determined by the assailant venomous animal and not by the size of the patient. There are no paediatric doses of antivenom; children require the same amount as adults. Determining how much antivenom to administer requires considerable clinical judgement. For some regions there are guidelines covering common species of venomous animal, notably snakes. Consultation with regional, national, or international experts is advised if the dose required is unclear. Most failures of antivenom therapy in the

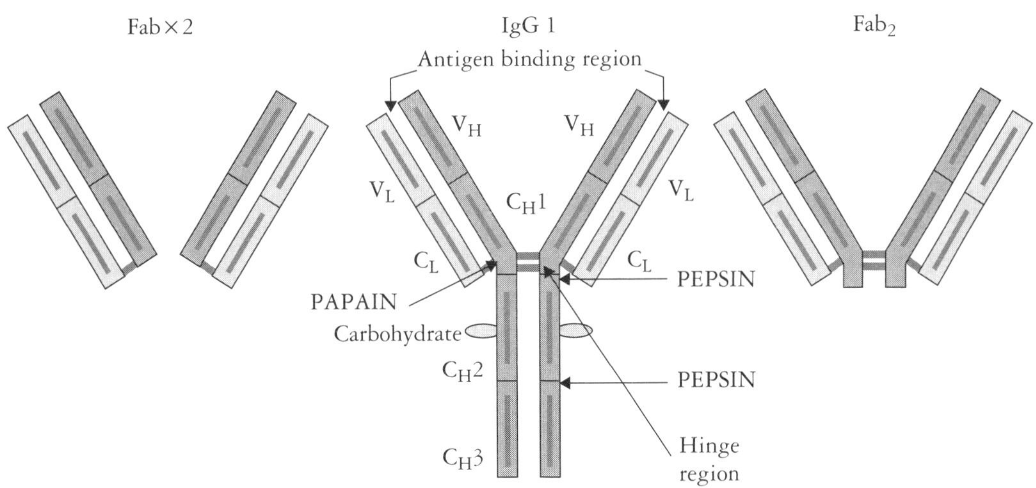

Figure 27.11 Basic types of antivenom. Illustration copyright Dr. Julian White.

Table 27.2 Characteristics of the major types of antivenom

Type of antivenom	Approximate molecular weight	Approximate half-life and distribution	Potential for adverse reactions
Horse IgG Unrefined	150 000+contaminants	24 h+ Intravascular	High
Horse IgG Refined	150 000	24 h+ Intravascular	Moderate to high
Horse F(ab)^2	90 000	24 h+ Mostly intravascular	Low to moderate
Horse Fab	45 000	<24 h Intra- and extravascular	Low to moderate
Horse F(ab)^2 Affinity purified	90 000	24 h+ Mostly intravascular	Minimal to low
Horse Fab Affinity purified	45 000	<24 h Intra- and extravascular	Minimal to low
Sheep IgG	150 000	24 h+ Intravascular	Low
Sheep F(ab)^2	90 000	24 h+ Mostly intravascular	Low
Sheep Fab	45 000	<24 h Intra- and extravascular	Very low to low
Rabbit IgG	150 000	24 h+	Very low to low
Dog IgG	150 000	24 h+	Moderate
Goat IgG	150 000	24 h+	Moderate

past can be attributed to inadequate dosage, or wrong choice of antivenom.

The second principle of antivenom therapy is to give as soon as possible, once it is indicated. From this it follows that in most situations of acute envenoming, the intravenous route is preferred, but there are exceptions, which will be noted for particular animals as they apply.

The third principle is to monitor carefully for the effect of antivenom therapy. This includes monitoring both effectiveness in counteracting envenoming and observing for adverse effects of therapy. It is frequently the case that an initial dose of antivenom may be insufficient and follow-up doses may be required. Some venom may be sequestrated at the bite site, being released over a period of hours or days, necessitating ongoing antivenom therapy.

Key point

- Tailor the dose of antivenom to the individual situation.
- Give as soon as possible.
- Monitor carefully.

Complications of antivenom therapy

The principle complications of antivenom therapy are:

- acute adverse reactions:
  - anaphylaxis and related early reactions
  - rash
  - febrile reactions (usually related to toxin contamination).
- delayed adverse reactions:
  - serum sickness.
- failure of efficacy:
  - incorrect antivenom
  - inadequate dose
  - inappropriate route of administration (intramuscuar or local when intravenous was required)
  - therapy commenced too late
  - out-of-date or poorly stored antivenom (i.e. refrigerated product that has been exposed to prolonged heat)
  - poor quality antivenom.

Several methods have been employed to minimize the chance of adverse effects from antivenom therapy.

- *Skin sensitivity testing before administration:* This method is flawed in both theory and practice. Such sensitivity testing will delay treatment, fail to reliably predict major adverse reactions (e.g. anaphylaxis), potentially sensitize the patient to antivenom should it be required in the future, and may precipitate an anaphylactic reaction. For these reasons skin sensitivity testing is not recommended, even though it is advised by a number of antivenom producers and is routinely used in some countries (e.g. the USA).
- *Premedication before antivenom therapy:* This is controversial and is not widely accepted or used. Antihistamines and steroids have been shown to have no real benefit in preventing acute antivenom reactions. In addition, antihistamines may induce drowsiness or occasionally, hyperexcitability, both potentially dangerous in major envenoming. Adrenaline (epinephrine) has been shown to reduce the likelihood of adverse reactions for certain high-risk antivenoms (those that are poorly refined, with a high rate of adverse reactions) in a single trial, but its benefit for other antivenoms is uncertain and it carries clear risks that may outweigh any potential benefits. This is particularly true if the envenoming causes increased bleeding, as seen with many snakebites. Premedication is not currently recommended by antivenom producers.

Future studies may better define its role, if any.

- *Use of diluted antivenom infusions:* Most antivenoms should be given intravenously. Many experts recommend dilution of the antivenom up to 1 : 10 in a suitable diluent for intravenous use, such as normal saline or Hartman's solution. The degree of dilution will be limited by the volume of antivenom and the size of the patient. Although this technique may be useful, it is not strictly necessary, as studies have shown that intravenous-push neat antivenom does not carry a higher incidence of acute adverse effects. In addition, the latter technique requires the doctor to stay with the patient throughout the antivenom infusion, which increases the chances of rapidly and effectively responding to acute adverse events.

Antivenom should always be given in the expectation that anaphylaxis may occur, even though this complication is rare with good quality antivenoms. Thus adrenaline (epinephrine) should always be ready in a syringe or set up as an infusion before antivenom therapy is commenced, and both staff and equipment for resuscitation should be on hand.

Non-antivenom treatments

Although antivenom is often the preferred treatment of significant envenoming, it is not available for all animals, nor in all areas of the world. Non-antivenom treatments may be effective as adjuncts to antivenom or as alternatives in some situations.

Pharmaceutical

Apart from the standard range of pharmaceuticals used in a wide array of diseases, a few agents have specific roles in certain forms of envenoming:

- *Anticholinesterases:* Useful for flaccid neurotoxic paralysis due to postsynaptic snake neurotoxins. They may be used as an adjunct to antivenom or as sole therapy where antivenom is unavailable. A tensilon test should performed first to determine efficacy.
- *Dapsone:* Potentially useful for reducing necrosis in known recluse spider bites, if used early, but toxic and controversial.
- *Fresh frozen plasma:* Of value in replacing depleted clotting factors after snakebite coagulopathy, but potentially hazardous if given before neutralization of all circulating antivenom.

Surgical

Surgical intervention is rarely appropriate in acute envenoming, with the exception of injuries causing acute significant local trauma, such as some stingray injuries or where a portion of the biting or stinging apparatus remains in the wound and requires urgent removal. Some surgical manoeuvres are worthy of particular comment.

- *Fasciotomy:* This technique for releasing local tissue pressure is generally only warranted to relieve proven compartment syndrome.
- *Bite or sting site wound excision:* There is no substantial evidence to suggest that excising the area of immediate envenoming is likely to be a useful procedure and it may often result in short-and long-term complications. For necrotic arachnidism it is clear that early debridement of the necrotic region (within the first 4–5 weeks) may actually extend the area of necrosis.

Other

Hyperbaric oxygen therapy has been used for necrotic arachnidism, both to reduce the associated pain and to accelerate healing. There is limited clinical evidence in support and the therapy is controversial, but may be useful in at least some patients. Guidelines for use in envenoming are not yet established.

Key point

- Surgical intervention is rarely appropriate.

Complications of envenoming

Of the many potential complications of envenoming that may occur, a few particularly common or important varieties are discussed here, most pertaining to snakebite.

Paralysis

The three principle manoeuvres available to manage significant paralysis are:

- *intubation and ventilation*
- *antivenom:* only effective for postsynaptic type paralysis
- *anticholinesterases:* only effective for postsynaptic type paralysis.

Myolysis

Major myolysis is particularly a feature of snakebite by some species (see Table 27.3). Myolysis is most problematic when systemic. Even late administration of antivenom may sometimes speed resolution. Early and maintained good renal throughput, by ensuring adequate hydration, may reduce the chance of secondary renal damage. Hyperkalaemia is always a risk in these cases and should be actively sought and vigorously treated if present. At least in the early stages, over the first 1–10 days, when muscle breakdown is peaking, it is advisable to avoid procedures that might increase muscle damage, such as active physiotherapy.

Table 27.3 Major groups of venomous animals likely to cause systemic myolysis

Type of animal	Examples
Elapid snakes	Sea snakes *Selected Australian snakes:* tiger snakes, rough scaled snake, taipans, mulga snakes, Collett's snake
Viperid snakes	Some South American pit vipers (*Crotalus* spp., selected *Bothrops* spp.) Sri Lankan Russell's viper

Coagulopathy

Although coagulopathy can be a secondary result of cardiovascular collapse after envenoming by a wide range of animals, by far the most common cause is snakebite (see Table 27.4). Antivenom is the preferred treatment, giving enough to neutralise expected venom load. In general, replacement therapy (fresh frozen plasma, cryoprecipitate) is unnecessary. Great care is required in avoiding iatrogenic bleeding, through injudicious insertion of cannulas. Beware femoral punctures, subclavian and jugular line insertions, and arterial blood gas sampling. For established coagulopathy, where repeat venous sampling is required to titrate antivenom therapy against response, an indwelling line, such as a long line through the cubital vein, may be advantageous.

Necrosis

The single most important aspect of care for necrotic bite wounds is good wound care; keeping the wound clean and elevated, and avoiding early surgical debridement (for a recluse spider bite). Particularly with necrotic arachnidism, ulcers may be indolent and slow to heal, suggestive of vascular impairment. A number of unfortunate patients have had limb amputations for intractable bite ulcers whose impaired healing is falsely ascribed to peripheral vascular disease. Early debridement and grafting most often fails and should generally be avoided. Infection should be treated with antibiotics targeted to the causative organism, so culture and sensitivity testing should be routine.

Table 27.4 Major groups of venomous animals likely to cause primary coagulopathy

Type of animal	Examples	Type of venom action
Colubrid snakes	Boomslang, vine snake	Procoagulant
	Yamakagashi, red necked keelback	Procoagulant
Elapid snakes	Selected Australian snakes; tiger snakes, rough scaled snake, taipans, brown snakes, broad headed snakes	Procoagulant
	Selected Australian snakes; mulga snakes, Collett's snake, Papuan black snake	Anticoagulant
Viperid snakes	Saw scaled or carpet vipers	Procoagulant, disintegrins, haemorrhagins
	Gaboon vipers and puff adders	Procoagulant, antiplatelet, disintegrins, haemorrhagins
	Russell's vipers	Procoagulant, haemorrhagins
	Malayan pit viper	Procoagulant, antiplatelet, haemorrhagins
	North American rattlesnakes	Procoagulant, fibrinolytic, antiplatelet, disintegrins, haemorrhagins
	North American copperheads	Procoagulant, anticoagulant, fibrinolytic, disintegrins
	South American pit vipers (selected *Bothrops* spp.)	Procoagulant, anticoagulant, fibrinolytic, disintegrins, haemorrhagins
	Asian green pit vipers (selected *Trimeresurus* spp.)	Anticoagulant, fibrinolytic, antiplatelet, disintegrins, haemorrhagins
	Eurasian vipers (selected *Vipera* spp.)	Procoagulant, disintegrins, haemorrhagins

Infection

Infection is always possible after any penetrating injury, such as a bite or sting. Though uncommon, tetanus does occasionally occur in venomous bites and stings, so tetanus prophylaxis should be routine. In snakebite, however, injections should be avoided until any coagulopathy is resolved. In most cases, prophylactic antibiotics are unnecessary. If secondary infection occurs, the organism should be cultured if possible so that antibiotic therapy can be targeted. If this is impractical, a wide variety of possible organisms should be assumed and an appropriate antibiotic combination used to provide wide coverage.

Follow-up

Mild envenoming without complications may not warrant follow up, but major envenoming usually does. In particular, patients who have received antivenom should be informed of the symptoms of serum sickness, so that they will report for early assessment should this complication arise.

Further reading

Venomous animals

Bawaskar HS, Bawaskar PH (1994) Vasodilators; scorpion envenoming and the heart (an Indian experience). *Toxicon* 32(9): 1031–1040.

Covacevich J, Davie P, Pearn J (1987) *Toxic plants and animals: a guide for Australia*. Queensland Museum, Brisbane.

Dehesa-Davila M, Possani LD (1994) Scorpionism and serotherapy in Mexico. *Toxicon* 32(9): 1015–1018.

Edmonds C (1995) *Dangerous marine creatures*. 2nd edition Best Publishing Company, Flagstaff, Arizona, USA.

Freire-Maia L, Campos JA, Amaral CFS (1994) Approaches to the treatment of scorpion envenoming. *Toxicon* 32(9): 1009–1014.

Gopalakrishnakone P, Chou LM (ed.) (1990) *Snakes of medical importance (Asia Pacific region)*. National University of Singapore, Singapore.

Gueron M, Sofer S (1994) The role of the intensivist in the treatment of the cardiovascular manifestations of scorpion envenomation. *Toxicon* 32(9): 1027–1029.

Habermehl G (1981) *Venomous animals and their toxins*. Springer-Verlag, Berlin.

Harvey A (ed.) (1991) *Snake toxins*. Pergamon Press, Oxford.

Howarth MH, Southee AE, Whyte IM (1994) Lymphatic flow rates and first aid in simulated peripheral snake or spider envenomation. *Medical Journal of Australia* 161: 695–700.

Ismail M (1994) The treatment of the scorpion envenoming syndrome; the Saudi experience with serotherapy. *Toxicon* 32(9): 1019–1026.

Ismail M (1995) The scorpion envenoming syndrome. *Toxicon* 33(7): 825–858.

Junghanss T, Bodio M (1996) *Notfall-Handbuch Gifttiere*. Thieme Verlag, Stuttgart, Germany.

Kamiguti AS, Hay CRM, Theakston RDG, Zuzel M (1996) Insights into the mechanism of haemorrhage caused by snake venom metalloproteinases. *Toxicon* 34(6): 627–642.

Kochva E, Bdolah A, Wollberg Z (1993) Sarafotoxins and endothelins; evolution, structure and function. *Toxicon* 31(5): 541–568.

Lalloo D, Trevett A, Black J *et al.* (1994) Neurotoxicity and haemostatic disturbances in patients envenomed by the Papuan black snake (*Pseudechis papuanus*). *Toxicon* 32(8): 927–936.

Markland FS (1998) Snake venoms and the hemostatic system. *Toxicon* 36(12): 1749–1800.

Mebs D (2000) *Gifttiere; Ein Handbuch für Biologen, Toxikologen, Ärzte, Apotheker*. Wissenschaftliche Verlagsgesellschaft, Stuttgart.

Meier J, White J (1995) *Handbook of clinical toxicology of animal venoms and poisons*. CRC Press, Boca Raton, Fla..

Miller MK, Whyte IM, White J, Keir M (2000) Clinical features and management of *Hadronyche* envenomation in man. *Toxicon* 38: 409–427.

Minton SA (1996) Bites by non-native venomous snakes in the United States. *Wilderness Environmental Medicine* 4: 297–303.

Murthy KRK, Hase NK (1994) Scorpion envenoming and the role of insulin. *Toxicon* 32(9): 1041–1044.

Rezende NA, Amaral CFS, Freire-Maia L (1998) Immunotherapy for scorpion envenoming in Brazil. *Toxicon* 36(11): 1507–1514.

Shier W, Mebs D (1990) *Handbook of toxinology.* Marcel Dekker, New York.

Sutherland S (1983) *Australian animal toxins*. Oxford University Press, Melbourne.

Theakston RDG, Warrell DA (1991) Antivenoms; a list of hyperimmune sera currently available for the treatment of envenoming by bites and stings. *Toxicon* 29: 1419–1470.

Tun-Pe, Aye-Aye-Mtint, Khin-Ei-Han, Thi-Ha, Tin Nu Swe (1995) Local compression pads as a first aid measure for victims of bites by Russell's viper (*Daboia russelii siamensis*) in Myanmar. *Transactions of the Royal Society of Tropical Medicine and Hygiene* 89: 293–295.

Warrell DA (1999) The clinical management of snake bites in the south east Asian region. *Southeast Asian Journal of Tropical Medicine and Public Health* 30 (Suppl 1): 1–85.

Warrell DA, Hudson BJ, Lalloo DG *et al.* (1996) The emerging syndrome of envenoming by the New Guinea small-eyed snake *Microechis ikaheka*. *Quarterly Journal of Medicine* 89: 523–530.

Weatherall D, Ledingham J, Warrell D (1996) *The Oxford Textbook of Medicine*, 3rd edition. Oxford University Press, Oxford.

Weinstein SA, Kardong KV (1994) Properties of Duvernoy's secretions from opisthoglyphous and aglyphous colubrid snakes. *Toxicon* 32(10): 1161–1186.

White J (1998) Envenoming and antivenom use in Australia. *Toxicon* 36(11): 1483–1492.

White J, Persson H (1996) Snakes. In: Descotes J (ed.) *Human Toxicology*. Elsevier Science, Amsterdam.

Williamson J, Fenner P, Burnett J, Rifkin J (eds) (1996) *Venomous and Poisonous Marine Animals: A Medical and Biological Handbook*. University of NSW Press, Sydney.

28

CHAPTER 28

Resuscitation and stabilization of the seriously injured child

GARY J BROWNE,
ROBIN K C CHOONG, AND
BARRY H WILKINS

CHAPTER 28

Resuscitation and stabilization of the seriously injured child

GARY J BROWNE, ROBIN K C CHOONG, AND BARRY H WILKINS

Perhaps no other emergency creates as much anxiety as that of a critically injured child, because the margin for error is so narrow. Children are not small adults, and although the approach to the injured child follows a similar framework to that of adults there are many differences.

An area of similarity between children and adults is the trimodal distribution of death.

- At the scene of the accident death usually occurs as a result of unsalvageable injuries such as massive head injury, high cervical spinal injury, major thoracic injury or major vessel disruption.
- During the first few hours (the 'golden hour' concept popularized by Trunkey—see Chapter 1) death and morbidity are potentially preventable if attention is directed to restoring airway, breathing, and circulation (ABC).
- Death in the days and weeks following the accident is usually secondary to sepsis and multisystem organ failure. These late deaths may be preventable if adequate resuscitation occurs in the first few hours.

Epidemiology

Trauma is the leading cause of death in children >1 year of age. Non-penetrating or blunt trauma is seen in >90% of cases, of which motor vehicle accidents and pedestrian injury account for 70% in western countries. Head injury accounts for 60–70% of total trauma cases and is the single most important cause of death and morbidity in children. Countries such as Australia and the UK are now experiencing an increase in penetrating injury from gunshots and stabbing, most cases relating to suicide or violence in adolescents (not dissimilar to the experience in the USA).

Aim of trauma care

An important principle in early trauma management is to get those most skilled in treating severely injured children in attendance as soon as possible.

The keys to good trauma care are:

- Focusing on the priorities of airway, breathing, circulation, and disability (ABCD).
- Paying attention to details.
- Re-evaluating the child frequently.
- Assuming that serious injuries do exist and then working systematically to exclude these injuries.

Important points include:

- A systematic, integrated and co-ordinated team approach. A senior medical officer acts as team leader to oversee assessment, resuscitation, and subsequent management. Each team member has a defined role, e.g. airway management, intravenous cannulation.

Table 28.1 Vital signs, measurements, and equipment

Age	Weight (kg)	Respirations (min–max)	Heart rate (min–max)	Systolic blood pressure (min–max)	Mid-trachea to teeth (distance in cm)	Endotracheal tube (uncuffed)	Laryngoscope blade	Suction catheter
Premature	1–2	30–60	90–190	50–70	8	2.5–3.0	0 straight	5.6 F
Newborn	3.5	30–60	90–190	50–70	10	3.5	1 straight	6 F
6 months	7	24–40	85–180	65–106	12	4.0	1 straight	8 F
1 year	10	20–40	80–150	72–110	12	4.5	2 straight	8 F
3 years	15	20–30	80–140	78–114	15	5.0	2 straight	8 F
6 years	20	18–25	70–120	80–116	16	5.5	3 straight	10 F
8 years	25	18–25	70–110	84–122	18	6.0 (cuffed)	3 straight/curved	10 F
12 years	40	14–20	60–110	94–136	20	7.0 (cuffed)	3 straight/curved	12 F
15 years	50	12–20	55–100	100–142	21	7.0 (cuffed)	3 straight/curved	12 F
18 years	65	12–18	50–90	104–148	22	7.0–8.0 (cuffed)	3 straight/curved	12 F

- Appreciation of the anatomical and physiological aspects of the paediatric patient (Table 28.1). These have implications for:
  - specific patterns of injury seen in children (frequently different from those in adults)
  - intravenous infusion rates and drug dosages (more often weight-related in children)
  - special equipment requirements for children.
- Because of their small size and elastic skeleton, children often sustain injuries to their internal organs with minimal or no external trauma.
- Consideration of the mechanism of injury: details of the accident frequently give important clues to the types and pattern of injury.
- Recognition that the response to trauma is a dynamic process. Regular monitoring of vital signs and repeated examinations are necessary if occult injuries are not to be missed.
- Consideration of the psychological impact. Trauma frequently places the child and their family under enormous psychological strain with possible long-term consequences. Clear communication, and allowing parents to see their child early and frequently, help to alleviate stress.
- Consideration of the possibility of child abuse (see Chapter 34). Important clues may be found in the history or the pattern of injury seen.

Classification

The majority of blunt injuries involve a localized area or single system. Children suffering from multiple injuries have often been exposed to critical forces distributed throughout all body regions, resulting in a high mortality rate.

The key to understanding traumatic injury, and therefore not missing injuries such as splenic trauma, is to understand the mechanisms of injury. Minimal forces will nearly always be associated with minor trauma that is often localized or single system in nature, whereas severe injury or multiple trauma must be considered when critical forces are involved. This is summarized in Table 28.2.

Table 28.2 Classification of injury

Blunt	Penetrating
Multiple	Local
Minor injury	Minimal force
Moderate injury	Significant force
Severe injury	Critical force

There are, however, circumstances that can lead to more serious injury although the forces involved may have been considered minimal. A child who falls from a low height such as a bed and hits a very hard surface such as a concrete or tiled floor may suffer a disproportionate injury. A skull fracture leading to an extradural haematoma may go unnoticed and the child discharged before the injury has evolved, with serious consequences. Additionally, if injuries are multiple and force is historically minimal, or explanation is unsatisfactory, then non-accidental injury must be considered.

The mechanism of injury is therefore just as important in children as it is in adults. A good history of the mechanism of injury will allow the treating clinicians to predict the potential problems that might arise before and during the initial resuscitation and stabilization of a trauma victim.

Definitions and scoring of trauma

Multiple trauma has been defined as substantial injury to more than one organ system or life-threatening injury to a single system. The recognized standards for describing injuries are the abbreviated injury score and its derivative the injury severity score (ISS), which classify injuries according to anatomical site and severity. Children with an ISS >15 are considered to have major trauma with

Table 28.3 Paediatric trauma score

Variable	+2	+1	−1
Airway	Normal	Maintainable	Unmaintainable
CNS	Awake	Obtunded/LOC	Coma
Body weightt	>20 kg	10–20 kg	<10 kg
Systolic BP	>90	50–90	<50
Open wound	None	Minor	Major
Skeletal injury	None	Closed	Open/multiple fractures

Table 28.4 Revised trauma score

Score	GCS	Systolic BP	Respiration rate
4	13–15	>89	10–29
3	9–12	76–89	>29
2	6–8	50–75	6–9
1	4–5	31–49	1–5
0	3	0	0

a high mortality and morbidity rate. Trauma scores were originally designed for rapid assessment and triage, for measuring progress of injury, for predicting outcome, and for assisting in quality assessment. They have proved to be useful in the overall management of the trauma patient, but less sensitive for severe injury to a single organ system.

Neither of these scores is used in the field by pre-hospital staff or in the emergency department. More useful tools for assessing the severity of injury are the paediatric trauma score (PTS) (Table 28.3) and the revised trauma score (Table 28.4). The PTS was developed to reflect the unique nature of injury patterns in children and to incorporate age. It is useful in triage and in predicting outcome in children. Children with a PTS <8 or a revised trauma score <11 should be treated in a designated trauma centre. Although these scores have a tendency to over-triage children with injury, there is no doubt that children with major trauma have a better outcome if managed in a designated trauma centre (see section on transfer, below).

Regardless of their trauma score, children who have sustained a high-energy impact should always be assessed carefully for possible life-threatening injuries.

Key points

- Children with an ISS >15 are considered to have major trauma with a high mortality and morbidity rate.
- More useful tools for assessing the severity of injury are the paediatric trauma score (Table 28.3) and the revised trauma score (Table 28.4)

Trauma team

Trauma management is a team activity that requires a co-ordinated approach, and much expertise channelled in a productive way for the optimal management of the patient. Most paediatric trauma centres have a team responsible for the initial care of children with a potential for major injury. Specialists in general surgery (often the team leader) and emergency medicine, intensive care, anaesthesiology, and radiology, and specialist trauma nurses are all involved. At our institution (the New Children's Hospital, Sydney) the emergency physician is often the first to respond, and leads the trauma team. The make-up of the trauma team is shown in Fig. 28.1.

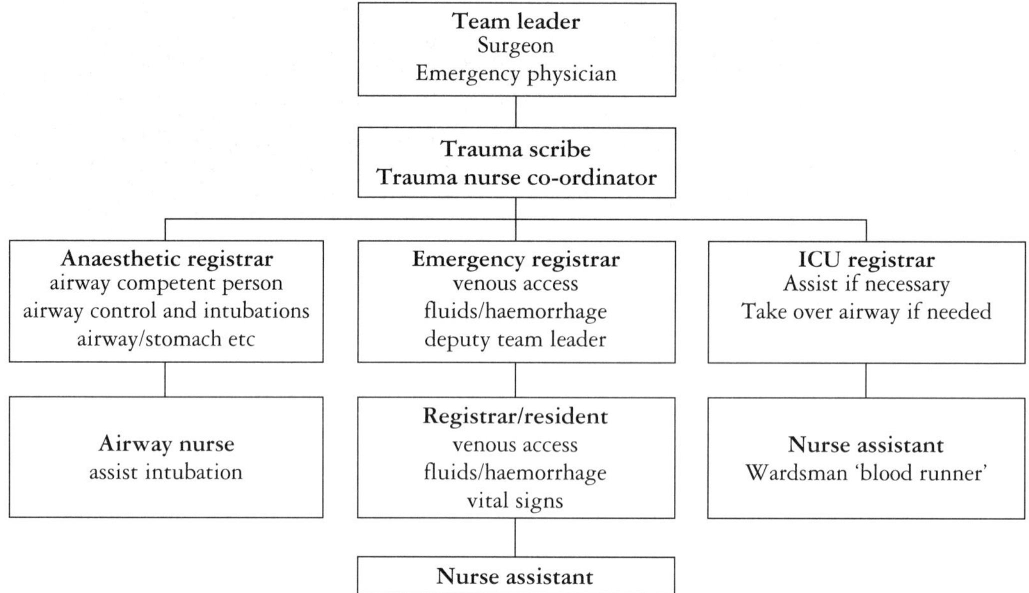

Figure 28.1 Trauma team.

It is important for smaller hospitals without a caseload large enough to warrant a trauma team to have protocols to define major trauma and for initial management, and criteria for transfer to a trauma centre.

Before arrival

Communication with the transporting pre-hospital service is vital in order to determine the extent of the child's injuries, the level of haemodynamic stability, and the current treatment of the child. The team can be prepare for the resuscitation by estimating the child's weight, and assembling age-appropriate equipment—laryngoscopes, endotracheal tubes, suction catheters, intravenous cannulae, and appropriate fluid delivering devices (see Table 28.1). Various support services such as the blood bank and operating theatres should be notified. If the child has suffered multiple injuries, ensure O-negative blood is on stand by for use immediately if necessary.

Primary survey and resuscitation

The key to successful resuscitation is to prioritize management according to injury severity. Attention should be paid first to life-threatening injuries; then limb-threatening injuries or high morbidity injuries; then minor injuries. Prioritization takes these steps:

- primary survey and resuscitation
- secondary survey
- definitive care.

The initial 5–10 minutes are spent evaluating and rapidly resuscitating vital signs, with immediate attention to life-threatening conditions. Resuscitation and monitoring continue throughout this process and through the child's stay in the emergency department. The secondary survey occurs during the next 20 minutes. These priorities are summarized in Fig. 28.2.

Vital functions should be rapidly assessed in order to identify life-threatening conditions and correct them. The priorities in order are:

A airway with cervical spine control

B breathing

C circulation with control of bleeding

D disability (brief neurological assessment)

E exposure; completely undress the child.

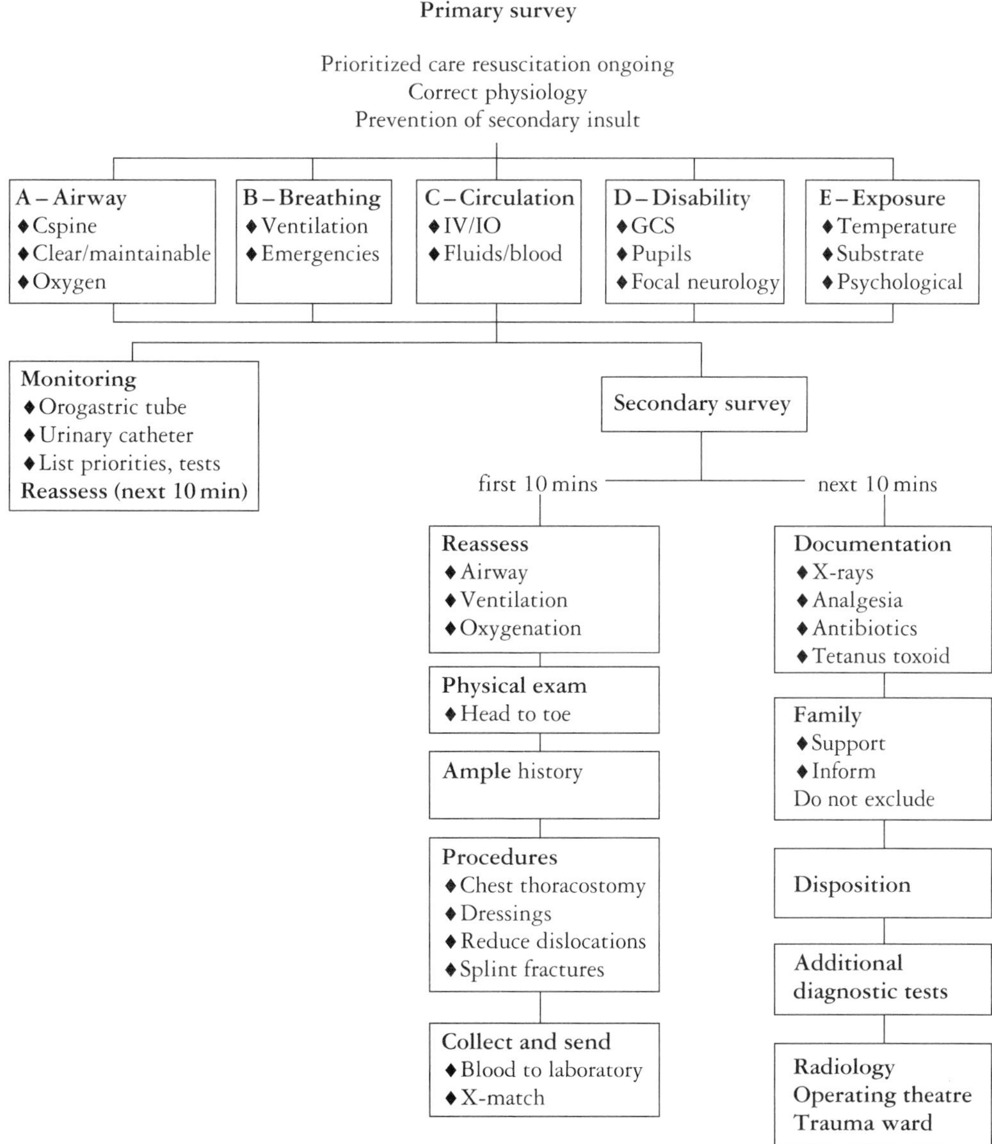

Figure 28.2 Priorities in trauma.

Details regarding the accident, vital signs, neurological status, and injuries can usually be obtained from the ambulance personnel while the patient is being transferred to a hospital bed.

Assessment

An older child should be asked, 'What is your name?' 'How old are you?', 'What happened?'. The child who answers has a patent airway, is breathing, and has adequate cerebral perfusion. It is important to check for cyanosis, stridor, hoarseness, and the free passage of air with each breath.

Intervention

Cervical spine injury should be assumed until proven otherwise by physical examination and radiology.

During airway control, the cervical spine should be protected by one or a combination of the following:

- in-line bimanual axial immobilization
- a hard cervical collar (of appropriate size)
- sandbags and adhesive tape (strapping the head and trunk to a spinal board will further assist to immobilize the cervical spine).

The principles of splinting involve immobilization of a body region above and below the injury. The neck should be kept in the neutral position.

Measures to establish an open airway

1 Chin lift (but excessive extension should be avoided if there is a risk of cervical spine injury) or jaw thrust (in spontaneously breathing, obstructed child). Undue force applied on the soft tissues under the chin may cause upper airway obstruction.

2 Suction (or manual removal of foreign material).

3 Oropharyngeal airway.

4 Orotracheal intubation.

5 Cricothyroidotomy.

If there is any difficulty, or problems are anticipated, senior help should be called for, but the establishment of a patent airway should not be delayed while assistance is awaited. Intubation is not immediately necessary if a patent airway and adequate ventilation are achieved. It should be remembered that infants (<6 months old) are obligate nasal breathers.

The initial hour of resuscitation for the injured child frequently involves attention to respiratory rather than circulatory problems. Injured children, particularly with head injury, may have altered consciousness or seizures, or may hypoventilate. Prompt assessment and rapid intervention are required to prevent hypoxia, secondary insult, and progression to cardiopulmonary arrest. The important anatomical

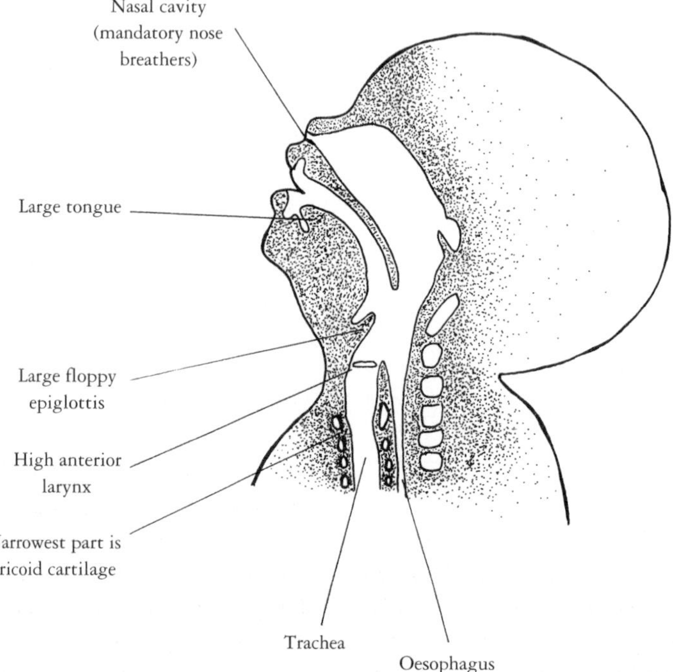

Figure 28.3 Anatomy of child airway.

(Fig. 28.3) and physiological aspects of the paediatric airway should be reviewed.

Key point

- The initial hour of resuscitation for the injured child frequently involves attention to respiratory rather than circulatory problems.

Equipment and assistance

All hospitals dealing with seriously injured children should have readily available basic monitoring equipment. This includes pulse oximetry, end-tidal carbon dioxide ($ETCO_2$), ECG, and non-invasive blood pressure (NIBP). It is essential that all equipment be checked on a daily basis and also immediately before use.

Minimum requirements for intubation are:

- oxygen (either cylinder or wall outlet) plus backup supply
- suction tubing, Yankauer sucker, Y-suction catheters
- paediatric breathing circuit: either bag–valve–mask of appropriate size or T-piece circuit (Ayre's or Jackson–Rees)
- face masks of various sizes according to age
- Guedel oropharyngeal airways
- nasopharyngeal airways, laryngeal masks (optional)
- full range of endotracheal tubes and tape for fixation
- laryngoscopes: standard Macintosh (curved) blade and infant blade (many variations of straight blade)
- Magill intubating forceps
- flexible introducers and stylets.

Injured children in emergency situations are often not co-operative patients: they may be distressed by their injury, by pain or anxiety related to the impending intervention, or by parental anxiety. When any airway intervention is required, skilled assistance must be available and dedicated to the operator attempting to secure the airway. There should be ready access to equipment without leaving the patient. Other staff may be required to restrain the child or assist with other procedures. In the event of suspected cervical spine injury an additional person must assist by immobilizing the neck. If there are any anticipated deviations from the usual procedure, then these should be outlined beforehand. In particular the assistant needs to be familiar with the technique of rapid sequence induction, endotracheal intubation, and the use of cricoid pressure to minimize the risk of pulmonary aspiration of regurgitated stomach contents.

Key point

- Many injured children in emergency situations are not co-operative and may be distressed by the injury.

Oropharyngeal (Guedel) airway

The size of the oropharyngeal airway is determined by placing flange adjacent to incisors; the tip of the airway should reach the angle of the mandible. An oropharyngeal airway should be insert directly in a child <1 year of age, using a tongue depressor, rather than upside down and rotating 180° as in adults, so that it follows the contour of the tongue. If it is too large, it may push the epiglottis over the larynx; if too small, it may obstruct against the back of the tongue. An oropharyngeal airway is only tolerated if consciousness and protective reflexes are impaired, otherwise gagging, coughing, or laryngeal spasm may occur.

Nasopharyngeal airway

The nasopharyngeal airway is a soft rubber or plastic, flanged tube that is gently inserted (well lubricated) via a nostril so that the tip lies above the laryngeal inlet. Great care is needed during insertion to prevent mucosal damage or adenoidal bleeding. A shortened endotracheal tube, suitably fixed, can be used as a substitute but must be clearly labelled as being nasopharyngeal rather than tracheal.

Bag–valve–mask ventilation

The self-inflating bag with valve attaches to an endotracheal tube or facemask. Remember to turn on the oxygen supply so that the reservoir bag is inflated (provides up to 80% F_IO_2). An adult bag (1600 mL capacity) can be used for children >5 years old and the paediatric bag (500 mL) for younger children and infants. Self-inflating bags should be fitted with a pressure release valve (30–40 cm H_2O pressure) that can be overridden if necessary. An anaesthetic breathing circuit (e.g. the Ayre's T-piece, Jackson–Rees circuit) should only used by personnel experienced with it. In certain difficult airway situations, in particular the obstructed airway, the T-piece circuit affords better airway control than the bag–valve–mask.

A clear airway should first be established, using head position, chin lift, or jaw thrust as necessary depending on the size and age of the child. The airway should be suctioned if blood or secretions are present. Infants will generally maintain a better airway with the head in a neutral position, whereas older children will require some extension of the atlanto-occipital joint. Gentle chin lift will usually clear the airway in a small child, providing the mouth is held open. In an older child more vigorous jaw thrust may be required, using support at the angle of the mandible. The face mask chosen, either a low dead-space Rendell Baker or the softer cushioned-type mask (easier for the inexperienced), should fit over the bridge of the nose and extend to the cleft between chin and lower lip. It is important that the thumb and index finger used to hold the mask remain at the top (where the mask connects to the bag-valve) so that pressure is distributed evenly around the base of the mask, maintaining a seal. The remaining three fingers are used to support the jaw or chin, taking care not to place any force on the soft tissues under the chin as this will tend to force the tongue up against the palate, obstructing the airway. ventilation should be commenced at a rate appropriate to the age of the child, achieving adequate chest movement.

Laryngeal mask airway

Widely used during anaesthesia, the laryngeal mask is useful for maintaining an airway especially where intubation is difficult or personnel are unskilled in intubation. It consists of a large-bore tube with elliptical cuffed 'mask' on the distal end which, after insertion, rests over the larynx. The cuff may be gently inflated to seal off the larynx, although this does not reliably prevent aspiration. Gentle ventilation may be performed, but care must be taken to prevent gastric distension. The airway requires care in insertion and fixation, as torsion will cause obstruction to airflow. It is not recommended if the operator is unfamiliar with its use. Use size 1 in infants <12 months, size 2 in 6 months–6 years, size $2\frac{1}{2}$ in 6–10 years and size 3 in >10 years.

Endotracheal tube

The endotracheal tube is the most practical way of establishing an artificial airway for ventilation or managing obstruction. However, in the injured child there may be other reasons why endotracheal intubation may be required, as outlined in Table 28.5.

The standard tube is soft, gently curved, and has an opening (Murphy eye) at one end to reduce the risk of lung collapse if inadvertent endobronchial placement occurs. The proximal end has a standard

Table 28.5 Indications for tracheal intubation

Inadequate ventilation by BVM device
Need for prolonged control of ventilation
Prevention of aspiration
Need for IPPV or controlled hyperventilation
Presence of flail chest
Shock unresponsive to volume
GCS <8
Facial injuries
Facial burns

15 mm adaptor, which will fit on to a breathing circuit or self-inflating bag. Most tubes have markings to indicate the length from the tip of the tube, which is bevelled to facilitate placement. In most cases there is a glottic marking. Shouldered tubes cause laryngeal trauma and are best avoided.

Tube size 2.5 mm internal diameter should be used in pre-term infants <1.5 kg, 3.0 mm in term infants, 3.5 mm in 3–9 months old, 4.0 mm in 9–24 months old. From age 2 years, the formula is:

$$\text{internal diameter (mm)} = \text{age}/4 + 4$$

but tubes one size smaller and larger should be available. Under the age of 8–10 years uncuffed tubes are used and there must be an audible leak around the tube to ensure there is not too much pressure on the subglottis. The optimal position for the tip of the tube is mid-trachea, as there is less likelihood of spontaneous extubation or endobronchial migration. This position is approximated using the formula:

$$\text{length (cm at incisor teeth)} = \text{age}/2 + 12 \text{ for an oral tube (age} + 10 \text{ for age } 1 - 5)$$

or

$$\text{length (cm at nostril)} = \text{age}/2 + 16 \text{ for a nasal tube (age} + 13 \text{ for age } 1 - 5)$$

The position should be confirmed by chest radiograph as soon as possible. The tip should be level with the body of T2, or between the clavicular heads.

At least two assistants are required. One should always assume that the child has a full stomach. Rapid sequence induction (using an anaesthetic induction agent and rapidly acting muscle relaxant, e.g. suxamethonium, rocuronium, or vecuronium) together with cricoid pressure, is performed to minimize the risks of vomiting and aspiration. Thiopentone (3–5 mg/kg) is the anaesthetic of choice but caution should be taken in hypotensive patients when lower doses (0.5–1.0 mg/kg) should be used. Alternatively, midazolam (0.1–0.2 mg/kg) or the dissociative anaesthetic ketamine (1–2 mg/kg) may be preferred if the patient is hypotensive.

Intubation

Endotracheal intubation provides the following advantages:

- ensures lungs are ventilated while minimizing gastric distension
- permits higher ventilatory pressures, hyperventilation, and use of postive end-expiratory pressure (PEEP)
- protects airway from aspiration of gastric contents, blood, or secretions
- allows endotracheal administration of drugs (adrenaline [epinephrine], atropine) if there is no intravenous access
- allows suction of airway to remove secretions
- frees up operator (less skill required to squeeze bag)
- allows access to head and neck, e.g. assessment, venous access
- humidification can be provided
- easy to induce anaesthesia.

Visualization of the larynx requires alignment of three axes—oral cavity, pharynx, and trachea—achieved by correct head positioning and then using a laryngoscope to displace the tongue and soft tissues while elevating the epiglottis to reveal the laryngeal inlet. For correct head position when a cervical spine injury is not a problem, the atlanto-occipital joint should be extended while flexing the lower cervical spine ('sniffing the morning air'), by placing a small pillow or folded towel under the head but not the shoulders. In infants who have a larger occiput this position is achieved without a pillow, providing the head remains in the neutral position. Older children will require manual extension of the head by placing a hand on the occiput; as the head is extended the mouth opens, allowing the laryngoscope to be inserted. Infants require the palm of the right hand to rest on the forehead, preventing excessive mobility, while the thumb and index fingers are used to open the mouth.

The technique for oral intubation in a trauma patient is somewhat different (Fig. 28.4). The child is supine on a spinal board with a semi-rigid collar in place. Drugs are given as needed. Before the patient is paralysed the anterior half of the collar is removed, and one assistant applies cricoid pressure as another holds the head in the neutral position. Positive pressure ventilation may be applied with bag, mask, and oxygen to pre-oxygenate in the unconscious child, with cricoid pressure applied to ensure ability to ventilate. Cricoid pressure will keep gas out of the stomach. The pressure required is quite firm, such that, if applied to the bridge of the nose, would cause some discomfort in an awake person. It is best applied using index finger and thumb (or one finger alone in an infant), pressed firmly backwards against the cricoid cartilage, but not so firmly that laryngeal anatomy is distorted. When muscle relaxation is achieved, oral intubation is performed, while in-line immobilization and cricoid pressure are maintained. Auscultation of both the axilla and over the epigastrium confirms correct endotracheal tube position. The cervical collar is reapplied, the tube taped, an oral airway can be inserted and positive pressure ventilation continued.

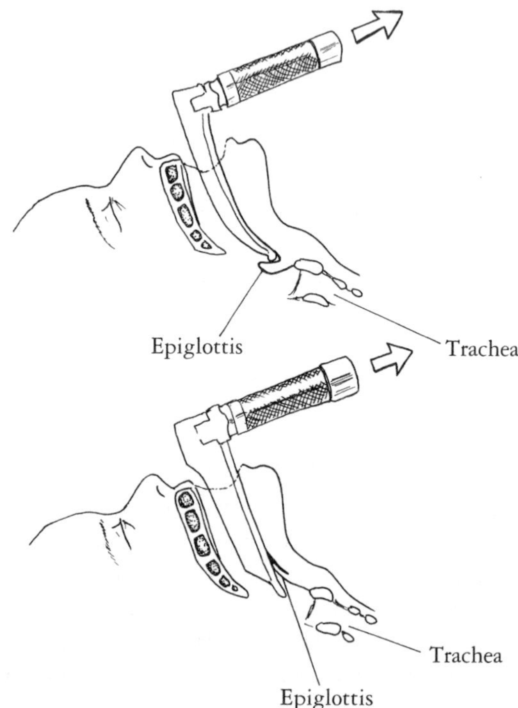

Figure 28.4 Intubation.

Key point

- The technique for oral intubation in a trauma patient is different from endotracheal intubation.

Rapid sequence intubation

In rapid sequence induction, anaesthetic and muscle relaxant are given and then airway is secured as rapidly as possible to minimize the risk of regurgitation and aspiration. It relies on the use of cricoid pressure to compress the oesophagus against the vertebral column. Cricoid pressure may also be used in unconscious patients during bag and mask ventilation to reduce gastric distension. This should not be confused with the use of laryngeal pressure to bring the vocal cords into view during a difficult intubation.

Key points

- Correct method for rapid sequence intubation:
  - Pre-oxygenate for 3 minutes. Have sucker working and next to patient's head.
  - Give atropine 20 μg/kg (minimum 100 μg) in children <8 years old.
  - Give thiopental/suxamethonium rapidly using precalculated dose, preferably into a running intravenous infusion to speed up onset.
  - Assistant applies cricoid pressure as consciousness is lost.
  - Intubation performed after suxamethonium fasciculation seen (noting that some infants may not fasciculate with suxamethonium) while cricoid pressure is maintained.
  - Once intubation accomplished and confirmed, release cricoid pressure and fix tube.

- If intubation is unsuccessful maintain cricoid pressure, oxygenate with bag and mask while allowing patient to wake up. Release cricoid only on return of reflexes or consciousness.
- Seek further expertise before attempting intubation again.
- Place gastric tube as soon as the endotracheal tube is in place and secured.

Nasotracheal intubation

Nasotracheal intubation is not routinely recommended for the injured child, although there may be occasions where this technique is preferred to secure the airway. Nasotracheal intubation requires considerable practice and experience, particularly when performed in smaller children. In the injured child with an undifferentiated head injury in whom a base of skull fracture with disruption of the cribriform plate has occurred but has not been identified, there is a small risk of passing the endotracheal tube into the cranial cavity.

The reasons for changing the tube are as follows:

- Long term fixation of a nasal tube is easier and more secure, especially when an intubated child requires transfer by air or road.
- Suction is easier via a nasotracheal tube, and the patient cannot bite on the tube.
- An awake patient, e.g. weaning prior to extubation, tolerates a nasal tube better.

In addition to equipment for oral intubation, a Magill forceps and tape pre-cut for fixation are required. Fixation is best achieved using two 5–10 cm × 2.5 cm tapes prepared as 'trouser legs', i.e. split longitudinally for half their length.

Intubation is accomplished in much the same manner as before.

Key points

- Correct procedure for nasotracheal intubation:
  - Ensure the patient is well sedated and muscle relaxed, and pre-oxygenate for a few minutes via the orotracheal tube (OTT). A nasogastric tube should be in place. Use cricoid pressure if there is any likelihood of a full stomach.
  - Inserted the (well lubricated) tube gently via the nostril (right side preferred) backwards not upwards until it lies in the nasopharynx before laryngoscopy. A nasal vasoconstrictor may be applied beforehand to reduce the risk of bleeding. Consider softening a PVC tube in warm water to minimize nasopharyngeal trauma.
  - Visualize the larynx and advance the tube to the larynx. Withdraw the OTT. Gentle manipulation of the laryngoscope can then be used to align the larynx with the advancing tube. It is important to maintain the head in a neutral, even slightly flexed, position at this stage. Excessive extension displaces the laryngeal axis upward, making alignment with the tube difficult.
  - If necessary, use the Magill forceps to grasp the distal end of the tube and assist its passage into the larynx. At this point the tube tip sometimes gets caught on the anterior commissure of the larynx, and slight flexion may assist in re-aligning the tube.
  - Once the correct position is established using the criteria previously mentioned, secure the tube using interlocking adhesive 'trouser leg' tapes after application of tincture of benzoin.
  - As with oral intubation, it is important to avoid hypoxia. Re-oxygenate with 100% oxygen and bag–valve–mask in the event that intubation is not successful.

Cricothyroidotomy

Cricothyroidotomy is the next option if intubation is not possible, e.g. because of massive facial fractures. Surgical cricothyroidotomy is restricted to children >12 years. Needle cricothyroidotomy, using a 14–18 gauge cannula, is indicated in younger children. Both procedures are temporizing measures. All children requiring a cricothyroidotomy should have a surgical tracheostomy within

2 hours. Disadvantages of this technique include difficulty in ensuring correct entry to trachea, damage to larynx or trachea, and insufficient exhalation in an obstructed patient. It may, however, be life saving while a tracheostomy is performed. It is of no use if the obstruction is below the cricoid level, e.g. a tracheal foreign body. As the cricoid is the narrowest part of the paediatric airway, it is quite possible that cricothyroidotomy will not provide access to the trachea if a foreign body is impacted at this level. If this occurs it is recommended that the patient be intubated and the endotracheal tube used to force the foreign body into a main bronchus. The tube can then be withdrawn to mid-trachea and ventilation can proceed on one lung pending urgent bronchoscopy.

Key points

- Correct procedure for cricothyroidotomy:
  - With neck extended, stabilize trachea using thyroid cartilage.
  - Locate cricothyroid space below lower border of thyroid cartilage.
  - Puncture cricothyroid membrane using large bore (14 or 16 gauge) intravenous cannula connected to a 2 mL syringe and inserted at 45° inferiorly and caudally.
  - Aspirate air to confirm correct placement; withdraw trocar from cannula.
  - Connect a T-piece circuit with oxygen (15 L/min) via a 3 mm endotracheal tube fitted directly into the intravenous cannula. Alternatively, cut off the end of an intravenous giving set, insert into the cannula, attach oxygen tube to the cut end and use the side injection port (also cut off) to administer intermittent positive pressure with your thumb on the cut end, 1 second on and 4 seconds off. Note that you still cannot ventilate adequately for long periods using such a small-calibre airway.

The technique is difficult to perform in a child <2 years old because of the shorter neck, and ventilation through small-bore cannulasmay be inadequate. Techniques using high-flow jet ventilators are unsuitable in this setting and generate very

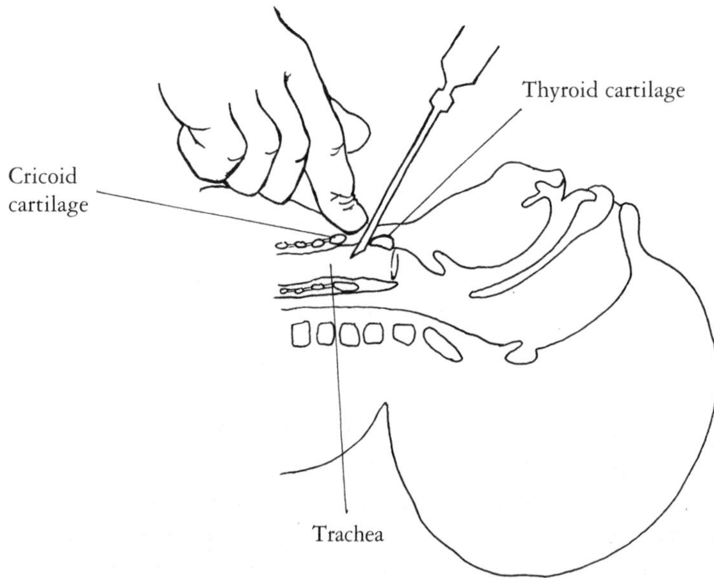

Figure 28.5 Cricothyroidotomy.

high pressures in the young child, with risk of barotrauma.

After age 12 years it may be easier and quicker to use a surgical approach (Fig. 28.5): using a scalpel to cut transversely through to the cricothyroid membrane, the space is opened up with the handle and an endotracheal tube of appropriate size inserted, although there may be small risk to deeper structures. This will also provide better gas exchange.

Key point

- Cricothyroidotomy is difficult to perform in a child <2 years old.

Airway problems in trauma management

Head injury is a leading condition requiring airway intervention (Hahn *et al.* 1988). Proper initial management of the airway is fundamental to improving outcome, in particular the early correction of hypoxia and hypercapnia and the ability to induce hypocapnia as method of reducing intracranial pressure (ICP). This almost always requires endotracheal intubation using a rapid sequence technique and then commencing ventilation to improve oxygenation and normalize carbon dioxide levels. Adequate anaesthesia must be provided to cover intubation in order to prevent a sudden increase in ICP. Muscle relaxation alone is inadequate. The possibility of cervical spine injury should be considered at all times: an assistant should maintain in-line cervical immobilization (in a neutral position) during intubation to avoid exacerbating spinal cord injury.

Cervical spine injury in children has a high mortality and morbidity. In general, children requiring intubation can be safely managed using the standard technique for rapid sequence induction, using in-line immobilization in the neutral position without traction. Although it may be preferable to intubate using an awake blind nasal or fibre-optic technique, this is rarely possible (or desirable) in the injured child. It is prudent to allow the most accomplished operator available to perform the procedure, and to avoid excessive movement or pressure on neck structures.

Faciomaxillary injury may require urgent intervention to secure the airway, as swelling may worsen if intubation is delayed. Blood in the airway may make visualization difficult, and the mobility of tissues and anatomical disruption will contribute to problems with ventilation using a bag and mask prior to intubation. In severe injury, e.g. LeFort III and bilateral mandibular fractures, airway obstruction may be improved by positioning the child on one side or semi-prone with traction on mobile structures. Once anaesthesia is induced it is usually possible to displace free-floating structures using the blade of the laryngoscope. There is usually the added problem of a stomach full of swallowed blood and the risks of cervical spine injury. If obstruction is severe it may be necessary to perform an urgent tracheostomy under local anaesthesia, unless expertise exists for other means of securing the airway.

Airway burns may contribute to respiratory problems in several ways: carbon monoxide poisoning, oedema of the upper airway, and direct thermal injury to the tracheobronchial tree from inhalation of hot gases. As a late development, eschar may cause chest wall contraction and impede ventilation. If carbon monoxide poisoning is suspected, 100% oxygen should be administered. Close observation is essential and if there is evidence of severe airway burns early intubation and assessment with fibre-optic bronchoscopy is mandatory, as swelling may preclude later intubation if obstruction becomes severe.

Key point

- Proper initial management of the airway is fundamental to improving outcome.

Breathing

Assessment

- *Expose* the chest and neck.
- *Look* for signs of respiratory distress such as cyanosis, tachypnoea, flaring of the alae nasi, use of accessory muscles. Observe the degree

and symmetry of chest wall excursion. Look for external signs of trauma such as contusions, abrasions or the paradoxical movement of a flail segment. Check the neck veins for distension.

- *Feel* for the trachea to assess its relationship to the midline. Palpate the chest for subcutaneous emphysema and areas of tenderness.
- *Listen* for breath sounds. Are they normal and symmetrical? Are the heart sounds normal? Listen for grunting, stridor, or wheeze.

Life-saving procedures

High-flow oxygen (12 L/min) should be administered via a reservoir facemask, or ventilation assisted with a bag–valve–mask if required. Nasal prongs do not deliver sufficient oxygen but may be a compromise in a distressed, combative child who does not allow a mask to be used.

Tension pneumothorax (Fig. 28.6) is a clinical diagnosis and should immediately be relieved by inserting a 14–18 gauge over-the-needle catheter into the second intercostal space in the midclavicular line. Subsequently, a chest tube should be inserted in the fourth or fifth intercostal space in the anterior axillary line. It must be remembered that once the chest has been needled to drain a pneumothorax, a chest drain is mandatory.

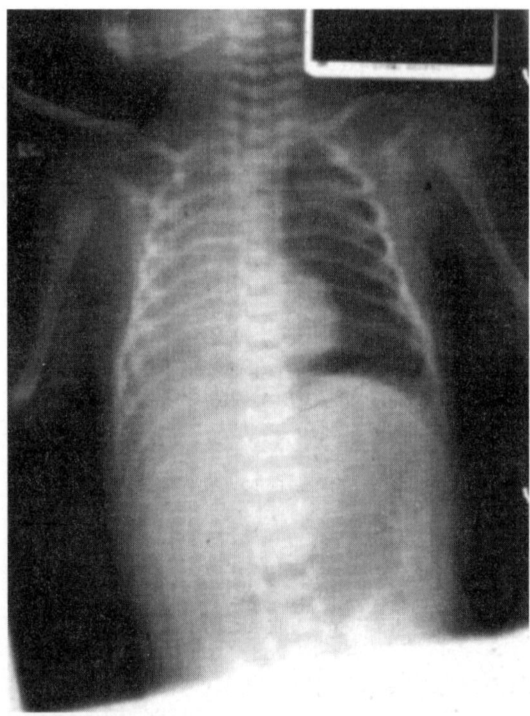

Figure 28.6 Tension pneumothorax.

A massive haemothorax should be relieved by inserting a chest tube and administering intravenous fluids for resuscitation.

A flail segment should be treated by inserting a chest tube, even if a pneumothorax is not initially seen on chest radiograph. Intubation may be required for associated pulmonary contusion. An open pneumothorax should be covered with an occlusive dressing that is taped on three sides; this produces a 'flutter-valve' effect which allows air to escape from the pleural cavity on exhalation, but prevents air from entering on inspiration. A chest tube should be inserted at a site remote from the open wound.

Appropriate sizes for chest tubes in children are:

- *infants:* size 30 cm (12 in)
- 2–10 year olds: sizes 40–50 cm (16–20 in)
- 11–16 year olds: sizes 60–70 cm (24–28 in).

The largest diameter tube that will pass through the intercostal space should be used when draining a haemothorax.

Assisted ventilation

If breathing is inadequate, ventilation can be assisted with a T-piece bagging circuit or self-inflating bag–valve device. For the experienced practitioner, a compressed gasdriven ventilator (e.g. Dräger Oxylog) may be used to ventilate children >1 year of age (a pressure-limiting valve is used when ventilating infants).

Key points

- Guidelines for assisted ventilation (Rubin and Sadonohoff 1996):
  - Start with tidal volume = 10 mL/kg.
  - Rate = 20/min (30/min for infants).
  - Peak airway pressure = 20 cm H_2O.

- Check arterial blood gases.
- Maintain $P_aCO_2 = 35–40$ mmHg (30–35 mmHg if head injury).
- Always exclude hypoxaemia or hypovolaemia if the child is agitated and/or confused.

Ventilation difficulties may be due to:

- a struggling child
- gastric distension
- airway obstruction
- massive aspiration
- direct laryngeal injury
- pneumothorax with increased airway pressure
- laryngospasm
- massive pulmonary artery obstruction.

Key point

- Always exclude hypoxaemia or hypovolaemia if the child is agitated or confused.

Circulation

Life-threatening injuries

Immediate life-threatening injuries are massive internal or external haemorrhage, cardiac tamponade, and tension pneumothorax. Cardiac output is the volume of blood pumped by the heart each minute (heart rate × stroke volume); stroke volume is the volume pumped with each contraction. In younger children the stroke volume is relatively fixed, with cardiac output primarily reliant on heart rate. Blood pressure is determined by cardiac output and peripheral vascular resistance. Normal blood pressure can be maintained (Fig. 28.7) as long as the circulation compensates adequately with vasoconstriction, tachycardia, and increased cardiac contractility. When compensation fails hypotension occurs. Tachycardia persists until pre-arrest.

Key point

- Immediate life-threatening injuries are massive internal or external haemorrhage, cardiac tamponade and tension pneumothorax.

If tachycardia in children is overlooked, then shock may go unrecognized. Although cardiac output falls in an almost linear fashion as blood volume is depleted, blood pressure remains initially unchanged because of increased vascular resistance. Hypotension is often a late and sudden sign of cardiovascular decompensation in seriously injured children and young adults. Even mild hypotension must be taken seriously and treated quickly and aggressively, since cardiopulmonary arrest is often

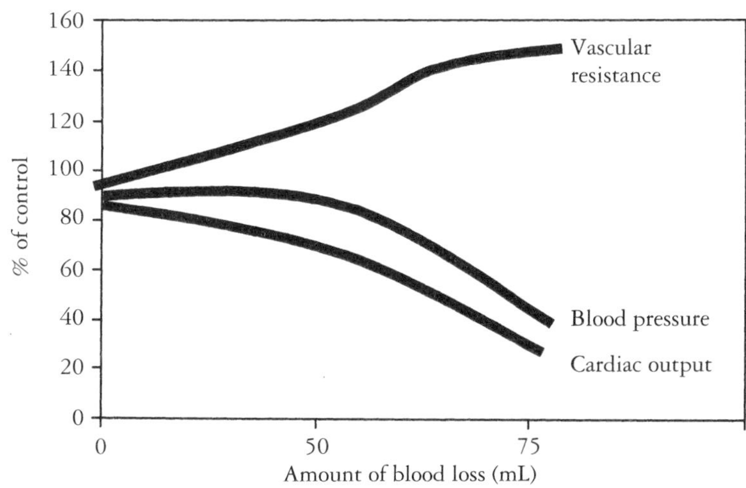

Figure 28.7 Cardiovascular response to haemorrhage. (Adapted from the American Heart Association—Paediatric Advanced Life Support.)

imminent. A further consequence of this robust cardiac response to haemorrhage in children is the degree of peripheral vasoconstriction that may occur. Many injured children in a compensated shocked state will be pale and shut down as a result of vasoconstriction. Capillary refill is often prolonged early on in seriously injured children who have compensated shock, provided ambient temperature is accounted for when assessed. This increase in peripheral vascular resistance and associated vasoconstriction makes intravenous access extremely difficult in seriously injured children.

Key point

- If tachycardia in children is overlooked then shock may go unrecognized.

Intravascular access

Drug administration requires access to the circulation. If no access is present or the cannula has extravasated or become blocked, then peripheral venous cannulation should be performed (Fig. 28.8). If peripheral venous cannulation attempts are unsuccessful within 90 seconds, then alternative vascular access is obtained via the intraosseous route. The anteromedial surfaces of the proximal or distal tibia are suitable sites. The needle is inserted perpendicularly to the bone surface and a screwing action is used to traverse the cortex. A loss of resistance is felt once the marrow is entered. Correct positioning of the needle, confirmed by aspiration of bone marrow or injection of saline without extravasation, is necessary to avoid compartment syndrome. When resuscitating through the intraosseous route it must be remembered that in order for fluids

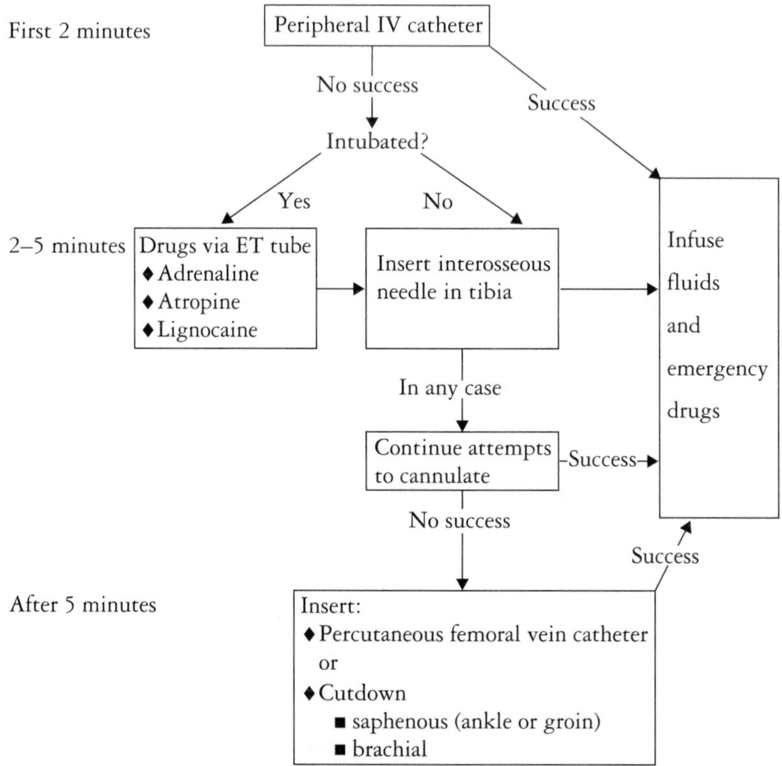

Figure 28.8 Emergency venous access in children.

to be infused they will need to be pumped through. Contraindications to the intraosseous route are few, although it should be avoided in the case of a significant or open fracture of the extremity (Rupert *et al.* 1994).

The 18 gauge needle is for use in infants and small children. The 16 gauge needle is suitable for older children. All drugs and resuscitative fluids may be given by the intraosseous route, but only adrenaline (epinephrine), atropine, lignocaine (lidocaine), and naloxone may be given via the endotracheal tube.

Central venous cannulation via the subclavian or internal jugular veins should be reserved for the post-resuscitation phase, but cannulation of the external jugular or femoral veins may be attempted during resuscitation. Surgical cutdown on to a vein remains an alternative but is also time consuming.

Assessment

- Shock (Fig. 28.9) is a clinical syndrome resulting from tissue perfusion that is inadequate to meet metabolic needs. Clinically, it is manifest by changes in haemodynamic measurements, tachypnoea and poor perfusion of the skin, brain, and kidneys. Shock can exist with a normotension, hypotension, or hypertension.
- Blood pressure, pulse rate, and respiratory rate are age dependent (Table 28.6). Systolic blood pressure = 80 + (2× age in years). Diastolic pressure is usually two-thirds of the systolic measurement. Children compensate extremely well for hypovolaemia. The first sign of hypovolaemia is narrowing of the blood pressure (rising diastolic pressure). Systolic hypotension occurs very late and indicates severe hypovolaemia (up to 40% of blood volume loss).
- Tachycardia is a very sensitive, but not specific, marker of shock. Assess pulse rate, pulse volume, and the presence of distal pulses. Bradycardia is a preterminal event.
- Assess skin for colour, temperature, clamminess, and capillary refill time (normal <2 seconds but varies according to the ambient temperature and is very observer dependent).
- Tachypnoea is frequently associated with hypovolaemia. Assess for 'air hunger' (hyperpnoea and tachypnoea).

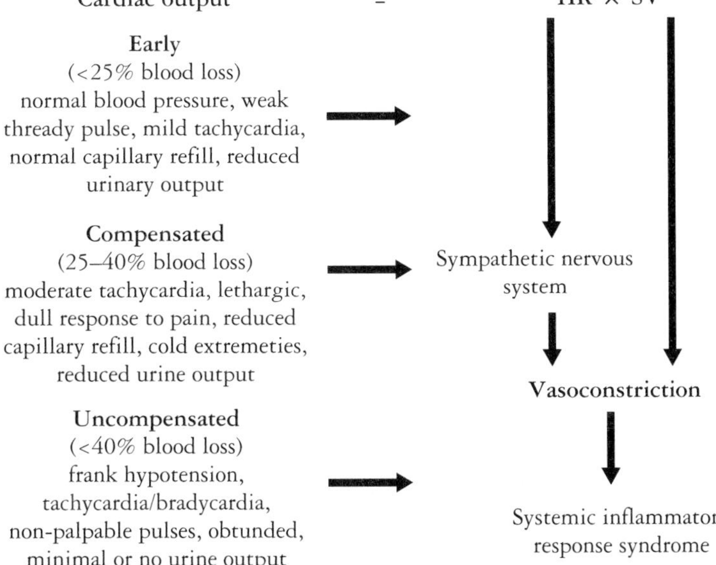

Figure 28.9 Stages of shock in children.

Table 28.6 Paediatric resuscitation chart

Endotracheal tube		Uncuffed					Cuffed		
Internal diameter (mm)		3.0	3.0–3.5	4.0	4.5–5.0	5.5	6.0–6.5	7.0–7.5	8.0
Length (cm) (OTT)		10	11	11–12	13–14	15	16–17	18	19–21
Length (cm) (NTT)		12	13	14	16	19	21	22	23
Age		Months		Years					
	Up to:	2	6	1	3.5	6	10	13	14
Length (cm)	Up to:	55	70	75	90	115	135	155	160
Weight (kg)	Up to:	5	7.5	10	15	20	30	40	50
Adrenaline									
Initial dose 1/10000		0.5	0.75	1	1.5	2	3	4	5
(0.1 mL/kg = 10 μg/kg)									
Subsequent doses and initial									
Endotracheal 1/1000									
(0.1 mL/kg = 100 μg/kg)									
Atropine (0.5 mg/mL)									
(0.04 mL/kg = 20 μg/kg)		0.2	0.3	0.4	0.6	0.8	1.2	1.6	2
Endotracheal dose		0.4	0.6	0.8	1.2	1.6	2.4	3.2	4
(0.08 mL/kg = 40 μg/kg)									
Bicarbonate (8.4%)									
(1 mL/kg = 1 mmol/kg)		5	7.5	10	15	20	30	40	50

Calcium chloride (10%)								
(0.2 mL/kg = 140 μmol/kg)	1	1.5	2	3	4	6	8	10
Diazepam (10 mg/2 mL)								
Intravenous (0.05 mL/kg = 0.25 mg/kg)	0.2	0.4	0.5	0.75	1	1.5	2	2
Rectal (0.1 mL/kg = 0.5 mg/kg)	0.5	0.75	1.0	1.5	2	2	2	2
Glucose (50%)								
(1 mL/kg = 500 mg/kg)	5	8	10	15	20	30	40	50
Lignocaine/lidocaine (1% = 10 mg/mL)								
(0.1 mL/kg = 1 mg/kg) (ETT)	0.5	0.75	1	1.5	2	3	4	5
Naloxone (800 μg/2 mL)								
(0.1 mL/kg = 40 μg/kg) (ETT)	0.5	0.75	1	1.5	2	3	4	5
DC shock (joules)								
SVT—1st shock	3–5	7	10	15	20	30	40	50
Defibrillation—1st shock	10	15	20	30	40	60	80	100
Subsequently	20	30	40	60	80	120	160	200
Initial fluid bolus (mL)								
(Colloid) (20 mL/kg)	100	150	200	300	400	600	800	1000

All doses are in millilitres, intravenous or intraosseous unless otherwise stated.

ETT, endotracheal tube; OTT, orotracheal tube; NTT, nasotracheal tube.

- Cerebral hypoperfusion may present as depressed consciousness, lethargy, agitation, or hypotonia.
- There may be thirst and poor urine output (<1 mL/kg per hour for infants, <0.5 mL/kg per hour for older children).
- Cardiac tamponade classically presents with Beck's triad, i.e. systolic hypotension, jugular venous distension, and muffled heart sounds. Symmetrical breath sounds and a midline trachea excludes tension pneumothorax.

Life-saving interventions

- High-flow oxygen, monitor continuous ECG, pulse oximetry, and continuous to 3 minutely non-invasive blood pressure monitoring (Table 28.7).
- Haemorrhage should be controlled by:
  - applying direct pressure to external bleeding sites; tourniquets should be removed as soon as possible
  - reducing fractures as soon as possible
  - recognizing haemorrhage that is uncontrolled or uncontrollable and arranging urgent intravascular access and surgery.
- Circulating volume must be restored. Two short-length, large-bore intravenous cannulas are inserted into a large proximal vein, e.g. the cubital fossa. Blood is collected for laboratory tests and cross-match. Warmed fluids should be administered immediately (colloid, e.g. Haemaccel 20 mL/kg or crystalloid, e.g. Hartmann's solution 20 mL/kg). If a patient fails to respond to a second bolus, then blood (whole blood 20 mL/kg or packed cells 10 mL/kg) is required (Table 28.8). In infants or small children with refractory shock a blood glucose level should be performed early on in the resuscitation.
- If packed cells are used, volume is made up using saline, plasma, or 5% albumin. If the child is stable and blood will be available within

Table 28.7 Trauma resuscitation guidelines

	Immediate life-threatening injuries	Life-saving procedures
Airway	Obstructed airway Laryngeal/tracheal trauma Faciomaxillary trauma	Oxygen Oropharyngeal airway Endotracheal intubation Cricothyroidotomy Tracheostomy
Breathing	Tension pneumothorax Flail chest Haemothorax Sucking chest wound (open pneumothorax) Central depression of respiration	Intercostal cannula Intercostal tube Endotracheal intubation Cover sucking chest wound on three sides
Circulation	Haemorrhage: Internal External Cardiac tamponade/rupture	 Pressure over bleeding sites Two large bore intravenous cannulas Intraosseous infusion Pericardiocentesis Emergency thoracotomy (penetrating trauma only)

10–15 minutes, fully cross-matched blood can be awaited. If unstable, type-specific blood may have to be used. If a delay of even a few minutes is critical, group O-negative blood is given.

- Cardiac tamponade unresponsive to fluid loading is treated with urgent pericardiocentesis. Rapid transfer to the operating theatre for urgent thoracotomy should be arranged.

Key point

- Technique for pericardiocentesis:
  - Place child supine and upright at 30–45°.
  - Ensure airway and ventilation are optimized. Continue volume loading.
  - Prepare with antiseptic solution and infiltrate the area just below the xiphoid process with 1% lignocaine (lidocaine).
  - Attach a 16–21 gauge cardiac or spinal needle to a stopcock and a 20–50 mL syringe.
  - Attach an alligator clip leading to a precordial lead of the ECG monitor to the needle's hub.
  - Insert the needle just below the xiphoid process at 60–70° to the horizontal, aiming at the left shoulder, advancing slowly while maintaining gentle suction to the syringe.
  - Advance until pericardial fluid is aspirated or epicardial contact is made as indicated by an injury pattern (ST or PR elevation or T-wave inversion). Withdraw the needle until the ECG pattern normalizes, and re-advance at a more medial angle.
  - Aspirate fluid to relieve tamponade and then insert a soft catheter via a guide wire to allow for continued drainage.
  - Complications of pericardiocentesis include myocardial penetration, coronary artery laceration, arrhythmias, pneumothorax, and infection.
- Military anti-shock trousers (MAST suits) are no longer recommended for use in the haemodynamically unstable patient. Their main use is pre-hospital splinting of pelvic and long-bone fractures. Occasionally, children arrive with a MAST suit on.
  - If the suit is deflated, is should be removed.

Table 28.8 Indications for blood products

1	Bleeding controlled, vital signs stable and further immediate bleeding unlikely: cross-match (45 min) if antibodies found (>60 min)
2	Bleeding caused hypovolemic shock but tissue oxygenation not critically affected: Support intravascular volume with colloid in aliquots of 20 mL/kg group specific blood Rh type-specific (15 min) cross-matched blood preferred
3	Bleeding with life-threatening hypoxia: Rh-negative administered in aliquots of 20 mL/kg. If a further 40 mL/kg has been administered this represents the whole blood volume of the child and serious consideration should be given to occult injury. If shock is refractory to adequate resuscitative effort also consider hypothermia, exclude hypoglycaemia and give more volume. In this situation operative intervention to exclude an abdominal or other injury should be strongly considered

- If one leg compartment is inflated to splint a fracture, it should be left inflated until the limb is examined. The suit should not be inflated for more than 90–120 minutes.
- If the suit is inflated for hypovolaemic shock, two large-bore intravenous cannulas should be inserted and volume replacement givem rapidly.
- The abdominal compartment should be slowly deflated, followed by lower limb compartments. About 1/3 of volume should be deflated at one time, then blood pressure rechecked.
- If systolic blood pressure drops by >10 mmHg deflation should be stopped and more volume replacement given.

Key point

- Military anti-shock trousers (MAST suits) are no longer recommended for use in the haemodynamically unstable patient.

Disability

- Level of consciousness may be assessed by use of the *AVPU mnemonic*:

  A alert and oriented

  V responds to verbal stimuli

  P responds only to painful stimuli

  U unresponsive
- Pupillary size and reaction to light should be noted. A unilateral, fixed dilated pupil may indicate the presence of an acute extradural or subdural haematoma. Bilateral, fixed dilated pupils indicate more serious traumatic or hypoxic brain injury.
- Any gross asymmetry in movement should also be noted. A more detailed neurological examination is performed in the secondary survey. Mentally alert or aware, pupillary activity and size should be noted.

Exposure

- The child should be fully undressed to allow examination of the entire body. Core temperature should be monitored via a rectal probe.
- The child should be exposed only as long as it takes to complete the physical examination. Normothermia should be maintained by using warmed intravenous fluids, blood warmers, warm blankets, and overhead heating lamps.
- By the completion of the primary survey and resuscitation the patient should be connected to the following 'lines' for monitoring and treatment:
  - oxygen via mask or endotracheal tube
  - end-tidal CO_2 monitor if ventilated
  - nasogastric or orogastric tube
  - large-bore intravenous cannula ×2
  - sphygmomanometer
  - pulse oximeter
  - ECG monitor
  - chest tube
  - rectal temperature probe
  - urinary catheter.
- The perineum and rectum should be examined for urethral trauma before a urinary catheter is inserted. Perineal haematoma, urethral meatal blood, or a high-riding prostate on rectal examination indicate likely urethral trauma and contraindicate urethral catheterization. Suprapubic catheterization would be required.

Secondary survey

The important aspects of the secondary survey are:

- *Continuing resuscitation and monitoring:* Any deterioration mandates immediate return to the airway, breathing, and circulation (ABC).

- *History:* An AMPLE history should be obtained from the child (if possible), family, ambulance personnel, friends, and bystanders:
  - A allergies
  - M medications, including tetanus immunization status
  - P past medical history
  - L last ate or drank (time)
  - E events/environment related to the injury
- *Head-to-toe examination:* A systematic head-to-toe, front-and-back examination should be perform to detect any injuries not noted in the primary survey. Each region of the body should be assessed including the ears, nose, mouth, rectum, and pelvis using the 'look, feel, listen' and 'tubes and fingers in every orifice' approach. In young children, if rectal or internal vaginal examination is required, then it may be prudent to have it performed once by the most senior clinician or while the child is under general anaesthesia. The sequence of examination is:
  - head
  - face
  - neck
  - chest and shoulder
  - abdomen
  - pelvis
  - lower limbs
  - upper limbs
  - central nervous system; include Glasgow Coma Scale (GCS) score (see Table 2.3, page 19)
  - back
  - perineum and rectum.

Secondary survey

- The ABCDE of the primary survey should be re-assessed regularly or as indicated.
- *Head:* Check pupillary size, conjunctiva, reaction of pupils, fundal appearance and vision. Examine face for maxillofacial trauma. Check dentition. Examine scalp for laceration of soft tissue injury. Look for signs of basilar skull fracture. Check for symmetry of voluntary movement and neurological function of facial muscles.
- *Neck:* Palpate cervical spine. Check for subcutaneous emphysema, abnormal tracheal position, haematoma, and localized pain. Evaluate neck veins for distension.
- *Chest:* Check for bilateral chest excursion, asymmetry of wall motion, and flail segment. Palpate trachea midline. Palpate chest. Auscultate lung fields and cardiovascular system.
- *Abdomen:* Repeated measurement of girth may help diagnosis of unsuspected bleeding. Inspect for ease of movement with respiration, bruises, lacerations, and bowel sounds. Palpate for localized findings. Observe and palpate flanks.
- *Pelvis:* Palpate bony prominences for tenderness or instability. Check for laceration, haematoma, and active bleeding. Check urethral meatus for blood.
- *Rectum:* Should be examined by a surgeon or a person responsible for the child's care only once, checking for sphincter tone. If urethral damage is considered then the level of the prostate should be noted.
- *Extremities:* Check for signs of fracture, dislocation, abrasion, contusion, and haematoma. Note bony instability.
- *Back:* Examine only if spinal cord injury is not suspected.
- *Skin:* Look for petechiae, burns, and contusions.
- *Neurological:* In-depth neurological examination, including a GCS score.

Explanatory notes for paediatric coma scale

Because the GCS is universally used and understood in adult emergency practice, in many cases in clinical practice this 3–15 score is extrapolated to children (see Table 2.3, page 18). The concern here is that such extrapolation is at best an approximation of the child's level of consciousness, rather than an objective representation of the child's clinical state. Although this score has not been validated we have found the modification of the GCS for children useful and highly accurate for use early on during resuscitation and stabilization.

Investigations

- *Laboratory tests*: Most of these specimens should already have been collected during the resuscitation phase.
  - full blood count
  - cross-match
  - coagulation studies
  - electrolytes, urea, creatinine
  - liver function tests (sensitive and specific for hepatic trauma)
  - amylase (not sensitive, not specific for pancreatic injury)
  - glucose
  - creatinine kinase (relevant for myocardial contusion, crush injury)
  - arterial blood gases
  - urinalysis for blood and myoglobin.
- *Radiology:* Trauma series. Most injured patients require three radiographs in the resuscitation room.
  - chest radiograph
  - lateral cervical spine radiograph. (A normal lateral radiograph does not exclude cervical spine injury. Other views are anteroposterior and odontoid. Immobilization of the spine must still be maintained until more definitive assessment.)
  - pelvis.

  Other radiological investigations that may be required in the trauma patient include:

  - CT scan, e.g. head, abdomen, chest, spine (Table 28.9)
  - full cervical spine series
    - radiographs of the extremities, thoracic spine, lumbosacral spine
    - skull radiograph
    - sternum radiograph
    - urethrogram (for suspected urethral injury)
    - cystogram (for suspected bladder injury).
  - angiogram (for suspected arterial injury; rarely, arch aortogram for suspected injury to the thoracic aorta).
- Special exams:
  - liver/spleen scan
  - pyelogram
  - compartment pressure measurement
  - echocardiogram
  - ECG in cases of chest trauma with suspected myocardial contusion.

Table 28.9 **CT imaging in acute trauma**
Gold standard for head trauma
Gold standard for abdominal trauma
Oral contrast via orogastric tube (visceral)
IV Contrast (Spleen, Liver, Pancreas, Kidney)
Useful in thoracic trauma

Definitive care

After completion of the secondary survey the following issues need to be addressed:

- *Response to resuscitation*
- *Prioritization of injuries* according to immediate threats to life and possible morbidity (in descending order of importance):
  - airway/breathing derangement
  - haemorrhage with shock

- intracranial space-occupying haemorrhage
- contained aortic disruption
- spinal cord compression
- vascular injury with distal ischaemia
- ruptured hollow viscus
- ocular injuries
- open or displaced fractures
- contaminated wounds
- other.

◆ *Analgesia:*

- *The cause of pain should be treated if possible*, e.g. finding a position of comfort for a fractured limb.
- Intravenous morphine titrated carefully will relieve severe pain. The intramuscular route should be avoided if possible as the absorption may be somewhat unpredictable and erratic in a seriously injured child. A suitable starting dose is 0.1–0.2 mg/kg; this does not usually mask clinical signs. Caution is required in hypotensive or lethargic children with head injury.
- Regional blocks can be very effective, e.g. femoral nerve block for femoral fracture.
- Nitrous oxide may be a useful adjunct, especially in orthopaedic injuries. It has been used in children as young as 16 months in the emergency department. Its use should be avoided in head injury, pneumothorax, or eye injuries.

◆ *Tetanus status (Table 28.10):* If the child has received three doses of diptheria, tetanus, pertussis vaccination (DTP) and the last dose was administered within 5 years, no further action is required. Otherwise, a tetanus toxoid booster is required. If the child has not been fully immunized, or there is a doubt about immunization status, then a tetanus immunoglobulin should be administered in addition to a tetanus toxoid (use separate syringes and inject at different sites).

◆ *Antibiotics:* A first-generation cephalosporin or penicillinase-resistant penicillin should be administered for open fractures, penetrating joint injuries, large contaminated soft tissue injuries, and penetrating eye injuries. If there is severe penicillin allergy, consider clindamycin or erythromycin. Penetrating abdominal injuries and perforated hollow viscera require broad-spectrum antibiotics, e.g. gentamicin, amoxicillin, and metronidazole.

Table 28.10 Guide to tetanus prophylaxis in wound management

History of tetanus vaccination		Type of wound	DTP, DT (CDT), Td (ADT) or tetanus toxoid as appropriate	Tetanus immunoglobulin
3 doses or more	If <5 years since last dose	All wounds	No	No
	If 5–10 years since last dose	Clean minor wounds	No	No
		All other wounds	Yes	No
	If >10 years since last dose	All wounds	Yes	No
Uncertain, or <3 doses		Clean minor wounds	Yes	No
		All other wounds	Yes	Yes

- *Fractures and dislocations:* Orthopaedic injuries should be splinted and, if necessary, reduced in the emergency department. Early reduction will be required, especially if there is neurovascular compromise.
- *Wound management:* Open wounds should be cleaned, dressed, and covered to reduce the likelihood of infection. Lacerations should be sutured as indicated.

Trauma arrest

The outcome from children with an out-of-hospital cardiopulmonary arrest remain poor (Basket 1989, Hazibnski *et al.* 1994). This is also true of children who have suffered blunt trauma and are in cardiopulmonary arrest from the time of the injury. Underlying conditions to exclude if an 'on the scene' arrest has occurred with a response to treatment in the pre-hospital setting include children with serious neurological injury from a major head injury or those having juvenile cervical spine injury or spinal cord injury without radiological abnormality (SCIWORA). These injuries are mostly associated with an extremely poor prognosis, and this issue should be addressed. In general, trauma patients who deteriorate to the point of cardiopulmonary arrest have a poor outcome (Schoenfield and Baker 1993). The only exceptions are young patients who have suffered penetrating trauma such as a stab wound to the chest who lose their vital signs in the emergency department or immediately before arrival.

Managing a trauma arrest follows the principles of advanced life support with a focus on volume replacement and controlling haemorrhage.

Key points

- Managing a trauma arrest (Goetting 1995):
  - Commence cardiopulmonary resuscitation (CPR).
  - Incubate and ventilate with 100% oxygen.
  - Insert two large-bore cannulas or intraosseous needles and rapidly infuse volume at 20 mL/kg aliquots.
  - Decompress both hemithoraces either by needle thoracocentesis followed by intercostal tubes or by intercostal tubes alone.
  - Assess the rhythm on the ECG and treat appropriately.

The most common underlying rhythm disturbances leading to cardiopulmonary arrest in children are asystole/bradycardia and electromechanical dissociation or pulseless electrical activity (Colucci and Somberg 1994, APLS 1996). The underlying cause in almost all cases is profound hypovolaemia due to multiple injury. Unexpected hypoxia due to poor airway control should never be a cause for cardiopulmonary arrest in children in this day and age. The treatment of these rhythm disturbances uses standard protocols (Fig. 28.10). If there is no response then volume should be given to a total of 20 mL/kg. If the neck veins are distended or there is a strong suspicion of tamponade, a needle pericardiocentesis should be performed, or thoracotomy or subxiphoid window. If the pericardiocentesis is successful, immediate transfer to surgery should be arranged. It is important to remember that fluid volume resuscitation throughout the management of the cardiopulmonary arrest with crystalloid or preferably whole blood must be aggressively pursued using two large-bore intravenous cannulas.

Key point

- The outcome from children with an out-of-hospital cardiopulmonary arrest remains poor.

Post-resuscitation stabilization

Post-resuscitation stabilization for an injured child will entail continued supportive therapy together with urgent transfer to the emergency operating theatre. This care will need to be continued in the operating theatre, which should be prepared at

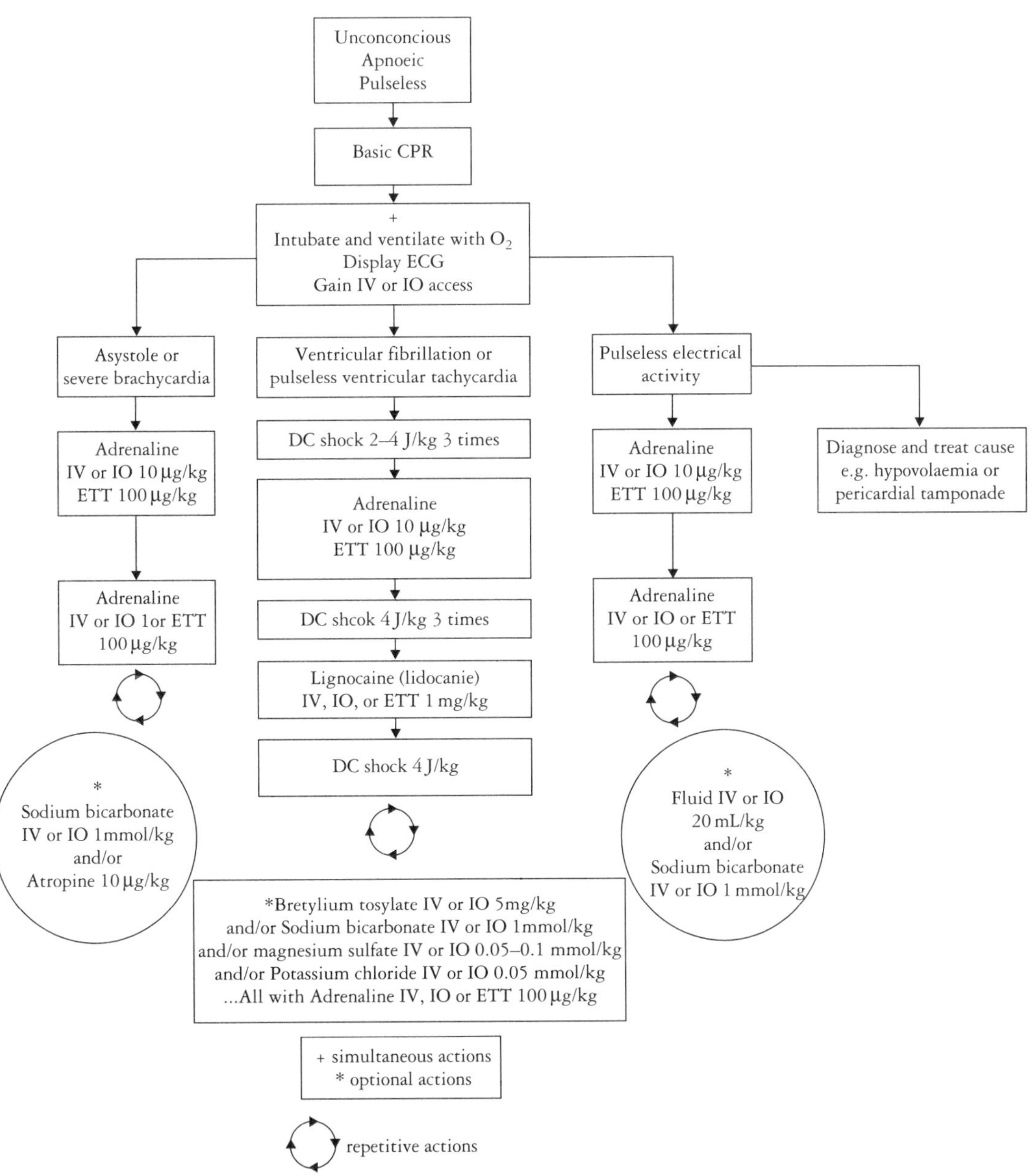

Figure 28.10 Protocol for management of cardiac arrest due to arrhythmia. (From the Australian Resuscitation Council Guidelines.)

the time the trauma call is put out. In most cases the cardiopulmonary arrest has occurred due to hypovolaemia as a result of near-fatal injuries and every member of the trauma team will need to be involved.

Once in the intensive care unit post-resuscitation stabilization will usually entail continued supportive therapy. Continuing support will usually include mechanical ventilation with supplemental oxygen, insertion of central and arterial lines, inotrope infusion, antiarrhythmic agents, fluid therapy, and possibly renal support (continuous veno-venous haemofiltration, peritoneal dialysis).

The cause of the cardiopulmonary arrest should be corrected if possible. Complications of resuscitation should also be sought, particularly if secondary deterioration occurs. A chest radiograph should be performed to check position of the ETT and the central venous catheter, to exclude pneumothorax, lung collapse or aspiration, and to check the cardiac outline. Investigations should include full blood count, arterial blood gas, and serum biochemistry.

As soon as possible, assessment of any neurological damage should be sought.

Emergency department thoracotomy

Emergency department thoracotomy as a technique for resuscitation of moribund thoracic trauma patients became popular in the 1960s. It is a controversial procedure in children and is not practiced at our institution. Enthusiasm for this procedure has waned as evidence has accumulated that patients do not benefit from it. In blunt trauma the evidence for any benefit is very scant indeed, with dismal survival rates of $<1\%$ in better studies (Balazs 1983). We believe that resources are best directed into areas where returns will be higher, such as better pre-hospital trauma care and improved trauma systems. The resources and organization that needs to be available to perform this technique 24 hours a day are often beyond even the financial scope of major trauma centres. It must be left up to the particular institution to weigh up the benefits of such an approach. If penetrating trauma makes up a large component of the daily trauma workload, benefits may occasionally be seen from emergency department thoracotomy.

Children with blunt trauma who sustain cardiopulmonary arrest at the scene of the injury and in whom CPR does not result in return of cardiac function are almost uniformly unsalvageable, and do not benefit from thoracotomy in the emergency department (Sheikh and Culbertson 1993). Children with penetrating trauma who suffer loss of vital signs at the scene, and have no electrical cardiac activity in the emergency department after standard CPR in the ambulance, do not benefit from thoracotomy either, especially if the pre-hospital time is >20 minutes (Millham and Gringlinger 1993). Paediatric trauma resources are better directed to other more productive areas such as injury prevention.

Cessation of resuscitation

Cardiac arrest in children has a poor outcome. The decision to stop resuscitation is based on a number of variables including the pre-arrest state, response to resuscitation, reversible factors, patient and parental wishes, likely outcome, and opinions of experienced staff. Senior medical staff are responsible for the decision to terminate resuscitation and should almost always be consulted.

Transfer of the injured child

Adequate attention at the referring hospital to the ABCs of resuscitation by those most experienced in paediatric care is more likely to reduce morbidity and mortality than rapid transfer to a tertiary centre (McNab 1991). Criteria for interhospital transfer are summarized in Table 28.11.

Reasons for transfer of children

- need for expert centralized care
- need for specialist services only available in a children's hospital
- remoteness of the referring hospital
- resources available in referral hospital
- type of service available in the referring hospital
- designated transfer criteria.

Some considerations in the transport of critically ill children

- patience and attention to detail will win the day
- transport methods

Table 28.11 Interhospital triage criteria: trauma

Central nervous system: head injury penetrating injury or depressed skull fracture open injury with or without CSF leak severe injury (GCS <10) or GCS deterioration lateralizing signs
Spinal cord injury
Chest: wide superior mediastinum major chest wall injury cardiac injury ventilated patient
Pelvis: pelvic ring disruption any pelvic injury with shock and evidence of continuing haemorrhage open pelvic injury pelvic visceral injury
Multiple system injury: severe face injury with head injury chest injury with head injury abdominal or pelvic injury with head injury burns with head injury
Evidence of high-energy impact: motor vehicle–pedestrian >40km/h motor vehicle accident with serious damage ejection of patient, or rollover death of occupant in same vehicle
Comorbid factors: extreme age <2 years underlying chronic disease
Secondary deterioration
Burns: 10% of body critical anatomical sites associated complications, pulmonary injury, carbon monoxide, cyanide poisoning

- types of transport teams, paramedic based, specialized, pressure to 'scoop and run'
- the 'golden hour' concept does not apply to the transport of critically ill children
- airway problems and respiratory compromise are the most common reasons for transport
- 50% of critically ill children require some form of airway intervention
- the airway needs to be either protected or stabilized
- accidental extubation should never occur.

Procedures performed prior to transport

- intubation 60%
- reintubation 30%
- repositioning ETT 50%
- ventilation 50%
- chest drain insertion 0.9%.

Ventilation of the transported patient

- For intrahospital transport, hand ventilation is acceptable. Use a ventilator (e.g. Oxylog) for all others.
- It is not easy duplicate mechanical ventilator settings using hand ventilation: there is a 75% incidence of changes in haemodynamic status and blood gases.

Mode of transport:

- *Ground transport:* Short to middle distance.
- *Helicopter:* Medium to long distances, limited room, ensure child stable, hypovolemia corrected, air collections drained.
- *Fixed wing aircraft:* Long journeys; need to ensure connectors are compatible, gas supplies adequate, and child stable. Factors to consider, space, speed of transport, cost, distance, severity of illness, safety of staff and patient.

Adverse events during transport

- *Respiratory events (64%):* Accidental tracheal extubation, occlusion of the ETT with secretions, secondary hypoxia from hypoventilation, acute airway obstruction other than secretions, acute gastric dilatation events during transport.
- *Cardiovascular events (24%):* hypertension, hypotension, cardiac arrest, hypothermia and related events.
- Central nervous system events (40%).
- Secondary brain insult, seizures (24%).

Transport within the hospital can be the greatest threat to the trauma patient (Wallen *et al.* 1995). Even in the best hands it can result in adverse events for the trauma patient, such as changes in vital signs, alteration in ventilation or oxygenation, equipment failure and—most important—the sequelae of unrecognized shock during a radiology procedure. The radiology suite is notorious in being the main area where an unstable or poorly differentiated trauma patient can come to grief, particularly if shock has not been anticipated or aggressively anticipated.

Key points

- Rules for transport within the hospital:
  - Pre-transport co-ordination/communication: have a plan, think in advance about what may go wrong, and formulate solutions.
  - Ensure personnel who accompany the patient are aware of potential problems and their solutions.
  - Ensure that the equipment to accompany the patient is in working order and fully charged, and that adequate oxygen and air is available. Always be a 'parasite' as far as electrical power and oxygen is concerned. Only use your own battery power or gases when absolutely necessary.
  - Monitoring during transport, pre-transport co-ordination, communication, accompanying personnel, equipment.
  - Constantly monitor the ABCs.

Key points

- Interhospital transport checklist:
  - Copy all patient records and radiographs.

- Obtain transport consent.
- Secure vascular access and ETT.
- Stabilize cervical spine and any fractures.
- Prepare blood products.
- If indicated, provide laboratory telephone number for pending laboratory results.
- Be aware of the capabilities of the transferring hospital.
- Be aware of the support services available.
- Ensure appropriate monitoring during transport.
- Constant clinical evaluation.

Key point

- Intrahospital transport can be the greatest threat to the trauma patient.

Conclusion

Trauma was the epidemic of the late twentieth century. Although it still accounts for a large number of paediatric deaths, these have reduced in many western countries over the last decade. This has come about through a number of factors including improved trauma care, trauma systems, and better pre-hospital care for injured children. However, one area that continues to be important in reducing morbidity and mortality from trauma in children is injury prevention. In many countries prevention strategies, such as wearing of cycle helmets and seatbelts to name just two, have made a significant impact on death rates and morbidity related to trauma.

However, despite the best prevention strategies, children will continue to be injured and therefore the knowledge, skills, and resources will always be needed to resuscitate and stabilize seriously injured children.

Key points

- Trauma is the leading cause of death in children >1 year of age.
- AIS, ISS, PTS and revised trauma score are classifications for describing site and severity of multiple trauma.
- Management of trauma is prioritized: primary survey (ABCDE) and resuscitation, secondary survey then definitive care.

References

APLS (1996) *Advanced Paediatric Life Support (APLS): The practical approach*. BMJ Publishing, London.

Balazs IM (1983) Emergency thoracotomy in the management of trauma. *JAMA* 249: 1891–1896.

Basket PJF (1989) *Resuscitation handbook*. Gower Medical Publishing, London.

Colucci RD, Somberg JC (1994) Treatment of cardiac arrhythmias. In: Chernow B (ed.) *The pharmacologic approach to the critically ill patient*, 3rd edn. Williams & Wilkins, Baltimore, Md.

Goetting MG (1995) Progress in pediatric cardiopulmonary resuscitation. *Emergency Medicine Clinics of North America* 13(2): 291–319.

Hahn YS, Chyung C, Barthel MJ *et al.* (1988) Head injuries in children under 36 months of age—demography and outcome. *Child's Nervous System* 4: 34–40.

Hazibnski MF *et al.* (1994) Outcome of cardiovascular collapse in pediatric blunt trauma. *Annals of Emergency Medicine* 23: 1229–1235.

McNab JM (1991) Optimal escort for interhospital transport of pediatric emergencies. *Journal of Trauma* 31: 205–209.

Millham FH, Gringlinger GA (1993) Survival determinants in patients undergoing emergency room thoracotomy for penetrating chest injury. *Journal of Trauma* 34: 332–336.

Rubin MA, Sadonohoff N (1996) Neuromuscular blocking agents in the emergency department. *Journal of Emergency Medicine* 14(2): 193–199.

Rupert JE, McCabe M, Thomas R (1994) Intraosseous infusion. *British Journal of Hospital Medicine* 51(4): 161–164.

Schoenfield PS, Baker MD (1993) Management of cardiopulmonary and trauma resuscitation in the pediatric emergency department. *Pediatrics* 91: 726–729.

Sheikh AA, Culbertson CB (1993) Emergency department thoracotomy in children: rationale for selective application. *Journal of Trauma* 34: 323–328.

Wallen E *et al.* (1995) Intrahospital transport of critically ill pediatric patients. *Critical Care Medicine* 23: 1588–1595.

Further reading

American College of Surgeons (1997) *Advanced trauma life support (ATLS) manual.*

Advanced Life Support Committee of the Australian Resuscitation Council (1996) Paediatric advanced life support—the Australian Resuscitation Council Guidelines. *Medical Journal of Australia* 165: 199–206.

Australian Resuscitation Council Policy Statements No. 4.4 (July 1988); No. 5.4 (July 1991); No. 7.1.2 (December 1990); No. 7.1.1 (March 1994); No. 12.1 (November 1995); No. 12.2 (November 1995); No. 12.3 (November 1995); No. 12.4 (November 1995); No. 12.6 (November 1995); No. 12.7 (November 1995); No. 12.8 (November 1995); No. 12.9 (November 1995).

Braman SS, Dunn SM, Amico CA, Millman RP (1987) Complications of intrahospital transport in critically ill patients. *Annals of Internal Medicine* 107(4): 469–473.

Brown TCK, Fisk GC (1992) *Anaesthesia for children*, 2nd edn. Blackwell Scientific, Oxford.

Chameides L (ed.) *Textbook of pediatric advanced life support.* American Heart Association, Dallas.

Duncan AW (1990) Acute respiratory failure in children. In: Oh TE (ed.) *Intensive care manual*, 3rd edn. Butterworths, Sydney, pp 634–643.

Gorback MS (1990) *Emergency airway management.* BC Decker, Philadelphia.

Graneto JW *et al.* (1993) *Transport and stabilisation of the pediatric trauma patient. Pediatric Clinics of North America* 40: 365–379.

Guidelines for cardiopulmonary resuscitation and emergency care (1992) Pediatric Basic Life Support. *JAMA* 268: 2251–2261.

Henning R (1992) Emergency transport of critically ill children: stabilisation before departure. *Medical Journal of Australia* 156: 117–124.

Hirschman AM, Kravath RE (1982) Venting vs ventilation. A danger of manual resuscitation bags. *Chest* 82: 369–370.

Horan MJ (1987) Report of the second task force on blood pressure in children. *Pediatrics* 79: 1–25.

Inaba AS, Seward PN (1991) An approach to pediatric trauma. *Emergency Medicine Clinics of North America* 9: 523–547.

Jaffe D, Wesson D (1991) Emergency management of blunt trauma in children. *New England Journal of Medicine* 324: 1477–1482.

Kanter RK (1987) Evaluation of mask-bag ventilation in resuscitation of infants. *American Journal of Diseases of Childhood* 141: 761–763.

Kisson N, Tepas JJ, DiScala C *et al.* (1996) Is the golden hour a valid concept for the injured child. 6th ICEM, 1996, Sydney, Australia, Paper 274.

MacKellar A (1995) Deaths from injury in childhood in Western Australia, 1983–1992. *Medical Journal of Australia* 162: 238–242.

Milner AD (1991) Resuscitation of the newborn. *Archives of Disease of Childhood* 66: 66–69.

Motoyama EK, Davis PJ (1990) *Smith's anesthesia for infants and children*, 5th edn. CV Mosby, St Louis.

Paediatric Life Support Working Party of the European Resuscitation Council (1994) Guidelines for paediatric life support. *BMJ* 308: 1349.

Peclet MH, Newman KD, Eichelberger MR (1990) Patterns of injury in children. *Journal of Pediatric Surgery* 25: 85–91.

Richmond CE, Bingham RM (1995) Paediatric cardiopulmonary resuscitation. *Paediatric Anaesthesia* 5: 11–27.

Rosen M, Laurence KM (1965) Expansion pressure and rupture pressures in the newborn lung. *Lancet* ii: 721–722.

Schafermeyer R (1993) Pediatric trauma. *Emergency Medicine Clinics of North America* 11: 187–204.

Tobias JD (1996) The laryngeal mask airway: a review for the emergency physician. *Pediatric Emergency Care* 12(5): 370–373.

Yamamoto LG (1991) Rapid sequence anaesthesia induction and advanced airway management in pediatric patients. *Emergency Medicine Clinics of North America* 9(3): 611–613.

Yamamoto LG, Yim GK, Britten AG (1990) Rapid sequence anesthesia induction. *Pediatric Emergency Care* 6: 200–213.

29

CHAPTER 29

Paediatric orthopaedics

NANNI ALLINGTON AND PETER TEMPLETON

CHAPTER 29
Paediatric orthopaedics

NANNI ALLINGTON AND PETER TEMPLETON

Children are not just small adults. Growth is a factor that is central to the problems and the solutions of paediatric fracture management. Growth can be an advantage by aiding in the correction of angular deformity or remodelling a fracture, but a disadvantage if growth arrest occurs. The initial work-up should eliminate the possibility of an underlying disease, and identify any associated injuries.

Management of childhood fractures is conservative in most cases and includes reduction, immobilization, and rehabilitation. Operative treatment is limited to specific fractures. Immobilization has to be adequate. Material that children can remove prematurely must be avoided: young children can easily remove short arm and short leg casts. Physical therapy after fracture immobilization is sometimes required. Physical examination, including neurovascular and soft tissue evaluation, is essential in the initial work-up of all fractures and will be mentioned in the text only if it is particular or special to the described fracture.

To keep the chapter succinct, classifications have been kept to a minimum. For some types of fractures where there is more than one good classification, only one will be used in this chapter for the same practical reasons.

Key points

- Growth is a major factor in the management of fractures in children.
- Management is usually non-operative.

Epiphyseal fractures

Growth plate

Epiphyseal fractures are potentially more severe than diaphyseal fractures because the epiphysis contains both the articular surface and the growth plate. The growth plate is made of several different layers of cells grouped into zones:

- The *resting zone* is adjacent to the epiphysis. Lipids and other nutritional elements are stored in this zone. The cells are sparse and the matrix is abundant. This zone is avascular.
- In the *proliferative zone*, cells multiply and matrix is formed. This zone is well vascularized.
- The *hypertrophic zone* is divided into the zone of maturation, the zone of degeneration, and the zone of provisional calcification. The chondrocytes change shape and the matrix slowly gets ready for calcification. Complex biochemical reactions are involved.

Any trauma to these layers will have a potentially damaging effect, and thus affect the harmonious growth of the involved bone.

There are several types of growth plates and most of them are responsible for the growth in length of the bone. The growth plate (physis) lies between the epiphysis and metaphysis in long bones. Any injury to the physis can result in growth arrest. The different growth plates contribute a different proportion to the growth of an individual bone. In the upper extremity the majority of growth comes from the proximal humerus and the distal radius and ulna. There is much less growth in length around the elbow. In the lower extremity the majority of growth is found around the knee, with the distal femur contributing about 1 cm per year.

Apophyses are similar to growth plates but are situated at the insertion of tendons into bone. An injury to these can be responsible for an abnormal shape of the bone. For example, an injury to the greater trochanter will result in a coxa vara and to the tibial tuberosity will result in genu recurvatum.

Key point

- Epiphyseal fractures are potentially deforming.

Classification

The most commonly used classification of fractures involving the growth plate is the one proposed by Salter and Harris (1963) (Fig. 29.1). In general the severity of the lesion increases from Salter I to V. This classification does not include all of the possible variants. Ogden (1982) proposed a more complex classification with further subgroups.

- *Salter–Harris type I fractures* affect the hypertrophic zone. This zone is avascular and the cells distally are intact, so there is a very low risk of growth arrest.
- *Salter–Harris type II fractures* also affect the hypertrophic zone but then go through a piece of the metaphysis. This is the most common Salter–Harris fracture and rarely causes growth arrest except in the distal femur.
- *Salter–Harris type III fractures* again affect the hypertrophic zone but then extend distally on to the articular surface.
- *Salter–Harris type IV fractures* are a combination of type II and III fractures. There is a great potential to develop an epiphyseodesis because of the possible malalignment of the physis. Perfect reduction is mandatory but does not guarantee absence of arrest.
- *Salter–Harris type V fractures* are compression injuries of the growth plate. They are the most serious type of injuries and are often only suspected with the discovery of growth arrest at a later date. This type of injury can also be seen as the result of chronic stress: injury to the distal radius growth plate in young gymnasts.

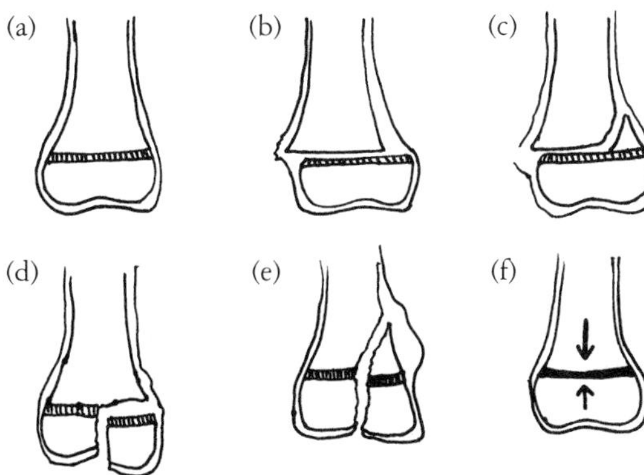

Figure 29.1 Salter–Harris classification of growth plate injuries: (a) normal; (b) type I; (c) type II; (d) type III; (e) type IV; (f) type V. See text for details.

Key point

- The Salter–Harris classification is the most widely used for fractures involving the growth plate.

Radiology

After good clinical evaluation, radiographs are the next basic investigation. It is important to image the entire bone in two orthogonal views, including the proximal and distal joints, to look for other potential injuries. Fractures can be overlooked in the younger child, as large areas are still cartilaginous. The presence of many secondary ossification centres can be particularly confusing, especially around the elbow. A traumatized young child may require sedation before an adequate evaluation can be performed. If the fracture is unusual or difficult to diagnose, it may be useful to image the other side for comparison. In the case of an intra-articular fracture, a CT scan will be helpful to determine the exact amount of displacement which is usually more than what is seen on plain films, e.g. triplane fracture.

Key point

- Radiographs of fractures in children may be difficult to interpret because large areas may be cartilaginous.

Complications

Growth arrest

The growth plates that are the most sensitive to trauma are the distal femur and the proximal tibia. The arrest can be symmetrical with leg-length discrepancy, or asymmetrical with a deviation of the involved bone. Any injury close to a growth plate will require a follow-up visit with radiograph 6–12 months after injury to verify the integrity of the growth plates. The discovery of an abnormality of the growth plate will require a work-up to determine whether the arrest is complete or if there is a partial bar. Radiography of the other side (to confirm that it is not naturally closing in the older child), tomograms, and CT scans will analyse the percentage of involved growth plate and map its location (Carlson and Wenger 1984).

If less than 50% of the growth plate is involved and there is still a significant amount of growth remaining, one can excise the osseous bridge. A direct approach can be performed if the bar is peripheral. Central bridges require a more complex approach via a transmetaphyseal window and the use of a dental mirror to visualize the bar and confirm its removal. The removal has to be complete. Fat or some other material has to be placed in the defect to keep it from tethering again. A non-weight-bearing cast is worn for a month in the lower extremity (Peterson 1984).

If the partial arrest has already produced axial deviation, an osteotomy can be added at the same surgical time. Close to the end of growth, an epiphyseodesis of the remaining part of the physis can be performed.

Conservative treatment is recommended if more than 50% of the growth plate is involved and the child is close to the end of growth. A minor discrepancy (up to 2 cm) of leg length is to be expected. Length discrepancy may be found in many normal children. A chart of leg-length discrepancy is compiled for each child from serial clinical examinations, scanograms, and bone age estimates. This will indicate the children who may require surgical correction (Moseley 1977). The younger the child, the greater the discrepancy. In the lower extremities use the following landmarks:

- <3 cm discrepancy at the end of growth: use a shoe lift.
- 3–5 cm: discuss epiphyseodesis of the longer extremity.
- >5 cm: propose lengthening procedures.

This will have to be adapted for the individual patient. A length discrepancy is much better tolerated in the upper extremity. The fractured extremity is usually stimulated, and an overgrowth of 1–2 cm is frequent. This rarely necessitates any type of treatment.

Intra-articular fractures

Fractures involving the epiphysis, such as Salter–Harris type III and IV fractures, will involve the articular surface and potentially damage the joint congruency. Tibia spine fractures are equivalent to anterior cruciate ruptures in adults and can cause instability.

Loss of motion

Children rarely develop permanent loss of motion and in general will not need any physical therapy after immobilization. Nevertheless, there are a few fractures (e.g. elbow, tibial, spine) that are more prone to loss of motion and, if it is still present after 6–12 months, a loss of motion may become permanent.

Treatment principles

Most epiphyseal fractures reduce by closed means but occasionally require open reduction. Intra-articular fractures require perfect reduction and possible internal fixation with wires or partially threaded screws. Since the osteosynthesis with pins is only used for alignment, immobilization in a cast is necessary until healing is complete. The vast majority of cases require only home exercises after removal of the cast.

Metaphyseal and diaphyseal fractures

Generalities

Metaphyseal and diaphyseal fractures are benign. In general:

- A thick periosteum and a good blood supply account for rapid healing (compared to the adult).
- The very thick cortex and the important periosteum also explain some particular type of fractures in the child: the torus (or buckle) fracture, the greenstick (or incomplete) fracture, and plastic deformation (Fig. 29.2).
- Complete fractures, as in the adult, are also seen.

Up to 15° of metaphyseal angulation will correct if there are 2 years of growth remaining in a child. Rotation or diaphyseal angulation will not correct significantly.

Key point

- Compared to epiphyseal fractures, metaphyseal and diaphyseal fractures are benign.

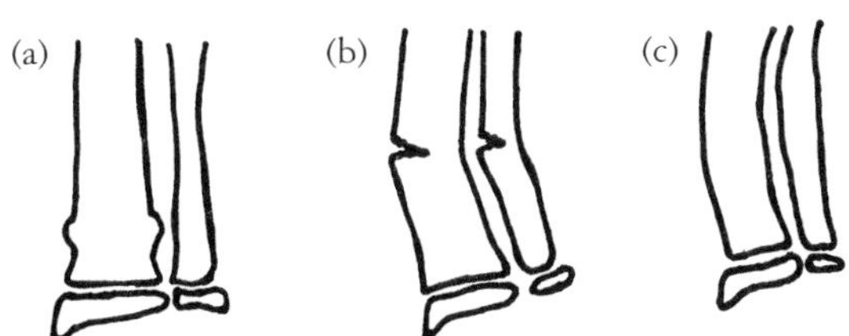

Figure 29.2 Fractures specific to children: (a) torus (buckle) fracture; (b) greenstick (incomplete) fracture; (c) plastic deformation.

Radiology

Good standard anteroposterior and lateral radiographs will usually be more than adequate to evaluate these fractures after a thorough clinical evaluation.

Treatment principles

Because of the potential of remodelling of these fractures, the vast majority of them can be treated conservatively in young children. Operative treatment is nowadays more often used in older children. This is mainly for social reasons. External fixation can be used in the child with multiple trauma, and in open fractures to facilitate nursing care (Hull and Bell 1997).

Complications

Incomplete reduction, hypertrophic callus, and malalignment will correct with time, especially in younger children. An overlap of the fracture could even be considered as favourable because of the natural stimulus of growth in the involved extremity.

Rotational malunion will not self-correct with time and can be responsible for loss of motion (decrease of pronation and supination of the forearm in a both-bone forearm fracture) or apparent angulation (elbow varus in a supracondylar fracture of the humerus).

Upper extremity

Shoulder

Clavicle fractures

A fracture of the clavicle is usually benign. Even if there is a large amount of displacement, surgery is not indicated. The basic treatment is a broad arm sling or a figure-of-eight bandage for 3–4 weeks. After application of the bandage, pulse and neurovascular status should be assessed, since compression can be seen with tight application. Parents have to be warned of the cosmetic issue of callus formation, and the slow remodelling. In the newborn, this fracture can be associated with brachial plexus palsy.

Very rarely the differential diagnosis of congenital pseudoarthrosis, must be considered. It is pain free and remains unchanged on serial radiographs. The right side is more often involved (Owen 1970).

Key points

- Clavicle injuries are treated non-operatively.
- Basic treatment is a figure-of-eight bandage for 3–4 weeks.

Shoulder dislocation

A traumatic dislocation in children <12 years of age is exceptional. An underlying disease (e.g. Ehlers–Danlos) has to be ruled out. Voluntary shoulder dislocation is seen in children and is very often related to psychological problems, which must be addressed (Rowe *et al.* 1973). One must refrain from surgery, even in the event of repeated dislocation in the child.

Acromioclavicular injury (Tolo 2000)

Injury to the acromioclavicular joint itself is rare and injuries in this location are often fractures of the distal clavicle. Treatment with a sling is best. Treat teenagers as adults (see Chapter 17, page 287).

Sternoclavicular injury (Tolo 2000)

Sternoclavicular injury is uncommon and the concerns are the same as in adults (i.e. anterior dislocation may become recurrent, posterior may impinge upon the mediastinum and require reduction. (See Chapter 17, page 288).

Proximal humerus fractures

Most fractures of the proximal humerus can be treated conservatively. For undisplaced fractures, or if the displacement is acceptable, a sling for 4 weeks will be sufficient. This growth plate is responsible for a great amount of growth and thus has a good potential for remodelling, especially in children <12 years (Dameron and Reibel 1969). The fracture may be reduced and placed in a thoracobrachial cast, or pinned and casted if the fractures are severely displaced. In exceptional circumstances, open reduction is required when reduction cannot be obtained. A common cause is incarceration of the biceps tendon in the fracture. This will leave a quite a visible incision. Proximal humeral epiphysis fracture can be seen in the newborn in association with a brachial plexus injury (Lemperg and Liliequist 1970).

Arm

Diaphyseal (shaft) humerus fractures

Diaphyseal fractures of the humerus are benign even if they look impressive clinically and on radiographs. If the fractures are due to direct trauma or twisting, beware of child abuse. Check distal neurological function. The parents will require much convincing that surgery is not needed. Treatment is conservative with a collar and cuff, swath, and Velpeau bandage. A coaptation splint is used if the fracture is situated in the midshaft and is displaced. A hanging cast is difficult to use in children. A thoracobrachial cast can be used if indicated. The younger the child, the faster the healing.

Surgery is indicated in open fractures or some multiple trauma. An external fixator or flexible intramedullary (IM) nails have been used for this purpose.

Radial nerve palsy maybe an indication for reduction and osteosynthesis (see Chapter 17, page 293). Consider exploration of the nerve at the 3–4 week stage.

Key points (Tolo 2000)

- An extension-abduction-external rotation injury in:
  - pre-teen produces a metaphyseal fracture
  - early teens produces a proximal physeal fracture
  - late teens produces an anterior shoulder dislocation.
- Note brachial plexus stretch injury.

- Treatment for all ages is closed reduction/sling/swath/Velpeau bandage.
- Remodelling occurs and open reduction and internal fixation is rarely indicated.
- Beware child abuse in diaphyseal fractures.

Elbow

Generalities

- The growth potential of the elbow is not great (about 20%) relative to the whole upper extremity and length discrepancy is thus not a major problem. The remodelling potential is low and reductions will have to be perfect. Early and late complications are frequent. Vascular complications are the most feared. They can be seen with any of the elbow fractures or dislocations and require frequent assessment to identify early compartment syndrome.
- Loss of motion is often seen and usually resolves on its own. Persistent stiffness of a joint is a rare occurrence in children, who in the majority of fractures recover their motion quite quickly after immobilization. The elbow is an exception, but improvement can be seen up to 1 year after the traumatic event. It is important to talk to parents about this problem. Loss of motion present 1 year after injury is permanent. A lack of extension <30° is quite well tolerated for everyday activity. Loss of motion in flexion is always limiting. Mobilization under general anaesthesia or other soft tissue releases do not give good results in children.
- Heterotopic ossification, especially brachialis muscle, can contribute to the loss of motion. In the majority of children, the deficit will heal and the ossification will slowly resorb. The child should avoid strenuous physical therapy.
- Rotational and angular deviations (cubitus varus or valgus) are mainly cosmetic problems and motion is usually satisfactory.
- Nerve palsies can be seen with Volkmann's syndrome but are also related directly to these fractures. Ulnar nerve palsy can also be secondary to cubitus valgus. The deficit is mainly sensory and resolution is the rule within 6–8 weeks. If the deficit is not resolving within 1 month, neurological evaluation by electromyogram should be performed.
- The diagnosis of elbow lesions in children is often underestimated because the cartilaginous structures are not visible on plain films. Contralateral films have their importance here. A strict anteroposterior and lateral view are also mandatory.

Key points

- The remodelling potential of the elbow is low, and reductions will have to be perfect.
- Be alert to complications, especially vascular.
- Loss of range of movement is common.

Supracondylar fractures of the humerus

A supracondylar fracture of the humerus is the most frequent fracture around the elbow (70%) and the one with the most complications. The most feared early complications are Volkmann's and acute arterial injury. Timely management and reduction will avoid dramatic situations. Fracture reduction will take care of most arterial compressions, but rare cases of arterial laceration will require exploration. Traction can be used as initial management in a very swollen elbow on occasions. Volkmann's ischaemia was more often seen with hyperflexion treatment, which is less commonly used nowadays.

Supracondylar fractures are classified into flexion and extension (95%) injuries. Depending on the degree of displacement, they are divided into three types:

- *type I:* undisplaced
- *type II:* displacement with intact posterior cortex
- *type III:* displacement with no cortical contact.

Treatment

- *Type I fractures* are treated by conservative means but immobilization has to be rigorous: long arm cast and sling strictly reinforced. In a turbulent child a thoracobrachial cast and coaptation splint might be necessary.
- *Type II and III fractures* require reduction, pinning, and cast immobilization for 3 weeks and an open reduction if appropriate reduction cannot be achieved by closed manipulation (Flynn *et al.* 1974, Wilkins 1997).

Technique: The elbow is reduced under general anaesthesia with use of fluoroscopy. First apply longitudinal traction to restore humero-ulnar angulation (i.e. align on anteroposterior view). Then your other hand hooks the olecranon and distal humerus onto the proximal end of the humerus. The elbow is gently hyperflexed to hold the position. Fluoroscopy is used to check the position.

- The goal is to restore Baumann's angle (the humeroulnar angle, 72 ± 4°).
- Note that if the fracture gap is obliterated, the fragment widths match, and Baumann's angle is restored then it can be assumed that the lateral view is also acceptable (Fig. 29.3).
- Two slightly divergent smooth pins may be inserted from the lateral side. Crossed pins are the most stable, but great care is required in placement of the medial pin to avoid damage to the ulna nerve. Remove pins at 3 weeks and leave out of cast.

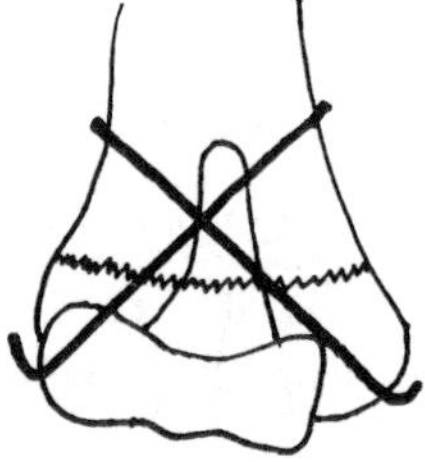

Figure 29.3 Osteosynthesis of supracondylar fracture.

Other techniques include:

- A Thomas splint where the arm is too swollen to flex; increase elbow flexion gradually over the following week. This is a cautious technique with good results.
- Trans-olecranon traction which allows gradual correction of deformity in all planes. After approximately 2 weeks, treatment can be changed to a cast once enough callus has formed.

Complications

- *Neurological (7%):* Radial nerve palsy is the most common and will recover in 6 months in most of the patients. A persistent dense median nerve palsy following fracture reduction may indicate entrapment of the nerve in the fracture necessitating exploration. The ulnar nerve is least likely to be involved.
- *Vascular (1%):*
  - If radial pulse present then lost after reduction, explore artery.
  - If radial pulse absent from injury and hand warm, observe.
  - If radial pulse absent from injury and hand cool, explore (Tolo 2000).
- *Stiffness* may limit elbow flexion. This restriction of movement is unlikely to improve with growth and will need surgical correction if disabling.
- *Late sequelae* are cubitus valgus (associated with tardy ulnar nerve palsy) or varus. Cubitus varus is a cosmetic problem secondary to inadequate reduction. Its incidence may be as high as 20% and is lowest with pinning. In the varus deformity, impaction of the medial portion of the growth plate can also be responsible. Varus deformity may require treatment with an osteotomy at any age after stiffness has resolved.

Key point

- Supracondylar fractures are the most common fracture around the elbow and have the most complications (including the most feared compartment syndrome or Volkmann's ischaemia and arterial injury).

Transphyseal fracture

Transphyseal fracture are seen in infants or toddlers. An arthrogram should be considered as the radiographs may be hard to interpret. There is medial displacement of the capitellar ossific nucleus.

This fracture is differentiated from a lateral condyle fracture by the presence of circumferential swelling and the fact that the ulna has shifted, unlike in lateral condyle fractures. It is treated with closed reduction and percutaneous pinning, otherwise cubitus varus may occur later. Elbow dislocations are rare in children <6 years of age.

Lateral condyle fractures of the humerus

Lateral condyle fractures of the humerus are often underestimated and are Salter III or IV intra-articular fractures.

Treatment

- Type I fractures are undisplaced and require long arm cast immobilization with weekly radiographs. There is a 10% chance of displacement of the fracture.
- Type II fractures show a lateral displacement and will need reduction and lateral pinning. Open reduction might be necessary. If an arthrogram shows that the articular surface is intact, then percutaneous pinning maybe possible after closed reduction (Tolo 2000).
- Type III fractures are completely displaced and rotated. They require open reduction and lateral pinning. Use 2–3 smooth Kirschner wires and remove pins at 3–4 weeks.
- Appropriate immobilization is required for 4 weeks. When performing an open reduction great care should be taken to avoid the posterior area where the vascular supply to the fragment lies.

Complications

Flynn (1989) describes the frequent complications of non-union and pseudarthrosis seen in the minimally displaced fractures. Non-union or pseudoarthrosis will require curettage, bone grafting, pinning, and immobilization. *In situ* cannulated screw fixation to compress the fracture is also a useful method.

Another complication is progressive cubitus valgus, with lateral growth arrest and possible secondary ulnar nerve palsy. This will require an osteotomy and an ulnar nerve transposition.

Fishtail deformity (seen on radiograph) and not clinically relevant. Avascular necrosis (AVN) is avoided by minimizing posterior soft tissue dissection.

Medial condyle fractures of the humerus

Medial condyle fractures of the humerus are intra-articular, rare, and severe. They require appropriate reduction and fixation (Fowles and Kassab 1980).

Medial epicondyle fracture of the humerus

Medial epicondyle fractures of the humerus are extra-articular (Fig. 29.4). Even significantly displaced fractures will heal well with conservative treatment. This includes temporary immobilization in a plaster backslab or sling until comfortable. The elbow must be mobilized early to prevent stiffness. If there is any valgus instability, open reduction and internal fixation (ORIF) is required. Incarceration of the medial epicondyle within the joint may occur and may be difficult to diagnose.

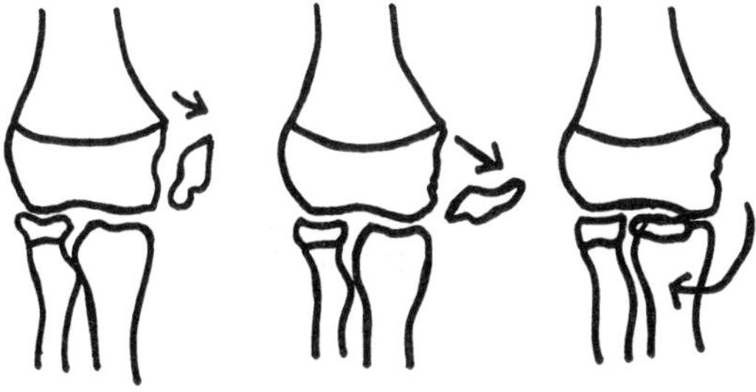

Figure 29.4 Medial epicondyle fractures of the humerus.

They require ORIF. Loss of elbow extension is frequently seen and parents should be warned of this possibility. Ulnar nerve palsies are also seen.

Lateral epicondyle fractures of the humerus

Lateral epicondyle fractures of the humerus are extra-articular and will require immobilization for about 3 weeks.

Posterior elbow dislocation

Posterior elbow dislocation is seen most commonly in males and is often associated with another fracture such as the medial epicondyle or radial head. In 10% of cases there is a nerve injury, but recovery is expected. Closed reduction is usually easy. If not, then suspect an entrapped medial epicondyle which will require open reduction. The elbow should be immobilized in 90° of flexion for a short period (1–2 weeks). Active movement should then be encouraged to prevent elbow stiffness. Ectopic calcification in the capsule is another problem that may result in stiffness.

Nursemaid or 'pulled' elbow

The nursemaid or 'pulled' elbow is seen in children between 1 and 5 years of age after a traction and forced pronation injury to the upper extremity. The child refuses to use the arm. The exact pathology of the injury is unknown, but plain films are always totally normal and the treatment is gentle passive forearm rotation and rest in a sling for 1–2 days.

Radial head and neck fractures

Fractures of the radial head and neck are quite frequent, and can be associated with elbow dislocation and other elbow fractures. Radial nerve palsy can be seen.

Treatment

- Undisplaced or displaced fractures with <35° of angulation have a good result with conservative treatment.
- Fractures that are significantly displaced with angulation >35° require reduction by manipulation.

Metaizeau *et al.* (1993) describe a technique where an IM wire is introduced distally and is used to reduce the displacement and to maintain it. Otherwise a percutaneous technique using the blunt end of a Kirschner wire to push the head back into position is usually successful. ORIF with a Kirschner wire via a lateral approach is rarely required. Transcapitellar wires should never be used as they usually break. Unsatisfactory results are often seen with open reduction due to AVN of the radial head.

Fully displaced fractures with a loss of contact between head and neck require surgery. Complication rates are high (about 30%). Radial head necrosis, cubitus valgus, radioulnar synostosis, and radial head overgrowth may occur. (D'Souza *et al.* 1993).

Olecranon fractures

Olecranon fractures are often associated with other elbow fractures, especially radial head fractures. They are often undisplaced and require immobilization. Rarely a displaced olecranon fracture might require open reduction, and the classical fixation with the figure-of-eight tension band wiring can be performed with the use of suture in the young child. Smooth Kirschner wires should be used in young children when the olecranon is less ossified.

Forearm

Two-bone fractures

Good anteroposterior and lateral radiographs are necessary and sedation may be required in the traumatized child. Care must be taken to always visualize both the wrist and the elbow, especially when only one bone is broken.

These fractures need adequate reduction. Rotational malunion will limit pronation and supination. Angulation often hides rotational malunion. Before the age of 10 years, 20° of pure angulation in the midshaft region is acceptable as this will correct with remodelling, but in older children reduction has to be perfect.

If reduction cannot be obtained or the fracture is unstable, surgery is indicated. Flexible IM nailing is a good alternative (Fig. 29.5) but technically

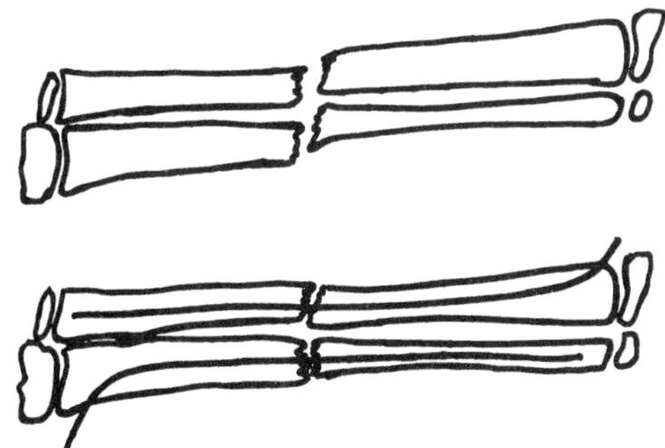

Figure 29.5 Midshaft radius and ulna fractures: flexible IM nailing.

demanding. In older children, reduction and plating as in adults is appropriate (Noonan and Price 1998). The plate length can be less than in adults as the fixation is protected with a cast (Tolo 2000).

These diaphyseal fractures may need 6–8 weeks of immobilization in a long arm cast. Refractures are frequent. Plastic deformation is a variant seen in children; it will not require any treatment in the child <4 years since it will remodel. In the older child it will require reduction under general anaesthesia and a gentle but firm continuous push of 5–10 minutes, to reverse the plastic deformation, followed by immobilization for 6–8 weeks (Sanders and Heckman 1984).

Key points

- Maintain interosseous separation, align rotation, mould ulnar border well.
- Repeat radiograph in first (and third) weeks to check for loss of reduction.
- Refractures occur.
- Beware plastic deformation.

Monteggia fracture

A Monteggia fracture is a fracture of the ulna associated with a dislocation of the radial head (Fig. 29.6). This fracture has a good prognosis when recognized and treated early. This is an often-missed fracture. Again good anteroposterior and lateral radiographs are needed with the elbow and wrist included in view. An isolated fracture of the ulna should not be missed (Bado 1967, Ring *et al.* 1998).

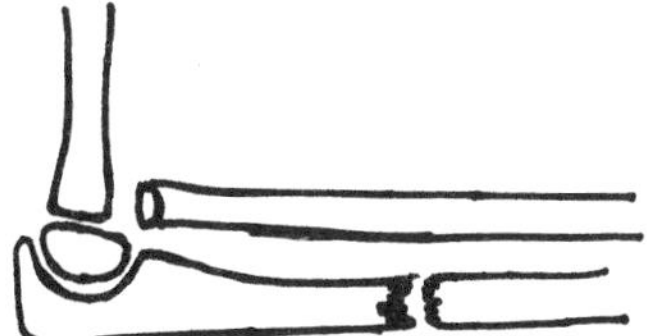

Figure 29.6 Monteggia fracture.

Classification

- *type 1 (60%):* anterior radial head dislocation with apex anterior proximal third ulnar fracture
- *type 2 (15%):* posterior radial head dislocation and apex posterior proximal third ulnar fracture
- *type 3:* lateral dislocation and proximal ulnar metaphyseal fracture
- *type 4:* anterior dislocation with proximal third radius and ulnar fractures.

Treatment

This fracture requires reduction under general anaesthesia and immobilization in a long arm cast for 6 weeks. The radial head typically relocates with reduction of the ulna. The proximal radiohumeral joint should be screened continuously during forearm supination and pronation to confirm the radial head's position. Irreducible radial head dislocations maybe associated with posterior interosseous nerve entrapment. Redislocation is associated with premature mobilization within 3 weeks of the injury and failure to reduce the original ulnar fracture.

If discovered within 3 months, non-operative treatment may be adequate. Many cases of late diagnosis require corrective osteotomy of the ulna and open reduction of the radial head with stabilization by the Bell-Tawse procedure (Bell-Tawse 1965). The results are often poor. It may be better to wait for the end of growth and deal with the prominent radial head by resection. Another sequela is limitation of pronation and supination. Late discoveries have to be differentiated from a congenital dislocation of the elbow. This abnormality might be unrecognized in a young child until a trauma occurs and the decrease in pronation and supination is noted. A radiograph of the other elbow will be help helpful if the condition is bilateral.

Key points

- Good prognosis if recognized and treated early.
- Monteggia fractures are often missed unless adequate radiographs are performed.
- Late discoveries have to be differentiated from a congenital dislocation of the elbow.

Galeazzi fractures

The Galeazzi fracture is a fracture of the radius associated with a dislocation of the distal radioulnar joint. This combination is rare, and good anteroposterior and lateral radiographic views are necessary in order to be able to make the diagnosis. Conservative treatment with reduction and immobilization in a long arm cast for 4–6 weeks is all that is required in the vast majority of patients (Walsh *et al.* 1987).

Greenstick fractures

This is a cortical compaction fracture on the concave side of the bone (Tolo 2000). Improve position by pronation and flexion to reduce volar angulation. Mould the cast into slight overcorrection and cast for 5–6 weeks.

Torus fracture

Torus fractures are low-impact fractures, seen in young children, and treated with short arm plaster backslab for 3 weeks.

Wrist

Distal fractures of the radius and ulna

A distal fracture of the radius or ulna is the most common childhood fracture. Fractures proximal to the growth plate are benign, and if displaced, will require reduction. Again some degree of displacement is acceptable. The younger the child, the closer to the growth plate, the more angulation is acceptable (Larsen *et al.* 1988); i.e. accept angulation in plane of motion and depending upon age:

- *age 4:* 30°
- *age 10:* 10°
- bayonet apposition is acceptable if <10 years old.

Immobilization in a long arm cast for 4–6 weeks is adequate. A short arm cast would theoretically be enough, but will be removed by young active children, or at least will not prevent them from using the involved upper extremity. This would increase the risk of secondary displacement and delayed union.

Fractures of the growth plate will need adequate reduction and might require pinning for stabilization. Salter I fractures can be mistaken for contusions or sprains. The distal growth plates are responsible for 80% of the growth, and an injury to one of the growth plates will give severe axial deviation. Clinical and radiological examination 6–8 months after the injury to verify adequate growth is recommended (Ray *et al.* 1996). Closed reduction will require overnight observation in the hospital. Median nerve palsies can occur. Growth arrest is rare (<1%).

Key point

- The most common childhood fracture.
- *Treatment:* long arm cast for 4–6 weeks.

Carpal fractures

Scaphoid fractures are rare and require conservative treatment.

Hand

Metacarpal fractures and phalangeal fractures

Metacarpal fractures and phalangeal fractures are often associated with more generalized hand injury (soft tissue injury, nerve and vascular injury) and require appropriate referral.

Acceptable angulation depends upon which metacarpal is fractured:

- accept up to 45° for the fifth metacarpal
- accept up to 10° for the second metacarpal.

Isolated metacarpal fractures require simple immobilization with the metacarpophalangeal joint in flexion. Reduction and pinning might be required for displaced fractures with rotation.

Open reduction for metacarpal fractures is required for:

- multiple fractures
- some oblique fractures with shortening (Tolo 2000).

Isolated phalangeal fractures will require adequate reduction; some angulation in the diaphysis will correct with growth.

A fracture through the growth plate will require perfect reduction, and pinning might be necessary. Rotational malalignment is a frequent complication and can be easily detected after reduction by flexing all the fingers together. Fingers should be immobilized by syndactylization or 'buddy strapping' with the adjacent finger for a maximum of 3 weeks. A short forearm cast with an aluminium splint is another alternative. Physical therapy might be necessary. In the younger child, more durable immobilization should be used to prevent the child from removing it (Barton 1979).

Open reduction for phalangeal fractures is required for:

- displaced intra-articular fractures
- oblique, shortened midshaft fractures.

Lower extremity

Pelvis

Pelvic fractures

Pelvic fractures are rare in children and are associated with severe trauma. Pedestrian–motor vehicle accidents are the primary cause. Thorough resuscitation is essential. Associated injuries to the head, chest, abdomen, and limbs must be ruled out.

Routine radiographs including anteroposterior, inlet and outlet views should be complemented by CT scan evaluation. CT scanning is most useful in studying breaks in the pelvic ring, evaluating displacement in acetabular fractures, revealing incarcerated fragments and incongruency, and following up the healing process.

Classifications of pelvic fractures are abundant and confusing in both the adult and the paediatric literature. A prognostic classification is advocated by Rang (1983):

- uncomplicated fractures
- fractures complicated by visceral injuries requiring surgical exploration
- fractures with immediate massive haemorrhage.

Key and Conwell (1951) proposed the following fracture classification. Only the fracture is described:

1 No break in the pelvic ring.
   a *Avulsion fractures:* Avulsions at the level of the anterior superior iliac spine, the anterior inferior iliac spine, and the ischial tuberosity can be seen in children during strenuous sporting activity. Conservative treatment is the rule.
   b *Pubis, ischium and iliac wing:* Pubic, ischial and iliac wing fractures in the child occur with severe trauma and any associated injuries will have to be managed. The treatment of these uncomplicated fractures is bed rest for a week, and then non-weight bearing for another 4–6 weeks.
2 Single break in the pelvic ring.
   a Fracture of two ipsilateral rami.
   b Fracture near or subluxation of the symphysis pubis.
   c Fracture near or subluxation of the sacroiliac joint.

The symphysis pubis and the sacroiliac joint have a certain degree of mobility, which explains the possibility of a single break in the pelvic ring, even with severe displacement. Associated lesions have to be ruled out, especially if the displacement is severe.

The treatment is conservative. Bed rest, associated with or without lower limb traction, application of a spica cast or pelvic sling in selected patients for 2–6 weeks, followed by non-weight-bearing for another 4–6 weeks. The different conservative modalities are chosen depending on the circumstances, the degree of reduction on radiographs and other conditions (e.g. abdominal trauma will hinder the use of a spica cast).

3 Double break in the pelvic ring.

  a Double vertical fractures or dislocation of the pubis.

  b Double vertical fractures or dislocation (Malgaigne).

  c Severe multiple fracture.

All these fractures are the result of very high-velocity trauma, e.g. a pedestrian struck by a motor vehicle. Associated injuries are almost always present.

In a child, especially a young one, significant remodelling will occur even in quite severe displacement. The management of the fracture is therefore conservative in most instances: bed rest associated with lower limb traction for 4–6 weeks, then non-weight-bearing for another 4–6 weeks. The older the child, the longer the treatment.

For double vertical fractures or dislocation, a reduction under general anaesthesia should be performed and a well-adjusted pelvic sling used. The pelvic injury may need an external fixator. Children rarely sustain severe multiple fractures. In these very rare cases, the management of the pelvic fracture is decided on an individual basis, either operative or non-operative treatment.

Key points

- In haemodynamically stable patients work-up thoroughly with CT or ultrasound scanning, peritoneal lavage, and, if necessary, mini-lapratomy.

4 Fractures of the acetabulum.

  a Small fragment associated or not with hip dislocation: Hip dislocation will dictate the treatment. After hip reduction, incarceration of a small bony fragment has to be ruled out. Simple small fragment fractures are treated with bed rest and non-weight-bearing ambulation.

  b Linear fractures associated with non-displaced pelvic fracture: Treatment again is conservative. Bed rest for 4–6 weeks followed by non-weight-bearing ambulation for another 4–6 weeks. Lower limb traction and a spica cast can also be used. CT scanning should be used to verify that there is no secondary displacement.

  c Linear fractures associated with hip joint instability: The treatment of these fractures is similar to the treatment in adults, and can usually be accomplished by traction on the involved extremity and bed rest for 6 weeks followed by non-weight-bearing ambulation. Surgical treatment should be reserved for the select group of patients where reduction can not be obtained. Poor results will occur in the more severe cases irrespective of whether surgery is performed or not.

  d Fractures secondary to central dislocation of the acetabulum: The management is the same as in adults and the results are poor. Any of these fractures may involve the triradiate cartilage. Triradiate cartilage fractures necessitate a perfect reduction. Growth arrest of the triradiate cartilage will affect hip joint congruity and may lead to hip subluxation and early arthrosis.

> Heeg *et al.* (1988) state that these fractures are often associated with multiple injuries, and are easily missed. Children with pelvic trauma should be followed for at least 1 year with clinical and radiological evaluation.

In summary, the vital prognosis of pelvic fractures in children depends on the associated lesion. The fracture will respond to conservative management of bed rest and traction until union in 4–6 weeks. Surgery might be required in very selected patients. In adolescents the management is similar to that of adults.

Key points

- Associated with severe trauma and other injuries.
- A CT scan is required.
- Classification by Key and Conwell (1951).
- Non-operative management in most cases.

Upper leg

Hip dislocation

Hip dislocation is rarely seen in a child, and is the result of very severe trauma. It can be isolated but is more often associated with pelvic, acetabular, or proximal femoral trauma. Posterior dislocation is the most frequent. Sciatic nerve palsy must be ruled out. Osteonecrosis of the head is the major complication. Reduction has to be performed as soon as possible (within 24 hours), and good anteroposterior and lateral radiographs have to be performed to check the head's position. A CT scan is required if there is any doubt. In young children, a spica cast should be applied for 4–6 weeks, followed by mobilization. Older children should stay in traction.

AVN of the femoral head is one of the major complications and can be seen up to 18 months after the injury. Regular clinical and radiological assessments are thus mandatory.

Key points

- Hip dislocation is associated with severe trauma.
- Rule out sciatic nerve injury.
- Reduce within 24 hours.

Proximal femur fractures (hip)

Fractures of the proximal femur are severe injuries resulting from high-energy trauma. The complication rate is high. Similar lesions as associated with pelvic fractures can be seen.

Delbet's classification is widely used (Colonna 1928):

- *type I:* transepiphyseal
  - A: without hip dislocation
  - B: with hip dislocation.
- *type II:* transcervical—most common
- *type III:* cervicotrochanteric—may drift into varus
- *type IV:* intertrochanteric—lowest risk of complications.

Treatment

- *Type I fractures* require reduction. Younger child may be immobilized in a cast. Older children may require cannulated screw fixation. Open reduction may be required if closed methods fail.
- *Type II fractures* require closed reduction and pinning with cannulated screws.
- *Type III fractures* should be gently reduced, if displaced, and fixed with cannulated screws to avoid further displacement.
- *Type IV fractures* require reduction and can be immobilized with a cast or skeletal traction. ORIF with a cannulated hip screw system should be considered for children with multiple injuries.

Complications

The sequelae are severe and frequent.

- *AVN* of the head is the most feared and frequent complication. It can be seen up to

18 months after the fracture. AVN can involve the head, neck, or both. Follow-up is thus critical, as well as explanation to parents. AVN is the norm in type I fractures (up to 100% according to some authors). It is seen in 50% of type II and 25% of type III, but is less frequent in type IV fractures (Canale and Bourland 1977). Significant displacement is more often associated with necrosis. Treatment of AVN is mainly conservative and consists of non-weight-bearing ambulation.

- *Delayed union:* These fractures have a high potential for delayed union. Non-union and pseudoarthrosis formation is uncommon. These complications may require better immobilization or bone grafting plus osteosynthesis.
- *Chondrolysis* causes stiffness and pain. Radiographs reveal a decreased articular distance. It can be caused by pin penetration of the joint space or AVN. Treatment is conservative and frustrating.
- *Coxa vara* is seen in 20% of these fractures and is often secondary to poor reduction, AVN or growth plate closure. It will require a valgus osteotomy if the neck-shaft angle is below 100°. Growth plate closure will lead to a leg length discrepancy; the contribution of the proximal femur physis to the growth of the lower extremity is 15%.

Key point

- Proximal femur fractures have a high complication rate.

Diaphyseal fractures

Diaphyseal fractures are frequent and mostly benign (Canale 1995). In the younger child (<2 years of age), child abuse or some other type of pathological cause has to be suspected.

Treatment

- *Newborn to 6 months:* Early hip spica with the hips in a flexed position. A Pavlik harness may be used for children <4 months of age (Toto 2000).
- *Young children from 6 months to 5 years of age:* The femoral fracture may be treated in an early hip spica or in traction for approximately 2 weeks followed by a spica cast (Irani *et al.* 1976). The classical overhead or gallows traction is useful for children <2 years of age but requires adequate neurovascular surveillance to avoid the development of skin sores or compartment syndrome. Simple longitudinal traction for 4–6 weeks with the hip in mild flexion will work just as well. Boman *et al.* (1998) describes the use of home traction for femoral fractures that reduces the length of hospital stay. This is a very interesting option, but not yet widely employed in many countries.

  Angulation as well as moderate overlapping of the fracture can be tolerated, as remodelling potential is great. Allow angulation up to 10° of varus or valgus and 20° of anterior bowing. Shortening of 1–1.5 cm is ideal because of average overgrowth of 1 cm from the femur and 0.2–0.5 cm from the tibia. Shortening >2–2.5 cm must be corrected before the fracture unites. Rotational malunion will not correct and must be avoided.
- In the older child (5–10 years of age), several options are available. Conservative treatment in traction will give good results but again for social and economic reasons is now frequently replaced or followed by one of the other options. A spica cast is fine but may not be practical in the older child, as a lengthy absence from school will result. Ante- or retrograde IM flexible nails, as described by Ligier *et al.* (1980), are the authors' favourite option.

  In this group of children it is unwise to use a reamed antegrade IM nail (Toto 2000) because of the risk of AVN. External fixation can be useful to stabilize a femoral fracture that is open or associated with multiple injuries in order to facilitate nursing. Reduction and plating can lead to significant overgrowth.

- The same treatment options are available for children >10 years of age. IM nailing can be performed in the adolescent, but there is a higher risk of AVN of the head. Beaty *et al.* (1994) reported one case of AVN (in a group of 30 patients) that was seen on radiograph 15 months after the injury and concluded that IM nailing is a reasonable alternative only in selected patients. Flexible IM nails can be used if the proximal physis is open, and reamed IM nails if the proximal physis is closed. In adolescents the entry point is close to the tip of the greater trochanter to reduce the risk of AVN.

Complications

Refracture is a particular problem with external fixation treatment and may occur in up to 10% of cases. Delayed union may occur with open fractures or after external fixation of transverse fracture. Overgrowth of 1–1.5 cm occurs in children aged 2–10 years. Much less overgrowth occurs after that. Internal rotational deformity of the distal fragment requires no treatment. Angular deformity is usually in varus and some remodelling occurs. Avoid AVN of the femoral head with antegrade IM nailing by using the tip of the greater trochanter.

Key points

- Most children with diaphyseal fractures do well with non-operative treatment.
- Recent trend towards use of IM nails.

Knee fractures

The growth plates around the knee are responsible for 70% of the growth of the lower extremity. Any growth plate injury can thus lead to a major leg length discrepancy. Severe genu valgum or genu varum is seen with asymmetrical growth arrest.

Supracondylar femur fractures

Supracondylar fractures proximal to the growth plate require a similar protocol to the diaphyseal fractures. Treatment with 90–90 skeletal traction followed by a spica cast is one option. Valgus or varus deformity is difficult to assess with the knee flexed; also the distal fragment tends to become flexed due to the pull from gastrocnemius.

Physeal fractures of the distal femur

Supracondylar fractures of the femur involving the growth plate have a high complication rate (Riseborough *et al.* 1983). Despite perfect reduction, with or without smooth pinning, growth arrest is frequent in up to 30–40% of patients and parents should be warned of this. Stress radiographs should be performed to show a Salter–Harris type I fracture or associated ligamentous injuries.

The distal femoral growth plate represents 70% of the growth potential of the femur. This represents about 1 cm/year, which is a useful figure to give parents. For instance, a full growth arrest in an 8 year old boy will give 8 cm of leg length discrepancy by the age of 16 when he becomes skeletally mature. If growth arrest is partial, angular deformity will result.

A vascular injury must excluded, particularly after an extension injury.

Key point

- Physeal fractures of the distal femur have a high incidence of growth arrest.

Treatment

Physeal fractures of the distal femur require anatomical reduction (Toto 2000).

- *Salter–Harris type I fractures* require closed reduction with smooth pin fixation.
- *Salter–Harris type II fractures:* If the metaphyseal fragment is small, then smooth crossed pins will provide adequate fixation. Where the metaphyseal fragment is large, then cannulated screws in the metaphysis may be used.
- *Salter–Harris type III fractures:* ORIF with one or two cannulated 4.5 mm screws provides adequate treatment.

- *Salter–Harris type IV fractures:* These fractures require ORIF with a cannulated screw in both the epiphysis and the metaphysis. All of these fractures will require immobilization in a long leg cast for 4–6 weeks.

Patella fractures

Patellar fractures are rare in children. Difficulties in diagnosis arise because there are numerous normal variants and chronic diseases; also, much of the patella is cartilaginous and invisible on radiographs. A direct blow is the usual mechanism. Undisplaced fractures require simple immobilization. Displaced fractures are treated with tension band wiring as in adults, although an absorbable suture may be used instead of wire.

The sleeve fracture in the child 8–12 years of age is especially difficult to diagnose. A little piece of bone is avulsed from the patella with a much larger surrounding portion of cartilage. The piece of bone can be very small and easily missed on plain radiographs. ORIF of displaced fractures is necessary.

Patellar dislocation

Dislocation of the patella is commonly associated with muscular deficiency, mainly the vastus medialis. Treatment consists of reduction and short immobilization followed by an intensive physical therapy programme to strengthen the muscles. If there is an associated avulsion fracture from the medial aspect of the patella then acute repair of the medial structures is recommended.

Lower leg

Tibial intercondylar eminence fractures

Tibial spine fractures are one variant, and are the equivalent to adult anterior cruciate ligament (ACL) injuries (Fig. 29.7). In children the ACL is commonly stretched as well. This injury is most common in the 8–14 age group. Half of these injuries are associated with bicycle accidents and are caused by hyperextension injuries to the knee.

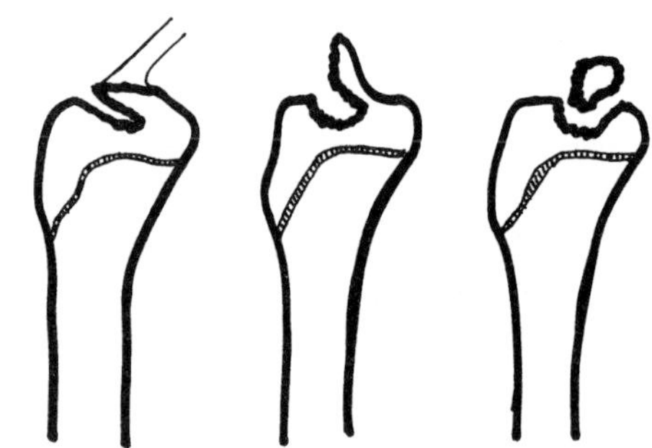

Figure 29.7 Tibial spine fractures.

Classification and treatment

There are three types, depending on the importance of the displacement. Good anteroposterior and lateral radiographs are necessary. CT scans may be required for displaced fractures to evaluate the importance and localization of the displaced fragment.

Type I: An undisplaced fracture should be treated by immobilization in a long leg cast with the knee 5° short of full extension.

Type II: Anterior portion is displaced but hinged posteriorly. Attempt closed reduction with hyperextension then cast in slight flexion. ORIF if required.

Type III: Fragment is completely separated. Internal screw fixation of the fragment with sutures or small screws via an arthroscope or small arthrotomy.

Late problems

The knee may have a persistent extension lag and mild ACL laxity, so great care has to be taken to establish normal tension in the cruciate ligament (Meyers and McKeever 1970).

Key point

- Great care has to be taken to establish normal tension in the cruciate ligament.

Tibial tuberosity fractures

Fractures of the tibial tuberosity fractures must be differentiated from Osgood–Schlatter disease, which is a predisposing factor in 50% of cases.

Classification and treatment

Type I: Across second ossification level. Closed reduction and application of a long leg cast in extension for 4–6 weeks followed by physical therapy is adequate.

Type II: Exits between primary and second ossification levels.

Type III: Intra-articular.

Treat displaced fractures with internal fixation using cannulated screws with washers (Ogden *et al.* 1980).

Proximal tibial physeal fractures

Proximal tibial physeal fractures may be caused by hyperextension. Displaced proximal fractures through the growth plate may compress or lacerate the tibial artery (Fig. 29.8). One has to be very careful even if the fracture is not displaced, as it might have been reduced during transport. These fractures have a high potential for growth arrest, and leg length discrepancy or angulation are possible complications.

Treatment

Careful evaluation for vascular injury or compartment syndrome is essential. Treat with anatomic reduction and fix with smooth crossed pins and a long leg cast.

Proximal tibial metaphyseal fractures

In the toddler one sees a particular variant of proximal metaphysis fractures, which is commonly treated for 4 weeks in a long leg cast moulded into varus. Over the next 18 months a valgus deformity may develop. This deformity can be quite significant but will correct itself with time in most patients. Parents should be warned about this, to avoid disappointment (Zionts and MacEwen 1986).

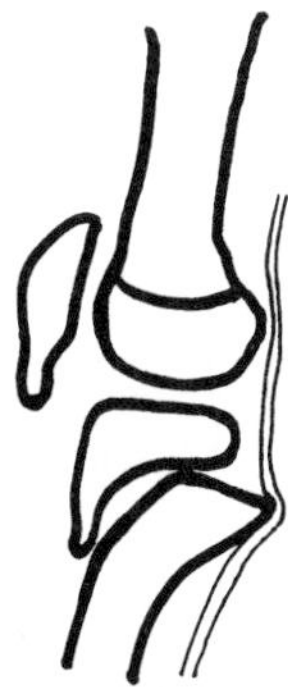

Figure 29.8 Vascular injury after proximal tibia fracture.

Key point

- Resultant valgus with proximal metaphyseal fractures will usually resolve over a few years.

Diaphyseal fractures

Lower limb fractures are commonly diaphyseal. Reduction is required if it is displaced and immobilization is best maintained with a long leg cast. They heal within 4–6 weeks in the young child but may require 8–12 weeks in the older child. No weight-bearing is allowed for 4–6 weeks. Surgical indications include external fixation for unstable or open fractures, and children who sustain multiple injuries.

Ankle

Distal tibia fractures

Fractures of the distal tibia are frequent and can be quite complex. If they involve the growth plate they can cause a leg length discrepancy. Partial arrest is more severe and results in ankle varus or valgus.

Fractures proximal to the growth plate require reduction and immobilization in a long leg cast until union. Reduction has to be perfect. Varus, valgus, and recurvatum deformity are seen with poor reduction and immobilization. All forms of Salter–Harris fracture types can be seen.

Treatment

- *Salter–Harris type I or II:* Usually closed reduction and immobilization in a cast is satisfactory. If the fracture will not reduce, open reduction is indicated to remove any periosteum infolded into the fracture site.
- *Salter–Harris type III or IV:* There require internal fixation with cannulated screws if

displaced. CT can be helpful to decide whether the fragments are displaced and where the cannulated screws should be placed.

Tillaux and triplane fractures

Both these forms of fracture of the distal tibia are often missed and underestimated. They are seen at the end of growth.

- The *Tillaux fracture* (Kleiger and Mankin 1964) is a Salter III fracture of the lateral portion of the distal tibia which requires CT scan evaluation. If the fracture does not reduce by closed methods, then open reduction and screw fixation is indicated. A non-weight-bearing long leg cast for 3 weeks followed by a short leg walking cast for 3 weeks more should be applied.
- The *triplane fracture* has a complex pattern (Fig. 29.9). The asymmetrical closure of the growth plate can explain the shape of the triplane fracture seen in the adolescent. CT scan evaluation will help to define the number of fragments and their displacement. A perfect reduction is mandatory because this is an intra-articular fracture. Displaced fractures require internal fixation with cannulated screws. A non-weight bearing long leg cast for 6 weeks followed by a short leg walking cast for another month should be applied (Cooperman *et al.* 1978, Ertl *et al.* 1988).

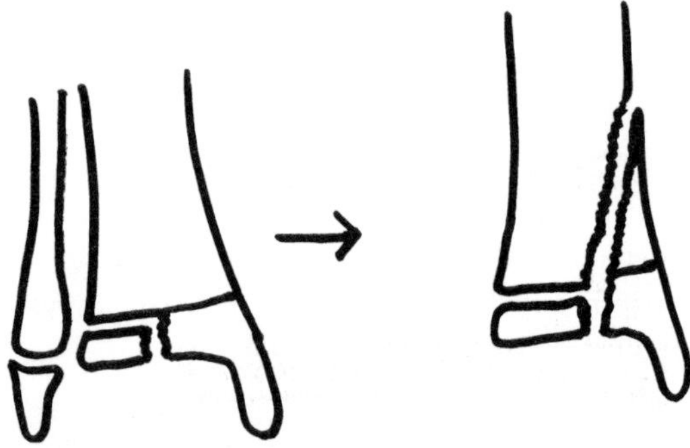

Figure 29.9 Triplane fracture.

Key point

- Late problems include asymmetric growth arrest and malunion.

Foot

Tarsal fractures

There are confusing normal variants, but clinical exam and radiographs of the other foot will allow comparison. Fractures of the talus are rare in the child, but the treatment and complications are the same as in the adult. Fractures of the calcaneus are also infrequent; they usually do fine in younger children (Schmidt and Wiener 1982). Bicycle spoke injuries, with or without fractures, have a benign appearance on first examination but may develop serious sequelae. These occur in children aged 2–8 years old and initially may look like superficial abrasions, but skin necrosis may develop within 24–48 hours. The child should stay in hospital for observation of the wounds. Debridement should be performed as necessary. Skin grafts are sometimes required. The parents should be told that healing takes 5–6 weeks (Felman 1973).

Lisfranc dislocation

Lisfranc dislocations are rare in children and management is the same as in the adult (see Chapter 23, page 412).

Metatarsal fractures and toe fractures

A fracture of the proximal fifth metatarsal is transverse, unlike the normal apophysis that is longitudinal in appearance. Metatarsal and toe fractures heal in 3 weeks. Displaced fractures are rare and may require reduction and pinning if necessary.

Spine

Cervical spine

Cervical spine injuries are rarer in children than in adults. The developing spine behaves quite differently. The adult configuration will be present at 8–10 years of age. Children <8 years of age will have a higher incidence of upper cervical spine lesions. Cervical spine or spinal cord injuries should be suspected in children who have been involved in road traffic accidents, or have suffered head, face, or multiple injuries.

The cervical spine is particularly challenging to analyse on radiographs in the young child where cartilaginous structures are abundant and normal variants confusing. Nevertheless, just as for adult patients, adequate anteroposterior and lateral cervical spine radiographs including the whole cervical spine are the basic first requirement after clinical examination. Odontoid, oblique views should be done whenever the clinical situation permits. Multiple-level injuries are frequent in children.

At birth the ring of the atlas and all the posterior arches are cartilaginous. Posterior arches will be ossified at the end of the first year, except for C2 (up to age 2) and C1 (up to age 4). The ring of the atlas will be ossified at the age of 1 year.

At birth the dens is made of two ossification centres, which give a normal V shape. Many variants in the normal formation of the dens are possible and the age of maturity is quite variable. The soft tissue space in front of C3 or C6 has no value in a crying child. Congenital anomalies and children with syndromes further complicate the issue.

The child's spine and ligamentous structures are much more flexible than in the adult and this explains the spinal cord injury without radiographic abnormalities (SCIWORA) seen on radiographs. This type of lesion is seen more often in the young child. One has thus to be very cautious even when the radiographs are normal (Pang and Wilberger 1982).

Occiput–C1 lesions are very rare and result from major trauma. They are usually fatal injuries. They are to be considered in the differential diagnosis of a 'floppy baby' at birth. C1–C2 instability is seen in numerous syndromes (e.g. Down's syndrome). Normal values of the landmarks are quite different in the child. An atlas–dens distance of 4 mm in flexion is normal. The average spinal canal diameter is 14 mm.

A hangman's fracture in a child is a rarity and treatment is conservative. Surgery might be required in selected patients. Another normal radiographic finding that can be confusing is the pseudosubluxation of C2–C3, described by Swischuk (1977).

Atlantoaxial rotatory subluxation is another childhood entity. It is associated with even minor trauma but has numerous other aetiologies, e.g. upper respiratory tract infection and dental sepsis. The child presents with a torticollis. Lateral radiograph can be impressive (mimics C1–C2 dislocation), but a good open-mouth view will show the asymmetry of the masses of the atlas. Treatment is conservative: cervical collar and anti-inflammatory medications, gentle cervical traction for more severe cases and arthrodesis for the child with chronic fixed subluxation.

Fractures of the dens exist. If found, treatment consist of gentle reduction and bed rest in extension followed by a Minerva. It heals in 6 weeks.

Children with suspected cervical spine injuries have to be positioned so that their head is a little lower than their trunk to prevent flexion of the upper cervical spine (Fig. 29.10). A rolled towel should be placed under their shoulders or a recess made in the backboard (Herzenberg *et al.* 1989).

Key point

- Spinal fractures are rare in children.
- In children <8 years the mechanism and types of injuries are different.

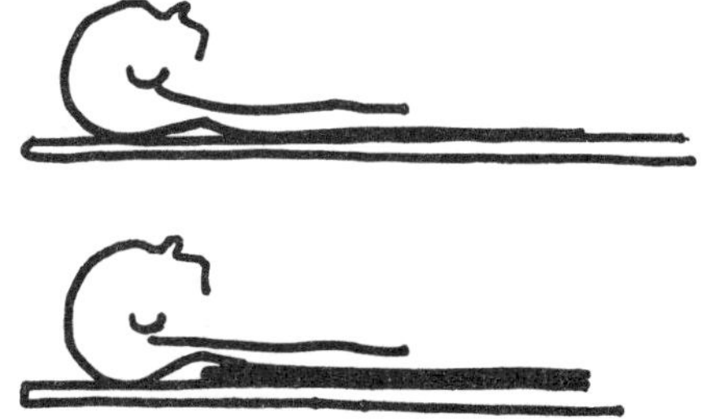

Figure 29.10 Position of child's relatively large head for transportation.

- May be difficult to diagnose on radiograph due to cartilage.
- SCIWORA is more common in children.

Thoracolumbar spine

Fractures of the thoracolumbar spine are even rarer than cervical spine injuries. By the age of 10 years, the adult pattern is found. Children often sustain multiple-level fractures. Radiographs of all the spine are indicated. A bone scan may help if there is concern despite normal radiographs. These fractures can be seen as a result of birth trauma, child abuse, motor vehicle accidents, or falls from a height.

Compression fractures due to hyperflexion are seen at multiple levels. Treatment is conservative and restoration of vertebral height is the rule with remodelling (6–8 weeks). Compression fractures can be seen in child abuse. Distraction shear is seen with violent trauma. The fracture is through the end plate apophysis and not through the disc.

Traumatic displacement of the vertebral ring apophysis will give symptoms similar to a prolapsed intervertebral disc. Chance fractures are seen with seatbelt injuries. They are associated with abdominal trauma. Treatment is conservative. Unstable lesions will require surgical stabilization as indicated.

Special conditions

These conditions can be the cause of a pathological fracture or the fracture can be the first sign of the disease. The fractures involve pathological bone and will contribute to the deformation of these already abnormal bony structures. The management of the fracture will be concurrent and/or followed by the treatment of the underlying condition. The list of pathological conditions is broad and just a few examples are given below.

Child abuse

Fractures can be one of the visible signs of child abuse (see Chapter 43). Always suspect this before the age of 4 years, and in particular in a child under the age of 2 years with multiple fractures of varying ages and an unclear history.

The child needs to be admitted to hospital. Physical examination may reveal bruises, burns, or other signs of abuse. A skeletal survey of the entire skeleton is necessary to identify new and healing fractures. A bone scan is useful if there is any doubt (Akbarnia and Akbarnia 1976).

Suspicion must be raised in children with lower extremity fractures before walking age, posterior rib fractures, or metaphyseal corner fractures (Kleinman *et al.* 1986).

Child abuse will have to be differentiated from a long list of other possible diagnoses—for example, milder forms of osteogenesis imperfecta and any of the diseases or disorders described below.

Fracture care is similar to that of other fractures, but the situation may be made more complex by the legal and social issues that will have to be raised.

Key point

- Be aware of child abuse especially if there are multiple fractures, fractures of varying ages, or a suspicious history.

Tumours

Pathological fractures can occur through tumours. The more common underlying malignancies include leukaemia, neuroblastoma, osteosarcoma, and Ewing's sarcoma. The treatment of malignant tumours by radiation or chemotherapy can weaken bones, leading to fractures.

Fracture can also occur in association with benign tumours or tumour-like lesions. Fractures through unicameral bone cysts are quite frequent, especially in the proximal humerus and femur. Other frequent benign tumours or tumour-like lesions associated with fractures are aneurysmal bone cysts, fibrous dysplasia, non-ossifying fibromas, enchondromas, and eosinophilic granulomas.

Metabolic bone disease

Although quite rare in developed countries, nutritional rickets is still frequent in the developing world. Rickets can also be seen in number of renal or metabolic diseases and in premature children. A radiograph of the wrist will typically show the widening of the growth plate. This entity has to be differentiated from child abuse. Rickets will facilitate slipped capital femoral epiphysis even in very young children. Other general metabolic diseases, such as Gaucher's disease, hyperparathyroidism, Cushing's syndrome, scurvy, and idiopathic juvenile osteoporosis also predispose to fractures.

Osteogenesis imperfecta

In many syndromes and conditions one can find a certain degree of osteoporosis. Typical osteogenesis imperfecta is easily recognized (Sillence 1981). Milder forms have to be differentiated from child abuse.

Cerebral palsy and other general disorders

Children with cerebral palsy can sustain fractures from minor trauma or regular physical therapy, or even spontaneously. These children are particularly susceptible to fractures if they are bedridden with quadriplegia, osteoporosis, and severe spasticity,

The same applies to severe arthrogryposis. In myelomeningocele and spinal cord injury, lack of sensitivity is another factor contributing to the fractures (Freehafer 1995). The diagnosis can be delayed because of the lack of pain; the initial symptoms are fever, swelling, and local heat, which might lead to the erroneous diagnosis of osteomyelitis.

Fracture management is essentially the same as described above. In debilitated patients a vicious circle can develop of fracture followed by immobilization, more osteoporosis, deformation, refractures and so on. Patients with severe head trauma, muscular dystrophy, and poliomyelitis also fit this description.

Haematological conditions

Leukaemia patients are prone to bone pain and fractures, which can be the first sign of the disease. Patients with haemophilia and sickle cell disease also experience bone pain.

Occult and stress fractures

Tibial and calcaneal stress fractures are seen in toddlers and are part of the differential diagnosis of the limping child. The history is not always clear, the radiographs are normal in the beginning but may show healing 3–4 weeks later. A bone scan can be performed to localize the fracture.

Stress fractures of the feet, tibia, and femoral neck are also be seen in athletic children. The differential diagnosis includes neoplasia, particularly if there is periosteal reaction (Engh *et al.* 1970).

Birth trauma

Birth trauma can be associated with normal childbirth, breech delivery, or difficult labour. It may be related to an underlying problem in the neonate such as osteogenesis imperfecta, numerous syndromes, or prematurity. Fracture of the clavicle is the most frequent fracture and does not require treatment. It can be associated with a brachial plexus palsy.

All other long-bone fractures are possible but rare. They are easily diagnosed and require a short period of immobilization (2–3 weeks). Epiphyseal fractures are seen in the proximal humerus, distal humerus, and distal femur. They may be difficult to diagnose and the differential will include osteomyelitis and septic arthritis.

Special problems

Open fractures and Volkmann's syndrome

These are treated in the same way as in adults and are just as dangerous (see Chapter 22).

Cast care

Since the treatment of children is mainly conservative, the treating clinician must have a thorough knowledge of good casting techniques. The same general cast care as in the adult applies, but an extra layer of padding in exposed zones can avoid compressions. Too much padding is not a good option since it will allow secondary displacement of a reduced fracture. An extra layer of cast material will prevent cast destruction.

Children are less tolerant to casting than adults are. In young children avoid short arm casts: they will be removed, or will not keep the child appropriately immobilized. Information booklets are a good source of information for parents.

Traction care

Traction care requires special attention in children. Two people are required to apply the traction and to take care of it. The skin of a young child does not have as much resistance as that of an adult. Regular application of 70% isopropyl alcohol on the buttocks and any other sensitive area 3–4 times a day will avoid blisters. Avoid lotions and creams that will soften the skin and facilitate breakdown. The traction should be placed on the whole leg from above the knee to divide the pull on the skin. Traction should be started at about 10% of body weight and increased to a maximum of 30% depending on position and reduction. The skin will not tolerate traction >5 kg, so skeletal traction is required. In selected patients, traction can be chosen for the full treatment of a femur fracture. This necessitates considerable adaptation, imagination and patience. Pelvic fractures will also require a long period of traction.

Conclusion

- In children the more obvious and spectacular diaphyseal fractures are usually the most benign ones.
- Great care must be taken to evaluate epiphyseal fractures because of the risk of injury to the growth plate or displacement of the fragments at the articular surface.
- Always keep in mind the possibility of an underlying bone disease or child abuse.

References

Akbarnia BA, Akbarnia NO (1976) The role of the orthopedist in child abuse and neglect. *Orthopedic Clinics of North America* 7: 733–742.

Bado JL (1967) The Monteggia lesion. *Clinical Orthopaedics and Related Research* 50: 71–86.

Barton NJ (1979) Fractures of the phalanges of the hand in children. *Hand* 11: 134–143.

Beaty JH, Austin SM, Warner WC, Canale ST, Nichols L (1994) Interlocking intramedullary nailing of femoral-shaft fractures in adolescents: preliminary results and complications. *Journal of Pediatric Orthopaedics* 14: 178–183.

Bell-Tawse AJS (1965) The treatment of malunited Monteggia fractures in children. *Journal of Bone and Joint Surgery* 47B: 718–723.

Boman A, Gardell C, Janarv PM (1998) Home traction of femoral shaft fractures in younger children. *Journal of Pediatric Orthopaedics* 18: 478–480.

Canale ST (1995) Fractures of the femur in children. *Journal of Bone and Joint Surgery* 77A: 294–315.

Canale ST, Bourland WL (1977) Fractures of the neck and intertrochanteric region of the femur in children. *Journal of Bone and Joint Surgery* 59A: 431–443.

Carlson WO, Wenger DR (1984) A mapping method to prepare for surgical excision of a partial physeal arrest. *Journal of Pediatric Orthopaedics* 4: 232–238.

Colonna PC (1928) Fractures of the neck of the femur in childhood. A report of six cases. *Annals of Surgery* 88: 902.

Cooperman DR, Spiegel PG, Laros GS (1978) Tibial fractures involving the ankle in children: the so-called triplane epiphyseal fracture. *Journal of Bone and Joint Surgery* 66A: 1040–1046.

Dameron TB Jr, Reibel DB (1969) Fractures involving the proximal humeral epiphyseal plate. *Journal of Bone and Joint Surgery* 51A: 289–297.

D'souza S, Vaishya R, Klenerman L (1993) Management of radial neck fractures in children: a retrospective analysis of one hundred patients. *Journal of Pediatric Orthopaedics* 13: 232–238.

Engh CA, Robinson RA, Milgram J (1970) Stress fractures in children. *Journal of Trauma* 10: 532–541.

Ertl JP, Barrack RL, Alexander AH, VanBuecken K (1988) Triplane fractures of the distal tibial epiphysis: long-term follow-up. *Journal of Bone and Joint Surgery* 70A: 967–976.

Felman AH (1973) Bicycle spoke fractures. *Journal of Pediatrics* 82: 302–303.

Flynn JC (1989) Nonunion of slightly displaced fractures of the lateral humeral condyle: an update. *Journal of Pediatric Orthopaedics* 9: 691–696.

Flynn JC, Matthews JG, Benoit RL (1974) Blind pinning of displaced fractures of the humerus in children. *Journal of Bone and Joint Surgery* 56A: 263–272.

Fowles JV, Kassab MT (1980) Displaced fractures of the medial condyle in children. *Journal of Bone and Joint Surgery* 62A: 1159–1163.

Freehafer AA (1995) Limb fractures in patients with spinal cord injury. *Archives of Physical Medicine and Rehabilitation* 76(9): 823–827.

Heeg M, Viiser JD, Oostvogel HJM (1988) Injuries of the acetabular triradiate cartilage and the sacroiliac joint. *Journal of Bone and Joint Surgery* 70B: 34–37.

Herzenberg JE, Hensinger RN, Dedrick DK (1989) Emergency transport and positioning of young children who have an injury of the cervical spine. *Journal of Bone and Joint Surgery* 71A: 15–22.

Hull JB, Bell MJ (1997) Modern trend for external fixation of fractures in children: a critical review. *Journal of Pediatric Orthopaedics* 6(1997): 103–109.

Irani RN, Nicholson JT, Chung SMK (1976) Long-term results in the treatment of femoral shaft fractures in young children by immediate spica cast immobilization. *Journal of Bone and Joint Surgery* 58A: 945–951.

Key JA, Conwell HE (1951) *Management of fractures, dislocations and sprains*. C.V. Mosby, St Louis.

Kleiger B, Mankin HJ (1964) Fracture of the lateral portion of the distal tibial epiphysis. *Journal of Bone and Joint Surgery* 46A: 25–32.

Kleinman PK, Marks SC, Blackbourne B (1986) The metaphyseal lesion in abused children: a radiologic-histopathologic study. *American Journal of Roentgenology* 146: 895–905.

Larsen E, Vittas D, Torp-Andersen S (1988) Remodelling of angulated distal forearm fractures in children. *Clinical Orthopaedics* 237: 190–195.

Lemperg R, Liliequist B (1970) Dislocation of the proximal epiphysis in newborns: report of two cases and discussion of diagnostic criteria. *Acta Orthopaedica Scandinavica* 59: 377–380.

Ligier JN, Métaizeau JP, Prévot L, Lascombes P (1988) Elastic stable intramedullary nailing of femoral shaft fractures in children. *Journal of Bone and Joint Surgery* 70B: 74–77.

Metaizeau JP, Lascombes P, Lemelle JL, Finlayson D, Prevot J (1993) Reduction and fixation of displaced radial neck fractures by closed intramedullary pinning. *Journal of Pediatric Orthopaedics* 13: 355–360.

Meyers MH, McKeever FM (1970) Fracture of the intercondylar eminence of the tibia. *Journal of Bone and Joint Surgery* 52A: 1677–1684.

Moseley CF (1977) A straight-line graph for leg length discrepancies. *Journal of Bone and Joint Surgery* 59A(1977): 174–179.

Noonan KJ, Price CT (1998) Forearm and distal radius fractures in children. *Journal of the Academy of Orthopaedic Surgeons* 6: 146–156.

Ogden JA (1982) Skeletal growth mechanism injury patterns. *Journal of Pediatric Orthopaedics* 2: 371–377.

Ogden JA, Tross RB, Murphy MJ (1980) Fractures of the tibial tuberosity in adolescents. *Journal of Bone and Joint Surgery* 62A: 205–216.

Owen R (1970) Congenital pseudoarthrosis of the clavicle. *Journal of Bone and Joint Surgery* 52B: 644–652.

Pang D, Wilberger JE (1982) Spinal cord injury without radiographic abnormalities in children. *Journal of Neurosurgery* 57: 114–129.

Peterson HA (1984) Partial growth plate arrest and its treatment. *Journal of Pediatric Orthopaedics* 4: 246–258.

Rang M (1983) *Children's fractures*, 2nd ed. J.B. Lippincott, Philadelphia.

Ray TD, Tessler RH, Dell PC (1996) Traumatic ulna physeal arrest after distal forearm fractures in children. *Journal of Pediatric Orthopaedics* 16: 195–200.

Ring D, Jupiter JB, Waters PM (1998) Monteggia fractures in children and adults. *Journal of the American Academy of Orthopaedic Surgeons* 6: 215–224.

Riseborough EJ, Barrett IR, Shapiro F (1983) Growth disturbances following distal femoral physeal fracture-separations. *Journal of Bone and Joint Surgery* 65A: 885–893.

Rowe CR, Pierce DS, Clark JG (1973) Voluntary dislocation of the shoulder: a preliminary report on clinical, electromyographic, and psychiatric study of twenty-six patients. *Journal of Bone and Joint Surgery* 55A: 445–460.

Salter RB, Harris WR (1963) Injuries involving the epiphyseal plate. *Journal of Bone and Joint Surgery* 45A: 587–622.

Sanders WE, Heckman JD (1984) Traumatic plastic deformation of the radius and ulna: a closed method of correction of the deformity. *Clinical Orthopaedics and Related Research* 188: 58–67.

Schmidt TL, Weiner DS (1982) Calcaneal fractures in children. *Clinical Orthopaedics and Related Research* 171: 150–155.

Sillence D (1981) Osteogenesis Imperfecta: an expanding panorama of variants. *Clinical Orthopedics* 159: 11–25.

Swischuk LE (1977) Anterior displacement of C2 in children: physiologic or pathological. *Pediatric Radiology* 122: 759–763.

Tolo VT (2000) Orthopaedic treatment of fractures of the long bones and pelvis in children who have multiple injuries. *Instructional Course Lectures* 49: 415–423.

Walsh HPJ, McLaren CAN, Owen R (1987) Galeazzi fractures in children. *Journal of Bone and Joint Surgery* 69B: 730–733.

Wilkins KE (1997) Supracondylar fractures: what's new? *Journal of Pediatric Orthopaedics* Part B 6: 110–116.

Zionts LG, MacEwen GD (1986) Spontaneous improvement in post-traumatic tibia valga. *Journal of Bone and Joint Surgery* 68A: 680–686.

Further reading

Rockwood CA Jr, Wilkins KE, King RE (1984) *Fractures in children*, vol. 3. J.B Lippincott, Philadelphia.

Epps CH Jr, Bowen JR (1995) *Complications in pediatric orthopaedic surgery*. J.B Lippincott, Philadelphia.

30

CHAPTER 30

Paediatric head and maxillofacial injuries

ERICA JACOBSON, MARK DEXTER, AND DANIEL T CASS

CHAPTER 30
Paediatric head and maxillofacial injuries

ERICA JACOBSON, MARK DEXTER, AND DANIEL T CASS

Head injuries

Injuries to the brain and spinal cord are a major cause of morbidity and mortality in children. The Traumatic Brain Injury Project (see web site) estimates that each year over 1 million children in the USA suffer some form of head injury. The majority of these will be mild injuries, but over 30 000 will lead to permanent disability. Spinal cord injury is less common in this age group, affecting around 1500 children in the USA per year (about 14% of all spinal cord injuries). The emotional, financial, and social burdens placed on the family and the community as a whole are enormous.

The principles of managing head and spinal cord injuries in children are essentially the same as those for adults. However, because of the physiological differences between these two populations, and even within the paediatric population itself, there are differences in the epidemiology, the presentation, and the complications that arise from head injury. It is these differences that are discussed here.

Aetiology

Overall, motor vehicle accidents account for the majority of head injuries in children (Chan *et al.* 1989). In children <2 years old, however, falls are the most significant cause of head injury. (Greenes and Schutzman 1997, Lavelle and Shaw 1998). These are often from low heights, such as beds and changing tables. Falls from greater heights become increasingly common as children learn to climb. Non-accidental injury is a cause of major head injury in this younger age group. In later childhood, pedestrian and bicycle accidents are also common causes of major injury. In adolescence attempted suicide is an increasingly important cause, particularly in boys.

Motor vehicle accidents are also the major cause of spinal injuries. However, in the paediatric population, one-third occur during play or sporting events. Diving into a shallow pool is a well-known cause of recreational accidents.

Key point

- Motor vehicle accidents and falls are the most common causes of head and spinal cord injuries in children.

Anatomy and biomechanics

In the neonate, the head is proportionately larger than in the adult, with underdeveloped neck muscles for its support. Despite this, it must accommodate considerable growth of the brain. The bone plates that make up the skull are not yet fused at the sutures. Thus, the volume of the skull is capable of increasing in size not only from increase in brain mass, but from an increase in any compartment of its contents. Because of this, an intracranial haemorrhage may reach considerable size before causing neurological symptoms.

The brain itself is still not fully developed. Myelinization is under way but far from complete, contributing to the lower fat and higher water contents of the neonatal brain. At this stage, both cerebral blood flow and metabolism are lower than in the adult.

With development of the brain, myelinization progresses to adult development by the age of 4 years. The cranial sutures fuse on average by 18 months old, though may still be patent at 3 years. Cerebral blood flow and metabolism increase and surpass adult levels by 3 years old, decreasing only in adolescence. By adolescence, the mechanics of the skull and brain are those of the adult.

Presentation

It is important to get a thorough history of events when a child has suffered a head injury, particularly as the child often cannot give one themselves. The velocity of the injury (high or low speed), the height fallen and the structure of the floor (carpet or stone), and events preceding and following (e.g. seizures), are all important in determining the possible severity of the injury.

As thorough a neurological examination as is possible, given the age of the child, should be performed. This should include palpation of the scalp for boggy swellings, palpation of the fontanel, measurement of head circumference for a baseline reading, and fundoscopic examination. When the neurological examination is normal and there are no outward signs of obvious trauma, and in the face of minor trauma such as a fall from a low height, the risk of intracranial injury may be low and the need for further investigation may be obviated (Fisher 1997, Strouse *et al.* 1998, Gruskin and Schutzman 1999). However, in children <12 months old, the absence of any outward signs of injury may be illusory. Up to 20% of intracranial injury may be occult in this age group (Greenes and Schutzman 1998).

When investigating suspected spinal cord injury, the examination should be aimed at determining the level of injury. Myotomal, dermatomal, and reflex changes may be used to assess the level of injury in the cord. This is particularly important as there may be no radiological findings to support the diagnosis.

Some clinical patterns are common in the presentation of paediatric head injury. The *paediatric concussion syndrome* occurs in about 10% of all admissions. It consists of pallor, drowsiness, and vomiting and may present some hours or even days after the injury. It usually causes concern regarding intracranial injury. In the infant, presentation may be vague. Drowsiness, poor feeding, and vomiting should make one suspicious if there is no good history of trauma.

Seizures are a common presentation, with head injury occurring in up to 30% of children with head injuries (Bruce 1996). Unlike in adults, early seizures are not a predictor of ongoing epilepsy, and if they settle, do not require ongoing management.

Coma scores, modified to suit the paediatric population, can be used to gauge the severity of the injury at presentation and to monitor the course of illness. It must be kept in mind, however, that the score is dependent on the child's development. For example, the neonate can score a maximum of 9 on the Paediatric Glasgow Coma Scale, with spontaneous eye opening (4), crying (2), and flexion to painful stimulus (3) (Simpson 1997).

Certain findings should alert the doctor to child abuse. A vague history, such as that of an unwitnessed fall, or variation in the story, plus signs of significant trauma, such as a scalp haematoma and retinal haemorrhages on fundoscopy, are highly suggestive of a non-accidental injury and follow-up is required.

Key points

- A thorough history and examination are vital.
- Myotomal, dermatomal, and reflex changes may give clues to the level of spinal cord injuries.
- Be alert to non-accidental injuries.

Classification of injuries

In older children, the patterns of injury are similar to those seen in adults. In young children (<2 years of age) the patterns of injury are not.

Birth injuries

Birth injuries account for less than 3% of all head injury admissions in children (Bruce 1996). The actual incidence of head injury at birth is unknown, thought it has declined significantly with improved

Table 30.1 Birth injuries

Scalp injuries	Caput succedanaeum[a] Subgaleal haematoma[a] Cephalhaematoma[a]
Skull injuries	'Ping-pong' fracture[a] Linear fractures[a] Occipital osteal diastasis
Intracranial injuries	Extradural haematoma Subdural haematoma Subarachnoid haemorrhage Intraventricular haemorrhage Parenchymal haemorrhage
Cord injuries	Distraction injuries, e.g. during breech birth

[a] Most common injuries.
Modified from Harpold *et al.* (1998).

obstetric practices and with the increase of caesarean section. A higher incidence of birth injuries is seen in primiparous births, precipitous labour, breech delivery, and forceps delivery (Harpold *et al.* 1998). A variety of injuries are seen, the majority of which can be managed conservatively. These are listed in Table 30.1. Spinal cord injuries are uncommon in this age group.

Injuries in the infant

Skull fracture is particularly common in this age group. Both linear and depressed fractures occur. The former is important for its risk of producing a 'growing' skull fracture. The latter is important for its cosmetic effect and slightly higher incidence of associated intracranial injury.

Intracranial injuries are less common in this age group. However, when present they are often associated with skull and scalp injuries. Intracranial injuries are often associated with more severe injuries. Extradural haematomas are usually located higher in the parietal area than those seen in adults. These may occur after a seemingly trivial accident, and in 85% there is no history of a loss of consciousness (McLaurin 1982). Acute subdural haematomas are less common than in adults. They are relatively common in child abuse, and if not detected early may progress to become chronic. Chronic subdural haematomas are relatively common in infancy. In these instances, there may be no obvious history of head injury. The presentation may be vague. McLaurin states that subdural haematomas are more likely to be acute in cases of child abuse.

Injuries in the child and adolescent

Once the sutures are closed, the mechanism and pathology of head injury more closely resemble those of adults. As with infants, intracerebral collections are associated with more severe head injuries.

Diagnosis

In assessing children with head injury, two issues need to be addressed.

- The severity of the injury may be difficult to assess, and the vomiting and drowsy child who looks as though they have a mass lesion may simply require observation.
- The question of abuse may arise.

Radiological assessment is important in answering these questions. Children at risk for later complications should be identified such that appropriate follow-up can be organized.

Skull radiographs

The use of skull radiography in controversial in assessing head injuries. In older children, as with adults, skull radiographs rarely add more information than has already been gleaned by a good neurological examination and is thus unnecessary (Grasso and Keller 1998). However, skull fractures are particularly common in children <1 year of age, as a result of even minor trauma (Bruce 1996). Further, it is this age group which is at risk for developing the 'growing' skull fracture, which may lead to delayed cortical damage and epilepsy. Thus, in infants, skull radiographs are useful in identifying those patients at risk of delayed complications.

Cervical spine radiographs

As with adults, the lateral cervical spine radiograph is important in assessing the trauma victim. However, one- to two-thirds of children presenting with a cord injury may have no radiological signs supportive of the diagnosis. This entity is named *spinal cord injury without radiological abnormality* (SCIWORA) (Pang and Wilberger 1982). Thus, the absence of radiographic evidence does not rule out cord injury.

CT scanning

CT is the imaging procedure of choice to investigate head injury in major centres. It is used to determine the presence of intracranial trauma, and sometimes to better delineate a fracture (e.g. a depressed skull fracture). A CT scan should be performed in any child with a depressed level of consciousness or other firm neurological signs after a head injury. In the alert child without neurological signs, a CT can be avoided (Fisher 1997).

Some CT findings may alert the doctor to child abuse. Subarachnoid haemorrhage associated with a posteriorly placed interfalcine acute subdural haematoma and basal ganglia oedema are all more common in abused children than in those suffering accidents (Bruce 1996, Hymel *et al.* 1997).

MRI

As with adults, MRI is rarely used in the acute setting. However, it may be useful for assessing children in whom a non-accidental head injury is suspected. It is also useful in the assessment of children with spinal cord injuries. MRI may reveal ligamentous damage, compression of the cord by soft tissue, or damage to the spinal cord itself. It is especially useful in the ongoing assessment of the child with SCIWORA (Grabb and Albright 1996).

Special note: investigating the child at risk

One of the most difficult issues in dealing with head injury in childhood is the issue of child abuse (see also Chapter 34). Identification of children at risk is important in preventing further injury, and minimizing the effects of the injuries which are often severe and warrant aggressive management.

As noted above, the doctor may be alerted to the possibility of child abuse during the initial history and examination. These include:

- a vague and inconsistent history
- outward signs of signficant head injury
- the presence of retinal haemorrhages on fundoscopy (Bruce 1996).

In these children, the clinical findings may be out of proportion to the history given. This may be supported by radiological evidence of severe head trauma. Common radiological findings include the presence of intracranial haemorrhages of varying age (chronic subdurals mixed with acute), acute subarachnoid haemorrhage in association with a posterior interhemispheric acute subdural, or the

Table 30.2 Clinical and radiological finding suggestive of child abuse

Clinical	Radiological
Vague or inconsistent history	Acute subdural haematoma, particularly interhemispheric
Signs of a significant head injury: racoon eyes Battle's sign scalp bruising retinal haemorrhages	Mixed subdural (blood of varying ages) Intracerebral hypodensities Oedema in the basal ganglia Skeletal survey demonstrating fractures of varying ages
Evidence of other injuries of different ages	

presence of intracerebral hypodensities such has basal ganglia oedema (Bruce 1996, Hymel *et al.* 1997, Dias *et al.* 1998). Radiological investigation should also include a full skeletal survey to identify other injuries. An urgent referral to the appropriate investigators is warranted. The clinical and radiological findings suggestive of child abuse are listed in Table 30.2.

Management

The principles of management are the same as those for adults. Acute trauma assessment following the well-known ABC rules should be followed. Secondary brain injury is as injurious in this age group as in adults, if not more, so hypoxia and hypotension should be aggressively avoided.

Children suffering minor head injuries without signs of neurological damage may be managed at home after a short period of observation in hospital. This includes infants with skull fractures in whom abuse is not suspected.

Any alteration in the level of consciousness or other signs of neurological injury warrants further observation and investigation.

Surgery is indicated in few situations. These include:

- *Elevation of a depressed skull fracture:* This should be performed when there is a significant (>0.5 cm) depression, where there are signs of dural laceration such as intracranial air, and when the injury has occurred in a cosmetically obvious location. Some fractures can be managed conservatively, particular in infants in whom skull growth may naturally remodel the fracture with time.
- *Evacuation of an intracranial haemorrhage:* This most commonly involves the evacuation of an extradural haematoma. Acute subdural haematomas are rare.
- *Intracranial pressure (ICP) monitoring:* This is imperative in the child with a head injury severe enough to warrant intubation and management in an intensive care unit. It allows aggressive cerebral perfusion pressure management, and is also important in the detection of malignant intracranial hypertension (see below) which may occur hours to days after the initial injury.

Complications

Malignant intracranial hypertension

Malignant intracranial hypertension is an early complication which is more common in children and may occur after significant head injury, even though apparently mild. It is associated with both subarachnoid and subdural haemorrhage. It cause is unknown, although increased cerebrovascular reactivity compared with adults is the favoured theory (Bruce *et al.* 1981). It may occur from 12 hours to several days after the injury.

Aggressive ICP management is required and, in desperate circumstances, bifrontal decompressive craniectomy may be performed, a procedure which has a greater success rate in children than in adults (Polin *et al.* 1997). Nevertheless, the usefulness of such a drastic surgical measure remains controversial.

Growing skull fractures

The growing skull fractures is an unusual complication almost unique to small children (<3 years of age). It presents as a swelling of the scalp or as a rapid increase in the child's head circumference. It is often asymptomatic, but seizures and signs of cortical dysfunction, such as hemiparesis, may occur. These lesions occur at sites of a previous linear skull fracture with an underlying dural tear of similar orientation to the fracture. Herniation of brain through the defect, which progressively enlarges, is the cause of the resulting defect (Pensler *et al.* 1996).

Management is surgical, with excision of gliotic brain tissue and repair of the dural defect. Because this is a disorder of infancy, cranioplasty, though an option, is not necessary, as new bone growth often results in complete remodelling.

Epilepsy

As with adults, late seizures requiring medical control are a complication of paediatric head injury. Lundar and Nestvold (1985) noted a 7% incidence of late seizure within 5 years of head injury caused by traffic accidents. Given that these include more severe injuries, the overall incidence is probably somewhat less. Unlike in adults, however, the occurrence of early seizures is not a predictor for later ones (Jennett 1997).

Cerebrospinal fluid

A leak of cerebrospinal fluid (CSF) commonly occurs after a base of skull fracture in which the overlying dura is disrupted. The main risk of CSF leak is meningitis, so it is important to identify and to manage. Watery fluid running from the nose or the ear after a head injury is the main sign of a leak. In general, management is initially conservative, with bed rest, and head elevation. The use of antibiotics is controversial in this setting.

Where there is no resolution, management involves localizing the leak if possible, using metrizamide cisternography. Lumbar drainage may help to settle the leak. If not, and rarely, open craniotomy and repair of the dural defect must be done.

Maxillofacial injuries

Maxillofacial injuries are extremely common in children, but fortunately most are minor injuries due to falls and sport. Severe maxillofacial injuries are less common and seen mainly in vehicle impacts with pedestrians.

Minor injuries

Mechanisms of injury

Falls are the most common mechanism of injury and cuts to the chin, lips, and tongue are the most frequent injuries.

The history of the mechanism of injury is the most important aspect of early management. If you are happy that the injury was a result of a very small force then you should be confident to treat it as an isolated injury and not concern yourself that there may be other injuries. In such situations of a single system injury there are rarely other significant problems which would put the child's life at risk, and the injury should be treated on its merits.

Treatment of lacerations

It is often difficult to decide whether to suture under local or general anaesthesia. There is subtle pressure of simple logistics and cost reduction to suture under local anaesthetic. Every child is different, and the clinician should discuss the options with the parents and the child. However, where there is doubt from the point of view of cosmetic result or the co-operation of the child, it is best to perform the procedure under general anaesthesia. Many children develop a phobia of hospitals that relates back to an unpleasant suturing experience. A timeless question is: how would you like your child treated?

- *Chin lacerations* can be treated by the use of glues or steristrips, or simple suturing under local anaesthetic. The wounds heal well with a good cosmetic result.
- Other *facial and scalp lacerations* are often deep, and the tissues can be painful to infiltrate with local anaesthetic. Also, seeing the needle come close to their eyes frightens the child. Overall, unless the child is co-operative, general anaesthetic is preferred.
- *Lip lacerations* require assessment as to whether the wound crosses the vermilion margin. Should this occur then it is important to get accurate apposition, as the cosmetic result can be unsatisfactory if the edges are not closely opposed. In such situations the use of general anaesthetic or nitric oxide is warranted so the child is kept still and the sutures can be placed with great accuracy. Sutures inside the mouth should be of chromic catgut and the knots buried to prevent the child chewing them out.
- *Lacerations to the tongue* are often treated by just giving the child mouthwashes and watching it heal. However, steps of over 1 cm or untidy

edges hanging free need to be sutured with chromic catgut with the knots buried.

Dog bites

Dog bites to the face are an extremely dangerous injury in that the deep structures can be damaged and there is a high risk of infection. The child should be taken to theatre and the wounds cleaned meticulously to remove any foreign body. The wound should be washed out with copious amounts of normal saline and the edges freshened up. Any devitalized tissue should be removed. In most instances it is possible to perform primary anastomosis with this regime.

A mistake made in dog bites is to clean the wound in the emergency department and place sutures. Such treatment will almost certainly result in a secondary infection.

The child that has been bitten by a dog has usually sustained some psychological trauma, and needs to be assessed regularly by the local doctor.

Prevention is the important part in the management of dog bites in children. Very young children and dogs do not mix, and they need to be supervised at all times. There are dangerous breeds of dogs, which should be outlawed in urban communities, but any dog can bite and children always need close supervision. A common problem is a child going to a neighbour's house with the parents being unaware that there is a dog there.

Moderate injuries

Common injuries of moderate severity include falls from moving bicycles, falls from a height of 1–2 m during play, and kicks from horses. In these situations there has been more force and the child needs careful assessment to ensure that there are no associated injuries. Skull radiographs and CT scans are warranted, as often a neurological examination is difficult and the child is unable to co-operate.

Injuries to look for are blowout fractures of the orbit and maxillary fractures and injuries to the dentition. These can be difficult to detect, as the facial bones of young children are difficult to interpret on readiographs. It is important to give the radiologist the maximum of clinical information to assist in interpretation of the images.

Severe injuries

Severe injuries occur predominantly in pedestrian–vehicle collisions, or to unrestrained or restrained car passengers. Crush injuries and some horse-kicking injuries can also be severe. In these situations the child needs a full emergency assessment with particular attention to airway and breathing management. Children, like adults, can suffer immense haemorrhage from the base of skull and from maxillofacial fractures. In the first instance attainment of an adequate airway is most important. In most instances an endotracheal tube can be placed, but if the situation demands, a tracheostomy can be performed. As in adults, the best way of reducing ongoing haemorrhage is to reduce the fractures.

In severe pedestrian injuries there are almost always associated thoracic injuries. These patients present a complex management problem and require a multidisciplinary approach.

Once the life-threatening injuries have been managed, the child needs a full craniofacial secondary survey. Every area of the head should be inspected and then the eyes, ears, and mouth examined. A common mistake, especially in the unconscious patient, is to concentrate on the prime injury such as a fractured base of skull and miss other injuries such as fractures to the mandible, nose, or orbits.

Child abuse

It is less common than one would think for the child to be hit about the face and head. A more common child abuse injury is for the child to be shaken, and present with neurological symptoms. The important feature of the examination in the child is to look for retinal haemorrhages. In some instances unusual burns around the face from cigarettes or to the ears can occur in situations of child abuse. If the history does not fit the injuries, or there are more than two injuries separated in time, then child abuse must be suspected.

Unusual injuries

In situations where there is an unusual history of injury, even a small entry wound warrants careful investigation. Often such children present with a small entry wound and an incomplete history. In such instances later evaluation shows that shotgun pellets, objects thrown by other children, or objects flung by lawn mowers have been involved.

If one is faced with a small penetrating wound and an incomplete history, careful physical examination, radiographs, and CT scans are warranted. The child's bony skeleton is thin, and together with the amount of cartilage, this allows significant penetrations of flying objects.

Paediatric features of emergency treatment

Airway

Details of features particular to children can be found in Chapter 28, 'Resuscitation and stabilization of the injured child'.

Breathing

Children who have severe maxillofacial trauma usually have other system injuries and a careful assessment needs to be made for the presence of an associated pneumothorax (see Chapter 11, 'Chest injuries').

Circulation

Children can exsanguinate from serious maxillofacial trauma. The same process of manual reduction of the injury applies as it does in adults. A child who has severe maxillofacial trauma is best taken to the operating theatre and anaesthetized. In this situation the operating theatre acts as the intensive care environment whereby manual reduction, followed by packing, followed by operative procedures, can be readily and sequentially instituted. Unfortunately, in the situation of severe maxillofacial trauma there is not sufficient time for investigative tests. The same principle as for other trauma management applies, in that a child who is unstable is best treated and managed in theatre. Tests should only be undertaken when the child remains stable for a half-hour period after a half blood volume resuscitation.

Specific injuries

Eyelid

Injuries to the eyelid need expert assessment, as they are often deeper than might appear.

Eye

One-third (33%) of severe eye injuries are in children, although only 8% of eye injuries occur in children. Sometimes the history is misleading, as the child may deny participating in a prohibited activity (playing with sticks, scissors, arrows, or pellet guns). The initial examining clinician needs a high index of suspicion. Where in doubt refer to a specialist paediatric eye clinic. It is far better to over-refer than to miss a treatable eye injury.

Fractured nose

The nose is the facial bone most commonly fractured. A fracture is often overlooked, and results in later deformity. As a general policy: any child with an injury sufficient to cause a 'bloody nose' or result in bruising or persisting pain needs a careful nasal examination. The septum should be midline without irregularity. If the septal mucosa has a bluish bulge; this may be a haematoma. The patient should be referred, as fractures will need reduction and haematomas may need drainage.

Mandibular fractures

These are important in children as fractures may involve growth plates and involve secondary teeth. Radiology can miss subtle fractures, but careful examination for malocclusion and painful points will reveal most fractures.

References

Bruce DA, Alavi A, Bilaniuk L (1981) Diffuse cerebral swelling following head injury in children: the syndrome of 'malignant' brain oedema. *Journal of Neurosurgery* 54: 170–178.

Bruce D (1996) Pediatric head injury. In: Regachary SS, Wilkins RH (ed) *Neurosurgery*, 2nd edn. McGraw-Hill, New York, pp 2709–2715.

Chan BS, Walker PJ, Cass DT (1989) Urban trauma: an analysis of 1,116 paediatric cases. *Journal of Trauma* 29(11): 1540–1547.

Dias MS, Backstrom J, Falk M, Li V (1998) Serial radiography in the infant shaken impact syndrome. *Pediatric Neurosurgery* 29: 77–85.

Fisher JD (1997) Syptomatic blunt head injury in children—a prospective, single investigator study. *Clinical Pediatrics (Philadelphia)* 36: 461–465.

Grabb PA, Albright AL (1996) Spinal cord injury without radiographic abnormality in children. In: Regachary SS, Wilkins RH (ed) *Neurosurgery*, 2nd edition. McGraw-Hill, New York, pp 2867–2870.

Grasso SN, Keller MS (1998) Diagnostic imaging in pediatric trauma. *Current Opinion in Pediatrics* 10: 299–302.

Greenes DS, Schutzman SA (1997) Infants with isolated skull fracture: what are their clinical characteristics and do they require hospitalization. *Annals of Emergency* Medicine 30: 253–259.

Greenes DS, Schutzman SA (1998) Occult intracranial injury in infants. *Annals of Emergency Medicine* 32: 680–6.

Gruskin KD, Schutzman SA (1999) Head trauma in children younger than 2 years: are there predictors for complications? *Archives of Pediatric and Adolescent Medicine* 153: 15–20.

Harpold TL, McComb JG, Levy ML (1998) Neonatal neurosurgical trauma. *Neurosurgery Clinics of North America* 9: 141–153.

Hymel KP, Rumack CM, Hay TC, Strain JD, Jenny C (1997) Comparison of intracranial computed tomographic (CT) findings in pediatric abusive and accidental head trauma. *Pediatric Radiology* 27: 743–747.

Jennett B (1997) Outcome after severe head injury. In: Reilly P, Bullock R (ed) *Head injury*. Chapman & Hall, London, pp 439–61.

Lavelle JM, Shaw KM (1998) Evaluation of head injury in a pediatric emergency depratment: pretrauma and posttrauma system. *Archives of Pediatric and Adolescent Medicine* 152: 1220–1224.

Lundar T, Nestvold K (1985) Pediatric head injuries caused by traffic accidents. A prospective study with 5-year follow up. *Child's Nervous System* 1: 24–8.

McLaurin RL (1982) Posttraumatic haematomas. In: *Paediatric neurosurgery. Surgery of the developing nervous system*. Grune & Stratton, New York, N.Y., pp 309–319.

Pang D, Wilberger JE Jr (1982) Spinal cord injury without radiographic abnormalities in children. *Journal of Neurosurgery* 57: 114–29.

Pensler JM, Ciletti SJ, Tomita T (1996) Late correction of sagittal synostosis in children. *Plastic and Reconstructive Surgery* 97(7): 1362–1367.

Polin RS, Shaffrey ME, Bogaev CA *et al.* (1997) Decompressive bifrontal craniectomy in the treatment of severe refractory posttraumatic cerebral edema. *Neurosurgery* 41: 84–92.

Simpson DA (1997) Clinical examination and grading. In: Reilly P, Bullock R (ed) *Head injury*. Chapman & Hall Medical, London, pp 145–165.

Strouse PJ, Caplan M, Owings CL (1998) Extracranial soft-tissue swelling: a normal postmortem radiographic finding or a sign of trauma? *Pediatric Radiology* 28: 594–596.

Web sites

Think First Foundation. Fact sheet: Brain Injury. Think First Foundation. http://www.thinkfirst.org/news3fs2.htm (accessed 10 March 2002).

Traumatic Brain Injury Project. http://www.sped.ukans.edu/spedprojects/tbi/FS.html (accessed 10 March 2002).

31

CHAPTER 31

Paediatric thoracic trauma

ANDREW J A HOLLAND AND
DANIEL T CASS

CHAPTER 31
Paediatric thoracic trauma

ANDREW J A HOLLAND AND DANIEL T CASS

Thoracic trauma is considered an infrequent problem in children, with an estimated incidence of 10% even in communities with a relatively high level of interpersonal violence (Stafford and Harmon 1993). This figure does not reflect the true significance of thoracic trauma. Detailed assessment of paediatric trauma deaths indicates that up to 27% will have thoracic injuries following blunt trauma (Eichelberger and Randolph 1981). As the quality and speed of pre-hospital care continues to improve, it seems likely that more of these children will reach hospital and require urgent management of their chest injuries (Allshouse *et al.* 1993, Sheikh and Culbertson 1993, Michaels *et al.* 1997, Mordehai *et al.* 1997).

In this respect chest trauma appears to act as a marker of injury severity (Peclet *et al.* 1990, Reilly *et al.* 1993). The mortality following blunt trauma increases to 25% in those children with a thoracic injury, compared to just 1.5% in those without (Allshouse *et al.* 1993). These injuries are rarely isolated, however, with children often sustaining additional injuries to the head, abdomen, and lower limb: the combination of thoracic and head injury is the most frequently associated with a fatal outcome (Peclet *et al.* 1990, Allshouse *et al.* 1993, Stafford and Harmon 1993, Wright 1995). Thoracic trauma may not be the presenting injury but should also be actively excluded in patients with injuries to adjacent systems, particularly in penetrating trauma of the neck and abdomen and blunt injuries to the larynx.

The distribution in severity of thoracic injuries in children is bimodal, with many injuries being minor such as bruises and simple abrasions of the chest wall. At the other extreme are high-speed road traffic accidents and injuries that include severe pulmonary contusions and pulmonary and tracheobronchial lacerations. A significant subgroup of patients is those with iatrogenic thoracic injuries, particularly those which occur during treatment of the trauma patient, such as haemothorax after insertion of an intercostal catheter or pnemothorax following insertion of central venous catheters (ACS 1997, Barrett *et al.* 1998).

Although most thoracic injuries are minor, the clinician assessing the child with chest trauma should not be lulled into a false sense of security by the initial haemodynamic stability of the child and the apparent lack of associated injuries. Rather, you should be extremely cautious of any thoracic trauma in a child, when cardiopulmonary reserve may mask the true severity of the injury and in a setting in which severe associated injury is common (Kissoon *et al.* 1990, Stafford and Harmon 1993, Lloyd-Thomas *et al.* 1996).

Key points

- Thoracic injuries account for 10% of all paediatric trauma but 27% of paediatric trauma deaths.
- Associated injuries, especially head injuries, are common.
- There is a bimodal distribution of severity of injury.

Pleuropulmonary injuries

Trauma to the pleura and underlying structures is indicated by a pneumothorax, haemothorax, or haemopneumothorax and is a common injury. There is a tendency to regard these terms as a diagnosis rather than a description of blood, air, or a combination of the two in the pleural cavity. Many may be adequately treated by insertion of an intercostal catheter in order to drain the pleural cavity and allow re-expansion of the lung, but do not lose sight of the true location of the injury. In addition to the pleura, there must have be damage to lung, chest wall or mediastinal structures.

- *Pneumothorax* is the most common finding in both adults and children, but the incidence of tension pneumothorax is much higher in children because of the increased mobility of the mediastinum (Eichelberger and Randolph 1981, Allshouse *et al.* 1993, Rowe *et al.* 1995). Rapid and definitive initial treatment with an intercostal catheter is therefore recommended. In the pre-school child breath sounds can be transmitted across the chest, so an increased percussion note and lack of chest wall movements on the affected side may be the only reliable indicators of a simple pneumothorax.
- *Haemothorax* is less common in children because of the lower incidence of rib fractures but may more frequently result from iatrogenic damage during chest drain insertion because of the smaller intercostal space. Haemothorax prior to insertion of a chest drain usually follows severe trauma in most children, and a significant underlying injury should be suspected (Allshouse *et al.* 1993). The thorax may also be a site of occult blood loss, in addition to the abdomen and pelvis, in a haemodynamically unstable child (Allshouse *et al.* 1993, Lloyd-Thomas *et al.* 1996). If a blood volume of >30% of the child's circulating volume is initially drained from the chest, or there is an ongoing loss equivalent to 20–30 mL/kg per hour for more than 2–4 hours, surgical exploration is indicated (Rowe *et al.* 1995). The blood should be drained from the pleural cavity once the diagnosis has been made: treatment delayed beyond 3–5 days may result in fibrinous adhesions and trapped lung with subsequent restrictive lung disease and a scoliosis as the child grows (Eichelberger and Randolph 1981, Allshouse *et al.* 1993).
- *Pneumomediastinum* is an uncommon finding following trauma but may represent a paramediastinal air cyst following pulmonary injury, an underlying tracheobronchial injury, or an oesophageal perforation (Bednarkiewicz *et al.* 1993). The difficulty is to distinguish the benign alveolar injury giving rise to paramediastinal air that may be treated conservatively, from the more serious trauma involving the oesophagus or respiratory tract. In this situation contrast studies, CT, or bronchoscopy may be required.
- *Pulmonary contusions* are the most common thoracic injury in children, but may be difficult to diagnose initially because of few signs and symptoms (Allen and Cox 1998). They represent a parenchymal injury to the lung characterized by haemorrhage and oedema, making the lung less compliant, increasing ventilation/perfusion mismatch because of arteriovenous shunting, impairing gas exchange, and predisposing to pneumonia and respiratory distress syndrome. The elasticity of the chest wall in children allows for highly effective transmission of the force of the trauma to the lung parenchyma with minimal or no external signs of injury (Rowe *et al.* 1995, Lloyd-Thomas *et al.* 1996, Tepas *et al.* 1996).

Although these injuries are usually eventually diagnosed with progressive opacification in the region of the injured lung on plain radiology, the initial chest radiograph may be completely normal even on subsequent review (Allen and Cox 1998). Early clinical signs include impaired oxygen saturation and mild tachypnoea, which may progress rapidly to severe hypoxia requiring ventilation. Plain radiographic changes lag behind the clinical progress of the contusion and frequently underestimate the extent of the injury (Allen and Cox 1998, Sivit *et al.* 1994). CT expedites diagnosis and allows for a more accurate assessment of the extent of the injury, but rarely directly influences clinical management (Sivit *et al.* 1989).

Treatment is supportive and involves the use of warmed, humidified supplementary oxygen, chest physiotherapy with incentive spirometry, and close observation in a high-dependency environment to monitor resuscitation. A paediatric intensive care physician should be involved early in the assessment and management of these patients, who should be reviewed at least 2 hourly in the first 12–24 hours. Those patients who continue to deteriorate should be transferred to an intensive care unit and mechanical ventilation introduced with positive end expiratory pressure (PEEP). Loop diuretics such as frusemide (furosemide) may be effective in reducing pulmonary oedema, but should only be used in conjunction with central venous pressure monitoring to avoid hypovolaemia. In a severe case refractory to conventional management, alternative ventilatory strategies may be required. Some of these, including oscillation and nitric oxide, are based on experience obtained in neonates with diaphragmatic hernia. The role of steroids in these injuries remains controversial (Allen and Cox 1998).

Pulmonary laceration is a rare injury in children as significant penetrating injuries, either from a foreign body or fractured rib, are uncommon. Clinically there is haemoptysis in addition to signs of local injury. There is usually evidence of haemopneumothorax on a chest radiograph, although this may be difficult to interpret on a supine film. Clinically, as haemorrhage continues, cardiovascular instability occurs. Treatment is surgical and involves thoracotomy and lobectomy in order to stem the blood loss. Autotransfusion may be a useful adjunct in the management of these rare patients (Kharasch *et al.* 1994).

Key points

- Pulmonary contusions are the most common injury.
- Tension pneumothorax more common than in adults due to mediastinal mobility.
- Haemothorax less common than in adults but blood loss may be haemodynamically significant in children.

Tracheobronchial injuries

It is fortunate therefore that tracheobronchial injuries are rare, as they are frequently associated with a fatal outcome (Stafford and Harmon 1993). There is some evidence, however, that bronchial injury may be more common in children than in adults because of differences in chest wall compliance (Mordehai *et al.* 1997).

Tracheobronchial injuries typically occur in children following rapid deceleration and severe blunt chest trauma in a road traffic accident or following penetrating chest trauma. These injuries are frequently difficult to diagnose, but should be suspected in a trauma patient with a pneumothorax that does not respond to an intercostal catheter (Rowe *et al.* 1995). The diagnosis should be confirmed by bronchoscopy and the treatment is usually primary repair via a thoracotomy, although an incomplete injury in a patient with blunt trauma that responds to the initial chest drainage may be treated conservatively.

Cardiovascular injuries

Significant cardiac injuries and trauma to the major vessels in the chest are rare following blunt trauma in children and may be difficult to diagnose even when there is clinical suspicion. In general the pattern of injury, diagnosis, and management are similar to those for adult patients.

Myocardial contusions are uncommon in children although this may be related to under-reporting, as there are no clearly defined diagnostic criteria (Langer *et al.* 1989). Certainly myocardial contusions requiring medical intervention or support for significant arrhythmias are rare, although minor ECG abnormalities and elevated cardiac enzymes may occur in up to a third of paediatric patients with blunt thoracic trauma (Stafford and Harmon 1993). This would seem plausible given the ability of the chest wall in children to transfer the energy associated with the injury to the lung parenchyma, resulting in a high incidence of pulmonary contusions. Thus the finding of severe pulmonary contusions or rib or sternal fractures should alert the clinician to the possibility of myocardial injury. Rarely, a powerful direct blow to the chest will result in refractory ventricular fibrillation (van Amerongen *et al.* 1997).

Other cardiac injuries that have been described include pericardial tamponade from air or blood, ruptured interventricular septum, papillary muscles damage leading to valvular disruption, and ventricular rupture (Harel *et al.* 1995, Michaels *et al.* 1997). Delayed pericardial tamponade may occur up to 2 weeks after blunt thoracic trauma in children (Bowers *et al.* 1994). Tamponade may now be rapidly diagnosed as part of the focused assessment for the sonographic examination of the trauma patient (FAST) examination in patients with multiple trauma (Wright 1995, Rozycki *et al.* 1998). More accurate imaging of the heart may be obtained via precordial or transoesophageal echocardiography, although in children the latter will require general anaesthesia (Wright 1995, Pretre and Chilcott 1997, Grasso and Keller 1998).

Major vessel injuries are probably as common in children as adults, after allowing for differences in number of journeys and speed of travel, although the greater mobility of the mediastinal structures in children increases the risk of major injury and most are dead at the scene (Eddy *et al.* 1990, Stafford and Harmon 1993). Aortic transection typically occurs as a result of rapid deceleration in road traffic accidents. Usually the patient is unrestrained in a motor vehicle accident at speeds >90 km/h (55 mph), or on a motorbike that hits a stationary object (Eddy *et al.* 1990). The diagnosis is suggested by the combination of an abnormal chest radiograph and an appropriate mechanism. Plain radiographic signs of aortic injury include widened mediastinum, tracheal or gastric tube deviation, a left apical cap, effusion or haemothorax, and depression of the left main bronchus (Stafford and Harmon 1993, Pretre and Chilcott 1997). The diagnosis is confirmed on aortography, although the use of magnetic resonance angiography or transoesophageal echocardiography has been described, with the latter perhaps more accurate in delineating intimal tears and flaps than aortography (Wright *et al.* 1995). In the patient with a suggestive mechanism of injury but a normal chest radiograph, a thoracic CT with intravenous contrast is the most appropriate investigation to exclude an aortic injury (Pretre and Chilcott 1997).

Other vascular injuries include subclavian vessel trauma in association with first rib fractures. This pattern of injury implies considerable force, and associated injuries are correspondingly severe (Harris and Soper 1990). The diagnosis may be suspected on the basis of neurovascular signs and symptoms in the upper limb of the affected side, but should be actively excluded by directed examination once a first rib fracture has been documented. The extent of the vascular injury should then be determined by angiography and a vascular surgeon involved in subsequent management.

Venous injuries most commonly represent iatrogenic injuries following operative intervention for insertion of a central venous catheter. These are usually identified at the time of insertion of the catheter, but occasionally the line may later migrate through the atrial wall to produce a haemopericardium (*Barrett et al.* 1998).

The thoracic duct may be injured during neonatal thoracotomy for repair of a tracheo-oesophageal fistula or patent ductus arteriosus, or rarely in a hyperextension injury to the cervical spine (Eichelberger and Randolph 1981). The result is a chylothorax that may initially be treated with an intercostal catheter and parenteral nutrition. If this treatment fails, open ligation of the duct is required.

Key points

- Cardiovascular injuries are rare in children and difficult to diagnose.

- Investigation and management similar to adults.
- Diagnosis of cardiac tamponade rapidly confirmed by FAST examination.

Oesophageal injuries

Oesophageal injuries occurring as a result of blunt or penetrating trauma to the thorax are rare. Perforation is usually seen following instrumentation or accidental ingestion of a sharp object (Rowe *et al.* 1995). The key to the diagnosis is the onset of moderate to severe chest pain in association with a combination of indicative history, pneumothorax, pneumomediastinum, surgical emphysema, or a pleural effusion. Chest pain in any child after oesophageal instrumentation should never be ignored.

Chest wall injuries

The high compliance of the chest wall in children, allowing transfer of energy to underlying structures, results in a relatively low incidence of rib and sternal fractures (Tepas *et al.* 1996). Correspondingly, when a fracture is identified, this usually implies that a considerably force has been applied and a significant intra-thoracic injury should be assumed. Isolated rib fractures following point application of a force, such as a fall on to the edge of an object, may not be associated with serious injury (Allshouse *et al.* 1993). Rib fractures are not infrequently seen in cases of child abuse, and the finding of multiple fractures of varying age should raise the index of suspicion (Carty 1997). First rib and scapular fractures, because of their location and surrounding musculoskeletal support, represent particularly severe injuries with a high likelihood of vascular and pleuropulmonary involvement (Harris and Soper 1990).

Multiple fractures leading to a flail segment are fortunately rare and usually associated with a crush injury from an object, such as a bookcase or heavy ornament, falling on to the child from a height (Tepas *et al.* 1996). The severe pulmonary contusions coupled with the flail segment inevitably result in hypoxia and respiratory failure requiring stabilization and mechanical ventilation. These patients routinely require admission to a paediatric intensive care unit.

Rib fractures may be diagnosed clinically and oblique view radiographs of the chest wall are not required for diagnosis or treatment. A chest radiograph is essential to help determine the presence of associated injuries. In the case of child abuse, a bone scan should be obtained to document the multiple fractures at different stages of healing.

Treatment of isolated rib fractures is supportive, with adequate analgesia and chest physiotherapy. A paediatric anaesthetist should be involved early to optimize the management of pain by appropriate use of non-steroidal anti-inflammatory analgesics and nerve blocks (Stafford and Harmon 1993). This enables effective chest physiotherapy and minimizes respiratory complications.

Key points

- Compliant paediatric chest wall results in low incidence of rib fractures.
- Force of injury in children is transmitted to underlying structures.
- First rib fractures are associated with neurovascular injuries.
- Multiple rib fractures of different ages are associated with non-accidental injury.

Diaphragmatic injuries

Diaphragmatic injuries following blunt trauma occur as a result of a direct blow to the lower chest or upper abdomen. This produces a rapid rise in intra-abdominal pressure, tearing the diaphragm and allowing the potential migration of abdominal contents into the chest. The injury is much more common on the left side, presumably because of splinting by the liver on the right. In part, however, this difference might represent underdiagnosis of right-sided defects that remain supported by the liver. Occasionally minor trauma may 'unmask' a small congenital diaphragmatic hernia previously plugged by the spleen or kidney.

The main difficulty in diaphragmatic injuries is in making the diagnosis. A chest radiograph may reveal disruption of the smooth contour of the diaphragm and the presence of abdominal viscera in the chest, but the appearance is rarely this obvious. Passage of a gastric tube and subsequent radiography will help reveal the site of the stomach, but its intra-abdominal location does not exclude a diaphragmatic tear. The diagnosis may be obtained by screening of the diaphragm fluoroscopically, ultrasound scanning, or CT. None of these modalities is specific, however, and the injury may even be missed at laparotomy.

If there is a high index of suspicion, an excellent view of the diaphragm is afforded by laparoscopy or thoracoscopy, with the option after confirming the diagnosis of performing the repair using these minimally invasive techniques (Graeber and Jones 1993, Liu *et al.* 1997). Most paediatric surgeons in the acute setting would favour performing a direct repair via the abdominal route as this allows easy reduction of viscera and inspection for associated intra-abdominal injuries.

Key points

- Diaphragmatic injuries may be difficult to diagnose by radiography or CT scan, and even at laparotomy.
- Laparoscopy/thoracoscopy are the diagnostic modalities of choice when there is high clinical suspicion as they afford the option of minimally invasive treatment after diagnosis.

Specific injury complexes

Penetrating trauma

Penetrating trauma as a result of interpersonal violence is rare in the UK and Australia, but is increasingly seen among older children and adolescents in the USA and South Africa. Children may be inadvertent victims of domestic violence, or civilian or wartime conflict. In these circumstances the potential for serious injury is obvious.

The much more common injury seen is the apparently minor penetrating wound resulting from a fall on to a piece of glass, or a twig breaking the skin after sliding down a tree. The chest wall is very thin in children, and any object that breaks through the skin should be assumed to have penetrated the chest cavity. These apparently minor wounds should not be simply closed directly in the emergency department. Formal exploration should be performed in a controlled environment in all cases (Wright 1995). As a minimum investigation a chest radiograph should be performed with subsequent treatment dictated by the result (Grasso and Keller 1998).

Traumatic asphyxia

Traumatic asphyxia is a specific and clearly defined injury complex seen relatively frequently in children (Eichelberger and Randolph 1981, Kissoon *et al.* 1990). The usual scenario is that of a vehicle backing over a pre-school child playing on the driveway at home. Because of the relatively low speed of the vehicle and the springy and compliant chest wall, rib fractures are uncommon. The lack of valves within the superior and inferior vena cavae allows the pressure rise to be transmitted to the head and neck area and the liver. This results in the appearance of multiple petechiae in the drainage area of the superior vena cava, with evidence of subconjunctival and retinal haemorrhages, and occasionally acute hepatomegaly.

The danger of these injuries is usually from the combination of cerebral oedema and secondary hypoxia as a consequence of pleuropulmonary injuries, typically pulmonary contusions or pneumothorax. Both give rise to confusion and disorientation that may make resuscitation of the child and its assessment difficult. Treatment is directed toward the underlying injury, but as these children usually require intensive monitoring they should be treated in a high dependency or intensive care area.

Burns

Burns are a common injury in childhood and the chest may be involved either directly as a result of burns to the chest wall or indirectly from an inhalational burn. In toddlers the most frequent injury is a burn to the upper chest and neck from a hot drink that the exploring child has pulled on to itself. These burns are often partial and infrequently compromise the airway. In older children, particularly boys experimenting with petrol or fire, major burns to the torso can occur. These injuries can severely compromise oxygenation as a result of an inhalational burn and splinting of the chest wall because of extensive cutaneous burns.

The key issues in the management of these patients are to establish the airway early, as this may rapidly deteriorate due to oedema, and to commence warmed humidified supplementary oxygen. The arterial blood gases should be checked and a carboxyhaemoglobin level obtained if carbon monoxide poisoning is suspected following burns in a confined space, such as a house fire. Respiratory distress syndrome may develop in children with inhalational burns, and there is some evidence in adults that exogenous surfactant may improve outcome (Pallua *et al.* 1998). In circumferential burns involving the upper torso, escharotomies to release the tourniquet effect of the burnt skin should be performed to allow adequate excursion of the chest wall for ventilation. These patients should be managed in a specialized paediatric burns unit with intensive care facilities, so that both the burn and the child can be optimally treated.

Early grafting minimizes the pain of multiple dressing changes, but the depth of the burn is often difficult to assess initially in children whose thin skin is more susceptible to thermal injury than adults. In patients who require grafting, great care should be taken to preserve the undeveloped breast bud during debridement, especially in girls (Garner and Smith 1992). Extended care is normally required in children with burns, in terms of both the functional result and scar management. Children are a dynamic platform because of growth and development, so regular re-evaluation of the result of burn management is required.

Summary

Thoracic trauma in children acts as a marker for severe injury and is usually associated with multisystem trauma, particularly head injuries. There is a potential for rapid deterioration that may initially be masked by the cardiovascular reserve of a normal child. Although severe injury is uncommon, it is a significant cause of mortality and morbidity. The majority of injuries may be managed by standard interventional measures with a successful outcome providing allowances are made for the differences in anatomy and physiology of children.

Key points

- Thoracic trauma is a marker for injury severity in children.
- It is usually associated with multisystem trauma.
- There is potential for rapid deterioration after cardiovascular reserve is exhausted.

References

ACS (1997) *Advanced trauma life support for doctors*, 6th edn. American College of Surgeons, Chicago.

Allen GS, Cox CS Jr (1998) Pulmonary contusion in children: diagnosis and management. *Southern Medical Journal* 91(12): 1099–1106.

Allshouse MJ, Rouse T, Eichelberger MR (1993) Childhood injury: a current perspective. *Pediatric Emergency Care* 9(3): 159–164.

Barrett AM, Squire R, Stringer MD *et al.* (1998) *Pediatric surgery and urology: long term outcomes.* 62, Vascular access. W B Saunders, London, pp 779–786.

Bednarkiewicz M, Pretre R, Huber O *et al.* (1993) Traumatic paramediastinal air cyst: report of two cases and review of the literature. *Journal of Trauma* 34(2): 305–308.

Bowers P, Harris P, Truesdell S, Stewart S (1994) Delayed hemopericardium and cardiac tamponade after unrecognized chest trauma. *Pediatric Emergency Care* 10(4): 222–224.

Carty H (1997) Non-accidental injury: a review of the radiology. *European Radiology* 7(9): 1365–1376.

Eddy AC, Rusch VW, Fligner CL, Reay DT, Rice CL (1990) The epidemiology of traumatic rupture of the thoracic aorta in children: a 13-year review. *Journal of Trauma* 30: 989–992.

Eichelberger MR, Randolph JG (1981) Thoracic trauma in children. *Surgical Clinics of North America* 61(5): 1181–1197.

Garner WL, Smith DJ Jr (1992) Reconstruction of burns of the trunk and breast. *Burns Rehabilitation and Reconstruction* 19(3): 683–691.

Graeber GM, Jones DR (1993) The role of thoracoscopy in thoracic trauma. *Annals of Thoracic Surgery* 56(3): 646–648.

Grasso SN, Keller MS (1998) Diagnostic imaging in pediatric trauma. *Current Opinion in Pediatrics* 10(3): 299–302.

Harel Y, Szeinberg A, Scott WA *et al.* (1995) Ruptured interventricular septum after blunt chest trauma: ultrasonographic diagnosis. *Pediatric Cardiology* 16: 127–130.

Harris GJ, Soper RT (1990) Pediatric first rib fractures. *Journal of Trauma* 30(3): 343–345.

Kharasch SJ, Millham F, Vinci RJ (1994) The use of autotransfusion in pediatric chest trauma. *Pediatric Emergency Care* 10(2): 109–112.

Kissoon N, Dreyer J, Walia M (1990) Pediatric trauma: differences in pathophysiology, injury patterns and treatment compared with adult trauma. *CMAJ* 142(1): 27–34.

Langer JC, Winthrop AL, Weisson DE *et al.* (1989) Diagnosis and incidence of cardiac injury in children with blunt thoracic trauma. *Journal of Pediatric Surgery* 24: 1091–1094.

Liu D-W, Liu H-P, Lin PJ, Chang C-H (1997) Video-assisted thoracic surgery in treatment of chest trauma. *Journal of Trauma: Injury, Infection and Critical Care* 42(4): 670–4.

Lloyd-Thomas AR, Anderson I, Skinner D, Driscoll P, Earlam R (1996) *ABC of major trauma*, 2nd edn. BMJ Publishing Group, London, pp 97–106.

Michaels A, Hirsh M, Maher T, McKenna C (1997) Survival following traumatic rupture of the heart in a child. *Pediatric Emergency Care* 13(1): 19–20.

Mordehai J, Kurzbart E, Kapuller V, Mares AJ (1997) Tracheal rupture after blunt chest trauma in a child. *Journal of Pediatric Surgery* 32(1): 104–105.

Pallua N, Warbanow K, Noah EM *et al.* (1998) Intrabronchial surfactant application in cases of inhalational injury: first results from patients with severe burns and ARDS. *Burns* 24: 197–206.

Peclet MH, Newman KD, Eichelberger MR *et al.* (1990) Thoracic trauma in children: an indicator of increased mortality. *Journal of Pediatric Surgery* 25(9): 961–966.

Pretre R, Chilcott M (1997) Blunt trauma to the heart and great vessels. *New England Journal of Medicine* 336(9): 626–632.

Reilly JP, Brandt ML, Mattox KL, Pokorny WJ (1993) Thoracic trauma in children. *Journal of Trauma* 34(3): 329–331.

Rowe MI, Fonkalsrud EW, O'Neill JA Jr *et al.* (eds) (1995) *Essentials of Pediatric Surgery*. 18, Thoracic Injuries. Mosby, St. Louis, Mo., pp 190–196.

Rozycki GS, Feliciano DV, Davis TP (1998) Ultrasound as used in thoracoabdominal trauma. *Surgical Clinics of North America* 78(2): 295–310.

Sheikh AA, Culbertson CB (1993) Emergency department thoracotomy in children: rationale for selective application. *Journal of Trauma* 34(3): 323–328.

Sivit CJ, Taylor GA, Eichelberger MR (1989) Chest injury in children with blunt abdominal trauma: evaluation with CT. *Radiology* 171: 815–818.

Sivit CJ, Taylor GA, Eichelberger MR (1994) Visceral injury in battered children: a changing perspective. *Radiology* 173: 559–561.

Stafford PW, Harmon CM (1993) Thoracic trauma in children. *Current Opinion in Pediatrics* 5(3): 325–332.

Tepas JJ III, Feliciano DV, Moore EE, Mattox KL (ed) (1996) *Trauma*, 3rd ed. Appleton and Lange, Stamford, Conn., pp 879–898.

van Amerongen R, Rosen M, Winnik G, Horwitz J (1997) Ventricular fibrillation following blunt chest trauma from a baseball. *Pediatric Emergency Care* 13(2): 107–110.

Wright MS (1995) Update on pediatric trauma care. *Current Opinion in Pediatrics* 7(3): 292–296.

32

CHAPTER 32

Paediatric abdominal injuries

ROY M KIMBLE AND
DANIEL T CASS

CHAPTER 32

Paediatric abdominal injuries

ROY M KIMBLE AND DANIEL T CASS

Around 8% of injured children will have an injury involving their abdomen; 9% of these end with a fatal result, of which 22% will be directly attributable to their abdominal injury (Cooper *et al.* 1994). Blunt abdominal trauma is seen with much greater frequency than penetrating trauma, but the latter is 1.4 times more likely to end in death (Cooper *et al.* 1994). Much progress has been made in the past two decades on the imaging of children with blunt abdominal trauma. This, along with a better understanding of the pathophysiology, has led to a sharp decline in the laparotomy rate. There are many differences in the assessment and management of abdominal trauma between adults and children, and these are the focus of this chapter.

Anatomy

Several anatomical factors combine to make a child more vulnerable than an adult to abdominal organ injury. The child's smaller size, thin abdominal wall, and cartilaginous ribs mean a greater force is transmitted to the abdominal organs. The close proximity of the abdominal organs also increases the chance of multi-organ injury. Also, the more horizontal position of the diaphragm in a child means that the liver and spleen lie lower and more anteriorly and are thus more vulnerable to injury. The thin abdominal wall also makes it prudent to assume that all penetrating injuries have entered the peritoneal cavity till proved otherwise.

Mechanism of injury

Blunt abdominal trauma remains the commonest cause of abdominal injury to the child. In the USA blunt trauma makes up 83% of all paediatric abdominal trauma (Cooper *et al.* 1994); in Australia it makes up 97%. Motor vehicle accidents are responsible for the majority of blunt abdominal injuries with slightly more occupant injuries (41%) than pedestrian (33%). Falls make up the next highest group (8%), followed by bicycle injuries (7%) (Cooper *et al.* 1994). Proper use of seatbelts with the use of car chairs and booster seats would reduce the injury rate significantly. Lap belt injuries are common in children and characteristically produce the triad of transverse abdominal wall ecchymosis, intestinal injury, and a flexion–distraction fracture to a lumbar vertebra (Chance fracture) (Newman *et al.* 1990). Handlebar injuries often cause severe organ damage because the force is applied through a small cross-sectional area. Commonly damaged organs from handlebar injuries include spleen, liver, pancreas, kidney, and intestine (specifically causing duodenal haematomas and bowel perforations) (Clarnette *et al.* 1997).

Penetrating injuries, although less common than blunt trauma, are associated with a higher mortality rate. In the USA penetrating injuries are usually the result of a stab or gunshot wounds, whereas in Australia most penetrating injuries are minor.

Child abuse is, unfortunately, very common and is the leading cause of trauma death in infants. Abdominal injury from child abuse carries a mortality rate as high as 45% (Cooper *et al.* 1988). These injuries are often the result of a punch or kick. A neglected infant who is the victim of child abuse can present moribund with rupture of intraabdominal organs. A high index of suspicion with a careful history and detailed examination is mandatory in any child suspected of being abused, to prevent repeated assault. The presenting problem is frequently minor, e.g. a finger injury, which can distract attention from a more serious abdominal injury.

Key point

- Anatomy and mechanism of injury lead to many differences in the assessment and management of abdominal trauma between adults and children.

General plan of management

The management of a child with abdominal trauma should follow the basic principals of any trauma resuscitation, i.e. a primary survey with treatment at each stage followed by the secondary survey. Abdominal examination normally comes into the secondary survey but may have to be included in the circulation phase of the primary survey if the child remains hypotensive after fluid resuscitation. A child is physiologically more resilient than an adult to blood loss. The first indication of hypovolaemia in the child is tachycardia, and hypotension may not become manifest until 45% of blood volume is lost. When intraabdominal haemorrhage from blunt trauma is suspected and the child is still unstable after 40–60 ml/kg crystalloid resuscitation, one should give 10 ml/kg of packed red cells, and a child who is still unstable should be taken immediately to theatre for laparotomy (ACS 1997). If the child is stable, or becomes stable after resuscitation, a non-operative approach can be undertaken. This approach followed the realization in the 1970s that most abdominal organ injuries in children stop bleeding spontaneously, and with time even the most severely damaged organs will usually heal. This approach depends on a surgeon being present and frequently re-examining the child. The child should be able to be taken to theatre immediately if they become unstable or develop signs of peritonitis signifying bowel perforation. Therefore the management of abdominal trauma in children should only be performed in institutions where the child can be fully managed, including laparotomy and aftercare.

Children will frequently swallow air when involved in trauma. This can lead to gastric distension, which not only impairs respiration but is also quite painful to palpate, making abdominal assessment difficult. In these children a gastric tube should be passed, remembering that it should be orogastric in the presence of cranial or facial injuries. A urinary catheter is helpful in the child sustaining major trauma, as urine output is a good indicator of haemodynamic status. A catheter should only be passed after you have checked that there are no signs of urethral injury (see Chapter 13, Urogenital injuries).

Key points

- Children are more resistant than adults to the effects of blood loss and the signs of hypovolaemia may not be apparent until 45% of blood volume is lost.
- Non-operative management may be possible in children even in severe organ trauma, but a child who becomes unstable should be taken to theatre.
- Gastric distension due to swallowed air can present a problem to assessment.

Investigations

Blood tests

Serum amylase measurement is useful because it rises not only in traumatic pancreatitis but also with small-bowel injuries. Beware that parotid trauma can also give an elevated serum amylase. Liver enzymes are usually elevated with hepatic damage (Hennes *et al.* 1990, Sahdev *et al.* 1991) and have been shown to be a useful indicator of occult hepatic injury in victims of child abuse (Coant *et al.* 1992).

Urinalysis

Microscopic and macroscopic haematuria, apart from being an indicator of urinary tract damage, are also an indicator of other intra-abdominal organ injury especially of the spleen and liver. However, this only remains true when there are other positive abdominal signs on examination (Taylor *et al.* 1988).

Plain radiograph

A plain abdominal film can be useful in detecting the presence of free gas signifying a bowel perforation. However, this investigation is only positive in 25–46% of perforations and should not be used to rule out the possibility of a visceral injury (Ulman *et al.* 1996, Ciftci *et al.* 1998). Other helpful signs on a plain abdominal film are loss of the psoas shadows, retroperitoneal gas (in the presence of a duodenal perforation), and bony injuries including lower rib, vertebral, and pelvic fractures. In the case of penetrating trauma a foreign body may be located.

Ultrasound

It has been shown in the paediatric trauma setting that free intraabdominal fluid correlates very well with organ injury (Taylor and Sivit 1995, Akgur *et al.* 1997). Ultrasound examination has been shown to be very reliable in detecting this free fluid and is being increasingly used as an emergency room screening tool (Katz *et al.* 1996, Patrick *et al.* 1998). The focused abdominal sonography in trauma (FAST) examination looks at pockets in the peritoneal cavity where blood will collect in the supine position, i.e. the retrovesical pouch or pouch of Douglas in males and females respectively, Morrison's pouch, the splenorenal recess, and right and left paracolic gutters. The advantage of this examination is that it can be performed in the emergency room, takes <3 minutes to perform, does not use ionizing radiation, and is repeatable. The FAST examination technique is fairly easy to learn (Ingeman *et al.* 1996) and is increasingly being used successfully by non-radiologists in the emergency room. Although this test is sensitive, it does not demonstrate the injured organ, so a positive test in a stable child is an indication that the patient requires a CT scan. It is also useful in the multiple trauma patient in whom initial resuscitation has not been successful and it is not certain where the bleeding source is. In this situation a FAST examination would rapidly confirm whether the bleeding was intraabdominal or not.

CT scan

CT scanning with the use of intravenous and oral contrast has become invaluable in the assessment of abdominal trauma (Graham and Wong 1996, Ruess *et al.* 1997). First reported by Rance and Bear (1980), the examination will usually demonstrate specific organ injuries, allowing for effective triage and a more focused plan of management (Neish *et al.* 1998). The main drawback of this examination is that it must be performed in the radiology department and therefore can only be done when the child is haemodynamically stable. Although CT will pick up many intestinal injuries, some will be missed and a negative examination is no substitute for frequent clinical assessment (Bensard *et al.* 1996, Akgur *et al.* 1997).

Diagnostic peritoneal lavage

The use of diagnostic peritoneal lavage (DPL) in children has greatly declined in popularity, mainly due to the realization that the majority of solid organ injuries can be managed non-operatively. Disadvantages include that it is a painful test and will cause distress to the conscious child, it can be the cause of intraabdominal trauma, and is non-specific when positive. The fact that fluid and gas are put into the peritoneal cavity makes interpretation of subsequent imaging difficult. The only area where DPL may have a role in children is in the situation where a child must be rushed to theatre for an extraabdominal injury a major abdominal injury must be ruled out. Emergency room ultrasound should make this last indication invalid.

Laparoscopy

The role and safety of laparoscopy for the diagnosis and treatment of intraabdominal trauma in children is controversial and a case has yet to be proven.

However, some preliminary studies have yielded promising results (Hasegawa *et al.* 1997).

Specific organ injury

Spleen

The spleen is the most commonly injured intra-abdominal organ in the child. The mechanism of injury is usually blunt trauma to the left upper quadrant, flank, or lower chest from a motor vehicle accident or fall. Physical examination will usually elicit tenderness in the left upper quadrant. Unlike adults with a splenic injury, rib fractures are unusual. A plain abdominal film may show the gastric bubble displaced to the right, but a CT scan is the investigation of choice. In most instances the spleen will bleed, resulting in either free intra-abdominal blood or bleeding contained within a subcapsular haematoma. The CT scan often looks dramatic but the key is to observe and act on the cardiovascular parameters, which allows over 90% of splenic lacerations to be successfully managed non-operatively. Delayed splenic rupture has only been very rarely reported. A vascular contrast blush seen on CT is, however, associated with arterial bleeding and may be an indication for early laparotomy in children (Cox *et al.* 1997).

In subsequent days with non-operative management the child is often difficult to manage with delayed re-establishment of normal feeding, some persistent abdominal pain, fever, and occasionally a pleural effusion. The main clinical concern is: could there be an associated intra-abdominal injury accounting for the persisting symptoms? If there is any doubt then a repeat CT scan is indicated. It has been shown that with selective non-operative management with careful observation the risk of missed associated injuries is minimal (Morse and Garcia 1994).

If operation is required, efforts are made to preserve the spleen which may include spenorrhaphy, partial splenectomy, or the use of an absorbable knitted bag to enclose the spleen (Aidonopoulos *et al.* 1995). This is important, as it has been shown that splenectomy caries a higher risk of death form overwhelming bacterial sepsis. This risk is highest in the paediatric population. In the situation where splenectomy has to be performed, there has been some success in splenic autotransplantation (Szendroi *et al.* 1997), although this does not guarantee protection from overwhelming sepsis (Moore *et al.* 1983), as to preserve splenic function 25% of the spleen has to remain. It is therefore prudent to immunize these children with polyvalent pneumococcal and *Haemophilus influenza* vaccine. It remains controversial whether children should be on long-term penicillin or have an adequate stock at home to be started as soon as any fever develops.

It is unclear how long one should restrict the physical activity of a child who has sustained splenic trauma. The rate of healing as determined on serial CT scanning seems dependent on the original grade of splenic injury; with grade 1 and 2 injuries healing within 4 months, grade 3 injuries taking up to 6 months and grade 4 injuries taking up to 11 months (Benya *et al.* 1995). An uncommon sequelae of splenic trauma is the formation of a splenic pseudocyst. Small cysts (<4 cm) often resolve spontaneously but larger cysts tend not to resolve and run the risk of infection, rupture, and haemorrhage. It is for these reasons that an operative approach be taken on large pseudocysts with the aim at splenic preservation. Techniques include enucleation, marsupialization, and partial splenectomy but sometimes these are not possible and splenectomy must be carried out (Teneriello *et al.* 1997).

Liver

In the last two decades the trend for children with liver injuries has also been to attempt non-operative management if possible. This is because in children most hepatic injuries, like splenic injuries, will stop bleeding spontaneously. Again the principles are of a detailed history working out the forces involved with intensive monitoring. It is important when reviewing the literature on the management of liver trauma to appreciate that the situation has changed in recent years, and with the advent of CT scanning many more minor liver injuries are being picked up. It is in such population groups that operative rates of 7% have been reported. The same basic rules apply for liver injuries as for any intrabdominal haemorrhage, i.e. if after a half blood volume replacement the child is still haemodynamically unstable then operative intervention is indicated. If one has to operate then same techniques as used in adults such as liver packing, blunt needle suturing, and partial hepatectomy are indicated. A rare long-term sequela of hepatic trauma in children is the formation of a hepatic cyst. Most of these are asymptomatic and can be managed conservatively, but occasionally they can become symptomatic and require surgical intervention (Chuang *et al.* 1996).

Pancreas

Pancreatic injuries are uncommon in children. They usually occur as a result of blunt trauma to the upper abdomen where an object has compressed the pancreas against the vertebral column. Common scenarios include injuries occurring from bicycle handlebars, go-kart steering wheels, and punch injuries (often, unfortunately, as a result of child abuse). Pancreatic injuries can present as a solitary finding or as part of multi intra-abdominal organ trauma. If occurring in isolation the presentation is often delayed a few days with the child eventually presenting extremely unwell with established pancreatitis. Trauma is responsible for 15–37% of all pancreatitis in children (Synn *et al.* 1987, Weizman and Durie 1988, Ziegler *et al.* 1988, Haddock *et al.* 1994, Yeung *et al.* 1996). The key to managing these injuries is to determine whether the main pancreatic duct is intact or not. When the duct is intact the management should be non-operative, but if it has been transected then distal pancreatectomy is indicated (McGahren *et al.* 1995). Endoscopic retrograde pancreatography has been shown to be safe in children and clearly defines the main pancreatic duct (McGahren *et al.* 1995, Richieri *et al.* 1994). CT scanning has improved the early detection of these injuries but often does not have the resolution necessary to demonstrate the status of the main duct. Serum and urinary amylase are elevated in pancreatic injury and levels are usually higher than found with isolated small-bowel injury.

Pseudocysts will complicate acute pancreatitis in children in 10–23% of cases, but the figure rises to 56% when the pancreatitis is due to trauma (Weizman and Durie 1988, Ziegler *et al.* 1988, Haddock *et al.* 1994, Yeung *et al.* 1996). When associated with trauma, up to 60% of pancreatic pseudocysts will require surgical intervention (Yeung *et al.* 1996). Surgical options for the management of pancreatic pseudocysts in children include percutaneous drainage and open procedures such as cyst-gastrostomy and cyst-enterostomy (Poston and Williamson 1990). Endoscopic drainage creating a cyst-gastrostomy with double pigtail catheters has been used successfully in the child with a post-traumatic pancreatic pseudocyst (Kimble *et al.* 1999).

Intestine

Injuries to the intestine are particularly problematic in children because they can be the result of minor abdominal trauma, and early physical examination and investigations may falsely reassure the clinician that there is no intraabdominal injury. The key to management is to suspect the injury and perform serial physical examinations, noting increasing abdominal tenderness, peritonism, tachycardia, and fever. The mechanisms of injury that suggest bowel trauma include seatbelt injuries (especially from lap belts), bicycle handlebar injuries, rapid deceleration, falls on to fences and rocks, and kicks or punches (Newman *et al.* 1990, Clarnette *et al.* 1997). Small-bowel injuries as a result of child abuse are particularly difficult as they frequently present late with peritonitis and the history of the injury is often hidden or confused. A left lateral decubitus abdominal radiograph is useful if it demonstrates free gas, but its absence does not exclude the possibility (Ulman *et al.* 1996, Ciftci *et al.* 1998). CT scanning will pick up many intestinal and mesenteric injuries (Graham and

Wong 1996, Ruess *et al.* 1997), but sometimes the signs are subtle such as focal bowel wall thickening, free peritoneal fluid, and non-progression of the contrast material without demonstrating a leak (Cox and Kuhn, 1996). However, the gold standard remains serial physical examinations and if perforated bowel is suspected then laparotomy is indicated (Albanese *et al.* 1996). Most bowel injuries can be managed with a primary anastomosis, but occasionally a defunctioning ostomy is required (Ciftci *et al.* 1998).

Duodenal haematomas are fairly common following blunt abdominal trauma and usually present with discomfort and bile-stained vomiting. Non-operative management, which is quite often prolonged, is usually successful.

Penetrating injuries

The abdominal wall of a child is very thin, so any object that penetrates through the skin must be assumed to have entered the peritoneal cavity. The non-operative approach that applies to adults is less indicated in children and should only be undertaken by experienced clinicians. All too often a small piece of glass, wood, or metal has penetrated the peritoneal cavity and it is a safe policy, if these injuries are seen infrequently, to explore the child and fully ascertain the extent of the damage.

References

ACS (1997) Pediatric trauma. In: *Advanced trauma life support instructor manual*. American College of Surgeons, Chicago, pp 360–362.

Aidonopoulos AP, Papavramidis ST, Goutzamanis GD *et al.* (1995) Splenorrhaphy for splenic damage in patients with multiple injuries. *European Journal of Surgery* 161: 247–251.

Akgur FM, Aktug T, Olguner M *et al.* (1997) Prospective study investigating routine usage of ultrasonography as the initial diagnostic modality for the evaluation of children sustaining blunt abdominal trauma. *Journal of Trauma* 42: 626–628.

Albanese CT, Meza MP, Gardner MJ *et al.* (1996) Is computed tomography a useful adjunct to the clinical examination for the diagnosis of pediatric gastrointestinal perforation from blunt abdominal trauma in children? *Journal of Trauma* 40: 417–421.

Bensard DD, Beaver BL, Besner GE *et al.* (1996) Small bowel injury in children after blunt abdominal trauma: is diagnostic delay important? *Journal of Trauma* 41: 476–483.

Benya EC, Bulas DI, Eichelberger MR *et al.* (1995) Splenic injury from blunt abdminal trauma in children: follow-up evaluation with CT. *Radiology* 195: 685–688.

Chuang JH, Huang SC (1996) Posttraumatic hepatic cyst—an unusual sequela of liver injury in the era of imaging. *Journal of Pediatric Surgery* 31: 272–274.

Ciftci AO, Tayel FC, Salman AB *et al.* (1998) Gastrointestinal tract perforation due to blunt abdominal trauma. *Pediatric Surgery International* 13: 259–264.

Clarnette TD, Beasley SW (1997) Handlebar injuries in children: patterns and prevention. *Australian and New Zealand Journal of Surgery* 67: 338–339.

Coant PN, Kornberg AE, Brody AS *et al.* (1992) Markers for occult liver injury in cases of physical abuse in children. *Pediatrics* 89: 274–8.

Cooper A, Barlow B, DiScala C *et al.* (1994) Mortality and truncal injury: The pediatric perspective. *Journal of Pediatric Surgery* 29: 33–38.

Cooper A, Floyd T, Barlow B *et al.* (1988) Major blunt abdominal trauma due to child abuse. *Journal of Trauma* 28: 1483–1487.

Cox CS, Geiger JD, Liu DC *et al.* (1997) Pediatric blunt abdominal trauma: role of computed tomography vascular blush. *Journal of Pediatric Surgery* 32: 1196–1200.

Cox TD, Kuhn JP (1996) CT scan of bowel trauma in the pediatric patient. *Radiology Clinics of North America* 34: 807–818.

Graham JS, Wong AL (1996) A review of computed tomography in the diagnosis of intestinal and mesenteric injury in pediatric blunt abdominal trauma. *Journal of Pediatric Surgery* 31: 754–756.

Haddock G, Coupar G, Youngson GG *et al.* (1994) Acute pancreatitis in children: a 15-year review. *Journal of Pediatric Surgery* 29: 719–722.

Hasegawa T, Miki Y, Yoshioka S *et al.* (1997) Laparoscopic diagnosis of blunt abdominal trauma in children. *Pediatric Surgery International* 12: 132–136.

Hennes HM, Smith DS, Schneiderk K *et al.* (1990) Elevated liver transaminase levels in children with blunt abdominal trauma: A predictor of liver injury. *Pediatrics* 86: 87–90.

Ingeman JE, Plewa MC, Okasinski RE, King RW, Knotts FB (1996) Emergency physician use of ultrasonography in blunt abdominal trauma. *Academic Emergency Medicine* 3: 931–937.

Katz S, Lazar L, Rathus V *et al.* (1996) Can ultrasound replace computed tomography in the initial assessment of children with blunt abdominal trauma? *Journal of Pediatric Surgery* 31: 649–651.

Kimble RM, Cohen R, Williams S (1999) Successful endoscopic drainage of a post-traumatic pancreatic pseudocyst in a child. *Journal of Pediatric Surgery* 34(10):1518–1520.

McGahren ED, Magnuson D, Schaller RT *et al.* (1995) Management of transected pancreas in children. *Australian and New Zealand Journal of Surgery* 65: 242–246.

Moore GE, Stevens RE, Moore EE *et al.* (1983) Failure of splenic implants to protect against fatal postsplenectomy infection. *American Journal of Surgery* 146: 413.

Morse MA, Garcia VF (1994) Selective nonoperative management of pediatric blunt splenic trauma; risk for missed associated injuries. *Journal of Pediatric Surgery* 29: 23–27.

Neish AS, Taylor GA, Lund DP *et al.* (1998) Effect of CT information on the diagnosis and management of acute abdominal injury in children. *Radiology* 206: 327–331.

Newman KD, Bowmen LM, Eichelberger MR *et al.* (1990) The lap belt complex: Intestinal and lumbar spine injury in children. *Journal of Trauma* 30: 1133–1138.

Patrick DA, Bensard DD, Moore EE *et al.* (1998) Ultrasound is an effective triage tool to evaluate blunt abdominal trauma in the pediatric population. *Journal of Trauma* 45: 57–63.

Poston GJ, Williamson RCN (1990) Surgical management of acute pancreatitis. *British Journal of Surgery* 77: 5–12.

Rance CH, Bear JW (1980) Computed tomography in the management of paediatric abdominal trauma. *Australia and New Zealand Journal of Surgery* 50: 506–512.

Richieri JP, Chapoy P, Bertolino JG *et al.* (1994) Endoscopic retrograde cholangiopancreatography in children and adolescents. *Gastroenterology and Clinical Biology* 18: 21–25.

Ruess L, Sivit CJ, Eichelberger MR *et al.* (1997) Blunt abdominal trauma in children: impact of CT on operative and nonoperative management. *AJR* 169: 1011–1014.

Sahdev P, Meadow E, Garramone RR (1991) Elevation of liver function tests in screening for intra-abdominal injuries. *Annals of Emergency Medicine* 20: 838–41.

Synn AY, Mulvihill SJ, Fonkalsrud EW (1987) Surgical management of pancreatitis in childhood. *Journal of Pediatric Surgery* 22: 628–632.

Szendroi T, Miko I, Hajdu Z *et al.* (1997) Splenic autotransplantation after abdominal trauma in childhood. Clinical and experimental data. *Acta Chirurgica Hungarica* 36: 349–351.

Taylor GA, Sivit CJ (1995) Posttraumatic peritoneal fluid: is it a reliable indicator of intraabdominal injury in children? *Journal of Pediatric Surgery* 30: 1644–1648.

Taylor GA, Eichelberger MR, Potter BM (1988) Hematuria: A marker of abdominal injury in children after blunt trauma. *Annals of Surgery* 208: 688–693.

Teneriello FL, Teneriello GF, Del Grande E *et al.* (1997) Non-parasitic splenic cysts. *Giornale di Chirurgia* 18: 222–228.

Ulman I, Avanoglu A, Ozcan C *et al.* (1996) Gastrointestinal perforations in children: a continuing challenge to nonoperative treatment of blunt abdominal trauma. *Journal of Trauma* 41: 110–113.

Weizman Z, Durie PR (1988) Acute pancreatitis in childhood. *Journal of Pediatrics* 113: 24–29.

Yeung C, Lee H, Huang F *et al.* (1996) Pancreatitis in children—experience with 43 cases. *European Journal of Pediatrics* 155: 458–463.

Ziegler DW, Long JA, Philippart AL *et al.* (1988) Pancreatitis in childhood. *Annals of Surgery* 207: 257–261.

33

CHAPTER 33

Paediatric burns

DANIEL T CASS

CHAPTER 33
Paediatric burns

DANIEL T CASS

Burns in a child are a triple tragedy. First is the injury, which requires prolonged, painful, and costly treatment. Secondly, the scars are visible and lifelong. Whereas a ruptured liver or spleen will heal to become normal tissue, deep burns to the skin—even with optimal treatment—heal to become unsightly fibrous scars. Thirdly, there are psychological problems. There is considerable parental guilt and the child has to endure the treatment and adjust to their new physical appearance. The tragedy is all the more poignant because it is so unnecessary: burns are the most preventable of injuries. Some communities (usually affluent) have significantly decreased burns, while the problem remains entrenched in others (usually deprived). It is not unusual to have almost no burns in some areas of a city but clusters in other areas. For example in Sydney (Australia), the eastern and northern suburbs have very few burns; whereas the western and southern suburbs have significant bunching of burns (often in the same street). Efforts to treat burns must focus not just on the surgery but also prevention.

Prevention

Most burns in children are scalds from kitchen and bathroom accidents, such as hot baths and spilt cups of tea or coffee (60%). Every effort should be made to educate the public about the hazards of these hot fluids, especially near toddlers. Regulating the temperature of the hot water system (or at least the taps) in the bathroom to 42°C can reduce injuries from bath scalds. Cold water should always be run in first, and then hot water, to bring up the temperature to the desired level. Epileptics always need to be supervised during baths and showers.

The other 40% of burns in children are due to flame (25%), contact (10%), and less commonly electrical, chemical and sun. Younger children are more likely to suffer scalds whereas older children suffer more flame burns. Open fires or radiators where a young child can put a piece of paper between the guards are known mechanisms that start devastating house fires. Similarly, allowing children to play with matches and cigarette lighters courts disaster. Many countries now outlaw easy-to-use cigarette lighters. Smoke detectors are a proven method of reducing mortality from fires. All houses should have them fitted, and there should be adequate checks to see they are being maintained and working well. Contact burns from barbecues are common in Australia and usually involve the palms of the hands in toddlers who do not realize the danger.

Fire-related risk-taking behaviour in adolescent boys has always been a problem, and they need to be forewarned about the dangers. This traditional high-risk group has been further stimulated by access to the Internet where irresponsible people have posted instructions on how make small incendiary devices from household products.

Physicians treating burns have an obligation to try to prevent further injury. Publicity for burns cases has a marked effect on public perception and is one of the main ways of further reducing the burden of burn injuries in the local community. Particular attention needs to be paid to deprived areas, where is it is difficult to get information across and poverty often leads to unsafe situations and a high risk of burns. It is a problem of a trilogy of 'not having', 'not knowing', and unfortunately at times 'not caring'. A low rate of childhood burns is an indicator of a community's sophistication.

The main differences between children and adults in the treatment of burns are:

- the difference in weight to body surface area, which produces a proportionately higher metabolic rate in a child than in an adult
- the thickness of the skin
- the differences in psychological status.

Key points

- Scalds from kitchen and bathroom accidents are among the most common mechanisms of burns in children.
- For the most part, burns are preventable: education is the key.

First aid

A key aim is to ensure that the harm is minimized. This can be achieved by ensuring that *all* clothing is removed immediately. When underwear is left on there is often accentuated burning where the material is thickest (pleats or seams).

The ideal treatment is to immerse the injured part in tepid water for 20–30 minutes. Temperatures of between 8°C and 25°C are satisfactory, with the optimum being 15°C. This is still useful up to 3 hours after the burn. A hand or foot is easy and safe to immerse, but if there is a burn to the trunk one needs to be careful of not inducing hypothermia. The use of ice, or meat from the freezer, is contraindicated as the very low temperature of these can produce further burns. A good indication that the first aid is working is the diminution of pain. If pain recurs when the burned area is removed from the fluid, it can be re-immersed. Such first aid can reduce the severity of pain and the degree of the burn.

Primary assessment

The key triage tool is the history.

Major burns

In the aftermath of a house fire, or where there is a risk of smoke inhalation in an enclosed area, one is dealing with an emergency. The early management of severe trauma must follow guidelines. Careful attention to the airway and early intubation if needed are mandatory. Precisely the same sequence of treatment must be instituted for an injured child as for an adult, as often more harm is done to the child by hesitating and not working through a set adult regime. If a situation exists that would necessitate intubation in an adult, then almost certainly a child would need to be intubated in the same situation. A similar mental priority list applies for decisions about the introduction of intravenous fluids and the need for escharotomy.

Scalds

Most burns are minor and involve the hands, feet, head, or trunk area. The common problems are to decide whether the child needs to be admitted to hospital, whether fluids should be introduced, and whether grafting is needed.

In general, burns to the hands, feet, face, and genital areas always require admission. Often a history is helpful, in that if the child has a simple splash injury and there is only erythema then the child can be managed as an outpatient. On the other hand, a child who has grabbed a hot iron and has burns to the flexor creases of the hand should be admitted and early grafting considered.

Fluid resuscitation

A child <1 year of age has a head and neck surface area equal to 18% of total body surface area, with each lower limb being 14%. Each year after this the head proportionally loses 1% and the lower limbs gain 0.5% each. Adult proportions are therefore reached at around 10 years of age. The estimation of the surface area and depth of burn is always difficult; more important than precise calculations is to start the appropriate fluids, insert a urinary catheter, and review the child regularly. The aim in children is to produce 1 mL/kg of urine per hour.

A starting resuscitation infusion is 4 ml of Ringer's lactate per kilogram body weight, for each percent of burns over the first 24 hours. Once the 24 hours fluid is worked out, one-half of the fluid is administered in the first 8 hours and the remaining half in the next 16 hours. It is important to remember that the above fluid requirement is for resuscitation, and maintenance fluids must be added. In young children glucose needs to be added to the solutions to maintain their blood sugar levels.

It must be stressed that the early calculations are only an approximation and the most important feature in the resuscitation of burns is frequent reassessment and adjustments of fluids depending on the urine output.

Key points

- Estimation of body surface area in children may be difficult.
- It is important to start fluid resuscitation early.

Burns care

The management of paediatric burns is a specialized area. As early as possible the child should be transferred to a burns unit for assessment by a paediatric burns surgeons. The reason for this is not so much the expertise in treating the burn *per se*, but rather the large team effort, which involves complex pain relief, specialist nurses, social workers, physiotherapists, nutritionists, and family therapists. Burns often occur in families where there has recently been some social disruption, and this, together with the guilt felt by the parents, greatly increases the difficulty in treating the burns. Contractures can occur quickly, and early movement with appropriate pain relief is essential.

Wound assessment (classification) (see also Chapter 14)

The initial assessment of wounds can be difficult both in estimating the fluid requirements and in assessing the ultimate need for grating.

- *Superficial burns:* The skin appear reddened and blistered.
- *Partial thickness burns:* These are often mottled with red and white patches interspersed which do not blanch on pressure. There are also areas of petechial haemorrhage.
- *Full thickness burns:* These appear much whiter and quickly go to a brown dry colour and are leathery on palpation. Thrombus veins may be visible in the base. There is a loss of pain sensation in the burned area.

Wound management

Pain relief

Morphine is the best agent for pain relief. The initial dose is 0.1 mg/kg but this may be increased to 0.2–0.3 mg/kg if necessary. The drug is given intravenously as a continuous infusion, but this necessitates meticulous respiratory monitoring in children. This will allow the initial cleaning of the wound, which allows more precise assessment.

The initial washing of the burn should be with tempered normal saline and performed in a warm environment. Any soot or other material should be gently removed. Blisters are best left intact.

Wound surgery

Opinions differ as to whether early grafting or observation with later grafting is preferable, and as to the precise technique of grafting. These controversies demonstrate that as yet we have not reached an optimal way of removing dead tissue and encouraging the regrowth of new skin. In many ways the techniques are the same as in adults, with refinements as to the depth of skin grafts taken. It is likely that in the future that the new technology of growing the patient's own skin will be a major contribution to the better care of paediatric burns.

Unusual burns

Electrical

Most electrical burn injuries to children are a result of exposure to electricity in the home. These injuries can easily be prevented by the use of blind plugs to cover electrical outlets and the installation of circuit breakers into the main switchboard.

A key message in electrical burns is that the degree of tissue injury is often much extensive than would be initially expected from the initial examination. Quite often vessels are thrombosed, muscles are hypoxic, and fractures may have occurred.

Face

Facial burns can lead to marked swelling that causes more alarm than is warranted by the end outcome. Although very swollen and blistered the skin often does recover well, although there is a tendency in many patients to keloid formation. When skin grating is needed it is important to colour match the area and to take thicker than normal grafts.

Eyes

When the eyelid is damaged there is often concern about direct damage to the cornea. However, this is very unlikely as the lids are often closed shut and there is relative protection of the eye. Early treatment should involve the use of chloroamphenicol eye ointment.

Hands

Burn injuries to the hands can be very difficult to manage as the ideal situation would be for the child to start early movement. Techniques such as putting the whole hand in a glove smeared with silver sulfadiazine (SSD) sometimes work, but the child may not co-operate and in that instance regular dressings are required. In general, early excision and grafting is used in the hand areas as it is important to get early mobility.

Feet

Burns to the feet can be deceptive. Splashes of hot liquid on to the feet may result in blistering and a very mild burn. In other instances, with the shoes on, or if fat falls on to socks, there can often be quite extensive localized burning. Very careful assessment and if necessary early excision and grafting is warranted. Keloid scars in this area are very difficult to treat as the child remains very active and resists pressure garments.

Perineum

Injuries to the perineum are difficult to manage because urine and faeces will interfere with the healing process. A urinary catheter is inserted and constipation induced by the use of codeine phosphate. This will allow up to 10 days of non-passage of faeces. If healing has not occurred in that stage, or the burn is more extensive and will not heal by that time, colostomy is warranted.

Infection

At the time of the burn all wounds will be sterile, but within 24–48 hours a flora partly from the patient and partly from the environment will cover the wound area. The key aim of treatment is not necessarily to pursue the impossible task of producing sterility, but rather preventing sepsis. Opinions continue to differ as to the value of various antiseptic agents and the place of antibiotics. For simple burns no treatment would be the best form of management, and for more extensive burns the use of SSD is practiced in most institutions. Antibiotics are reserved for episodes of sepsis or sometimes given prophylactically at the time of major grafting episodes.

Septicaemia when it occurs in children can be rapid and profound. Constant vigilance is required, and early aggressive treatment by both fluids and antibiotics is required once burns are suspected.

Further reading

Adamson JE (1985) Hand injuries. In: Mayer, TA (ed) *Emergency management of paediatric trauma*. Chapter 23, W B Saunders, London, pp. 390–405.

Raine PAM, Azmy AAF (1985) Burns and scald injuries. In: Raine PAM, Azmy AAF (ed) *Surgical emergencies in children*, Chapter 14,W B Saunders, London, pp. 272–285.

34

CHAPTER 34

Child abuse

NANNI ALLINGTON

CHAPTER 34
Child abuse

NANNI ALLINGTON

General issues

Historical background

Tardieu in 1860 (King 1988) described lesions such as burns found during the autopsy of children and associated these features with 'battered children'. In 1946, Caffey reported the association of subdural haematoma and long bone fractures (King 1988). Reports then became more frequent, but it was only after mainstream use of the definition by Kempe *et al.* (1962) of the term 'battered child syndrome' that the problem started to be debated in public, and legal measures put in place in various countries.

Key point

- Child abuse has been reported in the literature since the 1860s but it was not until the 1960s that there was public and legal awareness.

Definition

The initial definition by Kempe implied direct physical abuse and has since been broadened to psychological and sexual abuse and emotional and medical neglect. If a child is harmed by the lack of appropriate treatment for a specific condition (e.g. refusal of physical therapy and casting for a club foot), it is considered as medical neglect and necessitates the same general approach as direct physical abuse.

Key point

- Kempe's definition has been broadened to include psychological and sexual abuse, and emotional and medical neglect.

Epidemiology

The exact number of children being neglected or abused is impossible to determine, since numerous cases are undiagnosed or unreported. A general estimate is that 1–1.5% of all children are abused (Akbarnia 1996). Child abuse is universal and found in all races and classes. All children can be abused, but the majority are small children, especially below the age of 1 year. Boys and girls are equally affected. Stepchildren are at greater risk. Once abused there is about a 35% of chance of 'relapse' and 5% of death.

Diagnosis

The diagnosis and thus the management of child abuse is often delayed or undiagnosed.

Environmental elements

Doctors

Emergency department physicians, paediatricians, general practitioners, and orthopaedic surgeons are often in the first line in the discovery of an abused child. To be able to distinguish 'normal' physical injuries from neglect or abuse, the physician needs to first of all have a high level of suspicion in all injuries involving young children, especially if the caretaker gives no clear explanation. Less experienced physicians might also feel uncomfortable with these more 'general' and 'emotional' situations. Some physicians might be more reluctant to report cases from higher social classes. Overdiagnosis can bring conflicts in future patient–doctor relationships.

Despite the difficulties involved with even suggesting the possibility of an abused child, the orthopaedic surgeon must go further than simple fracture treatment. Each fracture in a child needs an appropriate explanation.

Medical history

There is no one simple clue, but again physicians need to have a level of suspicion when the trauma history given by the caretaker is vague, changes when repeated, or does not fit the lesions found. Caretakers can also report that they did not see the incident, or that the child just started to complain. They can also be reluctant to give explanations and delay bringing in the child for medical treatment. Another element of suspicion is if they come from outside the usual catchment area, as they may already be known to staff in their local hospitals (not because 'this hospital is better', which is the explanation they will give you).

Caretakers

Parents are the most common abusers, but any caretaker can be involved. Again, there is no single easily recognized pattern. The abuser can be aggressive towards the medical staff, raise lots of question, or refuse investigations on the child. They can also look unduly protective of the child and very concerned. Difficult social situations, disrupted families, drug or alcohol abuse, and disabilities can be involved but are not always present.

Key points

- Parents are the most common abusers.
- There are no simple patterns to recognize.
- Abusive parents may act over-concerned.

Child

The child also has different attitudes, from very compliant to aggressive. Girls and boys are equally affected. Stepchildren and handicapped children are more at risk. The abused child might show 'developmental delay' due to the abuse. In any one family, all children can be abused or only one of them.

The physician should be able to recognize any inappropriate behaviour in the caretakers or the child.

Clinical findings

The orthopaedic surgeon will be confined to examining the bony lesions, but will have to look for other 'clues' if an abused child is suspected.

Soft tissue lesions

Physical examination will reveal bruises, burns, lacerations, and scars. Again some of these have usual, normal explanations but it is important to make the distinction between 'normal' bruises from falls—often found on elbows, shins, knees—and inflicted ones—on buttocks, perineum, or trunk. The same is true for lacerations and scars. Cigarette burns are quite characteristic. Burns are seen in 10% of abused children, and some reports suggest as high as 20% (Galleno and Oppenheim 1982). It is also useful to determine the timing of the bruises and soft tissue lesions: one or more episodes?

Key point

- Photographs and appropriate documentation of suspicious lesions is crucial.

Head injuries

The head and face are often injured since they are quite easy targets. The usual weapon is the human hand.

Violent shaking of a baby or young child can be particular deleterious, with cerebral oedema or subdural haematoma, and is known as the *shaken baby syndrome*.

In any child where abuse or neglect is suspected, a good neurological examination is necessary. Conversely, in any child with unexplained neurological signs abuse has to be suspected. Skull radiography is part of the general skeletal survey, but quite often there are no skull fractures, only internal lesions. In the acute phase, CT scans will help and later on MRI will show the chronic neurological damage.

Internal injuries

Internal injuries are often the cause of death in child abuse. Younger children are more often affected. Death is due to the gravity of these lesions and the fact that the child is brought late to the emergency department. Any internal organ can be injured.

Bony lesions

Although some fracture types or patterns are more often seen in child abuse, there is no one 'absolute' sign of abuse. The other clinical and general findings must also be taken into account.

Fracture patterns: radiological findings

Multiple age fractures and an unclear history will raise suspicion. However, King (1988) reported that one single fracture was found in 50% of his series of abused children. Bone scintigraphy as well as radiographs of the entire skeleton need to be done to look for fractures (healed or not). These tests will be particularly helpful in young children who unable are express themselves (Akbarnia and Akbarnia 1976).

One has to suspect abuse in certain cases:

- fractures of the lower extremity in non-weight-bearing children
- the association of posterior ribs fractures with long bone fractures
- the metaphyseal 'corner fracture' (Kleinman *et al.* 1986).

All other combinations are possible. Some fractures are more specific: for example, a metaphyseal corner fracture is caused by forceful pulling on an extremity. They need good quality radiographs to be seen.

The list in Table 34.1 gives a summary of the degree of suspicion based on the type of fracture. Again, any of them can be seen, even the regular common fractures (but then with a suspicious history) (Kleinman 1987).

Table 34.1 Type of fracture and degree of suspicion

Highly suspicious fractures	Metaphyseal fractures Posterior rib fractures Scapular fractures Spinous process fractures Sternal fractures
Suspicious fractures	Multiple fractures Different age fractures Epiphyseal separations Vertebral body injuries Complex skull fractures
Regular common fractures	Clavicular fractures Long bone shaft fractures Linear skull fractures

Fracture dating

Although variations are of course present, it is quite helpful to date fractures. Table 34.2 gives a timetable of radiographic changes (Kleinman 1987).

Differential diagnosis

Child abuse will have to be differentiated from a long list of a possible other underlying pathology: milder forms of osteogenesis imperfecta (Sillence 1981), scurvy, rickets, leukaemia, septic arthritis, osteomyelitis, neurological disorders (osteoporosis in cerebral palsy, myelomeningocele, polyomyelitis), metastatic neuroblastoma, congenital indifference to pain, stress fractures, osteopetrosis, and congenital syphilis.

Treatment

Physical treatment

The child needs to be admitted to hospital for thorough work-up. The physical treatment of the different injuries is similar to the general practice for the same lesions. For example, fracture care is similar to that for regular fractures, but the situation might

Table 34.2 Timetable of radiographic changes

Lesion	Early	Peak	Late
Soft tissue	2–5 days	4–10 days	10–21 days
Periosteal new bone	4–10 days	10–14 days	14–21 days
Loss of fracture line definition	10–14 days	14–21 days	
Soft callus	10–14 days	14–21 days	
Hard callus	14–21 days	21–42 days	42–90 days
Remodelling	3 months	1 year	2 years till epiphyseal closure

be more complex with the legal and social issues that will have to be raised.

Legal and social issues

The management of child abuse involves the diagnosis, the medical treatment, and the appropriate social and legal measures. To be able to address the legal issues it is mandatory to document the lesion: good medical records with descriptions of the clinical examinations, social workers' reports, photographs, radiographs, CT scan, and bone scan are required.

Legal issues vary from country to country, but the primary goal is to protect the child from further abuse. Hospital stay will thus be necessary not only for the full work-up but also to give time to work out the situation with the social workers and the appropriate local 'teams' and legal system.

If possible the child will be returned to the family, with counselling for the abusive caretaker, but this will not always be possible and if necessary the child will be placed in a foster home.

Key point

- Legal issues vary from country to country, but the primary goal is to protect the child from further abuse.

Conclusion

The role of the physician and orthopaedic surgeon is to think of the possibility of child abuse in specific clinical conditions, to admit the child to hospital for work-up and treatment, and to alert the appropriate authorities.

References

Akbarnia BA (1996) The role of the orthopaedic surgeon in child abuse. In: Morrissy RT, Weinstein ST (ed.) *Lovell and Winter's pediatric orthopaedics*, Vol. II. 4th edn, Chapter 32. Lippincott-Raven, Philadelphia, Pa.

Akbarnia BA, Akbarnia NO (1976) The role of the orthopedist in child abuse and neglect. *Orthopedic Clinics of North America* 7: 733–742.

Galleno H, Oppenheim W (1982) The battered child syndrome revisited. *Clinical Orthopaedics and Related Research* 162: 11–19.

Kempe CH, Silverman FN, Steele BF, Droegemueller W, Silver NK (1962) The battered child syndrome. *JAMA* 181: 17–24.

King J, Diefendorf D, Apthorp J, Negrete VF, Carlson M (1988) Analysis of 429 fractures in 189 battered children. *Journal of Pediatric Orthopaedics* 8: 585–589.

Kleinman PKS (ed.) (1987) *Diagnostic imaging of child abuse*. Williams & Wilkins, Baltimore, Md.

Kleinman PK, Marks SC, Blackbourne B (1986) The metaphyseal lesion in abused children: a radiologic-histopathologic study. *AJR* 146: 895–905.

Sillence D (1981) Osteogenesis imperfecta: an expanding panorama of variants. *Clinical Orthopedics* 159: 11–25.

Further reading

Epps CH Jr, Bowen JR (ed.) (1995) *Complications in pediatric orthopaedic surgery*. J B Lippincott, Philadelphia.

Rockwood CA Jr, Wilkins KE, King RE (ed.) (1984) *Fractures in children*, vol. 3. J B Lippincott, Philadelphia.

35

CHAPTER 35

Child sexual abuse

JEAN R EDWARDS AND
DIANNA MILINKOVIC-BALOG

CHAPTER 35
Child sexual abuse

JEAN R EDWARDS AND DIANNA MILINKOVIC-BALOG

The growing body of literature and research on child sexual abuse that we witnessed in the latter part of the twentieth century was kindled primarily by adult women speaking out about their childhood experiences of sexual abuse. Despite significant numbers of documented cases and psychiatric discourse at the end of the nineteenth century about child sexual abuse, the issue was spoken about as if it were a rare problem. The 'battered baby syndrome' identified in the 1960s by Kempe drew attention to the issue of child physical abuse (Kempe *et al.* 1962). The women's movement in the 1970s lobbied to place the issue of child sexual abuse on the social, health, and political agenda. Retrospective studies of adults sexually abused as children revealed that 1 in 3–5 women experienced sexual abuse in childhood. These findings are well documented and have opened the door to a growing awareness that child sexual abuse is a significant problem affecting the lives of 1 in 3–5 girls and generally about 1 in 6–7 boys by the age of 18 years. In approximately 90% of cases, the offender is either a member of the child's family or is well known to the child and family.

Key points

- Kemp's definition of 'battered child syndrome' in the 1960s drew attention to child abuse and in the 1970s there was public awareness about child sexual abuse.
- 1 in 3–5 women and 1 in 6–7 men have experienced sexual abuse in childhood.
- In 9 of 10 cases the offender is known to child and family.

Definition

Though the laws on child sexual abuse vary in different jurisdictions, child sexual abuse is a crime, which occurs when an adult or older person uses his or her power, authority, or position to impose upon a child any sexual activity.

Features of child sexual abuse may include the following:

- Physical or psychological coercion which differentiates such abuse from consensual peer sexual activity (Tomison 1997).
- The dependency and immaturity of children is exploited by adults and adolescents who perpetrate child sexual abuse.
- The sexual activity may include sexual touching, masturbation, sexual penetration, and non-contact sexual acts such as exposing a child to pornographic material, exhibitionism, and voyeurism.
- The child is coerced to keep the sexual activity secret in order to prevent disclosure.
- Offenders commonly employ tactics to make the child feel responsible for the sexual activity.

Key point

- Child sexual abuse is a crime in any jurisdiction.

Nature of child sexual abuse

Prepubertal

- Sexual gratification of the adult by the use of the child's body.
- Commonly begins with touching of the genital area, making the child touch the adult's genitals, and may eventually progress to partial or full penetration.
- Commonly occurs over long period of time.
- The offender commonly employs a range of tactics to engage a child and involve the child in sexual activity, e.g. favouritism, bribery, tricks, threats, coercion.
- Child sexual abuse does not commonly present with concurrent physical violence.
- Most offenders are a member of the child's family or are known to the child and the family.
- Disclosure rarely occurs following a single incident, unless the offender is a stranger.

Postpubertal

- May be continuation of prepubertal abuse with increasing level of severity.
- Coercion may also involve the use of drugs, alcohol, and peer pressure.
- May resemble adult rape involving a single episode with an assailant of similar age to the victim.
- Commonly involves full penetration.
- May involve violence.

Key areas of consideration in managing a report of child sexual abuse

Child protection and welfare considerations

Safety of the child from further sexual abuse is of the highest priority. Notification to statutory authority vested with the legal responsibility of ensuring the safety of children, to investigate the report, is necessary to ensure the protection and safety of the child.

Legal considerations

Child sexual abuse is a crime. Since children do not have the capacity to consent to sexual contact, any person engaging in sexual activity with a child has committed an offence. Investigation by police and the laying of charges are possible following a report. Medical officers who receive a report and/or provide medical examination may be called to provide expert opinion on medical findings in criminal proceedings. Medical examinations should be carried out within the particular protocols and with an understanding of the interagency roles and policies.

Medical care and follow-up concerns

Physical trauma and medical needs, such as concerns about sexually transmitted diseases and pregnancy, must be addressed. Fears about permanent damage following sexual abuse need to be assessed, and the child and non-offending parent reassured.

Therapeutic and support considerations

Psychological and emotional impact on the child and non-offending parent need to be considered, and referral to specialist services should be offered where it is available. The disclosure of child sexual abuse often precipitates a crisis for which immediate counselling and support is strongly recommended. This counselling addresses practical issues, emotional impact and concerns, information, and support through legal proceedings if necessary.

Key point

- Psychological counselling should be offered to the child and the non-offending parent.

Responding to a report of child sexual abuse

Child sexual abuse requires an interagency approach that encompasses all the considerations outlined above. The child's future safety must receive priority and cannot be assumed because a disclosure has been made, or because the non-offending parent or offender gives assurances about the child's safety. It is crucial that child protection authorities are informed, and in many jurisdictions, medical officers are mandated notifiers of child sexual abuse. Child protection authorities, police, medical officers, and social workers all have a vital role to play in addressing the needs and concerns of the child sexual abuse victim and their non-offending parent.

Only a medical officer who has received specific training should be involved in the examination of a child where child sexual abuse is reported or suspected. Such training must include the normal and abnormal genital anatomy of children.

Key points

- The child's future safety is paramount—appropriate authorities should be notified.
- Only a medical officer who has received specific training should be involved in the examination.

Medical role in child sexual abuse assessments

Because of the sensitive nature of the material that needs to be explored, a child who has reported sexual abuse needs to be treated with sensitivity and respect. It is important that the doctor's intervention is not perceived by the child as a continuation of the abuse. Any examination that needs to be performed must be explained to the child in age-appropriate language, and must only be done with the consent and cooperation of the child.

The doctor has two major functions when involved in the assessment of a child or young person who has disclosed sexual abuse, or about whom there is a suspicion of sexual abuse:

- To inform, medically manage and reassure the child and it's parents about any medical concerns that they have.
- To document the assessment, including appropriate examination, for any medico-legal purposes that may arise.

Acute assessments

Children and young people who present within 72 hours of the reported abusive event must be seen immediately so that both medical and medico-legal issues can be dealt with. Because there is a possibility of pregnancy in postpubertal girls if there has been ejaculation near the genital area, the possibility of administering the 'morning-after pill' must be considered. Children should be offered a medical examination as soon as possible after their disclosure of sexual abuse, so the anxiety that they and their non-offending parents experience can be addressed.

Forensic evidence

In the medical assessment of children who have reported sexual abuse there may be forensic evidence to collect, particularly if the assessment is performed soon after the reported abuse.

The forensic evidence may consist of:

- physical evidence on the body of the child
- physical evidence on the clothing that the child was wearing
- physical evidence at the site of the sexual abuse such as stains on bedclothes, towels, etc.

The physical evidence on the child's body may be in the form of minor or major injuries consistent with the history of abuse. These must be documented on the body and genital diagrams of the child in the forensic protocol.

The other evidence present on the child's body may be the remains of seminal fluid if the offender ejaculated. Forensic specimens are taken from any parts of the body where traces of seminal fluid may remain and these specimens are retained in secure circumstances for future forensic examination.

The genital examination of young children who have been sexually abused is usually normal, due to the non-penetrative nature of the acts. Adams *et al.* (1994) summarize the physical findings of 236 children with conviction of the perpetrator for sexual abuse. The findings showed that there was clear evidence of abuse in only 9% females on the genital examination, and in 1% of males and females where the abuse was reported to be anal.

Disclosure of sexual abuse often creates an acute emergency within the family, even if the event occurred some time before and has occurred over a long period of time. These children should also be seen urgently so that assessment and reassurance can take place.

Investigation vs assessment

It is not the role of the doctor to investigate complaints of sexual abuse. The decision on whether abuse has occurred is a legal matter, which may be dealt with by a court. Depending on the circumstances the report of sexual abuse may be investigated by the police service or by the government department with the responsibility for child protection issues. It is the role of the doctor to assess, document findings, and treat these children.

The doctor should obtain the history of sexual abuse from the adult accompanying the child and from any referring agency. In the case of a very young child, only sufficient detail to ensure an adequate examination is necessary. The investigative interview with the child should be conducted by the police and child protection services. If a young child repeats the history to a large number of people, the evidence may become contaminated and unable to be used in legal proceedings.

Impact of sexual abuse of children

Child sexual abuse has been extensively documented since it was recognized as a significant clinical problem in the 1970s. Kendall-Tackett *et al.* (1993), reviewing 45 studies, found that 'sexually abused children had more symptoms with abuse accounting for 15–45% of the variants'. They also found that the following symptoms were most common:

- fears
- post-traumatic stress disorder
- behaviour problems
- sexualized behaviours
- poor self-esteem.

They also noted that approximately one-third of children had no symptoms, and that no one symptom characterized a majority of sexually abused children. Factors which affected the degree of symptomatology were:

- penetration
- duration and frequency of the abuse
- force
- the relationship of the perpetrator to the child
- maternal support.

Mullen and Fleming (1998), in their discussion of the long-term effects of child sexual abuse, noted that

> There is now an established body of knowledge clearly linking a history of child sexual abuse with higher rates in adult life of depressive symptoms, anxiety symptoms, substance abuse disorders, eating disorders and posttraumatic stress disorders.

Key point

- The long-term impacts of sexual abuse in childhood include a number of well-recognized effects.

Conclusion

The doctor who first assesses the child who has reported sexual abuse has a key role to play in the recovery process of this child and, by engaging in a multidisciplinary response, helps to ensure the child's future safety.

References

Tomison M. (1997) *Preventing child abuse and neglect in NSW: findings from a state audit*. NSW Child Protection Council, Sydney, Australia, p. 5.

Adams JA. Harper K. Knudson S. Revilla J (1994) Examination findings in legally confirmed child sexual abuse: it's normal to be normal. *Pediatrics* 94(3): 310–317.

Kempe CH, Silverman FN, Steele BF, Droegemueller W, Silver NK (1962) The battered child syndrome. *JAMA* 181: 17–24.

Kendall-Tackett KA, Meyer Williams L, Finkelhor D (1993) Impact of sexual abuse on children : a review and synthesis of recent empirical studies. *Psychological Bulletin* 113(1): 164–180.

Mullen PE, Fleming J (1998) Long-term effects of child sexual abuse. *Australian Institute of Family Studies Issues in Child Abuse Prevention*. No. 9, Autumn.

36

CHAPTER 36

The injured elderly patient

GREG B BENNETT AND
CAROLINE HOGAN

CHAPTER 36
The injured elderly patient

GREG B BENNETT AND CAROLINE HOGAN

Impact of ageing populations

Developed countries are continuing to age rapidly. By 2030, more than 25% of populations in the developed world will be >65 years of age (Mandavia and Newton 1998). This phenomenon will alter the face of healthcare. The developing world is also ageing rapidly. Patterns of health need are therefore changing dramatically across the whole world. In older people, injury generates a disproportionately greater amount of healthcare costs (Mandavia and Newton 1998). It is therefore imperative that the principles of effective care of older people are understood in trauma services and other healthcare services.

Interactions of multiple co-morbidities, disabilities, medications, undernutrition, psychosocial issues, environmental factors, and ageing *per se*, although unpredictable in the individual patient, are increasingly common with advancing age. The resultant effects on physiology and physiological reserves of many older people may render them more vulnerable to the effects of physical trauma and ensuing complications (Horan *et al.* 1992). Trauma or post-trauma care of older people therefore presents special challenges to clinicians involved at the various stages of care, from site of injury to rehabilitation.

Causes and patterns of injury in older people are quite different from those of younger people (Martin and Teberian 1990). Health and physiological changes of older people are heterogeneous and therefore unpredictable. Numerous studies of outcomes in older people indicate that co-morbidities and physiological changes are more important than age *per se* in predicting outcome from various medical and surgical conditions (Grisso and Kaplan 1994). Individualized assessment is always required. Management principles which guide the clinician are covered later in this chapter.

Epidemiology

Overview

Trauma facts: older versus younger people:

- Overall, falls are the most common cause of injury. Motor vehicle accidents predominate in younger people.
- Incidence of trauma is relatively less common.
- Recurrence of trauma is more likely.
- Trauma is relatively less severe.
- Consequences of trauma are more serious (Schiller *et al.* 1995).
- More injury occurs per unit force as age increases.
- Hospital stay is longer.
- Cost *per capita* is higher.
- Outcomes tend to be poorer in older people.

Currently the over-70s comprise over 11% of the US population. In Australia the over-65s are expected to increase to about 20% of the population in 2031, a 300% increase from 1986 figures (Kallman and Kallman 1989). As a group, older people are less likely to suffer trauma than younger people (van Aalst *et al.* 1991, Fildes 1994) and when they do suffer trauma it tends to be less severe (De Keyser *et al.* 1995).

In the USA, trauma is the fifth most common cause of death for people over the age of 65 (Martin and Teberian 1990). In Australia, 102 women and 141 men per 100 000 incur injuries over the age of 65 years (Fildes 1994). The death rate rises exponentially with age, increasing dramatically over the age of 75 years (Mandavia and Newton 1998). In the USA, although older people represent only 14% of the population, they account for 28% of fatalities and over 30% of trauma health costs (Oreskovich *et al.* 1984). Weingarten *et al.* (1982) report that trauma is usually less serious in older people but more costly. More over-85s die from falls than 18–19 year olds from motor vehicle accidents (Baker *et al.* 1992). Younger elderly people are much less likely to be injured by falls.

Overall, older people are less likely to be injured than younger people. In 1989 there were 16.5 episodes of injury per 100 people over the age of 65, compared to 23.8 per 100 people for all ages (Levy *et al.* 1993). However, injuries in this age group are more likely to have a fatal outcome. In the USA 30 000 older people die from trauma every year. A 12 month survey (Spaite *et al.* 1990) of all trauma admissions of a 370 000 population found that 30% of 1154 patients reviewed by trauma paramedics were over the age of 75 years. Women accounted for 65%. Of the 1154, 53% were aged 70–79 years, 39% were aged 80–89 years, and 7.6% were over 89 years. Trauma calls were 30% of all house calls for over 70s and 52.3% for younger people. Trauma cases >65 years old were more likely to be transported to hospital than cases under 65 years (75% vs 49%). Gerson and Skvarch (1982) reported that elderly people required advanced life support transport twice as often. Although the outcome after trauma is worse with increasing age, aggressive treatment in older people usually has a favourable outcome.

Under-reporting of injury-related death in elderly people appears to result from a bias to attribute death to medical conditions either contributing to or resulting from trauma-related death (Fife 1987).

Elder abuse, which is notoriously difficult to detect, is an under-reported cause of injury. Its prevalence is estimated at between 3% and 5% of the elderly population (Kurrle *et al.* 1991).

Trauma recurrence is high in elderly people (Gubler *et al.* 1996) and probably represents the recurrent nature of falls and falls injuries of those who have already fallen.

Key points

- Falls as compared to MVAs are the most common cause of trauma in elderly people.
- Trauma in elderly people is less severe, but the consequences are more serious including longer hospital stays.

Injury mechanisms

Causes of injury in usual order of prevalence are listed below. These are based upon surveys in western countries, which have used different methods, biased populations selection and different definitions and parameters (Preston Smith *et al.* 1990, van Aalst *et al.* 1991, Baker *et al.* 1992, Fildes 1994, Osler *et al.* 1998, Zietlow *et al.* 1994). Many trauma surveys followed patients through trauma retrieval systems and are therefore biased against detecting injurious falls in older people.

1 falls (40% to >80%; increasing percentage with increasing age)
2 motor vehicle accidents (>20%)
3 suicide (10%)
4 burns (10%)
5 assault/elder abuse (1–5%)
6 choking (about 2%)
7 self-induced poisoning (<2%)
9 miscellaneous (1–9%).

Most trauma is caused by falls and motor vehicle accidents (driver, passenger and pedestrian). The incidence of falls is increasing. This is probably related to the increasing proportion of older elderly who are more prone to falls and fractures than young elderly people. Elderly women have higher rates of fall injuries than elderly men. Older men have higher rates of injuries from burns and motor vehicle accidents, including pedestrian accidents.

They also have higher rates of death from these three categories. Among those aged 65–74 years, nearly one-quarter of deaths are due to falls and over one-third are due to motor vehicle accidents. By age 75, 50% of deaths from injury are due to falls and less than 20% due to motor vehicle accidents. Falls increasingly dominate injuries and injury deaths with advancing age (Baker *et al.* 1992). A survey of trauma indicated that 10% of falls in older people were caused by a specific medical diagnosis.

Outcomes

As the elderly population increases, we are faced with a greater number of injured elderly patients. Depending on the series, up to 40% of elderly trauma patients die (De Maria *et al.* 1987a, 1988, van Aalst *et al.* 1991, Baker *et al.* 1992, De Maria 1993, Fildes 1994, Schiller *et al.* 1995, Mandavia and Newton 1998). It is therefore desirable to be able to predict which patients will benefit from treatment, in order to avoid subjecting patients and their families to treatment in futile situations and—more importantly—to ensure that older people are not denied access to potentially useful treatment. For further discussion of trauma outcomes, see specific trauma types.

Outcome clearly depends on the individual's general health, the nature and severity of trauma, and the occurrence of complications. Little research has been undertaken in this field, and most studies have failed to include important risk factors for geriatric outcome such as pre-trauma co-morbidities, dementia, undernutrition, anthropometry, medication use, functional status, and combinations of risk factors. Study subject numbers have been too few to detect real and relevant associations. Trauma populations studied and definitions of trauma employed have varied significantly enough to produce results which are sometimes contradictory (De Maria 1993). Some facts appear to be reasonably clear, and are outlined below.

Morbidity in patients increases with injury severity (Knudson *et al.* 1994). In general, head injuries are related to a worse outcome than other types of injury in elderly people (Zietlow *et al.* 1994, van Aalst *et al.* 1991). Falls and pedestrian injuries and the presence of injury to the brain, chest, or abdomen are significantly associated with mortality (Knudson *et al.* 1994).

Mortality from a defined level of trauma increases as age does from about 10% at age 45, to 15% at age 55, and 20% at age 75 (Finelli *et al.* 1989). Studies defining elderly as either >65 or >75 report mortality rates ranging from 20% to 40% (van Aalst *et al.* 1991, Broos *et al.* 1993, Zietlow *et al.* 1994, Knudson *et al.* 1994). However, hospital mortality for fractured femur is only 5%. Trauma outcome is significantly poorer for older people over the age of 85 (Shabot and Johnson 1995). This undoubtedly relates to comorbidities, which predispose to complications. Elderly patients who are severely brain injured, with a Glasgow Coma Scale (GCS) of 5 or less, experience a higher mortality (up to 80%), die more frequently from secondary organ failure, have poorer functional recovery, and consume more resources per favourable outcome than younger injury-matched patients (Pennings *et al.* 1993). Although trauma mortality and recovery is significantly worse than that for younger people, several studies indicate that aggressive treatment of older trauma patients is warranted. Data from a number of studies suggest that 55–80% of older people survive serious trauma (De Maria *et al.* 1987a, Shapiro *et al.* 1994). The majority of severely injured geriatric patients who survive their injury return to some degree of independent living (De Maria *et al.* 1987a, van Aalst *et al.* 1991).

Pedestrian death rates rise with age. After controlling for injury severity, injury severity score, and mechanism of injury, the death rate rises from 10% after the age of 45, increasing to 20% at age 75. Interestingly, trauma outcome could not be correlated with pre-existing disease in a survey by Preston Smith *et al.* (1990). In their review of critical care outcome in the oldest old trauma patients, Shabot and Johnson (1995) state, 'decisions regarding outcome should be based on severity of illness rather than age, trauma type or injury severity'.

Physiological status in the emergency department appears to influence outcome. Mortality risk increases with decreasing admission trauma score using either the trauma score or the revised trauma score (Knudson *et al.* 1994). (The trauma score comprises systolic blood pressure, capillary refill, respiratory rate, respiratory expansion, and GCS; revised trauma score comprises systolic blood pressure, GCS, and respiratory rate.) Hypotensive shock on arrival is a poor prognostic indicator (Horst *et al.* 1986, van Aalst *et al.* 1991) and enhances mortality with increasing age (Osler *et al.* 1988). One study found a statistically significant relationship between hypotension in the emergency department and subsequent infection. Hypoventilation (respiratory rate of <10 per minute) also has a predictive value. Mortality increases as respiratory rate decreases. Patients over the age of 85 who have a respiratory rate of >30 have a poor prognosis. Requiring intubation upon admission is associated with poor outcome (Pellicane *et al.* 1992). Complications including infection and multiorgan failure are common in elderly people (occurring in up to one-third) and influence morbidity and mortality (De Maria 1993).

During admission, the following factors are associated with poor outcome: pulmonary infection, need for prolonged mechanical ventilation, central nervous system injury, burns, and hypovolaemic shock (De Maria *et al.* 1987b).

One complication will increase mortality from 5.4% to 8.6%. Two or more complications are associated with a mortality of 30% (Preston Smith *et al.* 1990), indicating that elderly patients do not tolerate complications well. Preventable complications in older patients with moderate degrees of injury warrant more aggressive care than that required by younger patients (De Maria *et al.* 1987a, Scalea *et al.* 1991, Pellicane *et al.* 1992, Broos *et al.* 1993).

In one study, preventable complications which contribute to death occurred in 32% of all deaths and 62% of organ failure deaths (Pellicane *et al.* 1992). The most common preventable complication was pulmonary aspiration of nasogastric or nasoduodenal feeds, despite chest radiograph confirmation of correct feeding tube position. The authors suggest admitting all patients with trauma score <15 to intensive care units. However, this accounts for 50% of all older trauma patients in his series.

Poor in hospital functional status at discharge has been associated with diabetes and dementia. Inpatient factors such as premorbid functional status, cognition, and nutritional status have not been included in most trauma outcome studies.

Marriage has positively associated with in hospital post-trauma functional outcome (Radke *et al.* 1992). Rehabilitation requirements are high. Many of the studies examining outcome have not included long-term rehabilitation outcome in detail, including quality of life issues.

Key points

- Head injuries have a poorer outcome than any other type of injury.
- Mortality from a defined level of trauma increases with age, trauma outcome is significantly poorer for those over age 85.
- Lower trauma scores on admission are correlated with increased risk of mortality.

Physiology

General

Summary of key features of physiology of ageing

- Causes of physiological decline:
  - genetically determined component
  - disuse (especially musculoskeletal and cardiovascular)
  - disease (obvious and occult).
- Heterogeneous—great variance of physiology of older populations
- Unpredictable in an individual
- Ageing *per se* does not cause disability
- Drugs commonly exacerbate impaired physiology.

Average ageing: an epidemiological concept

Many physiological changes have been described in aged populations (Rowe and Kahn 1987). As a population ages, there is increasing scatter around the mean of any particular physiological function. Elderly people are a heterogeneous group in whom chronological age may be a poor indicator of a patient's physiological status. Average population data do not always translate to clinical practice. Contributing multiple subclinical diseases impair the clinician's ability to predict physiological alterations in an individual. Cardiovascular impairment may not be apparent on initial assessment. The onset of sepsis or relatively minor blood loss may cause rapid decline in haemodynamic homeostasis, manifesting as precipitous and unexpected shock.

Ageing per se

Ageing itself does not cause physiological decline to the extent that an older person's ability to function and live independently is impaired (Rowe and Kahn 1987). Disability is always due to disease. Some older people have physiological performance exceeding that of some healthy younger individuals. The true contribution of the ageing process to physiological decline is less than previously thought (Bortz 1989). Many non-western cultures have demonstrated remarkable absence of degenerative diseases that were once thought to be part of the ageing process. Sensorineural hearing loss, systolic hypertension and subsequent left ventricular hypertrophy, arthritis, and coronary artery disease to name a few, seem to be degenerative consequences of western lifestyle superimposed upon the ageing process (Schneider and Rowe 1996, Svanberg and Selker 1994). Preconceived notions about ageing seem to have caused nihilistic approaches to care in some quarters and, not the least, affected the attitude of older people to themselves (Ogle 1998).

The demands that trauma places on physiological systems extends them to the maximum.

Relevance

In older trauma patient, physiological changes may have the following adverse effects (Horan *et al.* 1992), including:

- increased propensity to sustain trauma
- increased severity of injury per unit force
- disturbed maintenance of homeostatic mechanisms
- increased risk of complications, e.g. infections
- prolonged healing rate
- prolonged rehabilitation.

There is an increased probability of co-morbid disease processes and drug effects contributing to impaired physiological reserves in elderly patients.

Possibly the two most important factors which influence physiological processes in older people are nutritional status and physical activity. Both influence body composition (and therefore pharmocodynamics), cardiovascular function, immune function, thoracic muscle function, sarcopaenia development, osteoporosis, and thermoregulation. Nutritional status and physical activity are important in preventing trauma and rehabilitation after trauma.

Nutrition

Nutritional status is implicated in the aetiology of many chronic diseases. Undernutrition is a major predictor of poor outcome for older people in general (Lehmann 1989, Sullivan *et al.* 1990, 1991). Most surveys agree that about 50% (between 20–80%) of community-dwelling older people are undernourished, depending on the definition used (Lipski 1995). Undernutrition in residential care populations occurs in up to 80% of residents.

Assessment of nutritional status in the trauma patient is based on multiple measures, including

- estimates of usual dietary intake premorbidly (dietary history)
- evidence of recent weight loss
- anthropometric measures of fat and muscle

- laboratory measures of blood count, simple biochemistry, vitamin B_{12}, folate, iron, and serum proteins (albumin, retinol binding protein, and thyroxine binding protein), which can be used as nutritional indices in elderly people.

A medical history and examination may reveal causes of malabsorption or diseases causing increased nutritional requirements.

Undernutrition in the older trauma patient is a result of its adverse affect upon:

- fat and collagen integrity reducing soft tissue protection to the skeleton and internal organs
- capillary and small-vessel integrity and therefore propensity to bleeding
- immune function, especially cell-mediated immunity increasing susceptibility to infection
- thermoregulation (mild degrees of hypothermia in older people cause reduced balance coordination and impaired cognition which probably contribute to winter-time falls)
- possible increased risk of osteoporosis and therefore fractured femur
- muscle function pre- and post-trauma
- delayed wound healing (zinc and vitamin C are associated with improved wound healing rate)
- mortality, morbidity, domicile after hospital care and functional status (nutritional supplementation improves these outcomes) (Delmi *et al.* 1990).

In an individual patient with undernutrition, the cause is usually multifactorial. Contributing factors include:

- Increased nutritional requirements
    - infection
    - some drugs, e.g. corticosteroids, anticonvulsants, antibiotics
    - injury.
- Reduced intake
    - sub-optimal dietary choices
    - anorexia due to gut problems, sepsis, depression, narcotics, antibiotics
    - oral and chewing problems
    - impaired taste
    - swallowing problems
    - abdominal pain
    - diarrhoea (fear of).
- Poor digestion or assimilation
    - undernutrition
    - achlorhydria
    - antispasmodics, anticholinergic, anticonvulsants and other drugs
    - malabsorption.

Nutritional supplementation is associated with improved nutritional status, immune function, fewer infections, improved respiratory muscle function in chronic lung disease patients, and overall fractured femur outcome.

Optimizing nutritional status is best achieved by provision of small frequent meals rather than larger meals three times daily.

Key point

- Undernutrition is common and is an important aetiological factor in many chronic diseases in elderly people.

Body composition and sarcopaenia

Total body weight plateaus at age 40–60 then undergoes a gradual decline (Bennett and Gwinn 1998). The fat free (lean) mass tends to decline and body fat increases in a centripetal pattern. Many of the observed changes are reversible. Muscle is an important source of metabolic protein because the majority of hospitalized older trauma patients are unable to ingest adequate protein and other nutrients in the acute phase (Older *et al.* 1980, Delmi *et al.* 1990). Researchers have suggested that increased body fat is protective for hip fractures.

Sarcopaenia is a syndrome of ageing with a major contribution from disuse (LeBlanc *et al.* 1992, Bloomfield 1997), undernutrition, and age (Fiatarone *et al.* 1993).

The average 80 year old will demonstrate a 30–40% decline in voluntary strength of arm, leg, and back muscles compared to someone aged 30 years. A significant proportion of older people will experience greater declines from the average and can be said to define the *frail elderly.* This marked decline in muscle mass and strength not only impedes the older person's ability to participate in basic activities of daily living, it also predisposes them to falls and possibly other injuries due to reduced ability to protect themselves during falls. Muscle may also act to protect internal organs from injurious impact. Muscle weakness is also a significant predictor of mortality, self-reported disability and nursing home entry, and relevant to functional recovery after trauma (Bassey *et al.* 1992, Guralnik *et al.* 1994).

Bone mass is closely correlated with muscle mass. Risk of fractured femur is increased by both low bone mass and muscle mass. Increasing muscle mass seems to increase bone mass in older people (Nelson *et al.* 1994, Ryan *et al.* 1994).

Bed rest is associated with loss of up to 5% of lower limb muscle strength per day. For those who already have compromised strength, the consequences of bed rest may lead to inability to walk.

Immune function

The immune system comprises 8% of lean tissue mass. Involution of the thymus, beginning at puberty and complete by middle age, may represent the first age related decrements in the immune system. Although healthy older people have defects in both B and T cell activation, decline in cell-mediated function is the primary deficit in the older person's immune system (Adler and Nagel 1994, Schneider and Rowe 1996).

Protein calorie undernutrition and deficiencies in micronutrients (zinc, selenium, and vitamin B_6) result in decreased lymphocyte proliferation and decreased cytokine release (Lešourd 1997) closely resembling the defects associated with ageing *per se*. These act cumulatively to seriously compromise immune function. Older trauma patients, especially those who have suffered falls, commonly have borderline nutritional status. After trauma, nutritional requirements increase while nutritional intake or assimilation is commonly impaired.

Supplementation with micronutrients, including vitamin B_6, zinc, vitamin E, and β-carotene, is associated with improved immune function measures including immune cell cytokine production and response (Chandra 1992). Supplementation of elderly patients after fracture of the femur is associated with much improved clinical outcome, including a trend to fewer infections, improved functional status, and reduced morbidity and mortality at 6 months (Bastow *et al.* 1983b, Delmi *et al.* 1990). In community-dwelling elderly people, improved immune function is observed when intake of micronutrient exceeds the accepted required daily intake (RDI).

Nutritional status is also relevant to susceptibility to the development of decubitus ulcer and secondary infection of decubitus ulcers, which are common signs of malnutrition in institutionalized elderly patients.

Decreased particle clearance by the lung and poorer skin integrity with slower healing contribute to increased susceptibility to infection.

Key points

- Cell-mediated function is the primary deficit in an older person's immune system.
- Immune function is compromised by undernutrition but improves with supplementation.

Clinical relevance

Immune deficits are very common. Nutritional supplementation may reduce infection risk and skin breakdown.

Cardiovascular system

In older populations who have been screened to exclude cardiac disease, resting heart rate and cardiac output do not appear to change significantly (Lakatta 1990). However, at maximal exercise significant reductions of heart rate, cardiac output, and aerobic capacity occur with increasing age. In healthy older people, increases in left ventricular filling lead to an increase in stroke volume, thereby partly compensating for the effect lower maximum heart rate has on maximal cardiac output. With age, arterial compliance usually decreases, resulting in increased arterial peak systolic pressure. Mild left ventricular hypertrophy develops as a consequence and is associated with diastolic dysfunction. The heart becomes more reliant on atrial contraction to maintain ventricular filling and stroke volume. Diastolic blood pressure tends to fall in healthy older people, attenuating the increase in mean blood pressure.

There decreased chronotropic and inotropic response to catecholamine stimulation, due to decreased β-adrenergic modulation. According to cross-sectional studies, maximal oxygen uptake falls at about 1% per year (Fries 1980). Longitudinal studies demonstrate a non-linear decline, which is especially rapid in sedentary individuals. With regular endurance exercise the decline may by attenuated by about 50% (Buskirk and Hodgson 1987).

Clinical relevance

Coronary artery disease and cardiac dysfunction are common, occurring in up to 15% of over 70 year olds and in 20% of 80 year olds (Duncan *et al.* 1996). Cardiovascular and oxygen delivery responses to physiological stress are likely to be variable. Hypovolaemia and iatrogenic hypervolaemia may not be well tolerated. The increased dependence on left ventricular filling is accentuated in hypertensives and those with ischaemic heart disease due to diastolic dysfunction, the latter often being subclinical in many cases. Antihypertensive, antianginal, and diuretic drugs increase the propensity for hypotension. Clinical diagnosis of aortic stenosis and its severity is notoriously difficult in elderly people. Its presence will greatly impede the heart's ability to increase cardiac output and cope with reduced end-diastolic filling pressure in hypovolaemia or hypotension due to drugs. Afterload reductions may lead to reduced coronary artery flow and increase the risk of ischaemia. Septic endotoxaemia may precipitate injurious falls, and may also impede cardiac and peripheral circulatory function. Cardiac trauma causing contusion or pericardial effusion will be less well tolerated. Cardiac and haemodynamic monitoring should be considered for less severe degrees of trauma, especially where evidence of cardiovascular disease is present.

Respiratory system

Ageing is associated with:

- increased fibrous tissue in the lung parenchyma and bronchial tree
- reduced pulmonary elasticity
- decreased chest wall compliance
- reduced alveolar surface area, resulting in increased airflow resistance and reduced vital capacity and diffusing capacity (Tockman 1994, Ogle 1998).

The work of breathing is increased. Function of respiratory muscles is reduced, especially in sedentary and undernourished patients (Efthimiou *et al.* 1988). Compensation occurs through increased contribution from the diaphragm and abdominal muscles. An increased closing volume (increased volume at which small airways begin to close) results in increased residual volume (by 40–50% by age 70) and mild reduction of PO_2 (due to ventilation/perfusion mismatch in closed airways). Other changes include slowed clearance of particles from airways, decreased pulmonary afferent neural sensory function, and ventilatory response to hypoxia and hypercapnia. Gag and coughing reflexes may suffer some slowing. Diseases such as stroke, parkinsonism, and severe undernutrition exacerbate these problems.

Clinical relevance

Oxygen saturation should be monitored routinely in patients suffering relatively minor trauma (such as falls causing lower limb fractures), because narcotic analgesics, bed posture, cardiovascular deficits, and anaemia will impair oxygen transport. Tranquillizing drugs should be avoided in nearly all cases of delirium because they will exacerbate confusion and promote hypoventilation. Phenothiazines and butyrophenones cause drug-induced parkinsonism which can reduce ventilatory capacity. Pain management needs very close monitoring for efficacy and hypoventilatory effects.

Kidney and fluid electrolytes

The primary importance of progressive loss of glomerular filtration rate in older persons relates to drug excretion and adverse drug reactions which are common in older people (Beck 1994, Goldberg and Finkelstein 1987). Gradual glomerular sclerosis occurs with a 10% reduction in renal blood flow, and an 8 ml/min decrease in glomerular filtration rate for every decade after 40. How much of this renal decline is due to renovascular disease is unclear. Serum creatinine remains fairly constant due to declining muscle mass. Fluid and electrolytes remain relatively constant, however there is a decreased ability to maintain homeostasis in response to stress. There is evidence that antidiuretic hormone (ADH) may be excreted more readily in response to hypovolaemia and other stimuli causing the syndrome of inappropriate ADH secretion (SIADH) more frequently. As a result of defects in thirst, urinary concentrating ability, and free water excretion, elderly patients are prone to either hypernatraemia or hyponatraemia. Urine output is a less reliable sign of hypovolaemia because of the decrease in urine-concentrating ability. In patients with low muscle mass, serum creatinine may falsely underestimate renal function. Serum creatinine becomes unreliable as an accurate measure of renal function. Creatinine clearance equations based on serum creatinine and weight are better, although these may be unreliable measures in very old people.

Clinical relevance

In the context of serious trauma, older people are more prone to renal toxicity due to aminoglycoside antibiotics and acute renal failure due to drugs and diseases which affect:

- renovascular homeostasis (e.g. angiotension-converting enzyme inhibitors, non-specific anti-infalmmatory drugs, diabetes nephropathy, microvascular and macrovascular disease)
- plasma volume: (e.g. diuretics, reduced thirst sensation) and blood pressure (e.g. diuretics, antihypertensives and antianginals).

Measurement of blood levels of aminoglycosides is essential. Reduced thirst sensation places older people at greater risk of dehydration and prerenal failure.

Gastrointestinal system

Changes in the gut with ageing *per se* have relatively little effect on the ability to digest and absorb food and nutrients. In normal healthy older people, age does not appear to effect small-bowel mucosal morphology or absorption (Lipski *et al.* 1992). Pancreatic digestive activity is reduced. However, under normal conditions this decline still allows plenty of digestive reserve. Maximal fat absorption is mildly reduced in normal elderly people and significantly reduced in sick older people. This may present a problem when older people are unwell and have increased fat and energy requirements. Hypochlorhydria is a problem and may inhibit absorption of certain micronutrients such as iron, vitamin B_{12}, and folate. Folate deficiency is relatively common in older people. It induces small-bowel morphological changes and inhibition of folate absorption.

Clinical relevance

Chronic disease and disability are associated with poor digestion and undernutrition (Lehmann 1989). Frail and disabled older people are generally undernourished. Patients over the age of 75 years who have suffered a fall are at greater risk of being undernourished at the time of trauma. As a result of trauma and other factors associated with hospital admission, such as drug-induced anorexia, and sedation, their nutritional status may rapidly decline.

With increasing age, constipation is increasingly prevalent. Although ageing *per se* seems to have minimal effect upon colonic function (Melkersson *et al.* 1983), frail older people have a higher prevalence of chronic colonic hypomotility and are at risk of drug-induced hypomotility (usually anticholinergics) and the effects of immobility. Faecal impaction causes anorexia and is a precursor to ileus and colonic perforation. The latter may be relatively asymptomatic in the sick older patient, particularly if pain relief and sedatives are prescribed. Prevention is usually successful with adequate hydration, dietary fibre and appropriate use of aperients, suppositories and enemata.

Skin

The skin offers a barrier against trauma, infection, heat, and cold. Changes seen with age which compromise these functions represent the effects of sun damage as much as ageing itself (Kaminer and Gilchrist 1994). Flattening of epithelial layers, loss of collagen fibre strength and elasticity, and a decrease in subcutaneous fat contribute to thinner and more fragile skin and therefore to an increased likelihood of injury to ageing skin. Slower proliferation of keratinocytes and a decrease in blood supply result in slower healing after trauma to the skin. The dermis, being less vascular and supported by less subcutaneous tissue, offers inferior insulation especially in older women. Sweat gland numbers and function are decreased, thereby reducing evaporative heat loss.

Clinical relevance

Skin care requirements increase in frail older people. Decubitus ulcer prevention requires more frequent turning and increased use of specialized mattresses. Upper limb skin tears incurred during lifting are common and usually preventable. Preventable hypothermia may occur in hospitalized older people because of central temperature control impairment and reduced subcutaneous fat and impaired cold sensation.

Vision

The prevalence of visual problems among older people is very high (Grisso and Kaplan 1994, Schneider and Rowe 1996). Visual acuity, impaired adaptation to darkness, peripheral vision, depth perception, glare tolerance, contrast sensitivity, and accommodation may all be affected by age-related changes, cataracts, macular degeneration, glaucoma, and diabetic retinopathy.

Clinical relevance

Visual impairment has been associated with falls and fractured femur (Grisso and Kaplan 1994). Monocular vision and poor depth perception have been associated with increased risk of motor vehical accidents. Regular assessments should be performed in older drivers.

Balance

Increased body sway and a loss in righting reflex begin to occur in the sixth decade; see 'Pharmacodynamics', below). Maintenance of posture depends on co-ordination, central processing of inputs from vision, vestibular organs, proprioceptive pathways, muscle tone, and strength (Maki and McIlroy 1996). With increasing age, the frequency and amplitude of corrective movements involved in postural control have been shown to increase. Although the underlying mechanisms are complex and incompletely understood, the dopaminergic pathway may play a role, explaining why age-related reductions in dopamine-2 receptors in the striatum may contribute. Neuropathological studies indicate numerous additional age related brain changes including a significant reduction in cerebellar Purkinje cells. Muscle weakness due to disuse and undernutrition is common and reversible with physical therapy and exercise.

Clinical relevance

Drugs and other factors affecting any of the major components of postural control may increase falls risk. Examples include:

- central neural pathways: hypothermia, benzodiazepines, major tranquilizers: butyrophenones and phenothiazines (which have specific antidopaminergic activity and therefore may cause drug-induced

parkinsonism, appendicular tardive dyskinesia, risk of hypothermia, and reduced alertness)
- muscle function: disuse, undernutrition and benzodiazepines
- peripheral neural function: diabetes, drugs
- vision and vestibular function: drugs and degenerative diseases of the inner ear and eyes.

Thermal regulation

In normal ageing there is no clinically significant impairment of thermal control (Bastow *et al.* 1983a, Harchelroad 1993). However, thermal control is commonly abnormal in frail and unwell older people. Impairment of normal shivering responses, metabolic rate response to cold, vasoconstriction, and subjective appreciation of cold are common. Surveys of older people in winter-time have indicated that a significant number of older people living in the community were chronically hypothermic (Fox *et al.* 1973).

Clinical relevance

Reduction of temperature by as little as 0.5–1°C is associated with impaired alertness and postural control (Bastow *et al.* 1983a). Centrally acting drugs which have been implicated in impaired temperature control include alcohol, phenothiazines, and butyrophenones. These have also been implicated in reduction of sensory awareness, muscular activity, and vasoconstriction. Other drugs such as benzodiazepines, tricyclics, and narcotics may impair temperature homeostasis. Undernutrition, liver failure, and chronic renal failure are associated with impaired central control of temperature.

Clinical pharmacology and principles of drug treatment

Adverse drug reactions (ADRs) are common in older people confined to hospital. Contributing factors include polypharmacy, the presence of age-related alterations to pharmacokinetics and pharmacodynamics, disease alterations to physiology, and changes to body composition. The effects of trauma, operative procedures, and advancing undernutrition further compound these factors.

Relevance

Psychotropic drugs are the greatest single risk factor for falls in older people (Tinetti *et al.* 1988, Weiner *et al.* 1998). Falls have also been associated with polypharmacy, antihypertensives, and diuretics. Drugs most commonly affecting balance, righting reflexes, alertness and cognition, or precipitating delirium, include:

- narcotics, e.g. pethidine and morphine
- antipsychotics
- antidepressants, especially tricyclics
- anticonvulsants
- antiparkinsonians
- some NSAIDs e.g. indomethacin
- some Ca^{2+} channel blockers and beta-blockers, e.g. diltiazem

Newer generation antidepressants are not as sedating as many tricyclics, but they may all cause confusion and some cause postural hypotension (venlafaxine).

Psychotropic drugs are a risk factor for motor vehicle accidents in older people, especially those with dementia.

Sick older people are at greater risk of ADRs in hospital than any other group of patients. Great care in diagnosis and prescribing, followed by regular review of drug requirement and dose is warranted to avoid serious iatrogenesis.

For further reading see Montamat *et al.* (1989), Denham (1990), Fox and Auestad (1990), Meyer and Reidenberg (1992), and Ruiz and Lowenthal (1995).

Adverse drug reactions in inpatients

There are no specific studies of ADRs in older trauma patients. Several studies of older people in hospital have revealed high rates of ADRs, which increase with age (Duncan and Smith 1990). Approximate incidences are:

- >60 years: 5–15%
- >70 years: 10–20%
- >80 years: 15–20%.

ADRs directly account for about 3% of hospital admission. Geriatric medical unit admissions primarily due to ADRs have ranged from 15% to 30%. Elderly trauma patients are therefore at great risk of ADRs, especially in the presence of multiple organ problems and multiple medications.

Common drug adverse effects may present differently in older people. These include

- confusion/delirium
- incontinence of urine
- faecal impaction
- falls and gait disturbance
- anorexia (and poor nutrient intake).

For example, overdosing with narcotics may produce all these effects as well as ADRs typically described in younger patients, such as dry mouth.

Factors contributing to ADRs

General factors

General factors contributing to ADRs include being white and female, consuming multiple medications, medication dose, and a past history of ADR.

Multiple diseases

Ageing is associated with an increased incidence of treatable chronic disease. Diseases accompanied by organ impairment may alter drug disposal and tissue sensitivity to drugs. In this setting, multiple diseases and drugs increase the risk of drug interactions.

Inappropriate prescribing

Inaccurate diagnosis

Accurate diagnosis of symptoms is achieved by taking a relevant history and proper physical examination. Symptoms need to be regarded has having at least one underlying aetiology until proven otherwise. Two common examples of inappropriate diagnosis and prescribing are:

- Oedema treated with diuretics when the oedema is largely caused by immobility, a calcium channel blocker prescribed for hypertension. This treatment may precipitate postural hypotension, falls, and urinary incontinence.
- Dizziness due to postural hypotension treated with prochlorperazine (which is not a good treatment for any cause of dizziness in old people). This may result in drug-induced parkinsonism, tardive dyskinesia, and falls. Accurate history-taking and proper examination is essential in order to make reasonable diagnoses.

Excessive dose prescribed

In general, older people should be prescribed lower doses of drugs, which can be increased carefully and titrated according to desired or undesired effects. Emergency situations may demand aggressive drug doses, as in younger people.

The treatment of hypertension is a typical example, especially in the hospital setting. Antihypertensives are often used excessively with the aim of acutely reducing chronically elevated blood pressure to normal levels. This may lead to hypotensive symptoms even at normal or elevated blood pressure levels, shock, and cerebral ischaemia with brain damage if the duration is sufficiently long. Commonly the only symptom is postural hypotension with inability to walk. When treating the asymptomatic older person, gentle blood pressure reduction is required over a period of days to weeks.

Key point

- ADRs are common in elderly people.

Altered pharmacokinetics

Absorption

Absorption of drugs is mostly unchanged with age. Ageing *per se* alters many gut functions minimally.

A recent study has demonstrated that gut surface area is unchanged in healthy older people (Lipski *et al.* 1992). However, many older people have alterations to gastric acidity, delayed gastric emptying, increased intestinal transit time, decreased absorptive surface area, reduced gut blood flow, probable decreased gut active transport, and reduced liver size and liver blood flow. Despite these changes, it appears that nearly all drugs are absorbed normally. Levodopa is more rapidly and easily absorbed through the stomach than in younger patients, presumably owing to reduced dopa decarboxylase activity in the mucosa. Delayed gastric emptying, which occurs with anticholinergic drug use and in some diabetics, may reduce absorption rate and peak drug level. The rate of absorption of antibiotics (and possibly other drugs) from an intramuscular injection may be slowed in older people (Ruiz and Lowenthal 1995).

For further reading see Tregaskis and Stevenson (1990), Adler and Nagel (1994), and Schwartz (1994).

First-pass elimination

It is unclear whether ageing is solely responsible for the reported age-related reduction in first-pass metabolism of highly extracted drugs such as propranolol, verapamil, tricyclics, and prazosin. These drugs, and others, are affected by hepatic blood flow. Increased blood levels may occur in patients who have diseases or are taking drugs that affect hepatic blood flow, e.g. cardiac failure and beta-blockers. Hepatic function may vary greatly because of genetic and environmental factors such as nutrition, caffeine, nicotine, alcohol, disease, and ageing (Woodhouse and James 1990).

Drug distribution and body composition

Body composition determines volume of drug distribution. With age, fat volume increases and water volume (muscle mass) decreases. Increased fat volume will increase elimination half-life of fat-soluble drugs (e.g. diazepam, lignocaine, tricyclics). Reduced body water volume increases the potential for higher peak plasma level of water-soluble drugs (e.g. digoxin, ethanol, and paracetamol).

Protein binding

Protein binding may become clinically important if albumin levels are reduced during acute illness. In this circumstance, the free level of protein-bound drug increases. Tightly bound drugs are at most risk of being subject to or causing drug displacement, which increases the active free portion of the displaced drug. Examples of common drugs in which either avoidance or great care should be taken are aspirin, warfarin, phenytoin, and diazepam.

Renal function and drug excretion

For every decade of life after the age of 40, renal blood flow reduces by about 10%. Tubular urinary concentration function decreases by about 7% per decade. Serum creatinine is unreliable as an estimation of renal function in older people. It is better to estimate creatinine-clearance using the following formula:

creatinine clearance = [(140 − age) × weight (kg) × 0.85 for women]/[814− plasma creatinine (mmol/l)]

Dosage reduction is required for drugs with narrow therapeutic windows which are mainly renally excreted, such as digoxin and aminoglycosides. Because creatinine clearance estimation is still potentially unreliable using this formula, monitoring blood levels of these drugs is recommended (Beck 1994, Goldberg and Finkelstein 1987).

Altered pharmacodynamics

Older people have increased target organ sensitivity to psychotherapeutic drugs, digoxin, warfarin, and probably phenytoin also. There is evidence of age-related decrease in cholinergic activity (Albert 1994). In addition, people with Alzheimer's disease (which may otherwise be clinically occult) have even greater cholinergic loss. Anticholinergic drugs therefore commonly precipitate delirium in older people. People with Alzheimer's disease and other dementias are far more likely to suffer a drug-induced delirium.

It is quite likely that therapeutic levels of phenytoin and digoxin are lower than those quoted for younger people. Toxicity due to these two drugs seems to occur more frequently at so-called therapeutic blood levels.

Based on animal and human studies it is likely that older people generally have fewer and less responsive alpha- and beta-adrenergic receptors. Responsiveness to catecholamine administration is attenuated in older people (Lakatta 1990).

Altered homeostatic mechanisms of blood pressure control place older people at greater risk of postural hypotension. Drugs which reduce plasma volume, reduce sympathetic outflow, have secondary effects on the vascular tree, or blunt heart rate responsiveness may precipitate postural hypotension. Prolonged bed rest also seems to reduce responsiveness of homeostatic mechanisms to orthostasis.

For further reading see Schwartz (1994).

General clinical assessment and management

Providing optimal care requires an interdisciplinary approach involving ambulance and paramedical officers, emergency physicians, surgeons, geriatricians, other physicians, allied health personnel, and nursing staff.

Following are general considerations based on physiological, epidemiological, and pharmacological aspects discussed above.

General principles

Diagnostic principles in geriatric medicine

The traditional approach to diagnosis in medicine is based on finding a single unifying diagnosis, which explains all the patient's undiagnosed symptoms. In geriatric medicine, the paradigm is inverted. Multiple pathologies impinging upon a single symptom or physical manifestation becomes the dominating approach. Nonetheless, the wise clinician will attempt to use both approaches.

Altered disease presentation

Diseases in older people often present in typical ways. However, in many cases, especially the frail aged, diseases present atypically. For example, hyperthyroidism often presents as the 'apathetic thyroid' in older people. Pneumonia may present with few specific symptoms or signs other than weakness and confusion. Myocardial infarctions are commonly painless. The most common sign of digoxin toxicity in older people is a feeling of weakness, whereas nausea is most common in younger people. Many presentations are in the form of functional syndromes. Modern epidemiology has labeled these as *geriatric syndromes*.

Trauma and the geriatric syndromes

Several multifactorial syndromes have been well described in older people. Various contributing factors interact or combine to impinge upon a single body function. These syndromes may result in trauma or they may develop as a result of trauma and hospitalization. They include:

- falls
- gait disorders
- confusional states
- incontinence
- weight loss/undernutrition
- iatrogenesis—usually polypharmacy with ADRs.

Accurate diagnosis

Accurate diagnoses are essential in order to effectively reverse the reversible and prevent the preventable. For example, in an elderly trauma patient with confusion, narcotic dosage needs to be carefully determined. The pathologies contributing to delirium commonly include a combination of mild hypoxaemia due to hypoventilation and mild aspiration pneumonia, faecal impaction (due to narcotics and bed rest), and other drug side-effects. Narcotics will cause hypoventilation, exacerbate colonic dysfunction, and directly act on the brain to induce delirium. Oxygen therapy, ventilation monitoring, and measurement of oxygen saturation are especially important in older patients whether or not the chest has been involved in trauma. Temporarily discontinuing the patient's long-term drugs such as antidepressants should be considered. Accurate diagnosis of past diseases is required. After weighing risks and benefits in the individual, dosage may be reduced depending on the acute issues. Alternatively, analgesic drugs such as tramadol may be used with greater safety because they have minimal neurological and respiratory side-effects.

Management principles:

Acute phase—initial assessment and management

- *Determine mechanism of trauma*: Also consider whether 'elder abuse' has occurred (see below).
- *Determine immediate effects of trauma and institute resuscitation*: Close haemodynamic and pulse oximetry monitoring is associated with improved outcome in older patients with relatively mild injuries.
- If in doubt, admit the elderly patient to a *higher dependency unit* for the first 48 hours for relatively moderate trauma because of higher risk of acquiring complications early.
- *Determine possible medical problems precipitating injuries* e.g. arrhythmias, infections, hypothermia, pressure areas (long-lie). Urinary tract infection, pneumonia, faecal impaction, drug toxicity, alcohol, hypothermia, or a vascular event for example may have precipitated a fall.
- *Commence monitoring for delayed manifestations of trauma* which may present either typically or 'atypically', e.g. subdural, underlying infection, shock, hip fracture, and remediable complications such as circulatory shock and skin condition at vulnerable pressure points.
- *Identify, prevent, and manage undernutrition early, aggressively and carefully*: Nasogastric or nasoduodenal feeding carries significant morbidity, which can be minimized by careful tube positioning and posturing. Overnight feeding carries additional risk of aspiration. Percutaneous gastrostomy tube feeding has some advantages.
- *Review drugs that may be contributing* to underlying presentation or complications associated with bed rest, e.g. faecal impaction.
- *Look for and investigate geriatric syndromes*: These give clues to multiple underlying pathologies that may be reversible.
- *Prevention of pressure areas* begins at the scene of trauma. Decubitus ulcers commonly occur in busy emergency departments. Cutaneous and subcutaneous changes associated with age place frail older people at greater decubitus ulcer risk, especially if oxygen transport is impaired. Use of specialized mattresses with frequent turning or turning on an hourly basis is necessary.
- *Regular review* for other complications of trauma is particularly warranted in patients who arrive confused and in whom pain localization is poor. Brain CT scan is warranted in these patients, but confusion is commonly due to causes other than acute intracranial bleeding, cerebral contusion or concussion.

Subacute phase—manage and prevent secondary comorbidities

Prevent common problems found in hospitalized older people that have significant sequelae:

- *Undernutrition*: Give either nutritional supplements between meals or enteral feeding. Obtain dentures when the level of consciousness is adequate.
- *Venous thromboembolism*: prophylaxis.
- *Decubitus ulcers*: Frequent turning, avoidance of soiled bed linen, management of incontinence.
- *Contractures*: Early nursing and physiotherapy interventions.
- *Muscle wasting prevention*: Early mobilization and aggressive nutritional supplementation are nearly always required in elderly trauma patients. Early commencement of bed exercises.

- *Faecal impaction*: Aperients, suppositories, and close bowel chart monitoring.
- *Iatrogenesis*: Medication and procedure related, e.g. drug induced Parkinsonism.
- *Delirium* (see below): Avoid frequently moving patients from bed to bed or locating patient in a ward environment that is excessively stimulating. Both may precipitate delirium. Always obtain a premorbid cognitive history, from a relative if necessary. Obtain eyeglasses and hearing aids as these may reduce delirium and delirium-induced paranoia.
- *Remove indwelling catheters* as soon as reasonably possible, to avoid urinary sepsis and development of urethral stricture.

Recovery phase

- Early *mobilization and rehabilitation.*
- *Determine risk factors for trauma* (falls, driving risk, etc.) and the possibility of elder abuse.
- Continue nutritional supplementation.
- *Commence investigation of related conditions* such as falls, osteoporosis, and undernutrition.
- Be aware of *late complications* presenting as failure to rehabilitate.

Decubitus ulcer prevention

Pressure area care is of great importance in older people, who have a very high risk of acquiring decubitus ulcers. Significant morbidity and mortality is associated with their acquisition that may delay discharge by weeks or sometimes months. Management essentials include:

- Recognize that this is a medical responsibility.
- Titrate frequency of turning in bed according to skin thickness, vascular supply to heels, presence of diabetes or peripheral vascular disease, nutritional status.
- Commence nutritional supplementation early.
- Provide ripple or other mattresses for all at-risk patients.
- Increase skin and pressure prevention care for patients with hemiparesis or Parkinson's disease.

Delirium

Delirium or acute confusional state should not be confused with dementia, although delirium is more common in dementia sufferers. Dementia is a chronic multifocal disorder of brain function that usually progresses slowly. Delirium carries a very significant mortality risk that varies according to underlying disease processes.

Characterisitcs of delirium:

- primarily a disorder of attention or consciousness
- fluctuates in most cases ('lucid periods')
- may be 'quiet' or 'noisy' in manifestation
- is usually acute in onset
- occurs in older people with normal premorbid cognitive function
- is very common in dementia sufferers.

Delirium is very common in hospitalized older inpatients. Over one-third of elderly inpatients can be expected to suffer delirium in hospital. The aetiology is nearly always multifactorial and investigation for multiple causes is essential.

The causes of delirium are too long to list. Essentially, any medication and organ dysfunction including faecal loading can cause or contribute to delirium. Benzodiazepine or alcohol withdrawal should be considered. Stopping as little as one benzodiazepine sleeping tablet can trigger withdrawal. Early management with diazepam is very effective, but doses required in older people are much less than younger patients (diazepam having a half-life of up to 80 hours in older people). Reversing all these factors is essential. Underlying dementia or previously occult dementia may be associated with prolonged delirium. In older persons who were previously well cognitively the outcome is excellent if the underlying problem is reversible. Delirium is common after head injury.

Clinical surveys have repeatedly shown that physicians do not recognize many cases of delirium. Its manifestation may be subtle. Some patients present as passive, quiet, and incommunicative people; others present as unco-operative, or with urinary incontinence.

Management of delirium in the context of trauma consists of:

- Head CT scan (even if trauma is a minor fall).
- Reversing or treating maximally all underlying medical problems.
- Considering drug or alcohol withdrawal.
- Moving the patient to a quieter ward area.
- Avoidance of challenging the patient who appears unco-operative. Avoidance of sedation except when the patient is a danger to themself or others.
- Sedation with drugs such as haloperidol carries risk of causing drug-induced parkinsonism and therefore should be avoided unless the patient is a risk to themselves or others.

A geriatrician should be consulted. For further reading see Lipowski (1994).

The trauma patient with Parkinson's disease

Parkinson's disease is present in about 1% of older people. Immobility and muscle rigidity increase the risk of venous thrombosis and decubitus ulcers. Difficulty in eating, postural hypotension, and faecal impaction are more common. Early mobilization is and maintenance of levodopa is essential. Subcutaneous apomorphine is useful for patients who are nil by mouth. Relatively safe antiemetics such as domperidone that do not cause drug-induced parkinsonism are often needed. Drugs such as metoclopramide (Maxolon) and prochlorperazine (Stemetil) must be avoided absolutely. Sedation with phenothiazines or butyrophenones is potentially disastrous. Nutritional supplementation and early recommencement of antiparkinsonian treatment probably hasten recovery and reduce complications.

Blood pressure management

Rapid blood pressure reduction should be avoided in hypertensive patients, especially if it is asymptomatic. Rapid reduction is associated with brain ischaemia, falls, confusion, and probably stroke. Brain autoregulation requires time to accommodate to the reduced perfusion pressure. In the context of cerebral haemorrhage induced by blunt trauma, it is wise to reduce blood pressure. However, the risk of cerebral ischaemia to areas surrounding the haemorrhage is present with overzealous blood pressure reduction. Admission to high dependency or intensive care units is mandatory.

In older people, blood pressure <100 mmHg systolic peri-anaesthetic in older people is associated with postoperative delirium, implying brain ischaemia.

Carefully controlling pain or urinary retention may suffice to adequately reduce blood pressure.

Faecal impaction

Faecal impaction is a multifactorial disorder associated with the development of bowel obstruction and bowel perforation if left unattended. This condition is nearly always preventable.

Management principles

- Monitor bowel chart: No bowel movement, faecal incontinence (impaction with overflow), or faecal smearing, indicate a problem for further investigation.
- Examine abdomen and rectum if there has been no bowel movement for >2 days in hospital.
- If the rectum is empty a high impaction may be present and is assessed with an abdominal radiograph.
- Exclude electrolyte abnormalities (including serum magnesium and phosphate levels), narcotic, and other anticholinergic or antispasmodic medications.
- If treated with narcotics analgesics adequate use of prophylactic aperients should be considered.
- Intra-abdominal pathology should be considered including retroperitoneal haemorrhage and pancreatitis.
- If no intra-abdominal pathology is suspected, ensure adequate oral hydration, fibre in diet, stool softener e.g. coloxyl, and osmotic agent such as lactulose should be considered. Senna should only be used periodically as a rule.

Falls

Falls are the most common cause of trauma and trauma deaths in older people. About 75% of fall-related deaths occur in elderly people. Fall-related deaths are probably under-reported because complications are usually denoted as the cause of death. The majority of falls in older people, especially the old old, occur on the flat. About 30% of community dwelling people over the age of 65 fall each year; 24% of these result in serious soft tissue injury and 6% in fracture. About 1 in 40 fallers is hospitalized. Risk of falling increases dramatically after age 75. Falls are more common in mobile nursing home residents. One study found that 61% of subjects fell during their first year in the nursing home. Each year at least 10% of older patients suffer a serious injury from a fall such as fracture, dislocation or severe head injury. Evidence from Tinetti (1994), Tinetti and Williams (1997), and Tinetti *et al.* (1998) suggests that fear of falling is a risk factor for further falls by causing further physiological decline. Falls and injuries are associated with fear of falling, restricted activity, social withdrawal, pain, and increased risk of further falls. A retrospective review by Cummings *et al.* (1985) found that nearly 60% suffered non-syncopal falls, and 43% of older people have their accidents at home (Fildes 1994).

Falls in older people are significant because of their propensity to cause injury.

Risk factors for falls

Falls, like most geriatric problems, are multifactorial in nature. Risk factors for falls may be categorized into extrinsic and intrinsic factors.

- intrinsic (patient-related factors)
  - drugs affecting balance, alertness, movement
  - episodic problems—seizures, postural hypotension, cardiac syncope, vertigo
  - gait disorder—frailty, parkinsonism, neuropathy
  - painful arthritis or musculoskeletal pain
  - visual impairment.
- extrinsic (environment-related factors)
  - slippery surface
  - rugs, cords, footwear, clothes
  - poor lighting
  - pets, toys, etc.
  - steps
  - need for aids, e.g. toilet surrounds, rails.

Tinetti *et al.* (1988) calculated odds ratios (OR) for different risk factors in a study of 332 fallers. Psychotropic drugs carried the largest risk, (OR 28.3) followed by cognitive impairment (OR 5.0), lower extremity disability (OR 3.8), palmomental reflex (OR 3.0), foot problems (OR 1.8) and number of balance and gait problems; 0–2, (OR 1.0); 3–5 (OR 1.4); 6–7; (OR 1.9). The percentage increased risk due to falls increased as the number of risk factors increased. No risk factors carried 8% risk. Risk then rose linearly, the presence of four risk factors being associated with a falling risk of almost 80%.

Repeat fallers may be at lower risk because anticipation of falling and learned mechanisms of minimizing trauma may develop. Repeat fallers tend to avoid risks by restricting their activities.

Factors influencing fall injuries include:

- height of the fall
- velocity of impact and body weight
- hardness of surface
- soft tissue padding
- female gender
- presence of osteoporosis
- age >75
- slowed reflexes and protective responses.

Clinical assessment

Historical considerations

History is probably the most important diagnostic tool. Asking eyewitnesses to give descriptive accounts of falls is very useful. The possibility of elder abuse warrants vigilance. Falls are commonly under-reported by patients living in the community.

Assessment is often triggered by a concerned relative or an injury acquired from a fall.

Asking how, where, when, and what the patient was doing when they fell gives useful information, but non-specific symptoms usually mean multifactorial aetiology.

- Were there premonitory symptoms?
- How long did it take for the patient to get back to their feet?
- How did they feel immediately after the fall?
- Did they experience clamminess or nausea or were they incontinent?
- Did the fall occur while they were turning around or turning the head?
- Was there loss of consciousness?
- Did the patient have difficulty walking or suffer pain before the fall?

Patients will commonly say they felt either giddy, lightheaded, or dizzy. These statements must be followed by more specific questions to ascertain if possible, exactly what the patient experienced. These descriptions may mean they just felt unsteady. Did they experience any vertigo (suggesting an inner ear or brain problem), lightheadedness (suggesting a haemodynamic problem), darkening of vision (suggesting either haemodynamic or vascular problems), or a sense of unsteadiness on their feet (suggesting a balance problem)?

Falls at night may indicate poor lighting, or rushing to the toilet because of urge incontinence.

Dizziness may relate to postural hypotension. Enquire about the relationship of falls to meals or micturition, both of which are associated with increased postural hypotension. Symptoms relating to arrhythmias, ischaemic heart disease, stroke, or seizure should be asked specifically, although they are relatively uncommon causes of falls.

Occasionally a fractured femur may precede a fall. Pain in the hip may be noted first.

Undernutrition should be assessed through a diet history or nutritional screening tool such as the nutritional screening index (NSI) or Australian NSI, which if positive should lead to a full diet history and nutritional assessment.

Physical examination

First, exclude serious injury, then determine underlying medical problems precipitating and contributing to falls. If there has been serious injury, parts of the examination may have to be deferred to a later stage. Examination includes:

- Assess haemodynamics and orthostatic blood pressure responses (if no serious injury). Measure pulse rate and blood pressure at 0 minute after lying for at least 20 minutes and then at 1, 3, 5 minute intervals after standing and note any symptoms.
- Measure core body temperature (regarding fever or hypothermia).
- Assess skin pallor, tissue turgor (chest), and integrity, especially if patient suffered a 'long lie'.
- Neurological examination including alertness, mental state, cognitive function, extrapyramidal features, vision, hearing, gaze abnormalities, nystagmus, and strabismus.
- Examine the neck for reduced range of motion (if no acute neck trauma or acute pain without negative radiology), indicating degenerative spine disease and possible central cord syndrome vulnerability.
- Cardiovascular assessment—specifically looking for aortic stenosis, cardiac failure, rhythm disturbance, and carotid sinus sensitivity—which requires monitoring and firm pressure over the carotid sinus high in the neck deep to the angle of the jaw.
- Gait and balance analysis.

Initial investigations

Initial laboratory analysis should include a standard emergency department trauma screen. Thyroid function and additional parameters of nutritional status are warranted, e.g. transferrin, lymphocyte count, and total protein. Thyroid dysfunction is common in older people and subclinical disease may affect management.

Chest radiograph and ECG should always be performed. Serial ECGs and cardiac enzymes may detect painless myocardial infarction and should be ordered if there is suspicion.

The decision to order radiology is not significantly different in older people. Because pain perception may not be quite as reliable, radiographs should be ordered more readily.

Management

Diagnose and treat specific injuries, assess the aetiologies possibly causing the falls, assess potential environmental hazards, implement physical and nutritional rehabilitation programmes.

- Management is clearly determined by the contributing causes of the falls. Older people with balance impairment, muscle weakness, and sarcopaenia should be offered a trial of rehabilitation and strength training. Strength training is highly effective in improving most parameters of mobility, muscle strength, and general well-being. It is safe for frail older people and well tolerated.
- A high percentage of fallers and most frail fallers are undernourished. A nutritional supplementation programme is therefore appropriate. Several clinical trial studies in fractured femur sufferers have shown lasting benefits after one course of nutritional supplementation. Other studies have shown improved body composition and immune function indices.
- Associated problems such as social isolation and depression should be diagnosed in hospital. Management is commenced in hospital and is then addressed by the local aged care service and the patient's family practitioner in follow-up.
- Review of all medications is required in order to minimize falls risk. Sedatives should particularly be reviewed.
- Environmental hazards should be diagnosed through a home visit by either a geriatrician or a specialist occupational therapist.
- For patients with osteoporosis, hip protectors should be considered in order to prevent fractured femur.

Fractured femur

Fractured femur is the most common serious injury in older people and is a major cause of personal and health economic costs. In the USA over 500 000 femur fractures are predicted in the year 2040 (Cummings *et al.* 1990). Most occur in women who outnumber men and who have higher rates of falling and osteoporosis. An 80 year old woman has approximately a 15% chance of incurring a hip fracture before dying. Men have about half the risk. All patients with fractured femur following a low-velocity fall have osteoporosis.

Outcome

Mortality from hip fracture is about 5% in hospital (Jette *et al.* 1987). One year mortality is about 25–30%, which is 14–18% higher than their non-falling age peers (Mossey 1989, Parker and Palmer 1995). Disability after a fractured hip is common, about 50% not reaching premorbid level of ability to climb stairs and walk outdoors. About 65% do not regain all their prefracture activities of daily living (ADL) (Mossey 1989, Grisso and Kaplan 1994, Parker and Palmer 1995).

In the USA since the introduction of payment systems linked to diagnosis-related groups (DRG), more patients are being discharged to long-stay facilities without rehabilitation programmes.

Predictors of outcome

Predictors of outcome include age, prefracture functional status, number of prefracture medical conditions, mental status, depression, social factors, muscle strength, and serum albumin at admission. Fracture site, repair type, postsurgical complications, number of days in hospital, and discharge location have not been related to outcome. Interestingly, in most studies, age has not been positive as an independent predictor of outcome.

Specific management issues

It is our recommendation that hip fractures be operated on within 24 hours of arrival to hospital. Immobilization of patients causes increased mortality and morbidity. Before internal fixation, mortality rates were as high as 40%. Some studies have suggested that >48 hours to operation time is associated with poorer outcome.

Special care is required to prevent decubitus ulcers, which most commonly occur on the heel of the affected limb (especially if the patient has a hemiparesis on the fracture side). The unaffected limb may also be affected if sedation is used.

Secondary prevention of hip fractures

Little research has been undertaken in this field. Evidence to date and consensus point to the following:

- *Reduce the risk of falls*: Exercise has many benefits, including improved gait and ADL function. Some exercise trials have demonstrated significant reductions in falls risk. Optimal exercise prescription has not been demonstrated in this group. A trial assessing resistance exercise training is currently under way.
- *Treat osteoporosis* (Kanis 1997, Khaw 1998, Sambrook 1995): Although hormonal replacement therapy (Michaëlsson *et al.* 1998), bisphosphonates (Liberman *et al.* 1995), and other treatments can prevent non-vertebral fractures, it is unlikely that a trial of secondary prevention will soon be undertaken or completed specifically in a group of frail older people following hip fracture. Treatment of osteoporosis in this group seems appropriate, and likely to be of benefit to those who do not have severe underlying organ failure medically.

  Combination treatment may be more efficacious, including combining progestagins with oestrogen and bisphosphonates. Pretreatment dual energy X-ray absorptiometry (DEXA) is advised.

  Several studies have demonstrated the ability of strength training to increase bone mineral density in frail older people (Nelson *et al.* 1994, Ryan *et al.* 1994). It is our view that specific graduated strength training should be offered to all patients following hip fracture, until the results of current research trials into this treatment are available.

Hip protectors

Hip protectors have been shown to be efficacious in preventing hip fractures in nursing home residents (Lauritzen *et al.* 1997). Results from a community-based trial of elderly fallers are awaited. Hip protectors may increase the risk of other less serious injuries, but their outstanding results in the institutional setting allow us to strongly recommend their use.

Nutritional supplementation

Most fractured femur sufferers ingest inadequate calories during their stay inhospital (Older *et al.* 1980). Nutritional supplementation has shown very good results in three studies (Bastow *et al.* 1983a). Supplements should be given between meals. Unwell older people are unable to digest large meals fully, and smaller meals given more frequently are more likely to optimize nutritional status. Only one study so far has tested oral supplements (Delmi *et al.* 1990). Major benefits in mortality, complication rate, length of stay, and discharge destination were documented. The benefits were extended to the time of follow-up at least 6 months later. It is advisable to continue nutritional supplementation after discharge of older fractured femur patients. Supplements may need to be tailored to individual requirements and co-morbidities such as diabetes or renal failure.

Subdural haematomas and head injuries

Head trauma and dementia

Three case control studies have found an independent association between head trauma and Alzheimer's disease. Trauma probably causes brain impairment that hastens the presentation of the disease (Borenstein 1990).

Subdural haematomas

Subdural haematomas occur in older people with relatively trivial trauma or no history of trauma at all. The onset may therefore be insidious and its manifestations various. Subdural haematomas are known as neurological mimickers in older people, presenting as dementia, delirium, stroke, seizures, mood disturbances, or transient ischaemic attacks. Bilateral haematomas, metabolic derangement, and postoperative complications are more common in older people. Older men are more likely to acquire subdural haematomas than women. Mortality occurs in about 15% of sufferers. Neurological recovery is usually good in survivors who do not have suffer recurrence.

For furthere reading see Howard *et al.* (1989), Spallone *et al.* (1989).

Pathophysiology of subdural haematomas (Ellis 1990)

Subdural haematomas arise from bleeding bridging veins that are relatively intolerant of movement. Aged veins are generally more fragile and older brains are more likely to move within the cranium because of reduced brain size. The dura, which contains the bridging veins, is more adherent to the aged brain, explaining why brain movement is more likely to sever them, and why epidural haematomas are more uncommon in older people. Hence acceleration injuries may be sufficient to cause vein rupture. A direct blow to the head is not required. Haematomas tend to be larger in older people because of greater low-pressure space availability.

Diagnosis

Because trauma may be trivial, it is not always evident on history (30–50% of cases) (Spallone *et al.* 1989, Ellis 1990). Even acute haematomas may present relatively insidiously because of the increased size of the subdural space. A high index of suspicion should be held for any older person who may suffer from occasional falls and has some unexplained decline in function, cognition, language, or gait, especially if it fluctuates. Chronic subdurals may present with depression, confusion, dementia, stroke, headache, urinary incontinence, and behaviour change.

Acute subdural haematoma presentation symptoms include hemiparesis (50%), paraesthesias are common, dysarthria (25%), incontinence or vomiting (10–20%), seizures (<10%). Acute subdurals carry a worse prognosis, especially in the very old (35–50%) (Ellis 1990, Cagetti *et al.* 1992). Factors associated with poor outcome include reduced level of consciousness, extreme old age, acuity, and requiring craniotomy rather than simple drainage.

Treatment

Acute progressive subdurals require drainage quickly. Chronic subdurals require drainage if they are not spontaneously resolving or if disability is relatively severe. In some cases chronic subdurals are found incidentally and no treatment is required apart from monitoring. Craniotomy is required to treat symptomatic haematoma recollection.

Cervical injury

Older people tend to suffer less neurological damage from spinal injuries than younger people. This undoubtedly reflects the different mechanism of injury—usually a high-speed accident in the younger people and a fall in the old. Older people who do suffer major neurological damage have a very poor outcome, with a 60-fold mortality rate (Spivak *et al.* 1994). Cervical spondylosis is more common in older people, increasing the likelihood of central cord syndrome in people with relatively minor trauma such as a fall or whiplash injury (Lieberman and Webb 1994). New neurological deficits following falls in older people may be due to central cord syndrome. The prognosis for neurological recovery from this syndrome is reasonably good.

Of all spinal injuries attending a spinal unit, about 60% will have neurological deficit. Of these, odontoid fractures occurred in 33%. Neurological deficit recovery occurs in 80% of compression injuries and 60% of extension injuries.

Motor vehicle accidents

Older people have increased risk of being pedestrian victims (Kong *et al.* 1996). Pedestrian fatalities account for 28% of motor vehicle accident fatalities in older people, whereas 16% of MVA deaths are in pedestrians for all ages (Sattin and Nevitt 1992). Drivers over 75 have 25% more accidents per licenced driver and are more likely to have accidents at intersections than other ages. Accident rates per kilometre in over 75 year olds are second only to those for teenagers. Older people have greater injuries from similar accidents and take longer to recover (Sattin and Nevitt 1992).

Vision, especially night vision, neuromuscular reflexes, cognition, and adverse medication effects may explain the increased incidence of driver and pedestrian accidents.

Prevention involves clinician recognition of dementia and medication adverse effects. Screening of older driver performance because of age or illness may reduce injuries.

Elder abuse

The diagnosis of elder abuse should be considered, for example, in any patient with a delayed presentation of an injury (for example, fractures healing unset), when an implausible explanation for illness or injury is given, or if a patient is described as being accident prone. Neglect is more common than abuse, and this can contribute to injury in a number of ways. Neglect may be either passive, when a care provider is unable to provide care, or active, when a carer is actively withholding care. A carer may neglect to provide an elderly person with glasses, a walking aid, or a safe environment, thereby increasing their propensity to falls and possibly the severity of the injury sustained from a fall. Under- or over-medication may increase the likelihood of trauma, for example over-sedation due to inappropriate benzodiazepine use could contribute to falls, and over-medication with warfarin may mean that otherwise trivial trauma results in a severe bleed. If elder abuse or neglect is suspected the patient should be interviewed alone, and the history of abuse or neglect should be elicited sensitively. Determine the patient's functional status and the level of care required, and the level of care being provided by outside services. Carer support using existing aged care services probably averts further abuse in some cases.

In Australia there is no mandatory reporting of suspected elder abuse. Referral to the local aged care assessment team is advised.

For further reading see Jones *et al.* (1988), Kurrle *et al.* (1991), and Lachs and Fulmer (1993).

References

Adler HW, Nagel JE (1994) Clinical immunology and aging. In: Hazzard WR, Bierman EL, Blass JP, Ettinger WH Jr, Halter JB (eds) *Principles of geriatric medicine and gerontology*, 3rd edn. McGraw-Hill, New York, N.Y., pp 61–75.

Albert MS (1994) Cognition and aging. In: Hazzard WR, Bierman EL, Blass JP, Ettinger WH Jr, Halter JB (eds) *Principles of geriatric medicine and gerontology*, 3rd edn. McGraw-Hill, New York, N.Y., pp 1013–1019.

Baker SP, O'Neill B, Ginsburg MJ, Li G (1992) *The injury fact book*, 2nd edn. Oxford University Press, New York, N.Y.

Bassey EJ, Fiatarone MA, O'Neill EF, Kelly M, Evans WJ (1992) Leg extensior power and functional performance in very old men and women. *Clinical Science* 82: 321–327.

Bastow MD, Rawlings J, Allison SP (1983a) Undernutrition, hypothermia, and injury in elderly women with fractured femur: an injury response to altered metabolism? *Lancet* i: 143–145.

Bastow MD, Rawlings J, Allison SP (1983b) Benefits of supplementary tube feeding after fractured neck of femur: a randomised controlled trial. *BMJ* 287: 1589–1592.

Beck LJ (1994) Ageing changes in renal function. In: Hazzard WR, Bierman EL, Blass JP, Ettinger WH Jr, Halter JB (eds) *Principles of geriatric medicine and gerontology*, 3rd edn. McGraw-Hill, New York, N.Y., pp 615–24.

Bennett GB, Gwinn T (1998) Muscle weakness and high-resistance training in frail old people. In: Sherry E, Wilson S (eds) *Oxford handbook of sports medicine*. Oxford University Press, Oxford, pp 776–783.

Bloomfield SA (1997) Changes in musculoskeletal structure and function with prolonged bed rest. *Medicine and Science in Sports and Exercise* 29: 197–206.

Bortz WM (1989) Redefining human aging. *Journal of the American Geriatric Society* 37: 1092–1096.

Broos PLO, D'Hoore A, Vanderschot P, Rommens PM, Stappaerts KH (1993) Multiple trauma in elderly patients. Factors influencing outcome: importance of aggressive care. *Injury* 24(6): 365–368.

Buskirk ER, Hodgson JL (1987) Age and aerobic power: the rate of change in men and women. *Federation Proceedings* 46: 1824–1829.

Cagetti B, Cossu M, Pau A, Rivano C, Viale G. (1992) The outcome from acute subdural and epidural intracranial haematomas in very elderly patients. *British Journal of Neurosurgery* 6(3): 227–231.

Chandra RK (1992) Effects of vitamins and trace-elements on immune responses and infection in elderly subjects. *Lancet* 340: 1124–1127.

Cummings S, Kelsey J, Nevitt M, O'Dowd K (1985) Epidemiology of osteoporosis and osteoporotic fractures. *Epidemiological Reviews* 7: 178–208.

Cummings SR, Rubin SM, Black D (1990) The future of hip fractures in the United States. Number, costs, and potential effects of postmenopausal estrogen. *Clinical Orthopaedics and Related Research* 252: 163–166.

De Keyser F, Carolan D, Trask A (1995) Suburban geriatric trauma: the experiences of a level 1 trauma center. American Journal of Critical Care 4(5): 379–382.

De Maria EJ (1993) Evaluation and treatment of the elderly trauma victim. *Clinics in Geriatric Medicine* 9(2): 461–471.

De Maria EJ, Kenney PR, Merriam MA, Casanova LA, Gann DS (1987a) Aggressive trauma care benefits the elderly. *Journal of Trauma* 27(11): 1200–1206.

De Maria EJ , Kenney PR, Merriam MA, Casanova LA, Gann DS (1987b) Survival after trauma in geriatric patients. *Annals of Surgery* 206(6): 738–743.

De Maria EJ, Merriam MA, Casanova LA, Gann DS, Kenney PR (1988) Do DRG payments adequately reimburse the costs of trauma care in geriatric patients? *Journal of Trauma* 28(8): 1244–1249.

Delmi M, Rapin CH, Bengoa JM *et al.* (1990) Clinical practice, dietary supplementation in elderly patients with fractured neck of the femur. *Lancet* 335: 1013–1016.

Denham MJ (1990) Adverse drug reactions. In: Denham MJ, George CF (eds) *Drugs in Old Age:New Perspectives. British Medical Bulletin* 46, Churchill Livingstone, Edinburgh, pp 53–62.

Duncan G, Smith RG (1990) Geriatric medicine contribution in acute medical wards—a follow-up study. *Health Bulletin (Edinburgh)*, 48(1): 25–28.

Duncan AK, Vittone J, Fleming KC, Smith HC (1996) Cardiovascular disease in elderly patients. *Mayo Clinic Proceedings* 71: 184–196.

Efthimiou F, Fleming J, Gomes C, Spiro SG (1988) The effect of supplementary oral nutrition in poorly nourished patients with chronic obstructive pulmonary disease. *American Review of Respiratory Diseases* 137: 1075–1082.

Ellis GL (1990) Subdural hematoma in the elderly. *Emergency Medicine Clinics of North America* 8(2): 281–294.

Fiatarone MA, Evans WJ (1993) The etiology and reversibility of muscle dysfunction in the aged. *Journal of Gerontology* 48: 77–83.

Fife D (1987) Injuries and death among elderly persons. *American Journal of Epidemiology* 126: 936–941.

Fildes B (1994) *Injuries among older people: falls at home and pedestrian accidents*. Collins Dove, Victoria.

Finelli FC, Jonsson J, Champion HR, Morelli S, Fouty WJ (1989) A case control study for major trauma in geriatric patients. *Journal of Trauma* 29(5): 541–548.

Fox FJ, Austad AE (1990) Geriatric emergency clinical pharmacology. *Emergency Medicine Clinics of North America* 8: 221–239.

Fox RH, Woodward PM, Exton-Smith AN *et al.* (1973) Body temperature in the elderly: a national study of physiological, social and environmental conditions. *British Medical Journal* 1: 200–206.

Fries JF (1980) Aging, natural death, and the compression of morbidity. *New England Journal of Medicine* 303: 130–135.

Gerson LW, Skvarch L (1982) Emergency medical services utilisation by the elderly. *Annals of Emergency Medicine* 11: 610–612.

Goldberg TH, Finkelstein MS (1987) Difficulties in estimating glomerular filtration rate in the elderly. *Archives of Internal Medicine* 147: 1430–1433.

Grisso JA, Kaplan F (1994) Hip fractures. In: Hazzard WR, Bierman EL, Blass JP, Ettinger WH Jr, Halter JB (eds) *Principles of geriatric medicine and gerontology,* 3rd edn. McGraw-Hill, New York, N.Y., pp 1321–1327.

Gubler KD, Maier RV, Davis R *et al.* (1996) Trauma recidivism in the elderly. *Journal of Trauma: Injury, Infection and Critical Care* 41(6): 952–956.

Guralnik JM, Simonsick EM, Ferruci L *et al.* (1994) A short physical performance battery assessing lower extremity function: Association with self-reported disability and predition of mortality and nursing home admission. *Journal of Gerontology* 49: M85–M94.

Harchelroad F (1993) Acute thermoregulatory disorders. *Clinics in Geriatric Medicine* 9: 621–639.

Horan MA, Roberts NA, Barton RN, Little RA (1992) Injury responses in old age. In: *Oxford Textbook of Geriatric Medicine.* Oxford University Press, Oxford, pp 88–93.

Horst HM, Obeid FN, Sorensen VJ, Bivins BA (1986) Factors influencing survival of elderly trauma patients. *Critical Care Medicine* 14(8): 681–684.

Howard MA 3rd, Gross AS, Dacey RG, Winn HR (1989) Acute subdural hematomas: an age-dependent clinical entity. *Journal of Neurosurgery* 71(6): 858–863.

Jette AM, Harris BA, Cleary PD, Campion EW (1987) Functional recovery after hip fracture. *Archives of Physical Medicine* 68: 735–740.

Jones J, Dougherty J, Schelbe D, Cunningham W (1988) Emergency department protocol for the diagnosis and evaluation of geriatric abuse. *Annals of Emergency Medicine* 17(10): 1006–1015.

Kallman JL, Kallman S (1989) Accidents in the elderly population. In: Reichel W (ed.) *Clinical aspects of ageing*, 3rd edn. Williams & Wilkins, Baltimore, Md., pp 547–558.

Kaminer MS, Gilchrist BA (1994) Aging of the skin. In: Hazzard WR, Bierman EL, Blass JP, Ettinger WH Jr, Halter JB (eds) *Principles of geriatric medicine and gerontology*, 3rd edn. McGraw-Hill, New York, N.Y., pp 411–30.

Kanis JA (1997) *Osteoporosis*, revised edn. Blackwell Healthcare Communications, London.

Khaw K-T (1998) Hormone replacement therapy again. Risk-benefit relation differs between populations and individuals. *BMJ* 316: 1842–1844.

Knudson MM, Lieberman J, Morris Jr JA, Cushing BM, Stubbs HA (1994) Mortality factors in geriatric blunt trauma patients. *Archives of Surg*ery 129: 448–453..

Kong LB, Lekawa M, Navarro RA *et al.* (1996) Pedestrian–motor vehicle trauma: an analysis of injury profiles by age. *Journal of the American College of Surgeons* 182: 17–23.

Kurrle SE, Sadler PM, Cameron ID (1991) Elder abuse—an Australian case series. *Medical Journal of Australia* 155: 150–153.

Lachs MS, Fulmer T (1993) Recognising elder abuse and neglect. *Clinics in Geriatric Medicine* 9: 665–675.

Lakatta EG (1990) Heart and circulation. In: Schneider EL, Rowe JW (eds) *Handbook of the biology of aging*, 3rd edn, Chapter 10. Academic Press, London.

Lauritzen JB, Petersen MM, Lund B (1993) Effect of external hip protectors on hip fractures. *Lancet* 341: 11–13.

LeBlanc AD, Schneider VS, Evans HJ, Pientok C, Spector E (1992) Regional changes in muscle mass following 17 weeks of bed rest. *Journal of Applied Physiology* 73: 2172–2178.

Lehmann AB (1989) Review: undernutrition in elderly people. *Age and Aging* 18: 339–353.

Lešourd BM (1997) Nutrition and immunity in the elderly: modification of immune responses with nutritional treatments. *American Journal of Nutrition* 66: 478S–484S.

Levy DB, Hanlon DP, Townsend RN (1993) Geriatric trauma. *Clinics in Geriatric Medicine* 9(3): 601–20.

Liberman UA, Weiss SR, Broll J *et al.* (1995) Effect of oral alendronate on bone mineral density and the incidence of fractures in postmenopausal osteoporosis. *New England Journal of Medicine* 333: 1437–1443.

Lieberman IH, Webb JK (1994) Cervical injuries in the elderly. *Journal of Bone and Joint Surgery* 76B(6): 877–881.

Lipowski ZJ (1994) Delirium. In: Hazzard WR, Bierman EL, Blass JP, Ettinger WH Jr, Halter JB (eds) *Principles of geriatric medicine and gerontology*, 3rd edn. McGraw-Hill, New York, N.Y., pp 1021–1026.

Lipski PS (1995) The consequences of undernutrition in the elderly. *Proceedings of the Nutrition Society of Australia* 19: 146–151.

Lipski PS, Bennett MK, Kelly PJ, James OF (1992) Ageing and duodenal morphometry. *Journal of Clinical Pathology* 45: 450–452.

Maki BE, McIlroy WE (1996) Postural control in the older adult. *Clinics in Geriatric Medicine* 12: 635–657.

Mandavia D, Newton K (1998) Geriatric trauma. *Emergency Medicine Clinics of North America* 16(1): 257–274.

Martin RE, Teberian G (1990) Multiple Trauma and the elderly patient. *Emergency Clinics of North America* 8(2): 411–420.

Melkersson M, Andersson H, Bosaeus I, Falheden T (1983) Intestinal transit time in constipated and non-constipated geriatric patients. *Scandinavian Journal of Gastroenterology* 18: 593–597.

Meyer BR, Reidenberg MM (1992) Clinical pharmacology and ageing. In *Oxford textbook of geriatric medicine*. Oxford University Press, Oxford, pp 107–115.

Michaëlsson K, Baron JA, Farahmand BY *et al.* (1998). Hormone replacement therapy and risk of hip fracture: population based case-control study. *BMJ* 316: 1858–1863.

Montamat SC, Cusack BJ, Vestal RE (1989) Management of drug therapy in the elderly. *New England Journal of Medicine*, 321(5): 303–309.

Mossey JM (1989) Determinants of recovery 12 months after hip fracture. *American Journal of Public Health* 79: 279–286.

Nelson ME, Fiatarone MA, Morganti CM *et al.* (1994) Effects of high intensity strength training on multiple risk factors for osteoporotic fractures. A randomised controlled trial. *JAMA* 272: 1909–1914.

Ogle S (1998) The older athlete. In: Sherry E, Wilson S (eds) *Oxford Handbook of Sports Medicine*. Oxford University Press, Oxford, pp 746–774.

Older MWJ, Edwards D, Dickerson JWT (1980) A nutrient survey in elderly women with femoral neck fractures. *British Journal of Surgery* 67: 884–886.

Oreskovich MR, Howard JD, Copass MK, Carrico CJ (1984) Geriatric trauma: injury patterns and outcome. *Journal of Trauma* 24(7): 565–572.

Osler T, Hales K, Baack B *et al.* (1988) Trauma in the elderly. *American Journal of Surgery* 156: 537–543.

Parker MJ, Palmer CR (1995) Prediction of rehabilitation after hip fracture. *Age and Ageing* 24: 96–98.

Pellicane JV, Byrne K, DeMaria EJ (1992) Preventable complications and death from multiple organ failure among geriatric trauma victims. *Journal of Trauma* 33(3): 440–444.

Pennings JL, Bachulis BL, Simons CT, Slazinski T (1993) Survival after severe brain injury in the aged. *Archives of Surgery* 128: 787–794.

Preston Smith D, Enderson BL, Maull KI (1990) Trauma in the elderly: determinants of outcome. *Southern Medical Journal* 83(2): 171–177.

Radke MS, Flynn JPG, Smith M, Scott JC, Permutt T (1992) Functional improvement in geriatric trauma patients admitted to a dedicated rehabilitation hospital. *Maryland Medical Journal* 41(11): 981–987.

Rowe JW, Kahn RL (1987) Human ageing: usual and successful. *Science* 237: 143–149.

Ruiz JG, Lowenthal DT (1995) Geriatric pharmacology. In: Munson PL (ed.) *Principles of pharmacology*. Chapman & Hall, London.

Ryan AS, Treuth MS, Rubin MA *et al.* (1994) Effects of strength training on bone mineral density: hormonal and bone turnover relationships. *JAMA* 272: 1909–1914.

Sambrook PM (1995) Treatment of postmenopausal osteoporosis. *New England Journal of Medicine* 333: 1495–1496.

Sattin RW, Nevitt MC (1992) Epidemiology and environmental aspects. In: *Oxford textbook of geriatric medicine*. Oxford University Press, Oxford.

Scalea TM, Simon HM, Duncan AO *et al.* (1991) Geriatric blunt multiple trauma: improved survival with early invasive monitoring. *Journal of Trauma* 30(2): 129–136.

Schiller WR, Knox R, Chleborad W (1995) A five-year experience with severe injuries in elderly patients. *Accident Analysis and Prevention* 27: 167–174.

Schneider EL, Rowe JW (1996) *Handbook of the biology of aging*, 4th edn. Academic Press, London.

Schwartz JB (1994) Clinical pharmacology. In: Hazzard WR, Bierman EL, Blass JP, Ettinger WH Jr, Halter JB (eds) *Principles of geriatric medicine and gerontology*, 3rd edn. McGraw-Hill, New York, N.Y., pp 259–275.

Shabot MM, Johnson CL (1995) Outcome from critical care in the 'oldest old' trauma patients. *Journal of Trauma, Injury, Infection and Critical Care* 39(2): 254–260.

Shapiro MB, Dechert RE, Colwell C, Bartlett RH, Rodriguez JL (1994) Geriatric trauma: aggressive intensive care unit management is justified. *American Surgeon* 60(9): 695–98.

Spaite DW, Criss EA, Valenzuela TD, Meislin HW, Ross J (1990) Geriatric injury: an analysis of prehospital demographics, mechanisms, and patterns. *Annals of Emergency Medicine* 19: 1418–1421.

Spallone A, Giuffre R, Gagliardi FM, Vagnozzi R (1989) Chronic subdural hematoma in extremely aged patients. *European Neurology* 29(1): 18–22.

Spivak JM, Weiss MA, Cotler JM, Call M (1994) Cervical injuries in patients 65 and older. *Spine* 19(20): 2302–2306.

Sullivan DH, Walls RC, Lipschitz DA (1991) Protein-energy undernutrition and the risk of morality within 1 year of hospital discharge in a select population of geriatric rehabilitation patients. *Americal Journal of Clinical Nutrition* 53: 599–605.

Svanberg A, Selker L (1994) Ageing in different cultures: implications for postponement of aging. In: Hazzard WR, Bierman EL, Blass JP, Ettinger WH Jr, Halter JB (eds) *Principles of geriatric medicine and gerontology*, 3rd edn. McGraw-Hill, New York, N.Y., pp 177–85.

Tinetti ME (1994) Falls. In: Hazzard WR, Bierman EL, Blass JP, Ettinger WH Jr, Halter JB (eds) *Principles of geriatric medicine and gerontology*, 3rd edn. McGraw-Hill, New York, N.Y., pp 1313–1320.

Tinetti ME, Williams CS (1997) Falls, injuries due to falls, and the risk of admission to nursing homes. *New England Journal of Medicine* 337: 1279–1284.

Tinetti ME, Speechely M, Ginter SF (1988) Risk factors for falls among elderly persons living in the community. *New England Journal of Medicine* 319: 1701–1707.

Tockman MS (1994) Aging of the respiratory system. In: Hazzard WR, Bierman EL, Blass JP, Ettinger WH Jr, Halter JB (eds) *Principles of geriatric medicine and gerontology*, 3rd edn. McGraw-Hill, New York, N.Y.

Tregaskis BF, Stevenson IH (1990) Pharmacokinetics of old age. In: Denham MJ, George CF (eds) *Drugs in old age new perspectives. British Medical Bulletin* 46, Churchill Livingstone, Edinburgh, pp 9–21.

van Aalst JA, Morris JA, Yates HK, Miller RS, Bass SM (1991) Severely injured geriatric patients return to independent living: a study of factors influencing function and independence. *Journal of Trauma* 31(8): 1096–1102.

Weiner DK, Hanlan JT, Studenski SA (1998) Effects of central nervous system polypharmacy on falls liability in community dwelling older people. *Gerontology* 44: 217–221.

Weingarten MS, Wainwright ST, Sacchetti AD (1982) Trauma and aging effects on hospital costs and length of stay. *Annals of Emergency Medicine* 17: 10–14.

Woodhouse KW, James OF (1990) Hepatic drug metabolism and ageing. In: Denham MJ, George CF (eds) *Drugs in old age new perspectives. British Medical Bulletin* 46, Churchill Livingstone, Edinburgh, pp 22–35.

Zietlow SP, Capizzi PJ, Bannon MP, Farnell MB (1994) Multisystem geriatric trauma. *Journal of Trauma* 37(6): 985–988.

37

CHAPTER 37

The injured pregnant woman

BRIAN SPURRETT AND HENRY MURRAY

CHAPTER 37

The injured pregnant woman

BRIAN SPURRETT AND HENRY MURRAY

Although trauma in some form occurs in 6–7% of all pregnancies (Hoff *et al.* 1991), severe trauma occurs in about 1/200 pregnant women, the common causes being motor vehicle accidents and physical abuse (Rothenberger *et al.* 1978, Fries and Hankins 1989). In such severe cases, maternal mortality is 10% and fetal loss can be as high as 15% (Kissinger *et al.* 1991). Lesser degrees of trauma pose a smaller risk to the mother. However, fetal loss, even from the most minor of physical blows, can be significant. It is, therefore, important that the carer of first contact, who may not have advanced training in obstetrics, understands maternal indicators—especially in the first 24 hours after the trauma—that may predict preventable fetal demise.

The fact that maternal mortality from trauma has not altered over 20 years and that trauma is a major cause of mortality in the first four decades of life shows that a pregnant woman is vulnerable. The gravid uterus is mobile and vascular and a potential source of haemorrhage after trauma. Physiological changes in other organs increase the vulnerability and may also mask or mimic abnormality in vital signs. In developed countries, trauma is a significant cause of maternal mortality. The fetus has special risks because blood loss may not be immediately obvious. Careful and specialized assessment over a 72 hour period following injury is, therefore, essential.

Key points

- Severe trauma occurs in about 1/200 pregnant women.
- In such severe cases, maternal mortality is 10% and fetal loss can be as high as 15%.

Mechanism of injury and physiological changes in pregnancy

Anatomical and physiological changes in pregnancy are enormous. Only those relevant to trauma are described here.

Blood vessel wall changes

Changes in the collagen of vessel walls in pregnancy leaves them softer, distensible, and more susceptible to damage.

Placentation

The formation of the placenta from the earliest weeks of pregnancy is a complicated process enabling fetal and maternal circulations to be separated by cellular membranes, thus allowing an exchange of gases, nutrients, and waste products. As a result of this, fetal haemorrhage into the maternal circulation is common and may be augmented by even minor trauma.

Rapid enlargement of the uterus

The enlargement of the uterus makes it susceptible to direct trauma as it becomes an abdominal rather than a pelvic organ protected by the bony pelvis.

Cardiovascular changes

There is a 30% increase in blood volume by 28 weeks gestation. This allows women to tolerate up to 1.5 L of blood loss before a change in routine vital signs occurs (Dilts *et al.* 1969). Pulse rate is increased by 10–15 beats/minute in pregnancy and this may mimic haemodynamic instability.

Presentation and triage

The triage of the injured pregnant woman and her immediate management is dependent on damage to organs other than those related to the pregnancy. Severe neurological, limb, and vascular damage will clearly take priority. These will interact with her pregnant state, especially in later pregnancy when the fetus is viable (after 23 weeks gestation) and may create a dilemma between saving the fetal life by caesarean section and compromising maternal stability when the mother is badly or fatally injured. It is important that non-obstetric surgery is not withheld for the sake of the fetus. If surgery is undertaken such procedures will enhance the thrombophilic changes of pregnancy and will induce the output of endogenous prostaglandins. Prophylactic methods to decrease the risk of venous thrombosis should be adhered to, and the use of an antiprostaglandin such as indometacin should be considered. Intraoperatively, fetal hypoxaemia should be diagnosed early by the use of cardiotocograph if that is logistically possible.

Key point

- It is important that non-obstetric surgery is not withheld for the sake of the fetus.

Severe injury

The decision for caesarean section in the living but severely injured woman, or postmortem caesarean section, is always difficult. Time may not permit the ideal of consultation with anaesthetists, intensive care physicians, neonatologists and skilled obstetricians. Fetal compromise is often rapid when the mother is haemodynamically unstable, which raises the following questions in the management of a severely injured mother with a viable fetus:

- when to deliver the baby
- where to deliver the baby
- how to deliver the baby.

The answers to all three questions may be immediately obvious, e.g. when the mother is dead or about to die, the fetal heart is audible, but signs of fetal hypoxia are present and the gestational age of the fetus is >23 weeks. In this situation, the fetus must be delivered immediately and the courageous decision in a medical world of criticism and litigation must be dealt with wherever the situation arises. All that is required is a scalpel, a midline incision, and a classical caesarean section. A Pfannensteil incision and lower-segment caesarean section is quick in the hands of a trained registrar in a hospital, who is the usual person called upon to make such decisions. Transfer from the emergency department to an operating theatre may be a death sentence for the fetus, so occasionally, the correct decision is to carry out a postmortem caesarean section in the emergency department.

Less severe injury

Much more judgement than courage is necessary in the second category of injured pregnant women, that is, when the injuries are life threatening but not immediately a problem. The principles in these situations are:

- adequate maternal fluid replacement and oxygenation
- monitoring by cardiotocography
- exclusion of fetal haemorrhage
- nursing with a 15° lateral tilt
- constant review by the perinatal team
- monitoring of the maternal serum bicarbonate level.

Apart from death, the most common indicator of a poor fetal outcome is the degree of trauma (Dilts *et al.* 1969). Nevertheless, even the most severely traumatized women may have a live fetus. Maternal tissue hypoperfusion leading to fetal hypoxia is the commonest mechanism of fetal death. It has been shown that the variable most commonly associated with fetal loss is maternal serum bicarbonate on admission (Dilts *et al.* 1969). Keeping the mother in optimum fluid and blood gas equilibrium is not only best for her but crucial to fetal survival. Meticulous care of these factors in the injured pregnant women is critical because the mother may compensate by vasoconstriction at the expense of the fetus. Vasoconstriction can also occur as a result of a release of thromboxane and prostaglandins, leading to cerebral ischaemia.

Slight injury

The third category of injured pregnant women is where the injury has been slight. These women are often sent home or relegated to a ward where there is no obstetrical expertise. All injured pregnant women must be carefully monitored for 72 hours by as expert a team as the hospital has available. Slight injuries to the abdomen, especially seatbelt injuries, may result in delayed or undiagnosed fetal haemorrhage.

Steroids to hasten lung maturation should be considered even if delivery can be predicted 6 hours before the event. Intravenous steroids may be of use at an appropriate gestational age. This decision must be discussed with the obstetrician and neonatologist. A single intravenous injection of 12 mg of dexamethasone 6 hours before surgery may be useful in avoiding later pulmonary complications in the neonatal intensive care unit.

Key point

- Steroids to hasten lung maturation should be considered even if delivery can be predicted 6 hours before the event.

For women in early pregnancy, the avoidance of unnecessary radiographic examination is important. Drost *et al.* (1990), in the examination of a series of pregnant women suffering major trauma, noted that 92% underwent at least one diagnostic radiographic examination. Most underwent multiple studies. There is a teratogenic potential with radiation doses >10 rads (Mossman and Hill 1982) and also an increase in the incidence of childhood cancers. For these reasons, and especially in women in early pregnancy, selecting imaging methods such as ultrasound which do not involve radiation, positioning patients optimally, questioning critically the usefulness of the anticipated procedure, and careful shielding of the abdomen with lead aprons should be carried out. In most trauma cases it is possible, using these means, to keep the total radiation dose to the gravid uterus below 10 rads. Table 37.1 gives a guide to radiation doses from common radiological studies in injured patients.

Key point

- In women in early pregnancy, the avoidance of unnecessary radiographic examination is important.

Women in early pregnancy (<12 weeks gestation) rarely have direct trauma to the uterus because it is protected by the pelvis. The large mobile organ can, however, undergo 'whiplash' injuries with consequent rupture of the relatively softer vessels in the broad ligament. This should be considered when unexplained blood loss is encountered.

Key point

- The large mobile uterus can undergo 'whiplash' injuries.

Diagnosis of fetoplacental trauma

Trauma during pregnancy is associated with a high rate of fetal death (Kettel *et al.* 1988). This is mostly associated with occult fetal haemorrhage and may occur with even minimal maternal injury. Early diagnoses and constant effective surveillance in the 72 hours after trauma to the pregnant woman are the important issues for maximizing fetal well-being.

Key point

- Trauma during pregnancy is associated with a high rate of fetal death.

Clinical examination

The medical officer in the emergency department, who is often the first doctor to see the patient, may

Table 37.1 Absorbed radiation dose to the unshielded gravid uterus from common radiological studies often performed during trauma resuscitation and evaluation

Study	Unshielded uterine dose range (rads)
Cervical spine	No detectable contribution
Chest (AP)	0.0003–0.0043
Pelvis (AP)	0.142–0.486
Abdomen (AP)	0.133–0.451
IVP	0.202–0.815
Full spine (AP)	0.154–0.527
Femur (AP)	0.0016–0.012
Humerus (AP)	<0.000 001
Cystography	0.135–0.441
CT scan	
Head	<0.05
Thorax	<1
Upper abdomen	<3
Cumulated dose (without CT scans)	0.768–2.736
Cumulated dose (with CT scans)	>0.768–6.786

AP, anteroposterior.

have only rudimentary training in obstetrics. It is important that the following are noted and recorded:

- bruises on the abdomen, especially from seatbelts
- the presence and severity of uterine tenderness
- the presence of uterine contractions
- the vaginal passage of blood, liquor, and liquor containing meconium
- the presence of a fetal heart beat and its rate.

Cardiotocography

In the second half of pregnancy, this is the most rapid way of accurately assessing fetal well-being. With rapidly changing haemodynamic events in severely injured women, the question of how long should monitoring occur or how often it should be repeated must be carefully assessed. In the 72 hours after trauma, the acceptable minimum is monitoring for 1 hour every 8 hours. The use of cardiotocography in observing uterine activity is useful.

Diagnostic ultrasound

A simple ultrasound examination with a small portable machine will be able to confirm fetal cardiac activity when there is clinical doubt about the presence of a fetal heart beat. It can also be used to assess liquor volume. More detailed examinations requiring movement of the patient may be useful in diagnosing subplacental or broad ligament haematoma and fluid in the pouch of Douglas.

More sophisticated studies which are usually only available in specialized perinatal units may be of great use in monitoring patients whose trauma has caused occult placental haemorrhage. Flow studies in the umbilical artery and peak systolic velocity in the fetal middle cerebral artery flow may give accurate knowledge of fetal anaemia as result of haemorrhage.

Key point

- A simple ultrasound examination with a small portable machine will be able to confirm fetal cardiac activity when there is clinical doubt.

Kleihauer–Betke count

Alkaline elution of haemoglobin F and the ratio of stained (fetal) red cells to unstained (maternal) red cells in a peripheral maternal blood smear is the basis of this simple test. This test of fetal haemorrhage into the maternal circulation and an estimate of its extent is a good alert mechanism. Once it has been established by this test that significant fetal haemorrhage has occurred, it is pointless repeating it. The test has significant problems of sensitivity. Close observation of fetal welfare by other mechanisms is preferable to repeating the test. If the test is negative, the fetus must still be carefully observed. Haemorrhage of the fetus into the mother's circulation is common. Rhesus-negative women with a positive Kleihauer count have a special significance and require anti-D gamma-globulin administration.

Maternal serum bicarbonate

The data of Scorpio *et al.* (1992) have shown that maternal serum bicarbonate level correlates well with fetal loss and is more accurate than blood pH or PCO_2 as an indicator of poor maternal tissue perfusion. A 30% reduction in fetal blood flow can occur before changes in pulse or blood pressure are present (Griess 1966). Serum bicarbonate levels will then give the earliest indicator of poor tissue perfusion. It should be performed on all pregnant accident victims as soon as possible and repeated especially in category 1 and 2 patients (Table 37.2).

Key point

- Maternal serum bicarbonate level correlates well with fetal loss and is more accurate than blood pH or PCO_2 as an indicator of poor maternal tissue perfusion.

Table 37.2 Triage of the injured pregnant woman

Category		Salient management points
1	Severe injury/death >23 weeks gestation	Consider immediate delivery
2	Moderate to severe injury >23 weeks gestation	Perform and repeat maternal serum bicarbonate Monitor the fetus Exclude fetal haemorrhage Nurse 15° lateral tilt Review frequently
3	Mild injury >23 weeks gestation	Do not send home Exclude fetal haemorrhage Review for 72 hours to eliminate fetal haemorrhage.
4	Injured pregnant woman <23 weeks gestation	Avoid unnecessary radiographic examination Exclude uterine/broad ligament rupture

The treatment of uterine contractions

Tocolysis in traumatized pregnant women is controversial. Pearlman *et al.* (1990) found uterine activity common in these situations but contractions ceased in 90% of women with 'frequent uterine contractions'. Two factors must be kept in mind:

- Premature birth and abortion can occur following trauma.
- The uterine activity may result from occult placental abruption, which may be augmented by tocolysis.

Summary

The injured pregnant woman presents diagnostic challenges because of the physiological changes of pregnancy which may both mask and mimic signs of shock. Meticulous care of the mother prevents fetal death and prolonged fetal observation is necessary to diagnose and accurately manage fetal hypoxia. One injured patient can be difficult; managing the mother and fetus can be extremely challenging.

References

Dilts PV, Brinkman CR, Kirschbaum TH *et al.* (1969) Uterine and systemic haemodynamic inter relationships and their response to hypoxia. *American Journal of Obstetrics and Gynecology* 103: 138–157.

Drost TF, Rosemurgy AS, Sherman HF, Scott LM, Williams JK (1990) Major trauma in pregnant women: maternal/fetal outcome. *Journal of Trauma* 30: 574–578.

Fries MH, Hankins GD (1989) Motor vehicle accident associated with minimal trauma but subsequent fetal demise. *Annals of Emergency Medicine* 18: 301–310.

Griess F (1966) Uterine vascular response to haemorrhage during pregnancy. *Obstetrics and Gynecology* 27: 408–411.

Hoff WS, D'Amelio LF, Tinkoff GH *et al.* (1991) Maternal predictors of fetal demise in trauma during pregnancy. *Surgery, Gynaecology and Obstetrics* 172: 175–180.

Kettel LM, Branch DW, Scott JR (1988) Occult placental abruption after maternal trauma. *Obstetrics and Gynecology* 71: 449–453.

Kissinger DP, Rozycki GS, Morris JA Jr *et al.* (1991) Trauma in pregnancy—predicting pregnancy outcome. *Archives of Surgery* 126: 1079–1086.

Mossman KL, Hill LT (1982) Radiation risks in pregnancy. *Obstetrics and Gynecology* 60: 237–240.

Pearlman MD, Tintinnali JE, Lorenz JP (1990) A prospective controlled study of outcome after trauma during pregnancy. *American Journal of Obstetrics and Gynecology* 162: 1502–1507.

Rothenberger D, Quattlebaum FW, Perry JF *et al.* (1978) Blunt maternal trauma: a review of 103 cases. *Journal of Trauma* 18: 173–179.

Scorpio RJ, Esposito TJ, Smith LG *et al.* (1992) Blunt trauma during pregnancy: factors affecting fetal outcome. *Journal of Trauma* 32: 213–216.

38

CHAPTER 38

Psychiatric trauma

ALISON L S CHIU AND
MICHAEL D ROBERTSON

CHAPTER 38

Psychiatric trauma

ALISON L S CHIU AND MICHAEL D ROBERTSON

Psychiatric disorders are characterized by patterns of abnormal or deviant behaviour and psychological signs and symptoms that result in dysfunction. Psychiatric disorders can commonly generate the need for attention in the trauma care setting. This may involve addressing the management of intercurrent psychopathology in a trauma victim or the detection and management of the psychiatric sequelae of trauma.

Psychiatric disorders which present in the trauma situation, and may possibly result from trauma itself, include:

- delirium
- substance-related disorders (drugs and alcohol)
- acute or persisting organic brain syndromes
- major depressive disorder
- adjustment disorders with associated depression or anxiety
- anxiety disorders (including acute stress disorder and post-traumatic stress disorder)
- suicidality
- other disorders including cognitive impairment, psychotic disorders, personality disorders, and relational disorders.

Individuals with altered or disturbed mental states also require specialized management in the pre-, peri- and postoperative stages. Management of psychiatric disorders in the trauma patient requires collaboration among the primary physician, psychiatrist, and surgeon.

Psychiatric disorders have complex biological, psychological, and social aetiologies. Frequently, traumatic injuries may precipitate a psychiatric illness or may be the initial presentation of an underlying psychiatric disorder.

Psychological responses to trauma

The ways in which individuals respond to a traumatic event, such as a motor vehicle accident, vary with the trauma itself and the individual patient. Many authors have tried to characterize a typical pattern of psychological response to trauma, and most models emphasize the role of acute psychological processes such as dissociation and denial, followed by attempts to adapt to the physical and psychological sequelae.

In essence, most people proceed through a process of acute distress followed by psychological numbing, which may persist for days to weeks. The development of some degree of psychological re-experiencing is common and leads to the eventual processing of the event. In most cases, people deal with traumatic events by mobilizing their available social and family resources, but there are some circumstances where a patient may persist in a particular stage of the process leading to the development of psychopathology. When a patient's responses are atypical or unexpected, it is usually prudent to request some form of psychological assessment by a psychiatrist or skilled trauma counsellor.

Key points

- The trauma setting may bring to light a psychiatric disorder resulting from the trauma itself, or a pre-existing psychiatric disorder.
- The individual response to trauma is highly variable.

Emergency issues

Occasionally, severe psychiatric disturbance necessitates urgent intervention by the trauma clinician. This is particularly the case when a patient is potentially harmful to themselves or, far less frequently, to others. It is also important to acknowledge that acute severe mental disorder may be the result of life-threatening illness (e.g. severe sepsis), also requiring urgent attention.

Control of aggressive behaviour and initiating management of symptoms

Physically combative patients are not commonly encountered on general medical or surgical wards, but are more likely to appear in the emergency department. A number of serious or life-threatening illnesses may at first appear as inappropriate behaviour. If the patient must be transferred to another hospital for management, then diagnostic evaluation must be completed in the emergency room.

A previous history of aggressive behaviour is the best predictor of potential violence. Psychiatric disorders in which aggressive behaviour may be a problem in an acute or critical care setting are usually those associated with disinhibition such as delirium, intoxication, or dementia. Persecutory delusions arising from psychotic disorders such as schizophrenia may also increase the likelihood of aggression. Irritability may also be a feature of hypomania or depressive illnesses, and may lead to aggression. In attempting to control aggressive behaviour, the following points should be considered:

- If a patient is brought to the emergency department in physical restraints, they should not be removed until a careful evaluation has been completed (regardless of whether the patient appears relaxed and co-operative).
- If restraints are required after arrival in the emergency department, a minimum of four people and preferably five should be used to apply appropriate restraints to ensure the safety of the patient and others. It must be acknowledged that physical restraint in itself can so distress the patient as to lead to agitation and distress. Moreover, the use of restraints may be complicated by physical injury, e.g. after spinal trauma.
- Frequently, situations involving potentially aggressive patients can be defused with a calm, non-confrontational approach.

Clinicians should give continuous reassurance:

- Explain the need for any planned procedure (physical examination, giving medication, etc.).
- Ask repeatedly if the patient is able to co-operate with the next step to be taken.

Medication (for rapid sedation)

The clinical objective is to reduce agitation, rather than produce sedation. Several approaches to medication exist and these will be dependant on institutional protocol and physician preferences. All following recommendations are given as a guide.

Hypnosedatives

If the patient is too agitated to co-operate, give lorazepam (1–4 mg oral) or diazepam (5–10 mg oral or intravenous). Repeat every 20–30 minutes if necessary, until the patient is able to co-operate, to a maximum of four doses. Care must be taken to avoid respiratory suppression or evidence of a paradoxical reaction. It takes 5–10 minutes for these agents to enter the central nervous system (CNS), so patience in waiting for a response to medication is vital to avoid overdosing.

Non-specific sedatives such as barbiturates or benzodiazepines may promote further disinhibition unless the cause of the situation is alcohol or sedative withdrawal.

Neuroleptics

For agitated psychotic or delirious patients a high-potency antipsychotic such as haloperidol (5–10 mg oral or intramuscular) at 30–60 minute intervals, until the patient becomes manageable. For elderly patients, use only incremental doses of 1–2 mg (Motto 1990). In general, most patients respond before a total dose of 15–20 mg is given. Relative to the oral or intramuscular route, intravenously administered haloperidol has a lower incidence of extrapyramidal side-effects (Menza *et al.* 1987). Droperidol 2.5–10.0 mg intravenous infusion is more sedating, but may cause hypotension via marked alpha$_1$-adrenergic blockade. Chlorpromazine is often given intramuscularly but this is no longer considered good practice, as its absorption is unpredictable and there may be abscess formation at the injection site.

The clinician must be aware for the potential of extrapyramidal side-effects to appear particularly within the first 24 hours after rapid sedation, and although side-effects are rare they should not be overlooked. Specifically, these include:

- *Acute dystonia:* Abnormal posture characterized by a persistent increase in tone, usually of truncal musculature, but rarely can occur in the upper airway leading to acute upper airway obstruction. This is treated by rapid administration of benztropine mesylate 1–2 mg intravenously (Motto 1990) as needed to minimize such symptoms, or diphenhydramine 50 mg intravenously as well as oxygenation.
- *Akathisia:* A syndrome of acute motor restlessness or mental perturbation. This is best managed by cessation or reduction of the dose of antipsychotics. Benzodiazepines such as diazepam are often helpful in relieving the symptoms.
- *Neuroleptic malignant syndrome:* Characterized by fever (>40 °C or 140 °F), rigidity, cardiovascular instability, and delirium. A raised CPK (i.e. >1000 Units/L) may be helpful in the diagnosis but can also be raised with multiple trauma surgical procedures that are prolongued or involve tourniquet use, or in individuals struggling against restraints. This condition has a 5–10% mortality rate and requires management in a critical care setting.

Diagnosis

Obtaining a complete history in an emergency situation may be impossible. Accurate psychiatric diagnosis is difficult and critical for appropriate management, but a few clinical situations require prompt recognition and intervention; for example, behavioural disturbances in severely injured or medically ill patients, or symptoms such as excitement or aggression. In these cases, precise diagnosis is often less important than determining the principal symptom complex. Emergency use of psychotropics is often necessary even before a diagnosis is made.

Aggressive behaviour arising from an organic cause includes:

- alcohol and sedative intoxication or withdrawal
- amphetamine intoxication
- thyroid dysfunction
- hypoglycaemia
- temporal lobe epilepsy.

Functional causes include:

- psychoses with persecutory delusions
- catatonic excitement
- disorders of impulse control, e.g. borderline personality disorder
- antisocial personality.

A detailed medical history may make the diagnosis obvious (e.g. drug ingestion, previous psychiatric diagnosis), but supplemental sources of information may be necessary (family, friends, police, employer, therapist, or physician).

Physical examination

A physical examination may aid in identifying factors underlying altered mental state:

- blood pressure, pulse, temperature
- evidence of head trauma, e.g. laceration, or rhinorrhoea of cerebrospinal fluid
- evidence of intravenous drug use, e.g. needle tracks, pupillary constriction or dilation
- evidence of intoxication e.g. alcoholic fetor, vasodilation suggesting atropinic intoxication
- hyperplasia of the gums, suggesting long-term use of phenytoin and a possible postictal state
- stigmata of long-term alcohol abuse, e.g. hepatomegaly, capillary distension, spider angiomas, etc.
- Medic-alert tag (possible diabetes).

Recognition of medical illness or intoxication

Recognition and treatment of any medical illness is crucial. Virtually all behavioural disturbances can be caused by an organic process or toxic condition. A thorough organic screen would include:

- arterial blood gases
- serum electrolytes
- serum calcium
- liver and renal function tests
- blood glucose
- thyroid function tests
- urine or blood toxicology screen for phencyclidine (PCP), amphetamines etc
- imaging of the head (e.g. CT brain) may also be indicated.

The mental state examination

Frequently, the mental state examination (MSE) must be performed on the basis of observation rather than interview. A thorough MSE would include:

- level of arousal, orientation and attention
- evidence of psychotic symptoms such as perplexity, distraction, talking to self
- presence of disorganized thought or behaviour
- abnormal involuntary movements
- suicidal thinking
- malevolent intent to others
- presence of insight and the capacity for sound judgement
- impairment of judgement.

In an emergency situation, a thorough MSE may not be possible.

The role of a consultation/liaison psychiatrist

In most circumstances, a specialist psychiatric consultation should be sought for a patient who presents with abnormalities of mental state, particularly if it is felt that persisting psychopathology is present and likely to require ongoing use of psychotropic medication. Most large centres now have access to consultation/liaison psychiatrists specializing in the psychological care of medical patients. Joint management may be required where the behaviour is caused as a result of a medical condition (e.g. delirium).

Management focuses on ensuring safety for the patient and staff, making a complete diagnostic formulation, devising a treatment strategy that addresses short and long-term issues, providing a supportive environment for the patient and their family or friends, and providing clarification and explanation.

The general principles of psychopharmacology for the medically ill revolve around the appropriate use of psychotropics in this patient population, with careful considerations of altered pharmacokinetics, the potential for drug interactions and the problems of side-effects. Care must also be taken to ensure that informed consent from the patient or family is obtained where possible. Psychological treatments also have a place in the management of mental illness and are best provided by trained mental health professional. Table 38.1 gives a guide to psychotropic drugs and their use in the treatment of psychiatric disorders.

Key points

- Potentially aggressive patients are rarely harmful to others—more frequently they are harmful to themselves.
- Consider medical causes for psychiatric presentations (e.g. sepsis, hypoglycaemia, thyroid dysfunction, temporal lobe epilepsy, head trauma, substance intoxication or withdrawal).
- Beware of extrapyramidal symptoms as a side-effect of rapid sedation. Treat with benztropine mesylate (1–2 mg, IV or IM), or diphenhydramine (50 mg IM or IV).
- Effective management requires a multifaceted approach with collaboration between the primary physician, psychiatrist, and surgeon.

Table 38.1 Uses and common side-effects of psychotropic drugs

Medication	Class	Uses	Side effects
Antipsychotics (e.g. chlorpromazine, haloperidol, flupenthixol)	Neuroleptics	Psychotic disorders Control of agitation Delirium	Extrapyramidal (e.g. dystonia) Anticholinergic Antiadrenergic Sedation Weight gain
Lithium	Mood stabilizer	Acute and maintenance management of mania Augmentation of antidepressants	Thirst Weight gain Skin eruptions Thyroid suppression Renal impairment
Tricyclic antidepressants (e.g. dothiepin [dosulepin], amitriptyline)	Antidepressants	Major depression Anxiety disorder Obsessive compulsive disorder	Antihistaminergic Anticholinergic Antiadrenergic Cardiotoxicity
Fluoxetine Sertraline Citalopram	Selective serotonin reuptake inhibitors	Major depression Anxiety disorder Obsessive compulsive disorder Dysthymia	Nausea Insomnia Sexual dysfunction
Carbamazepine Sodium valproate Lamotrigine	Anticonvulsants	Mood stabilizers Aggression management Seizure control	Nausea Rash Hepatotoxicity Blood dyscrasia

Delirium

The core feature of delirium (or acute confusional state) is grossly impaired attention, presenting as disorientation or inability to maintain communication. Psychotic features such as persecutory delusions or frightening visual hallucinations are often present, particularly at night.

Delirium is usually multifactorial in origin. In a patient who has sustained trauma, there are a number of common factors predisposing to the development of delirium.

Pre- and postoperative factors

Pre- and postoperative 'organic' CNS disorders should be addressed with an appropriate search for specific aetiology such as underlying metabolic, infectious, and neurological causes of altered mental state. Cognitive impairment is an important medicolegal issue when obtaining informed consent to operative procedures, and frequently this may be required from next of kin or other appropriate statutory body. Postoperatively, anaesthetic agents or intolerance to specific analgesic agents or their metabolites e.g. norpethidine (Eisendrath *et al.* 1987) or intolerance to other drugs should be suspected as causes of delirium. In other cases depression of CNS function may be evidence of postoperative cardiopulmonary, metabolic or infectious complication. Impaired cognition on a surgical service is frequently a result of sepsis. These are often sicker patients with increased postoperative morbidity.

The principals of management of postoperative delirium include:

- prompt recognition and diagnosis (often EEG will be helpful if the disturbance is subtle)
- detection and treatment of underlying aetiologies
- judicious use of psychotropics—low-dose haloperidol and lorazepam for agitation are the most frequently used
- environmental interventions including use of single room, minimal transfers to and from wards, regular nursing contact and orientation, and optimal lighting in the ward.

Table 38.2 lists causes of delirium.

Fat emboli syndrome

Fat emboli syndrome is most often seen in fractures of the long bones or pelvis. A confusional state is probably more common than reported (Murray 1991). Early recognition is important in preventing morbidity and mortality of patients (ten Duis 1997).

Table 38.2 Causes of delirium

Drug intoxications
Other withdrawal states (particularly alcohol withdrawal delirium)
Sepsis (especially urinary tract infections)
Dehydration and electrolyte imbalance
Undiagnosed head injury
Pulmonary embolism or other causes of hypoxia
Ictal or postictal states
Metabolic derangement
Paraneoplastic syndromes (especially hypercalcaemia)
Cardiac disease (including acute myocardial infarction and congestive cardiac failure)
Hypothermia
Sleep deprivation and severe constipation in the elderly
Other underlying medical problems
Frequent environmental changes (e.g. frequent transfers from wards)

Alcohol abuse

Alcohol is the most commonly abused agent in the community and is frequently a factor in sustaining trauma. Alcohol abuse exists as a spectrum from social drinking, to hazardous use, to dependence. Apart from dealing with acute intoxication in the emergency department, the emergence of alcohol withdrawal in a medical setting is the most problematic alcohol-related problem.

Alcohol intoxication

An acutely intoxicated patient presents a management dilemma for a trauma team. Restraint and, in some circumstances, use of rapid sedation may be required in order to manage intoxicated patients properly. Judicious use of psychotropics is required given the potential for interaction with alcohol, as well as the possibility of hepatic or renal impairment altering metabolism of medications. It is also important to note that several life-threatening medical emergencies may mimic intoxication, e.g. closed head injury or diabetic ketoacidosis. Patients who abuse alcohol are also more prone to sustain intracerebral bleeding, especially subdural haematoma.

Alcohol dependence

The core features of alcohol dependence include a stereotypical pattern of drinking, primacy of drinking over other activities, the presence of increased tolerance to alcohol, and the appearance of withdrawal phenomena after cessation of drinking. All acutely intoxicated patients should immediately receive a dose of parenteral thiamine 100 mg by intramuscular injection prior to any glucose containing solutions.

Alcohol withdrawal

Withdrawal from alcohol exists as a spectrum from mild agitation and autonomic arousal to the rarer syndrome of delirium tremens. Withdrawal often appears 12–24 hours after the last drink and is often subtle. This time frame frequently corresponds with the immediate postoperative period.

Preoperative detoxification is best, whenever possible. In the surgical setting, prevention of withdrawal is a primary goal. Supplemental nutritional support should be instituted and full doses of chlordiazepoxide (50–100 mg oral or intravenous) initiated at 4–6 hour intervals (maximum 300 mg/day) or diazepam (10–20 mg oral) every 2 hours in those patients suspected of being candidates for alcohol withdrawal. Identifying the minority of high-risk patients who require medically supervised and pharmacologically assisted intervention for detoxification is often clinically challenging (Halla and Zadorb, 1997).

Management

Treatment requires administration of parenteral thiamine 100 mg by intramuscular injection, hydration, and the use of benzodiazepines to avert the development of an acute withdrawal syndrome. Chlordiazepoxide or diazepam are the commonest agents used, but oxazepam or lorazepam are better if hepatic impairment is suspected. Adequate hydration and maintenance of serum potassium and magnesium levels is important. The severity of alcohol withdrawal symptoms can be monitored using standardized clinical rating scales and scores can be used to guide clinical intervention e.g. The Clinical Institute Withdrawal Assessment for Alcohol (revised) (CIWA-Ar) (Sullivan et al. 1986)

Mortality from delirium tremens is approximately 15% and usually results from sepsis or acute renal failure. In a small proportion of patients the delirium may evolve into Korsakoff's psychosis, with permanent cognitive impairment.

Substance abuse

Stimulants

The signs and symptoms of acute stimulant intoxication such as amphetamine or cocaine are physiological over-arousal, agitation, aggression, and frequently paranoid psychosis without delirium. Hypertension and tachycardia are also common, but not specific. Seizures and arrhythmias may predispose to the development of confusional states.

Seizures can be treated with diazepam 5–10 mg (iv) every 10–15 minutes until symptoms resolve, not to exceed 30 mg. For acute psychotic states halopendol can be used (5 mg, iv/1 m) titrated to effect, with initial dose up to doubled after 20–30 minutes.

Opioids

Heroin is usually ingested by intravenous injection, smoking, or inhalation. Psychosis is uncommon, but agitation may occur during the characteristic withdrawal phase.

In managing acute intoxication (overdose characterized by abnormal mental status, respiratory depression and miotic pupils), naloxone, an opioid antagonist, 0.4–0.8 mg intravenously is often life saving, and frequently given in the field. A subsequent intramuscular injection is usually required. Patients resuscitated from opiate overdose may be agitated or aggressive. Heroin overdoses frequently represent suicidal acts, and this must be explored with the patient after medical stabilization.

Opiate abuse frequently occurs against a background of severe personality disorder and, occasionally, treatable serious mental illness such as mood disorder and psychotic illnesses.

Benzodiazepines

Up to 45% of patients receiving stable, long-term doses of benzodiazepines will show evidence of physiological withdrawal, particularly those who use agents with short half-lives such as temazepam. This is relevant in surgical patients where medication may have been halted in the preoperative period. Withdrawal symptoms are usually the same in both high- and low-dose patients, and include anxiety, insomnia, irritability, depression, tremor, nausea or vomiting, and anorexia. Seizures and psychotic reactions have also been described.

The management of benzodiazepine withdrawal requires stabilization on an equipotent dose of diazepam and a gradual reduction over a period

Table 38.3 Dose equivalents for benzodiazepines

Drug	Dose equivalent (mg)
Diazepam	5
Lorazepam	0.5
Oxazepam	15
Nitrazepam	5
Flunitrazepam	1
Clonazepam	0.5
Temazepam	10
Alprazolam	0.5

of weeks, preferably under close medical supervision. See Table 38.3 for equivalent doses of benzodiazepines.

Phencyclidine

Phencyclidine (PCP) intoxication frequently involves the development of paranoid psychosis, agitation, and delirium. Patients intoxicated with PCP are often extremely agitated and hostile, and often require high doses of neuroleptics for tranquillization. Rhabdomyolysis may occur as a result of intoxication or trauma and may lead to acute renal complications.

Key points

- Delirium should be treated with low-dose haloperidol and lorazepam. Intolerance to norpethidine postoperatively (causing myoclonus and/or anxiety) is one example of many causes, most of which are of multiple organic or psychogenic aetiology.
- Alcohol is responsible for more psychiatric syndromes in general hospitals than all other substances combined.
- Alcohol withdrawal symptoms are delayed beyond the usual textbook limits by previous sedation and anaesthesia. Administration of thiamine, 100 mg IM is vital. Neuroleptic medication is not recommended as a first-line approach since impairment in temperature regulation is a possibility.
- Benzodiazepine withdrawal manifests in up to 45% of patients receiving stable, long-term doses, especially with short-acting agents (e.g. temazepam). This may be relevant in the trauma patient where medication is ceased e.g. preoperatively.
- Narcotic overdose should be treated with naloxone 0.4–0.8 mg IV.

Major depressive disorder

Depressive illnesses occur in 15–30% of medically ill patients and frequently affect the prognosis of the underlying condition. Many neurovegetative depressive symptoms of depression may be the product of underlying medical illnesses or their treatment. Acute despondency and dysphoria are also quite common among surgically and medically ill patients.

Depressive symptoms have been reported in most medical conditions, particularly illnesses involving the CNS, e.g. stroke, cancer, renal impairment and cardiac disease. It is acknowledged that depression in a medical or surgical setting is under-recognized and undertreated (Rodin and Voshart 1986).

Diagnosis

The DSM-IV-TR (APA 2000) criteria for major depressive disorder should be applied to the patient with medical illness in the same way as they are to a primary psychiatric patient. To diagnose a major depression at least five of the following nine symptoms must be present for most of the day, nearly every day, include either depressed mood or loss of interest or pleasure, and almost always result in impaired interpersonal, social and occupational functioning:

- depressed mood, subjective or observed
- markedly diminished interest or pleasure in all, or almost all, activities most of the day

- significant (more than 5% of body weight per month) weight loss or gain
- insomnia or hypersomnia
- psychomotor agitation or retardation
- fatigue or loss of energy
- feelings of worthlessness or excessive or inappropriate guilt
- diminished ability to think or concentrate, or indecisiveness
- recurrent thoughts of death or suicide.

The distinction between depression as a symptom and as a clinical syndrome may be difficult to make in the medically ill, and there is frequently overlap between the symptoms of depression and those of physical illness. Not only can depression mimic symptoms of a medical illness, e.g. unexplained pain or weight loss, but also medical illness may produce symptoms that are identical to the symptoms of depression. There are certain circumstances when a clinician may suspect an underlying depressive episode e.g. non-compliance or refusal of treatment, or irritable or difficult interactions with staff, that prompt request for psychiatric consultation.

Depression may be the result of a medical condition e.g. stroke or malignancy. Occasionally medications can lead to iatrogenic depression. Table 38.4 lists drugs more commonly associated with the development of depression.

The depressed surgical patient may therefore be irritable, agitated, or withdrawn. They may not co-operate with treatment and occasionally try to discharge themselves against advice. A higher level of postoperative morbidity for depressed patients has been reported as postoperative mobilization is a challenge, and impaired nutrition undermines the process of surgical repair. There may also be a tendency for medical or surgical staff to overlook or exclude certain treatment options on the basis of difficult interactions with a depressed patient or their family.

Care must also be taken to differentiate depression from an acute delirium, as the two conditions often present in a similar way in a medical setting.

Table 38.4 Drugs commonly associated with a depressive syndrome

Antihypertensives
reserpine
methyldopa
thiazides
spironolactone
clonidine hydrochloride
Oral contraceptives
Steroids and adrenocorticotropic hormone
Opiate analgesics (especially pentazocine)
Cimetidine, ranitidine
Barbiturates
Benzodiazepines
Beta-blockers (esp. propranolol hydrochloride)
Metoclopramide hydrochloride
Cocaine
Amphetamine
Antineoplastics (especially vinca alkaloids)

Management

Specialist psychiatric intervention is essential in treating depressive states. All of the psychological, social, and biological forms of treatment available for depression are applicable to depressed medically ill patients. Antidepressant pharmacotherapy—tricyclics, monoamine oxidase inhibitors (MAOIs), selective serotonin reuptake inhibitor (SSRIs)—is of proven efficacy in the treatment of serious mood disorders, although special attention must be given to altered pharmacokinetics, drug interactions, and greater potential for drug toxicity in medically ill patients.

Side-effects can be problematic in medically ill patients and may produce life-threatening complications. Drug interactions with some antidepressants, particularly the SSRI group, must be considered in prescribing for the medically ill. Tricyclic antidepressants have a class IA anti-arrhythmic or 'quinidine-like' effect and may produce arrhythmias in those patients thus predisposed. Moreover, tricyclic antidepressants produce side-effects such as dry mouth or constipation that may predispose surgical patients to complications such as mucosal candidiasis.

In the surgical patient, the anaesthetist and surgeon should be informed of medication requirements in all instances. Appropriate antidepressant medication should be continued through the preoperative period and resumed postoperatively as soon as the patient can take medication orally. If a patient is taking or prescribed irreversible MAOIs, e.g. phenelzine, care must be taken to avoid pethidine and caution required in prescribing opiate analgesics. Phenelzine inhibits the metabolism of suxamethonium and possibly barbiturates. Rarely, a 'cheese reaction' may occur whereby life-threatening hypertension develops when tyramine is ingested. Similarly the 'serotonin syndrome' characterized by tremor, autonomic instability, delirium, gastrointestinal symptoms, and seizures may present in patients taking MAOIs, particularly when they are co-administered with other antidepressants.

Adjustment disorder with depressed mood

Adjustment disorder is the second most common psychiatric diagnosis, after delirium, among patients admitted to hospital for medical and surgical problems. Adjustment disorder is a short-term maladaptive response to psychosocial stress. It is precipitated by one or more stressors with resulting emotional or behavioural symptoms appearing within 3 months of the onset of the stressor. Adjustment disorder tends to remit after the stressor ceases or, if the stressor persists, a new level of adaptation is achieved. The response is maladaptive because of impairment in social or occupational functioning or because of symptoms or behaviours that are beyond the normal, usual, or expected response to such a stressor. In adjustment disorder with depressed mood, the predominant manifestations are depressed mood, tearfulness, and hopelessness. Adjustment disorder with depression or anxiety can present with aggressive behaviour or self-harm.

Key points

- Depressive illness occurs in a significant number (15–30%) of medically ill patients.
- Depression in the medical and/or surgical setting is underdiagnosed and therefore undertreated.
- Medical conditions or medications can lead to depressive symptoms.
- Postoperative morbidity is higher in depressed patients.
- Depressed patients may have increased postoperative analgesic requirements.

Anxiety disorders

Anxiety is a common response to trauma or medical illness. The presence of anxiety may represent the patient's reaction to the meaning and implications of medical illness or the medical setting or a manifestation of a physical disorder itself, or may arise from an underlying psychiatric disorder.

Anxiety in the surgical patient

Anxiety may result from poor understanding of the surgical condition or its treatment. Often, time spent clarifying these matters will significantly alleviate the patient's distress. Some personality types are more prone to experience anxiety in a medical setting, such as patients who are excessively controlling or obsessive. Moreover, the absence of anxiety in a traumatized or surgically ill patient may be suggestive of problematic coping mechanisms such as denial or repression. In either case, there may be implications for compliance with treatment and longer-term implications for the development of persisting psychopathology.

The treatment of perioperative anxiety may be merely to provide reassurance and clearer communication. In some circumstances, judicious use of benzodiazepines such as lorazepam 0.5–1 mg or diazepam 5–10 mg for a few days may alleviate excessive distress in this patient group.

Adjustment disorder with anxiety

Symptoms of anxiety, such as palpitations, jitteriness, and agitation, are present in adjustment disorder with anxiety, which must be differentiated from anxiety disorders.

Post-traumatic stress disorder

Acute stress disorder

Post-traumatic stress disorder (PTSD) and acute stress disorder (ASD) are characterized by the development of a characteristic group of psychological symptoms following exposure to a traumatic event. The stressor is the prime causative factor of PTSD and ASD. Such trauma may include armed combat or terrorist attacks, violent assaults, rape, incarceration, and/or torture (prisoners of war, concentration camp survivors, refugees), natural catastrophes, serious accidents, or being diagnosed with a life threatening illness. The traumatic event may be directly experienced or simply witnessed. Not every individual responds to such trauma with a PTSD. A variety of factors in clinical combination are required to produce the pathologic state, including a person's subjective response to trauma.

Posttraumatic stress disorder and acute stress disorder consist of:

- the persistent re-experiencing of the trauma (e.g. flashbacks, nightmares)
- persistent avoidance of stimuli associated with the trauma (e.g. panic attacks)
- persistent hyperarousal (e.g. anxiety, hyperalertness, insomnia)
- a general numbing of emotions (e.g. decreased interest in previously enjoyable activities, feelings of detachment or estrangement from others, and a restricted range of affect).

The onset of symptoms of PTSD typically occurs a few days to a few weeks after the trauma, but the delay in onset may last several years. Symptoms usually persist for at least 1 month. Acute stress disorder is characterized by symptoms similar to those of PTSD that occur immediately (within 1 month) after exposure to an extreme traumatic stressor. Symptoms may fluctuate over time and may be most intense during periods of stress.

Management

The provision of debriefing, counselling, and support networks after a traumatic event is essential for prevention or amelioration of post-traumatic psychopathology. It is of vital importance to provide adequate debriefing for staff and other professionals involved in a traumatic event.

There is limited data available as to which pharmacotherapeutic or psychotherapeutic interventions are efficacious in PTSD. Accumulating evidence supports the use of SSRI medications, but it is important to vigorously treat co-morbid conditions such as depression or substance abuse. Frequently, referral to a specialized service is required.

Key points

- Anxiety can be a component of many medical conditions.
- Anxiety symptoms should be differentiated from anxiety disorders.
- Post-traumatic stress disorder or acute stress disorder can result from exposure to a traumatic event.
- Post-traumatic stress disorder can be highly resistant to treatment.

Suicidal states

Suicide represents the commonest cause of death in 15–24 year olds and suicidal behaviour is the commonest reason for psychiatric consultation in the acute care setting. Frequently, traumas represent attempted suicide and trauma specialists must carry a high index of suspicion of suicidal behaviour, particularly in young males.

Classically, distinction is drawn between serious suicide attempts and deliberate self-harm or so-called parasuicide. In practice, such distinctions are arbitrary and misleading as a significant percentage of parasuicide attempters go on to complete suicide subsequently. It is sound clinical practice for the trauma or emergency physician to regard all self-harming behaviour as serious and refer for specialist psychiatric care.

A number of demographic factors predisposing to suicidal behaviour include male gender, substance abuse, physical or mental illness, low socio-economic status, recent loss or interpersonal stress, unemployment, and access to means (e.g. firearms or dangerous drugs). The most reliable predictor of suicidal behaviour is previous attempts.

In evaluating the suicidal patient the clinician must establish:

- the degree of intent to die
- whether provision was made for death (including wills, notes, telephone calls to friends)
- what steps were taken to avoid discovery or prevention
- what degree of remorse or relief exists in the patient
- whether acute psychosocial stressors exist.

In virtually all instances, the clinical situation should be discussed with a psychiatrist. Infrequently, self-harming behaviour may occur in response to psychotic symptoms such as hallucinations commanding the patient to do so. Enquiries must be made to exclude the presence of such phenomena.

Key points

- Suicidal behaviour is the most common reason for psychiatric consultation in the acute-care setting.
- All suicidal gestures and attempts should be taken seriously.
- Patients must be asked about suicidal thoughts, intents, and plans.
- The most reliable predictor of suicidal behaviour is previous attempts.

Other areas

Frequently, clinicians working in trauma settings are required to deal with patients who are difficult or exhibit problematic personality and do not appear to suffer from a diagnosable psychiatric disorder. Such behaviour may indicate acute distress leading to maladaptive coping mechanisms, disordered personality, or simple interpersonal deficits. Cultural factors may also play a role. Often such difficult interactions can be avoided by the observance of professional courtesy, clear communication, and patient acknowledgment of the individual's concerns.

References

APA DSM-IV-TR (2000) *Diagnostic and Statistical Manual of Mental Disorders*, 4th edn. Text revision American Psychiatric Association, Washington DC.

Eisendrath SJ, Goldman B, Douglas J, Dimatteo L, Van Dyke C (1987) Meperidine-induced delirium. *American Journal of Psychiatry* 144(8): 1062–1065.

Halla W, Zadorb D (1997) The alcohol withdrawal syndrome. *Lancet* 389 (9069): 1897–1900.

Menza MA, Murray GB, Holmes VF, Rafuls WA (1987) Decreased extrapyramidal symptoms with intravenous haloperidol. *Journal of Clinical Psychiatry* 48(7): 278–280.

Motto JA (1990) Psychiatric emergencies. In: Ho MT, Saunders CE (ed) *Current emergency diagnosis and treatment*. Prentice-Hall, London.

Murray GB (1991) Confusion, delirium, and dementia. In: Cassem NH (ed) *Massachusetts General Hospital handbook of general hospital psychiatry*. Mosby Year Book, St Louis.

Rodin G, Voshart K (1986) Depression in the medically ill: an overview. *American Journal of Psychiatry* 143(6): 696–705.

Sullivan JT, Sykora K, Schnerderman A, Naranjo CA, Sellers EM (1989) Assessment of alcohol withdrawal: the revised clinical institute withdrawal assessment for alcoholic scale (CIWA-Ar). *British Journal of Addiction* 84(11): 1353–1357.

ten Duis HJ (1997) The fat embolism syndrome. *Injury* 28(2): 77–85.

39

CHAPTER 39

HIV and other infections

JAMES BRANLEY AND
JENNY MA WYATT

CHAPTER 39

HIV and other infections

JAMES BRANLEY AND JENNY MA WYATT

Control and prevention of infection in a multiply traumatized patient involves ensuring that the infectious risk is minimized both for the patient and for the healthcare workers involved. Trauma provides a major insult to the first line defences against infection, resulting in the development of acute and chronic infections. The acute management of trauma also exposes those caring for the patient to potential infection hazards, and in particular to blood-borne pathogens.

Although preventing contact with blood and body fluids by the implementation of universal precautions remains the primary method of preventing occupational exposure to blood-borne agents, the use of post-exposure prophylaxis is recommended for significant exposures to HIV and in some situations to the hepatitis viruses. The HIV epidemic has focused attention on the risk of transmission of blood-borne agents in the healthcare setting. Although HIV has been the headline infectious agent, the infectivity of HIV is considerably less than that of hepatitis B and or hepatitis C. The hepatitis viruses now include A, B, C, D, E, G (GBV) with B, C, D, and G being blood-borne. Rarely, blood products have been known to transmit a range of infectious agents, including the above viruses, HIV-2, parvovirus, malaria and babesiosis, EBV, CMV, and leptospirosis. Other human-derived medical products have transmitted the agent responsible for Creutzfeld–Jacob disease (CJD) and there is a growing unease about the ability of blood to transmit prion diseases such as CJD and variant CJD. As was learnt from the HIV epidemic, there is always the potential for blood to transmit an unknown or undetectable agent. This should continue to remind the health profession that exposure of one human to another's blood carries the risk of transmitting infections.

Key point

- Control and prevention of infection in a multiply traumatized patient involves ensuring that the infectious risk is minimized for patients and healthcare workers.

Universal precautions

Universal precautions were initially devised as a response to the HIV/AIDS epidemic in the mid 1980s by the US Centers for Disease Control and Prevention (CDC). This approach emphasized for the first time the importance of avoiding contact with blood and body fluids regardless of the presumed infectivity status. Body fluids include blood-stained fluids; semen; vaginal secretions; cerebrospinal, pericardial, pleural, peritoneal, synovial, and amniotic fluids; and saliva. There have been differences internationally with regard to the status of some body fluids such as saliva, sweat, tears, urine, and faeces that did not contain visible blood. Although these fluids have never been shown to transmit HIV to healthcare workers, some countries chose to regard all body fluids as potentially infectious.

When a patient is known or suspected to be infected with an epidemiologically important or highly transmissible agent, additional precautions are required. Hence agents spread by airborne transmission (*Mycobacterium tuberculosis*, varicella zoster virus), or by contact with dry skin (methicillin-resistant *Staphylococcus aureus* [MRSA], vancomycin-resistant enterococci [VRE]) require a further level of vigilance or isolation in addition to universal precautions.

Despite the introduction of universal and standard precautions, transmission of blood-borne infections (patient to patient, patient to healthcare worker, and healthcare worker to patient) continues to occur. This has led to changes in work practices such as the abolition of multidose vials and significantly, standards for sterilization in office/surgery practice, greater awareness that medical equipment (e.g. anaesthetic circuitry) may be a means of transmitting infection, and the introduction of a range of safer equipment. Requirements have also changed for those involved in exposure-prone surgery. In general terms, this is the subset of surgical procedures where the potential exists for transmission of blood-borne agents from the operator to the patient. Specifically, exposure prone surgery is any invasive procedure where there is potential for contact between the skin of the healthcare worker and sharp surgical instruments, needles, or sharp tissues (spicules of bone) in body cavities or poorly visualized or confined body sites (e.g. the mouth). Some countries place an obligation on practitioners of exposure-prone surgery to know and update their serological status to HIV and hepatitis B and C (NHMRC 1996).

Key point

- Agents spread by airborne transmission (Mycobacterium tuberculosis, varicella zoster virus), or by contact with dry skin (MRSA, VRE) require a further level of vigilance or isolation in addition to universal precautions.

Occupational exposure to blood-borne infections

An occupational exposure is an incident in which a healthcare worker has a percutaneous injury (e.g. needlestick), contact with a mucosal membrane or non-intact skin, or contact with intact skin that is prolonged or extensive, with blood, tissue, or a body fluid. The risk associated with an occupational exposure depends on the source material, the type of exposure, the volume and the severity of the injury, and the infectivity status of the source. If the source material is not contaminated with body fluid, there is no risk of transmission of a blood-borne infectious agent. There is the risk of bacterial wound infection, and wound cleaning is appropriate. Such an injury may also provide a valuable educational opportunity to review technique and vaccination status. The risk associated with a percutaneous exposure is also dependent on the type of injury sustained experimentally. Hollow-bore needles present a higher risk than solid (suture) needles (Mast *et al.* 1993). The risk of transmission of HIV varies with the inoculum of blood as evidenced by visible blood on the needle or device and depth of the injury, and an injury during procedures involving placing a needle directly into an artery or vein (Cardo *et al.* 1997). The risk also appears to be greater when the source patient has terminal HIV disease, presumably related to the high viral load in this setting. The infusion of infected blood by transfusion, such as occurred prior to the routine screening of blood donors for HIV and viral hepatitis, is the most efficient mode of transmission with seroconversion rates close to or equalling 100%. A superficial scratch with a solid needle is a low-risk injury, with minimal seroconversion observed.

Key point

- With percutaneous exposure, hollow-bore needles present a higher risk than solid (suture) needles.

HIV

The risk of acquiring HIV from a percutaneous exposure is 0.3% (Bell 1997) or 1 in every 300 exposures. The risk following skin or mucous membrane contact is 0.09% (<1 in 1000) (Ippolito *et al.* 1993). Of 52 US healthcare workers with documented occupationally acquired HIV, 47 were exposed to blood, 1 to visibly blood-stained body fluid, 1 to unspecified fluid, and 3 in laboratory exposure. Of these exposures 45 were percutaneous and 5 mucocutaneous, with 1 case of dual exposure. In 41 cases the exposure involved a hollow-bore needle, in 2 a broken glass vial, in 1 a scalpel and in 1 case an unknown sharp object (Centers for Disease Control).

The median interval for seroconversion after occupational exposure is 46 days, with an estimated 95% of those infected seroconverted by 6 months (Busch and Satten 1997).

The risk of exposure to HIV in the management of trauma depends on the underlying prevalence of infection in the population. In developing nations, including African countries, the population prevalence of HIV in some groups can be as high as 30% (Ansaloni *et al.* 1996, Pearn 1996). The widespread nature of the infection, with heterosexual and vertical transmission, means that some individuals in all sections of society are potentially infected. The occurrence of war and social unrest in many of these countries makes the treatment of HIV-infected trauma patients a daily occurrence. This, combined with often primitive working conditions and lack of basic resources such as protective and non-reusable equipment, means that healthcare workers in these environments are at significant risk of occupationally acquired HIV infection.

The epidemiology of HIV in the developed world is markedly different. Risk groups include men who have sex with men, intravenous drug users, and their sexual partners. The spread of HIV into the drug using population has been variable within the developed world, perhaps because the early introduction of needle exchange programs prevented spread in some countries. Prevalence figures in the general population in developed countries range from 0% to 5.8% (Short and Bell 1993), with the higher figures being found in some inner city populations. This urban population is also more at risk of trauma. Several studies have defined the seroprevalence of blood-borne infectious agents in the trauma population. Within urban populations in the USA, the prevalence of HIV in the trauma population varies considerably. In Baltimore, Maryland, HIV prevalence rates among patients presenting to emergency were 5.2–6% (Kelen *et al.* 1988). In Detroit, the code 1 trauma population had a prevalence of 0.52% (similar to the general population) (Henein and Lloyd 1997). Prevalence in other high-risk areas ranges up to 8.9%. Hepatitis B is present in up to 3.1% (Sloan *et al.* 1995) and hepatitis C in up to 14% (Henein and Lloyd 1997). Historical factors associated with infection include penetrating trauma (Kelen *et al.* 1988), age between 20 and 49 years, a history of intravenous drug use, a history of sexually transmitted disease, being a city resident, and being non-white (Sloan *et al.* 1995). In most of these populations there is an over-representation of HIV and hepatitis in the trauma population. This may represent the dual risks of infection and trauma in the drug-using population. Hepatitis C infection in long-term users is common. with >80% infected (Chetwynd *et al.* 1995).

Key point

- The risk of acquiring HIV from a percutaneous exposure is 0.3% or 1 in every 300 exposures.

Hepatitis B

Hepatitis B is about 100 times more infectious than HIV and is preventable. It is transmitted vertically, sexually, and through blood and body fluid (including saliva) contact. Infectivity is marked by the presence of hepatitis B surface antigen (HbsAg) and more specifically by the presence of e antigen. The presence of both of these markers conveys a 30% risk of seroconversion after a percutaneous exposure (Shapiro 1995). Hepatitis B is more common within the intravenous drug-using population, sex workers, and some ethnic groups including Asians, Pacific Islanders, and people from the Mediterranean and Middle East. After acute infection, immunity and viral clearance or chronic viral carriage with the risks of cirrhosis and hepatocellular carcinoma may result. Hepatitis B is a significant risk to healthcare workers and is responsible for between 100 and 200 deaths annually in the USA (Shapiro 1995). Before the introduction of vaccination it is estimated that 40% of American surgeons became infected during their career (Stafford *et al.* 1995). It is entirely preventable and a responsibility lies with both the individual and the employer to ensure all healthcare workers are adequately vaccinated and know their immune status. For those (5–10%) who fail to seroconvert with vaccination, attempted revaccination should be undertaken. If the healthcare worker is persistently seronegative after vaccination, they should be made aware of their status and encouraged to report all occupational exposures and to present for post-exposure prophylaxis (with hepatitis B immunoglobulin) if the source is hepatitis B positive or indeterminate.

Hepatitis C

Hepatitis C is an RNA virus discovered by molecular methods and is responsible for most cases of non-A non-B hepatitis. It is spread efficiently by parenteral exposure, with the major risk groups for infection being recipients of blood transfusions (before the introduction of blood product screening) and others with percutaneous risk factors (intravenous drug use, tattoos, etc.). Vertical and sexual transmission is inefficient, with transmission rates of about 5%. In most developed countries the prevalence varies between 0.3% and 1.2% of the population (Liddle 1996). However in parts of Japan, the Middle East, and Mediterranean Europe, the prevalence is much higher. Approximately 20% of hepatitis C carriers have no identifiable risk factors, again highlighting the need for universal precautions. Up to 14% of trauma patients are hepatitis C positive (Caplan *et al.* 1995, Henein and Lloyd 1997). Needlestick injury is approximately 10 times more likely to transmit hepatitis C than HIV, with overall rates ranging from 1% to 10% (CDC 1998a).

Although not a direct measure of viral activity, the presence of antibody to hepatitis C is a surrogate marker of infectivity as most (79%) of those with antibody to hepatitis C also have viral RNA detectable by polymerase chain reaction (PCR) (Cuthbert 1994). This is currently the gold standard for infectivity. At present the only recognized treatment for hepatitis C infection is interferon, although combination therapy with other antivirals (e.g. ribavirin) is likely. The role of post-exposure prophylaxis or early treatment of hepatitis C with interferon has been examined in a small number of studies with evidence that treatment commenced during or shortly after acute hepatitis produced a better long-term response than prolonged therapy in chronic hepatitis C infection (Quin 1997). Any healthcare workers suffering an occupational exposure from a patient positive for hepatitis C should be referred for assessment of suitability for early treatment.

Key point

- Hepatitis C is an RNA virus discovered by molecular methods and is responsible for most cases of non-A non-B hepatitis.

Other infectious agents

New blood-borne infectious agents continue to be described. Hepatitis D and the hepatitis G viruses are both spread through percutaneous exposure. Hepatitis D is spread only to those already infected with hepatitis B, and is preventable by hepatitis B vaccination. The epidemiology and implications of hepatitis G and related viruses (GBV) are still being determined but risk factors appear to be similar to those for hepatitis C. Rarely blood may also transmit malaria, syphilis, toxoplasmosis, cytomegalovirus, HIV-2, and potentially prion diseases such as Creutzfeldt–Jakob and its newly described variant. There are emerging infectious diseases such as the new herpesviruses (human herpesviruses 6–8) and highly infectious non-blood-borne agents such as tuberculosis, drug-resistant strains of which represent a significant hazard to all healthcare workers. There is the ever present risk of an unknown or new agent being acquired by percutaneous exposure, again emphasizing the need for universal procedures regardless of the perceived risk.

Management of an occupational exposure

In the event of an occupational exposure, a detailed assessment of the type of exposure, the source patient, the potential inoculum, and the infectious agent needs to be made. The aim is to assess the level of risk and to reach a decision with the healthcare worker as to the benefit of post-exposure prophylaxis.

Immediately after exposure to blood or body fluids, the area should be washed with soap and water and irrigated with large amounts of water. For eye or mucosal exposure, water or sterile saline should be used. Where possible, blood should be drawn with consent, from both the source patient and as a baseline from the recipient. In a high-risk situation, the exposed healthcare worker should be assessed as soon as possible, often necessitating their replacement on the treating team pending an assessment for post-exposure prophylaxis. If there is doubt or delay in establishing the HIV status of a high-risk patient, the option to commence antivirals pending results should be available.

In a retrospective review of occupational exposure, zidovudine (AZT) prophylaxis decreased the risk of seroconversion to HIV following percutaneous exposure to seropositive patients (CDC 1998b). Zidovudine also decreases maternal infant transmission (Connor *et al.* 1994). Protection is far from complete, with many questions remaining including the optimum drug regimen, the duration of treatment, and the optimum timing of commencement.

With the development of new antivirals including protease inhibitors, the treatment of HIV has been significantly advanced with major measurable effects on viral load obtainable by using combination therapy with three or more drugs of different classes. The marked reduction in viral load seen in HIV infection using combination therapy has been extrapolated to the post-exposure prophylaxis setting. Current recommendations include the use of more than one antiviral agent, and often triple therapy (two nucleoside reverse transcriptase inhibitors and a protease inhibitor) for moderate and high-risk exposures. The exposed patient and the physician should discuss the balancing of risk between the level of exposure and the potential toxicity of prophylaxis. Common toxicities include gastrointestinal (nausea, vomiting, diarrhoea), bone marrow toxicity (anaemia, neutropenia) for the nucleoside reverse transcriptase inhibitors (zidovudine, lamivudine) and metabolic and drug interactions with the protease inhibitors. Post-exposure prophylaxis options include no prophylaxis, a basic regimen of two reverse transcriptase inhibitors (zidovudine 600 mg daily and lamivudine 150 mg twice daily) and an expanded regimen of the above plus a protease inhibitor (indinivir 800 mg every 8 hours or nelfinivir 750 mg every 8 hours). Prophylaxis should ideally be commenced within hours of exposure and the option to take prophylaxis presumptively, before full assessment is completed, is available in many centres. Delayed presentation within 14 days should not preclude post-exposure prophylaxis. The duration of therapy is usually 4 weeks provided it is tolerated. Healthcare institutions should provide a mechanism for timely access to post-exposure prophylaxis for all staff.

Post-exposure prophylaxis for hepatitis B and C has already been discussed. In addition to baseline serology it is important that healthcare workers are follow up with repeat serology usually at 3, 6 and 9 months, particularly if the source patient is unknown. This is also an opportune time to ensure adequate immunity to hepatitis B and to review and reinforce safe work practices.

Key points

- Post HIV exposure prophylaxis options include:
  - no prophylaxis
  - a basic regimen of two reverse transcriptase inhibitors (zidovudine 600 mg daily and lamivudine 150 mg twice daily)
  - an expanded regimen of the above plus a protease inhibitor (indinivir 800 mg every 8 hours or nelfinivir 750 mg every 8 hours).

- Start within hours of exposure, consider before full assessment, and even in delayed presentation (within 14 days). Continue for 4 weeks.

Prevention of occupational infection

The acute management of trauma involves one of the highest risk situations for needlestick injury or body fluid exposure. These are potentially life and death situations where work proceeds in a highly charged atmosphere, involving numerous staff members performing simultaneous procedures on an unstable and often grossly blood-contaminated patient. The situation is by its nature less controlled than in the operating theatre, where a patient is anaesthetized and usually more stable. In the emergency department a patient may be semiconscious and combative, or several patients may arrive together and numerous procedures involving sharp implements must be undertaken quickly in an often cramped environment. Uncontrolled bleeding may result in aerosolized blood. The infectivity status of the patient is seldom known, and an accurate history of risk factors is usually unavailable. Preparation and training are essential to the avoidance of injury in this setting. Hospitals have a responsibility to ensure that staff are adequately trained and that environment and equipment minimize the chance of occupational exposure, and to assess and treat staff who are exposed. Staff have an individual responsibility to their own and colleagues' health.

When it is known that a trauma patient is on the way, staff should ensure they are dressed in protective clothing before the patient's arrival. All too often safety issues are ignored once an unstable patient arrives. Clothing should include a water-impermeable underlayer, gowns, gloves, and eye protection. These items should be changed if breached. Sharp instruments and needles should be handled with deliberation and care. A sharp should never be advanced toward a passive hand (e.g. in re-sheathing needles or using fingers to hold tissue while it is being sutured). Sharps should be passed in a rigid tray (e.g. kidney dish) and disposed of in an appropriate, rigid sharps disposal container which should be readily and conveniently accessible in the trauma room.

Manufacturers of medical equipment continue to redesign sharps with occupational safety in mind. There is a wide range of products including needleless systems, blunt needles, and retractable and protected needles. It is important that an advocate for occupational safety be involved in equipment purchasing decisions.

Key point

- All too often safety issues are ignored once an unstable patient arrives.

Infection in the traumatized patient

Trauma patients are at risk of infection for a number of reasons. Many of the body's first line defences are violated both at the moment of impact and subsequently. The skin is often broken. There may be trauma and soiling of the peritoneal cavity if bowel is damaged. Foreign material, dirt, and debris may be implanted in normally sterile and sometimes vascularly compromised tissue. Head injury may result in decreased level of consciousness and compromised ability to protect the respiratory tract from aspiration of oral secretions or vomitus. Loss of skin from a burn may result in loss of a major defence against infection. Shortly after the arrival of medical assistance, several other barriers will be breached. Intravenous cannulation, chest tubes, urinary catheters, endotracheal tubes, and wound drains all act as foreign bodies and conduits to normally sterile sites. Each of these will become colonized with the prevailing microflora of the patient and the hospital or ward where they are accommodated. The use of antibiotics will transiently change this flora, with reduction in some highly virulent organisms and concomitant overgrowth of resistant flora. The more severe the injury and the longer the normal barriers are breached, the higher the chance of nosocomial infection. If this occurs in a setting of poor infection control and high rates of antibiotic-resistant nosocomial organisms, there is a significant impact on morbidity and mortality. Trauma significantly impacts immune function, causing abnormalities in macrophage and neutrophil function, activation of complement, and complex cytokine interactions including alterations in levels of tumour necrosis factor and prostaglandins. This has been implicated in the development of adult respiratory distress syndrome (ARDS). The use of steroids (e.g. for head injury) and blood transfusions may further alter immune responses. Nosocomial infection in the traumatized patient may be difficult to separate from the systemic inflammatory response which occurs in many seriously ill patients. Fever leukocytosis and haemodynamic instability may reflect tissue destruction, brain injury, or a response to multisystem damage and haemorrhage. Equally, infection is a common and severe problem in these patients and antibiotic therapy must often be commenced empirically. Four sites account for 60% of nosocomial infections in traumatized patients—vascular lines (14%), respiratory tract (15%), urinary tract (17%), and wounds (12%) (Stillwell and Caplan 1989). Less commonly, central nervous system infections, intra-abdominal infection, and sinusitis occur. Antibiotics are widely used to prevent infection in the trauma setting but, except for a few specific settings, there is little or no evidence that prophylactic antibiotics are of benefit. Clearly, where there is gross contamination of a normally sterile site, antibiotics should be given. Rupture of a hollow abdominal viscus, open fracture, and penetrating injuries are all indications for antibiotics. Because an inoculum of infectious material has been implanted in a normally sterile site, this usage amounts to early (presumptive) treatment of infection rather than prophylaxis. Use of antibiotics may also be considered in facial fractures and basilar skull fractures, although clear evidence for benefit is lacking (Choi and Spann 1996, Brodie 1997).

In general terms, where prophylaxis is used, it should primarily be aimed at *Staphylococcus aureus*. Most antistaphylococcal agents in sufficiently high dosage will also cover the important β-haemolytic streptococci, and additional prophylaxis for these organisms is not required. Where devitalized tissue is present, additional cover for anaerobes (e.g. metronidazole), or clostridia (high-dose penicillin) may be added. For the injury sustained in contaminated water or potentially contaminated with bowel flora, cover should be broadened to include the relevant Gram-negative organisms. The duration of antibiotic therapy should be limited to the minimum possible to minimize the chance of colonization with resistant organisms. Most studies have shown that 24 hours is as effective as longer periods. In a dirty injury, presumptive therapy of 1–3 days is usually recommended.

There is a common perception that antibiotics do no harm. The increase in nosocomial infections due to highly resistant organisms and the subsequent rise in morbidity and mortality dispels this myth. MRSA is now widespread in hospital environments throughout the world. The spread of VRE and vancomycin-insensitive *Staphylococcus aureus* (VISA) means that the pool of virtually untreatable infectious agents is growing. Numerous resistant nosocomial Gram-negative organisms have also been problematic, particularly in the intensive care setting. It is clear that overuse of antibiotics combined with failure of basic infection control standards is responsible for major epidemics of resistant organisms over the last two decades. It is important that these issues are not overshadowed by the immediacy of acute patient management.

Key points

- Trauma patients are at risk of infection.
- In general terms, where prophylaxis is used, it should primarily be aimed at *Staphylococcus aureus*.

Care of the HIV-infected trauma patient

HIV/AIDS is a condition of progressive immune suppression, brought about by virally induced reduction in the number of CD4 lymphocytes (T helper cells). This results in a complex diminution in cell-mediated immunity combined with a dysregulation in humoral (B cell) immunity. Contrary to first expectations it does not appear that HIV/AIDS patients suffer a higher rate of wound infection following surgery than the normal population (Davidson *et al.* 1991, Deziel *et al.* 1990). Data on trauma patients is limited. AIDS patients may have complicating medical conditions on arrival, thrombocytopaenia, chronic infections (e.g. cytomegalivirus, mycobacterial infections) or neoplasms (lymphoma, Kaposi's sarcoma). They may be taking a range of medications including antivirals and other anti-infectives, some of which may have significant side-effect profiles. They may have co-morbidity from drug use or malnutrition. T lymphocyte subset analysis (CD4 count), although a good marker of immune status in AIDS patients, is not a useful predictor in acute illness as an unpredictable and profound decrease may occur (Feeney *et al.* 1995). It is important that an HIV physician be involved in management and that staff appreciate that, although HIV remains a terminal condition, the prognosis has improved considerably since the introduction of the new treatment regimens.

Acknowledgment

The authors wish to thank Dr Michael Whitby, Director of Infectious Diseases, Infection Control and Sexual Health, Princess Alexandra Hospital, Brisbane, Australia and Dr Roger Wilson, Director of Pathology, Nepean Hospital, Sydney, Australia for their assistance in the preparation of this chapter.

References

Ansaloni L, Acaye GL, Re MC (1996) High HIV seroprevalence among patients with pyomyositis in Northern Uganda. *Tropical Medicine and International Health* 1(2): 210–212.

Bell DM (1997) Occupational risk of human immunodeficiency virus infection in healthcare workers: an overview. *American Journal of Medicine* 102 (Suppl 5B): 9–15.

Brodie HA (1997) Prophylactic antibiotics for posttraumatic cerebrospinal fluid fistulae. A meta-analysis. *Archives of Otolaryngology and Head and Neck Surgery* 123(7): 749–752.

Busch MP, Satten GA (1997) Time course of viraemia and antibody seroconversion following human immunodeficiency virus exposure. *American Journal of Medicine* 102 (Suppl 5B): 117–124.

Caplan ES, Preas MA, Kerns T *et al.* (1995) Seroprevalence of human immunodeficiency virus, hepatitis B virus, hepatitis C virus and rapid plasma reagin in a trauma population. *Journal of Trauma, Injury, Infection and Critical Care.* 39(3): 533–537.

Cardo D, Culver DH, Ciesielski CA *et al.* (1997) A case control study of HIV seroconversion in health care workers after percutaneous exposure. *New England Journal of Medicine* 337: 1485–1490.

CDC (1998a) Guideline for infection control in healthcare personnel, 1998. *Infection Control and Hospital Epidemiology* 19(6): 420–423.

CDC (1998b) Public health service guidelines for the management of health care worker exposures to HIV and recommendations for post exposure prophylaxis. *Morbidity and Mortality Weekly Reports* 47(RR-7): 1–33.

Chetwynd J, Brunton C, Blank M *et al.* (1995) Hepatitis C seroprevalence amongst injecting drug users attending a methadone programme. *New Zealand Medical Journal* 108(1007): 364–366.

Choi D, Spann R (1996) Traumatic cerebrospinal fluid leakage: risk factors and the use of prophylactic antibiotics. *British Journal of Neurosurgery* 10(6): 571–575.

Cuthbert J (1994) Hepatitis C: progress and problems. *Clinical Microbiology Reviews* 7(4): 505–532.

Davidson T, Allen-Mersh TG, Miles AJG *et al.* (1991) Emergency laparotomy in patients with AIDS. *British Journal of Surgery* 78: 924–926.

Deziel DJ, Hyser MJ, Doolas A *et al.* (1990) Major abdominal operations in acquired immune deficiency syndrome. *American Surgeon* 56: 445–450.

Feeney C, Bryzman S, Kong L *et al.* (1995) T-lymphocyte subsets in acute illness. *Critical Care Medicine* 23(10): 1680–1685.

Henein MN, Lloyd L (1997) HIV, Hepatitis B and Hepatitis C in the code one trauma population. *American Surgeon* 63: 657–659.

Ippolito G, Puro V, De Carli G, Italian Study Group on Occupational Risk of HIV Infection (1993) The risk of occupational human immunodeficiency virus infection in health care workers. *Archives of Internal Medicine* 153: 1451–1458.

Kelen GD, Fritz S, Qaqish B *et al.* (1988) Unrecognised human immunodeficiency virus infection in emergency department patients. *New England Journal of Medicine* 318: 1645–1650.

Liddle C (1996) Hepatitis C. *Anaesthesia and Intensive Care* 24(2): 180–183.

Mast ST, Woolwine JD, Gerberding JL (1993) Efficacy of gloves in reducing blood volumes transferred during simulated needlestick injury. *Journal of Infectious Diseases* 168: 1589–1592.

NHMRC (1996) *Infection control in the health care setting*. Australian Government Publishing Service, Canberra.

Pearn J (1996) Viewpoint war zone paediatrics in Rwanda. *Journal of Paediatric and Child Health* 32: 290–295.

Quin JW (1997) Interferon therapy for acute hepatitis C viral infection—a review by meta-analysis. *Australian and New Zealand, Journal of Medicine* 27: 611–618.

Shapiro CN (1995) Occupational risk of infection with hepatitis B and hepatitis C virus. *Surgical Clinics of North America* 75: 1047–1056.

Short LJ, Bell DM (1993) Risk of occupational infection with blood borne pathogens in operating and delivery room settings. *American Journal of Infection Control* 21: 343–350.

Sloan EP, McGill BA, Zalenski R *et al.* (1995) Human immunodeficiency virus and hepatitis B virus seroprevalence in an urban trauma population. *Journal of Trauma, Injury, Infection and Critical Care* 38(5): 736–741.

Stafford MK, Kitchen VS, Smith JR (1995) Reducing the risk of blood borne infection in surgical practice. *British Journal of Obstetrics and Gynaecology* 102: 439–441.

Stillwell M, Caplan ES (1989) The septic multi-trauma patient. *Infectious Diseases Clinics of North America* 3: 155.

40

CHAPTER 40

Organ and tissue donation

RAY F RAPER AND
PAULA J MOHACSI

CHAPTER 40
Organ and tissue donation

RAY F RAPER AND PAULA J MOHACSI

Introduction

Organ and tissue transplantation saves and enhances lives. It provides enormous benefit to individuals and society in general. Donation of organs and tissues usually involves the death of a person, hence transplantation cannot be seen as a right ascribable to a potential recipient. Nevertheless, it seems reasonable to attempt to maximize donation if this can be achieved in a fashion that is commensurate with the dignity of the individual. This is especially so since it seems most unlikely that the demand will ever be met from the potential supply.

A number of strategies to maximize cadaveric donation have been explored. These include the 'Spanish model' (Miranda *et al.* 1999, Matesanz and Miranda 2001), which has produced the highest organ donation rate in the world. This is not a legislative model but involves active donor identification and management, and aggressive seeking of consent. Different legislative models of consent have been developed. These include 'opting-in', 'opting-out', or required request models. Other systems have relied upon health care professional education and support. The relative merit of these various approaches is yet to be determined.

Early identification of potential organ donors greatly facilitates the process. The subsequent medical management of the potential donor and the communication with and consideration for the needs of the patient's family greatly influence the experience of the family and their subsequent support for organ donation. The most common preventable source of under-utilization of donation is the failure to request. This is particularly so for tissue only donation (Riker and White 1991, Kennedy *et al.* 1992).

Most patients can donate tissue after death. The potential for solid organ donation is much less. Organ donation usually occurs from patients who have been certified dead based on a brain function criterion ('brain death'). This occurs in less than 1% of hospital deaths and as high as 12% of ICU deaths (personal data), and results from a severe brain injury. This constitutes the subject matter of this chapter. Live donation of regenerative or paired tissue or organs will not be discussed. Neither will supplementary or alternative treatment modalities for people with end stage organ failure or disease.

Duty of care to patients

Organ and tissue donation is not usually the initial focus of the care and management of patients with acute brain injury and other trauma. However, donation may be a component of the continuum of care delivered to the patient admitted for acute hospital management.

Traditionally, organ and tissue donation has been viewed as a clear break in the continuum of care of a patient with an acute brain injury, representing a shift from the interests of the patient to those of the recipients. Patient-orientated management is aimed at recovery and ultimate hospital discharge with return to a 'normal' life. If in the course of active management the patient loses all brain function, in spite of all efforts to prevent this, then the focus changes to managing them as a source of potential organs and tissues. Rather than a cessation of the care of the patient, enabling donation should be seen as a duty of care to the patient if it reflects their actual or projected wishes. Care of the family, for the same reason that it reflects the wishes and hence interests of the patient, can also be included under the rubric of duty of care. Most (though not all) donor families gain considerable solace and benefit from their generosity reflected in the process of donation.

In support of this view, transplantation and donation are generally well supported by the community in many Western countries. A national Australian marketing survey (Australian Coordinating Committee on Organ Registries and Donation 1995) of 1213 adult respondents indicated 90% supported transplantation and organ donation. In a 1999 national survey (Australian Bureau of Statistics 1999) of approximately 30,000 respondents, 46% reported having taken steps to be identified as an intending donor. Of the remainder, more than half (56%) were willing to donate some organs and tissues.

Recognition of a donor

All deceased patients are potential donors. Cadaveric donation can be undertaken from in-hospital patients legally declared dead based upon *either* irreversible loss of circulation (non-heart beating donor—NHBD), or irreversible loss of brain function (beating heart donor—BHD). Most deceased patients can donate eyes for corneal transplantation, heart valves, bone, and skin. However, very few deceased patients can donate solid organs such as heart, lungs, liver, pancreas, and intestine for transplantation. These are beating-heart donors who are also preferred for kidney donation, although occasionally kidneys are retrieved from NHBD. Not all countries or centres undertake donation of all of the above, as the scope of transplantation varies both among and within countries. Organs and tissues that can be donated by BHDs and NBHDs are summarized in Table 40.1.

Table 40.1 Summary of donatable organs and tissues in non-beating and beating heart donors

Cadaveric donor				Live donor	
BHD (death certified by no brain function)		NBHD (death certified by no cardiac function)		BHD (alive and well)	
Donation of	**Retrieval in**	**Donation of**	**Retrieval in**	**Donation of**	**Retrieval in**
Bone	OT or mortuary	Bone	Mortuary	Blood	Hospital, clinic
Eyes (corneas)	OT or mortuary	Eyes (corneas)	Mortuary	Bone	OT
Heart	OT	Heart valves	Mortuary	Bone marrow	OT
Heart valves	OT or mortuary	Kidneys	OT	Cord blood	Delivery room
Intestine	OT	Skin	Mortuary	Kidney	OT
Kidneys	OT			Partial intestine	OT
Liver	OT			Partial liver	OT
Lungs	OT			Partial lung	OT
Pancreas	OT			Partial pancreas	OT
Skin	Mortuary				

OT = operating theatre.

Beating heart donors are always mechanically ventilated in Emergency or Critical Care departments. All patients with severely impaired and deteriorating brain function should be considered as potential organ donors (Buckley 1998). Brain trauma and cerebrovascular accident/stroke account for approximately 85% of all actual donors in the USA and Australia (ANZOD Report 2000, UNOS 2000). However, the importance of trauma as a major cause of death varies from country to country (Table 40.2), and with donor age. Clearly, trauma centre hospitals (O'Brien *et al.* 1996) and those with neurosurgical facilities, have a greater potential to contribute to organ donation. This does not, however, preclude small, rural, or urban hospitals from offering the option of donation to relatives of deceased patients.

Early donor recognition is important because evidence indicates that the loss of brain function usually leads to haemodynamic instability and cardiac arrest, even when cardio-respiratory support is maintained (Tropman and Dunn 1999). Early recognition and appropriate management of patients with loss of brain function reduces loss of transplantable organs, which can result from haemodynamic instability, excessive inotrope administration, serious nosocomal infections, and complications related to intensive care. For instance, there is a negative correlation between the duration of mechanical ventilation and lung donor suitability. Early contact with the local procurement agency is beneficial in shortening the entire process and in initial assessment and management of the potential organ donor.

All medically suitable deceased patients can become tissue donors. Criteria for specific tissue donation should be ascertained from the local procurement agency or tissue bank. These will vary. For example, for heart valve donation the upper age limit is 55 years in one State in Australia, and 60 years in another.

If at any time there is uncertainty concerning the medical suitability of a possible donor, contact with the local procurement agency is advised. Acceptance criteria change with transplant techniques, treatment advances, and experience. There are very few absolute or even relative contraindications to donation. These are listed in Table 40.3 and vary among countries and local donation and transplantation programmes.

The medical and nursing staff caring for the patients are best placed to recognize potential donors. This should be a routine part of best practice and the care of all dying patients, but especially those suffering trauma and other causes of acute brain injury.

Table 40.2 Donor cause of death

	Australia	USA
Number of cadaveric donors (1999)	164	5824
Cause of death	%	%
CVS/stroke	54	43
Head trauma	33	42
Anoxia	8	11
Other	3	3
CNS tumour	2	1

Source: ANZOD Report 2000.

Table 40.3 General contraindications for organ and tissue donation

Absolute	Relative
Malignancy other than primary intracerebral and non-melanotic skin cancers	Unknown cause of death
HIV infection, TB, septicaemia, fungaemia, disseminated viral infection	High risk behaviour group HIV, HBV, HCV HBV and/or HCV infection
Creutzfeld–Jacob disease	Previous treatment with human pituitary hormone extract; family history early dementia

'Brain death'

A brain function criterion for the determination and certification of death has become well established in both medical practice and statute in many countries throughout the world. Particularly in English-speaking countries, the sentinel steps in the evolution of the concept of 'brain death' included the report of the *ad hoc* committee of the Harvard Medical School (1968) and the statement on the 'diagnosis of brain death' by the Medical Royal College of the UK (1976). These and other initiatives including the report of the Law Reform Commission in Australia (1977) have seen death equated with the irreversible loss of brain function. Although now inexorably linked to organ donation for transplantation, the original motivation in developing the brain function criteria was partly to recognize a state of irreversible coma to facilitate the withdrawal of apparently futile treatment (Mollar and Goulon 1959).

The acceptance of a brain function criterion for the determination of death recognizes the central importance of brain function to the collective understanding of what it is to be a human being. In this framework, human life is not merely the sum of the lives of the component human parts. While consciousness is probably the most important brain function, other relevant functions include the ability to breathe (Pallis 1983) and the integrative function of the brain.

Definition

The precise definition of death based on a brain function criterion varies slightly around the world. In the UK, brain stem death is equated with death whereas in Australia and the USA it is the loss of the function of the entire brain which is required. In practice, this distinction is mostly moot since the loss of brain stem function is usually caused by supra tentorial pathology and is thus associated with loss of higher centre function as well. Whatever the legal definition, clinical, and diagnostic criteria vary very little and are commonly determined by practice guidelines. The legal requirements for certification of death, however, vary considerably throughout the world and may be quite specific. Familiarity with local statutory requirements is essential. For instance, in New South Wales, Australia, death based on the brain function criterion must be certified independently by two registered practitioners who have practiced medicine for 5 of the past 8 years. One of the two must be a specialist doctor, specifically designated for the purpose.

Pathophysiology

The irreversible loss of all brain function usually results from a combination of primary and secondary brain injury. Occasionally, an insult is so severe that it immediately stops all intracranial blood flow. More commonly, an initial brain injury results in brain oedema with subsequent compromise to brain perfusion causing secondary, ischaemic insult with further oedema and ischaemic injury eventually resulting in the interruption of all cerebral blood flow. The causes of loss of brain function are listed in Table 40.2.

Recognition and diagnosis

'Brain death' usually evolves in the context of the management of severe brain injury, the aim of which is generally the prevention of secondary injury. Occasionally the initial injury appears rather trivial and the progressive loss of brain function is unexpected. More often, it is somewhat predictable and may occur in spite of aggressive, brain-protective management. Recognition depends on regular clinical assessment and an awareness of the diagnostic criteria.

There are two aspects to the diagnostic criteria—preconditions and clinical features. The preconditions include the presence of an injury of sufficient severity to account for the loss of brain function. This usually requires the demonstration of a severe structural brain injury on brain imaging (CT or MRI). Further, it must be clear that the loss of brain function cannot be attributable to reversible factors such as electrolyte disturbances, drugs, hypothermia, or other metabolic abnormalities such as severe renal or hepatic failure. Acceptable levels of abnormality are generally not defined. Neither are criteria for excluding drug effects although some guideline documents provide relatively specific information.

Clinical assessment involves examination of brain stem function as outlined in Table 40.4. Assessment should follow a suitable period of observation during which there has been no evidence of any brain function. Some guidelines are very specific with regard to the timing of the clinical examinations. This aspect is generally not covered by statute and it is important for local practice to be conducted in a way which is consistent with local laws and which has the confidence of the profession and the local population.

Table 40.4 Determination of death based on brain function criteria

Diagnostic criteria

Preconditions

- Irremediable, structural brain injury
- Exclusion of potential reversible factors
  - Hypothermia
  - Significant electrolyte or metabolic abnormality
  - Drug induced coma or paralysis

Clinical assessment

- No response to pain in cranial nerve distribution
- Absent reflexes
  - Gag
  - Cough
  - Corneal
  - Papillary
  - Occulomotor (vestibulo-ocular)
  - Apnoea in the presence of acidosis and hypercapnoea

Ancillary or confirmatory test*

- Absent intracranial blood flow
  - Radionuclide scanning
  - 3 or 4 vessel cerebral angiography
- Absent brain electrical activity
  - EEG
  - Evoked response testing

* These are only essential when the diagnostic criteria cannot be fulfilled.

Irreversibility of the loss of all brain function is established by observation over time and by an understanding of the severity of the brain injury. Formal repetition of brain functional assessment is a common feature of practice guidelines. The recommended temporal separation between formal examinations varies from 2 to 24 h.

Confirmatory test such as EEG, evoked electrical responses, and cranial blood flow studies are used with widely varying frequency. In some jurisdictions, confirmatory testing is the norm. The absence of intracranial blood flow can be used to establish the irreversible loss of all brain function where sedative administration or facial damage precludes full clinical assessment. Absent intracranial blood flow has no independent legal standing. It is an alternate way of determining the irreversible loss of brain function. The certification standards are the same as for clinical assessment. It is generally appropriate that the practitioner performing and reporting the blood flow study not also certify the irreversible loss of all brain function.

Controversies

Although now widely accepted, 'brain death' remains a somewhat controversial subject (National Health and Medical Research Council 1997). The absence of brain function is not universally accepted as death. Certainly, it is not empirically satisfying as 'brain dead' patients appear asleep rather than dead. The status of the warm, pulsatile, functional body left behind after 'brain death' is also problematic.

Beyond these largely empirical concerns, it has been intimated that the clinical criteria used for assessment do not establish the irreversible loss of all brain function. It would appear that the clinical criteria do not absolutely preclude some spontaneous or inducible electrical activity and diabetes insipidus (DI), while very common, is not universally observed. However, affording clinical significance to minor electrical activity employs a far more reductionist definition of 'brain function' than can be inferred from the President's Commission Report (1981) which drew a distinction between function and activity and offered that relevant function is that which is clinically assessable. There have been occasional reports of patients apparently recovering from the loss of all clinically detectable brain function. This can occur when the preconditions, especially the exclusion of drug-induced coma, have not been fulfilled.

A brain function criterion for the determination of death has become widely accepted and is rarely controversial at the bedside. Nevertheless, empirical and philosophical concerns with 'brain death' dictate that practitioners should be alert to and accommodating of divergent views.

Management of the potential organ donor

The loss of all brain function usually leads to haemodynamic instability and generalized organ system dysfunction (Prager 1991, Scheinkestel *et al.* 1995, Novitzky 1997a,b, Buckley 1998, Troppmann and Dunn 1999). Resuscitated trauma patients with loss of all brain function often have functional damage of their organs, as reflected in organ-specific biochemical parameters (Werkman *et al.* 1991). A recent addition to the management of potential organ donors has included the use of high dose methylprednisolone resulting in a significant increase in the number of successful procurements (Follette *et al.* 1999). As well, aggressive multidisciplinary management can increase, for example, lung procurement rates (Follette *et al.* 1999).

As donor exclusion criteria have been liberalized, donation is now rarely precluded on the basis of abnormal biochemical results alone. Each case is reviewed individually. Abnormal parameters may be relatively insignificant or reversible. The anticipation and treatment of potential problems can greatly enhance opportunity for donation for patients and their families, and can also affect subsequent transplant outcome. Potential problems and management options are summarized in Table 40.5.

Table 40.5 Summary of the management of the potential organ donor

Problem	Management options
Arrhythmias	◆ Minimize risk with correction of electrolyte and biochemical problems ◆ Achieve fluid management, minimal inotrope use, ventilation, and normal temperature
Coagulopathy	◆ Monitor and replace clotting factors as required
Diabetes insipidus (DI)	◆ Establish DI, then give DDAVP 1–3 mcg to keep the urine output <150 ml/h ◆ Sub-massive DI, fluid, and electrolyte replacements (avoid hyperglycaemia)
Electrolytes	◆ Regular and frequent monitoring ◆ Correct as required
Endocrine disturbances	◆ Monitor and observe
Hyperglycaemia	◆ Keep dextrose infusions <200 ml/h ◆ Glucose level persistently >15 mmol/L, commence insulin infusion
Hypertension	◆ Aggressive management usually counter-productive ◆ If considered essential, use short acting agents
Hypotension	◆ Fluid replacement ◆ Metaraminol (0.5–5 mg bolus, infusion 40 mg/100 ml) ◆ Noradrenaline infusion 4–6 mg/100 ml ◆ Dopamine infusion 200 mg/100 ml
Hypothermia	◆ Warming blanket, warmed fluids, etc.
Respiration	◆ Positive end expiratory pressure (PEEP) with mechanical ventilation

Hypertension and catecholamine surges

For approximately 1–2 h around the time of brain-stem herniation, an intense sympathetic 'storm' is frequently observed. This is associated with significant increases in circulating catecholamines, which may cause severe peripheral vasoconstriction, and may cause acute left ventricular failure and pulmonary oedema (Scheinkestel *et al.* 1995). The final loss of all brain function is commonly preceded by a period of hypertension and tachycardia, which may be brief or last a few hours. Hypertension helps preserve cerebral blood flow in the presence of intracranial hypertension. Aggressive management may therefore be counter-productive. Moreover, as hypotension often rapidly ensues, the use of short acting agents is generally recommended if anti-hypertensive therapy is deemed essential.

Hypotension

The increased blood pressure associated with increased intracranial pressure is commonly followed by hypotension, which may be abrupt and profound. Vasodilatation is an important physiological factor. Hypovolaemia or left ventricular dysfunction may be contributory. The prevention and management of hypotension help preserve kidney and other organ function and thus improve later graft function.

Resuscitation (including volume replacement) should follow standard guidelines and practices. As for all patients, hypothermia and electrolyte abnormalities should be avoided. Not only are these potentially hazardous to the patient but also significant abnormalities may preclude the certification of death based on a brain function criterion.

Fluids should be warmed as sometimes large volumes are required. Fluid overload may be detrimental to hepatic and pulmonary function (Robertson and Cook 1990). Frequent biochemical assessment is indicated to maintain electrolyte and glucose homeostasis.

Inotropes and vasoconstrictors are frequently required to maintain adequate blood pressure. Most guidelines recommend maintenance of a systolic pressure of 100 mmHg or a mean arterial pressure of 70 mmHg. Options include Metaraminol (0.5–5 mg bolus or infusion 40 mg/100 ml), or a Noradrenaline infusion (4–6 mg/100 ml). Intravenous Dopamine (200 mg/100 ml) may also be added, or used as an alternative to Metaraminol or Noradrenaline. Intravenous Adrenaline and Dobutamine are best avoided due to the excessive beta stimulation of the heart and down regulation of beta-receptors, resulting in depletion of energy stores.

Diabetes insipidus (DI)

Loss of secretion of antidiuretic hormone (ADH) will result in an inappropriate and often massive urine output that has no relationship to the intravascular fluid volume. Haemodynamic instability can occur if hypovolaemia or electrolyte disturbances develop. Correction may be difficult but essential both for patient management and for certification of death. A sudden, inappropriate polyuria after deterioration of neurological function is strongly suggestive of DI, especially when accompanied by low urinary sodium (<10 mmol/L), hypernatraemia, increased plasma osmolality (>300 mosmol/L), and low urine osmolality (<300 mosmol/L) or urine SG (<1.005).

Management of DI requires frequent measurement of serum electrolytes and glucose, and of urine output and electrolytes. Management suggestions include:

1. For established DI, administer DDAVP 1–3 mcg as required to maintain urine output less than 150 ml/h.
2. For sub-massive diuresis or when diagnosis is in doubt, careful fluid and electrolyte re-placement with attention to the potential for hyperglycaemia may suffice.

Hyperglycaemia

This is multifactorial and probably relates to a combination of insulin resistance as a consequence of stress and inotropic infusions (catecholamine effect), and rapid infusions of glucose containing fluids to replace DI losses. Hyperglycaemia increases osmolality and causes an osmotic diuresis with further loss of water and electrolytes. This can be avoided by keeping dextrose infusions <200 ml/h. Glucose levels persistently >15 mmol/L should be treated with an insulin infusion.

Electrolytes

Frequent measurement of plasma electrolyte levels is recommended. Electrolyte abnormalities caused by fluid or DI mismanagement can lead to hypernatraemia, hypomagnesaemia, hypokalaemia, hypocalcaemia, and hypophosphataemia. Hyponatraemia is uncommon. Correction of any significant electrolyte abnormality is required before undertaking the brain function assessment for death certification. It also optimizes organ function and viability.

Temperature

Hypothermia is very common and can have serious consequences. Prevention or correction of hypothermia is required for patient management and for brain function assessment. Prevention of hypothermia is preferred, as correction can be slow and difficult. Temperature must be measured centrally with a cold responsive thermometer.

The consequences of hypothermia include coagulopathy, cold diuresis, reduced tissue oxygen delivery (due to altered oxyhaemoglobin dissociation), myocardial depression, hypotension, progressive bradycardia, cardiovascular instability, and ultimately cardiac arrest. Temperature <28°C is associated with ventricular arrhythmias and irritability, often refractory to treatment. If cold related dysrythmias occur, Bretylium is the drug of choice.

Increased temperature is a common problem in brain injury and should be managed actively. However, it becomes less problematic as brain function is progressively lost.

Arrhythmias

Delays in organ retrieval following death certification should be minimized as haemodynamic instability may jeopardize organ viability. Potentially correctable contributing factors may include electrolyte disturbances (especially in the context of DI), hypovolaemia, hypotension, secondary myocardial ischaemia, acidosis secondary to hypoperfusion and anaerobic metabolism, hypoxia, hypothermia, and inotrope side effect. These variables should be monitored and corrected or optimized where possible. Coincident patient disorders such as myocardial contusion may also contribute to haemodynamic instability.

Respiration

Hyperventilation is now rarely employed as part of a brain protective strategy. Certainly, when brain function ceases hyperventilation should be discontinued since hypocapnoea may be detrimental to organ function. Pulmonary oedema may develop for several reasons. It may be hydrostatic from fluid overload, or result from capillary or acute lung injury (neurogenic or adult respiratory distress syndrome). Management is not specific for the brain-injured patient.

Coagulopathy

Disseminated intravascular coagulopathy (DIC) may develop from releases of fibrinolytic agents from ischaemia or necrotic brain tissue. Administration of clotting factors, platelets, and blood transfusions may be required as part of active patient management but is probably not indicated when brain function has ceased.

Endocrine disturbances

With the irreversible loss of all brain function, hypothalamic-pituitary function is usually lost. This may result in deficiencies of several critical hormones including cortisol, thyroxine, and ADH. ADH should be administered if DI develops, and cortisol will be required if plasma cortisol levels fall to critical levels. Precise indications for the administration of cortisol and T3 are not clear, but hormone replacement should be considered if haemodynamic instability occurs, especially where support will be required for long periods after brain function has ceased.

Organization

The optimal organization of donation requires an understanding of the local legal framework, together with knowledge of processes and practices required for donation. The organization may therefore be peculiar in some aspects to particular regions or countries, but always needs to be structured to be responsive to the many and varied needs of the many people involved in the process.

There are variable legal frameworks that support practices associated with organ donation and transplantation. There are several consent models for instance. 'Opting-in' legislation is in place in the UK, Australia, and Singapore, and 'opting-out' is more usual in European countries. 'Opting-in' requires people to have chosen to donate after they die and to have informed their relatives of this decision, or have noted this choice on a driver's license or donor registry. 'Opting-out' legislation assumes that all citizens are donors after death unless the individual has dissented and has made this decision known to relatives or a donor register. In practice, approaching and obtaining permission from relatives is virtually always undertaken prior to removal of any organs or tissues for transplantation, irrespective of the local legislative requirements.

Discussion of donation with bereaved relatives should be undertaken with great sensitivity, appropriate support, and a focus on the known or projected wishes of the deceased. Training for those who make this approach is advisable. Training initiatives include the European Donor Hospital Education Program; 'Making the Critical Difference' in the USA, or the Australasian Donor Awareness Programme in Australia and New Zealand. The person making the request should have knowledge of the process of donation, and be able to answer at least simple questions. Some important features are summarized in Table 40.6. The separation of the communication and explanation of death from the request for donation has been found to be beneficial for relatives (Garrison *et al.* 1991). Bereavement support and follow-up information on transplant outcomes to relatives and others involved in the donation process may be provided by the local procurements agency.

Table 40.6 Facts to be conveyed to organ donor families

- Time of death is the time when loss of brain function is certified
- Consent is required for donation of each specific organ and tissue for transplantation or research
- Routine potential donor blood testing includes HIV, HBV, HCV, CMV, and tissue typing
- All donation and retrieval are done with care and respect for the deceased
- Organ retrieval happens in the operating theatre under normal surgical conditions (specialist surgeon, anesthetist, scrub, and scout nurses)
- Donation does not disfigure the deceased, and viewing after donation is encouraged
- Donation and autopsy have separate purposes, processes, and procedures
- Donation does not interfere with normal funeral arrangements
- There is no financial cost to the family after death is declared for ongoing management for donation

Where the death is subject to coronial or similar legal scrutiny, care must be taken to obtain the appropriate coronial permission and to complete all the legal requirements. This may involve local police for instance.

The process of donation involves several steps and is multidisciplinary. Timely involvement of the local procurement agency can be beneficial. The efficient organization of a donation with sensitivity to the needs and wishes of the donor's relatives and staff in the donor hospital is essential (Mohacsi and Thompson 1992).

Conclusions

Donation and transplantation are beneficial to donor families, recipients, and the society in general. Most deceased patients can donate tissues, though few can donate organs after death. However, all dying patients are potential donors.

There is a need to be proactive in the identification and management of profoundly brain-injured patients if the wishes of the patient with respect to organ and tissue donation are not to be left unfulfilled. Medical and nursing practitioners attending to such patients need to be aware of issues related to donation if the benefits of donation are to be realized. Training, organization and structures need to be in place to support the process and, most especially, the people involved in this delicate and sometimes difficult, but highly rewarding, aspect of the management of critically ill patients.

References

ANZOD Report (2000) Australian and New Zealand Organ Donation Registry, Adelaide, South Australia.

Australian Bureau of Statistics (1999) ABS Population Survey Monitor 1999. Australian Bureau of Statistics, Canberra.

Australian Coordinating Committee on Organ Registries and Donation (1995) Public Awareness and Attitudes Towards Organ Donation. Frank Small & Associates Pty Ltd, Sydney.

Australian Law Reform Commission, ALRC 7 (1977) Report of the Law Reform Commission on Human Tissue Transplants. Australian Government Publishing Service, Canberra.

Buckley TA (1998) Management of the multiorgan donor. In: Oh TE (ed.) *Intensive care manual*. Reed Educational and Professional Publishing Pty Ltd, Great Britain, pp 795–801.

Diagnosis of Brain Death (1976) Statement issued by the Honorary Secretary of the Conference of Medical Royal Colleges and their Faculties in the United Kingdom on 11 October 1976. *British Medical Journal* ii: 1187–1188.

Follette D, Rudich S, Bonacci C, Allen R, Hoso A, Albertson T (1999) Importance of an aggressive multidisciplinary management approach to optimize lung donor procurement. *Transplantation Proceedings* 31: 169–170.

Garrison RN, Bentley FR, Paque GH, Polk HL, Sladek LC, Evanisko MJ *et al.* (1991) There is an answer to the shortage of organ donors. *Surgery Gynecology and Obstetrics* 173: 391–396.

Harvard Medical School (1968) A definition of irreversible coma. *Journal of the American Medical Association* 205(6): 85–88.

Kennedy AP Jr, West JC, Kelley SE, Brotman S (1992) Utilization of trauma-related deaths for organ and tissue harvesting. *Journal of Trauma* 33: 516–519.

Matesanz R, Miranda B (2001) Expanding the organ donor pool: The Spanish Model. *Kidney International* 59: 1594.

Miranda B, Fernandez Licas M, de Filipe C, Naya M, Gonzales-Posada JM, Matesanz R (1999) Organ donation in Spain. *Nephrology, Dialysis, Transplantation* 14(Suppl 3): 15–21.

Mohacsi PJ, Thompson JF (1992) The organization of cadaveric multiple organ donation: a critical issue for establishing and maintaining successful transplantation programs. *Transplantation Proceedings* 24: 2046.

Mollar P, Goulton M (1959) 'Le coma dépassé' (mémoire préliminaire). *Revista de Neurologia* 101: 3–15.

National Health and Medical Research Council (1997) Certifying death: the brain function criterion. Ethical issues in organ donation—Discussion Paper no. 4. Commonwealth Department of Health and Family Services, Canberra.

Novitzky D (1997a) Detrimental effects of brain death on the potential organ donor. *Transplantation Proceedings* 29: 3770–3772.

Novitzky D (1997b) Donor management: state of the art. *Transplantation Proceedings* 29: 3773–3775.

O'Brien RL, Serbin MF, O'Brien KD, Maier RV, Grady MS (1996) Improvement in the organ donation rate at a large urban trauma center. *Archives of Surgery* 131: 153–159.

Pallis C (1983) *ABC of brain stem death*. British Medical Journal, London.

Prager MC (1991) Care of organ donors. In: Lebowitz PW (ed.) *International anesthesiology clinics*. Little, Brown and Company, Boston, pp 1–16.

President's Commission Report (1981) *Study of ethical problems in medicine and biomedical and behavioural research, defying death: medical, legal and ethical issues in the definition of death*. US Government Printing Office, Washington.

Riker RR, White BW (1991) Organ and tissue donation from the emergency department. *Journal of Emergency Medicine* 9: 405–410.

Robertson KM, Cook DR (1990) Perioperative management of the multiorgan donor. *Anesthesia Analog* 70: 546–556.

Scheinkestel CD, Tuxen DV, Cooper DJ, Butts W (1995) Medical management of the (potential) organ donor. *Anaesthesia Intensive Care* 23: 51–59.

Tropmann C, Dunn DL (1999) Management of the organ donor. In: Irwin RD, Cerra FB, Rippe JM (eds) *Irwin and Rippe's intensive care medicine volume II*. Lippincott-Raven Publishers, USA, pp 2184–2202.

UNOS (2000) www.unos.org/frame_default.asp?category=data

Werkman HA, Pruim J, ten Vergert EM, ten Duis HJ, Sloof MJH (1991) Organ donation from trauma victims. *Transplantation Proceedings* 23: 2553–2554.

41

CHAPTER 41

Sexual assault

JEAN R EDWARDS AND DIANNA MILINKOVIC-BALOG

CHAPTER 41
Sexual assault

JEAN R EDWARDS AND
DIANNA MILINKOVIC-BALOG

The terms 'rape' and 'sexual assault' are often used interchangeably. Historically, the legal definition of rape was understood as the penile penetration of the vagina without the consent of the woman.

Societal awareness, legislative frameworks, and the development of specialized responses (medical, counselling, police) and services (crisis centres) were significantly broadened as a result of the women's movement in the 1970s, which advocated strongly for the needs of victims and highlighted the absence of an appropriate societal response to a significant and serious issue.

A woman or a man who has suffered a sexual assault has suffered a severe personal invasion with varying degrees of emotional, physical, and genital injury. For this reason they need meticulous care and attention, with respect for their trauma and preferably a multidisciplinary response, which may involve medical, social work, and investigative support.

Definition

Legal terminology varies from jurisdiction to jurisdiction, but essentially sexual assault or rape is any sexual act which is non-consensual. It may involve penetration of the genitalia, mouth or anus by any part of the body of another person or an object. The non-consensual act may be enforced by physical violence, the threat of physical violence, or coercion. Certain groups in the community are particularly vulnerable, such as people with physical or intellectual or psychological disability.

Key points

- Sexual assault or rape is any sexual act which is non-consensual.

Prevalence

Reported incidence figures vary greatly from one country to another and do not provide a true indication of the extent of the problem. It is widely thought that sexual assault is severely under-reported; study estimates vary from 10% to 25% of cases being reported. It is believed that male sexual assault is even more seriously under-reported.

Medical role

Victims' responses to sexual assault may vary greatly, and medical practitioners coming into contact with these victims need to ensure that personal judgements are suspended and that their response is empathic. Knowledge of the medical, psychosocial, and legal needs of the victim is important.

The medical officer seeing a patient reporting a recent sexual assault has a dual role:

- *A care-giving therapeutic role* at the time of the acute assessment of the victim of sexual assault, looking at immediate medical concerns, providing information and referral to specialist services where available as well as follow-up services if required.
- *A role as the collector of forensic evidence*. In this forensic role the medical officer does not act as an

advocate for the patient nor as an investigator, but as an impartial observer and recorder.

The *primary function* of the medical officer who examines a patient in an emergency department of a hospital or a sexual assault centre immediately or soon after a report of sexual assault is to *satisfy the medical needs of that patient*. This should include:

- asking them what their primary concerns are (e.g. fears about safety, pregnancy, or sexually transmitted infections)
- ascertaining the patient's needs for a support person to be present throughout interview or examination
- offer to provide referral for counselling to specialist services if available.

The *secondary function* of the medical officer is to offer to conduct a *forensic examination* and explain what this involves. The purpose of the forensic examination is for the medical officer to observe and record the history and examination of the patient. It is also to collect any samples from the patient which may contain the DNA of the assailant. Following this, the medical officer should be able to express an opinion, based on these observations, of the likely causation of any recorded injuries or of the possible reasons for the absence of injuries. This may then be considered, together with all the other evidence, in the subsequent investigation of the reported sexual assault. Medical officers involved in forensic examination should follow correct guidelines for documentation of findings as well as the collection and storage of forensic samples.

The choice of course of action must lie with the patient presenting after a sexual assault. They may want:

- to leave without any medical or counselling assistance
- counselling only
- immediate medical attention with no examination
- medical examination but no forensic examination.

If the patient is considering legal action or is undecided, they need to be made aware of the option of having a full medical and forensic examination, together with counselling.

Key point

- Only the patient should decide whether a forensic examination is to be done.

It is important that the patient feels in control of what is happening to them while in the sexual assault centre, hospital or other medical facility. It is possible that they will perceive persuasion as coercion and it is very important that the medical examination is seen as part of the healing process and is not remembered as a continuation of the assault.

Patients who refuse a forensic examination should be given information about the time limits of the examination and should be invited to re-present if they change their minds. If a forensic examination is to be performed, it should preferably be performed as close as possible to the time of the reported assault and preferably within 72 hours. A forensic examination with documentation of injuries can be performed up to a week after the sexual assault, but the likelihood of the forensic examination providing useful information is lessened the longer after the sexual assault that it takes place. It is unlikely that an assailant's DNA will be found on swabs longer than 72 hours after the sexual assault, but bruising and signs of resolving injuries may still be present. It may be remotely possible to obtain the assailant's DNA from a cervical swab up to 7 days after the assault.

The protocols for recording the examination of a patient with a history of sexual assault vary from place to place but should contain the same basic components, concerning consent, history, examination, and specimen collection.

Consent to forensic examination

Based on the request by the patient for a forensic examination, the first concern is to obtain the informed consent of the patient. Since a forensic examination is not a therapeutic procedure, informed consent is essential. This means explaining to the patient the nature and purpose of the examination. It is necessary for the examining doctor to check with the patient that they understand the implications of the examination.

Key point

- Forensic examination is not a therapeutic procedure.

Problems arising around consent

The problems that may arise include:

- Treatment of a severe medical problem and stabilization of the medical condition must take priority over the forensic examination.
- In the case of intoxication by alcohol or other drugs, the effect of the intoxication must wear off before the consent to perform the forensic examination is obtained.
- In the event that it is not possible to obtain informed consent due to the medical condition of the victim, it may be possible to obtain consent from the next of kin, a previously appointed guardian, or a tribunal with the power to give consent.
- Appropriate language interpreters should be made available to patients where necessary, and signing interpreters should be available to a patient who is hearing impaired.
- The legal framework and authority available to intervene where there is a problem in obtaining consent will vary throughout countries. Medical officers need to be aware of the appropriate authorities and policies within their jurisdiction.
- In New South Wales, Australia, the circumstances where the guardianship tribunal may be involved in giving consent to a forensic examination are:
  - an unconscious patient where there is a suspicion of sexual assault and the patient's condition is too serious to wait for her/him to regain consciousness
  - a patient with a psychiatric condition who has complained of sexual assault and who is willing to be examined but who (owing to thought disorder) does not have the capacity to consent to the forensic examination
  - a patient with an intellectual disability who has complained of sexual assault and who does not have the capacity to give informed consent
  - the next of kin or a previously appointed guardian is unavailable or unwilling to give consent to the forensic examination.

Key point

- Since a forensic examination is not a therapeutic procedure it should never be performed on anyone who indicates that they are unwilling to have it done.

History

Because of the stigma that sexual assault victims often experience, it is important that the medical officer takes the history in a sensitive, non-judgmental, and respectful manner. Medical officers need to be mindful that some aspects of the detail of the sexual assault may be difficult for the patient to provide, as they may see it as shameful or culturally inappropriate to discuss. Similarly, male victims of sexual assault may be very apprehensive to discuss aspects of the sexual assault that they found shameful.

It is necessary to note and record the following:

- date and time, if known, of the assault
- date and time of the arrival of the patient at the emergency department or sexual assault centre

- date and time of the commencement and conclusion of the examination.

These details, which should be obtained and recorded by the doctor, will confirm the contemporaneous nature of the notes which is important in subsequently writing a statement and giving evidence in court.

Note the following information:

- changed clothes
- showered or bathed
- eaten or drunk fluids
- used toilet
- last menstrual period
- last date of any sexual intercourse within 1 week of the examination
- use of condoms, by assailant and other partners.

Brief details of the assault should be obtained and recorded. It is important to take sufficient history to ensure an adequate examination, but a detailed history of the circumstances surrounding the assault should be left to the investigating police officer. It is not necessary to record the exact words of the patient, but if a particular phrase is used by the patient a number of times and is obviously distressing to them, the phrase can be recorded using the exact words and it should be put into inverted commas to distinguish it in the record of the assault.

Ensure the history includes details of the contact between the patient and the assailant and include any threats or force used. It should also include:

- where the assault took place
- nature of physical contact in detail
- if hit, what with e.g. fist, hand, object
- what part of the body was involved.

Details of the sexual contact must be specified. It is also important to use language that the patient understands. If the patient says 'he had sex with me', remember that they often find it difficult to give a history of oral penetration and even more difficult to give a history of anal penetration. Men can be sexually assaulted too and will require the same level of sensitive understanding as women. Confirm the following:

- did the penis go into the genital area or the vagina
- any other genital contact, e.g. penis with mouth or anus
- awareness of ejaculation
- any injury the patient may have caused to the assailant.

General examination

The medical officer must:

- offer a clear explanation of what the examination involves at every step as the examination proceeds
- be sensitive to the patient's emotional state, suspending the examination if necessary
- be sensitive to issues related to the gender of the medical officer
- be aware that some patients may want a support person throughout the examination.

General assessment of presentation using descriptive instead of diagnostic terms:

- tearful rather than depressed
- frowning and shaking rather than anxious
- describe stains and damage of clothing, e.g. white stains, brown or red stains.

The final analysis of the stains as blood or semen is microscopic analysis by the forensic laboratory. The appearance of any damage of clothing should be noted, e.g. frayed, torn, cut, burnt, etc.

Each part of the body needs to be uncovered individually and examined. A good light source is important so that the colour and nature of all injuries seen can be accurately described and they can be measured and drawn on a body chart and described briefly in words. If there are a lot of individual injuries, number them for easier inclusion in a report.

Note any of the following:

- Frequently facial injuries are accompanied by buccal trauma corresponding to the tissues being forced against the teeth.
- Scalp injuries may occur from the hair being pulled, and the presence of large numbers of loose hairs with roots attached should be noted.
- Fingertip bruising of the arms and inside thighs is typical of the type of trauma caused by manual restraint of the patient and forcing the thighs apart.
- Larger bruises may be due to punches, kicks, or being hit by objects.
- Red marks around the wrists and ankles are typical of marks caused by being tied up.
- Sand and grass seeds may be found in the hair or may stick to parts of the body and the clothing.
- Multiple fine abrasions on the lumbar and sacral region may be caused by the assault taking place on a rough surface such as concrete.
- Weapons such as knives may leave fine lines or small abrasions when held against the skin.
- Broad abrasions may be caused by dragging the patient from one place to another in the course of the assault.

Inconsistencies between the history and examination may be due to the following:

- part of the assault was forgotten by the patient when they gave you the history
- a previous assault
- prior accidental injury
- self-inflicted injuries prior to or after the reported assault.

Genital examination

The anogenital area is the last part of the body to be examined. There may be no physical injuries to be seen, or there may be minor injuries that are not specific to sexual assault. The time that has elapsed from the reported time of sexual assault and the time of examination is critical in assessing the appearance of these injuries. Note in particular:

- Due to the excellent blood supply to the genital area most minor injuries are likely to be well healed after a few days.
- Minor abrasions of the tissues of the introitus or opening of the vagina may be consistent with consensual sexual intercourse, but if it is associated with other minor body trauma indicative of restraint and the use of force then the patient's history of assault is partially substantiated.
- Digital assault, particularly when described as rough by the patient, may lead to a midline furrowing type of abrasion on the posterior wall of the vagina from the posterior commissure below the entry of the vagina to just inside the entry into the vagina.
- Sometimes bruising or bite marks can be seen.
- Women who have not previously had sexual intercourse may have tears in the tissue of the hymen that can extend into the vaginal wall.
- Tears in the vaginal wall may also be seen when objects have been used, when the woman has been abstinent from sexual activity for a prolonged period, or when the woman is postmenopausal.
- Bright bleeding from the vagina that continues for some time after a sexual assault must be looked at very carefully and the source found and controlled.
- Anal injuries may be seen in both male and female patients after sexual assault and may include bruising of the anal verge, bright bleeding, fissure formation, and extreme anal pain with spasm.
- If lubricant has been used there may be no physical signs at all, and minor anal injuries may heal extremely quickly.

- The presence of an anal fissure may not necessarily be due to sexual assault as the commonest cause of anal fissure is constipation.

In assessing both genital and anal injuries very soon after a sexual assault, the insertion of objects such as a speculum or a proctoscope should be considered very carefully. It will certainly increase the trauma of the examination for the victim and should only be done if there is a medical reason, such as the need to identify the source of bright bleeding or the extent of an injury. If the patient is unable to tolerate the insertion of a speculum or a proctoscope, their general condition should be assessed. If they appear well they should be given the option of returning for further assessment in a few days. If their condition is unstable, and particularly if there is substantial bright bleeding from the anus or the vagina, consideration should be given to examination under general anaesthetic. This is for clinical reasons, not forensic reasons, but the results still need to be recorded in a forensic report.

Specimen collection

The last part of the examination is the collection of material for forensic examination in the laboratory. Many jurisdictions require that the forensic specimens are collected according to a specific protocol and you should familiarize yourself with such protocols before the need to use them occurs in order to minimize technical errors.

Note the following:

- Collect any foreign material in the hair such as vegetation, both in the scalp hair and in the pubic area.
- Swabs and slides should be collected from all parts of the body where there has been penile contact, even if there is no history of ejaculation.
- From every place that a swab has been taken, a corresponding dry slide should be made.
- It is possible to obtain vaginal swabs by separating the labia and without inserting a speculum.
- Swabs and slides must be taken from any area where there is a history of ejaculation onto the skin.
- Swabs may also be taken if there is the likelihood of obtaining saliva samples, such as over a bite mark or when there is a history of sucking of the breasts or genital area.
- A blood sample or a buccal smear should be collected from the patient for identification purposes.
- The only reason for using a speculum to obtain a forensic endocervical swab and slide is if the patient is not seen until several days after the assault when it may be possible to obtain sperm from the endocervical canal—the patient must have the reason for the examination explained to her and must feel able to refuse the examination if unable to tolerate speculum insertion.
- If there appear to be loose hairs lying on the genital area the pubic hair can be combed and possible hairs from an assailant may be collected.
- There is no need to collect pubic hair from the patient as a collection of blood or a buccal smear will give all the identifying DNA information required about the patient.
- If there is a history of the patient scratching the assailant, swabs should be taken from under the fingernails and fingernail clippings should be collected.
- The underwear worn immediately after the assault should be spread out to dry and placed in a paper bag.
- All of these specimens should be handled and labelled by the examining medical officer only and must not be left unattended between collection and storage.
- The swabs, slides, blood collected from the patient, underwear, and all other specimens should be placed in an envelope by the examining medical officer, together with a copy of the relevant notes of the forensic examination.

- The envelope should be sealed and the medical officer should sign over the sealed flap.
- The sealed envelope should be placed in a locked refrigerator with the details entered into a forensic register.
- The clothing of the patient should be retained for forensic examination if they are still wearing the clothing in which the assault took place.
- Each item should be bagged separately in a paper bag to prevent cross-contamination of any evidence from one item to another.

Key point

- Local protocols should be followed for forensic specimen collection.

Release of the forensic specimens

The preferred option is that the forensic specimens are retained securely in the medical facility so that a decision about further legal action is delayed until after the immediate effects of the sexual assault have settled. Since the cross-examination of a victim of sexual assault in a court room can be difficult for the victim, the patient needs to consider this before the specimens are handed over, but you will need to follow the protocol of the particular service in which you are working.

It is essential that there is provision for an unbroken chain of evidence from the collection of the specimens to their reception in the analytical laboratory, and the medical officer is responsible for ensuring their part in the secure sealing and storage of the specimens. If secure storage to ensure an unbroken chain of evidence is not available in the medical facility, the sealed envelope must be handed over to the accompanying police officer, who must also sign over the seal. The medical officer must record in the notes what happens to the forensic specimens.

Medical report

At the conclusion of the forensic assessment, the medical officer should re-read their notes and check that all the necessary information has been documented. Depending on the practice of the place where the assessment was performed, the medical officer may draft a medico-legal report immediately or when requested by the police service. The medico-legal report must conform to the legal requirements of the jurisdiction in which the examination was performed and must arise directly from the original notes, recorded contemporaneously with the forensic examination. It must contain the following:

- adequate identification of the patient
- adequate identification of the medical officer performing the examination
- a brief CV confirming the medical officer's qualifications and expertise
- details of the time and place at which the examination took place
- details of the history of the sexual assault as recorded in the forensic examination
- details of the physical and genital examination conducted with a description of any injuries observed
- your opinion on whether these examination findings are consistent with the account of the sexual assault given to you by the patient.

Giving evidence in court

The above statement, together with the original examination records, will form the basis of any evidence you may need to give in subsequent legal proceedings. As an expert witness, you are entitled to give opinion evidence, which is your opinion of the nature and causation of any observed injuries, or the absence of injuries.

You are an independent witness whose responsibility is to inform the court of the results of your examination. You do not determine whether a sexual assault has taken place. That decision is made by the court. Your examination is only part of the evidence, which will also include the evidence of the complainant, the investigating police officer, and any other person who can give evidence in the matter.

The more objective you are in your evidence, the better you help the court to determine the facts of the matter.

Conclusion

The medical officer involved in forensic examinations of patients reporting sexual assault has two distinct roles to fulfil. The primary role is to satisfy the medical needs of the patient, such as dealing with their fears about injury, pregnancy and infection. The secondary role is to conduct a non-traumatic, efficient forensic examination which collects all necessary evidence from the patient. From the record of this examination a statement can be prepared documenting any injuries and commenting on the likely causes of such injuries. The efficient conduct of the forensic medical examination and the subsequent evidence in court may be the most valuable help that the medical officer can provide if the patient subsequently decides to make a statement to the police and a trial takes place.

The successful management of reported sexual assault should involve a multidisciplinary response. The use of specialized sexual assault services, which include counselling, support during the legal process, and medical follow-up will help to reduce the severity of long-term effects commonly resulting from the trauma of sexual assault.

42

CHAPTER 42

Rehabilitation of trauma

STEPHEN F WILSON, JAMES MIDDLETON, CLAYTON KING, AND IAN D CAMERON

CHAPTER 42
Rehabilitation of trauma

STEPHEN F WILSON, JAMES MIDDLETON, CLAYTON KING, AND IAN D CAMERON

General principles of rehabilitation

Patients suffering major trauma require an integrated interdisciplinary approach across the continuum of care from early injury management to later community reintegration, and beyond, to achieve the best outcome for quality of life and independence. Rehabilitation commences on the first day of injury and requires development of a good understanding by all members of the treating team of the person's personality, lifestyle, interests, and motivation, as well as family situation and social support network.

Key point

- Rehabilitation commences on the first day of injury.

Definitions

Rehabilitation is a process of restoration to achieve maximum physical, social, psychological, vocational and recreational functioning following injury or illness. As well as primary restoration, rehabilitation also places a strong emphasis on secondary prevention through identification of the causative or risk factors and provision of education and appropriate interventions to maintain future health and well-being.

Rehabilitation after traumatic injury can be divided into four overlapping phases:

- *Acute:* Stabilization of injury with surgical and medical management, early rehabilitative measures to prevent secondary impairments and initial remobilization (acute hospital).
- *Subacute:* Comprehensive assessment and intensive inpatient rehabilitation to enhance level of functional independence and psychological adjustment, prescribe appropriate prostheses, orthoses, aids, and equipment and assess necessary home modifications in anticipation of discharge (rehabilitation centre).
- *Community:* Resettlement into a safe independent living environment with continuation of therapeutic input as an outpatient to achieve patient's optimum recovery and potential. Also covers further education and retraining if required, return to work and leisure pursuits (day therapy/day hospital/outreach).
- *Maintenance:* Ongoing management of disability and maintenance of support network (outpatient clinics).

Developing a framework for rehabilitation requires an understanding of some basic concepts (ICF-2001). Impairment relates to the injury at the tissue level and the *body*. In the case of a compound lower limb fracture a possible impairment may be vascular insufficiency and amputation of the limb. The resulting disability would cause a limitation to activities at the level of the *person*. In this case there would be a limitation to activities such as walking. This limitation to activities would affect the person's participation in *society*, involving psychological aspects and choices for work and leisure.

Team approach

The rehabilitation team must always recognize the involvement of the patient and family as the key to successful rehabilitation. Self-implemented programmes are preferred, as rehabilitation is an active rather than passive process.

Consulting and participating members of the team include the doctor, nurse, physiotherapist, occupational therapist, social worker, speech pathologist, psychologist, and recreation therapist.

Key point

- The rehabilitation team must always recognize the involvement of the patient and family as the key to successful rehabilitation.

Rehabilitation planning

A problem list is prepared and goals set as part of a rehabilitation plan. The goals may be medical or therapy based and must be negotiated with the patient to be achievable within a set time frame. Regular case conferences and review of goals is essential.

Rehabilitation plan checklist:

- impairment/diagnosis
- functional score (e.g. Functional Independence Measure or Barthel Index)
- problem list
  - medical/surgical
  - physical and therapeutic
  - functional
  - psychosocial
  - avocational
  - vocational
  - educational
- rehabilitation goals
  - problem oriented
  - specific, achievable, time limited
  - negotiated patient goals
- review date.

Components of rehabilitation

Measurement in rehabilitation

Functional

Rehabilitation and its progress can be monitored to assess improvement and response to treatment. Although most rehabilitation centres have developed local measures of function, a number of activities of daily living (ADL) scales have become internationally accepted. These measures provide a useful checklist of basic functions such as self-care, bladder control, bowel control, transfer, and locomotion, and assist the team in goal setting. They are regularly reviewed at a case conference and provide a basis for clinical decision-making regarding treatment strategies and care requirements. It is important to remember when setting goals that performance may be influenced by numerous factors other than impairment alone, including adaptive equipment, suitable environment, social supports, time and energy required, and safety.

A simple and reliable measure of activities of daily living is the Barthel index (Mahoney and Barthel 1965). Another more comprehensive ADL scale developed by the State University of New York is the Functional Independence Measure (FIM) (Keith *et al.* 1987). The FIM records communication as well as social cognition items. Examples of data collection sheets are shown in Tables 42.1 and 42.2.

Key point

- A number of ADL scales have become internationally accepted (the Barthel Index and the FIM).

Physical

Serial measures of muscle strength and recording on a *muscle chart* will assist in monitoring the progress of exercise programs. Grading of muscle strength from 0 to 5 has been widely accepted. Grading movement against slight, moderate and strong

Table 42.1 Barthel Index

		With help	Independent
1	Feeding (if food needs to be cut up = help)	5	10
2	Moving from wheelchair to bed and return (includes sitting up in bed)	5–10	15
3	Personal toilet (wash face, comb hair, shave, clean teeth)	0	5
4	Getting on and off toilet (handling clothes, wipe, flush)	5	10
5	Bathing self	0	5
6	Walking on level surface	10	15
	(or if unable to walk, propel wheelchair)	0[a]	5[a]
7	Ascend and descend stairs	5	10
8	Dressing (includes tying shoes, fastening fasteners)	5	10
9	Controlling bowels	5	10
10	Controlling bladder	5	10
Score	(maximum 100)		

[a] Score only if the patient is unable to walk.

From Mahoney FI and Barthel DW (1965) Functional evaluation: the Barthel index. *Maryland Medical Journal*. With permission.

Table 42.2 Functional Independence Measure (FIM)

FIM™ instrument

LEVELS		
	7 Complete Independence (Timely, Safely) 6 Modified Independence (Device)	**NO HELPER**
	Modified Dependence 5 Supervision (Subject = 100%+) 4 Minimal Assist (Subject = 75%+) 3 Moderate Assist (Subject = 50%+) **Complete Dependence** 2 Maximal Assist (Subject =25%+) 1 Total Assist (Subject = less than 25%)	**HELPER**

Self-Care	ADMISSION	DISCHARGE	FOLLOW-UP
A. Eating			
B Grooming			
C. Bathing			
D. Dressing - Upper Body			
E. Dressing - Lower Body			
F. Toileting			
Sphincter Control			
G. Bladder Management			
H. Bowel Management			

Table 42.2 Continued

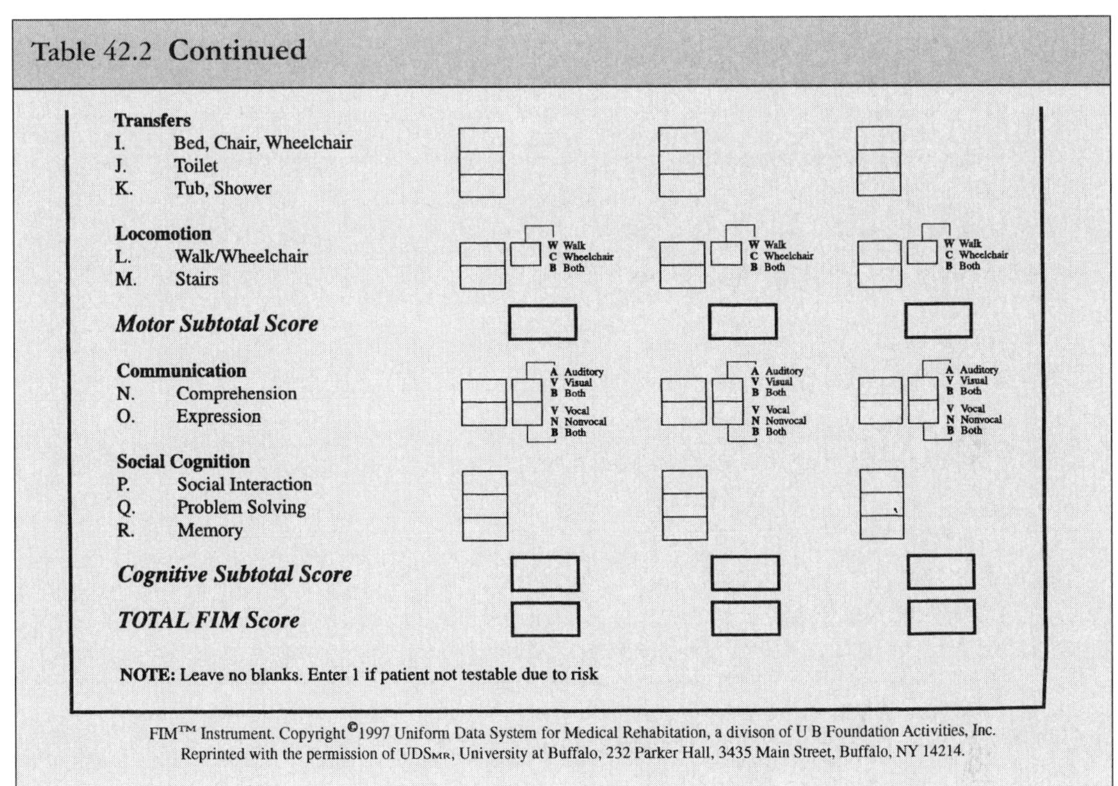

Transfers
I. Bed, Chair, Wheelchair
J. Toilet
K. Tub, Shower

Locomotion
L. Walk/Wheelchair (W Walk, C Wheelchair, B Both)
M. Stairs

Motor Subtotal Score

Communication
N. Comprehension (A Auditory, V Visual, B Both)
O. Expression (V Vocal, N Nonvocal, B Both)

Social Cognition
P. Social Interaction
Q. Problem Solving
R. Memory

Cognitive Subtotal Score

TOTAL FIM Score

NOTE: Leave no blanks. Enter 1 if patient not testable due to risk

resistance as 4, −4 and +4 is sometimes a useful variation to the original scale (MRC 1976).

0 no contraction

1 flicker or trace of contraction

2 active movement with gravity eliminated

3 active movement against gravity

4 active movement against gravity and resistance

5 normal power.

Measures of mobility such as the motor assessment score add extra detail to the less sensitive FIM and Barthel index in neurological disorders. Other tests of mobility may be very simple, such as a 6 metre (20 feet) walking speed or the timed 'Up and Go' test (Posiadlo and Richardson 1991). In this test the patient is observed as they rise from an armchair and walk 3 metres, turn, walk back, and sit down again.

Checking and recording the range of motion (ROM) at hip for patients in bed requires flexing of the contralateral hip and straightening the lumbar spine (Thomas test). Assessment of ROM at the knee and ankle should also be routine for non-ambulant patients.

Cognitive

Traumatic brain injury is often associated with impaired cognition. This can be initially assessed on admission by the *Glasgow Coma Scale (GCS)* (Teasdale and Jennett 1974) (see Table 2.3, page 00). However, patients with a GCS score of 15/15 may still have significantly impaired cognition and be suffering *post-traumatic amnesia* (PTA) (Table 42.3). Monitoring the period of PTA in which the injured person has no reliable short-term memory, and particularly recovery from PTA, is extremely valuable in the management of a head-injured

Table 42.3 Westmead PTA scale

Date								
1. How old are you?	A							
	S							
2. What is your date of birth?	A							
	S							
3. What month are we in?	A							
	S							
4. What time of day is it?	A							
(morning, afternoon or night)	S							
	A							
5. What day of the week is it?	S							
	A							
6. What year are we in?	S							
	A							
7. What is the name of this place?	S							
	A							
8. Face	S							
	A							
9. Name	S							
	A							
10. Picture I	S							
	A							
Picture II	S							
	A							
Picture III	S							
Total								

A, answer; S, score (1 or 0).

PTA may be judged to be ended on the first of 3 successive days of a recall of 12.

Reproduced with permission from Shores EA, Marosszeky JE, Sandanam J, Batchelor J (1986) Preliminary validation of a scale for measuring the duration of post-traumatic amnesia. *MJA* 144: 569–572.

patient. Once a patient is capable of remembering from one day to the next, then they can actively participate in a rehabilitation programme. A scale which is easily applied is the Westmead Post Traumatic Amnesia Scale (Shores *et al.* 1986) (Table 42.3).

Basic screening tests of cognitive function such as the Mini-Mental State Examination (Folstein *et al.* 1975) test orientation, short and long-term memory, and language. It is essential to establish rapport and leave the patient relaxed and comfortable. The patient must have adequate hearing and vision to respond to questions. This is only a screening instrument for cognitive dysfunction. A low score (<24) indicates a need for more detailed evaluation, rather than establishing a diagnosis of permanent cognitive impairment.

More detailed neuropsychological assessment must be performed by a neuropsychologist. A variety of scales and batteries are available to examine a wide range of cognitive abilities, including concentration, attention, planning, problem solving, judgement, and other executive functions. Tests of learning use diagrams such as the Rey–Ostereith complex figure, card sorting, mazes, and trail-making tests. Standard texts contain more detailed explanations (Deutsch Lezak 1995). Results from such tests prove most helpful when determining issues such as a patient's competency to handle financial affairs, ability to drive a motor vehicle safely, or return to work, and may assist choices for employment.

Key point

- Traumatic head injury is often associated with impaired cognition.

Passive physical modalities

Heat, cold, and electricity are adjuvants to active physical therapy. There effects are only short term. A knowledge of the risks and benefits may add substantially to the safe design of a rehabilitation programme.

Heat

Superficial heat can be applied by conduction such as a hot pack, radiant heat, or paraffin bath, or by convection as occurs in hydrotherapy or moist air (sauna). Conversion of non-thermal to thermal energy occurs in deep heat modalities such as microwave and ultrasound.

Contraindications to the application of heat include:

- acute trauma, haemorrhage, and oedema
- anaesthetic areas where burns may occur
- vascular insufficiency, particularly feet and hands
- bleeding disorders
- sepsis
- unreliable or cognitively impaired patient
- pregnancy
- in the region of the gonads
- altered thermoregulation (precaution depending on modality).

Benefits of the application of heat include:

- increase inextensibility of collagen, aiding stretching of ligaments, and musculotendinous unit
- decrease in joint stiffness
- decrease in pain
- decrease in muscle spasm by an effect on the muscle spindle
- increase of superficial blood flow through arteriolar and capillary dilatation
- increase in tissue metabolism
- consensual response in opposite limb or deeper structures
- psychological benefits.

Recommended selective heating of skin and subcutaneous tissues should be within the therapeutic range of 40–45°C for no longer than 30 minutes. Prolonged heating should be avoided as core temperature will eventually rise.

Applications of heat that are commonly used:

- *Hot packs*, hydrocollator, and Kenny packs: Usually applied wrapped in towelling for 10 minutes repeated 2–3 times.
- *Infrared* lamps provide superficial heating only and carry the risk of superficial burns.
- *Paraffin baths* or wax baths consist of heated melted mixtures of oil (usually one part mineral oil to 6–7 parts paraffin wax). It can be applied to the skin despite the high temperature of 52°C because of the low specific heat. Application is by dipping 3–4 times and wrapping in a towel, or by brushing or immersion. Open wounds are a specific contraindication. This treatment is specifically used for joint stiffness and for mobilization after hand trauma.
- *Contrast baths* consist of alternate immersion in hot (40–43°C) and cold water (15–18°C) for 4 cycles of 4 minutes and 1 minute durations respectively, ending in hot water. This produces a hyperaemia and maybe useful in regional pain management.
- *Ultrasound* produces high frequency sound above the audible range (0.8–1.0 MHz) causing heating at the interface between tissues of differing density, typically at fascial planes and bone. Ultrasound is produced by a piezoelectric transducer in the applicator or head of the machine. The intensity may vary from 0.5–2 W/cm^2 area applied for 5–10 minutes duration. The head is applied to the skin with a coupling medium of gel or water if the treated part is submerged. This medium is necessary to provide efficient energy transmission. Although non-thermal effects may be beneficial in certain situations, those arising from gaseous *cavitation*, caused by alternating compression and rarefaction where gas bubbles form, may have a destructive effect on tissues. To avoid overheating of tissues and gaseous cavitation, ultrasound should never be applied over large fluid-filled areas such as the eyeball, amniotic sack, or larger effusions. Ultrasound should also not be applied over nerve roots following laminectomy, implants, or devices, and epiphysis in growing children. The transducer head is continually moved with a stroking technique by the operator to avoid local damage.
- *Hydrotherapy* in heated pools and spas allows a patient to exercise in a non- or partial weight-bearing environment. This is particularly useful in the rehabilitation of lower limb fractures. Pool temperatures vary from around 28°C for recreational activities to 31°C for therapeutic sessions of less than 30 minutes.

Cold therapy (cryotherapy)

Cold therapy is used for a variety of acute ligament and muscle trauma and superficial burns and analgesia. The *benefits* are:

- reduction of swelling and bleeding by vasoconstriction
- pain reduction by slowing nerve conduction in peripheral nerve fibres
- muscle relaxation by reducing muscle spindle activity.

Contraindications to the application of cold include:

- peripheral vascular disease, Raynaud's phenomenon/disease
- anaesthetic areas where cold burns may occur
- severe cardiovascular disease (pressor response if large area).

Application of ice for cooling deep tissues may be as:

- crushed ice in plastic bag
- ice with dry towel
- ice via wet towels
- immersion in iced water with or without movement
- gel pack.

The cooling medium should be kept in close contact with the treated area. It is best to bandage the bag of ice or gel pack on to the limb. The period of application will depend on the thickness of subcutaneous fat. Ice packs are usually applied for 15–20 minutes 3–4 times daily for the first 48–72 hours after injury. If acute trauma is being treated, cold is usually combined with compressive bandaging and elevation using the rest, ice, compression, elevation (RICE) regime (Johannsen and Langberg 1997).

Key point

- For acute trauma use RICE.

Electrical therapy

Laser

Low intensity laser can non-destructively alter cellular function without significant heating. Its use affects muscle skelation and soft tissue conditioning (Basford 1993).

Transcutaneous electrical nerve simulation

Direct application of electricity to the strain (TENS) has been used to relieve acute and chronic pain. Two or four electrodes are applied in the pain-related segment with a frequency of 75–100 Hz for >20 minutes. Narcotic analgesics should be stopped while therapy is tried. Contraindications include:

- cardiac pacemaker
- cardiac disease or arrythmias
- pregnancy
- larynx/pharynx/eye.

Active physical therapy

After major injury or illness, in addition to the directly related impairments to neurological, musculoskeletal, and cardiovascular systems, prolonged bed rest and immobility lead to deconditioning with reduction in strength, endurance, and fitness. Physical therapy and exercise aims to increase ROM and muscle strength and endurance, improve balance, motor control and co-ordination, teach important functional skills, and upgrade physical fitness to enhance overall performance and independence.

Broadly, therapeutic exercise can be divided into the following components:

- strengthening and endurance
- stretching
- balancing, motor control and co-ordination
- cardiovascular fitness.

Strengthening and endurance

The principle of 'overload' generally used in strength training is not entirely applicable to major trauma without judicious modification of the programme to avoid producing further injury or delaying healing while promoting progressive physiological and psychological adaptation.

Exercise prescription entails specification of the following:

- type of exercise
- intensity
- number of repetitions and sets
- recovery interval.

Traditionally, different guidelines have been used for muscle strengthening (high resistance, low repetitions) and training endurance (low resistance, high repetitions), although there are crossover effects. Exercises may be performed either concentrically or eccentrically, with the former more usual early after traumatic injury.

The different types of exercise used for muscle strengthening and training endurance are isometric, isotonic, and isokinetic:

- *Isometric* exercises contracting muscles without joint movement can be used when joint motion is painful or contraindicated, but are of limited value due to angle specificity. A maximal contraction is held for 5 seconds with 5–10 repetitions. Care must be taken with individuals with a high resting blood pressure or underlying cardiovascular disease, owing to pressor response.
- *Isotonic* exercises are the most commonly used during rehabilitation after serious injury. As already mentioned, the exercise programme

should be customized to the clinical situation, carefully monitored, and progressively upgraded as possible. An arbitrary starting intensity must be chosen, for example 3 sets of 10–15 repetitions at 40–65% of 1 repetition maximum (1RM). This endurance type of programme (low/medium resistance, low/medium repetitions) allows the patient to become familiar with exercises and provides a stimulus to improve motor unit recruitment. The range provided allows some flexibility and ability to progressively upgrade the programme. When muscle strength in particular is a limiting factor (e.g. to lift body weight against gravity to transfer independently) a predominant strength programme, for example 1 set of 6–8 repetitions at 85–100% of 1 RM, may be used. Care must be taken when prescribing exercises not to generate excessive torsional forces around injured joints and bones.

- *Isokinetic* exercise using a dynamometer such as TM after Orthoton, Cybex, or Kincom allows maximum tension to be safely exerted throughout complete range of movement, but is generally only used for rehabilitation after traumatic injury to larger joints, e.g. knee.

As strength and endurance improve in individual muscle groups, the exercise programme will progressively incorporate more functional activities involving combined patterns of movement.

Flexibility

Extended periods of bed rest and non-weight-bearing will result in muscle shortening and contracture. This is most common at the hip, knee, and ankle. Maintenance stretching regimes range from 30 to 60 seconds, three repetitions twice daily. Self-implemented slow stretch and techniques progressing to the level of discomfort can be demonstrated to the patient (Fig. 42.1) (Sherry and

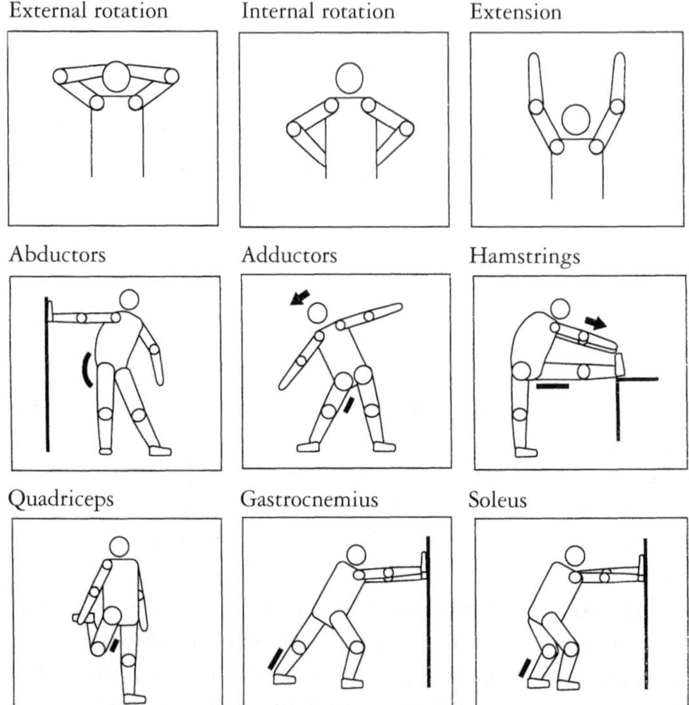

Figure 42.1 Muscle stretching exercises.

Wilson 1998). Ballistic (bouncing) exercises should be avoided because of the risk of muscle tears.

In established contractures, longer and more frequent stretching is required to restore muscle length. These passive techniques should be administered by a physiotherapist. Passive stretching may be combined with the use of mechanical devices and serial splinting.

Proprioception

Ligaments, tendons, and joints are involved in determining position sense of limbs. Rehabilitation for damage to these structures should include retraining for balance and co-ordination. Supervised balance exercises on one or two legs involve distractions of visual cues, e.g. blindfold bouncing or throwing of balls. The patient progresses from static to dynamic exercises to mobility on flat and rough or undulating surfaces or a moving surface (wobble board). Proprioception may be temporarily enhanced by use of taping around joints due to increased sensory input.

Cardiovascular fitness

Exercise prescription for cardiovascular conditioning entails specification of the following:

- type of exercise
- frequency
- intensity
- duration
- length of programme
- interval/rest interval (if continuous exercise not possible).

The type of exercise prescribed (e.g. cycling, arm ergometry) will depend to some extent on the clinical situation. A frequency of 3–4 times per week is usually recommended. Intensity must be adjusted to 40–70% of heart rate reserve (HRR). HRR is calculated by subtracting resting heart rate from age-predicted or observed peak heart rate. Standard formulas to determine maximum heart rate (e.g. 220 − age) are not reliable when a patient is significantly impaired and deconditioned after injury. Under these circumstances, peak heart rate is best determined using a progressive stress test (e.g. cycling, arm ergometry). Exercise duration should be a minimum of 20 minutes lasting up to 40 minutes. A programme should run for a minimum of 8 weeks to provide a benefit. If someone is unable to perform continuous exercise for at least 20 minutes, then interval training can be used instead. Exercise for a period of 5–7 minutes is undertaken followed by a rest interval of half the exercise time or when HRR drops below 40%. Like other therapies, an individually tailored programme can be provided by consultation with an exercise specialist.

Key points

- The principle generally used in strength training of 'overload' is not entirely applicable to major trauma.
- The type of exercise prescribed (e.g. cycling, arm ergometry) will depend to some extent on the clinical situation.

Checklist for major injury

Reflex sympathetic dystrophy (also known as complex regional pain syndrome, type 1)

This is covered in Chapter 16 (page 279).

Rehabilitation after amputation

Overview

Amputations due to trauma have been reported to account for over 20% of all amputations (Goldberg 1985). This percentage is dropping in developed countries as a result of better road safety, industrial standards, and advances in replantation surgery (Ebskov 1992).

The causes for traumatic amputation in developing countries are quite different. In India, train accidents are a frequent cause. In Africa and South-East Asia, war and unexploded landmines contribute to the problem. Estimations for traumatic amputation may be as high as 1 amputee per 256 people in Cambodia and 1 per 470 in Angola, compared to a figure of only 1 per 22 000 in the USA (Staats 1992).

Lower limb trauma is a far more frequent cause for amputation than upper limb, with a ratio of approximately 11 : 1. Overall figures (from all causes) for amputation levels reflect the trend to preserve the knee for proprioceptive input and length for biomechanical efficiency. Published figures (Fyfe 1990) show: above knee 38%, below knee 54%, through knee/Gritti–Stokes 6%, Symes (through ankle) 1%, forefoot 1% (Lisfranc, Pirigoff, Chopart).

Key point

- Amputations due to trauma have been reported as accounting for >20% of all amputations.

Key issues in the rehabilitation of the lower-limb amputee

Surgery

Preservation of limb length has implications for prosthetic fitting and the eventual energy cost of ambulation. Increased energy costs of ambulation are reflected in the comfortable walking speed of amputees compared to normal. A study of traumatic amputees demonstrated a velocity of 87% of normal at the below-knee level and 63% at the above-knee level when using a prosthesis. An even greater effort is required when using crutches (Waters *et al.* 1976).

Balance and stability of joints of the required residual limb will result in better prosthetic outcome and activity for the amputee in above-knee transfemoral amputees. This is achieved by myodesis of the adductor magnus to the remaining femur. In transtibial amputation the musculotendinous portion of the gastrocnemius is tethered to the anterior distal tibia as a posterior flap. It is desirable to achieve skin closure without tension (Bowker and Michael 1992).

Key point

- Preservation of limb length has implications for prosthetic fitting.

Stump care

Early amputation stump management is essential as a means of hastening prosthetic rehabilitation. A variety of methods are used postoperatively with the same intention:

- rapid resolution of stump oedema
- prevention of stump fibrosis
- promotion of would healing
- wound protection
- desensitization and pain management
- reduction of infection
- early mobilization and weight bearing
- muscle strengthening and stability
- anticontracture treatment.

Key points

- Early amputation stump management is essential.

The following techniques are currently in use:

- The non-removable rigid dressing is applied in the operating theatre and maintained until removal of sutures at about 2 weeks postoperatively (Jones and Burniston 1970). The advantages are early (7–14 days) weight bearing through the plaster of Paris dressing and early mobilization with a temporary prosthesis applied at the end of week 2–3 postoperatively when the dressing is removed. This technique is used in only 8% of centres in the USA because of the need for access for inspection of the surgical incision.
- The removable rigid dressing can be applied postoperatively and used continuously until a temporary or definitive prosthesis is fitted (Yeongchi and Krick 1987). The advantages are that the wound may be inspected as required and stump socks may be applied as the stump shrinks. The additional use of a supporting strap allows patients to perform quadriceps exercise, anticontracture, and antioedema

movement while sitting in a wheelchair (Hughes *et al.* 1998).

- Elastic bandaging, stockingette, and support stockings (shrinkers) are the most commonly used techniques. Stump compression may commence within 1–3 days postoperatively, depending on wound condition and pain tolerance. Bandaging techniques should provide more distal than proximal compression. Correct bandaging and avoidance of a tourniquet effect is essential. Stump compression with bandaging or stocking usually continues for 12–18 months postoperatively at times when the prosthesis is not in use.

Contractures

Contractures at the hip and knee form quickly with the loss of the limb as a lever. An anticontracture programme should start within the first postoperative week. This programme involves lying prone for 30 minutes twice daily to encourage extension at the hip. Knee exercises involve 10 second isometric quadriceps exercises 10 repetitions every hour. An extension *stump board* should be attached to the wheelchair for below-knee amputees.

Mobilization

Mobilization should occur as soon as tolerated. Partial weight transference through a rigid dressing should be attempted after the first postoperative week with full weight bearing as tolerated after sutures are removed. After the third week an interim prosthesis should be considered to commence gait training. The choices are either a polypropylene patellar tendon bearing socket for the below-knee amputee or a quadrelateral ischial weight-bearing socket for the above-knee amputee. Modular aluminium tubing shanks or pylons with solid ankle cushion heel (SACH) feet are commonly used, and in the above-knee amputee a single-axis semi-locking *safety knee* may be fitted. Because of the need for socket changes over the first weeks or months, some centres use other alternatives until fitting of the definitive prosthesis. Sockets for interim prostheses may be fabricated in plaster of Paris, or a variety of resin wraps. Pneumatic weight-bearing temporary prostheses utilize an air splint inflated around the stump and enclosed in a metal frame (Little 1971). They have been used from day 6 postoperatively and, as with other interim methods, aid in reduction of oedema, maturation, and shaping of the above- or below-knee stump (Redhead *et al.* 1978).

Pain management

Pain management is necessary to reduce the incidence of postoperative phantom pain. Postoperative pain relief may be achieved by narcotic analgesics, spinal anaesthesia, or local anaesthetic infusions into sensory nerves. Narcotic analgesics and other methods usually cease by day 5–7 when simple analgesia (i.e. paracetamol) is adequate for treating stump and wound pain. Phantom sensation occurs in nearly all patients. Phantom pain often commences as stump pain and subsides in the second or third postoperative week. The pain may be episodic and stabbing, or of a constant and burning nature. Adequate stump compression bandaging, massage, physical, and diversional therapy may be useful in the daytime. Often the pain is worse at night, with the patient finding it difficult to sleep. Simple analgesics with an adjuvant medication may assist sleeping and reduce phantom pain. Medications often used are tricyclic antidepressants such as amitriptyline and doxepin. Sometimes an antiepileptic medication is added or used as an alternative, e.g. carbamazepine. TENS has been reported to reduce pain when applied to the amputation stump or on the contralateral limb (Carabelli 1985).

Psychological adaptation

Psychological adaptation to the loss of a limb is associated with grief and mourning (Elberlik 1980, Furst and Humphrey 1983). The phases of denial, anger, depression, and acceptance may continue over months or years after amputation. There is a functional impairment which can be compensated for by fitting of a prosthesis. This is not always accompanied by an adjustment of body image. Counselling with patients and family adjustment to disability, body image, and roles in the family and society is integral to the rehabilitation process. Relaxation and pain coping techniques are useful skills.

Rehabilitation of traumatic spinal cord injury

Overview

Traumatic spinal cord injury (SCI) has an incidence of approximately 15–30 per million population. Young males between 16–30 years of age are at greatest risk, with motor vehicle-related injury the most common cause, followed by falls, sporting/recreational accidents, and violence in some countries (Go *et al.* 1995). Improved survival after injury has resulted from better roadside resuscitation, rapid retrieval to specialized trauma centres, and intensive medical care. Likewise, advances in rehabilitation and management of complications after SCI, as well as long-term medical follow-up by dedicated spinal cord injury specialists have lead to improved life expectancy and quality of life for individuals with SCI.

Key rehabilitation issues

Successful rehabilitation after severe SCI involves not only developing as much functional independence as possible through physical training, adaptive techniques, and specialized aids (Fig. 42.1), but also adjusting to disability and ultimately re-establishing a fulfilling lifestyle in the community with satisfying roles and interests. Intensive, interdisciplinary rehabilitation as an inpatient provides the initial stepping stones for reintegration into the community, but in many ways rehabilitation only really begins once the person has returned home.

The purpose of this section is not to provide a comprehensive coverage of all aspects of rehabilitation after SCI, but rather to highlight some key issues and the importance of early rehabilitation to prevent complications and achieve the best functional outcome.

Skin

After SCI patients are at great risk of developing skin complications due to factors such as immobility, loss of protective sensation, weight loss, and altered tissue viability. The injured patient should be transferred off the spinal board immediately on arrival in hospital and the skin over entire body including the back must be inspected for evidence of injury or pressure as soon as possible (Mawson *et al.* 1988). Nutritional status must be closely monitored with the aid of a dietitian and enteral or parenteral nutrition considered early to avoid later complications of altered body composition such as decubitus ulceration secondary to poor coverage of bony points.

Patients should be managed on an appropriate mattress, such as a convoluted foam mattress initially and later a ripple mattress, and must be turned or lifted and repositioned every 2 hours by a team of four trained staff with the skin checked. Sheepskins may also prove helpful. Particular attention must be given to areas at greater risk overlying any bony prominence, such as the sacrum and heels when lying supine or greater trochanter, medial aspect of knee, and lateral malleolus if lying on one side.

Essential measures to avoid pressure problems in the longer term include the following:

- Appropriate prescription of equipment such as mattress overlay, commode chair, or toilet seat cover and pressure-relieving cushion for wheelchair (such as air floatation, gel, or cut-out foam design).
- Regular pressure relief when sitting by lifting, leaning forward or to one side, or tilting motorized wheelchair in space for 15–30 seconds 2–3 times an hour.
- Self-inspection of skin (with assistance if necessary) using a mirror to monitor for pressure marks twice daily.

Key point

- After SCI patients are at great risk of developing skin complications.

Pain

Pain frequently accompanies SCI and can significantly affect a person's functional ability, ability to return to work, psychological well-being, and quality of life. At present there are no clear links between acute pain management and longer-term outcomes. However, some evidence is emerging from studies in other areas such as phantom limb pain after amputation to suggest that early treatment may be helpful for preventing later development of chronic pain. Pain should therefore be vigorously treated during the acute period. Patients are more likely to be actively involved in rehabilitation when pain is adequately controlled.

The most important issue in the treatment of pain is to correctly classify the type of pain, which most commonly is either musculoskeletal or neuropathic (Siddall *et al.* 1997). Classification is crucial in terms of determining the appropriate treatment. As with other types of acute musculoskeletal pain, opioids are effective. In contrast, the management of neuropathic pain remains difficult. There are currently no available treatments that consistently and effectively alleviate this problem, although a number of treatments are in current use (Siddall *et al.* 1998).

In the acute phase, local anaesthetics such as lignocaine (lidocaine) administered subcutaneously or intravenously may be useful and, if effective, followed by mexiletine orally. Anecdotally, ketamine infusion has also been described, although side-effects may be limiting. With chronic pain, a tricyclic antidepressant such as amitriptyline alone or in combination with an anticonvulsant such as carbamazepine or sodium valproate is commonly used. More recently, anecdotal reports suggest the effectiveness of gabapentin in treating intractable neuropathic pain.

Other techniques which have proved helpful in some cases include anaesthetic blockade at various levels—sympathetic, epidural, or spinal blockades—and intrathecal administration of baclofen, clonidine, and morphine via an implanted pump.

Physical treatments including exercise and hydrotherapy programmes, postural re-education, wheelchair and seating adjustments, and possibly other physical modalities are often helpful in managing pain resulting from a mechanical cause. It should never be forgotten that pain is a complex phenomenon and that emotional, behavioural, and environmental factors may contribute to the experience of pain. Therefore, attention should always be paid to psychological factors and the use of cognitive-behavioural techniques and strategies such as relaxation and distraction.

Key point

- Correctly classify the type of pain.

Positioning and contracture prevention

Contractures may develop as the result of immobilization and poor positioning, spasticity, or muscle imbalance around a joint, and interfere with later rehabilitation. During the acute phase, it is important to ensure that all joints are correctly positioned, rested in mid-position of function and regularly moved passively through a full ROM at least once daily.

Problems due to shortening of shoulder capsule can be prevented by daily positioning of shoulders in abduction and external rotation (the crucifix position). Foot drop can be prevented with a pillow or bolster at the foot of bed maintaining the ankle in neutral position.

In the individual with C5 or partial C6 tetraplegia without antigravity strength wrist extension, splinting of fingers and hand at rest with a long opponens wrist–hand orthosis is used to maintain wrist in 15–30° extension, metacarpophalangeal (MCP) joints in 60° and thumb in abduction. Particular attention in the tetraplegic hand must be given to prevention of clawing (intrinsic-minus hand posture) and MCP joint, proximal interphalangeal joint (apart from functional finger flexor tightness for tenodesis), and thumb adduction contractures. Presence of such contractures can ultimately limit effectiveness of tenodesis grasp (natural finger flexion with wrist extension), use of a wrist-driven flexor-hinge splint, and potential for later tendon-transfer surgery (Keith and Lacey 1991).

Spasticity

Spasticity is a common problem in SCI patients with upper motor neurone lesions after spinal shock and tends to increase in severity during the first few months after injury. Severe spasticity during the early phase after injury may exacerbate pain, predispose to pressure sores, and contribute to development of contractures. Spasticity which is evident early and very pronounced or not symmetrical may indicate an incomplete lesion.

Treatment should usually be instituted if spasticity interferes with functional independence, endangers safety when transferring, causes pain, or places skin at risk from shearing. Management is normally approached using a hierarchical model of care, beginning with the simplest and least invasive measures and progressing to more invasive methods as required (Merritt 1981).

When the degree of spasticity increases significantly without obvious explanation, consideration must always be given to looking for aggravating factors such as:

- urinary tract infection
- renal or bladder calculi
- constipation
- skin ulceration
- ingrown toenails
- less commonly, intra-abdominal or pelvic problems.

Key point

- Spasticity is a common problem in SCI patients.

Regular stretching is important to maintain muscle length, particularly hip flexors and plantar flexors. Medications commonly used include baclofen (10–25 mg four times daily) and diazepam (5–7.5 mg three times or four times daily). Other medications less commonly used include dantrolene sodium and clonidine. Motor point injections with botulinum toxin, phenol, or alcohol, or more definitive surgical approaches such as tendon lengthening, tenotomy and/or neurectomy, may be used for localized spasticity, and intrathecal management (Penn *et al.* 1989) with baclofen may be used for more difficult generalized spasticity. Surgical techniques such as rhizotomies, myelotomies, and cordotomies are rarely if ever indicated.

Neurogenic bladder

Overdistension of the neurogenic bladder during the acute period should be avoided until after the post-injury diuresis has occurred by indwelling urethral catheter or percutaneous suprapubic drainage (e.g. Cystocath) on continuous drainage. Catheter clamping for 2 hours twice daily may help to maintain bladder capacity and compliance. After this period, regular intermittent catheterization by an attendant may be commenced with appropriate fluid restriction.

Choice of definitive bladder management will be influenced by factors such as:

- type of bladder impairment
- functional ability (particularly mobility, sitting balance and hand function)
- patient's motivation and lifestyle.

The types of bladder impairment occurring after SCI may be classified as:

- *suprasacral* or reflex (upper motor neurone type)
- *infrasacral* or acontractile (lower motor neurone type)
- *mixed* (conus lesions).

It is important to remember that different underlying impairments may lead to similar outward appearance of bladder dysfunction, e.g. detrusor hyperreflexia, poor bladder compliance, or bladder neck insufficiency all cause storage failure, while similarly detrusor–sphincter dyssynergia (DSD), acontractile bladder or myogenic insufficiency from chronic overdistension may cause voiding failure (Wein 1981). Common clinical presentations of DSD include high residuals and recurrent urinary tract infections, autonomic dysreflexia on voiding, increased spasticity, posture-related difficulty in voiding, and upper tract deterioration. Urodynamic assessment (cystometry/anal sphincter EMG or X-ray videocystography) is performed after passage of spinal shock to help to classify bladder type (Watanabe *et al.* 1996).

Goals for bladder management include:

- *protecting* upper urinary tracts from sustained high pressure (<40 cm H_2O)
- *minimizing* post-void residual volumes (ideally <50 mL)
- *preventing* urinary tract infections
- *ensuring* social continence.

In both male and female patients with paraplegia or males with tetraplegia and sufficient hand function, clean intermittent self-catheterization (CISC) every 4–6 hours with anticholinergic medication such as oxybutynin hydrochloride (5 mg three times daily) or propantheline bromide (15–30 mg three or four times daily) to relax the bladder is the preferred method.

In males with tetraplegia and insufficient hand function to perform CISC, drainage by reflex voiding with tapping, Valsalva or Credé manoeuvre using an external collection device or indwelling urethral or suprapubic catheter is possible. If employing bladder training to achieve balanced reflex voiding, use of short-term cholinergic medication such as bethanecol (10–20 mg three times daily) to enhance detrusor tone with an alpha-adrenergic blocker such as phenoxybenzamine (10 mg three times daily) to reduce internal sphincter spasm is frequently required. In addition, a sphincterotomy or urethral wall stent may also be required to help manage DSD. Urinary antiseptic medications to lower pH of urine, such as hippuric acid and vitamin C or cranberry juice/tablets, which in addition appears to inhibit bacterial adhesion, are often prescribed particularly in patients using reflex emptying or CISC. In female tetraplegic patients either suprapubic or indwelling urethral catheter is most common because of the greater difficulty of management.

Urinary tract calculi are a common complication that should be suspected when difficulty clearing or recurrent urinary tract infections with the same or different organisms, particularly urea-splitting *Proteus*. These will require removal by lithopaxy, lithotripsy, or (rarely) open methods.

Regular follow-up by ultrasound examination or intravenous pyelogram every 2 years unless indicated more frequently because of previous abnormal study is recommended, particularly in those patients using reflex voiding/expression techniques to monitor for early signs of hydroureter/hydronephrosis (Staskin 1991).

Key point

- Overdistension of the neurogenic bladder during the acute period should be avoided.

Neurogenic bowel

Patients should be kept nil by mouth initially until bowel sounds return. A nasogastric tube is required to decompress the stomach and reduce abdominal distension until ileus resolves to prevent vomiting and risk of aspiration as well as respiratory compromise due to diaphragmatic splinting. H_2 receptor antagonists should be used to combat low pH and stress ulceration. Initially, the neurogenic bowel is emptied with assistance by an attendant, usually daily.

Later bowel management (Banwell *et al.* 1993, Stiens *et al.* 1997) will involve:

- Developing a regular bowel routine (daily or every second day).
- Adequate fluid intake (approximately 2000 mL/day).
- Healthy eating habits with a well-balanced diet high in fibre, such as from whole grain breads, cereals, fruits, and vegetables.
- Stool bulking agents such as psyllium and softening agents such as dioctyl sodium sulphosuccinate (commonly used to increase water content and volume of stool, soften and

regulate stool consistency, and promote intestinal evacuation).

- Avoidance of irritant laxatives such as senna and bisacodyl if possible (these may be used in the short term to help establish a satisfactory bowel programme, but are best avoided in the longer term due to unpredictability of results, tolerance, and potential long-term side-effects).
- Bowel emptying timed 20–30 minutes after a meal (to utilize gastrocolic reflex).
- Rectal emptying achieved using an enema, suppositories, digital stimulation and/or manual evacuation; the latter is particularly helpful in lower motor neurone type bowel dysfunction.

Psychological issues

The reality of a sudden traumatic SCI with the inherent disbelief, fear, sadness, and uncertainty about the future places enormous stress on both the injured individual and their family. In this setting, anxiety and depression are common after SCI (Craig *et al.* 1994). Post-traumatic stress disorder may also occur early after injury in which the injured individual re-experiences the traumatic event with distressing flashbacks or nightmares often associated with a variety of physical symptoms and increased arousal (APA 1994).

In the past perhaps insufficient attention has been paid to psychosocial assessment and adjustment after injury, but their importance to the overall success of rehabilitation (Trieschmann 1988) and the value of specific interventions such as cognitive-behavioural therapy are now well recognized (Craig *et al.* 1997). The very specialized area of psychosocial rehabilitation following SCI requires intensive and co-ordinated input from an experienced psychologist and social worker.

Key point

- The reality of a sudden traumatic SCI with the inherent disbelief, fear, sadness, and uncertainty about the future places enormous stress on the injured person and their family.

Fertility

Infertility is common in males after SCI due to anejaculation or poor semen quality. Since the majority of spinal injuries occur to young, single men this is an important issue. Two methods of semen retrieval are commonly used, vibroejaculation and electroejaculation (Linsenmeyer 1993). Vibroejaculation is the most frequently used method in patients with lesions above T11 level. However, electroejaculation may be used in the acute phase for collection of semen, when vibroejaculation will be unsuccessful in the presence of spinal shock (Mallidis *et al.* 1994). When this technique is performed within 7–10 days after injury, semen quality is usually normal and can be cryopreserved for future use. Problems with reduced sperm quality later can be overcome using assisted reproductive technologies, such as *in vitro* fertilization (IVF) and micromanipulation techniques (Linsenmeyer 1993).

Key point

- Infertility is common in men after SCI.

Autonomic dysreflexia (hyperreflexia)

Autonomic dysreflexia is peculiar to individuals with SCI above the splanchnic outflow (lesion generally above the T6 level) and is the result of dissociation from higher centres. A triggering sensory stimulus initiates excessive reflex activity of the sympathetic nervous system below the level of injury, causing vasoconstriction and a rapid rise in blood pressure, which is uncontrolled due to isolation from the normal regulatory response of vasomotor centres in the brain. Parasympathetic activity occurs when the rise in blood pressure is sensed by baroreceptors in the aortic arch and carotid bodies resulting in compensatory slowing of the heart and dilatation of blood vessels above the level of injury. If not recognized or treated promptly the blood pressure may rise to dangerously high levels and precipitate intracranial haemorrhage, seizures, or a cardiac arrhythmia (Braddom and Rocco 1991, Colachis 1992).

Common symptoms and signs are:

- sudden hypertension (Remember blood pressure for these individuals is usually around 90/60–100/60 mmHg lying down and possibly lower while sitting, so patients may become symptomatic with blood pressure in the normal range for population. If untreated this can rapidly rise to dangerously high levels.)
- pounding headache
- bradycardia
- flushing/blotching of the skin
- sweating above spinal injury level
- goose bumps
- chills without fever
- nasal stuffiness
- blurred vision (dilatation of pupils)
- shortness of breath and associated anxiety.

Common causes include:

- *bladder:* distended or severely spastic bladder, urinary tract infection, urological procedure, or even inserting a catheter
- *bowel:* distended rectum, enema irritation
- *skin:* pressure sores, burns, ingrown toenails, tight clothing
- *other:* any irritating stimulus, including fracture, renal stones, epididymo-orchitis, distended stomach, labour, severe menstrual cramping.

It is vitally important to remember that autonomic dysreflexia is a *medical emergency* requiring urgent treatment (detailed in Table 42.4).

Key point

- Autonomic dysreflexia (hyperreflexia) is a medical emergency.

Rehabilitation after traumatic brain injury

Overview

Traumatic brain injury (TBI) affects predominantly males under 40 years of age (Lyle *et al.* 1986, Jennett 1996). Long-term disability and handicap issues relate to cognitive and behavioural impact on social role, with little correlation with physical disability (Jennet *et al.* 1981, Oddy 1984, Oddy *et al.* 1985, Tate *et al.* 1989, Powell and Wilson 1994). In particular, disrupted families and social contacts and poor work return are prevalent. These are significant issues even for people who have made a good recovery and require long-term strategies implemented by a team working with the patient and their family.

Most recovery and most rapid changes in terms of Glasgow Outcome Score (GOS) (Table 42.5) occurs in the first 6 months (Jennett *et al.* 1981, Multi-Society Task Force on PVS 1994). Of those who have good recovery or are moderately disabled at 12 months, almost two-thirds are already at that level at 3 months and 90% at 6 months.

However, recovery significant to the individual can be seen over 3–4 years after accident, particularly in people with more severe disability (Powell and Wilson 1994). This highlights the requirement for adequate follow-up.

Key point

- Traumatic brain injury (TBI) affects predominantly males under 40 years of age.

Pathology and outcomes

Poorer prognosis is associated with older age (Vollmer *et al.* 1991); forces of injury; evidence of hypoxia or hypotension; acute subdural haematoma; widespread contusions; raised intracranial pressure; low GCS in the first 24 hours after resuscitation and longer duration of PTA.

Diffuse axonal injury is usual and may have few changes on acute CT scan. Low GCS and duration of PTA may be better indications. The characteristic frontal and temporal distribution of contusions (Courville 1937) is associated with planning, organizing, and executive impairments, personality and behaviour control changes, and memory impairments (Oddy *et al.* 1985). These deficits have been associated with unemployment levels

Table 42.4 Treatment protocol for autonomic dysreflexia

1	Initial steps	Elevate the patient's head and lower the legs Ask patient if they suspect a cause Loosen any constricting clothing Check bladder drainage equipment for kinks or other causes of obstruction to flow (such as clogging of inlet to leg bag or overfull leg bag) Monitor BP every 2–5 minutes Avoid pressing over the bladder
2	Further treatment	If symptoms persist or BP remains elevated following the above efforts or a cause cannot be quickly identified, antihypertensive treatment (see 5) should be commenced whilst searching for and treating the noxious stimulus
3a	For a person with an indwelling catheter	If a blocked catheter is suspected, empty the leg bag and estimate volume. To help determine if bladder is empty or not, consider patient's fluid intake and output earlier that day and normal pattern of drainage. If catheter seems blocked, irrigate the bladder *gently* with no more than 30 mL of sterile normal saline. If urine does not drain after irrigation, recatheterize using a generous amount of lubricant containing a local anaesthetic, e.g. lignocaine (lidocaine) gel
3b	For a person wearing a uridome or doing intermittent self-catheterization	If bladder is distended and patient is unable to void in their usual manner, lubricate the urethra with a generous amount of lignocaine (lidocaine) gel, wait 2 minutes and then pass a catheter to empty bladder Leave catheter *in situ* until reason for retention is identified and remedied NB: If BP declines after bladder is empty, the person still requires close observation as the bladder can go into severe contractions causing hypertension to recur (see pharmacological treatment)
4	For faecal evacuation	If you are sure the bladder is empty and symptoms persist, gently insert a generous amount of lignocaine gel into the rectum. Wait 5 minutes before gently inserting a finger to remove faecal matter NB: Monitor BP closely during digital stimulation and if it increases significantly, cease digital stimulation and only recommence under cover of nifedipine (see below)
5	Pharmacological treatment	Nifedipine should be given by puncturing a 10 mg capsule (or 2×5 mg capsules) and squeezing contents into mouth from capsule and swallowing. The dose may be repeated after 10 minutes. Glyceryl trinitrate (GTN) is an alternative, preferably as a sublingual spray.

Table 42.4 Continued

	If hypertension is not relieved by nifedipine or glyceryl trinitrate, then administration of parenteral antihypertensive medications will be required in an acute hospital setting Where control of the noxious stimulus is difficult, regional epidural anaesthesia may be appropriate
If hypertension recurs in the presence of an indwelling catheter	Instil lignocaine (lidocaine) for injection (10 ml of 1% solution) via a catheter, flush with a further 10 ml of saline and clamp for 5 minutes. This can be repeated 2-hourly for 6 doses if necessary Administer an oral anticholinergic eg. Oxybutynin.

Modified from Patient Emergency Treatment Card, Royal North Shore Hospital, Sydney, with permission of S Rutkowski, J Middleton and G Bashford.

Table 42.5 Glasgow Outcome Scale (GOS): a global measure of outcome in five categories

Group	Characteristics
Dead	
Vegetative	Prolonged unconsciousness with no verbalization, no following of commands, and no meaningful interaction with the environment
Severely disabled	Presence of residual disabilities that prevent the patient from independent function for any 24 hour period (both physical and cognitive deficits are included)
Moderately disabled	Residual deficits that, although significant, do not prevent an independent lifestyle
Good recovery	Minor or no residual deficits.

Reproduced with permission from Jennett B, Bond M (1975) Assessment of outcome after severe brain damage. *Lancet* i: 480–487.© The Lancet Ltd.

(Brooks *et al.* 1987, Crepeau and Scherzer 1993). Penetrating injury, haematomas, and infarction superimpose focal syndromes on the diffuse and polar injuries. Hypoxia, subdural haematoma, vascular spasm with subarachnoid haemorrhage, cerebral oedema, and hydrocephalus may all complicate the presentation. The multiple pathologies overlap to cause individual clinical presentation and may place significant caveats to functional prognostication for the individual (Choi *et al.* 1988).

Mild head injury (GCS 13–15 or PTA <1 hour), which accounts for 70–90% of admitted TBI, can have an appreciable incidence of sequelae including headaches, memory changes, and unemployment after several months (Rimel *et al.* 1981).

Key point

- Poorer prognosis is associated with older age.

Coma and poor responsiveness

Plum and Posner (1980) characterized coma by:

- unarousable psychological unresponsiveness
- closed eyes
- no psychologically understandable response to external stimulus or inner need
- neither producing understandable words nor accurately localizing noxious stimuli with discrete defensive movements.

This is a feature of acute injury and is self-limiting, rarely lasting longer than 4 weeks.

Duration of coma is associated with outcome, with only one third or less of those in coma longer than 2 weeks or more making a good to moderate recovery (on the GOS), in comparison with 80–90% of those with coma <2 weeks (Lyle *et al.* 1986).

Pathophysiology

The content of conscious behaviour is a reflection of arousal and cognitive behaviour. Arousal is a product of the brainstem reticular system interacting with the cerebral cortex. Loss of consciousness occurs with dysfunction either of upper brainstem structures or diffusely of the cortex. The upper brainstem and cortical connections seem particularly liable to injury where the head is free to move on the trunk (Gennarelli *et al.* 1982).

Coma should be distinguished from brainstem death, persistent vegetative state, locked-in syndrome, and severe disability with minimal responsiveness.

Management

Progress is monitored clinically, including the GCS, to identify complications. Exacerbating factors are excluded, particularly hydrocephalus or intracranial space-occupying lesion; Electrolyte disorders; sepsis; drug toxicity; seizures. Medications are critically reviewed, minimizing those associated with adverse central nervous system effects or negative effects on recovery, particularly sedatives, anticonvulsants, anticholinergics, and sympatholytic agents.

- *Nutrition:* Energy requirements are usually underestimated by calculation of the Harris–Benedict equation (Wilson and Tyburski 1998), because of the significant catabolic state associated with TBI. Management requires regular review of nutrition parameters and adjustment of intake. Gastrostomy feeding may not necessarily prevent aspiration, being associated with an appreciable risk of reflux aspiration (Finucane and Bynum 1996). Indication for gastrostomy feeding include agitation and risk of inappropriate removal in post-coma recovery.
- *Bowel care:* Regular enema and aperient regimen with the aim of establishing predictable evacuation, promoting good nursing care, hygiene, and skin care.
- *Bladder:* Early removal of urinary catheter and management with a collection device is preferable, to minimize the risk of infection and bladder dysfunction. Monitoring for urinary retention is required initially.
- *Immobility:* Skin management, management of hypertonia, and maintenance of joint ROM require appropriate bed, seating system, splinting materials, pharmacotherapy, and staff expertise. A programme of positioning, maintained stretching, seating, and splinting needs to be managed.
- *Respiratory:* Clinical monitoring, tracheostomy, and airway management require attention to chest physiotherapy, posturing, and oral care.

Family knowledge and education are addressed and as are issues such as emotional support, income support, and access to community assistance.

After the period of coma (rarely >4 weeks after onset), the person establishes a new state in recovery. The key issues after emergence from coma are the need to identify the degree of the person's ability to interact with their surroundings and the setting up of programmes to promote their participation and skills acquisition.

For people thought to be suffering from the vegetative state, it is important to distinguish this from severe disability with minimal responsiveness (Table 42.6). Misdiagnosis remains a risk. Recent reviews of referrals to two specialist units showed 30–40% or more of people incorrectly diagnosed as having persistent vegetative state. Visual impairment was common.

Post-traumatic amnesia

PTA is a self-limiting confusional syndrome characteristically following closed head injury in which new memories are unable to be reliably established, often associated with agitation. It is distinct from retrograde amnesia in which memory is lost for events occurring before the incident. Inasmuch as it is defined by being self-limiting, it is can only be confirmed retrospectively.

The patient is inattentive and distractible, unable to orientate to the environment or recent events. They are unable to learn to compensate for other

Table 42.6 Differential diagnosis of minimal responsiveness after traumatic brain injury

Condition	Features	Key points
Brainstem death	Loss of brainstem function, with inability to maintain homeostasis Irremediable structural damage	Assessment of brainstem physiology Exclude remediable causes
Coma	Eyes closed Unarousable unresponsiveness no psychologically understandable response to external or internal stimulus	Ventilation/sedation/ paralysis and facial injury interfere with assessment GCS monitoring
Persistent vegetative state	Complete unawareness of the self or environment No evidence of attention, intention or learning Cyclical sleeping and awakening Autonomic function permits survival Bowel and bladder incontinence Any activities are part of 'subcortical, instinctively patterned, reflexive response to external stimuli' (Multi-Society Task Force on PVS, 1994)	Persistent' = more than 1 month post injury Persistent not the same as permanent Diagnosis after recurrent assessment in a variety of situations by several observers Risk of misdiagnosis (Andrews *et al.* 1996, Childs *et al.* 1993)
Locked-in syndrome	Retained consciousness and cognition Quadriparesis and brainstem motor impairment	Rare Usually vascular aetiology (rarely traumatic)
Severe disability with minimal responsiveness	Cognitive and motor impairment so severe that the presence of awareness may have been in doubt	

sensory, language, or cognitive deficits related to injury and unable to recall explanations for injuries. Agitation, confabulation, disinhibition, or uncharacteristic behaviour may occur. Patient safety and avoidance of elopement may be prominent management problems, with lack of insight into safety or requirements for injury healing.

Problems of retrospective assessment of PTA duration lead to development of prospective measures such as the Galveston Orientation and Amnesia Test (Levin *et al.* 1979), Westmead PTA Scale (Shores *et al.* 1986) and the Oxford PTA scale. The latter provide a hierarchy of orientation and recent memory tasks.

Key point

- PTA is a self-limiting confusional syndrome.

Russell and Nathan (1946) related PTA to return to full duty by military servicemen (Table 42.7). Jennett and Teasdale (1981) noted the relationship between PTA and outcome in terms of GOS for a group of patients admitted with severe head injuries (GCS 8 or less), adding an 'extremely severe' category for PTA >4 weeks duration (Table 42.8).

Management

Monitoring progress of PTA helps identify patients in whom exacerbating factors should be sought, and identifying when resolution of PTA allows benefit from education and strategies in rehabilitation.

Careful clinical survey is required to avoid additional morbidity from mismanagement of associated injuries, particularly when agitation is a prominent feature. Particular attention is required to managing sources of pain and impairments of vision and hearing, often needing serial evaluation and observation over time.

Other causes of delirium need to be excluded (Table 42.9).

Key elements in orientation in a suitable environment include:

- Limit conflicting sensory stimulation and noise.
- Provide clear cues to time and place, including items of personal relevance, familiar photographs, and possessions.
- Minimize changes of location.
- Establish regular daily routine with rest periods.
- Train family and staff to deal consistently with the person. Consistency in communication may be enhanced by use of a communication log book and timetable.

Table 42.7 Relationship between PTA and return to full duty by military servicemen

PTA	Percent of work return	Classification
Nil	85	No injury
<1 hour	85	Mild injury
1–24 hours	75	Moderate injury
1–7 days	60	Severe injury
>7 days	<20	Very severe injury

Table 42.8 Relationship between PTA and outcome for patients with severe head injury (GCS <8)

PTA (days)	n	Severely disabled	Moderately disabled	Good recovery
<14	101	0%	17%	83%
15–28	96	3%	31%	66%
>28	289	30%	43%	27%

Table 42.9 Typical causes of delirium complicating PTA

Intracranial lesions	Hydrocephalus, chronic subdural haematoma, empyema
Hyponatraemia	Syndrome of inappropriate ADH, cerebral salt wasting, dilutional
Hypercalcaemia	Immobilisation in young males with fractures
Medication toxicity	Anticonvulsants; anticholinergic effects; sedatives; psychotropics; non-steroidal anti-inflammatories
Thromboembolic disease	DVT, pulmonary embolism
Seizures	Complex partial seizures
Infection	Urinary, respiratory, venous access site, wound; other, especially sinusitis, parotitis, dental

- Limit visitor numbers at any one time.
- Limit duration and scope of activities within the patient's agitation and fatigue.
- Recognize the patients inability to incorporate strategies.

Agitation is best managed without use of restraints. Environment modification and problem-solving triggering factors are a priority. Monitoring and control of the environment requires appropriate ward design with sensitivity to noise, patient interactions, and safety. Nursing on mattresses on the floor or a modified, low bed may be best for the markedly agitated patient with impaired balance. Formal behaviour control programmes are not indicated.

Where agitation cannot be managed by other means, physical restraint may be required.

Key points

- Agitation is best managed without use of restraints.
- Restraint tends to exacerbate agitation.
- Use the least restrictive option for a minimum duration at any one time.
- Be justifiable on a risk–benefit basis.
- A clear plan of management is documented.
- Regular observation, evaluation of suitability of the particular form of restraint, its effectiveness and continued necessity.
- Attend to legal obligations in the local jurisdiction (may require reference to a guardianship board or similar).

Communication and support of family and staff requires regular review. Medication management needs to observe the following principles:

- Withdraw any potentially exacerbating medications.
- Trial adequate analgesia.
- Medication in management of extreme or persistent agitation may be needed to avoid unacceptable morbidity.
- Document baseline target behaviour, trial of medication with titrated dosage, regular review of effectiveness, and trial of withdrawal.
- Minimum dosage for shortest period.
- Most medications are associated with negative effects on cognition and perhaps recovery of function, with the exception of adrenergic agonists.
- Not clear that any particular symptom complex may respond to a particular therapy and management is empirical.
- Paradoxical exacerbation as well as withdrawal effects need to be appreciated.

It seems likely that haloperidol, although used by some as initial therapy, has no specific effect on agitation or aggressive behaviour. Care in use of

Table 42.10 Heterotopic ossification

Causes	Local soft tissue or bone injury Burn of overlying skin Tumours Post joint arthroplasty Post CNS injury 'neurogenic heterotopic ossification'
Incidence	61–77% (by radiological screening) in those in coma or vegetative state 1 month or longer (Hammond and Francisco 1996) 11% of all patients have clinically significant HO (with pain or decreased range of motion): of these 33% lost ROM; ankylosis in 16%
Characteristic distribution (in order of frequency)	Hip: inferomedial (adductor spasticity) most frequent; anterior (ASIS to femur); posterior Elbow: anterior (if flexor spasticity present); posterior (if extensor spasticity); most likely joint to ankylose; a combination of trauma and spasticity at the elbow can increase incidence of HO to 89%. Shoulder: inferomedial, associated with internal rotator spasticity Knee: unusual, may be seen in distal femur or about knee
Presentation/ history	About 2 months after injury Acute inflammatory signs Limitation of range of motion Firm mass Decubitus ulceration Loss of function Secondary nerve palsies (particularly ulnar, sciatic)
Diagnosis/ investigation	Clinical suspicion in differential diagnosis of localized inflammation ^{99m}Tc-labelled methylene diphosphonate scan positive up to 4 weeks before radiographic evidence Serum alkaline phosphatase usually elevated CT may assist later management.
Management	Symptomatic treatment—analgaesia Maintain joint range of movement with physical therapy (Daud *et al.* 1993) NSAIDs: indomethacin, ibuprofen, aspirin Diphosphonates: disodium etidronate (Hammond and Francisco 1996, Glenn 1993) Radiotherapy: in association with resection of HO in those with a high risk of recurrence or where adverse effects of other modalities are limiting (Ayers *et al.* 1991, McAuliffe and Wolfson 1997) Resection: Considered where functional gains are likely to be achieved and pathological process controlled, at 14–18 months after injury. Earlier resection with radiotherapy may be considered. Requires assessment of neuromuscular function, clarification of associated joint function and pathological anatomy and strategy to control the HO

neuroleptics is indicated by their effect on memory and mobility, risk of epileptogenesis, and tardive symptoms in management of a transient condition. Care of withdrawal agitation is necessary, particularly with less potent agents.

Sedation with benzodiazepines may be helpful, particularly if sleep disturbance is an associated feature, although this does not establish a normal pattern. They may also be useful where acute control is required.

Tricyclic and other antidepressants (including doxepin), beta-blocking agents (particularly propranolol), and anticonvulsants (valproate and carbamazepine) may be effective.

Key point

- It seems likely that haloperidol has no specific effect on agitation or aggressive behaviour.

Rehabilitation after fracture

Heterotopic ossification

Heterotopic ossification (Table 42.10) is true bone formation by intramembranous ossification (Keenan and Haider 1996) at an abnormal site, usually in soft tissues surrounding joints. Neurogenic heterotopic ossification is most associated with traumatic brain

Table 42.11 Management of spasticity and tone-related disorders

Action	Detail	Comment
Exclude exacerbating factors	Sources of pain managed, especially urinary tract infection and stones; decubitus ulceration; local infection; fracture; heterotopic ossification; orthosis/cast fit. Adequate analgaesia: codeine	High level of suspicion especially with behaviour disorder and where an exacerbation of tone occurs Modifies spinal reflexes
Maintain muscle length	Stretching program twice daily; positioning and seating regimen; casting and orthosis management	Labour intensive; requires trained staff; early intervention, when prognosis for recovery unclear
Modify tonic influences	Muscle: dantrolene Neuromuscular junction: botulinum toxin injection Nerve: alcohol/phenol Spinal GABA agonists: baclofen; diazepam oral Baclofen infusion pump Spinal α_2 agonists: clonidine; tizanidine Spinal/surgical: selective dorsal rhizotomy; selective dorsal root entry zone-otomy	Marginally effective; Well tolerated; dose limits restrict muscle numbers; limited duration; Local problem management; expensive. Destructive; pain SE risk; local problem management; inexpensive Less effective in cerebral hypertonicity than spinal injury; cognitive SE Lower limb management; flexible titration; Surgical procedure; expensive Cognitive/other SE Destructive; highly selected situations
Manage deformity	Joint and tendon surgery Orthoses, aids, footwear, training	Later intervention; functional goals pursued Continued follow-up required

SE, state examination.

or spinal cord injury and may be distinguished (Garland 1988) from 'traumatic' heterotopic ossification (without neurological injury). Local trauma, surgical intervention, or decubitus ulceration increase risk of heterotopic ossification in TBI. Spontaneous regression is described (Hammond and Francisco 1996). Incidence is increased in people with more severe neurological injury, affecting the limbs with hypertonia.

Spasticity and related disorders of tone and posture

Spasticity is primarily related to loss of descending inhibition on polysynaptic reflex pathways. Secondary viscoelastic changes in muscle and joint contribute. Nociceptive and other sensory stimulation modulates responses, including complex postural reflexes.

- *Positive effects* may include maintaining muscle bulk over pressure-prone areas (especially buttocks); facilitating transfers; allowing ambulation.
- *Negative effects* may include pain/spasm; mobility/ function; posture; hygiene; decubitus ulceration.

Management (Table 42.11) requires a focus on the goals of the intervention. Combination therapy is usually required.

References

APA (1994) *Diagnostic and statistical manual of mental disorders: DSM-IV*. American Psychiatric Association, Washington, DC, pp 424–429.

Andrews K, Murphy L, Munday R, Littlewood C (1996) *Misdiagnosis of the vegetative state: retrospective study in a rehabilitation unit*. BMJ Publishing, London, pp 13–16.

Ayers DC, Pellegrini VD Jr, Evarts CM (1991) Prevention of heterotopic ossification in high-risk patients by radiation therapy. *Clinical Orthopaedics and Related Research* 263: 87–93.

Banwell JG, Creasey GH, Aggarwal AM, Mortimer JT (1993) Management of the neurogenic bowel in patients with spinal cord injury. *Urology Clinics of North America* 20(3): 517–526.

Basford JR (1993) Laser therapy: scientific basis and clinical role. *Orthopedics* 16(5): 541–547.

Bowker JH, Michael JW (1992) *Atlas of limb prosthetics: surgical, prosthetic and rehabilitation principles*. Mosby Year Book, St. Louis, Mo.

Braddom RL, Rocco JF (1991) Autonomic dysreflexia: a survey of current treatment. *American Journal of Physical Medicine and Rehabilitation* 70: 234–241.

Brooks DN, McKinlay W, Symington C, Beattie A, Campsie L (1987) Return to work within the first seven years of head injury. *Brain Injury* 1: 5–9.

Carabelli RA, Kellerman WC (1985) Phantom limb pain: relief by application of TENS to contralateral extremity. *Archives of Physical Medicine and Rehabilitation* 66: 466–467.

Childs NL, Mercer WN, Childs HW (1993) Accuracy of diagnosis of persistent vegetative state. *Neurology* 43: 1465–1467.

Choi SC, Narayan RK, Anderson RL, Ward JD (1988) Enhancing specificity of prognosis in severe head injury. *Journal of Neurosurgery* 69: 381–385.

Colachis SC (1992) Autonomic hyperreflexia with spinal cord injury. *Journal of the American Paraplegia Society* 15: 171–186.

Courville CB (1937) Pathology of the central nervous system, cited in Adams RD *et al., Principles of Neurology* 6th edn, McGraw-Hill, New York, 1997.

Craig AR, Hancock KM, Dickson HG (1994) A longitudinal investigation into anxiety and depression over the first two years of spinal cord injury. *Paraplegia* 32: 675–679.

Craig AR, Hancock K, Dickson H, Chang E (1997) Long-term psychological outcomes in spinal cord injured persons: results of a controlled trial using cognitive behavioural therapy. *Archives of Physical Medicine and Rehabilitation* 78: 33–38.

Crepeau F, Scherzer P (1993) Predictors and indicators of work status after traumatic brain injury: a meta-analysis. *Neuropsychological Rehabilitation* 3: 5–35.

Daud O, Sett P, Burr RG, Silver JR (1993) The relationship of heterotopic ossification to passive movements in paraplegic patients. *Disability and Rehabilitation* 15(3): 114–118.

Deutsch Lezak M (1995) *Neuropsychological assessment*, 3rd edn. Oxford University Press, Oxford.

Ebskov LB (1992) Level of lower limb amputation in relation to etiology: and epidemiological study. *Prosthetics and Orthotics International* 16: 163–167.

Elberlik K (1980) Organ loss, grieving and itching. *American Journal of Psychotherapy* 34(4): 523–533.

Finucane TE, Bynum JP (1996) Use of tube feeding to prevent aspiration pneumonia. *Lancet* 348: 1421–1424.

Folstein MF, Folstein SE, McHugh PR (1975) 'Mini-mental state'. A practical method for grading the cognitive state of patients for the clinician. *Journal of Psychiatric Research* 12: 189–198.

Furst L, Humphrey M (1983) Coping with the loss of a leg. *Prosthetics and Orthotics International* 7: 152–156.

Fyfe NCM (1990) An audit of amputation levels in patients referred for prosthetic rehabilitation. *Prosthetics and Orthotics International* 14: 67–70.

Garland D (1988) Clinical observations on fractures and heterotopic ossification in the spinal cord and traumatic brain injured populations. *Clinical Orthopaedics and Related Research* 233: 86–101.

Gennarelli TA, Thibault LE, Adams JH, Graham DI, Thompson CJ, Marcincin RP (1982) Diffuse axonal injury and traumatic coma in the primate. *Annals of Neurology* 12: 564.

Glenn MB (1993) Etidronate sodium: effects on heterotopic ossification and osteoporosis. *Journal of Head Trauma Rehabilitation* 8(3): 99–102.

Go BK, DeVivo MJ, Richards JS (1995) The epidemiology of spinal cord injury. In: Stover SL, Delisa JA, Whiteneck GC (eds) *Spinal cord injury: clinical outcomes from the model systems*. Aspen, Gaithersburg, MD, pp 21–55.

Goldberg RT (1985) New trends in the rehabilitation of lower extremity amputees. *Orthotics and Prosthetics* 39(1): 29–40.

Hammond FC, Francisco GE (1996) Should we use etidronate disodium as prophylaxis in patients with brain injury at risk for heterotopic ossification? *Journal of Head Trauma Rehabilitation* 11(6): 80–88.

Hughes S, Ni S, Wilson S (1998) Use of removable rigid dressing for transtibial amputees rehabilitation; A Greenwich Hospital experience. *Australian Physiotherapy* 44(2): 135–137.

ICF (2001) International classification of functioning, disability and health. WHO, Geneva

Jennett B (1996) Epidemiology of head injury. *Journal of Neurology, Neurosurgery and Psychiatry* 60: 362–369.

Jennett B, Bond M (1975) Assessment of outcome after severe brain damage. *Lancet* i: 480–487.

Jennett B, Teasdale G (1981) *Management of head injuries*. F A Davis, Philadelphia, Pa.

Jennett B, Teasdale G, Braakman R, Minderhoud J, Heiden J, Kurze T (1979) Prognosis inpatients with severe head injury. *Acta Neurochirgurgica Supplementum* 28: 161–164.

Jennett B, Snoek J, Bond M, Brooks N (1981) Disability after severe head injury: observations on the use of the Glasgow Outcome Scale. *Journal of Neurology, Neurosurgery and Psychiatry* 44: 293.

Johannsen F, Langberg H (1997) The treatment of acute soft tissue drams in Danish emergency rooms. *Scandinavian Journal of Medicine and Science in Sports* 7(3): 178–181.

Jones RF, Burniston GG (1970) A conservative approach to lower-limb amputations. *Medical Journal of Australia* 2: 711.

Keenan MAE, Haider T (1996) The formation of heterotopic ossification after traumatic brain injury: a biopsy study with ultrastructural analysis. *Journal of Head Trauma Rehabilitation* 11(4): 8–22.

Keith MW, Lacey SH (1991) Surgical rehabilitation of the tetraplegic upper extremity. *Journal of Neurological Rehabilitation* 5: 75–87.

Keith RA, Granger CV, Hamilton BB, Sherwins FS (1987) The Functional Independence Measure. *Advances in Clinical Rehabilitation* 1: 6–18.

Levin HS, O'Donnell VM, Grossman RG (1979) The Galveston orientation and amnesia test. *Journal of Nervous and Mental Disease* 167: 675–684.

Linsenmeyer TA (1993) Male infertility following spinal cord injury. *Journal of the American Paraplegia Society* 14: 116–121.

Little JM (1971) A pneumatic weight-bearing temporary prosthesis for below-knee amputees. *Lancet* i: 271–273.

Lyle DM, Pierce JP, Freeman EA *et al.* (1986) Clinical course and outcome of severe head injury in Australia. *Journal of Neurosurgery* 65: 15–18.

Mahoney FI, Barthel DW (1965) Functional evaluation: the Barthel index. *Maryland State Medical Journal* 14: 61–65.

Mallidis C, Lim TC, Hill S *et al* (1994) Collection of semen in acute phase of spinal cord injury. *Lancet* 343: 1072–1073.

Mawson AR, Biundo JJ Jr, Neville P *et al* (1988) Risk factors for early occurring pressure ulcers following spinal cord injury. *American Journal of Physical Medicine and Rehabilitation* 67: 123–127.

McAuliffe JA, Wolfson AH (1997) Early excision of heterotopic ossification about the elbow followed by radiation therapy. *Journal of Bone and Joint Surgery* 79A(5): 749–755.

Merritt JL (1981) Management of spasticity in spinal cord injury. *Mayo Clinic Proceedings* 56: 614–622.

MRC (1946) *Aids to the examination of the peripheral nervous system*. Memorandum No. 45, Medical Research Council, London, p 1.

Multi-Society Task Force on PVS (1994) Part Two. Medical aspects of the persistent vegetative state. *New England Journal of Medicine* 330: 22.

Oddy M (1984) Head injury and social adjustment. In: Brooks N (ed) *Closed head injury: psychological, social and family consequences.* Oxford University Press, Oxford, pp. 108–122.

Oddy M, Coughlan T, Tyerman A, Jenkins D (1985) Social adjustment after closed head injury: further follow-up seven years after injury. *Journal of Neurology, Neurosurgery and Psychiatry* 48: 564–568.

Penn RD, Savoy SM, Corcos D *et al* (1989) Intrathecal baclofen for severe spinal spasticity. *New England Journal of Medicine* 320: 1517–1521.

Plum F, Posner J (1980) *The diagnosis of stupor and coma*, 3 edn. F A Davis, Philadelphia, Pa.

Posiadlo D, Richardson S (1991) The timed 'up and go': a test of basic functional mobility for frail elderly persons. *Journal of the American Geriatics Society* 39: 142–148.

Powell GE, Wilson S (1994) Recovery curves for patients who have suffered very severe brain injury. *Clinical Rehabilitation* 8: 54–69.

Redhead RG, Davis BC, Robinson KP, Vitali M (1978) Post-amputation pneumatic walking aid. *British Journal of Surgery* 65: 611–612.

Rimel RW, Giordani B, Barth JT, Boll TJ, Jane JA (1981) Disability caused by minor closed head injury. *Neurosurgery* 9: 221–228.

Russell WR, Nathan PW (1946) Traumatic amnesia. *Brain* 69: 280–300.

Sherry E, Wilson S (1998) *The Oxford Handbook of Sports Medicine.* Oxford University Press, Oxford, p 656.

Shores EA, Marosszeky JE, Sandanam J, Batchelor J (1986) Preliminary validation of a scale for measuring the duration of post-traumatic amnesia. *Medical Journal of Australia* 144: 569–572.

Siddall PJ, Taylor DA, Cousins MJ (1997) Classification of pain following spinal cord injury. *Spinal Cord* 35: 69–75.

Siddall PJ, Taylor DA, Cousins MJ (1998) Mechanisms and treatment of spinal cord injury pain: an update. In: Ashburn MA, Fine PG, Stanley TH (eds) *Pain management and anesthesiology*. Kluwer, Dordrecht, pp. 247–262.

Staats TB (1992) The rehabilitation of the amputee in the developing world: a review of the literature. *Prosthetics and Orthotics International* 20: 45–50.

Staskin DR (1991) Hydroureteronephrosis after spinal cord injury: effects of lower urinary tract dysfunction on upper tract anatomy. *Urology Clinics of North America* 18(2): 309–316.

Stiens SA, Bergman SB, Goetz LL (1997) Neurogenic bowel dysfunction after spinal cord injury: Clinical evaluation and rehabilitative management (Focused review). *Archives of Physical Medicine and Rehabilitation* 78: S86–S102.

Tate RL, Lulham JM, Broe GA, Strettles B, Pfaff A (1989) Psychosocial outcome for the survivors of severe blunt head injury: The results from a consecutive series of 100 patients. *Journal of Neurology, Neurosurgery and Psychiatry* 52: 117–126.

Teasdale G, Jennett B (1974) Assessment of coma and impaired consciousness. *Lancet* ii: 81–84.

Trieschmann RB (1988) *Spinal cord injuries: psychological, social and vocational rehabilitation*, 2nd edn. Demos, New York.

Vollmer DG, Torner JC Charlebois D (1991) Age and outcome following traumatic coma: why do older patients fare worse? *Journal of Neurosurgery* 75: S37–S49.

Watanabe T, Rivas DA, Chancellor MB (1996) Urodynamics of spinal cord injury. *Urology Clinics of North America* 23(3): 459–473.

Waters RL, Perry J, Antonelli D *et al.* (1976) Energy cost of walking of amputees: the influence of level of amputation. *Journal of Bone and Joint Surgery* 58A(1): 42–51.

Wein AJ (1981) Classification of neurogenic bladder dysfunction. *Journal of Urology* 125: 605–609.

Wilson RF, Tyburski MD (1998) Metabolic responses and nutritional therapy in patients with severe head injuries. *Journal of Head Trauma Rehabilitation* 13(1): 11–27.

Yeongchi W, Krick H (1987) Removable rigid dressing for below-knee amputees. *Clinical Prosthetics and Orthotics* 11(1): 33–44.

43

CHAPTER 43

Diagnostic and therapeutic techniques

ROBERT KIRBY, SAMEER VISWANATHAN, AND ROLAND JIANG

CHAPTER 43

Diagnostic and therapeutic techniques

ROBERT KIRBY, SAMEER VISWANATHAN, AND ROLAND JIANG

Techniques for investigation of abdominal trauma

Accurate assessment and investigation of the injured or potentially injured abdomen may be the initial key to successful management of the injured patient. Resuscitation room screening radiographs including plain views of pelvis and chest may alert the receiving clinician to the possible presence of abdominal trauma. Plain abdominal radiographs may be of benefit in demonstrating gross changes such as damage to transverse processes of lumbar vertebrae or increases in the psoas shadow (suggestive of bleeding), but these signs are inaccurate and should not be relied upon.

Further investigations may be non-invasive (abdominal ultrasound or CT) or invasive (paracentesis, diagnostic peritoneal lavage [DPL], or laparoscopy). Adequate treatment should not be delayed for the purposes of investigation. At times the injury is so obvious (e.g. penetrating trauma or peritonitis) and the patient so unstable that immediate transfer for laparotomy is the only alternative.

Indications for further investigation include an equivocal abdominal examination, haemodynamically unstable patient (hypotension or drop in haematocrit/haemoglobin level), and altered mental status due to a closed head injury or intoxication with alcohol or drugs. Other indications include spinal cord injury and patients who cannot be examined serially because of other diagnostic procedures.

Paracentesis (four-quadrant tap)

Many clinicians will have gained experience of paracentesis in patients with ascites. The indication for paracentesis in trauma is very limited. The procedure may confirm an obvious diagnosis of major intra-abdominal bleeding, but it has a high false negative rate (Credi 1994), and negative findings carry little clinical relevance. Its use should be limited to the situation when a DPL (see page 215) cannot be carried out owing to time constraints and bedside ultrasound is not available. Paracentesis is contraindicated when the abdomen is both distended and tympanic, possibly secondary to dilated bowel. In this situation a blind tap might perforate or tear bowel and cause leakage of bowel contents under pressure. A distended but non-resonant abdomen may well be full of blood, although the presence of other fluids such as urine should also be considered (in the event of possible bladder perforation).

Key point

- The indication for paracentesis in trauma is limited to the situation when a DPL (see page 215) cannot be carried out because of time constraints.

Procedure

- Expose the entire abdomen and prepare it with antiseptic (e.g. povidone-iodine).
- Choose the site in each of the four quadrants of the abdomen (Fig. 43.1). Areas which are dull

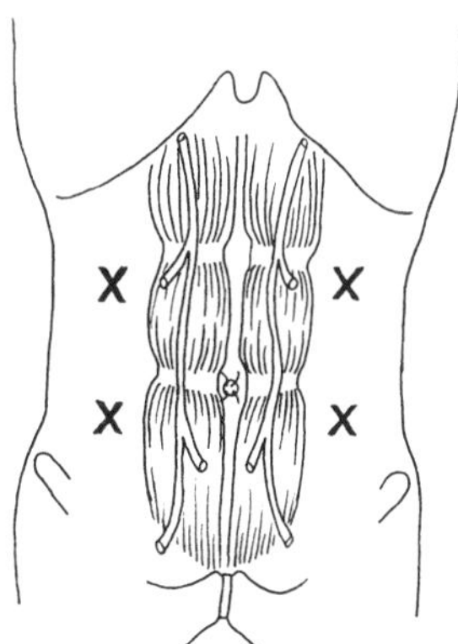

Figure 43.1 Sites for paracentesis.

to percussion may contain fluid or blood. Old scars should be avoided, because bowel may be adherent internally. The site of puncture should be lateral to the rectus abdominis muscle to avoid injury to the epigastric vessels.

- Infiltrate local anaesthetic (1% lignocaine [lidocaine] with adrenaline) in each site. *In extreme situations the use of local anaesthetic may be deferred.*
- Attach a 20 mL syringe to an 18G bevelled needle. Insert the needle into the abdomen, aspirating once the needle has penetrated the abdominal wall.

Notes

- A positive result is obtained when non-clotted blood is aspirated. This is an indication for a laparotomy.
- Penetration of non-dilated bowel by the (18G) needle is usually non-consequential because it should seal quickly causing no leakage.

Diagnostic peritoneal lavage

DPL is used in many units as a first line investigation for possible or suspected intra-abdominal bleeding. It is extremely sensitive to the presence of intraperitoneal bleeding, being able to pick up just 20 mL of blood (Day *et al.* 1992) (sensitivity 85–98%), but because of this laparotomies may be carried out for minor injuries which would not have in themselves needed surgery, leading to a non-therapeutic laparotomy rate of 20–40% (Bilge and Sahin 1991, Fryer *et al.* 1991).

Relative contraindications to DPL include near-term pregnancy (DPL should be carried out supraumbilically in this situation), presence of a coagulopathy, cirrhosis, and multiple prior abdominal operations.

Key points

- The indications for a DPL are:
  - equivocal abdominal examination
  - haemodynamically unstable patient (hypotension or drop in haematocrit)
  - altered mental status due to a closed head injury or intoxication with alcohol or drugs
  - spinal cord injury
  - patient who cannot be examined serially because of other diagnostic procedures.

Procedure

Prepare the patient

- Insert a urethral catheter and also a nasogastric tube if there is a chance that the stomach may be full.
- Prepare the abdomen with antiseptic (e.g. povidone-iodine) and drape aseptically.

Open technique for DPL

- Infiltrate local anaesthetic into the selected site (usually below the umbilicus but supraumbilical in pregnant patients).
- Make a 4–5 cm midline incision through skin and subcutaneous tissue till the linea alba is revealed.
- Incise the linea alba to expose the peritoneum.

- Secure the peritoneum with haemostats and incise to achieve access to the peritoneal cavity.
- Insert a peritoneal dialysis catheter into the peritoneal cavity, advancing it towards the pelvis.
- Attach a syringe to the catheter and aspirate.
- If there is no blood in the aspirate, the fascia should be closed using Vicryl sutures. At least 1 L of warmed normal saline is then instilled via the catheter into the peritoneal cavity. The catheter should be attached to an empty peritoneal dialysis bag.
- The abdominal cavity should then be agitated by gently rolling the patient from side to side.
- After 5 minutes place the bag below the level of the patient and allow the instilled fluid to drain.
- At least 750 mL of dialysate fluid should be collected and sent for analysis.

Notes

- Red cell and white blood cell counts should be carried out on the fluid collected, as well as tests for amylase and bilirubin concentration. Microscopy is also performed, along with a Gram stain.
- A DPL is deemed positive if blood or bowel contents are aspirated from the abdomen. It is also determined to be positive if, on analysis of the dialysate, $>$100 000 RBC/mm^3 or 5000 WBC/mm^3 are found. If laboratory analysis of the returned dialysate is likely to be delayed, an inability to read newsprint through the fluid bag is often regarded as 'positive'! The presence of bile, bacteria, or faecal matter in the dialysate suggests bowel damage.
- There are variations on the open technique as described above, including the semi-open technique and the closed technique. The *semi-open technique* involves blind insertion of a catheter through the fascia, preperitoneal fat, and peritoneum after the skin and subcutaneous fatty tissue is incised. In the *closed technique*, an 18G needle is passed into the peritoneal cavity and a guide wire passed through the needle. A dilator is then introduced over the guide wire and removed. A catheter is then passed over the guide wire in the peritoneal cavity, after which the guide wire is removed. In both cases the remainder of the procedure follows the technique described above.
- If necessary the catheter may be left *in situ* in order to allow repeat lavage after a suitable time interval.
- DPL should not be carried out prior to planned abdominal ultrasound or CT scanning, in order to reduce risks of false positive findings on scanning.
- False positives on DPL may occur from abdominal wall bleeding from a traumatic catheter placement, or from pelvic fractures.

Laparoscopy

Although laparoscopic investigation was first mooted by Sherwood *et al.* (1980), the revolution in general surgical laparoscopy in the 1990s led to only a relatively limited use of the technique for both investigation and sometimes treatment of the injured abdomen. Laparoscopy has been used in both blunt and penetrating trauma, although it may be risky if diaphragmatic injury is a possibility because of the effects of the pneumoperitoneum on the pleural cavity. It is, however an excellent method of accurately identifying and assessing such injuries. 'Bedside' use of laparoscopy under local anaesthetic is possible, although most reports have concerned procedures carried out under general anaesthetic in the operating theatre.

This technique should only be carried out by experienced surgeons with laparoscopic practice in the non-injured abdomen. The advantages of laparoscopy are that intra-abdominal bleeding may be identified, minor injuries may be identified without recourse to full laparotomy, and some minor therapeutic procedures may be carried out without the need to inflict a major laparotomy scar. Anterior penetrating injuries can be evaluated well (Rossi *et al.* 1993). Laparoscopic treatment may lead to less postoperative chest complications and earlier discharge form hospital. The drawbacks to the procedure are

- It is highly invasive.
- The retroperitoneum and some of the bowel are not amenable to easy inspection.
- The patient needs to be haemodynamically stable.

At present the use of laparoscopy for assessment of the injured abdomen should continue to be evaluated in experienced centres in trial settings to allow full assessment of safety and accuracy. (Rossi *et al.* 1993, Leppaniemi and Elliott 1996, Zantut *et al.* 1997)

Abdominal ultrasound

Abdominal ultrasound (ultrasonography) can identify both free fluid (>70 mL) in the abdominal cavity with a sensitivity of over 95% and also solid organ injury, although with less accuracy. Ultrasound examination is a non-invasive procedure and can be carried out at the patient's bedside or in the resuscitation room. The procedure can take only about 2–3 minutes to carry out and can be repeated as necessary. For this reason ultrasound examination is becoming a first line investigation in many centres (Bain *et al.* 1998), especially those dealing with paediatric trauma (Akgur *et al.* 1993, Rossi *et al.* 1993, Corbett *et al.* 2000). The major drawback of the procedure is that it is observer dependent, requiring an operator with experience of the scanning equipment and with experience of abdominal scanning. Use of colour Doppler scanners in the assessment of internal organs may improve accuracy (Nilsson *et al.* 1999) by demonstrating non-perfused tissue, but this practice has not yet gained wide enough use to establish the routine need for such equipment in the recovery area. Some centres are now introducing focused abdominal sonography for trauma (FAST) where limited structured examinations are carried out by non-radiologists to identify free abdominal fluid. Such identification equates with the discovery of blood on DPL. Initial results of studies looking at the accuracy of FAST appear encouraging (Boulanger *et al.* 1999, Yeo *et al.* 1999, Lingawi and Buckler 2000).

Because ultrasonic evaluation of the injured abdomen relies on the presence of free blood for a positive result, very early examination may lead to false negative findings. Re-examination after a short period of resuscitation is worthwhile in case of continuing intraperitoneal haemorrhage.

Hand-held scanning devices are being developed, and may lead to greater versatility in the use of trauma ultrasonography (Wherry 1998).

The role of CT scanning and MRI in trauma

CT scanning

CT scanning has become established as a diagnostic tool of choice in the assessment of head trauma and pelvic fractures. It may also be invaluable in the assessment of abdominal, thoracic, and spinal injuries. Like MRI scanning, CT scanning requires patients to be haemodynamically stable for a period of time. Spiral CT scanning has allowed the scan times to be reduced, but the patient still needs to be stable enough for transfer to a CT suite.

Abdominal trauma

CT scanning of the injured abdomen is often claimed to be the 'gold standard' in abdominal trauma investigation (Corbett *et al.* 2000) because it is not only sensitive, but also has a high specificity. In addition to being able to identify the presence of intra-abdominal fluid, individual organ damage can be identified. Retroperitoneal trauma may be identified and trivial trauma not requiring laparotomy may be diagnosed as such. Active decisions can be made regarding non-operative treatment of these patients with view to repeat examinations as necessary.

More information can be gained with the use of both oral and intravenous contrast agents. An oral agent (e.g. Gastrograffin) can be drunk sufficiently prior to the scan by the patient or instilled via a nasogastric tube. This is not always practical in severely injured patients. Intravenous contrast agent may be injected at the time of the scan. This helps not only to identify the major vascular structures, but also to confirm the vascular integrity of major abdominal organs such as the liver or kidneys. Individual organ injuries can be initially assessed and if necessary, repeatedly monitored, allowing closely controlled conservative management such as non-operative treatment of paediatric splenic injuries.

Patients with stab wounds to the back and flank can be evaluated with triple contrast enhanced CT scans. Retroperitoneal structures can be evaluated with the administration of contrast material orally, rectally, and intravenously.

Head trauma

CT scanning is the diagnostic modality of choice in the evaluation of head trauma. The presence of intracranial haemorrhage is usually well demonstrated. CT scanning can also detect oedema, mass effects (hemispheric shifts) on brain matter, brain infarction, foreign bodies, skull fractures, and hydrocephalus.

A fresh bleed in the brain usually appears white on scanning, whereas cerebrospinal fluid looks black. Oedema in brain matter appears darker than non-oedematous brain. Most studies in head trauma do not need contrast enhancement unless a tumour or abscess is suspected.

Normal scan findings despite severe neurological changes would normally require serial scans.

Epidural haematoma

An epidural haematoma can occur as a result of skull fractures, which classically occur in the petrous temporal bone causing laceration of the posterior branch of the middle meningeal artery. The injury causes stripping of the dura from the inner table of the skull, creating a potential space into which the lacerated artery bleeds. The expanding extradural haematoma can cause compression of the brain.

The classical finding on CT scanning is a biconvex (or lentiform) lesion, which does not cross suture lines.

Subdural haematoma

Subdural haematomas are common in trauma. They are caused by injured bridging veins. These normally drain blood from the cortex to the dural sinuses. Lesions may be small or may present with catastrophic symptoms. Subdural haematomas are classically seen in the elderly.

The findings on CT scanning include crescenteric collections, which conform to the surface to the brain. Other CT findings include oedema, brain shift, and loss of gyrae. Repeat CT scans with enhancement and coronal views can often pick up atypical haematomas.

Subarachnoid haemorrhage

Subarachnoid haemorrhage is usually detected on a non-contrast CT scan. It is commonly detected in the basal cisterns.

Other head injury

CT scanning has a crucial role in the evaluation of orbital fractures with the detection of haematomas (and subsequent evacuation under CT guidance). It also has a role in the evaluation of maxillofacial fractures. Three-dimensional reconstruction of axial sections can be used to accurately elucidate midface fractures. Diffuse axonal injury can also be picked up CT scanning although MRI is a better diagnostic tool for this purpose.

Traumatic injury of the larynx

CT scanning is particularly useful in the detection of fractures of the thyroid cartilage and other injuries of the larynx including haematomas, arytenoid cartilage dislocation, and injuries to the trachea.

Spinal trauma

CT scanning of spinal injuries provides good visualization of soft tissue damage. There is also better visualization of the C7–T1 junction than might be obtained in standard radiographs. The scans are usually thin cuts in the axial plane. MRI provides better images of the spinal cord, but CT scanning is preferred for bony tissue.

The cervical spine should be protected and immobilized in a hard cervical collar if the level of damage to the spine is unknown.

Chest trauma

Thoracic CT scanning is more accurate than plain chest radiographs in demonstrating trauma in the chest. Chest wall, pulmonary, mediastinal, or pulmonary damage may be accurately assessed. CT scanning is particularly useful when pulmonary contusion, pneumomediastinum, or haemomediastinum is suspected. In addition, diaphragmatic and pleural injuries may be visualized by CT scanning.

- In the case of suspected oesophageal injury, CT scanning can be used to detect signs of mediastinitis.
- Intrathoracic fluid collections may be drained under CT guidance (by experienced interventional radiologists).
- In the case of aortic injury, CT scanning has made rapid advances and in conjunction with transoesophageal echocardiography is becoming important in the evaluation of blunt injury to the chest (Patel *et al.* 1998). However, thoracic aortography remains the reference standard for the diagnosis of aortic injury.

Pelvic trauma

CT scanning has become an invaluable tool in the assessment of pelvic trauma. It is particularly good for imaging the sacroiliac joints and the sacrum itself, and may also demonstrate femoral head or acetabular fractures, joint instability, and pelvic ring disruption.

Key point

- CT scanning has become established as an early diagnostic tool in head trauma and pelvic fractures.

MRI scanning

There are potential roles for MRI as a diagnostic tool in trauma. It is particularly useful in injuries to the spinal cord and vascular injury. One major advantage of MRI is that there is no need for a contrast agent; another advantage is the ability to obtain images in other planes such as sagittal and oblique.

There is a need for a co-operative patient, ideally not connected to monitoring equipment, which may cause interference with the scanner itself. Other problems include the presence of pacemakers or prostheses in the patients, which precludes the use of MRI. In the future there may be a role for MRI in assessing aortic injury, myocardial injury, and brain or spinal cord trauma.

Key points

- Advantages of MRI are:
  - no need for a contrast agent
  - useful in spinal cord and vascular injuries
  - images can be obtained in other planes such as sagittal and oblique.

Local wound exploration for stab wounds

Local exploration of stab wounds is carried out to determine the end point of the tract. The following procedure is not appropriate for assessment of gunshot wounds. The critical determinant is whether the posterior fascia has been penetrated (Markovchick *et al.* 1985). If there has been no penetration then the patient can be discharged with local wound treatment. The decision to proceed to laparotomy is more complex, with some surgeons choosing to operate with evidence of fascial penetration while others opt for laparotomy only on evidence of peritoneal penetration (Cameron and Civil 1998). There is consensus, however, on the decision to proceed to a laparotomy if there is any indication of peritonism or haemodynamic instability.

Procedure

- The area around the wound should be prepared with antiseptic (e.g. povidone-iodine).
- The wound should then be infiltrated with local anaesthetic, such as 1% lignocaine (lidocaine) with adrenaline.
- The wound should be lengthened with a scalpel along its longitudinal axis and exposed with surgical retractors.
- Exploration of the wound should be continued until the end of the tract can be seen or if evidence of penetration of fascia or peritoneum is obtained.

Notes

- A negative test is obtained when the tract is seen to end in subcutaneous tissue.
- A positive test is obtained if in abdominal stab wounds the posterior rectus fascia or transversus abdominis fascia is penetrated.
- Positive test criteria for lower chest wound involves a penetration of the intercostal muscles in the mid axillary line below the fifth intercostal space. Exploration of lower chest wounds may result in an iatrogenic pneumothorax.
- If on local exploration the end point of the wound cannot be determined, DPL may then be carried out for lower chest wounds, anterior abdominal wounds, and anterior flank wounds. A CT scan is recommended for posterior flank wounds and back wounds.

Key point

- Local exploration of stab wounds is carried out to determine the endpoint of the tract.

Urinary catheters

Catheterization of the bladder (indwelling catheter, IDC) is usually performed in trauma to monitor urine output and to relieve urinary retention. It is also performed before surgery (for the same reasons) and also used to obtain urine for analysis. Other indications include decompression of the bladder before DPL, and on the discovery of haematuria to diagnose trauma to the urinary tract.

Insertion of a catheter should be avoided if there is any evidence of urethral injury such as the presence of blood on the urethral meatus, and scrotal or perineal haematomas. An IDC should also be avoided if the prostate is found to be high-riding on rectal examination, or in the presence of a complex pelvic fracture. Infection of the lower urinary tract is a relative contraindication.

The most commonly used catheter is the Foley in sizes 16–18F. This is a double-lumen tube with the larger lumen draining urine and the smaller lumen inflating the balloon. The size of the balloon should be noted before insertion. Other types of catheter include the straight (Robinson) catheters, the Coudé catheter (which has a curved tip and is used if an obstruction is found), and the three-way bladder irrigation catheter.

Procedure in the male

- The patient should be positioned supine. Aseptic technique should be used. Gowns and sterile gloves should be worn.
- Materials needed include a Foley catheter (size 16F to start with), standard sterile dressing pack, aqueous chlorhexidine, sterile drapes and sterile gauze swabs with plastic forceps, lignocaine (lidocaine) gel in a syringe and nozzle, and a standard 10 mL syringe (to inflate the balloon). A collection bag should be available to connect up to the IDC.
- A sterile drape with a hole cut in the middle is used, with the shaft of the penis threaded through the hole.
- The penis is held in the operator's non-dominant hand and the foreskin retracted (in uncircumcized males). The dominant hand remains sterile while the non-dominant hand is now considered non-sterile and should not touch the catheter.

- Swabs soaked in aqueous chlorhexidine are used to clean the glans. Each swab is used only once. At least 4–5 swabs should be used in the manner described.
- The lignocaine (lidocaine) gel is injected into the urethra with the use of the special nozzle. If the patient is awake he should be warned of a slight stinging sensation. If there is no urgent requirement for immediate catheterization in a conscious patient, a delay of 2–3 minutes at this stage will allow the local anaesthetic to take more effect.
- The penis is first held perpendicular and the catheter is inserted, gently advancing without forcing the passage at any stage.
- If any resistance is encountered the penis shaft should be manoeuvred to the horizontal plane first and then in other directions with gentle pressure exerted until the catheter passes to its hilt.
- When the catheter enters the bladder there will be a gush of residual urine (the volume of which should be measured). Continue to pass the catheter up to the hilt.
- The balloon should then be inflated (noting the balloon size of the catheter before insertion) with normal saline or sterile water. Always ask a conscious patient if he is experiencing any pain during this step. If excessive pain is experienced then this is an indication that the balloon might still be within the prostatomembranous urethra.
- The catheter should then be withdrawn until it catches against the bladder neck.
- The foreskin should be replaced.
- The IDC should be connected to the collecting bag.

Procedure in the female

As above with the following points of difference:

- Wash the labia majora and labia minora with gauze swabs soaked in aqueous chlorhexidine in a anteroposterior direction, with each swab (grasped with forceps) being used in one downward motion only. The labial folds should be held apart with the operator's non-dominant hand. The non-dominant hand is hence considered non-sterile and should not touch the catheter.
- The catheter should be lubricated with the lignocaine (lidocaine) gel. There is no need to inject the gel into the urethra.

Notes

- As a general rule of thumb, if resistance is encountered, a larger size catheter should be tried.
- Other types of catheter are designed for prostatic obstruction. Consultation with a senior urology resident/registrar is recommended, to exclude the need for insertion with a catheter introducer or even a suprapubic catheter.
- Consider the presence of a female chaperone if the catheter is to be inserted in a female patient by a male health professional.
- If the catheter cannot be inserted consider urethral oedema from multiple insertion attempts, or removal of the IDC without deflating the balloon as a cause. Other serious causes include carcinoma of the prostate, urethral stricture, or urethral diverticulum. False passage is also a rare occurrence. Urethral oedema is countered by using a smaller catheter (this is the only indication for a smaller catheter), and a Coudé catheter or a suprapubic catheter considered in cases of severe retention.
- Complications that can arise from the insertion of a urinary catheter include infection of the urinary tract (urethritis, epididymitis, bacteraemia), trauma (false passage, stricture), paraphimosis, and haemorrhage.

Nasogastric tubes

The primary use of nasogastric tubes in trauma is to decompress the stomach in order to prevent aspiration of gastric contents. A secondary use is to exclude the presence of blood which otherwise might signify upper gastrointestinal trauma.

The use of a nasogastric tube should be avoided when there is trauma to the face or neck. A fractured cribiform plate can result in the nasogastric tube tracking into the cranial vault. An orogastric tube is an alternative in such a situation. With injuries to the neck, damaged vessels can rupture and bleed if there is an increase in intrathoracic pressure induced by coughing or vomiting which in turn is caused by the insertion of the nasogastric tube.

There are various types of nasogastric tubes with single or double lumens. If the tube is placed beyond the pylorus it can be used for feeding in patients with depressed level of consciousness. Larger-diameter lumen tubes are used for decompression and smaller or fine-bore lumen tubes are used for feeding purposes.

Key point

- The primary use of a nasogastric tube in trauma is to decompress the stomach.

Procedure

- The tube chosen is lubricated with lignocaine (lidocaine).
- With the patient supine the tube is inserted heading posteriorly. It is important that the tube is not guided in a superior direction.
- The patient is asked to make vigorous swallows as the tube passes through the pharynx and oesophagus.
- The position of the tube can be confirmed by injecting air through the tube and auscultating over the stomach. Alternatively, gastric contents may be aspirated and the acidity checked on pH indicator paper. An radiograph confirming the position of the nasogastric tube may be requested.

Notes

- On insertion the nasogastric tube can enter the trachea or can curl up on itself in the mouth. Such situations are characterized by a failure to hear the air which is injected, or a failure to aspirate any stomach contents. In this case the tube will have to be removed and a new one inserted.
- Nasogastric tubes can be blocked by debris or blood clots. Regular flushing of the tube may prevent blockage and subsequent vomiting with aspiration of stomach contents into the lungs.

Chest tubes

Chest tubes (closed-tube thoracostomy) are used to drain air (pneumothorax), blood (haemothorax), pus (empyema), or fluid (pleural effusions) from the pleural cavity. In the case of a pneumothorax, a chest tube is life saving. In trauma, the decision to insert a chest tube can be made clinically with the findings of shortness of breath, reduced air entry and increased percussive note. Radiographs of the chest should be ordered to confirm the presence of the pneumothorax. The finding of hypotension and tracheal shift from the midline should alert to the possibility of a tension pneumothorax, which should be treated immediately with a needle thoracocentesis. The chest tubes are connected to an underwater drain and might be left to suction drainage or gravity drainage.

Procedure

- The site of insertion is usually the fifth or sixth intercostal space in the midaxillary line. The patient can be positioned with the arm of the affected side raised and the fingers placed behind the head. The head should be slightly elevated and the body of the patient tilted away slightly with a pillow. Tubes should not be inserted through wounds (Fig. 43.2).
- The skin should be prepared with antiseptic (e.g. povidone-iodine) and sterile drapes.
- The site chosen for insertion should be anaesthetized with lignocaine (lidocaine) taking

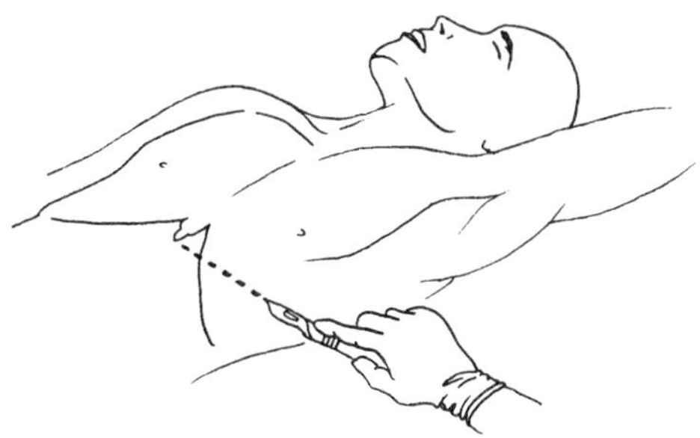

Figure 43.2 Closed-tube thoracostomy: positioning the patient and choosing the site of insertion.

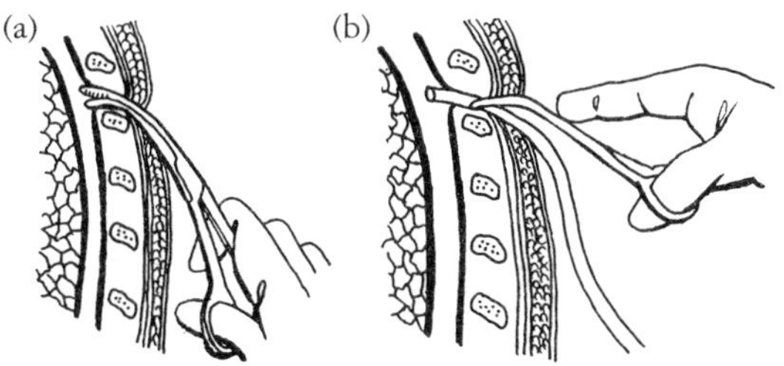

Figure 43.3 Closed-tube thoracostomy: method of insertion: (a) Dissect over rib. (b) Insert chest tube into pleural space.

care to infiltrate the local anaesthetic to skin, intercostal muscles, and pleura.

- An incision (4–5 cm) is made over the intercostal space below the chosen site. Using a curved haemostat, a tunnel is made to the chosen intercostal space. The curved haemostat is guided to the upper edge of the rib (Fig. 43.3a). This creates a cover, which occludes the hole created when the tube is removed.
- The intercostal muscles are dissected over the selected rib and opened to expose the parietal pleura.
- The parietal pleura over the rib is punctured (associated with a rush of air) and a gloved finger is inserted. A sweeping motion with the finger confirms that the pleural space has been reached and that any adhesions are removed. The finger can also be used to feel the diaphragm and detect if there is a diaphragmatic tear.
- The finger is then used to guide the chest tube (size for adults 28–32 Fr or children 16–24 Fr) into the pleural space. Then using a curved forceps (Fig. 43.3b) over the distal end the tube is guided apically for a pneumothorax or posterolaterally for a haemothorax. The tube should be clamped at this stage.
- The tube is then observed for 'fogging' with expiration, which is an indication of correct placement.
- The tube is connected to the underwater drain, unclamped and observed for bubbling and 'swinging' of the fluid. The fluid should 'swing' (fluid column variation) with each respiration. If the fluid column does not swing, advance the tube further or withdraw a little. Ask the patient to cough and look for bubbles in the column. If there is no movement in the column despite these measures, the tube will need reinsertion.
- The tube should be secured to the chest wall with a suture (2–0 silk or nylon) and the incision dressed.
- Obtain a chest radiograph to determine the position of the chest tube.

Notes

- Removal of the chest drain involves first removing the dressing and sutures. The patient is then asked to inspire deeply and hold, while the tube is rapidly removed. A gauze dressing should then be placed over the wound and a mattress suture used to close it. A plain chest radiograph should then be performed.
- Administration of prophylactic antibiotic in patients who receive a chest tube lowers the rate of infective complications (Gonzalez and Holevar 1998).
- If there is persistent bubbling or a failure of re-expansion, ensure that all the holes of the

intercostal catheter are in the pleural cavity. In addition, the tube should be checked to ensure that it is not kinked. Other possibilities include loculation of air, or an air leak from traumatized lung leading to a bronchopleural fistula or a ruptured oesophagus.

Key point

- In the case of a pneumothorax, a chest tube is life saving.

Central venous catheterization

Central venous access following trauma can be life saving for resuscitation purposes. Other indications for central lines include central venous pressure monitoring, pacemaker insertion, and infusion of irritant or concentrated solutions such as dopamine or hyperosmolar saline (Stevenson 1988). The use of a guide wire through a needle followed by the catheter (also known as the Seldinger technique) has made central venous access commonplace and safe. Central venous access can be obtained via the subclavian vein or the internal jugular vein. Contraindications to insertion include distorted local anatomy and an agitated patient.

Key points

- Central access is very helpful because the rates of flow that can be achieved by the larger catheters can be life saving for resuscitation purposes.
- It is particularly useful for:
  - central venous pressure monitoring
  - pacemaker insertion
  - infusion of irritant or concentrated solutions such as dopamine or hyperosmolar saline.

Subclavian vein access

Access to the subclavian vein allows the measurement of the central venous pressure and subsequent catheterization of the pulmonary artery. It also provides direct access to the superior vena cava and allows easy access to the subclavian vein. Problems that can arise with subclavian vein catheterization include pneumothorax, arterial puncture, and damage to the superior vena cava (which can be life threatening). There is also an increased risk of pneumothorax and phrenic as well as brachial plexus trauma.

Procedure

Infraclavicular approach

- Aseptic technique is used for this procedure.
- The patient is positioned in the Trendelenburg position and the skin widely prepared with antiseptic (e.g. povidone-iodine).
- The skin and the periosteum of the clavicle is anaesthetized with 1% lignocaine (lidocaine).
- With one finger placed on the suprasternal notch as a reference point the needle is inserted below the clavicle (at the junction of the medial third and the middle third of the clavicle) and guided towards the finger placed on the reference point. As the needle advances, the plunger on the syringe is withdrawn until blood is aspirated.
- When free blood flow is achieved into the syringe the needle is advanced a further 1 mm, and then the guide wire is advanced slowly.
- If the guide wire inserts without any resistance, the needle is removed and an incision made with a skin knife. A dilator and a catheter sheath are inserted into the incision over the guide wire. The dilator may be removed before insertion of the catheter (in standard catheters; however, in those with an introducer sheath, the catheter may be passed over the dilator).
- The catheter is then advanced over the guide wire into the subclavian vein. Free backflow of blood into a fluid bag connected to the catheter which is lowered below the bed is an indication of a properly placed catheter.

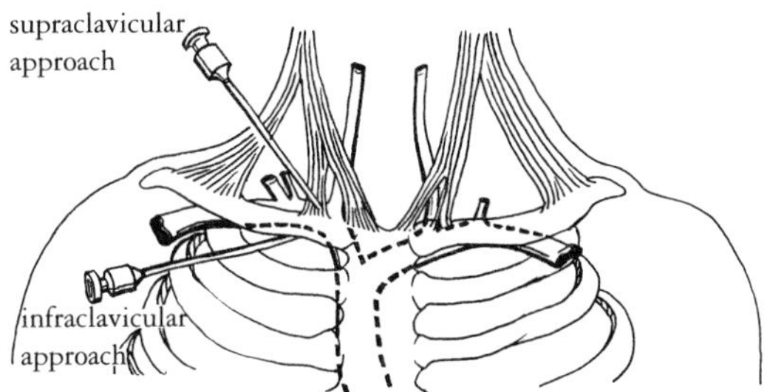

Figure 43.4 Supraclavicular and infraclavicular approaches.

Supraclavicular approach

The supraclavicular approach is an alternative to the infraclavicular approach (Fig. 43.4).

- The insertion point is 1 cm posterior the clavicle and 1 cm lateral to the sternocleidomastoid (clavicular head) (Terracina 1994). The needle is aimed towards the contralateral nipple and the rest of the procedure is as described above.

Internal jugular central venous access

The technique used is essentially similar to the technique described above. The central approach uses the two heads of the sternocleidomastoid as an anatomic landmark. The advantages of this procedure include a lower rate of malposition, and a lower incidence of pleural puncture. However, it has a higher failure rate than the subclavian catheters.

- Insertion is usually in the supraclavicular triangle, the apex of which is formed by the two heads of the sternocleidomastoid muscle (Fig. 43.5).
- While palpating the carotid pulse with the free hand and retracting it away from the insertion site, the needle is directed at an angle of 40° aiming for the nipple on the same side.
- The needle should not be advanced more than 4–5 cm for fear of causing a pneumothorax.
- Once the vein is accessed the procedure is followed as described above.

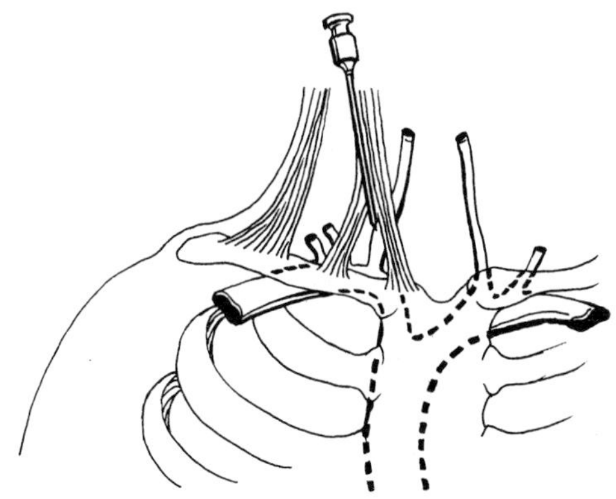

Figure 43.5 Internal jugular vein approach.

- In addition to the central approach to the internal jugular vein there is also an anterior approach and a posterior approach. The anterior approach uses the midpoint of the medial border of the sternocleidomastoid muscle. The posterior approach utilizes the lateral border of the this muscle at the level of the apex of the two heads of the muscle, aiming the needle towards the sternal notch.

Femoral vein access

Access to the femoral vein may be used for resuscitation purposes. The anatomical landmark is the femoral artery with the vein lying 1 cm medial to the arterial pulse and below the inguinal ligament. The technique of insertion is largely the same as that described above. The landmarks for the femoral vein are shown in Fig. 43.6.

Notes

Complications from central lines are numerous, ranging from the already mentioned (pneumothorax, haemothorax, and damage to vascular and neural structures), to tracheal perforation, sepsis, cellulitis, osteomyelitis, air embolus, pericardial tamponade, arteriovenous fistulae, thrombosis of the superior vena cava, arrhythmias, and ascites (Terracina 1994).

Saphenous cutdown

A cutdown may become necessary for the resuscitation of patients. It is also useful in obtaining access

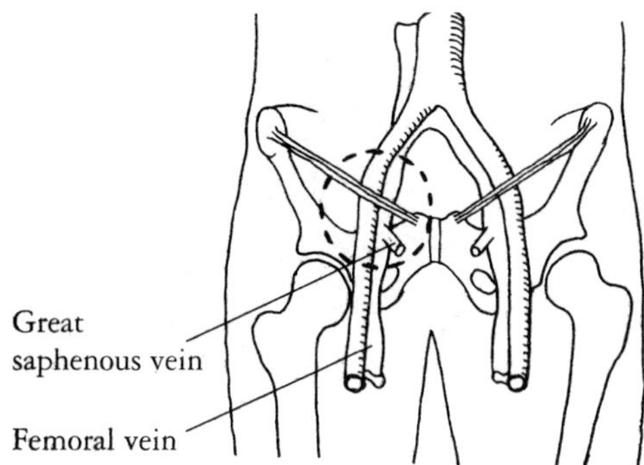

Figure 43.6 Landmarks of the femoral vein.

to the peripheral venous system in people whose veins may be difficult to cannulate. The long saphenous vein may be used for cutdowns.

Procedure

- The site of the cutdown (e.g. 1 cm anterior and proximal to the medial malleolus) is prepared with antiseptic (e.g. povidone-iodine) ointment and surgical drapes.
- The skin is anaesthetized with local anaesthetic, e.g 1% lignocaine (lidocaine).
- A transverse incision is made and the subcutaneous fat and tissue is retracted longitudinally.
- The vein is isolated and secured with forceps.
- At this point two sutures (silk) are slung under the vein with the distal suture tied off and the proximal suture looped and held with tension.
- A small incision is made in the vein and a catheter is inserted into this venotomy.

Other sites for cutdowns include:

- The proximal long saphenous vein 5 cm below the inguinal ligament using the femoral artery as a landmark (vein is medial to the artery).
- The antecubital fossa: It is best to choose a proximal site, with the basilic vein (2 cm proximal and 2 cm medial to the medial epicondyle) being the best option (to avoid damage to the median nerve and the brachial artery).
- The cephalic vein (which is 2 cm proximal and medial to the lateral epicondyle).

Arterial catheters

Arterial catheters are primarily used to obtain frequent blood samples (such as frequent sampling of arterial blood gases), and to allow continuous blood pressure monitoring (which is particularly useful in the haemodynamically unstable patient),

Arteries that are most commonly chosen for catheterization include the radial and femoral, but use of the axillary, dorsalis pedis, and brachial arteries has also been documented. The use of the latter arteries is more problematic.

Procedure

There are three ways described of which two utilize a catheter-over-needle approach and a third uses a guide wire passed through a needle, followed by a dilator and catheter (modified Seldinger) method, as described above.

Catheter-over-needle method

- The site of insertion is carefully chosen (by palpation of the maximum pulsation).
- The site is prepared with povidone-iodine, sterile drapes, and local anaesthetic (which helps counteract vasospasm).
- The needle and catheter is advanced into the skin at an angle of 45°. The needle is guided further until there is a flashback (with pulsation) into the apparatus.
- At this point either of two methods can be used. The first method involves advancing the catheter and the needle through the superior and inferior walls of the artery. The needle is then withdrawn, and following this the catheter is gradually withdrawn till pulsatile flow results. At this point the catheter is advanced through the artery. The alternate method is similar to cannulation of a peripheral vein. After the skin is punctured at an angle of 45°, and pulsatile flashback is obtained, the

apparatus is dropped to an angle of 10° and advanced 2 mm, after which the catheter is advanced into the artery.

- After the catheter has been introduced into the artery, it is connected up to an infusion of heparinized saline and sutured into position.

Notes

- Complications of this procedure include haematomas (most commonly), cellulitis, nerve injury, and embolus. Arterial lines appear to have a lower infection rate than central lines (Samsoondar *et al.* 1985).
- The brachial artery appears to have a higher complication rate than the radial artery.
- Allen's test should be performed on elderly patients. Patients with a positive Allen's test have an increased risk of ischaemia due to ulnar artery insufficiency. The test involves simultaneous occlusion of both the radial and ulnar arteries. The patient is asked to open and close their hands till there is palmar pallor. At this point the ulnar artery is released and a palmar 'blush' is looked for. If this is delayed (longer than 7 seconds) or fails to occur then the test is deemed positive.

References

Akgur FM, Aktug T, Kovanhkaya A, Erdag G, Olguner M, Hosgor M, Obuz O (1993) Initial evaluation of children sustaining blunt abdominal trauma: ultrasonography vs. diagnostic peritoneal lavage. *European Journal of Pediatric Surgery* 3(5): 278–280.

Bain IM, Kirby RM, Tiwari P *et al.* (1998) Survey of abdominal ultrasound and diagnostic peritoneal lavage for suspected intra-abdominal injury following blunt trauma. *Injury* 29(1): 65–71.

Bilge A, Sahin M (1991) Diagnostic peritoneal lavage in blunt abdominal trauma. *European Journal of Surgery* 157: 449–451.

Boulanger BR, McLellan BA, Brenneman FD, Ochoa J, Kirkpatrick AW (1999) Prospective evidence of the superiority of a sonography-based algorithm in the assessment of blunt abdominal injury. *Journal of Trauma* 47(4): 632–637.

Cameron P, Civil I (1998) The management of anterior abdominal stab wounds in Australia. *Australian and New Zealand Journal of Surgery* 68(7): 510–513.

Credi RG (1994) Diagnostic peritoneal lavage. In: Lopez-Viego MA (ed) *The Parkland Handbook trauma handbook*. Mosby, St. Louis, Mo.

Corbett SW, Andrews HG, Baker EM, Jones WG (2000) Evaluation of the pediatric trauma patient by ultrasonography. *American Journal of Emergency Medicine* 18(3): 244–249.

Day AC, Rankin N, Charlesworth P (1992) Diagnostic peritoneal lavage: integration with clinical information to improve diagnostic performance. *Journal of Trauma* 32: 52–57.

Fryer JP, Graham TL, Fong HM, Burns CM (1991) Diagnostic peritoneal lavage as an indicator for therapeutic surgery. *Canadian Journal of Surgery* 34: 471–476.

Gonzalez RP, Holevar MR (1998) Role of prophylactic antibiotics for tube thoracostomy in chest trauma. *American Journal of Surgery* 64(7): 617–621.

Leppaniemi AK, Elliott DC (1996) The role of laparoscopy in blunt abdominal trauma. *Annals of Medicine* 28(6): 483–489.

Lingawi SS, Buckley AR (2000) Focused abdominal US in patients with trauma. *Radiology* 217(2): 426–429.

Markovchick VJ, Moore EE, Moore J, Rosen P (1985) Local wound exploration of anterior abdominal stab wounds. *Journal of Emergency Medicine* 2(4): 287–291.

Nilsson A, Loren I, Nirhov N, Lindhagen T, Nilsson P (1999) Power Doppler ultrasonography: alternative to computed tomography in abdominal trauma patients. *Journal of Ultrasound Medicine* 18(10): 669–672.

Patel NH, Stephens KE Jr, Mirvis SE, Shanmuganathan K, Mann FA (1998) Imaging of acute thoracic aortic injury due to blunt trauma: a review. *Radiology* 209(2): 335.

Rossi P, Mullins D, Thal E (1993) Role of laparoscopy in the evaluation of abdominal trauma. *American Journal of Surgery* 166(6): 707–710.

Samsoondar W, Freeman JB, Coultish I, Oxley C (1985) Colonization of intravascular catheters in the intensive care unit. *American Journal of Surgery* 149(6): 730–732.

Stevenson N (1988) Procedures in emergency medicine. In: Fulde GWO (ed) *The principles of practice*. MacLennan Petty, Artamon, NSW, pp 393–404.

Sherwood R, Berci G, Austin E, Morgenstern L (1980) Minilaparoscopy for blunt abdominal trauma. *Archives of Surgery* 115(5): 672–673.

Terracina A (1994) Diagnostic peritoneal lavage. In: Lopez-Viego MA (ed) *The Parkland Handbook trauma handbook*. Mosby, St. Louis, Mo.

Wherry DC (1998) Potential of a hand-held ultrasound in assessment of the injured patient. *Cardiovascular Surgery* 6(6): 569–572.

Williams RD, Zolliner RM (1959) Diagnostic and prognostic factors in abdominal trauma. *American Journal of Surgery* 97: 575.

Woods SD (1995) Assessment of blunt abdominal trauma. *Australian and New Zealand Journal of Surgery* 65(2): 75–76.

Yeo A, Wong CY, Soo KC (1999) Focused abdominal sonography for trauma (FAST). *Annals of the Academy of Medicine, Singapore* 28(6): 805–809.

Zantut LF, Ivatury RR, Smith RS *et al.* (1997) Diagnostic and therapeutic laparoscopy for penetrating abdominal trauma: a multicenter experience. *Journal of Trauma* 42(5): 825–829; discussion 829–831.

44

CHAPTER 44

Drugs (formulary) for trauma

EMMA GREEN AND ROSLYN CRAMPTON

CHAPTER 44
Drugs (formulary) for trauma

EMMA GREEN AND ROSLYN CRAMPTON

See list of abbreviation and symbols on page 743.

Drugs	Dosage	Drug type	Used for	Comments
Adenosine	*Adult:* 6 mg rapid IV bolus If ineffective in 2 min increase to 12 mg rapid IV bolus If ineffective in 2 min increase to 18 mg rapid IV bolus	Blocks conduction AV node	Reversion of supraventricular tachycardia	Extremely short half-life May cause brief flushing and apprehension
Adrenaline (epinephrine)	1 : 1000 (1 mL=1 mg) for SC/IM may be repeated every 15 min prn 1 : 10 000 (1 mL=0.1 mg) for IV administration *Severe anaphylaxis or asthma:* adult initially 0.1–1.0 mg IV *Child:* 10 μg/kg/dose; max single dose 500 μg *Adjunct in cardiac arrest,* IV: adult: initial 1 mg bolus repeat every 3–5 min during CPR *Child:* 10 μg/kg/dose q3-5 min prn Infusion for above or for *Hypotension*: 0.1 μg/kg/min by continuous IV infusion. Increase by 0.1 μg/kg/min up to a maximum of 20 μg/kg/min as required	Inotropic and chronotropic agent mixed α- and β-stimulating effects	Ventricular asystole Severe hypotension not due to hypovolaemia Acute asthma Anaphylaxis	IV duration 5–10 min *Contra*: hypovolaemic shock; interarterial administration; when using non-selective β-blockers *Adverse*: cerebral haemorrhage, cardiac arrhythmias Effective given via endotracheal tube at twice the dosage in 10 mL of normal saline Effective intra-osseous
Amiodarone	*Adult:* loading dose 5 mg/kg over 30 min *Child:* 25 μg/kg/min for 4 h	Class III anti-arrhythmic agent	Ventricular tachycardia Reversion of atrial fibrillation	Extremely long half life Caution in hepatic disease
Amoxicillin/ potassium clavulanate (co-amoxiclav)	*Adult:* 500/125 mg *Child:* (40/10 mg/kg per day up to adult dose, in 3 divided doses) orally, 8-hourly for 5–10 days	Broad-spectrum penicillin antibiotic with resistance against most β-lactamases	Bites and clenched-fist injuries where antibiotic therapy is necessary (with penicillin sensitivity—see metronidazole)	*Contra:* jaundice, hepatic dysfunction *Prec:* renal, severe hepatic impairment; prolonged use; infectious mononucleosis; lymphatic leukaemia; pregnancy *Adverse*: sensitivity phenomena; superinfection; pseudomembranous colitis; hepatic disturbances *Interact:* allopurinol alcohol

Drugs	Dosage	Drug type	Used for	Comments
Atropine sulfate	May be given endotracheally *Pre-op:* adult—300–600 mg IV immediately before anaesthesia; infants, Child*:* 15–20μg/kg *CPR:* adult*:* 0.4–1 mg IV q5 min prn; (3 mg results in complete vagal blockade)	Anticholinergic Antiarrhythmic	Ventricular asystole and symptomatic bradycardia (due to vagotonic states e.g. in inferior AMI).Atropine accelerates the H and raises the BP Infants <6 months with heart rate <80 should be treated	*Contra:* prostatic hypertrophy; closed-angle glaucoma; obstructive GIT gravis; CNS toxicity May induce ventricular irritability or increase magnitude of MI (accelerates sinus rate)
Benzylpenicillin	*Compound fractures:* 1.2 g (120 mg/kg/day up to adult dose in 4 divided doses) IV, q6 h, 3–10 yr*:* 150–300 mg q6 h <3 yr: 60 mg q6 h *Neonate:* 30–60 mg q12 h	Penicillin antibiotic	Antibacterial prophylaxis (*Clostridium perfringens*) after compound fractures with wound soiling or severe tissue damage or devitalized tissue present	*Prec:* renal impairment; CHF; high doses
Bupivacaine hydrochloride (0.125% and 0.25%)	*Without adrenaline:* max. 2 mg/kg *With adrenaline:* max. 2.6 mg/kg	Local anaesthetic prolonged anaesthesia	Infiltration anesthesia Peripheral, sympathetic nerve, epidural anesthesia	*Not for IV infusion block* (Biers block); would lead to seizure, cardiovascular collapse *Contra:* severe shock; uncorrected hypotension *Adverse:* CNS, cardiovascular, respiratory, GIT disturbances
Calcium chloride	Slow IV into large vein (10% soln contains 6.8 mmol/10 mL) *Hypocalcaemia:* adult: load: 10 mL slowly; infusion: 40 mL 10% Ca gluconate in 500 mgL saline over 2–8 h; adjust according to serum Ca estimations; child: 0.2 mL/kg IV over 5 min; then 0.5–2.0 mmol/kg/day infusion *Severe hyperkalaemia:* 5–10 mL of 10% (3.4–6.8 mgmol); monitor ECG during admin; adjust accordingly *CPR:* 0.5–1 g IV over 1–2 min; 100 mg/mL	Divalent cation	Hypocalcaemic tetany Severe hyperkalaemia (adjunctive); Magnesium toxicit Cardiac resuscitation [its use in ventricular fibrillation and electromechanical dissociation is not supported by experimental studies]	*Contra:* IM, SC, hypercalcaemia, hypercalciuria; severe renal disease; ventricular fibrillation (in cardiac resuscitation) *Adverse*: peripheral vasodilatation, hypotension, bradycardia, arrhythmias, syncope, cardiac arrest *Interact*: cardiac glycosides; Ca channel blockers, carbonates, phosphates, sulfates, tetracyclines Do not put in IV line with bicarbonate solutions and never inject into tissues as will cause sloughing Do not give as oral or scalp vein administration in infants
Cefotaxime or ceftriaxone	*Cefotaxime:* 1 g (150 mg/kg/day up to adult dose in 3 divided doses) IV, q8 h or *Ceftriaxone:* 1 g (75 mg/kg/day up to adult dose) IV, once daily for 5–10 days. Ceftriaxone can be given IMI in lignocaine hydrochloride 1%	Cephalosporin antibiotics	Injuries where antibiotic therapy is necessary and penicillin sensitivity is present	*Cross sensitivity to penicillins* *Prec*: renal or hepatic impairment; pregnancy, lactation *Adverse:* superinfection; pseudomembranous colitis; sensitivity phenomena; local reactions
Cephalothin or cephazolin	Cephalothin 2 g (100 mg/kg/day up to adult dose in 4–6 divided doses) IV, q6 h or cephazolin 1 g (40 mg/kg/day up to adult dose in 3 divided doses) IV, q8 h; for at least 5 days [Used in conjunction with metroidazole]	Cephalosporin antibiotics	Antibacterial prophylaxis (for broad-spectrum antibacterial activity) after muscular, skeletal and soft tissue trauma, crush injuries and stab wounds Compound fractures	*Adverse*: superinfection; pseudomembranous colitis; thrombophlebitis; sensitivity phenomena

Drugs	Dosage	Drug type	Used for	Comments
	Compound fractures: cephalothin 1 g (child: 15 mg/kg up to 1 g) IV, q6 h *or* cephazolin 1 g (child: 15 mg/kg up to 1 g) IV or IM, q8 h; 1-3 days treatment is standard; if wound soiling or tissue damage is severe and/or devitalized tissue is present, add gentamicin and benzylpenicillin			
Clonazepam	*Initial:* 0.25–0.5 mg IV bolus Adult 1 mg IV Slow infusion: 2–3 mg/12 h	Benzodiazepine Anticonvulsant	Status epilepsy	*Contra:* CAL with incipient respiratory failure *Adverse:* cerebral, respiratory and cardiac depression, and hypotension [More profound respiratory depressant than diazepam]
Codeine (methyl-morphine) phosphate	Oral administration *Adult:* 10–60 mg q4-6 h *Child:* >1yr: 1–3 mg/kg q4-6 h; extreme care needed when giving to newborn or premature infants	Opioid analgesic; antitussive; antidiarrhoeal	Mild to moderate pain	*Contra:* respiratory depression; after biliary tract operations; head injuries, raised intracranial pressure; bronchial asthma; heart failure secondary to chronic lung disease; with MAOIs *Adverse:* constipation, nausea, vomiting, sedation
Co-trimoxazole (trimethoprim and sulpha-methoxazole)	160/800 mg (8/40 mg/kg/day up to adult dose, in 2 divided doses) orally, q12 h for 5–10 days. [Used in conjunction with metronidazole]	Antibiotics	Bites and clenched-fist injuries where antibiotic therapy is necessary and penicillin sensitivity is present	*Contra*: marked liver parenchymal damage; blood dyscrasia; severe renal insufficiency; infants *Adverse*: superinfection; systemic reactions; senstivity phenomena; GIT and haemotological disturbances *Interact*: numerous
Dexamethasone	*Acute adrenocortical insufficiency*: 10 mg IV; then continue with hydrocortisone *Reduction of cerebral oedema*: initially, 4–10 mg q4–6 h; titrate to response *Child* 0.1–0.25 mg/kg IV IM or PO	Steroid	Reduce cerebral oedema, acute adrenocortical insufficiency	*Contra*: uncontrolled infections *Adverse*: fluid and electrolyte, musculoskeletal, GI, skin, neurological, haematological endocrine, ocular, metabolic disorders *Interact*: numerous
Diazepam	Give slow (5 mg/min) IV *Adult:* 2–10 mg IV *Anticonvulsant*: 5–10 mg IV q10–15 min to max 30 mg, repeat in 2–4 h if necessary; follow with IV phenytoin *Child:* ≤0.20 mg/kg IV, titrate to response	Benzodiazepine Anticonvulsant Sedative	Status epilepsy, alcohol withdrawal	*Contra:* CAL with incipient respiratory failure *Adverse:* cerebral and cardiac depression, hypotension [only to be used when ventilatory facilities are available]; thrombophlebitis if injected into peripheral veins

Drugs	Dosage	Drug type	Used for	Comments
Dicloxacillin	500 mg–1 g every 6 h	Penicillin	Treatment or prophylaxis against infections caused by staphylococci in elderly people at risk of hepatotoxicity with flucloxacillin	Risk of marked thrombophlebitis
Dobutamine hydrochloride	2.5–20 μg/kg/min as continuous IV infusion via an infusion pump [Dilute: 250 mg in 100 mL dextrose 5% in water (2.5 mg/mL) before admininstration]	β_1-selective agonist: inotrope and reduces preload and afterload	Short-term treatment of cardiogenic shock secondary to acute MI or cardiac surgery Low dose: increased CO with minimal increase in H or change in BP Synergistic effects with dopamine (more potent than dopamine but without renal and mesenteric vasodilatory effects)	Idiopathic hypertrophic subaortic stenosis
Dopamine hydrochloride	Initial dose 2–5 μg/kg/min; titrate for desired response; give as continuous IV infusion via an infusion pump. [Dilute: 200 mg in 100 mL dextrose 5% in water (2 mg/mL) before admin.] Low dose = 2–5 g/kg/min Higher dose = 5–20 g/kg/min	Inotropic agent	Cardiogenic shock due to MI, trauma, endotoxic septicemia, open heart surgery, renal failure and chronic cardiac decompensation as in CHF Low dose: improves renal and mesenteric blood flow Higher dose: increased β-adrenergic stimulation (inotropic effects) >20 μg/kg/min: more β-adrenergic stimulation and vasoconstriction Synergistic effects with dobutamine	*Contra:* hypovolaemia; dilution with alkaline soln; hypertensive states
Doxycycline	100 mg orally, daily for 5–10 days (not in child <8 yr, nor in pregnant or breast-feeding woman) [Used in conjunction with metronidazole]	Tetracycline antibiotic	Bites and clenched-fist injuries where antibiotic therapy is necessary and penicillin sensitivity is present	*Contra:* concomitant vitamin A, retinoids; pregnancy, lactation, child *Adverse:* photosensitivity; superinfection; pseudomembranous colitis *Interact:* anticoagulanta; penicillins; antacids; retinoids; Ocs
Fentanyl citrate	Individualize dosage IV; adult: 50–200 g; Child μ2 yr: 1–5μg/kg Infusion 2–10 μg/kg/h	Opioid analgesic in anaesthesia	Induces analgesia and unconsciousness: useful for its short duration of action (1–2 h)	*Contra:* Bronchial asthma; coma; myasthenia gravis; with monoaminoxidases High doses lead to muscle rigidity

Drugs	Dosage	Drug type	Used for	Comments
Flucloxacillin	*Muscular, skeletal and soft tissue trauma, crush injuries and stab wounds:* 1 g (child: 75–100 mg/kg/ day up to adult dose in 4 divided doses) IV, q6 h; [Used in conjunction with gentamicin and metronidazole] *Compound fractures:* 1 g (child: 75–100 mg/kg/day up to adult dose in 4 divided doses) IV, q6 h (as alternative use cephalothin); if wound soiling or tissue damage is severe and/or devitalized tissue is present, add gentamicin and/or benzylpenicillin	Penicillinase-resistant penicillin antibiotic	Antibacterial prophylaxis (for penicillinase-producing penicillin-resistant staphylococci) after muscular, skeletal and soft tissue trauma, crush injuries and stab wounds Compound fractures	*Contra:* history of jaundice ot disturbed liver function Caution in patients >60 yr *Adverse:* superinfection; pseudomembranous colitis; GI upset; sensitivity phenomena
Flumazenil	*Reversal:* 0.05–0.1 mg initially; titrate to response	Antidote to benzodiazepine overdose; BDZ antagonist	Deterioration in consciousness or respiration thought to be due to diazepam or related drugs; short duration of action	*Contra:* symptomatic mixed BDZ/cyclic antidepressant intoxication Must have adequate monitoring due to unpredictable antagonism of respiratory depression and re-sedation
Frusemide (furosemide)	*Adult:* *Cerebral oedema:* 20–40 mg IV *Acute pulmonary oedema:* 40–80 mg slow IV then 40 mg after 1 h prn *Child:* 1 mg/kg IV max. dose 6 mg/kg	Loop diuretic	Oedema Rapid diuresis	*Contra:* prerenal or renal failure; hepatic coma; sulfonamide sensitivity Ototoxic Do not give to infants with or prone to jaundice
Gentamicin	*Adult:* 5–7 mg/kg/day IV, as a single daily dose; subsequent doses adjusted after measuring trough level 20 h after 2nd dose *Child:* >10 yr: 1.7 mg/kg IV, q8 h 5–10 yr: 2 mg/kg IV, q8 h 1mo-5 yr, 2.5 mg/kg IV, q8 h [Used in conjunction with flucloxacillin and metronidazole]	Aminoglycoside antibiotic	Antibacterial prophylaxis (for gram-negative organisms) after muscular, skeletal and soft tissue trauma, crush injuries and stab wounds; and for compound fractures with wound soiling or severe tissue damage or devitalized tissue present	*Caution needed due to its narrow therapeutic index* *Contra:* myasthenia gravis *Adverse:* ototoxicity and renal toxicity: need regular blood assays; superinfection
Glyceryl trinitrate	Infusion 50 mg in100 mL 5% dextrose. Commence at 3 mL/h Titrate to effect	Arteriolar dilator	Pulmonary oedema Myocardial ischaemia Hypertensive emergencies	Use non-PVC IV tubing Close monitoring of BP
Hydrocortisone	*Acute severe asthma:* 200 mg q6 h IV *Adrenal crisis:* after dexamethasone administration; 100 mg q6 h *Child:* 5 mg/kg IV	Corticosteroid	Acute severe asthma Acute respiratory failure Adrenal crisis	Unproven usefulness in cerebral oedema associated with head trauma

Drugs	Dosage	Drug type	Used for	Comments
Ibuprofen	Oral administration *Adult:* 200–400 mg q4–6 h *Child:* not recommended	Non-steroidal anti-inflammatory	Acute or chronic pain states in which there is an inflammatory component	*Contra:* hypersensitivity to ibuprofen, aspirin or other NSAIDs; active GIT bleeding or peptic ulceration; pregnancy or lactation *Adverse:* nausea, vomiting, indigestion, diarrhoea, constipation, abdominal bloating/ flatulence; tinnitus; oedema; dizziness, headache, nervousness, rash, pruritis; hepatotoxicity Caution with concurrent anticoagulation
Isoprenaline hydrochloride/ Isoproterenol	*Adult:* IV 200 μg [in 100 mL 5% dextrose], followed by titrated rate infusion: 30μg/h and increase by 30μg/h according to pulse rate and BP; adjust dosage q5 min *Child:* 0.1–0.5 μg/kg/dose, followed by titrated rate infusion: 0.1 μg/kg/min (= 1 mL/h) [mix 0.6 mg/kg in 100 mL of 5% dextrose in water]; increase by 0.1 μg/kg/min prn	Potent β_1 and β_2 agonist; inotrope and chronotrope	Haemodynamically significant bradycardia unresponsive to atropine Heart block Stokes Adams attacks Torsades des pointes Cardiac arrest Bronchospasm during anaesthesia Adjunctive with shock; β blocker overdose (with severe haemodynamic compromise)	*Contra:* tachycardic states; recent MI; angina; heart block secondary to digoxin toxicity *Interacts:* adrenaline; cyclopropane, digitalis
Ketamine	Induction 1–2 mg/kg IV over 1–2 min	Rapidly acting anaesthetic induction agent	Can be used IM at 10 mg/kg	Maintains airway reflexes May cause increased pulse and BP May cause vivid emergence phenomena
Lignocaine (lidocaine) hydrochloride	*Adult:* *Antiarrythmic in cardiac arrest:* 1–1.5 mg/kg IV bolus slowly, then 0.5 mg/kg q5 min, until a max of 3 mg/kg has been given. *Do not exceed 1.5 mg/kg* in patients with metabolic acidosis, liver disease or congestive cardiac failure. *Antiarrythmic in noncardiac arrest:* 1–1.5 mg/kg bolus, then 2–4 mg/min by continuous IV infusion. [For the IV infusion: load 4 g lignocaine into 500 mL of 5% dextrose] *Child:* Initial bolus of 1 mg/kg, then 20–50 mg/kg/min by continuous IV infusion [120 mg in 100 mL of 5% dextrose in water, i.e. 1% solution] *Local anaesthetic:* max: 4 mg/kg (plain solution) or 7 mg/kg (containing adrenaline)	Potent antiarrhythmic (type I_B), esp. in AMI Local or regional anaesthetic	Ventricular tachycardia or ventricular fibrillation Local/regional anaesthetic	*Side-effects* [toxic level ≥9 mg/L; therapeutic serum level = 2–6 mg/L]: *CNS* (esp. with shock, CCF, or severe liver disease)—seizures, psychosis, disorientation, confusion, paraesthesias, drowsiness, agitation, twitching, decreased hearing *CVS*—myocardical depression; hypotension, AV block, sinus arrest *Contra:* hypotension (systolic ≤90), local inflammation; supraventricular arrhythmias; Stokes–Adams syndrome; severe S-A, A-V, intraventricular block, severe shock *Interact:* antiarrythmics, anticonvulsants

Drugs	Dosage	Drug type	Used for	Comments
Mannitol (20%)	*Adult:* *Diuresis:* 1–2 g/kg over 30–60 min *Reduction of intracranial and intraocular pressure*: 0.5–2 g/kg IV over 30–60 min *Child:* 0.5–1 g/kg/dose	Osmotic diuretic	Raised intracranial and intraocular pressure Acute haemolysis Acute renal failure	*Contra:* anuria; pulmonary congestion or oedema; dehydration
Metronidazole	500 mg (15 mg/kg loading dose followed by 25 mg/kg/day up to adult dose in 3 divided doses) IV q12 h. [Used in conjuction with flucloxaciilin and gentamicin or in conjunction with cephalothin or cephazolin]	Antibiotic	Antibacterial prophylaxis (for anaerobic bacteria) after muscular, skeletal and soft tissue trauma, crush injuries and stab wounds Bites and clenched-fist injuries where antibiotic therapy is necessary and penicillin sensitivity is present Amputation, especially of an ischaemic leg	*Contra:* blood dyscrasias; CNS disease; pregnancy, lactation *Adverse:* superinfection; GI upset; leucopenia; neurological disturbances; sensitivity *Interact:* alcohol; warfarin
Midazolam	0.5–5.0 mg IV; titrate to effect Child sedation 0.1–0.5 mg/kg	Short-acting sedative	Useful prior to intubation, minor procedures	*Contra:* airway compromise; shock, coma; acute alcohol intoxication; narrow-angle glaucoma; rapid or bolus IV
Morphine sulphate	*Pain relief:* incremental doses of 2.5–5.0 mg up to 20 mg then constant infusion at 2.5–10 mg/h; use with antiemetic. *Child:* 0.1–0.2 mg/kg IV or IM	Opioid analgesic sedative	Analgesic for severe pain Sedative Pulmonary oedema	*Contra:* respiratory depression; acute alcoholism; biliary tract surgery; MAOIs; premature infants *Adverse:* biliary spasm Effects can be reversed with naloxone
Naloxone	*Adult:* 0.1–2 mg; titrate to effect IV, IM; repeat q2–3 min prn to max. 10 mg *Child:* Initially 0.01 mg/kg IV, repeat with 0.1 mg/kg if necessary	Opioid antagonist	Reversal of narcotic depression induced by opioids	*Prec:* rapid reversal, pregnancy *Adverse:* hypertension, pulmonary oedema, arrhythmias, seizures
Nitrous oxide 50% + oxygen 50%	Self-inhaled prn	Analgesic	Analgesic for conscious, co-operative patients, short, but painful interventions	*Contra:* altered consciousness, airway/ ventilation problems; chest injuries/ pneumothorax; bowel obstruction
Noradrenaline (norepinephrine)	0.2–1 μg/kg/min; increase as needed. [Dilute in glucose 5% in saline for continuous IV infusion]	Potent α-agonist—powerful generalized vasoconstrictor	Shock, i.e. acute hypotension Adjunct in treatment of cardiac arrest	*Contra:* pregnancy; hypovolaemia; mesenteric or peripheral vascular thrombosis *Adverse:* decreases renal perfusion; visceral ischaemia Interactions: MOAIs, tricyclics. *Must monitor BP;* if extravasation occurs: give phentolamine, 5–10 mg in 10–15 mL of saline, in same IV catheter
Pancuronium*	0.04–0.1 mg/kg IV	Non-depolarizing muscle relaxant	Skeletal muscle relaxation in surgical anaesthesia Artificial respiration support	*Prec:* depolarizing drugs; myasthenia gravis; electrolyte imbalance, dehydration; hypo/hyperthermia

Drugs	Dosage	Drug type	Used for	Comments
Paracetamol (acetaminophen)	Oral administration *Adult:* 0.5–1 g q4–6 h (max: 4 g/day) *Child:* 15–20 mg/kg q4 h max. 100 mg/kg/24 h 7–12 yr: 250-500 mg q4–6 h (max. 2 g/day)	Analgesic; antipyretic	Mild to moderate pain or fever	*Contra:* Known hypersensitivity to paracetamol; care needed with impaired renal function *Adverse:* rare—allergic and haematological reactions, dyspepsia, nausea, skin eruptions *Hepatotoxic in overdosage levels* (c. 10–15 g for adult)
Penicillin Procaine	4.8 g (50 mg/kg up to adult dose) IM, as a single dose (followed by amoxicillin/potassium calvulanate)	Sparingly soluble salt of benzylpenicillin	Bites and clenched-fist injuries where antibiotic therapy is necessary (with penicillin sensitivity—see metronidazole)	*Prec:* IV administration *Adverse:* superinfection; sensitivity phenomena
Pethidine hydrochloride	*Adult:* 1 mg/kg IM or incrementally up to 1.5 mg/kg IV q3-4 h *Child:* 0.5–2 mg/kg (max. 100 mg) IM or SC q3–4 h or 1 mg/kg (max. 50 mg) *slow* IV q4 h	Opioid analgesic	Moderate to severe pain unresponsive to non-opioids	*Contra:* respiratory depression; severe hepatic disease; head injury, raised ICP (intracranial pressure); cardiac arrhythmias; convulsive states; acute alcoholism *Interact:* phenothiazines; CNS depressants, e.g. alcohol; MAOIs; phenytoin *Adverse:* convulsions; psychosis; hypotension
Phenytoin sodium	*Status epilepsy*: *Adult:* Load: 10–15 mg/kg slow IV (max. 50 mg/min); then 100 mg orally or IV q6–8 h *Child, neonate:* Initially 10–20 mg/kg by slow IV over 30 min, max. 1-3 mg/kg/min; then maintenance dose *Arrhythmias*: 3–5 mg/kg slow IV; repeat if necessary	Anticonvulsant with antiarrthymic properties	Seizures (partial, tonic clonic and status)	*Contra:* sinus bradycardia; heart block; rapid IV admin. *Adverse:* CNS disturbances; GI upset; rash; haemopoietic complications; hyperglycemia; hypersensitivity reactions; hepatic failure; hypotension and cardiac arrhythmias; numerous drug interactions Preferably use central vein for IV administration as it is very alkalotic BP and ECG monitoring during infusion is important Not stable in dextrose solutions; stable in saline for 30 min; do not give IM in emergencies because absorption is unpredictable
Prilocaine	Maximum dose: plain 4 mg/kg with adrenaline 6 mg/kg	Amide local anaesthetic	Local anaesthesia Intravenous regional anaesthesia (upper limb)	CNS toxicity with excess dose Methaemoglobinaemia can occur
Promethazine	10 mg –25 mg slow IV or IM	Antihistamine (H_1 blockadge)	Adjunctive treatment for anaphylactic reactions	Causes sedation and may cause extrapyramidal symptoms
Propofol* (1% emulsion)	*Adult:* *Induction*: 2–2.5 mg/kg, titrate to response *Maintenance*: admin. by continuous infusion or repeat bolus inj.; 1–3 mg/kg/h	Short-acting IV anaesthetic	Induction and maintenance of anaesthesia; rapid emergence from sedation Short-term sedation of ventilated child ⩾ 3 yr; rapid emergence from sedation	*Prec:* cardiac, renal, respiratory or hepatic impairment; hypovolaemia; epilepsy *Adverse:* hypotension, hypersensitivity; apnoea; bradycardia; seizures

Drugs	Dosage	Drug type	Used for	Comments
	Child: *Induction*: >8 yr: 2.5 mg/kg; 3–8 yr: usually >2.5 mg/kg *Maintenance:* >3 yr: usually 9–15 mg/kg/h as IV infusion or repeat bolus injection			*Child:* death from MI and metabolic acidosis; neurological disorders, so should not be used by infusion in children
Salbutamol	*IV:* *Adult:* 100–300μg bolus [5 mg in 100 mL Dextrose 5% in water *i.e.* 50μg/mL]: 5–20μg/min; *Child:* 10μg/kg bolus infusion,: 1–10μg/kg/min *Inhalation:* *Adult:* 5 mg q4 h; *Child:* 4–12 yr: 2.5 mg q4–6 h; *status asthmaticus:* nebulize with O_2 as 0.05 mg/kg of 0.5% solution diluted to 4 mL with sterile water, q 2–4 h initially, then prn	Selective β_2 agonist; bronchospasm relaxant	Relief of bronchospasm (asthma, chronic bronchitis, emphysema)	*Adverse:* tremor; tachycardia, palpitations; headaches; nausea; hypokalaemia *Interact:* sympathomimetics; β-blockers; digoxin; steroids; diuretics
Sodium bicarbonate (8.4% solution)	*Adult:* slow IV, 50–100 mmol as guided by ABG measurements when available *Child:* 1–2 mL/kg immediately then 1 mL/kg/10 min arrest time [In infants, dilute 1 : 1 with 5% dextrose in water.]	H^+ neutralization	Severe persistent metabolic acidosis e.g. pH <7.0 (due to renal tubular acidosis and GIT bicarbonate loss; not recommended when due to diabetes or cardiac arrest) Antidote to poisoning by membrane depressant cardiotoxic drugs, e.g. tricyclic antidepressants, quinidine Life-threatening hyperkalaemia Routine use during CPR is not justified (only in prolonged arrest)	Do not give in same IV line as any other medication, especially catecholamines or calcium *Contra:* renal failure; metabolic or respiratory alkalosis; hypertension; oedema; CHF; hypoventilation; chloride, calcium or potassium depletion; hypernatraemia *Adverse:* alkalososis; hypokalamia; tetany
Suxamethonium chloride* (succinylcholine)	*Adult:* 1 mg/kg IV bolus	Depolarizing muscle relaxant (5–10 min of duration of action)	Muscle relaxant in anaesthesia Emergency induction with rapid sequence intubation	*Contra:* inability to intubate; head injuries, open eye injuries, hyperkalaemic; severe burns; trauma; non-traumatic rhabdomyolysis, spinal cord injuries with paraplegia or quadriplegia; muscular dystrophies *Adverse:* cardiac arrhythmias; bradycardia if second dose given malignant hyperthemia
Tetanus toxoid	*Tetanus prone wound* either with full immunization but >2 yr since last tetanus toxoid (when >10 yr since last tetanus toxoid, also give TIG) toxoid 0.5 mL	Vaccine against tetanus; active immunization against tetanus	Tetanus-prone wound with full immunization but >2 yr since last tetanus toxoid	*Contra:* acute respiratory infection (booster dose) *Prec:* immunosuppressive therapy; intra-arterial/venous injection

Drugs	Dosage	Drug type	Used for	Comments
	Clean, minor wound but 10 yr since last tetanus toxoid: 0.5 mL *Immunization schedule*: 3 doses of 0.5 mL IM; 2nd dose after 6–12 weeks; 3rd dose 6–12 months after 2nd dose; booster every 10 yr			
TIG (tetanus immuno-globulin)	*Clinical tetanus*: 4000 IU by slow IV infusion *Tetanus prone wounds* with dubious history: 250 IU IM *Grossly contaminated wound or if ≥24 h since injury*: 500 IU IM	Human immunoglobulin for tetanus	Management of clinical tetanus tetanus-prone wounds where immunization history dubious	*Contra:* isolated IgA deficiency *Prec:* pregnancy; renal failure; rapid infusion *Interact:* live attenuated virus *Adverse:* abdominal pain; headache; chest tightness; pyrexia; dyspnoea rash; hypotension; nausea, vomiting; aseptic meningitis syndrome
Thiopentone sodium* (2.5% in aqueous solution)	2–5 mg/kg slow IV; may need <1 mg/kg when hypotension is a risk; *Prolonged seizures*: as above, then 1–5 mg/kg/h by IV infusion into a central vein when other measures insufficient	Ultrashort-acting barbiturate; anaesthetic induction agent	IV induction anaesthetic for short-duration operations; uncontrolled seizures; refractory elevated ICP	*Contra:* status asthmaticus; porphyria; constrictive pericarditis; shock *Prec:* extravasation, intra-arterial inj. *Interact:* numerous *Adverse:* respiratory, myocardial depression; hypotension; cardiac arrhythmias; anaphylactoid reactions *Necessitates endotracheal intubation* and mechanical ventilation and possibly inotropic drugs (counters myocardial depressant effects); monitor blood concentrations during prolonged use
Vancomycin	1 g IV q12 h *Child:* 40 mg/kg/day in 2–4 divided doses	Glycopeptide antibiotic	Severe infection with gram-positive organisms in penicillin-allergic patients	Must be administered over 1 h to avoid anaphylactoid reactions Monitor plasma levels Impaired renal function
Vecuronium*	0.08–0.1 mg/kg IV; additional doses of 0.01–0.015 mg/kg prn	Short acting non-depolarizing muscle relaxant	Skeletal muscle relation in surgical anaesthesia; emergency endotracheal intubation	*Contra:* cross-sensitivity with pancuronium *Prec:* neuromuscular syndromes; impaired renal or hepatic function; electrolyte disturbances Not to be used in neonates or premature babies

Classified index to formulary

acute haemolysis
mannitol
adrenal
dexamethasone
hydrocortisone
alcohol withdrawal
diazepam
anaesthetics
general induction
thiopentone sodium
propofol
midazolam
fentayl citrate
ketamine
emergency induction
suxamethonium chloride
muscle relaxants
pancuronium
suxamethonium chloride
vecuronium
local anaesthetics
bupivacaine hydrochloride
lignocaine (lidocaine)
prilocaine
sedatives
midazolam
diazepam
analgesics
severe pain
morphine sulphate
moderate to severe pain
pethidine hydrochloride
mild to moderate pain
nitrous oxide
anaphylaxis
adrenaline
hydrocortisone
promethazine
antibiotics
amoxycillin
benzylpenicillin
cefotaxime/ceftriaxone
cephalothin/cephazolin
co-trimoxazole
doxycycline
flucloxacillin
gentamicin
metronidazole
penicillin procaine
vancomycin
anticonvulsants
clonazepam
diazepam
phenytoin sodium
thiopentone sodium
antidotes
benzodiazepine overdose—flumazenil
opioid overdose—naloxone
cardiotoxic drugs—sodium bicarbonate
calcium chloride
cardiac arrest
adrenaline (epinephrine)
atropine sulphate
dobutamine hydrochloride
dopamine hydrochloride
isoprenaline hydrochloride
lignocaine (lidocaine)
cerebral oedema
dexamethasone
mannitol
renal
sodium bicarbonate
calcium chloride
mannitol
frusemide
respiratory
adrenaline (epinephrine)
hydrocortisone
salbutamol
hydrocortisone
tetanus prophylaxis
tetanus toxoid
TIG (tetanus immunoglobulin)

Abbreviations and symbols

Contra	contraindications
Prec	special precautions
Adverse	adverse reactions
Interact	drug interactions
IM	intramuscular
IMI	intramuscular infusion
IV	intravenous
PO	*per os* (by mouth)
SC	subcutaneous
prn	*pro re nata* (as required)
*	for use only by experienced anaesthetic staff
/	may be repeated every 15 min

45

CHAPTER 45

Trauma resources online

LAWRENCE TRIEU

CHAPTER 45
Trauma resources online

LAWRENCE TRIEU

In the fields of trauma and orthopaedic surgery there has been an explosion of information available on the Internet. Initially used by university academics to communicate via e-mail, the Internet is now being used as a vast interactive multimedia library that is accessible 24 hours a day and transcends national as well as geographical boundaries. Available resources for trauma surgeons include bibliographical and statistical databases, literature reviews, discussion groups, press releases, newsletters, drug information, self-assessment questionnaires, drug information, clinical decision aids, patient simulations, multimedia textbooks, interactive discussion forums, and much more (Klemenz and McSherry 1997).

This chapter provides a detailed discussion on searching for trauma information on the World Wide Web—one of the most widely used and useful components of the Internet—followed by a brief description of currently available online trauma resources. Detailed discussion on mailing lists, newsgroups, file transfer protocol (ftp), and gopher are beyond the scope of this text. Details of these may be found in a general computing text such as Kent (1999).

The Internet and the World Wide Web

The Internet is a global network of thousands of smaller networks of computers used by millions of people to communicate and share information. The Internet began in 1969 as a project of the United States Department of Defense. They were investigating methods of connecting different local area networks (LAN) and wide area networks (WAN) of computers to each other. These various networks were often incompatible in terms of software and hardware. This revolutionary method of linking disparate networks of computers was constructed, as the Department of Defense wanted the information stored in these computers to survive a nuclear strike and be accessible in other parts of the country if such an eventuality did occur. In order to construct the Internet special computers called routers had to be built, which connected the various LANs and WANs, and a special protocol of data transmission (TCP/IP) was designed (Leow 1996).

The World Wide Web is the latest and most useful service to appear on the Internet and has contributed enormously to the rapid growth of the Internet. It was established by the CERN European Particle Physics Laboratory in Switzerland. Workers there designed HTML, the scripting language that forms the basis of the World Wide Web. This scripting language instructs the *browser* (a special program needed to access the web) to display text, graphics, sound, and video in the desired format. The most widely used browsers are Netscape Navigator and Microsoft Internet Explorer. The multimedia nature of the World Wide Web (also known simply as the 'web') has contributed greatly to its user-friendly nature and hence its popularity. This particular feature makes the Internet an attractive medium as a teaching resource. Other features of the Internet include e-mail (electronic mail) and ftp (file transfer protocol), which allows transfer of computer files between two computers, as well as newsgroups, gopher, and many other such formats.

Finding trauma resources on the web—search engines and directories

The World Wide Web contains huge amounts of information and is growing exponentially (it is anticipated to expand 1000% over the next few years). Finding information on the World Wide Web can often be a difficult task. Because of the exponential growth in information available, and the disorder in which it is accumulating, there is no reliable or comprehensive way to find all of the information available on a given topic. Unlike paper journal articles where there are *de facto* standard indices such as Medline, there is no official central index of the web. Several strategies, however, have been developed to help people find what they are looking for on the Internet—*search engines* such as such as Google (http://www.google.com) and AltaVista (http://www.altavista.com), and *directories* such as Yahoo! (http://www.yahoo.com) These two paradigms are the Internet equivalent of a contents page and the index of a book respectively, although the analogy is not quite perfect in that book indexes only allow querying of a single term, whereas the search engine paradigm also allows construction of complex queries of multiple terms.

With directories like Yahoo! the content of the Internet is divided into topics and subtopics. Human intervention is required in creating these categories and subcategories and in the allocation of websites to them. By selecting from a list of top-level subject headings, then from a series of lists of increasingly more specific subcategories, the user is guided to a list of websites that offer information relevant to the topic of interest (Kastin and Wexler 1998). A short summary of each website, written either by the directory administrator or by the creator of the website, assists the user in selecting websites. The categories are arbitrary and the user must discover the correct one before the information is accessible. Directories can also be searched by keyword, but keyword searching only retrieves word occurrences either in the category/subcategory listing or the summary of the website. Because directories do not index word occurrences on the website of interest itself, it is imperative that the categorization of the site is correct. Keyword searching will fail if the chosen keyword is replaced by a synonym or is spelt differently. Also, because the scope of general directories is not limited to medical information, an unrestricted search is likely to retrieve a lot of irrelevant information.

Search engines, unlike directories, do attempt to categorize information and their index is automatically generated. The advantage of a search engine over a directory is comprehensiveness—search engines can index every word on every web page of a given list of websites (Spooner 1996, Kastin and Wexler 1998). Search engines build their indices using programs called crawlers, spiders, or robots. These programs note the address or URL (universal resource locator) of the web page, scan, and store all or part of the contents (some crawlers index only the header information or summary, whereas others index every word on every page), and follow all the links found on that site; then the process is repeated on web pages of those links. With this comprehensiveness though, there comes a loss of specificity. It is not unusual for a search engine to return a list of tens of thousands of web pages for one search. Because the Internet is not static, crawlers must revisit sites to update the search engine index. The frequency that this occurs varies, from monthly to longer, so out-of-date links can be returned. This is another disadvantage of search engines.

Centralized versus distributed search engines

Search engines can be further divided into centralized and distributed approaches (see Table 45.1). The centralized approach is the conventional one, and is epitomized by the general-purpose Internet search engines described earlier. It involves attempting to create a single index for all existing Internet content, and consequently has enormous demands on running times and storage requirements. This is because Internet content approximately triples in size each year, thus requiring a centralized search engine to similarly triple in storage capacity and indexing speed each year in order to guarantee the same degree of comprehensiveness and freshness of links. This is an exponentially difficult task, and as a result, the leading general search engines only index approximately a third of indexable Internet content

Table 45.1 Comparison of directories and search engines

	Directories	Search engines
Organization	Organized as a hierarchical directory of topics	Organized as an index—essentially a database containing a dictionary that maps terms to resource locations.
Access	Accessed by top-down navigation of the classification tree, with minimal or no searching facilities	Accessed by querying, returning a set of results that match a given set of criteria, i.e. contain a certain combination of words
Granularity	Granularity at the level of resources, with each link describing a single Internet site or section	Granularity at the level of words, with the ability to locate individual occurrences of a given word
Compilation	Manually compiled by human evaluation and classification of each resource	Automatically compiled by a crawler

(Lawrence and Giles 1998). Distributed search engines create indexes only of specific subsets of Internet content, and where queries span more than one subset, perform separate queries on each subset and assemble the results. This distribution/assembly process can be repeated recursively.

OrthoSearch—an integrated directory/search engine specific to orthopaedic and traumatic surgery

The directory and search engine paradigms both serve a complementary function—the directory paradigm is easier to use, but for large resource sets is less powerful than indexing because of the labour-intensiveness of both compilation and navigation. However, the search engine paradigm can yield an extremely large result set that is difficult to navigate, and often contains many irrelevant matches. Existing centralized Internet search engines try to sort the result set by using a relevance algorithm, usually by counting the number of occurrences, and whether occurrences are in a heading or a paragraph body. However this is still imperfect, being opaque and difficult for users to understand, and often arbitrary in the final ordering of resources.

OrthoSearch (http://www.orthosearch.com) is a search engine/directory implemented specifically for the retrieval of orthopaedic and trauma data on the Internet. OrthoSearch is an integrated search engine/directory using a distributed approach in that, firstly it indexes only orthopaedic content, and secondly, it uses the OWL (Orthopaedic Web Links, http://owl.orthogate.org) directory classification system to distribute this orthopaedic content into sub-indexes—one for each OWL category. Much effort was made to integrate these two paradigms as this integration permits seamless transitions between searching and browsing. A search can be performed at any sub-section in the OWL hierarchy, and the result set in turn is displayed hierarchically using OWL as the classification/ordering system. Seamless two-way transition is thus possible between the directory paradigm of OWL, and the indexing paradigm of a term occurrence-based search engine. Even very large sets of results are presented in an order that is easy to understand, with OWL descriptions used throughout to describe sections of the result set. In essence, the result set is no longer linear as with other search engines but hierarchical, permitting the user to examine an overview, or zoom in on any part of it, all the way down to the granularity of individual occurrences.

Both parallel indexing and parallel querying are permitted. The integrated approach also permits efficient querying of sub-sections of the OWL hierarchy, as well as independent re-indexing of each sub-section. Use of a distributed design raises a number of design and implementation issues. It requires specification of crawling constraints to prevent the crawler from indexing content outside it's content subset. This is achieved through associating each OWL link with a crawler indexing level parameter that can vary from page-only, or up to any level of directory, with the entire site being the limiting case. Links between sites are not followed, as such site-granularity links are handled by OWL rather than the OrthoSearch crawler. Co-ordination between crawlers of each subindex is required to prevent duplicate indexing of the same content. A metaindex of the OWL links, sorted by physical resource location, is compiled to permit such coordination, and is the only centralized data structure.

Because of the smaller index that results in the distributed approach, re-indexing is permitted at a greater frequency than that of a general search engine. Whereas general search engines like AltaVista re-update their indices on a monthly or longer frequency, the smaller index of OrthoSearch can be re-updated weekly.

The full power of a search engine can often be difficult to exploit because construction of complex queries requires understanding of Boolean logic, and knowledge of the query language syntax. OrthoSearch solves this by the use of a graphic user interface for the construction of such advanced queries, dramatically reducing the users learning curve. The other difficulty in query construction is with synonyms (such as 'orthopaedic' versus 'orthopedic'), and with terms that are sub-concepts of other terms (for example simply searching for cancer may miss occurrences of osteosarcoma). This can be overcome through the use of a dictionary of such synonyms and sub-concepts. Each term in a given query can then be looked up, and related terms found and also included in the query. Construction of such a dictionary is being incorporated into OrthoSearch.

As the Internet multiplies in size each year, the specialized approach that OrthoSearch uses will increasingly be more relevant, up-to date, and comprehensive within a given topic than general Internet search engines. The model pioneered by the OrthoSearch will also be applied across other medical and surgical specialties with a research and marketing arm, MedPacific, acting as a conduit. Thus, a wide range of health content can be browsed, indexed and searched in a powerful yet highly consistent manner.

Essential online resources

The following websites provide a great starting point for the trauma and orthopaedic surgeon into the wealth of trauma resources available online. Other relevant sites can be found by following hyperlinks provided on these websites whilst specific information can be searched using the OrthoSearch search engine.

General trauma and orthopaedic resources

OrthoSearch (http://www.orthosearch.com)

As described above, OrthoSearch is the leading orthopaedic and traumatic surgery search engine. Relevant, comprehensive, and intelligent.

WorldOrtho (http://www.worldortho.com)

WorldOrtho is one of the first truly comprehensive orthopaedics and trauma websites online. This site features over 2000 slides of patients with traumatic injuries and orthopaedic conditions with relevant lecture notes. It also includes an interactive clinico-pathological quiz, an electronic textbook of orthopaedic surgery, a large bank of exam questions with answers and abstracts from landmark trauma and orthopaedic literature. It is accompanied by a companion CD ROM (Sherry and Huckstep 1999).

Trauma.org (http://www.trauma.org)

Trauma.org is a comprehensive trauma site which aims to promote and disseminate the knowledge and practice of injury prevention and trauma care, provide accurate, current information in the field of trauma, and present an interactive forum for trauma care providers throughout the globe. An outstanding feature of this site are the excellent trauma moulages.

Liverpool Trauma Home Page (http://www.swsahs.nsw.gov.au/livtrauma)

Website of the Trauma Department of Liverpool Hospital, a tertiary referral hospital in Sydney, Australia. This large unit co-ordinates the EMST course. Special features of this site are the interactive resources including a discussion forum, MCQ questions, and clinical cases. The site itself is comprehensive and easy to navigate.

Orthogate (http://www.orthogate.org)

Orthogate was formed in 1998 by an amalgamation of the 12 most prominent sites on the Internet. It is an ambitious non-profit Internet project to provide unity to the provision of orthopaedic information on the World Wide Web.

The Orthogate Project is overseen by a learned society, the Internet Society for Orthopaedic Surgery (http://www.isost.org), and aims to:

- Provide a guide to where to find orthopaedic information on the Internet, offering comments on the validity of the information where appropriate.
- Educate orthopaedic surgeons concerning the potential benefits of collaboration via the Internet.
- Enlist the co-operation of each and every orthopaedic society and association around the world.
- Encourage the transition of existing traditional information resources towards electronic distribution and facilitate new mechanisms for making these resources available online.
- Support the research and development of innovative new concepts in the distribution of orthopaedic information and the utilization of the Internet in the delivery of orthopaedic care.

Orthopod (http://www.mailbase.ac.uk/lists/orthopod/)

Orthopod is the leading international academic mailing list for discussion, collaboration, sharing ideas and the dissemination of research in orthopaedics and trauma surgery for orthopaedic surgeons, allied professionals, and students.

OWL (Orthopaedic Web Links) (http://owl.orthogate.org)

Founded by Myles Clough, a Canadian orthopaedic surgeon, OWL was initially a personal collection of orthopaedic and trauma web links which he updated regularly. OWL has now grown to become the largest collection of links and is edited by multinational group whose aim is finding and evaluating available information online.

Wheeless' Textbook of Orthopaedic Surgery (http://www.medmedia.com)

A well-written, comprehensive and authoritative textbook available free online.

Medical Multimedia Group (http://www.sechrest.com/mmg)

The most comprehensive collection of trauma and orthopaedic patient education material available online.

e-hand (http://www.eatonhand.com)

The Electronic Textbook of Hand Surgery; a comprehensive online textbook of hand surgery.

Belgian Orthoweb (http://www.belgianorthoweb.be)

An international online service whose mission statement is to 'stimulate the communication among orthopaedic surgeons and residents in training and spread detailed information on modern surgical techniques, communicate new developments, principles of treatment, job opportunities, fellowships and awards, data on orthopaedic conferences and courses and interesting new products.'

Trauma societies online

British Trauma Society (http://www.trauma.org/bts)

An international society advancing and promoting education and research in the treatment of trauma.

American Association for the Surgery of Trauma (http://www.aast.org)

AAST's charter is to promote the exchange of scientific information regarding all phases of the care of the trauma patient.

American Trauma Society (http://www.amtrauma.org)

The American Trauma Society is a nationwide, non-profit, voluntary organization dedicated to the prevention of trauma and improvement of trauma care.

Eastern Association for the Surgery of Trauma (http://www.east.org)

A not-for-profit organization aiming to furnish leadership and foster advances in the care of injured patients. Members are located east of the Mississippi River in the USA.

References

Kastin S, Wexler J. (1998) Bioinformatics: searching the net. *Seminars in Nuclear Medicine* 28(2):177–187.

Kent P (1999) *The complete idiot's guide to the internet*, 6th edn. McMillan Computer Publishing, Indianapolis.

Klemenz B, McSherry D (1997) Obtaining medical information from the Internet. *Journal of the Royal College of Physicians of London* 31(4): 410–413.

Lawrence S, Giles CG (1998) Searching the World Wide Web. *Science* 280: 98–100.

Leow CK (1996) Internet and surgery. *Australian and New Zealand Journal of Surgery* 66: 655–658.

Sherry E, Huckstep RL (1999) *WorldOrtho on CD-ROM*. ISBN: 0646372610 (available from amazon.com).

Spooner SA (1996) The pediatric Internet. *Pediatrics* 98(6): 1185–1192.

Appendices

APPENDIX A

*Sample trauma flow sheet**

Name:

Date:

Arrival Time:

CHIEF COMPLAINT:

PREHOSPITAL TRANSPORT INFORMATION

❑ Scene ❑ Ambulance ❑ Helicopter

❑ Police ❑ Private vehicle ❑ Ambulatory

❑ Wheelchair ❑ Other ______

❑ Referring Doctor ______

❑ Referring Hospital ______

❑ Other information ______

______

______

______

PROCEDURES BEFORE ARRIVAL

❑ Oral airway ❑ Nasal airway ❑ EOA / PTL

❑ ETT # ❑ NTT # ❑ RSI

❑ Crico # ❑ O_2 @ ______ L /min via ______

Breath sounds: L: R:

❑ IVs # ❑ Peripheral ❑ Central ❑ Intraosseous

❑ IV fluids 1 2 3 4 5 6 ❑ Blood 1 2 3 4 5

❑ CPR ❑ PASG: ❑ Legs ❑ Abdomen

❑ Urinary cath ❑ Gastric tube

❑ Chest tube: ❑ R ❑ L ❑ Both

❑ C-spine protection ❑ Spine protection, Time on:

❑ Splints Type: ______

❑ Medications: ______

______

❑ Other procedures: ______

______

______

OTHER SERVICES CONTACTED (Time called and arrived)

______

______

______

______

______

______

______

MECHANISM OF INJURY

❑ MCV: ❑ Driver ❑ Passenger: ❑ Front ❑ Back

❑ Seat belt on ❑ Airbag inflated

❑ MCC: ❑ Driver ❑ Passenger

❑ Helmet worn ❑ Protective clothing worn

❑ Pedestrian vs vehicle

❑ Vehicle speed ______ mph / kph

❑ Fall ______ feet / meters

❑ GSW ❑ Stab ❑ Crush ❑ Burn / Cold

❑ Assault ❑ Hypothermia ❑ Other

AMPLE HISTORY

Allergies: ______

Medications: ______

______

Past Illnesses: ______

______

Last Meal: ______ Last-Tetanus: ______

Events: ______

______

Pregnant? ❑ Yes ❑ LMP ______ ❑ No

Spine protection device removed @ ______

PERSONNEL RESPONSE

SERVICE	NAME	CALLED	ARRIVED
ED Doctor			
Trauma Surgeon			
Neurosurgery			
Orthopedics			
Anesthesia			
Pediatrics			
ENT/OMFS			
Plastics, Burns			
Urology			
Nurse			
Nurse			
Other			

*Reproduced from *Advanced Trauma Life Support® Student Manual*, 1997 edition, pp. 467–470, by permission of the ACS Committee on Trauma.

INITIAL ASSESSMENT	IDENTIFY INJURY SITE BY NUMBER

INITIAL ASSESSMENT

AIRWAY / BREATHING

❑ Patent ❑ Obstructed ❑ Symmetrical

❑ Asymmetrical ❑ Unlabored ❑ Labored

Trachea midline? ❑ Yes ❑ No

Breath Sounds:			
	Present	❑ Right	❑ Left
	Clear	❑ Right	❑ Left
	Decreased	❑ Right	❑ Left
	Absent	❑ Right	❑ Left
	Rales/rhonchi	❑ Right	❑ Left

Crepitus? ❑ Yes ❑ No

CIRCULATION

Skin/mucous: ❑ Pink ❑ Pale

Membrane color: ❑ Flushed ❑ Jaundiced

❑ Ashen ❑ Cyanotic

Pulses: ❑ Normal, Site

❑ Bounding, Site

❑ Weak, Site

❑ Absent, Site

Rate ________ /minute Rhythm ___________

Skin temp: ❑ Warm ❑ Hot ❑ Cool/cold

Skin moisture: ❑ WNL ❑ Dry ❑ Moist

DISABILITY

GCS Score: Eye opening score_______

Verbal score___________

Best motor score________

TOTAL GCS SCORE:_____________

RTS Score: Respiratory score_______

Systolic BP score_______

GCS Score____________

TOTAL GCS SCORE_____________

Pupil Reaction	OS Size	OD Size
❑ Brisk	_____mm	_____mm
❑ Constricted	_____mm	_____mm
❑ Sluggish	_____mm	_____mm
❑ Dilated	_____mm	_____mm
❑ Nonreactive	_____mm	_____mm

2 3 4 5 6 7 8 9

IDENTIFY INJURY SITE BY NUMBER

1. Laceration	6. Open fx	11. Edema
2. Abrasion	7. GSW	12. Amputation
3. Hematoma	8. Stab	13. Avulsion
4. Contusion	9. Burn	14. Pain
5. Deformity	10. Cold	

Head: ______________________

Maxillofacial: ______________________

C-spine/neck: ______________________

Chest: ______________________

Abdomen: ______________________

Perineum: ______________________

Musculoskeletal: ______________________

(Graphics used with permission from LifeART Collection Images, Copyright © 1989–1997, by TechPool Studios, Cleveland, OH.)

TRAUMA RESUSCITATION ORDERS

TIME	LABORATORY	TIME	X-RAYS	TIME	PROCEDURES
	Type/cross # units		Chest:		O_2 @ L min via
	Type/hold		Pelvis		ETT # by:
	CBC Screen		Lateral c-spine		NTT # by:
	ETOH		Swimmers		Crico # by:
	Drug screen		Odontoid		Needle thoracostomy by:
	PT/PTT		Thoracic spine		Chest tube # by
	ABGs		Lumbar spine		R return: L return:
	Urinalysis		Skull		ED thoracotomy by:
	DPL Fluid		Facial series		Autotransfuser
	Pregnancy test + −		Mandible		RIV Site: Size:
	HIV + −		Abdomen		RIV Site: Size:
			Extremity: LUE/RUE		LIV Site: Size:
	Other:		Extremity: LLE / RLE		LIV Site: Size:
			IVP		CVP Site: Size:
			Cystogram		Pericardiocentesis by:
			Urethrogram		ECG
			Arteriogram/Aorto		Gastric tube # by:
			CT Head		Return:
			CT Chest		Color:
			CT Abdomen		Rectal tone:
			CT Pelvis		Rectal blood:
					Urinary cath #
					Return:
					Color
					Urine dip + −
					Spont void dip + −
					DPL: + 1 by;
					Sonography: by
					Results:
					Suturing by:
					Restraints: UE LE

FLUID INTAKE/OUTPUT

INTAKE	OUTPUT
Total fluids prehospital _____mL	Urine________mL
ED: Total fluids___________	Gastric_______mL
Total blood prehospital______mL	Blood________mL
ED: Total PRBCs__________ml	TOTAL_______mL
FFP Total______________mL	
Platelets_______________mL	
Other:	
TOTAL:_______________ mL	

ABGs

O_2 LPM	pH	Pco_2	Po_2	TIME

MEDICATIONS

MED	DOSE	BY	ROUTE/SITE	TIME
Tetanus				

TIME									
CUFF BP	/	/	/	/	/	/	/	/	/
Pulse									
Rhythm									
Respirations									
Temperature									
MAP line									
O_2 / Hgb Sat									
Carboximetry									
CVP									
Urinary output									
Blood output									
GCS Score									
1. Eye opening score									
2. Verbal score									
3. Best motor score									
TOTAL (1 + 2 + 3)									
R pupil size and reaction									
L pupil size and reaction									

TIME	**NOTES**

DISPOSITION: ❑ Alive; Time out: ________ To: ________________ Service: ________

❑ Dead: Time out: ________ To: ________________

❑ Operative permit signed ❑ Family notified ❑ Pastoral service notified ❑ Social service notified

Valuables / clothing: ________________________ Forensic evidence ________________

Doctor's Signature: ____________________________________

*NOTE: This flow sheet is only an example of information that may be required. All institutions that receive trauma patients should develop a form that meets the needs of the institution.

APPENDIX B
*Air Medical Transport**

ERICA DAVIS AND MICHAEL RHODES

I. General

A. Based on the experience of the Korean and Vietnam Wars, air medical transport has grown to become a major part of trauma care in the United States. Approximately 250 hospital-based and military air medical helicopter programs transport nearly 160 000 patients annually, 48% of whom are trauma-related patients. Two thirds of the transports are interhospital, whereas one third are transported directly from the scene. Forty percent of the flights occur during the hours of darkness.

II. Equipment

A. Most air medical transport today is done with twin-engine helicopters specifically configured for advanced life support. Most aircraft allow up to two-patient transport and two flight crew members in addition to the pilot.

B. Once in flight, the environment is noisy, rendering auscultation of blood pressure and breath sounds difficult. Therefore, nonaudible dependent monitoring is employed (by palpation or automated blood pressure cuffs). Most transports are limited to flying approximately 2000 feet above the ground, with only a minor impact on pressure changes such as exacerbation of pneumothorax or change in the military antishock trousers (MAST) inflation pressure.

C. The flight crew communicate with each other through headsets and may be able to communicate with the receiving hospital. Advance notification of patient assessment allows the receiving Trauma Center to be better prepared.

III. Triage

A. Interhospital transport by helicopter versus direct on-scene transport remains an area of controversy. Several studies have suggested that direct from-scene transport for trauma patients may be more cost-effective than interhospital transport when compared for hospital length of stay and resource utilization. However, this is geographic-specific, and undue delay of transport to the closest hospital while waiting for the helicopter should be avoided. This transport decision should be supported by the medical command physician, based on factors of time, distance, patient stability, and resources.

B. Interhospital transport of trauma patients is usually done to move a patient to a higher level of care. Multiple studies have shown that the skill of the flight crew is more important in patient outcome than the speed and size of the helicopter.

*Reproduced with permission from Peitzman AB *et al.* (ed.) (1998) *The Trauma Manual.* Lippincot-Raven, Philadelphia, pp. 61–64.

Table B.1 On-scene helicopter triage
Trauma center candidate based on triage criteria
>15 minutes to the trauma center by ground
>20-minute extrication time
Local ambulance out of service
Difficult patient access
Wilderness rescue
Multiple victims
No advanced life support available

C. The National Association of emergency medical service (EMS) Physicians has recommended triage guidelines for on-scene helicopter transport (Table B.1).

D. The final authority on patient transport lies with the pilot. Weather, geography, logistics, or other factors determine flight suitability.

IV. Flight Crew

A. Most helicopter transport is done with single pilot using visual flight rules (VFR). Some aircraft in specific geographic locations are used in the two-pilot or single-pilot instrument flight rules (IFR) mode.

B. More than 70% of the medical flight crews consist of a nurse-paramedic team. Approximately 20% of programs use two nurses, and only 3% of programs use a flight physician.

V. Interventions

A. In general, most therapeutic interventions such as endotracheal intubation, chest decompression, intravenous (IV) access, and external control of hemorrhage are done prior to lift-off.

B. Monitoring of hemodynamics, pulse oximetry, end-tidal CO_2, and ventilation is available in flight.

C. IV analgesia, sedation, and chemical paralysis as well as administration of vasoactive substances and blood products can be done in flight. These interventions must be under strict medical control or predetermined approved protocols.

VI. Helipad Access Team

A. A landing team trained in helicopter safety is usually designated to assist the flight crew in unloading and transporting the patient from the helicopter to the emergency department. With helipads in close proximity to the resuscitation area, the need for therapeutic intervention on the helipad is minimal.

B. With helipads remote from the resuscitation area (e.g., rooftop with elevator or corridor transport), occasional therapeutic intervention, such as establishing an airway in a compromised patient, may be required on the helipad. In these circumstances, the responding team will depend on institutional protocols.

C. Only a limited number of resuscitative procedures should be performed on the helipad or areas leading to the emergency and trauma department. Focus should be on identifying the need for immediate life-saving procedures; establishment of an airway, decompressing a tension pneumothorax, applying direct pressure to an open bleeding wound, or administration of resuscitative drugs and countershocks for dysrhythmias. Other interventions, such as IV catheter placement for volume therapy or thoracotomy, are best performed in the Emergency Department or Trauma Center unless the helipad is located at a prohibitive distance that could impede the success of these procedures.

VII. Safety

A. Air medical transport is primarily an aviation event with a medical component. Air medical safety has substantially improved over the past decade (Fig. B.1).

B. In general, a 500-foot ceiling and 2-mile visibility are required for flight. This may be geographic-specific, depending on the presence of mountains and pockets of fog.

C. The pilot's decision to complete a mission should be based on aviation factors and not influenced by patient criteria.

D. Comprehensive orientation programs for ground personnel for helicopter communication, setting up landing zones, patient preparation, and conduct around the aircraft are an essential part of any EMS air medical system.

E. Table B.2 outlines safety conduct around the helicopter either at the scene or on a hospital helipad.

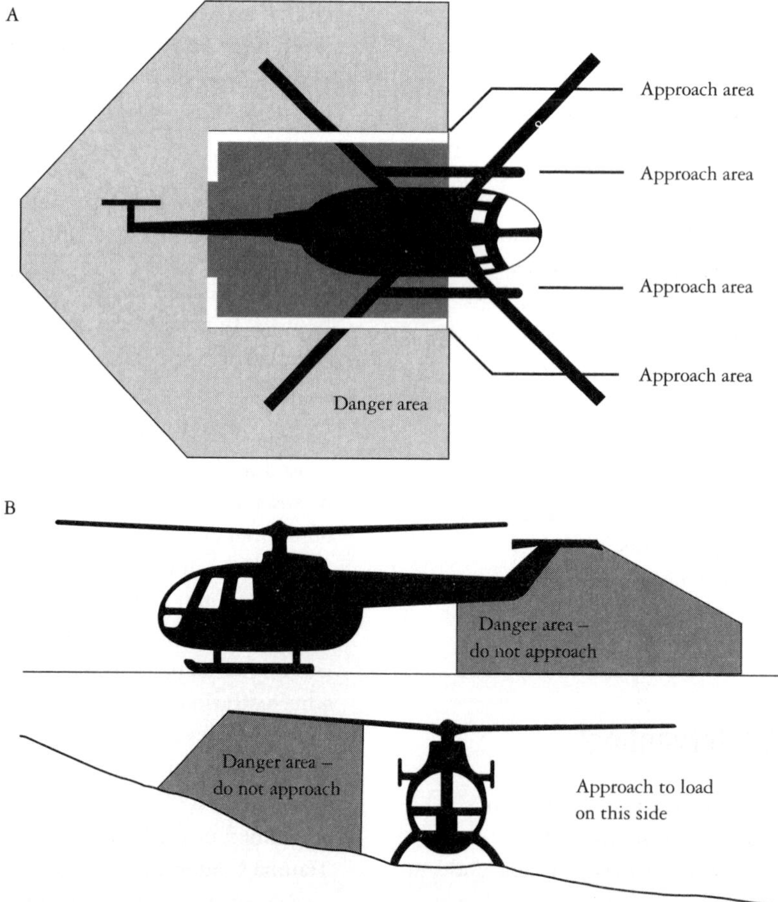

Figure B.1 (A) Air view and (B) ground view of safe approaches.

Table B.2 Safety around the helicopter

The same safety standards should be practiced whether the helicopter's engines are running or shut down. To ensure the safest operation, good habits should be established for working around the helicopter:

- Do not approach the helicopter after landing unless signalled to do so by a flight team member.
- Remain clear of the helicopter at all times unless accompanied by a flight team member.
- When approaching the helicopter, always approach from the front of the aircraft and move away in the same direction.
- When approaching the helicopter on a slope, *never* approach from the uphill side. Always approach from the downhill side because the main rotor to the ground clearance is much greater. Always be aware of the blade clearance. (See Fig. B.1B).
- *Never* walk around the tail rotor area. (See Fig. B.1).
- No unauthorized personnel within 100 feet of the aircraft.
- No smoking within 100 feet of the aircraft.
- No traffic within 100 feet of the aircraft.
- No ambulances within 50 feet of the aircraft.
- No IVs or other objects should be carried above the head, and long objects should be carried parallel to the ground.

Axioms

- The outcome of air medical transport for trauma patients is dependent on appropriate triage and the skill of the flight crew.
- Air medical transport is primarily an aviation event with a medical component.
- Never approach a helicopter without the assistance of the flight crew.

APPENDIX C
*Specific radiographic views for specific injuries**

Injury/location	Eponym/description	Technique
Hand and wrist		
Hand injuries		AP/lat./obl., digit: dental film
4th & 5th MC	Reverse obl.	Hand placed 45° tilted
MC head	Brewerton	30° pronated from full supination
Gamekeeper's thumb	Robert	Stress view (with anesthesia); AP hypersupinated (dorsum on cassette)
1st MC-trapezium	Burnam	Robert with 15° cephalic tilt
Hamate hook/CT	CT view	Tangential through carpal tunnel
Dorsal carpal chip	Dorsal tangential	Tangential of dorsal carpus
Wrist—ulnar var.	Zero rotation	AP, shoulder and elbow at 90°
Carpal instability	Motion	Cineradiography
Radial wrist	Pronation oblique	AP with 45° pronation
Ulnar wrist	Bura	Sup. obl.; AP with 35° supination
Scaphoid	Series	PA/lat./obl. fist, PA in ulnar deviation
Forearm and elbow		
Forearm	Tuberosity	AP elbow with 20° tilt to olecranon
Radial head		45° lateral of elbow, magnification
Elbow		Check fat pad, ant. humeral line, radius-capitellum
Elbow contracture	AP/lateral	AP humerus, AP forearm
Shoulder		
Shoulder	Trauma	True AP (scapula—45°obl.), scapular lat. (Y)
Shoulder	Axillary lateral	Through axilla with arm abducted
Tuberosities	AP ER/IR	AP with arm in full extension and internal rotation
Impingement	Caudal tilt	AP with 30° caudal tilt
Impingement	Supraspinatus outlet	Scapula lat. with 10° caudal tilt
Hill Sachs	Stryker notch	Supine, hand on head, 10° cephalic tilt
Bankart	West Point	Prone axillary lat. with 25° lat. and post. tilt
Bankart	Garth	Apical obl. with 45° caudal and AP tilt
AC injury	Stress	AP both AC (large cassette) with 10 pounds *hanging* weight
AC injury	Alexander	Scapular lat. with shoulders forward
AC arthritis	Zanca	10° cephalic tilt of AC
SC injury	Hobbs	PA, patient leans over cassette
SC injury	Serendipity	40° cephalic tilt center on manubrium
Clavicle		AP 30° cephalic tilt

*Reproduced with permission from Miller MD (ed.) (1996) *Review of Orthopaedics*, 2nd edn. W.B. Saunders, Philadelphia, p. 352.

Spine		
C-spine	Series	AP/lat./obl., open-mouth odontoid
C7	Swimmers' view	Lat. through maximally abducted arm
Instability	Flex/Ext	AP with flexion and extension
L-spine	Series	AP/lat./obl. (foramina), L5/S1 spot lat.
Pelvis and hip		
Pelvic injury	Inlet	45–50° caudad (assess AP displacement)
Pelvic injury	Outlet	45° cephalad (assess SI superior displacement)
Pelvic injury—Judet	Iliac obl.	Oblique on ilium (*post, column, ant. acetabulum*)
Pelvic injury—Judet	Obturator obl.	Oblique on obturator (*ant. column, post. acetabulum*)
Pelvic injury	Push-pull	Outlet view with stress (assess stability)
SI injury		Judet views centered on SI joints
Hip	Surgical lat.	Lat. from opposite side with that hip flexed
Femoral neck		AP with 15° internal rotation
Knee		
Knee AP & lat.		AP with 5° flexion, lat. with 30°' flexion
Osteochondral Fx	Notch	Prone 45° from vertical
Knee DJD	Rosenberg	Weight-bearing PA with 45° flexion
Patella	Merchant	45° flexion, cassette perpendicular to tibia
Tibial plateau		AP with 10° caudal tilt
Tibial plateau		Internal and external obl. views
Foot and ankle		
Ankle	Mortise	AP with 15° internal rotation
Ankle	Stress	AP with lat. stress, lat. with drawer
Foot	Weight bearing	AP and lat. weight bearing
Midfoot		Include obliques
Talus	Canale	AP with 75° cephalic tilt, pronate 15°
Talar neck		AP with 15° pronation
Subtalar	Broden	45° rotation lat. with varying tilts
Calcaneus	Harris	AP standing, 45° tilt
Sesamoid		Tangentials with dorsiflexed toes

APPENDIX D
*Surgical approaches**

Table D.1 Summary of popular orthopeadic surgical approaches: upper extremity

Region	Approach	Eponym	Muscular interval 1 (nerve)	Muscular interval 2 (nerve)	Dangers
Shoulder	Anterior	Henry	Deltoid (axillary)	Pec. major (med./lat. pectoral)	MC N/cephalic V
	Lateral		Deltoid (splitting) (axillary)	Deltoid (splitting) (axillary)	Axillary N
	Posterior		Infraspinatus (suprascapular)	Teres minor (axillary)	Ax. N/post. cir. hum. A
Prox. humerus	Anterolateral	Deltoid (axillary)	Pec. major (med./lat. pectoral)	Radial and axillary N/ant circ. hum. A	
Distal humerus	Anterolateral		Brachialis (musculocutaneous)	Brachioradialis (radial)	Radial N
	Lateral	Triceps (radial)	Brachioradialis (radial)	Radial N	
Humerus	Posterior	Lat. triceps (radial)	Long triceps (radial)	Radial N/brachial A	
Elbow	Anterolateral	Henry	Brachialis/pron. teres (musculocut./median)	Brachioradialis (radial)	Lat. ABC N/radial N
	Posterolateral	Kocher	Anconeus (radial)	Ext. carpi ulnaris (PIN)	PIN (diss. to ann. lig.)
	Medial		Brachialis (musculocutaneous)	Triceps/pron. teres (radial/median)	Ulnar N
Forearm	Anterior	Henry	Brachioradialis (radial)	Pronator teres/FCR (median)	PIN
	Dorsal	Thompson	ECRB (radial)	EDC/EPL (PIN)	PIN
	Ulnar		ECU (PIN)	FCU (ulnar)	Ulnar N and A
Wrist	Dorsal		Third compartment (PIN)	Fourth compartment (PIN)	
Scaphoid	Volar	Russe	FCR or through sheath (median)	Radial A	Radial A
	Dorsolateral	Matti	First compartment (PIN)	Third compartment (PIN)	Sup. rad. N/radial A

N, nerve; A, artery; V, vein; PIN, posterior interosseous nerve; ABC, antebrachial cutaneous.

*Reproduced with permission from Miller MD (ed.) (1996) *Review of Orthopaedics*, 2nd edn. W.B. Saunders, Philadelphia, pp. 422–423.

Table D.2 Summary of popular orthopeadic surgical approaches: lower extremity

Region	Approach	Eponym	Muscular interval 1 (nerve)	Muscular interval 2 (nerve)	Dangers
Iliac crest	Posterior		Gluteus maximus (inferior gluteal)	Latissimus dorsi (long thoracic)	Clunial N, SGA, Sciatic N
	Anterior		TFL/glut. med. & min. (superior gluteal)	Ext. abd. Oblique (segmental)	ASIS/LFCN
Hip	Anterior	Smith-Peterson	Sartorius/rectus fem. (femoral)	TFL/gluteus medius (sup.(sup. gluteal)	LFCN, Fem. N, Asc. br. LFCA
	Anterolateral	Watson-Jones	Tensor fasciae latae (sup. gluteal)	Gluteus medius (sup. gluteal)	Fem. NAV/Profunda A
	Lateral	Hardinge	Splits glut. med. (sup. gluteal)	Splits vastus lat. (femoral)	Femoral NVA/LFCA (transverse br.)
	Posterior	Moore-Southern	Splits glut. max. (inf. gluteal)	N/A	Sciatic, inf. glut. A
	Medial	Ludloff	Add. longus/add. brevis (ant. div. obt.)	Gracilis/add. magnus (obt./tibial)	Ant. div. obt. N/MFCA
Thigh	Lateral		Vastus lateralis (femoral)	Vastus lateralis (femoral)	Perf. br. profundus
	Posterolateral		Vastus lateralis (femoral)	Hamstrings (sciatic)	Perf. br. profundus
	Anteromedial		Rectus femoris (femoral)	Vastus medialis (femoral)	Med. sup. geniculate A
Distal femur	Posterior		Biceps femoris (sciatic)	Vastus lateralis (femoral)	Sciatic/N PFCN
Knee	Med. parapatellar		Vastus medialis (femoral)	Rectus femoris (femoral)	Infrapatellar br. saphenous N
	Medial		Vastus medialis (femoral)	Sartorius (femoral)	Infrapatellar br. saphenous N
	Lateral		Iliotibial band (sup. gluteal)	Biceps femoris (sciatic)	Peroneal N/popliteus ten.
	Posterior		Semimem./lat. gastroc. (tibial)	Biceps/lat. gastroc. (tib.)/(tib.)	Med. sural cut. N/tib. N/ peroneal N
	Lateral		Vastus lateralis (femoral)	Biceps femoris (sciatic)	Peroneal N/lat. sup. gen. A
Tibia	Posterolateral		GS, soleus, FHL (tibial)	Peroneus brevis/longus (sup. peroneal)	Sm saph. V/post. tib. A
	Anterior		Tibialis anterior (peroneal)	Periosteum	Long saph. V
Ankle	Anterior		EHL (deep peroneal)	EDL (deep peroneal)	S and D peroneal N/ant. tib. A
Med. Malleolus	Posterior		Tibialis posterior	FDL	Saphenous N and V
Ankle	Posterolateral		Peroneus brevis (sup. peroneal)	FHL (tibial)	Sural N/sm saph. V
Distal fibula	Lateral		Peroneus tertius (deep peroneal)	Peroneus brevis (sup. peroneal)	Sural N
Ankle	Anterolateral		Peroneal muscles (sup. peroneal)	EDC and per. Tertius (deep peroneal)	Deep per. N/ant. tib. A
	Posteromedial		TP or FDL	FDL or FHL	Post. tib. A/tib N

A, artery; V, vein; N, nerve; S, superficial; D, decr; LFCA, lateral femoral circumflex artery; MFCA, medial femoral circumflex artery; SGA, superior gluteal artery; PFCN, posterior femoral cutaneous nerve; LFCN, lateral femoral cutaneous nerve.

APPENDIX E
Application of traction[*]

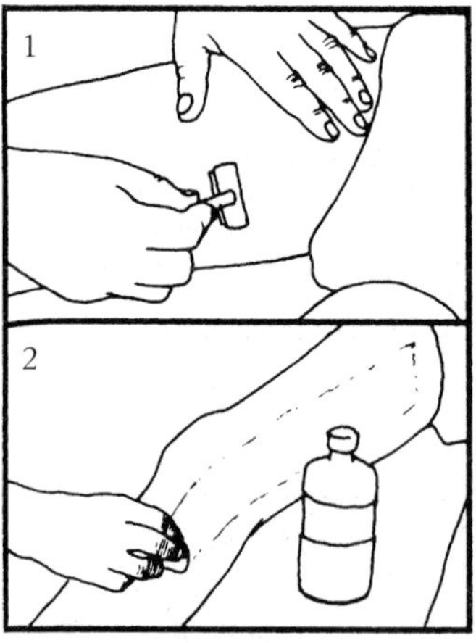

1. Applying skin traction (1): With the exercise of care and gentleness this can usually be done without an anaesthetic. (1) Begin by shaving the skin. (2) It is then traditional to swab or spray the skin with a mildly antiseptic solution of balsam of Peru in alcohol. This may facilitate the adhesion of the strapping.

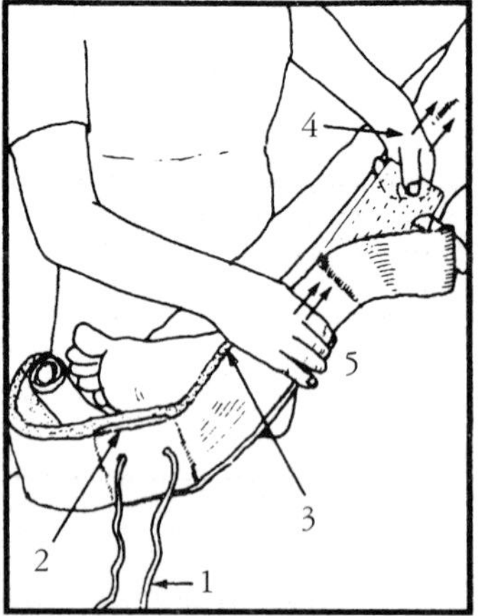

2. Applying skin traction (2): Commercial traction sets use adhesive tapes which can stretch from side to side but not longitudinally. They come supplied with traction cords (1) and a spreader bar (2) with foam protection for the malleoli (3). Begin by applying the tape to the medial side of leg—do this by peeling off the protective backing with one hand (4) while pressing the tape down and advancing the other (5).

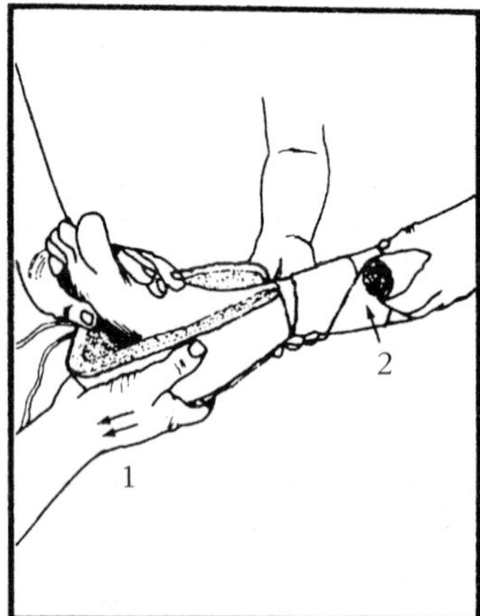

3. Applying skin traction (3): The leg is internally rotated and the tape applied to the outside of the leg, preferably a little more posterior than on the medial side. The tapes should extend up the leg as far as possible, irrespective of the site of the fracture. Now apply traction to the leg (1) and finally secure the tapes throughout their length with encircling crepe bandages (2).

[*]Reproduced with permission from McRae R (1994) *Practical Fracture Management*, 3rd edn Churchill Livingstone, Edinburgh, pp. 271–81.

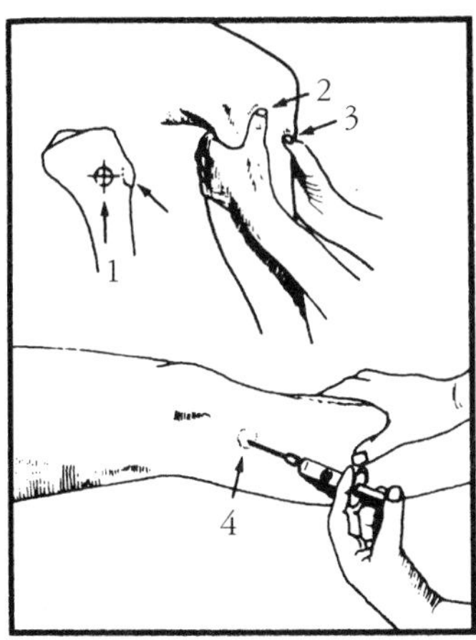

4. Applying skeletal traction (1): The preferred site is the upper tibia a little under 2 cm (1″) posterior to the prominence of the tibial tuberosity (1). It is important to avoid the knee joint, and the growth plate in children: so begin by carefully identifying it by flexing the knee (2), noting its relationship to the tuberosity (3). If a general anaesthetic is not employed, infiltrate the skin and tissue down to periosteum with local anaesthetic (e.g. 2–3 ml of 1% lignocaine) (4).

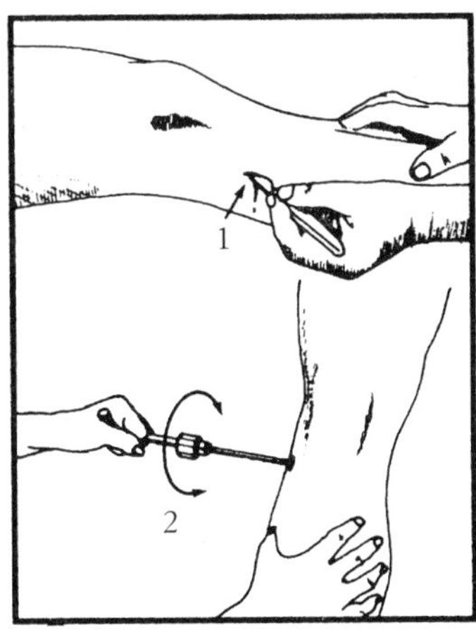

5. Skeletal traction (2): Now make a small incision in the skin (1) enough to take the traction pin only; inset it until the point strikes bone. Drive the pin through the lateral tibial cortex by applying firm pressure and twisting the chuck handle (2). You should feel it penetrate the outer cortex and pass quickly with little resistance till it meets the medial cortex. Stop at this stage.

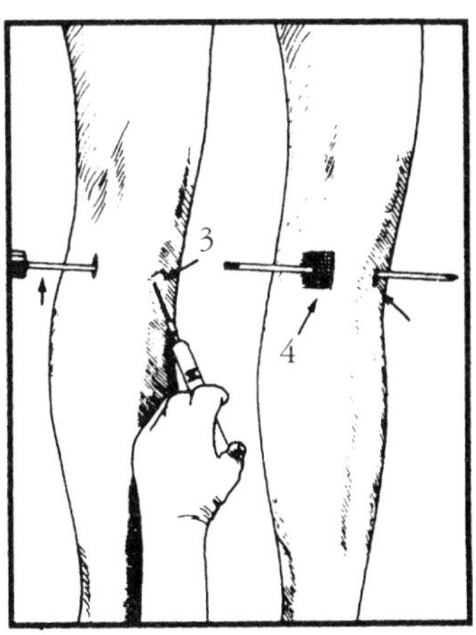

6. Skeletal traction (3): Infiltrate the skin down to periosteum on the medial side, using the lie of the pin to guide you to the expected exit area (3). Drive the pin through the medial cortex, and make a small incision over the tenting skin to allow it to come through. Protect the openings with gauze strips soaked in Nobecutane® or a similar sealant (4). Try to inset the pin at right angles to the leg.

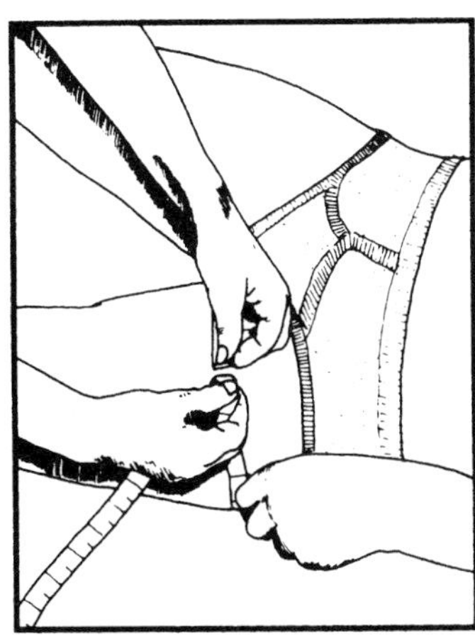

7. Traction systems (A): Skin traction in a Thomas splint (1): The most important decision in selecting a Thomas splint is the ring size. To save time (e.g. before anaesthesia) the uninjured leg may be measured, and an allowance made for swelling, present and anticipated. It is nevertheless wise to have readily available a size above and below the estimate in case of inaccuracies.

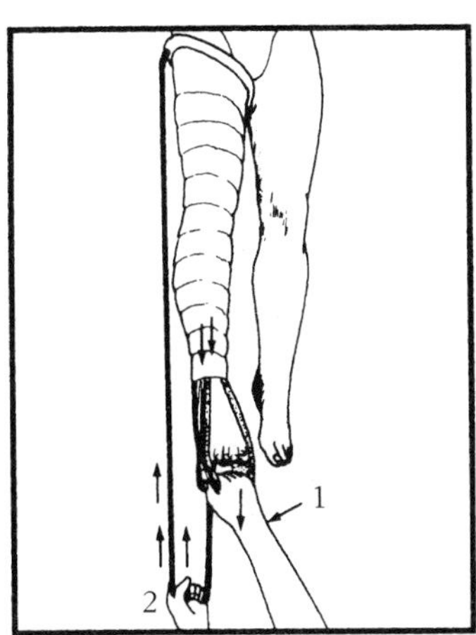

8. Thomas splint (2): Applying traction with one hand on the spreader bar (1) the selected splint is pushed up the leg (2). It should reach the ischial tuberosity (or more likely the perineum) and it should be possible to pass one finger beneath the ring round its complete circumference. If the ring is too large or too small, maintain traction while the next size is tried.

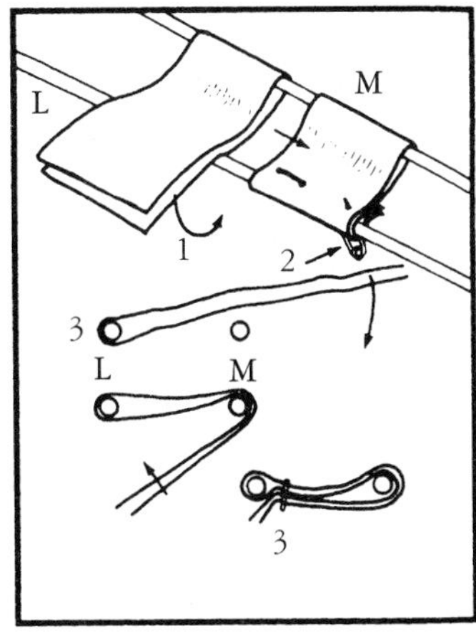

9. Thomas splint (3): The choice of soft furnishings and their method of application is often made with a fanaticism that may amaze the uncommitted. Slings to bridge the side irons may be formed from strips of 15 cm (6″) wide calico bandage (1). It is traditional to secure these with large safety pins inserted from below, close to the outer iron (2). Sometimes spring clips are used. A double bandage thickness ensures greater rigidity (3).

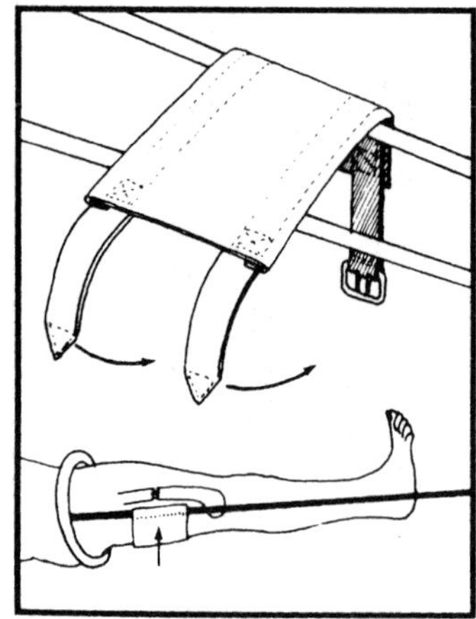

10. Thomas splint (4): The sling placed directly beneath the fracture should preferably be unyielding, and one of canvas with web and buckle fastenings is often favoured in this situation. It is customary to apply the splint with the master sling in position; the other slings are then attached and adjusted to the contours of the limb. Less satisfactorily perhaps the splint is applied with all the slings already in position.

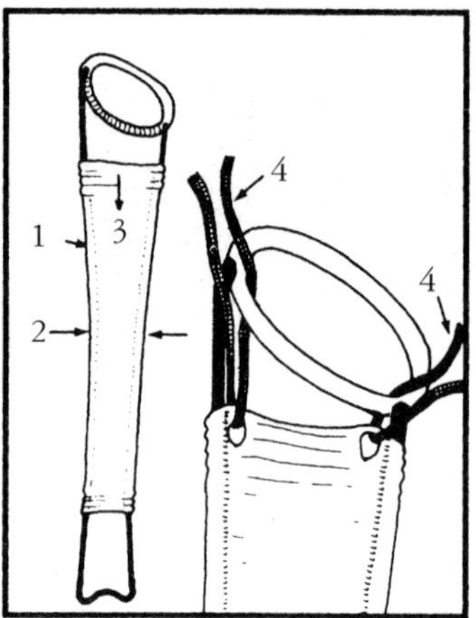

11. Thomas splint (5): Calico and canvas slings can drift, separate, or ruck, and many prefer the smoothness of an unbroken circular bandage, stretched in double thickness over the splint (e.g. Tubigrip®) (1). This has the disadvantage of 'waisting' the splint (2), being less than firm under the fracture and tending to drift distally (3). The last may be prevented by anchoring it to the ring with ribbon gauze or bandage (4).

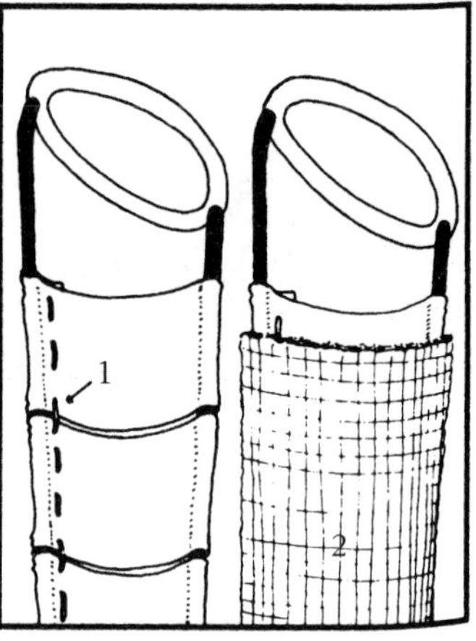

12. Thomas splint (6): If separate slings are used, their tendency to separate may be minimised by pinning each to its neighbour (1). Nevertheless, a layer of wool should be placed between them and the limb to smooth out any unevenness (2) (not necessary with circular woven bandage). In all cases, a large pad (e.g. of gamgee) should be placed directly beneath the fracture to act as a fulcrum.

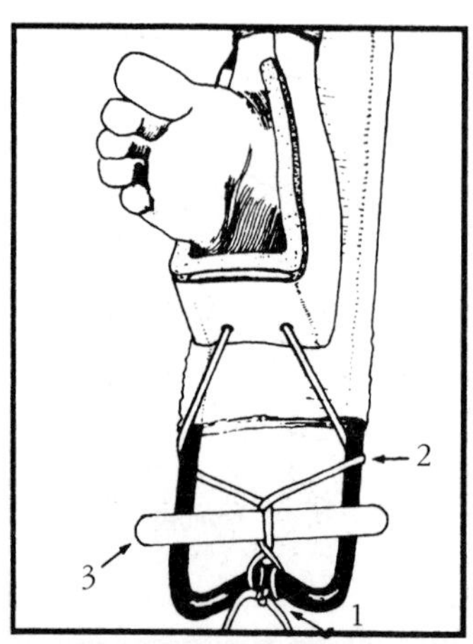

13. Thomas splint (7): In long oblique fractures and those with apposition no manipulation will be needed and the traction system may be completed by, for example, tying the cords to the end of the splint (1). The convention of passing the medial cord under the corresponding iron helps to control the tendency to lateral rotation (2). A Chinese windlass (of spatulae or a metal rod) may be used to take up slack (3).

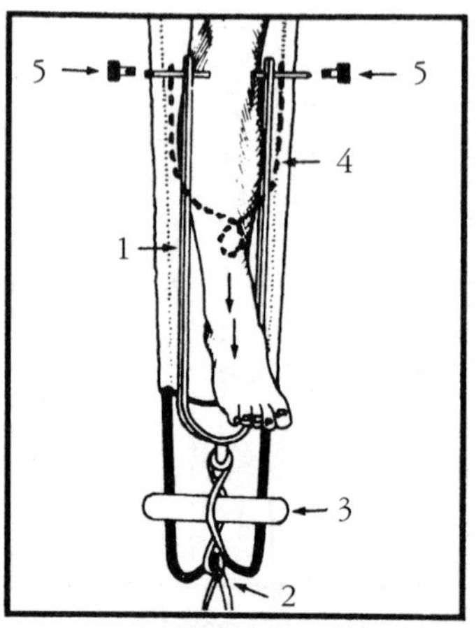

14. Thomas splint (8): Where skeletal traction is being used a metal loop (1) (Tulloch–Brown loop) allows a direct pull to be made in the line of the limb. The loop may be tied to the end of the Thomas splint (2) and tensioned with a windlass as previously described (3). A stirrup may be employed to prevent springing of the loop (4). Protect the sharp ends of the pin with caps (5).

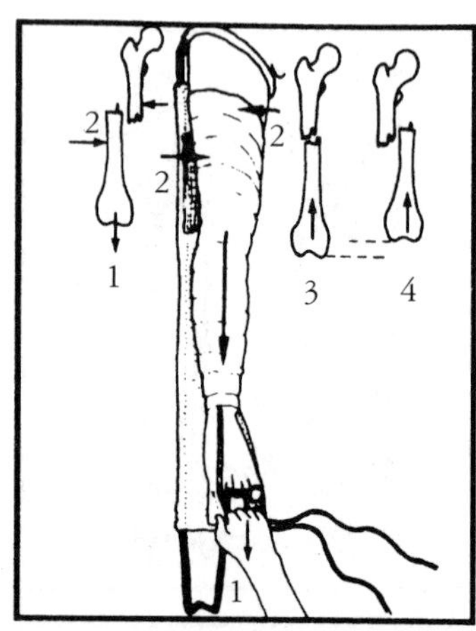

15. Thomas splint (9): Manipulation: With the exception of the young child, manipulation is advisable if there is loss of bony apposition. With the splint in position, but unattached, an assistant applies strong traction (1) while pressure is applied in the directions deduced from the radiographs (2). When the traction is eased off, the limb remains the same length if a hitch has been obtained (3) but telescopes if not (4).

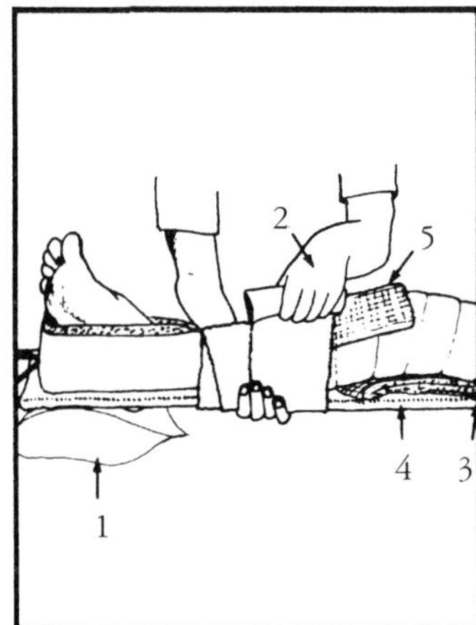

16. **Thomas splint (10):** After the traction cords have been attached, the end of the splint can be raised temporarily on a pillow (1) while the limb is bandaged to the splint, using for example 15 cm (6″) crepe bandages (2). Note gamgee or wool padding behind the fracture to act as a fulcrum (3), behind the knee to keep it in slight flexion (4), and along the shin to avoid sores (5).

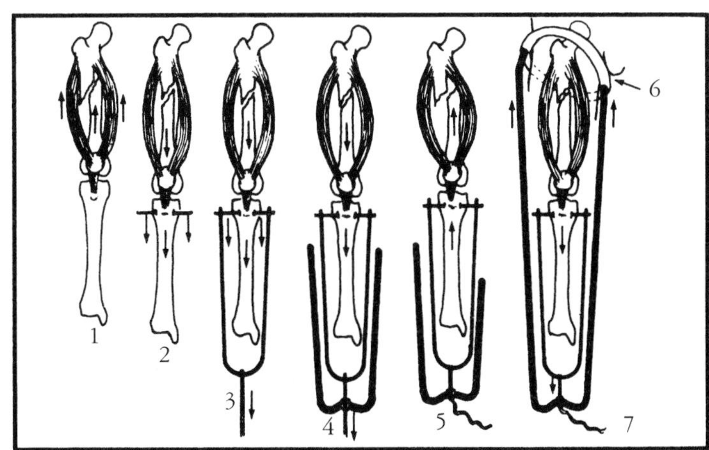

17. **Thomas splint (11):** The system described is normally referred to as fixed traction in a Thomas splint. The basic principles are straightforward, but it is important that they are thoroughly understood. Muscle tension (mainly quads and hams) tends to produce shortening (1): this can be overcome by traction, for example through a Steinman pin (2) aided by a loop and traction cord (3). If the traction cord is tied to a ringless Thomas splint, the reduction is maintained so long as a pull is kept on the cord (4); redisplacement occurs if the cord is released (5). This proximal migration is normally prevented by the ring (6) so that the reduction is maintained even when the traction cord is released (7). Note that muscle tone = tension in traction cord = ring pressure.

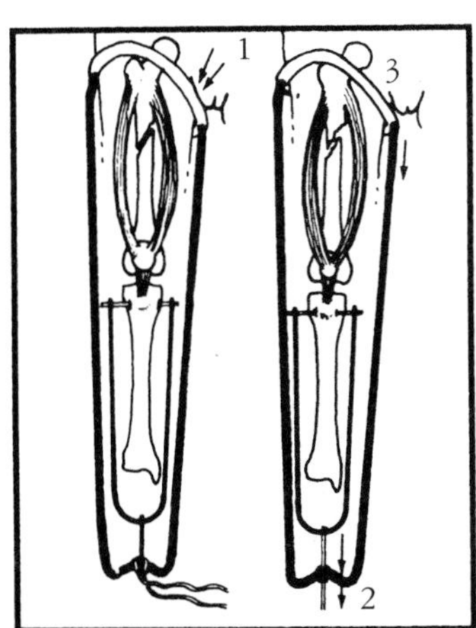

18. **Thomas splint (12):** This pressure of the ring of the Thomas splint tends to produce sores (1) (especially in the perineal, groin and ischial tuberosity regions) and must be relieved (3). This is done by applying traction (*c.* 3 kg/8 lb) to the anchored cords (4). If ring pressure is unrelieved, *increase the traction weights*.

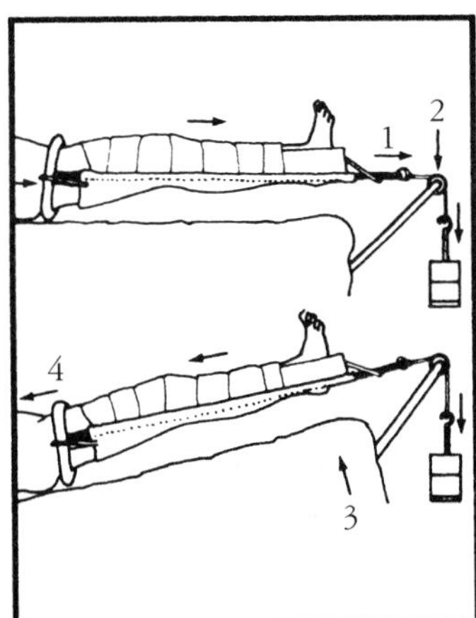

19. **Thomas splint (13):** The traction weights have a tendency to pull the patient down towards the foot of the bed (1). This may continue till the splint comes to rest on the traction pulley (2). This may be countered if it becomes a problem by raising the foot of the bed (3), when the traction weight is balanced by the upward component of the patient's body weight (4).

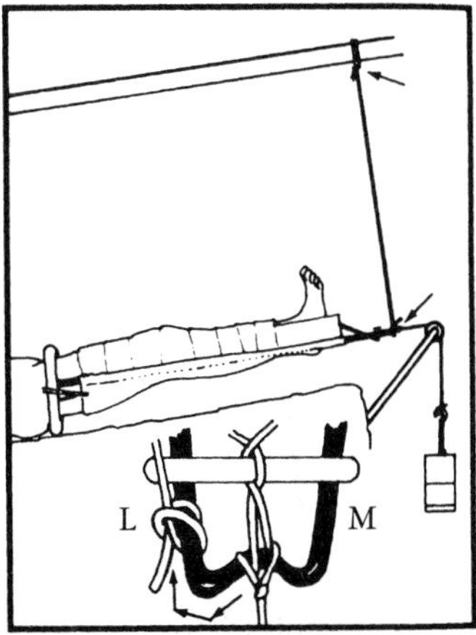

20. **Thomas splint (14): Supporting the limb and the splint (1):** To allow the patient to move about the bed and prevent pressure on the heel, it is desirable to support the splint; this may be done most simply by tying a cord from the end of the splint to an overhead bar of the Balkan beam bed. The position of the suspension cord may be adjusted from near the midline to either side, (Illus.: lateral attachment to control external rotation.)

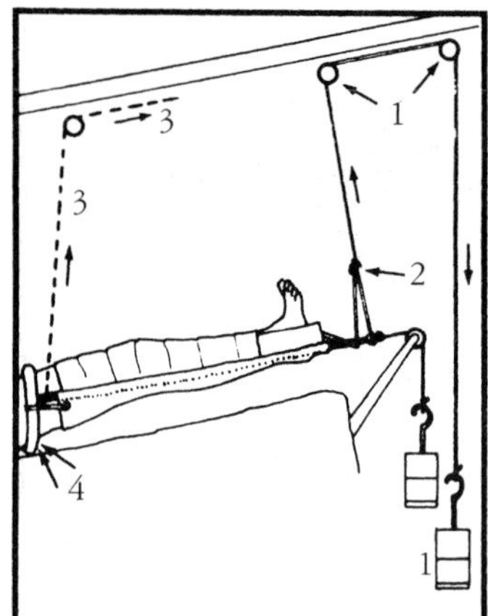

21. **Thomas splint (15): Supporting the splint (2):** Some prefer a lively system which can be achieved in various ways, e.g. by weights and a system of pulleys (1). The suspension cord may be arranged in Y-fashion to straddle both irons of the Thomas splint (2). Support for the proximal end of the splint (3) is less clearly an advantage although often pursued—it may cause extra pressure beneath the ring (4).

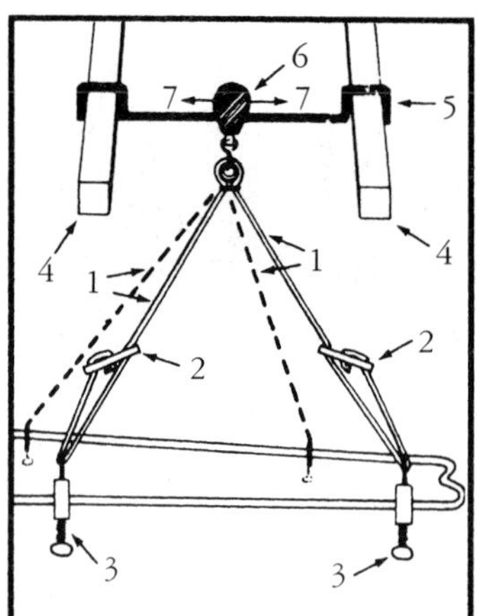

22. **Thomas splint (16): Supporting the splint (3):** Another form of lively splint support ('octopus') consists of elastic Bunjee cord (1), which can be adjusted with tensioners (2). The cords are attached to the splint with G-cramps (3) and to cross members of the Balkan beam (4) by means of a bar (5) along which a pulley (6) is free to move, allowing easy movement up and down the bed (7).

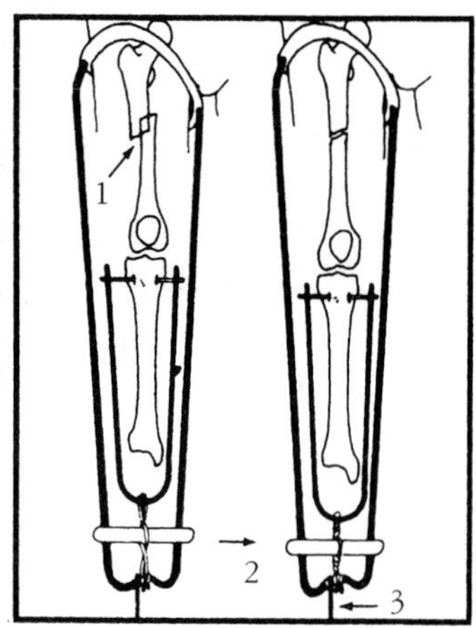

23. **Thomas splint (17):** Check radiographs should be taken after the application of a Thomas splint, after any major adjustment, and thereafter at fortnightly intervals till union.

Corrections: (a) If there is persistent shortening (1) tighten the windlass in a fixed traction system (2). This will inevitably increase ring pressure, and must be compensated by increasing the traction weight (3). (Soft tissue between the bone ends may nevertheless thwart reduction.)

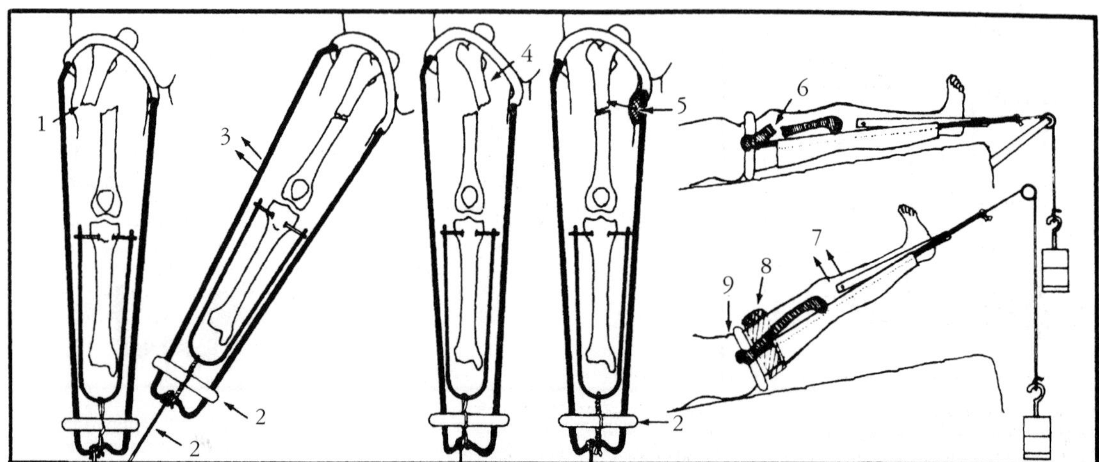

24. **Thomas splint (18): Corrections:** (b) Where the proximal fragment is abducted (1) the position may be improved by increasing the traction (2) and abducting the leg (3). The position of the ring traction pulley and the splint supports will require corresponding adjustment. (c) If the proximal fragment is adducted (4) increase of traction alone (2) may lead to an improvement in the position. It may be helpful to apply side thrust with a pad (5) Between the leg and the medial side iron, (d) Flexion and/or abduction of the proximal fragment (6) due to unresisted psoas and gluteal action is frequently a very painful complication. In the young patient, raising the splint (7) and/or abducting the leg and bandaging a local pad in position (8) may bring the fragments into alignment, but this manoeuvre is less certain in the older patient where internal fixation is frequently advisable for femoral fractures at this level and of this type. In any patient in whom this conservative technique is practised, care must be taken to avoid pressure in the region of the anterior superior iliac spine (9).

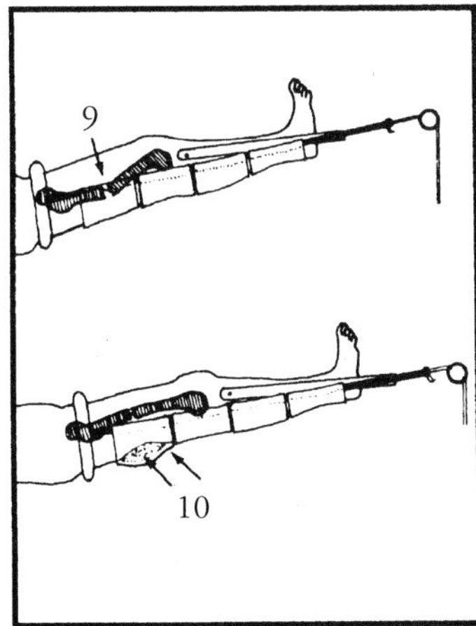

25. Thomas splint (19): Corrections: (e) Perhaps the commonest residual deformity requiring and amenable to correction is backward sag at the fracture site (9). If a continuous posterior support is used, the padding behind the fracture should be increased in thickness. If separate slings are used, the sling behind the fracture should be tightened and/or the padding behind the fracture increased (10).

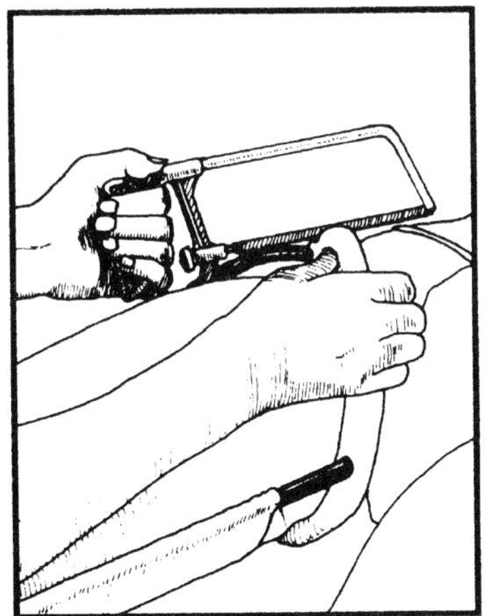

26. Thomas splint (20): After care (1): During the first 72 hours following fracture, swelling of the thigh from haematoma and oedema may render the ring tight round its circumference. (Normally it should be easy to put a finger under the ring at any point.) To avoid changing the splint, split the ring with a hacksaw, ease the ends apart, and protect them with adhesive strapping.

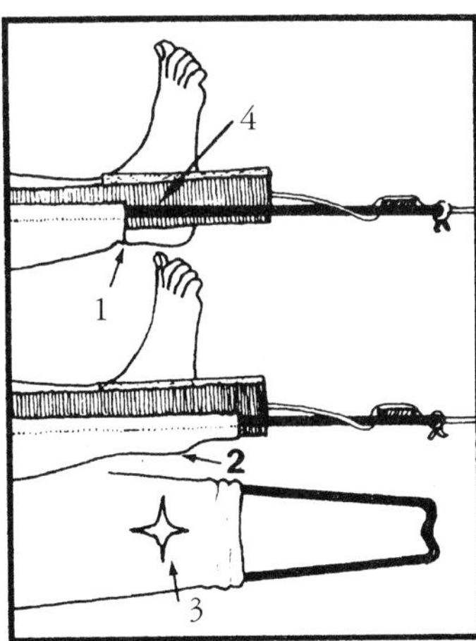

27. Thomas splint (21): After care (2): The following items should be checked daily. Look for impending pressure sores (and take appropriate action). (a) *In the Achilles tendon region* if the slings stop at this level (1); (b) *Under the heel*, if the heel is included (2); If a circular woven support is used, a cruciate incision in it at heel level is prophylactic (3); (c) *Over the malleoli* (4).

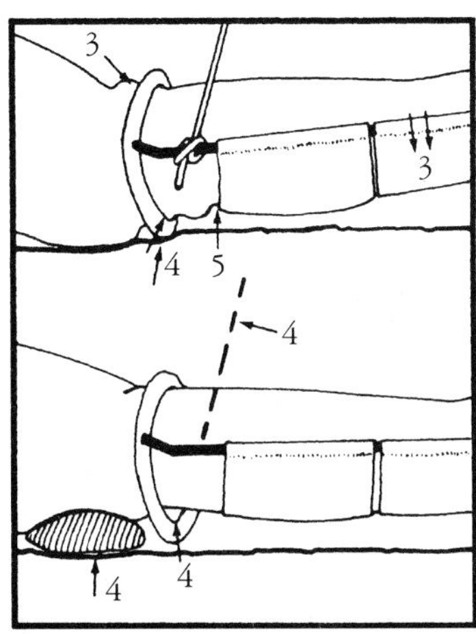

28. Thomas splint (22): After care (3): (d) *The ring area:* Good nursing care is vital to avoid skin breakdown. In addition for: (1) circumferential tightness—split the ring; (2) perineal pressure—increase the ring traction weight; (3) anterior spine pressure—lower the splint; (4) pressure behind the ring—decrease or remove any support weight and place a pillow above the ring (4); (e) pad the edge of the sling if needed (5).

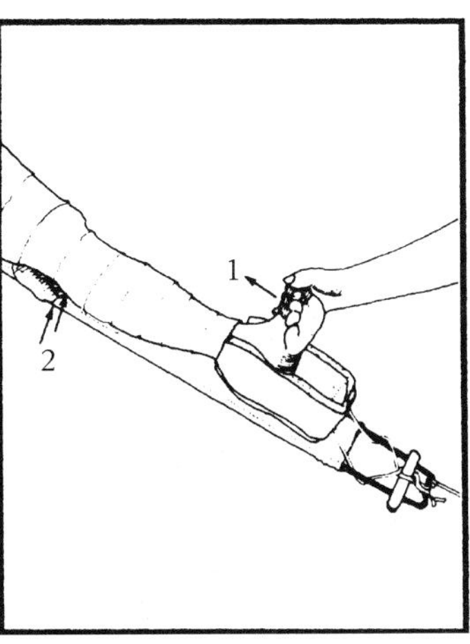

29. Thomas splint (23): After care (4): Check daily for weakness of ankle dorsiflexion (1) indicative of common peroneal nerve palsy and necessitating careful inspection of the neck of the fibula where the cause is generally felting of the wool padding, transmitting pressure from the side iron (2). Repad and fit a Sinclair foot support if the palsy is complete: expect recovery in 6 weeks.

30. Thomas splint (24): After care (5): In those cases where skeletal traction is employed, look for: (i) Loosening of the Steinman pin; this may require recentring; other treatment is seldom required, so that traction may be continued, (ii) Pin-track infection; a wound swab should be sent for bacteriological examination and the appropriate antibiotic administered. If infection is marked, the traction site may have to be abandoned, (iii) Shifting and digging-in of the loop; adjust with padding.

During the period a patient spends in bed he should practise quadriceps and general maintenance exercises. Splintage in children should be continued till union (6–12 weeks). In adults, mobilisation of the knee joint and/or the patient may be possible before union is complete.

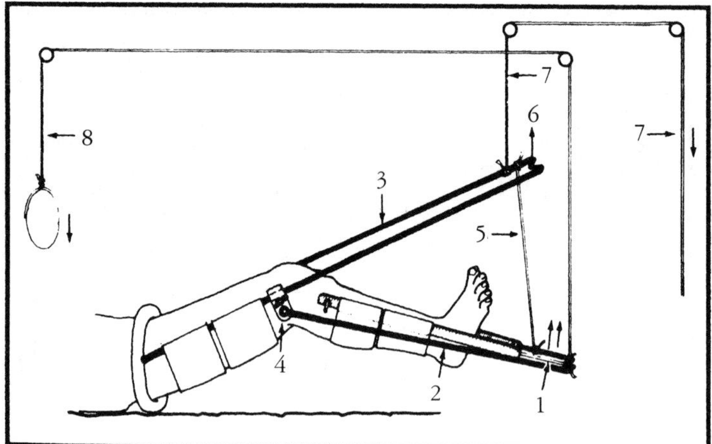

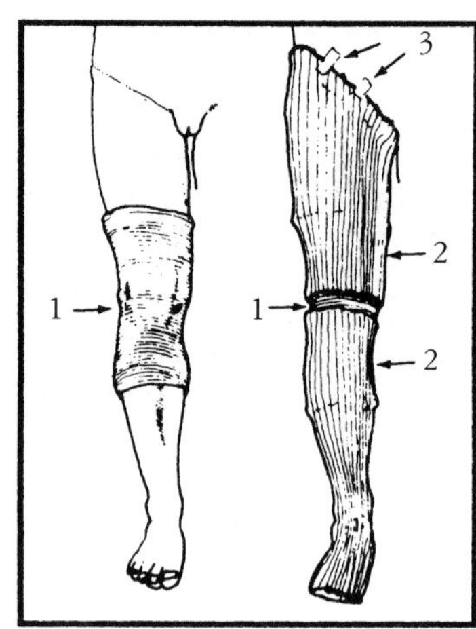

31. **Early mobilisation techniques:** *(i)* Where there is abundant callus and the fracture cannot be sprung, splintage may be discarded and the knee mobilised till there is sufficient mature callus to allow weight bearing. *(ii) The Pearson knee-flexion piece*: this may be used as soon as some stabilising callus appears at the fracture site.

Method: The traction cord (1) is transferred to the Pearson attachment (2) which is fixed to the Thomas splint (3) and hinges at the level of the knee axis (4). An adjustable cord (5) may be used to gradually advance the range of permissable knee flexion. The end of the Thomas splint is raised (6) and supported (7) while a cord (8) may allow the patient to assist his knee extension manually.

32. **Early mobilisation techniques: (iii) Cast bracing (1):** After 4–8 weeks in a Thomas splint, cast bracing may be considered, especially in fractures of the distal half. Many techniques are practised. In a typical procedure the patient is sedated with diazepam, a sandbag placed under the buttocks, and a cast sock drawn over the knee (1). Circular woven bandages (stockingette) encase the limb in two sections (2) and are taped in position (3).

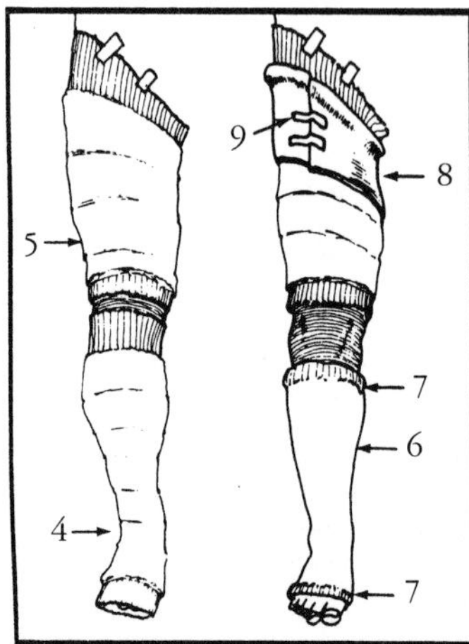

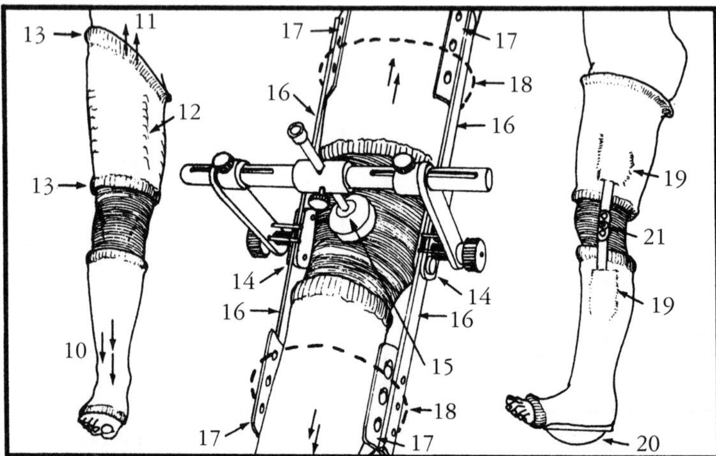

33. **Cast bracing (2):** A layer of wool roll is used to protect the bony prominences below the knee (4) and as a single layer of padding in the thigh (5). A below-knee plaster is then applied (6) and completed by turning back and incorporating the circular woven bandage (7). An appropriately sized bucket top of polythene is selected (8), trimmed as required and taped in position (9).

34. **Cast bracing (3):** Traction is applied to the leg (10), the bucket is pulled well into the groin (11), a plaster thigh piece applied, moulded in a quadrilateral fashion (to prevent rotation) (12) and completed (13). Maintaining traction in 10° flexion, polycentric hinges (14) are carefully positioned with a jig which is centered on the patella (15). The side-stays (16) are adjusted until the fixation plates (17) lie snugly against the upper and lower plaster components. Large encircing jubilee clips (18) may be used to hold the hinges in position while the jig is removed and flexion function checked. The hinges are plastered in position (19) and a rocker or boot applied (20). The hinges can be unlocked by removal of 2 set screws (21).

35. Cast bracing (4): The cast brace affords moderate support of the fracture, and mobilisation of the patient may be commenced at first using crutches and with the hinges locked. After 1–2 weeks or as progress determines, flexion can be permitted and the crutches gradually discarded. The brace is worn until union is complete.

A number of commercially produced cast-bracing kits are available using materials other than plaster of Paris (e.g. the bucket may be formed from pre-cut plastic sheet which can be temporarily softened by heating and moulded to shape: resin plaster bandages and polyethylene hinges can be employed). In many cases these render the technique comparatively simple, with the result that the so-called weight-relieving calliper, tubed into the patient's shoe, is now much less frequently employed for early mobilisation than in the past.

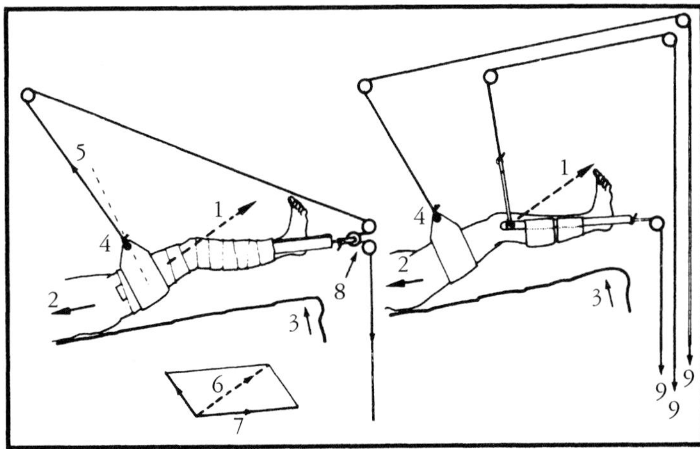

36. Other methods of treating fractures of the femur: (1) Hamilton–Russell traction: This is particularly applicable in the conservative treatment of bilateral fractures; it is a form of balanced traction where the pull on the limb (1) is countered by the body weight (2) through the bed being raised (3). The fracture and distal fragment are supported by a padded canvas sling (4), angled slightly towards the head (5) to counter a tendency to distal drift. The theory behind the classical arrangement is that the line of pull on the femur is the resultant (6) of a parallelogram of forces, where the horizontal component (7) is doubled because of the pulley arrangement (8). Friction losses spoil the theory, and many prefer direct control of all forces (9). This method of treatment, although often useful, gives restricted support to the fracture. Note that balanced traction can be carried out using a Thomas splint bandaged to the limb, but unattached to any of the traction cords.

APPENDIX F
*Trauma rules**

- Anxiety provokes memory loss: so learn a system and stick to it.
- Save yourself before casualty.
- Assume the worst and proceed accordingly.
- Do a frisk or take a risk.
- Don't let the obvious distract from the occult.
- The trauma team can only look or listen, not both.
- All trauma patients are dying for oxygen.
- The airway is more important than the cervical spine.
- It is not lack of intubation that kills, it is lack of oxygenation.
- Do not delay with a burned airway.
- Think of cricothyrotomy when all else fails.
- Look at the neck three times in the primary survey.
- A hard collar does not protect the cervical spine.
- All Trauma surgeons Occasionally Miss Cervical Fractures:

All	Airway obstruction
Trauma surgeons	Tension pneumothorax
Occasionally	Open pneumothorax
Miss	Massive haemothorax
Cervical	Cardiac tamponade
Fractures	Flail chest

- When patients with facial injuries look up at heaven they will soon be there.
- Blood on the floor is forever lost to the patient
- Short and thick does the trick.
- Hidden blood loss will CRAMP your resuscitation:

Chest	Do a chest radiograph
Retroperitoneum	Test the urine
Abdomen	Do a diagnostic peritoneal lavage
Missed long bone fracture	Examine the limbs
Pelvis	Do a pelvic radiograph

- Surgery does not follow resuscitation, it is part of resuscitation.
- O negative is good, but you can have too much of a good thing.
- The stabbed stay stabbed until they reach theatre.
- An injury above and below the abdomen implies an injury in the abdomen.
- A penetrating wound below the nipple involves the abdomen.
- Examination of the abdomen is as reliable as flipping a coin.
- Neurogenic shock is hypovolaemic shock until proved otherwise.
- Think of the EMD causes or your patient is for *THE CHOP*
- Head injury alone does not cause hypotension.
- Resuscitate the mother and the baby will look after itself.
- Children are not small adults.
- Limp splintage is part of resuscitation.
- The Glasgow Coma Scale does not measure prognosis.
- A patient has a front, a back, two sides, a top, and a bottom.

*Reproduced with permission from Hodgetts T, Deane S, Gunnng K (eds) List of 60 trauma rules. In: *Trauma Rules* © BMJ Publishing Group, 1998.

- Put a finger in before putting a tube in.
- The agitated patient will calm down whilst deteriorating.
- You are not dead until you are death warmed up.
- The golden rule is golden fluid in the golden hour.
- It does not hurt to give analgesia.
- The team leader is always right.
- If in doubt, call the trauma team.
- The golden hour belongs to the patient.
- You can assess vision with the eyes closed.
- You may read the newspaper, but not read the DPL.
- A tension pneumothorax cannot be diagnosed on the chest X-ray.
- A supine chest X-ray may be worse than no chest X-ray.
- Investigation must never impede resuscitation.
- Serial blood gases are the signposts on the road to resuscitation.
- The radiology department is a dangerous place.
- Patients are transferred, not their injuries or investigations.
- Never believe a transferring hospital.
- Better a negative laparotomy than a positive postmortem.
- Go down the middle and be liberal.
- Fix the pelvis to fix the bleeding.
- Biology is the mother of all fixation.
- The solution to pollution is dilution.
- It doesn't pay to be complacent about an elderly fracture of the rib.
- A missed tertiary survey is a missed injury.
- With multiple casualties do the most for the most.
- Black is beautiful, and some things are never as black as they seem.
- Rehabilitation begins at the roadside.
- Death is the only certainty in life.

Index